MW01257023

Atlas of Gastrointestinal Pathology

A Pattern Based Approach to Neoplastic Biopsies

DORA M. LAM-HIMLIN, MD
Associate Professor
Department of Laboratory Medicine and Pathology
Mayo Clinic
Scottsdale, Arizona

ELIZABETH A. MONTGOMERY, MD
Professor of Pathology, Oncology, and Orthopedic Surgery
Department of Pathology
Division of Gastrointestinal and Liver Pathology
Johns Hopkins Medical Institutions
Baltimore, Maryland

CHRISTINA A. ARNOLD, MD
Associate Professor
Department of Pathology
Division of Gastrointestinal and Liver Pathology
The Ohio State University Wexner Medical Center
Columbus, Ohio

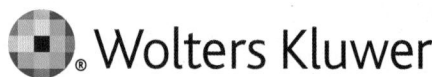

Philadelphia • Baltimore • New York • London
Buenos Aires • Hong Kong • Sydney • Tokyo

Acquisitions Editor: Ryan Shaw
Editorial Coordinator: Lindsay Ries
Marketing Manager: Julie Sikora
Production Project Manager: Linda Van Pelt
Design Coordinator: Holly McLaughlin
Manufacturing Coordinator: Beth Welsh
Prepress Vendor: TNQ Technologies

Copyright © 2019 Wolters Kluwer

All rights reserved. This book is protected by copyright. No part of this book may be reproduced or transmitted in any form or by any means, including as photocopies or scanned-in or other electronic copies, or utilized by any information storage and retrieval system without written permission from the copyright owner, except for brief quotations embodied in critical articles and reviews. Materials appearing in this book prepared by individuals as part of their official duties as U.S. government employees are not covered by the above-mentioned copyright. To request permission, please contact Wolters Kluwer at Two Commerce Square, 2001 Market Street, Philadelphia, PA 19103, via email at permissions@lww.com, or via our website at shop.lww.com (products and services). 1V2018

9 8 7 6 5 4 3 2

Printed in China

Library of Congress Cataloging-in-Publication Data

Names: Lam-Himlin, Dora M., author. | Montgomery, Elizabeth (Elizabeth A.), 1958- author. |
   Arnold, Christina A., author.
Title: Atlas of gastrointestinal pathology : a pattern based approach to neoplastic biopsies / Dora M. Lam-Himlin,
   Elizabeth A. Montgomery, Christina A. Arnold.
Description: Philadelphia : Wolters Kluwer Health, 2019. | Includes bibliographical references and index.
Identifiers: LCCN 2018046981 | ISBN 9781496367549 (hardback)
Subjects: | MESH: Gastrointestinal Tract–pathology | Gastrointestinal Diseases–pathology | Biopsy | Atlases
Classification: LCC RC802.9 | NLM WI 17 | DDC 616.3/307–dc23
LC record available at https://lccn.loc.gov/2018046981

This work is provided "as is," and the publisher disclaims any and all warranties, express or implied, including any warranties as to accuracy, comprehensiveness, or currency of the content of this work.

This work is no substitute for individual patient assessment based upon healthcare professionals' examination of each patient and consideration of, among other things, age, weight, gender, current or prior medical conditions, medication history, laboratory data and other factors unique to the patient. The publisher does not provide medical advice or guidance and this work is merely a reference tool. Healthcare professionals, and not the publisher, are solely responsible for the use of this work including all medical judgments and for any resulting diagnosis and treatments.

Given continuous, rapid advances in medical science and health information, independent professional verification of medical diagnoses, indications, appropriate pharmaceutical selections and dosages, and treatment options should be made and healthcare professionals should consult a variety of sources. When prescribing medication, healthcare professionals are advised to consult the product information sheet (the manufacturer's package insert) accompanying each drug to verify, among other things, conditions of use, warnings and side effects and identify any changes in dosage schedule or contradictions, particularly if the medication to be administered is new, infrequently used or has a narrow therapeutic range. To the maximum extent permitted under applicable law, no responsibility is assumed by the publisher for any injury and/or damage to persons or property, as a matter of products liability, negligence law or otherwise, or from any reference to or use by any person of this work.

shop.lww.com

CCS0120

To my family:
Matt: For being my rock.
Madeline: Stay brave. Stay curious.
Matthew: Always have the heart of a gentleman.
Tommy: Yes, I'd rather be outside, too.
Dora M. Lam-Himlin, MD

To all the colleagues who love gastrointestinal pathology as much as we do.
Elizabeth A. Montgomery, MD

To my loving family:
Mary and Andy: Mike and I didn't realize how much we needed parents, until we became parents ourselves.
Thank you for always being there for us, and for reminding us about the importance of family, love, and laughter.
Mom: Thank you for being my first best friend, believing in me always, and teaching me the value of hard work.
Our Wednesday afternoon brownies are some of my favorite memories.
Jackson and Madelyn: Objects in the mirror are sometimes closer than they appear. If it is important,
NEVER give up—hunker down and dig in!
Mike: The keys to a good road trip are fun, excitement, danger, and Johnny Cash.
OGN: This book and my career would not be possible without you. Although I don't deserve you,
I thank the heavens for you every day. Here's to Baltimore, the Inca trail, and all of tomorrow's
mischievous adventures.
Christina A. Arnold, MD

Diagnosis and reporting of neoplastic GI biopsies is a complex moving target, as evidenced by evolving nomenclature, updates in society guidelines, recognition of new therapeutic targets, and increasing requirements for prognostic elements and ancillary testing interpretation. This follow-up textbook on GI neoplasia is the highly anticipated companion volume to *Atlas of Gastrointestinal Pathology: A Pattern Based Approach to Non-Neoplastic Biopsies*. This new book applies the now-familiar method of pattern based learning to GI neoplasia and provides a systematic algorithm for tackling common and uncommon interpretation challenges. Mirroring the previous text, this book highlights tell-tale "red flags" found in the clinical chart, hidden clues in the slides, and how to discern an exact diagnosis despite sometimes disabling artifacts.

New topics covered include a simple approach to the endoscopic mucosal resection (EMR) specimen, the latest definition of Barrett esophagus and its reporting, an algorithmic approach to serrated polyps, instructions for decoding the alphabet soup of colorectal cancer molecular testing, the latest consensus guidelines on approaching anal dysplasia and dysplasia arising in inflammatory bowel disease, and a handy guide to syndromic polyps with emphasis on morphology, clinical considerations, genetics, and practical reporting.

The illustrations extend beyond a handful of classic examples for each entity, and more than 1600 images cover the full morphologic spectrum of the major patterns of GI neoplasia. The sessile serrated adenoma/polyp, for example, is illustrated in more than 50 figures that include direct comparisons with differential diagnoses and borderline cases, and each image is captioned with a careful description. The corresponding text details information on how to classify the polyp, minimum diagnostic criteria, clinical implications of surveillance intervals, and sample sign-out notes.

In this book, disease processes are grouped by their histologic patterns—an approach that echoes the first volume and closely approximates the method by which experienced pathologists mentally approach daily sign-out. Organized by these major patterns, each chapter details neoplastic considerations for the esophagus, stomach, small intestine, colon, anus, and soft tissue.

The text is high yield and focused on checklists, key features, diagnostic pearls and pitfalls, frequently asked questions, and sample notes—see the following descriptions. We hope this collective experience leaves the reader with a familiarity of the major patterns of GI neoplasia and confidence in navigating through the clinicopathologic clues and pitfalls to arrive swiftly at the correct diagnosis. Select structural elements are briefly introduced as follows.

- Each chapter opens with a "Chapter Outline" that outlines the enclosed structure and allows the reader to quickly hone in on select patterns and pertinent differential diagnostic considerations. Similar checklists are found throughout the chapter to neatly organize complicated topics.

- "The Unremarkable X": Normal histology is sometimes overlooked in textbooks because it is assumed to be widely understood, much to the frustration of junior trainees. A firm understanding of normal is essential to recognizing subtle injury patterns. As such, each chapter begins with a brief discussion of normal histology to contrast to the succeeding mucosal injury patterns and to highlight helpful diagnostic clues.

- The "Pearls & Pitfalls" boxes include lessons from real life sign-out experience with an emphasis on important diagnostic clues, mimics, and hazards.

- The "Frequently Asked Questions" sections stem from our busy consult service and teaching sessions. In these sections, we discuss real-life diagnostic dilemmas and offer diagnostic tips and tools to sort through commonly encountered sign-out challenges.

- All major topics close with a "Key Features" section that summarizes the essential elements of the subtopic for handy reference.

- A "Sample Note" section accompanies the more challenging topics. In these sections, an example pathology report is included with the top-line diagnosis, pertinent discussion, and salient references. These notes offer a template of how to synthesize complicated topics and are based on real-life cases and interactions with clinicians. The select references are included for those interested in further reading but also can be included in pathology reports to help guide clinical management.

- Each chapter features a corresponding "Quiz" section in the appendix to emphasize important teaching points. These sections offer the reader experience and confidence with high-yield teaching topics. Questions are in the format of the board type examinations and can also serve as useful board preparatory materials.

ACKNOWLEDGMENTS

We thank our institutions, colleagues, and trainees for invaluable resources and support. We are indebted to our inquisitive trainees and clinicians whose fresh perspectives and lively discussions drove the direction of this book. We particularly thank our families for understanding the numerous late night, early morning, and weekend marathon writing sessions.

We thank our Acquisition Editor, Ryan Shaw, for taking a chance on this project, and our Editorial Coordinator, Lindsay Ries, for working diligently with us to ensure timely completion. We thank Frank M. Corl, MS, for the custom medical illustrations; Rick Marshall for computer assistance in identifying pertinent teaching material; and Shawn Scully for photography editing on select topics.

Lastly, we thank the production team led by Ramkumar Soundararajan for their careful attention to detail.

CONTENTS

CHAPTER OUTLINE

THE UNREMARKABLE ESOPHAGUS

Normal esophageal mucosa is a common sample in the practice of gastrointestinal pathology, and most of us are familiar with squamous mucosa on biopsies. Mucosa consists of epithelium (stratified squamous), lamina propria, and muscularis mucosae. Beneath those structures are the submucosa and muscularis propria. Assessing resections and endoscopic mucosal resections (EMRs) helps us learn about these layers.

The layers matter and there are some pitfalls! Cancers that invade only the lamina propria are staged as T1a, whereas those that extend into the submucosa are T1b neoplasms.[1] There are some issues that can arise and result in confusion. In general, mucosal biopsies grasp some epithelium and a little bit of lamina propria. Many biopsies contain only squamous epithelium and lack even lamina propria; normal squamous mucosa is slippery, and it is difficult for the endoscopist to easily grasp it to obtain a large "bite," so abundant lamina propria and/or muscularis mucosae tend to be present in biopsies from damaged mucosa. Most biopsies do not grasp submucosa.

Note the indicated layers in the samples in Figs. 1.1 and 1.2. The layer just under the epithelium is the lamina propria rather than the submucosa. This is easy to spot on well-oriented samples such as the one seen in Fig. 1.1 but not so obvious at times on samples such as those seen in Fig. 1.2. Furthermore, once the esophagus is damaged and the epithelium is replaced by columnar epithelium, as in Fig. 1.3, the muscularis mucosae becomes thick and disorganized, sometimes even forming two (duplicated) or three (triplicated) layers with bits of lamina propria between them.[2] The tissue between these sloppy smooth layers is all lamina propria, not submucosa! The irregularities in the muscularis mucosae following mucosal damage are further discussed in the section concerning EMRs. In Fig. 1.3, there is a clue (in addition to the squamous epithelium) that the sample is from the esophagus; an esophageal submucosal gland is present at the lower right of the image, and a duct that is intended to lead from the submucosal gland to the surface is indicated. The presence of esophageal submucosal glands and ducts in a sample confirms that the sample is derived from the esophagus, but this is not a common finding in mucosal biopsies.

The presence of so-called multilayered epithelium,[3,4] discussed later, is also a clue that a specimen is derived from the esophagus. Figure 1.4 shows a mucosal biopsy that contains a submucosal gland, but this is unusual.

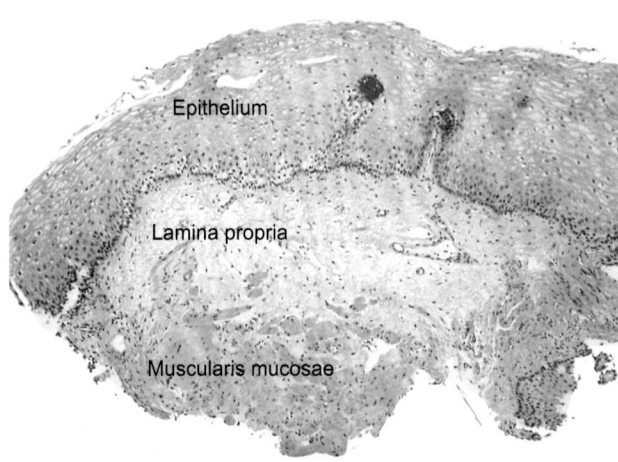

Figure 1-1. Esophageal mucosal biopsy. This sample is slightly tangentially embedded. Note that the biopsy contains all three layers of the mucosa, namely, the squamous epithelium, the loose lamina propria with a few delicate blood vessels, and the muscularis mucosae (this is Latin for the muscle of the mucosa). The epithelium has only a few layers of the darker basal cells, and the more superficial cells are pink (eosinophilic), with their long axes arranged parallel to the basement membrane, which is normal polarity for squamous epithelium. For columnar epithelium, the long axes of the nuclei are normally arranged perpendicular to the basement membrane. This sample is essentially normal and fairly well oriented.

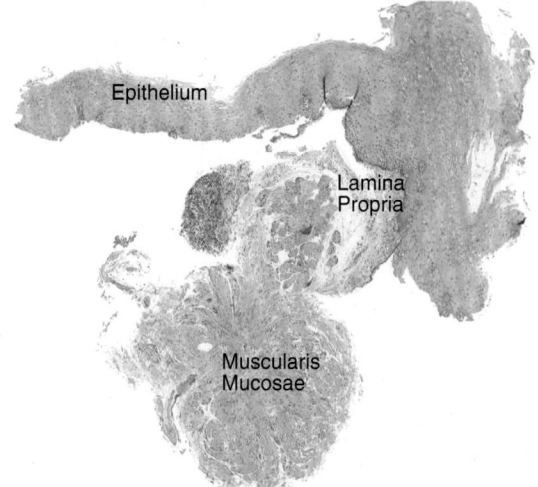

Figure 1-2. Esophageal mucosal biopsy. This mucosal biopsy has been embedded in a disorderly fashion such that it is a bit trickier to interpret than the sample shown in Fig. 1.1 There is a lymphoid aggregate at the left. The muscularis mucosae is tangentially embedded and appears thick, but this is not muscularis propria. The loose connective tissue at the upper right is lamina propria rather than submucosa.

Pancreatic acinar cell heterotopia is also common in esophageal biopsies and resections and is an incidental finding. The resection images shown in Figs. 1.5 and 1.6 highlight this finding and compare it with the appearance of submucosal glands. Pancreatic acinar heterotopia of the esophagus is generally encountered in the mucosa, whereas submucosal glands, of course, are in the submucosa.

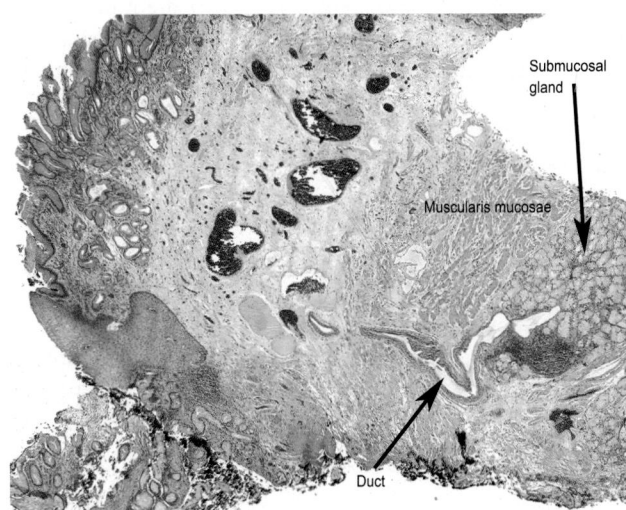

Figure 1-3. Endoscopic mucosal resection. Even though this specimen is not well oriented, it shows the layers that can be seen. Submucosa appears at the lower right of the field, and a submucosal gland is indicated. To the left of the submucosal gland, a thickened portion of muscularis mucosae courses across the sample. A duct, which transports secretions from the submucosal gland to lubricate the surface, is seen piercing through the muscularis mucosae. The zone to the left beneath the mucosa is the lamina propria and not the submucosa. Epithelium is seen at the left. Note that in the columnar cardiac mucosa portion, lamina propria invests individual glands, whereas it is under the squamous epithelium in the zone with squamous epithelium.

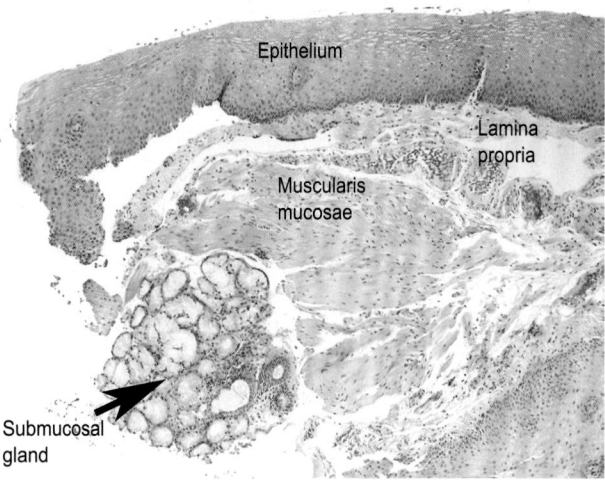

Figure 1-4. Biopsy of esophagus. This is an unusual case in that a submucosal gland is present such that a small portion of submucosa is clearly present in the specimen. However, the loose connective tissue in between the epithelium and the muscularis mucosae is lamina propria rather than submucosa.

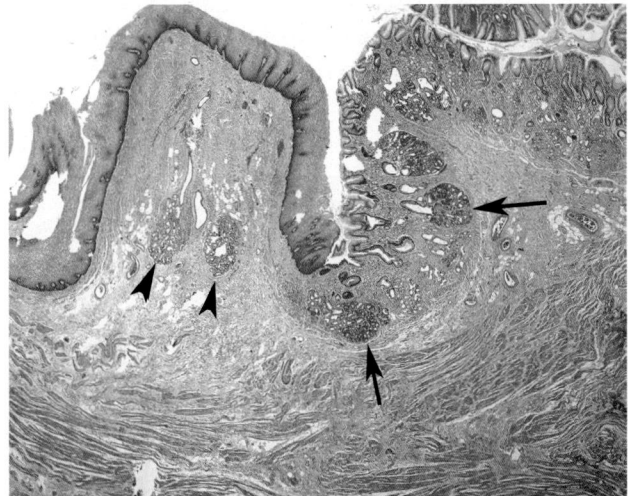

Figure 1-5. Gastroesophageal junctional tissue, resection specimen. In this resection specimen, the muscularis propria curves across the bottom of the field, and an area of squamous epithelium at the left coats the lamina propria, muscularis mucosae, and submucosa, where two submucosal glands are marked with *arrowheads*. At the center and right, the mucosa is of the cardiac type and cardiac glands are present as well as foci of pancreatic heterotopia that are within the mucosa, and a delicate cord of muscularis mucosae is beneath these foci of pancreatic heterotopia marked by the *arrows*.

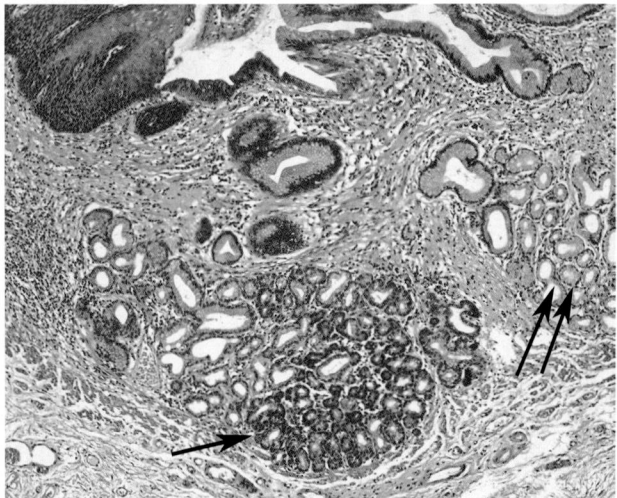

Figure 1-6. Gastroesophageal junctional tissue. This is a high-magnification image of one of the foci of pancreatic heterotopia that are indicated in Fig. 1.5. A nodule of pancreatic heterotopia is indicated by a *single arrow* and wisps of muscularis mucosae are beneath it. The *double arrows* mark gastric cardiac glands, which produce mucin.

SOME ESOPHAGEAL POLYPS

GRANULAR CELL TUMOR

Granular cell tumors of the esophagus account for about 1% to 2% of all granular cell tumors,[5] and the esophagus is the most common gastrointestinal tract site.[6] Most esophageal granular cell tumors arise in the distal esophagus and about 5% to 10% are multicentric. There is a female predominance, and these tumors are more common in African-Americans than in whites. Occasional large examples require radical surgery, and malignant examples are rare.[7,8] Most esophageal granular cell tumors appear as well-marginated masses on imaging studies such that they are interpreted as gastrointestinal stromal tumors (GISTs). The important thing with granular cell tumors is that they can be foolers. Do not be the next victim!

It is not clear why granular cell tumors are prone to elicit a pseudoepitheliomatous reactive response in the overlying squamous epithelium (Fig. 1.7). "Epithelioma" is an old term for carcinoma, so "pseudoepitheliomatous hyperplasia" simply means "pseudocarcinomatous hyperplasia." This benign response of squamous epithelium occasionally leads to a misinterpretation of squamous cell carcinoma if the granular cell tumor is not spotted. This phenomenon also applies to anal canal granular cell tumors. Of course, pseudoepitheliomatous hyperplasia can be found on top of carcinomas as well as other processes. Figs. 1.8 and 1.9 show pseudoepitheliomatous (squamous) hyperplasia overlying an adenocarcinoma of the esophagus.

Like granular cell tumors in the skin and elsewhere, esophageal granular cell tumors show strong S100 protein expression (Fig. 1.10). Remember that a high-quality S100 protein preparation should display both nuclear and cytoplasmic labeling.

LEIOMYOMA

Leiomyoma is by far the most common spindle cell tumor of the esophagus, but it is still uncommon. Esophageal leiomyomas arise in young patients (well, at least compared with one of the authors—median age, 35 years),[9] with a male predominance. They consist of cells with eosinophilic cytoplasm (Fig. 1.11) and express desmin and alpha-smooth muscle actin, but not CD117 and CD34. The important pitfall to be aware of in diagnosing gastrointestinal tract leiomyomas is that, if one performs immunolabeling for CD117 and DOG1, these stains label Cajal cells that are either entrapped in or proliferating along with the lesion (Fig. 1.12). For this reason, confident morphologists avoid these stains. Esophageal leiomyomas are easy to diagnose on staining with hematoxylin and eosin (H&E)—they are hypocellular, pink, and benign.

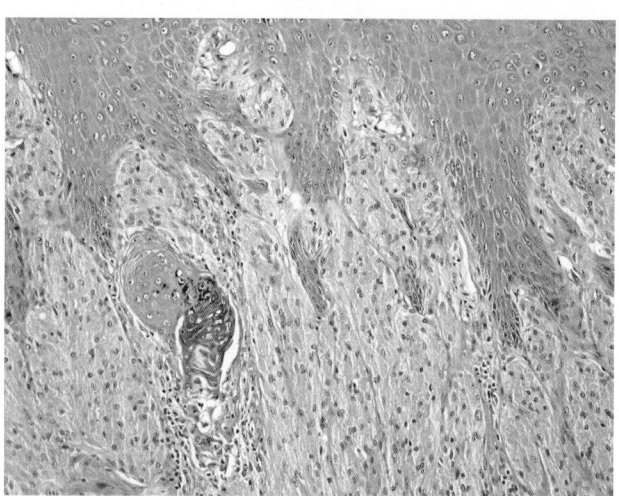

Figure 1-7. Granular cell tumor. The tumor consists of plump eosinophilic cells with granular cytoplasm and small nuclei. This type of tumor is notorious for stimulating hyperplasia of the overlying squamous epithelium (so-called pseudoepitheliomatous hyperplasia), which can be mistaken for carcinoma.

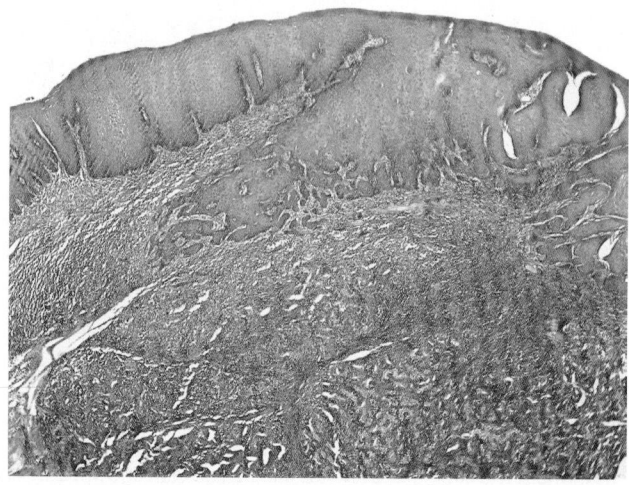

Figure 1-8. Pseudoepitheliomatous hyperplasia associated with an adenocarcinoma. The adenocarcinoma at the bottom of the field has undermined the squamous epithelium at the top of the field. The squamous process is benign and reactive.

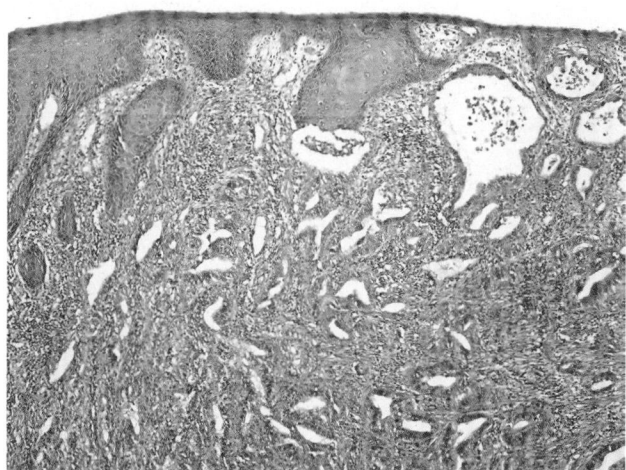

Figure 1-9. Pseudoepitheliomatous hyperplasia associated with an adenocarcinoma. This is a high-magnification image of the same lesion as that seen in Fig. 1.8. The surface squamous component is benign and simply reacting to the adenocarcinoma beneath it.

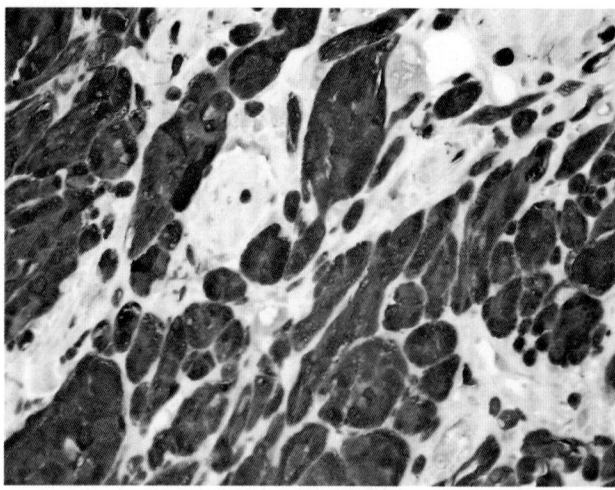

Figure 1-10. Granular cell tumor. This stunning S100 protein immunohistochemical stain shows striking nuclear and cytoplasmic expression.

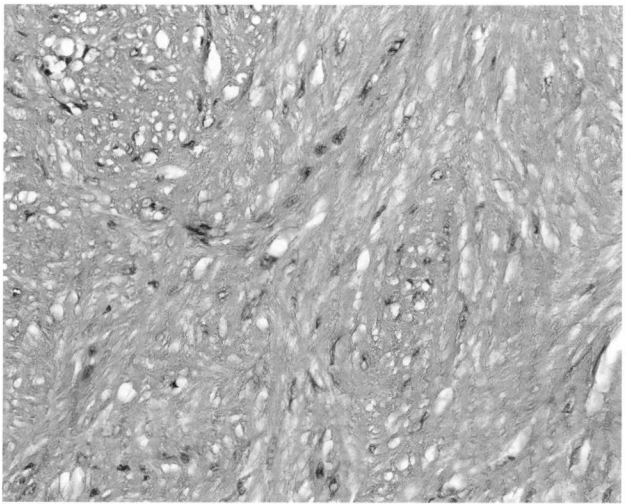

Figure 1-11. Esophageal leiomyoma. The lesional cells are brightly eosinophilic, and the tumor has low cellularity. The cytoplasm is fibrillary, and paranuclear vacuoles are present.

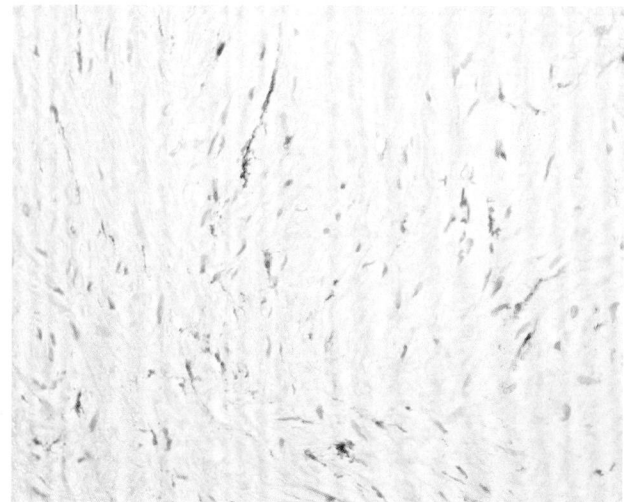

Figure 1-12. Esophageal leiomyoma. This is a CD117/KIT stain. Do not be fooled by the scattered labeled cells. Whether these are entrapped Cajal cells or an integral part of the leiomyoma is not clear, but they should not result in an interpretation of gastrointestinal stromal tumor.

GASTROINTESTINAL STROMAL TUMORS OF THE ESOPHAGUS

GISTs predominate in the stomach and intestines, but they are vanishingly rare in the esophagus. Even the combined files of the former Armed Forces Institute of Pathology and the Haartman Institute of the University of Helsinki yielded only 17 examples of esophageal GISTs![9] They arose in the lower third of the esophagi of adults (12 men and 5 women), with a median age of 63 years). Patients most commonly presented with dysphagia. Compared with leiomyomas, GISTs have an overall basophilic appearance and combinations of solid, myxoid, and perivascular collarlike patterns (Figs. 1.13–1.15). GISTs are discussed in "Stomach" and "Mesenchymal Lesions" chapters in more detail, but those in the esophagus are truly rare.

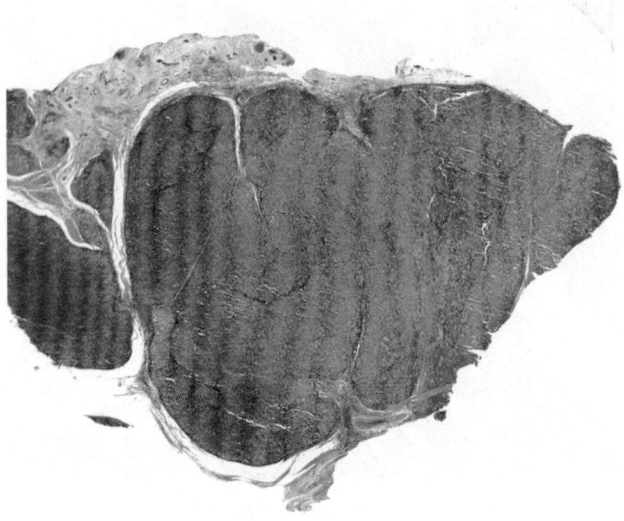

Figure 1-13. Esophageal gastrointestinal stromal tumor. These lesions are rare in contrast to gastric gastrointestinal stromal tumor. Note the prominent cellularity, a striking difference from the cellularity of the leiomyoma in Figs. 1.11 and 1.12.

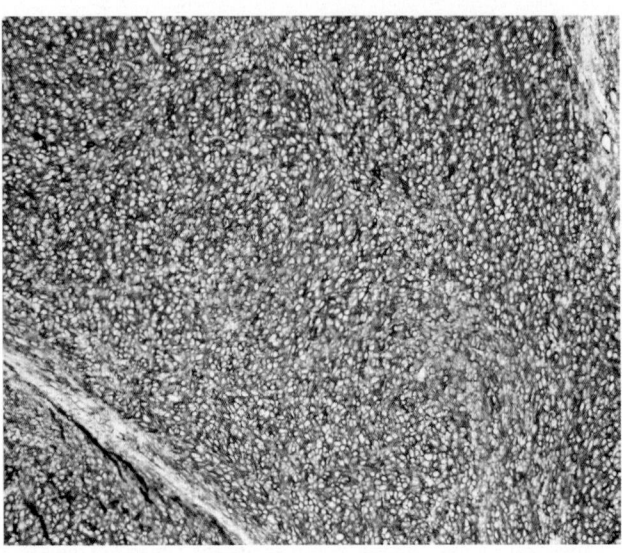

Figure 1-14. Esophageal gastrointestinal stromal tumor. This is a CD117/KIT stain.

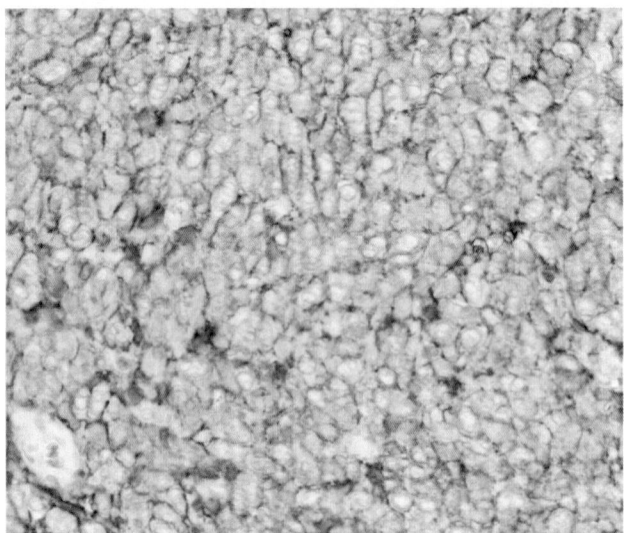

Figure 1-15. Esophageal gastrointestinal stromal tumor. This is a DOG1 stain.

Most patients in Miettinen's early series died of their tumors, but the study was from the era before targeted therapy. Regardless, in contrast to GISTs of the stomach, esophageal examples should be considered aggressive.

BARRETT ESOPHAGUS

Evaluating for Barrett esophagus and the neoplasia associated with it is a large part of the practice of Western pathologists. Columnar metaplasia in the esophagus is the source of anxiety for patients and pathologists alike. This section is approached with a short list of questions before dysplasia is discussed.

FAQ: How is Barrett mucosa defined?

Answer: It depends on whom you ask! In the United Kingdom and Japan the definition differs from that in the United States, and at this writing, there is some flux at play in the United States.

British (and Japanese) definition of Barrett mucosa 2014:

- Columnar epithelium with or without goblet cells extending ≥1 cm above the gastric folds[10]

American Gastroenterological Association definition of Barrett mucosa 2011:

- Columnar epithelium in the esophagus that contains goblet cells—no length requirement[11]

American College of Gastroenterologists' definition of Barrett mucosa 2016:

- Columnar epithelium with goblet cells extending ≥1 cm above the top of the gastric folds[12]

The last definition (the 2016 one from the American College of Gastroenterologists) makes the life of the pathologist challenging. In some instances, we have a good idea about the length of a segment of columnar epithelium in question, whereas in others, the only information we have is "esophagus." Obviously, if we have a sample labeled "esophagus, 40 cm" and we see intestinal metaplasia and we have a second sample that is labeled "esophagus, 34 cm" and we see intestinal metaplasia, it is clear that the affected segment of lesion measures at least 1 cm. Interestingly, the gastroenterology colleagues who compiled the recommendations even went so far as to caution our endoscopy colleagues to refrain from biopsies of the gastroesophageal junction unless there was a visible alteration. At least in our hospitals, there seems to be little compliance with the latter suggestion. The American College of Gastroenterology suggested the term "specialized intestinal metaplasia of the esophagogastric junction" for lesions that contain goblet cells but do not satisfy the requirement for the mucosal irregularity to extend at least 1 cm above the top of the gastric folds.[12]

To get around the length issue, we have developed two notes that we find useful for situations for which (1) we see intestinal metaplasia and we do not know the segment length or (2) the sample is labeled "gastroesophageal junction" and we see intestinal metaplasia.

SAMPLE NOTES: Barrett Mucosa

Situation A: Barrett Mucosa, Negative for Dysplasia. See Note

Note: The diagnosis of Barrett esophagus is made owing to the presence of goblet cells (intestinal metaplasia), with the assumption that the biopsies were obtained from columnar mucosa in the distal esophagus and the mucosal irregularity extends at least 1 cm above the top of the gastric folds as per 2016 American College of Gastroenterology (ACG) guidelines.

Reference:
Shaheen NJ, Falk GW, Iyer PG, Gerson LB; American College of Gastroenterology. ACG clinical guideline: diagnosis and management of Barrett's esophagus. *Am J Gastroenterol.* 2016;111(1):30-50.

Situation B: Cardiac Mucosa With Intestinal Metaplasia. See Note

Note: This biopsy shows gastric-type mucosa with scattered goblet cells. The diagnosis in this case depends on the location of this biopsy. If this biopsy was taken from the tubular esophagus and the mucosal irregularity extends at least 1 cm above the top of the gastric folds, the diagnosis is Barrett mucosa of the distinctive type. If this biopsy was taken from the gastric cardia, the diagnosis is intestinal metaplasia of the gastric cardia.

Reference:
Shaheen NJ, Falk GW, Iyer PG, Gerson LB; American College of Gastroenterology. ACG clinical guideline: diagnosis and management of Barrett's esophagus. *Am J Gastroenterol.* 2016;111(1):30-50.

FAQ: The ACG 2016 criteria state: *BE should be diagnosed when there is extension of salmon-colored mucosa into the tubular esophagus extending ≥1 cm above the top of the gastric folds with biopsy confirmation of IM (strong recommendation, low level of evidence).* So, if there is a 0.5-cm island that is >1 cm above the top of the gastric folds that contains intestinal metaplasia, is it Barrett esophagus?

Answer: This is a contentious area in gastroenterology circles. The ≥1 cm length of mucosal irregularity rule was created to differentiate irregular Z lines with intestinal metaplasia in cardiac mucosa from true Barrett mucosa, which is a lesion of the tubular esophagus. By the rules of the ACG, the described 0.5-cm island >1 cm above the top of the gastric folds is "intestinal metaplasia in the esophagus" and not Barrett mucosa. This is in fact a shortcoming of the Prague classification as well. By common sense, such an island is biologically Barrett mucosa, but it is not formally recognized as such according to the newest guidelines. However, recent data suggest that such a lesion should be managed as per Barrett esophagus.[13] As such, report what you see on the slide and work with your endoscopist to plan follow-up.

FAQ: Why do some observers want to eliminate the requirement for goblet cells for a diagnosis of Barrett mucosa in the United States?

Answer: There are some studies that suggest that most esophageal adenocarcinomas that are detected arise in the absence of intestinal metaplasia. In one of them, the authors used EMR samples and found adjoining intestinal metaplasia in less than half of the samples with early cancers.[14] However, these colleagues did not attempt to learn if the patients had separate samples that contained intestinal metaplasia. In two West Coast US studies, intestinal metaplasia essentially always accompanied high-grade columnar epithelial dysplasia and carcinomas.[15,16] We found similar results in an East Coast study[17] and would endorse retaining the requirement for goblet cells, but others have suggested eliminating the requirement.[18] Regardless, there are a few cases of esophageal adenocarcinomas that are unassociated with intestinal metaplasia, but they are not numerous in our Western population. Elimination of the requirement for goblet cells to diagnose Barrett esophagus in the United States would even further reduce the cost-effectiveness of surveillance of patients with Barrett esophagus because it would open the floodgates to patients with reflux. A key issue is that, when cardiac mucosa is found (without intestinal metaplasia), it could be a normal finding, so the presence of intestinal metaplasia offers some assurance that at least abnormal tissue has been biopsied.

FAQ: Which histologic patterns can mimic Barrett mucosa?

Answer: This topic has been addressed in the non-neoplastic volume preceding this volume (*Atlas of Gastrointestinal Pathology. A pattern based approach to non-neoplastic biopsies*), although we have changed our practice patterns. We performed up front periodic acid–Schiff/alcian blue staining on upper gastrointestinal tract samples (including all biopsies of the esophagus) in the past; we no longer follow this practice, but there are occasional cases for which it is instructive. Both pancreatic acinar heterotopia (Figs. 1.5, 1.6, 1.16, and 1.17) and some gastric foveolar cells (Figs. 1.18 and 1.19) can suggest intestinal metaplasia. Pancreatic heterotopia contains cells with granules, so these cells can be easily distinguished from goblet cells, but some gastric foveolar cells can take on a bluish hue or show weak alcianophilia on alcian blue staining. These latter cells lack the true intestinal differentiation that we will see later.

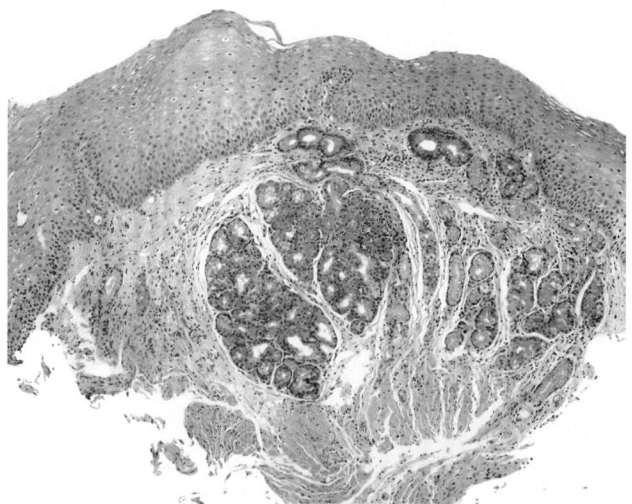

Figure 1-16. Pancreatic acinar cell heterotopia. This image allows us to further consider the layer in which pancreatic acinar cell heterotopia is found. In this case, there is squamous rather than cardiac-type mucosa associated with the pancreatic acinar cell heterotopia. Note that it is found in the lamina propria. There is squamous epithelium over it, cardiac glands to the right, and muscularis mucosae below it.

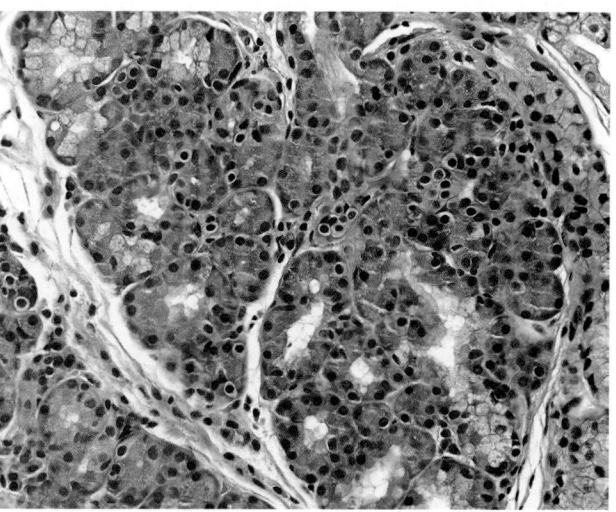

Figure 1-17. Pancreatic acinar cell heterotopia. This high-magnification image shows zymogen granules in the cells to full advantage.

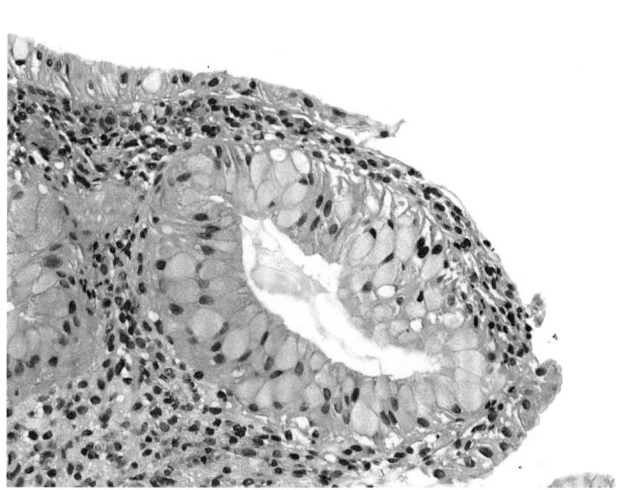

Figure 1-18. "Fake" goblet cells. A few of the cells in this cardiac gland have a bluish tint but lack the demarcation of goblet cells.

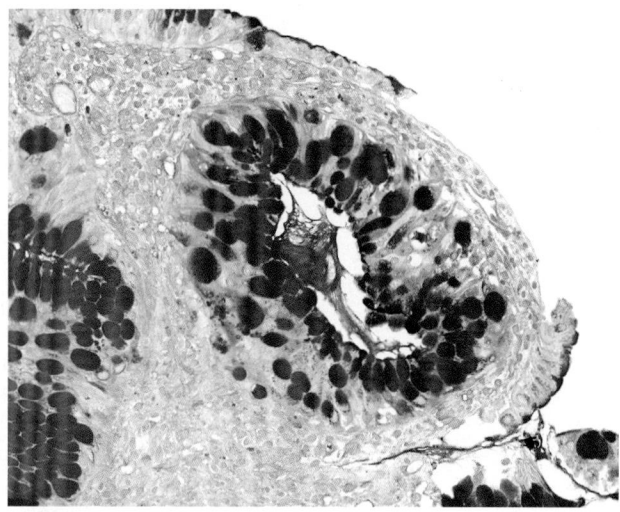

Figure 1-19. "Fake" goblet cells. This is a periodic acid–Schiff/alcian blue stain. It shows a bit of nonspecific alcianophilia, but no goblet cells are present. This does not qualify as Barrett mucosa.

FAQ: What is the difference between complete and incomplete intestinal metaplasia and do they matter?

Answer: Complete intestinal metaplasia indicates that the metaplasia perfectly recapitulates intestine in that there are goblet cells separated by absorptive cells that have a brush border but not any cytoplasmic mucin. Incomplete intestinal metaplasia has only incompletely converted from gastric cardiac mucosa to intestinal-type mucosa. As such, there are goblet cells separated by cells that resemble gastric foveolar cells. An example of a sample with both types juxtaposed is shown in Figs. 1.20 and 1.21. The complete type is far more likely to be found in gastric mucosa than in intestinal metaplasia of the esophagus, and its presence can suggest that the sample is from the stomach rather than from the esophagus. However, complete intestinal metaplasia is not specific for gastric intestinal metaplasia. The incomplete type, epidemiologically, is more likely to progress to adenocarcinoma than the complete type, but reporting it is not particularly relevant in any given patient, and it is not necessary to report which type is seen unless the purpose is a study protocol.

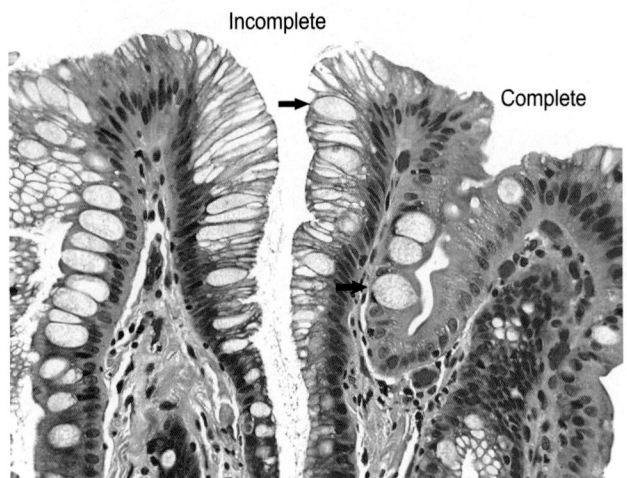

Figure 1-20. Barrett esophagus with complete and incomplete intestinal metaplasia. In incomplete intestinal metaplasia, the mucosa has incompletely transformed from gastric cardiac type to an intestinal phenotype such that there are goblet cells (see the *arrow* beneath the "incomplete" annotation) interspersed with gastric foveolar cells with apical mucin. In contrast, the complete type of intestinal metaplasia fully recapitulates intestinal epithelium and cells with brush borders are seen between goblet cells (a goblet cell is marked with an *arrow* underneath the zone marked as "complete").

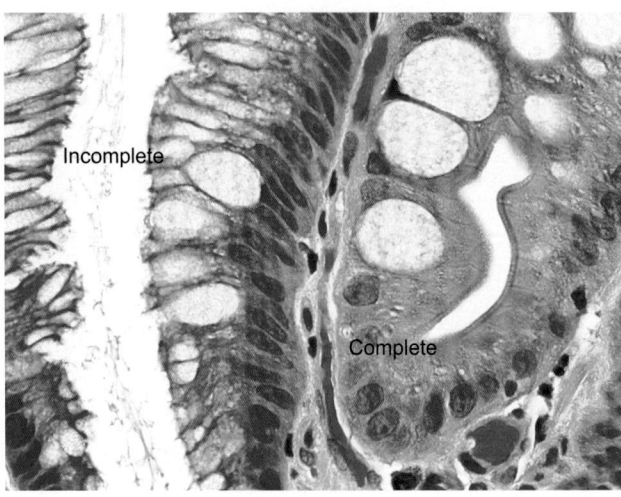

Figure 1-21. Barrett esophagus with complete and incomplete intestinal metaplasia. This is a high-magnification image of the area shown in Fig. 1.20. It is not necessary to specify the type of metaplasia in reports unless there is a specific protocol, but, on epidemiologic grounds, the incomplete type is more likely to progress to carcinoma. In the individual case, it is not an important factor.

FAQ: What is multilayered epithelium?

Answer: Multilayered epithelium is a type of epithelium that is associated with gastroesophageal reflux and that has some properties of intestinal-type epithelium and some properties of squamous epithelium.[3,4,19,20] Because of these features, many observers have suggested that it is a precursor to Barrett mucosa (a precursor to a precursor).[21] Essentially, it is only important to avoid diagnosing it as dysplasia and not worry too much about it! Because it correlates with clinical reflux disease and can be found in association with Barrett mucosa, it is a topic of interest. In addition, the presence of multilayered epithelium is a clue that a sample has come from the esophagus rather than from the stomach. For those who use special stains to detect Barrett mucosa, some examples of multilayered epithelium react with these stains, including CDX2 and MUC2, but not diffusely. There is no need to either use these stains or be concerned about the labeling if you do.

The multilayered epithelium has an appearance similar to that of immature squamous metaplasia in the uterine cervix. The surface has a few cells that have a blush of mucin, and the base has a squamous appearance. The mucin can have a basophilic appearance akin to that of goblet cells but is not crisply delineated like that in goblet cells. An example is seen in Figs. 1.22 and 1.23.

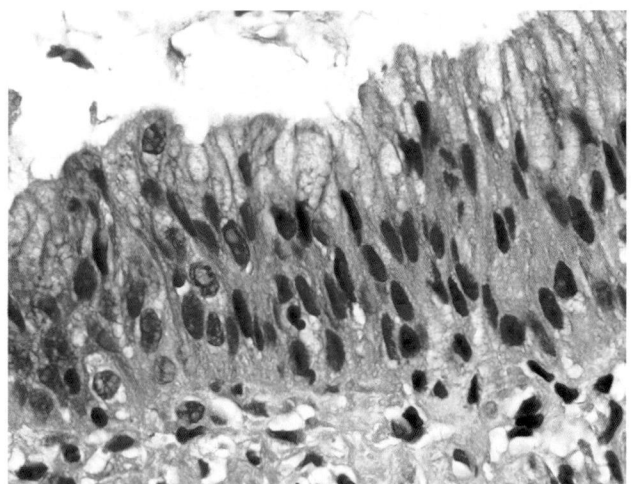

Figure 1-22. Multilayered epithelium. This is a high-magnification image showing epithelium and a tiny sliver of lamina propria at the bottom of the image. At first glance, the basal cells appear hyperchromatic, but a quick glance at the lymphocytes at the lower right is reassuring. The epithelial cell nuclei are only slightly larger than the lymphocyte nuclei, so this is not squamous dysplasia. Note that the cells at the surface contain bubbly mucin-filled cytoplasm that is bluish, a feature similar to the mucin in goblet cells, but the mucin does not form a single discreet droplet in the manner of goblet cells. The appearance of esophageal multilayered epithelium is similar to that of immature squamous metaplasia of the uterine cervix. This type of epithelium is found in patients with reflux and can also accompany conventional Barrett mucosa. There is also some experimental evidence that this type of epithelium gives rise to conventional Barrett mucosa.[21] We do not currently report this finding.

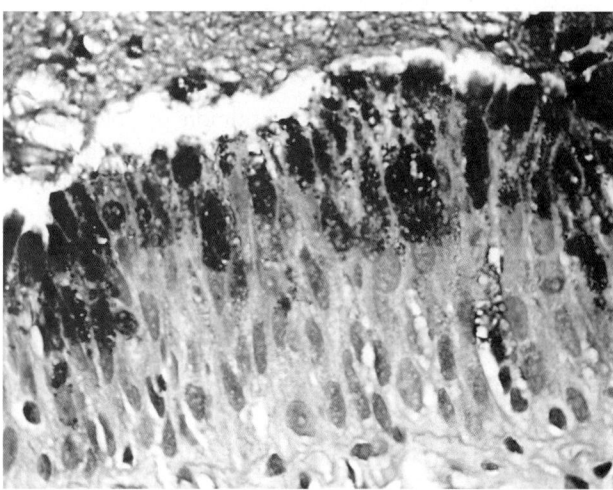

Figure 1-23. Multilayered epithelium. This is a periodic acid–Schiff/alcian blue stain. Some of the mucin-laden cells display alcianophilia (have a *blue* appearance), but their morphology is different from that of actual goblet cells like those seen in Fig. 1.21.

FAQ: How does Barrett mucosa appear endoscopically?

Answer: Barrett mucosa appears as velvety "salmon-colored" epithelium that extends as "tongues" above the gastric folds (Figs. 1.24 and 1.25). When an area of Barrett mucosa is encircled by squamous mucosa, the columnar zone is referred to as an "island."

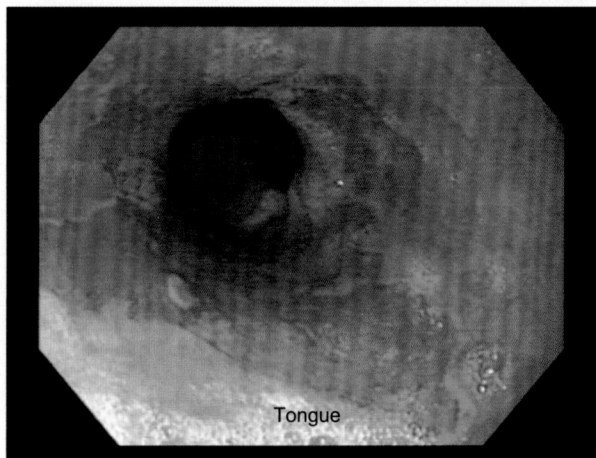

Figure 1-24. Barrett esophagus, endoscopic image. There is a tongue at the lower right, which means an extension of columnar epithelium above the gastric folds into the tubular portion of the esophagus. In this image, we are looking down from the incisors and the dark area at the left center of the image is the stomach. The gray mucosa at the lower left of the image is squamous mucosa. The word "tongue" is written on the squamous epithelium to indicate the tongue of columnar epithelium just to the right of the word.

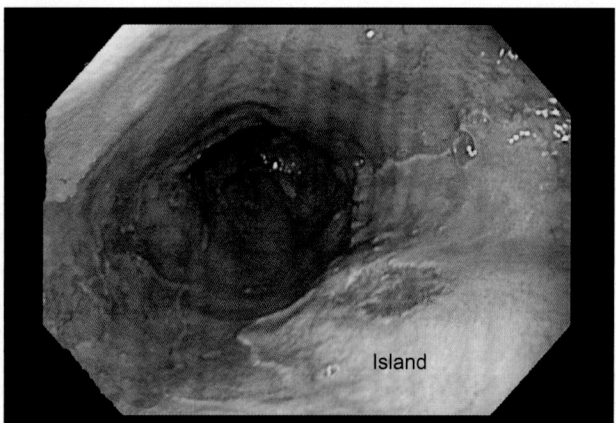

Figure 1-25. Barrett esophagus, endoscopic image. There are tongues of salmon-colored columnar mucosa at the top, lower center, and lower left of the image. The gastric folds can be seen in the center of the image. One area of columnar epithelium is present at the lower right. It is salmon colored but surrounded on all sides by gray pearly squamous mucosa. This is referred to as an "island" of columnar epithelium. A biopsy is needed to learn whether this area has intestinal metaplasia.

Our endoscopy colleagues use a wonderful system to describe the extent of Barrett esophagus called the Prague system (of course they got to have a fancy meeting in Prague, probably with nice concerts and fancy food and a posh hotel, whereas we have to meet in Baltimore or Columbus, but that is fine because we get to sit down when we do our daily work) in which the distance of the circumferential length of Barrett mucosa (C) and the maximum length (M) are recorded.[22] This method has allowed standardization of endoscopy reports and is important for pathologists to also understand. When these data are provided to us, they can help us understand whether the samples are from long-segment of short-segment Barrett mucosa—long segment means more than 3 cm. This scheme is seen in Fig. 1.26.

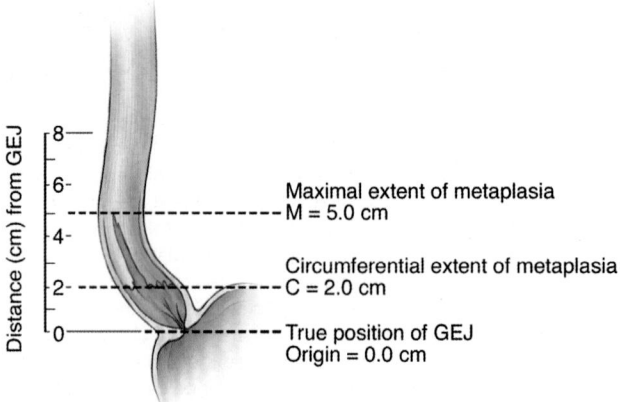

Figure 1-26. Schematic for the Prague classification for Barrett mucosa. In this scheme, which is used worldwide by endoscopy colleagues, the distance of the circumferential length of Barrett mucosa (C) and the maximum length are recorded (M). If the information is provided to the pathologist, it can be used to decide whether the findings in any given case meet criteria for Barrett mucosa because a minimal length criterion has been introduced.

FAQ: Are special stains needed to diagnose Barrett esophagus?

Answer: The short answer is "nope," but, of course, we all occasionally need a bit of help. However, we would note that, when Panarelli and Yantiss reviewed the topic, they concluded that neither histochemical nor immunohistochemical stains add value over H&E stains because they tend to produce false-positive results.[23]

In the past, the idea that CK7/CK20 stains could be used to differentiate esophageal intestinal metaplasia from gastric cardiac intestinal metaplasia was entertained but did not really catch on.[24,25] Long-segment Barrett esophagus cases (>3 cm) were characterized by superficial and deep CK7 immunoreactivity in the intestinalized mucosa, with only superficial CK20 staining in the intestinalized zones. In contrast, distal gastric intestinal metaplasia was characterized by patchy, superficial, and deep CK20 staining in areas of incomplete intestinal metaplasia; strong, superficial, and deep CK20 staining in areas of complete intestinal metaplasia; and patchy or absent CK7 staining in either type of gastric intestinal metaplasia. Many other immunostains have been studied, including mucin core (MUC) polypeptides, to better characterize gastric cardiac versus esophageal intestinal metaplasia. The MUC polypeptides seem to be of little practical value in any given patient and are presently of academic interest only. They include MUC5 (gastric foveolar mucin), MUC6 (cardiac glands, antral glands, Brunner glands), and MUC2 (goblet cells). Some have used CDX2 staining to label areas of intestinal metaplasia.[26] Others have used it to note that some cases lacking goblet cells express these markers (illustrated later) anyway to make the point that the United States should drop the requirement for goblet cells to diagnose Barrett esophagus.[27] Others have suggested that hepatocyte antigen (Hepar-1, carbamoyl phosphate synthetase 1) is helpful in detecting intestinal metaplasia or processes that are intestinalized in the absence of goblet cells.[28] It seems more practical to simply search for goblet cells because that can be done consistently in any laboratory without the added costs of immunolabeling. In fact, none of the immunostains intended to detect goblet cells offers added value over H&E stains.[23] Fig. 1.27 was prepared from a consultation case. It is a CDX2 stain of Barrett mucosa in which every single nucleus is labeled, including both those of goblet cells and those of gastric foveolar cells.

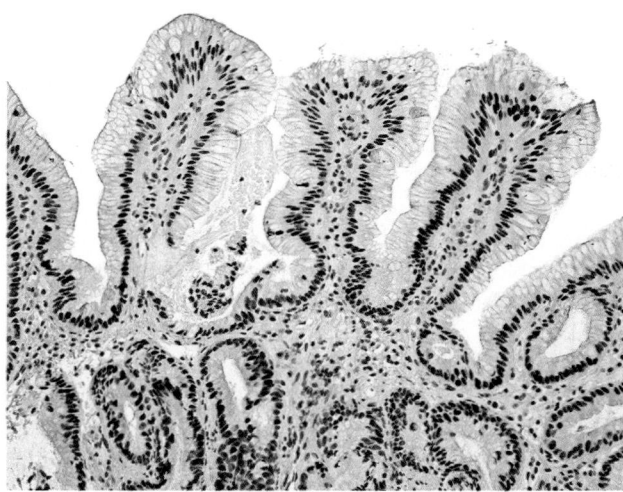

Figure 1-27. Esophageal columnar mucosa with scattered goblet cells, CDX2 stain. This is interesting in that cells that are clearly goblet cells, such as the one near the tip of the villuslike structure at the upper left, and all other columnar cells are reactive. This finding suggests that the cardiac-type epithelium already has some traits that overlap with those of the intestinal-type epithelium. However, at least in a US population, goblet cells are probably a better marker for patients who require surveillance than columnar epithelium alone.[17]

GRADING BARRETT DYSPLASIA

This should be a piece of cake and easy, right? In fact, most of the time it is easy because most samples from Barrett lack dysplasia! However, it is not always easy and knowing a few tricks and tips can help. It is well known that observer variation is an issue,[29] but we can take steps to reduce this. In the past, at least in Johns Hopkins, we have reported low-grade dysplasia and "indefinite for dysplasia" too liberally but have been able to tighten our criteria in the last few years and this has not resulted in patient harm by missing important lesions (Data unpublished at presstime; search Waters et al.), but as a general rule, an institution should not be reporting more than 5% low-grade dysplasia in patients presenting to clinic. However, clinics devoted to dysplasia would be expected to have a higher percentage of dysplasia cases. Here are the categories that are used on biopsies[30]:

Negative for dysplasia
Indefinite for dysplasia
Low-grade dysplasia
High-grade dysplasia
Adenocarcinoma (intramucosal carcinoma for the purpose of this discussion)

In evaluating Barrett mucosa, it is a good idea to have a systematic approach. Finding goblet cells is important and then the epithelial changes can be studied. Check for surface maturation and glandular crowding, examine the cytologic features, and decide if inflammation is an obscuring factor before making a diagnosis.

Barrett Esophagus, Negative for Dysplasia

Nondysplastic Barrett mucosa should feature surface maturation, which can be difficult to assess in badly embedded samples. It is normal to encounter some degree of nuclear alterations in the bases of the metaplastic pits and this can be ignored. Remember not to focus too much on these pits when you see surface epithelium on all sides of a biopsy fragment and the center portion shows areas with larger nuclei. This is normal for nondysplastic Barrett mucosa. Ignore it!

The best way to add confidence to diagnosing dysplasia in Barrett mucosa is to always think about the polarity of the epithelial cells and how they are arranged with respect to their neighbors. An extremely useful indication of maintained overall cellular polarity can be referred to as "the four lines." This appearance indicates preserved polarity of epithelial cells in both gastric cardiac mucosa and in Barrett mucosa (with goblet cells). Figs. 1.28–1.30 show cardiac mucosa (Fig. 1.28) and Barrett mucosa (Figs. 1.29 and 1.30) annotated to demonstrate the four lines at high magnification, but they can be spotted easily at 4X. The top line consists of the apical mucin cap of neutral mucin typical of Barrett mucosa (with incomplete intestinal metaplasia) and cardiac mucosa. The second line is formed by the bases of the mucin caps. The third line is formed by the aligned cytoplasm and the fourth line by the row of nuclei. These lines are not the same in the rare cases of complete intestinal metaplasia in the esophagus, but these lesions are generally readily classified for the purposes of grading dysplasia. Complete intestinal metaplasia has two lines, one for the cytoplasm and one for the row of nuclei. Awareness of these patterns makes it easy to dismiss many cases as reactive. Figs. 1.31–1.33 show cardiac mucosa with nuclear stratification that can be regarded as reactive. This same principle applies to Figs. 1.34–1.36, a Barrett case (negative for dysplasia). There is surface maturation, and the lines are preserved despite nuclear stratification. Using the magic lines as a criterion can help reduce the use of indefinite for dysplasia and overdiagnosis of low-grade dysplasia.

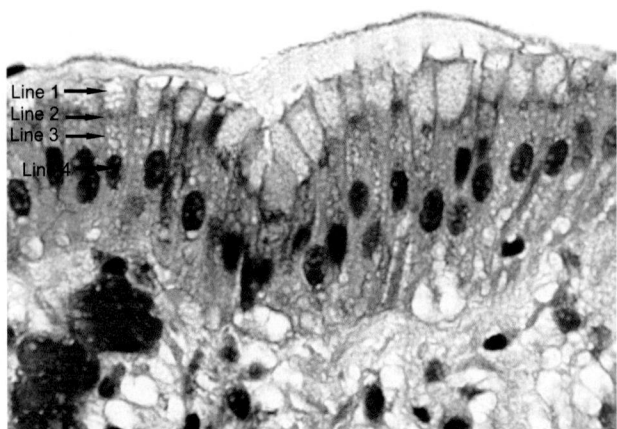

Figure 1-28. Gastric cardiac epithelium, high magnification. This image shows the four lines. Their presence indicates that the cells are arranged in an orderly fashion with respect to one another. This concept is also shown in "Colon" chapter. The top line or row consists of the apical cap of neutral mucin that characterizes gastric foveolar-type cells. The second line is the base of the cap, the third line is the row of cytoplasm, and the fourth is the row of well-aligned nuclei.

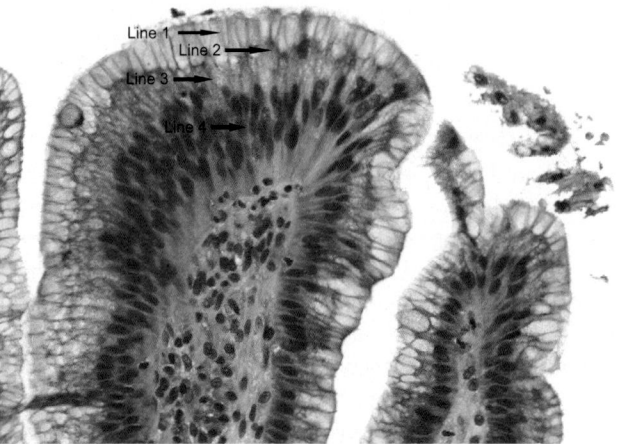

Figure 1-29. Barrett mucosa. There is a goblet cell at the upper left of the left villiform structure and another one at the left side of the villiform structure on the right. Nondysplastic Barrett mucosa retains the same overall cell-to-cell polarity as that seen in gastric cardiac mucosa. Again, the top line is the apical mucin cap of the foveolar cells, the second line is the base of this mucin vacuole, the third line is the cytoplasm, and the fourth line is the row of nuclei. The goblet cell cytoplasm punctuates but does not disorder this basic polarity.

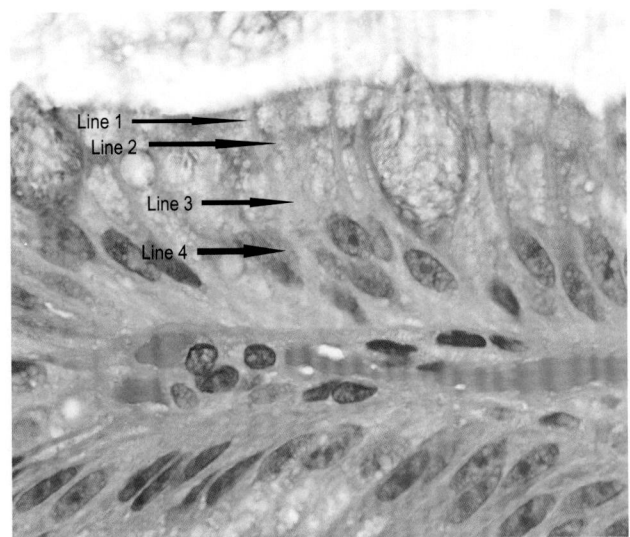

Figure 1-30. Barrett mucosa. Despite some tangential embedding, the lines are all present, even though they are broken up into dashed lines by goblet cells. Between the goblet cells, line one consists of the droplet of gastric foveolar mucin, line two consists of the base of the mucin cap, line three consists of the cytoplasm of the foveolar-type cells, and line four consists of the row of nuclei. This is nondysplastic Barrett mucosa. The nuclei appear a bit reactive, as evidenced by the presence of perfectly round nucleoli, but these nuclei are not hyperchromatic and their nuclear membranes are smooth.

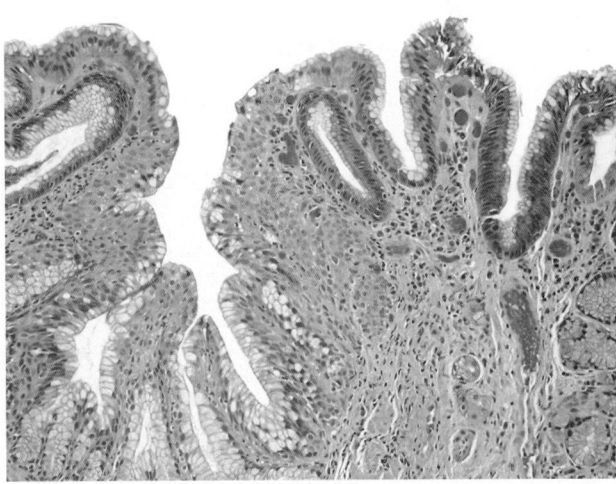

Figure 1-31. Reactive gastric cardiac mucosa adjoining multilayered epithelium. There is a lot of multilayered epithelium at the left of the image. Some of the basal zone cells in this area have an appearance like that of squamous epithelium, but there are surface columnar characteristics. The cardiac epithelium contains cells with mild nuclear enlargement, but it is easy to spot the four lines, especially at the right side of the image. This epithelium can confidently be regarded as reactive.

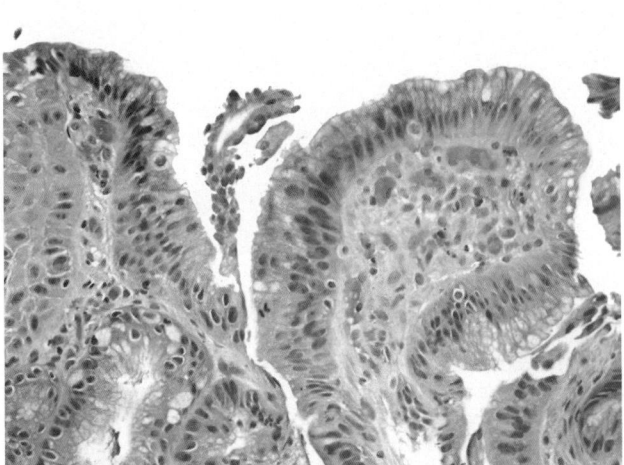

Figure 1-32. Reactive columnar mucosa. There appear to be a few goblet cells in the gland at the lower left, so this could be Barrett mucosa or intestinal metaplasia of the cardia depending on the endoscopic appearance. Importantly, although the nuclei are slightly stratified, the lines are intact. This is reactive mucosa.

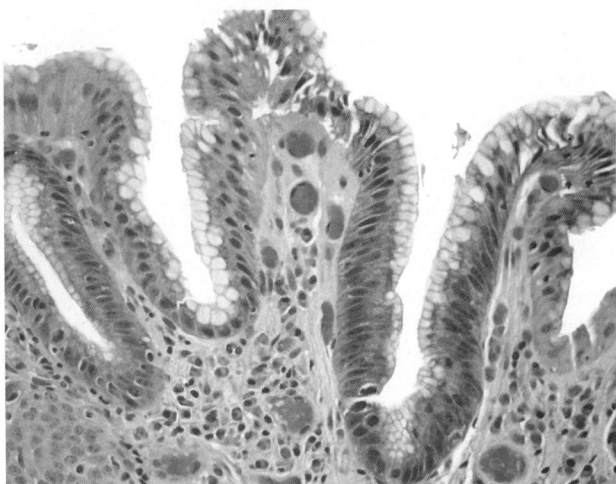

Figure 1-33. Reactive gastric cardiac mucosa. Although some of the nuclei are elongated and have nucleoli, the cells have preserved relationships to one another and the four lines are intact. This focus can be regarded as reactive. Note that there is some mitotic activity in the deep part of the gland at the right. This is acceptable, especially because the nuclei gradually mature (become smaller) toward the surface.

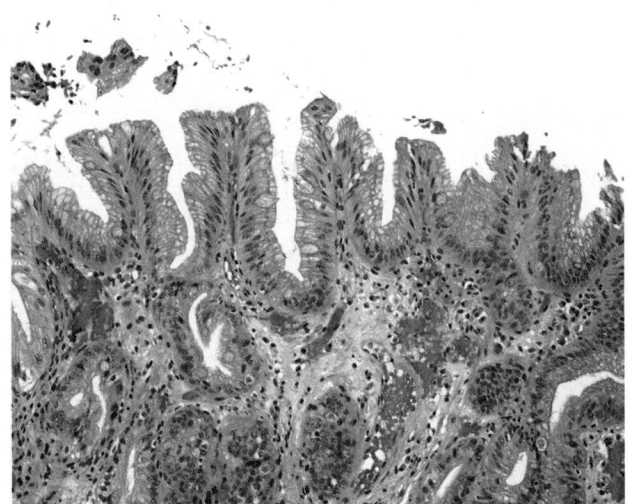

Figure 1-34. Barrett mucosa, negative for dysplasia. There is plenty of lamina propria between the glands. The glands at the deep part of the sample have larger nuclei than those seen at the surface. This is perfectly acceptable. Notice that the four lines are perfectly seen at the surface. However, note that where there is tangential sectioning, they are more difficult to make out.

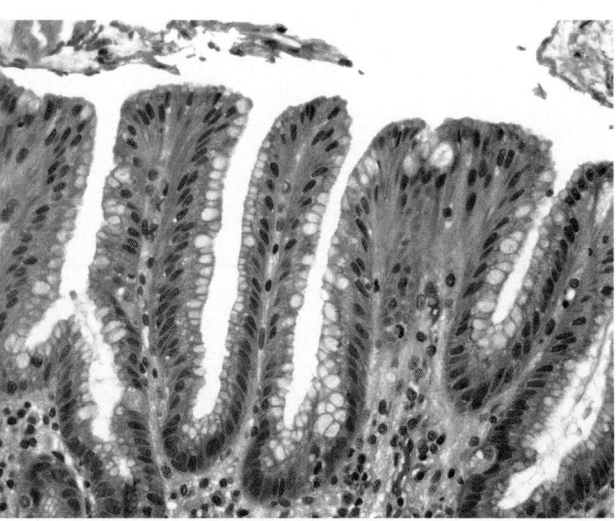

Figure 1-35. Barrett mucosa, negative for dysplasia. The lines are essentially intact. The nuclei become smaller and a bit less open at the surface, where slight tangential embedding slightly obscures the lines. However, the lines are easy to see on the sides of the glands in this image.

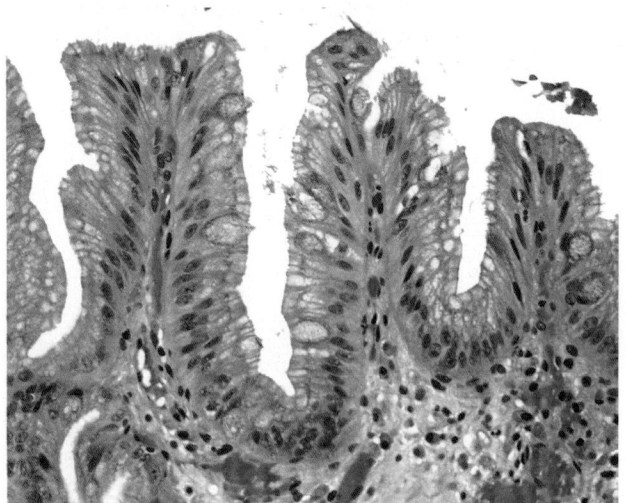

Figure 1-36. Barrett mucosa, negative for dysplasia. Note that the nuclei are smaller and more condensed at the surface, as they prepare to slough into the lumen.

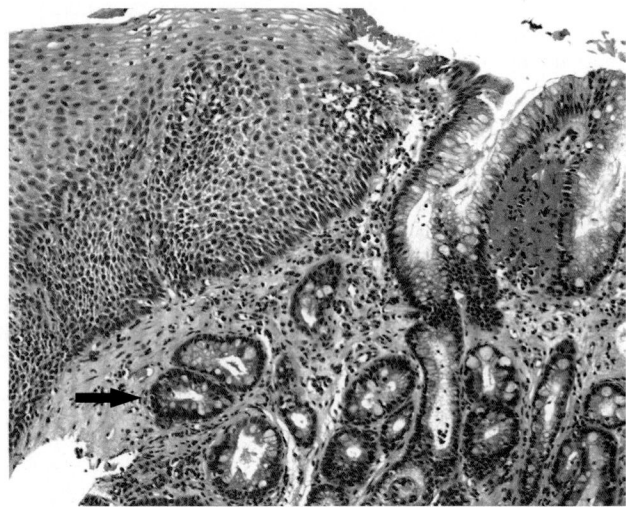

Figure 1-37. Barrett mucosa with reactive changes and inflammation, negative for dysplasia. This image shows a few tricks! The findings are all reactive. Note at the surface that the columnar epithelium directly adjoining the squamous component is typically a bit hyperchromatic and slightly disorderly, but as the surface is scanned in the image, the lines are present everywhere that the epithelium is well oriented. The *arrow* indicates a deeper gland that displays slight nuclear enlargement, but it does not "jump out" from the other deep glands. Spending a lot of time looking at such glands at very high magnification can quickly lead to an overinterpretation as basal pattern dysplasia.

The case shown in Figs. 1.37–1.40 has reactive features and illustrates another pitfall. The deep glands have slightly enlarged hyperchromatic nuclei in a context of inflammation and gradual surface maturation. A TP53 (P53) stain is also shown for this case and shows a wild-type pattern. Many laboratories endorse the use of TP53 immunolabeling in all Barrett cases, and this is a common practice in Europe. We have not adopted this practice, but if P53 labeling is always used in your practice, it is important to think before reacting to light staining. This protein is a tumor suppressor protein, and thus it is active during cell proliferation and has a quick half-life. Because it is busy preventing cancer during cell

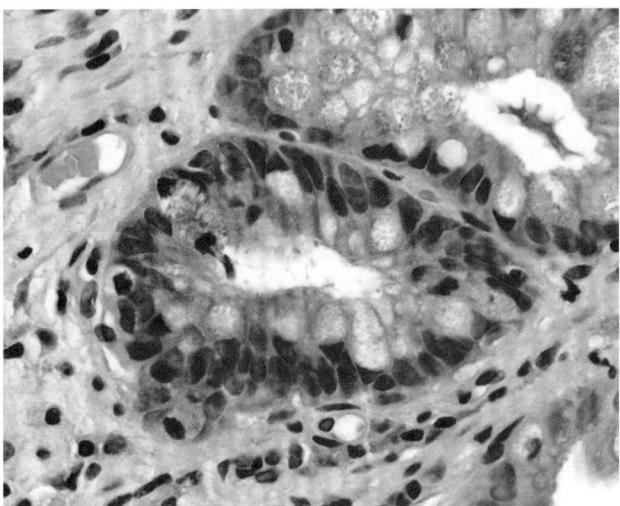

Figure 1-38. Barrett mucosa with reactive changes and inflammation, negative for dysplasia. This is a very-high-magnification image of the gland indicated in Fig. 1.37. This was not a good idea! Mitoses are present (acceptable in deep glands), and the nuclei appear somewhat jumbled and hyperchromatic out of context.

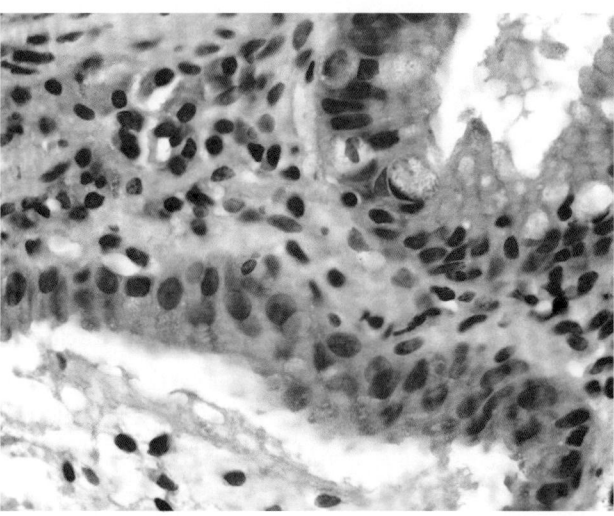

Figure 1-39. Barrett mucosa with reactive changes and inflammation, negative for dysplasia. This is another high-magnification image of some of the deep glands in the case seen in Fig. 1.37. The nucleoli in the gland with cells containing abundant eosinophilic cytoplasm and a somewhat syncytial arrangement have all of the features of a reparative process. This sort of appearance can be seen after any type of injury (including mucosal ablation). This field shows reactive nuclei rather than dysplastic ones.

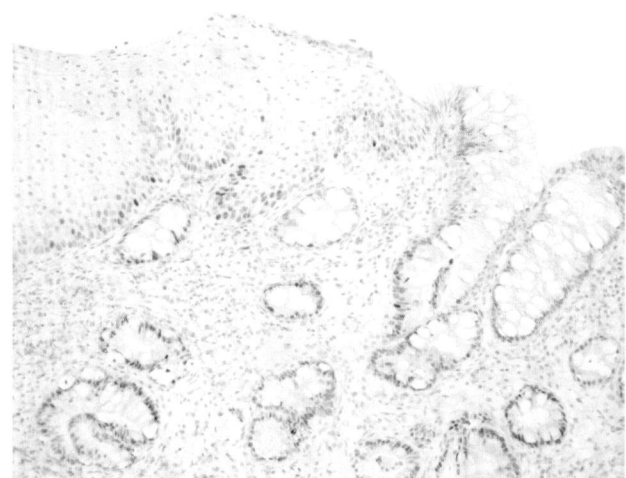

Figure 1-40. Barrett mucosa with reactive changes and inflammation, negative for dysplasia. This is a TP53 (P53) immunohistochemical stain. It shows a wild-type (not mutated) pattern that would be expected in mucosa with reparative/reactive changes. The P53 protein is a tumor suppressor protein encoded by a tumor suppressor gene. Its job is to suppress neoplastic transformation while cells are going through the proliferation process every time our mucosa is made and remade. As such, there should be a little of this protein in cells that are proliferating or regenerating an area (our mucosa turns over constantly). As such, there is staining in the basal layer of the squamous epithelium and in the deeper glands. The normal gene produces a protein that has a short half-life, so we just see just a little bit of it accumulate in proliferating nuclei. Notice that there is none at the columnar surface, and only the basal squamous nuclei are labeled. A few of the lymphocyte nuclei are also labeled lightly. When the TP53 gene is mutated, it produces a protein that is not properly degraded and has a longer half-life, so the cells with mutant TP53 show prominent nuclear labeling. Do not equate light labeling such as that in this image as evidence of dysplasia.

proliferation, a bit of labeling is to be expected in the proliferative compartment of the mucosa. As such, there is always a bit of nuclear labeling in the basal layer of the squamous epithelium and in the pits of the stomach. When the *TP53* gene is mutated, this results in a TP53 protein with an extra-long half-life, so it accumulates in the nuclei of the cells and can be detected by immunolabeling and is a wonderful marker for dysplasia, but intense staining should be used to confirm dysplasia. Fig. 1.41 shows an area of intense labeling in a zone that could be interpreted as basal pattern dysplasia (basal crypt dysplasia[31]), which is discussed later. The so-called null pattern of P53 labeling is discussed in the "High-Grade Dysplasia" section.

Barrett Esophagus Indefinite for Dysplasia

This is everyone's least favorite category. The term was introduced in a 1983 study of epithelial changes in inflammatory bowel disease that is further discussed in "Colon" chapter (which concerns the colon) and was a radical change[32] because it was baffling to our clinical colleagues that sometimes we simply have no idea whether epithelial changes are dysplastic/neoplastic or not. The term was later used in evaluating columnar epithelial changes in Barrett mucosa,[29,30] and until recently, gastroenterology societies did not even mention how to address it in guidelines. This category can be regarded as a holding diagnosis until the findings in the patient are sorted out by a course of treatment to reduce any inflammation followed by repeat sampling.[12]

No matter which images we show to illustrate our conception of cases that we would regard as indefinite for dysplasia, some colleagues will dismiss the illustrated changes as reactive and others will be concerned that dysplasia has been overlooked. That is the entire point of this category. It merits follow-up, but the patient should not receive definitive treatment (mucosal ablation therapy) until the findings are clarified.

Because, by definition, the indefinite category indicates that the pathologist is uncertain whether the area in question manifests reparative changes or dysplastic/neoplastic ones, it is difficult to write criteria. However, one can view cases that show glands with nuclear alterations in the pits that are concerning for dysplasia but that mature toward the surface as indefinite for dysplasia or lesions that lose the four lines at the surface but lack nuclear hyperchromasia as indefinite for dysplasia. When the issue concerns epithelial changes restricted to the bases of the pits, the question always concerns whether to regard the changes as those of basal pattern dysplasia (discussed later) or to diagnose them as indefinite for dysplasia. However, the main issues revolve around inflamed samples with nuclear alterations or poorly embedded samples showing diathermy (cautery) artifact.

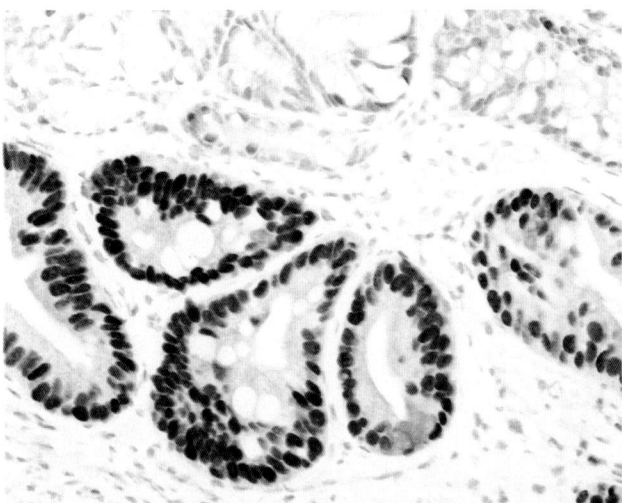

Figure 1-41. Basal pattern dysplasia, P53 immunostain. There is strong nuclear labeling, support for dysplasia, in five glands in the lower half of the image. Those in the upper half show a wild-type pattern. This is from a case of basal pattern dysplasia and included at this point to compare and contrast with Fig. 1.40.

Figs. 1.42–1.45 are images taken from biopsies from a single patient. Are the features reactive? In some areas the four lines are present, but in other areas these lines are jumbled and some of the surface nuclei are arranged in a disorderly fashion. Are the nuclei hyperchromatic? Maybe. In one area a deeper gland appears hyperchromatic but perhaps it is crushed. Based on the uncertainty, this process was interpreted as indefinite for dysplasia. Figs. 1.46–1.51 show similar alterations in the setting of inflammation that were interpreted as indefinite for dysplasia. There is no shame in diagnosing lesions as indefinite for dysplasia, but the number can be reduced by showing colleagues the case, and sometimes the presence of a wild-type P53 immunolabeling pattern can be reassuring. Sometimes fresh eyes can clarify the findings! This diagnosis should be used in only a small percentage of cases (up to 3% to 5%). Some colleagues (personal communications) essentially never use this category. Perhaps these colleagues are very good and always know. We wish we were that good!

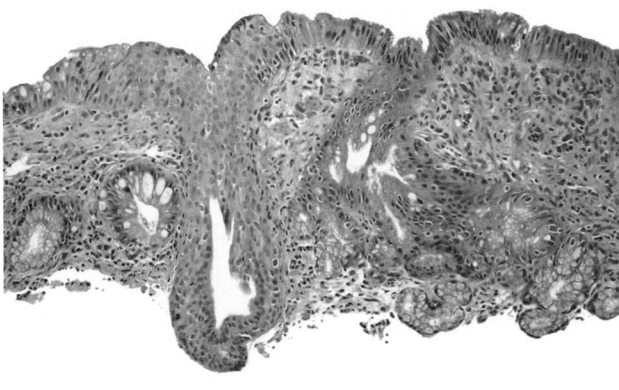

Figure 1-42. Barrett esophagus, indefinite for dysplasia. In this case, the findings are difficult to interpret. There is a large complex gland at the right and adjoining squamous epithelium at the left. Many of the nuclei on the surface at the right are hyperchromatic, but it is not clear if they are reactive. The lines are obscured at the upper right, but the nuclei are not particularly enlarged. Perhaps this is all reactive, but it is difficult to be entirely certain.

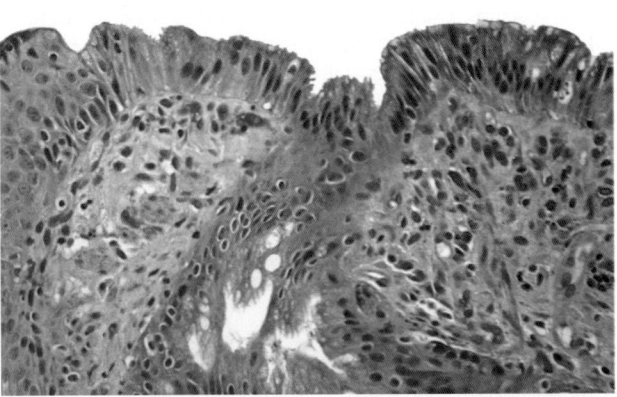

Figure 1-43. Barrett esophagus, indefinite for dysplasia. This is from the same case as that seen in Fig. 1.42. One could argue that the lines are intact at the upper right and assume that the findings at the upper left reflect tangential embedding. However, the image seen in Fig. 1.44 is from the same case as well.

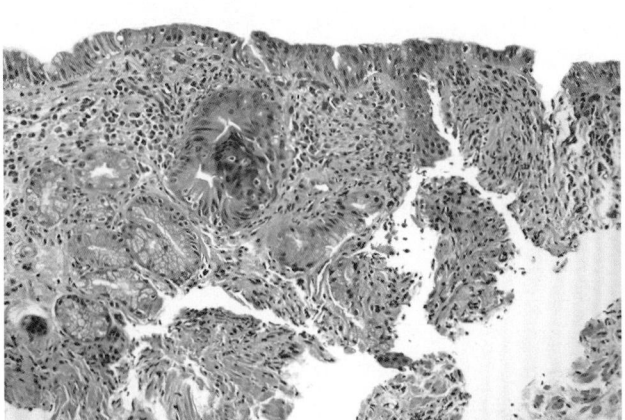

Figure 1-44. Barrett esophagus, indefinite for dysplasia. There is an atypical gland at the left of center, but the section appears thick in that focus. The overlying nuclei are not particularly enlarged, but the lines are obscured. Is this reactive? Not sure. Is this dysplastic (adenoma like)? Not sure.

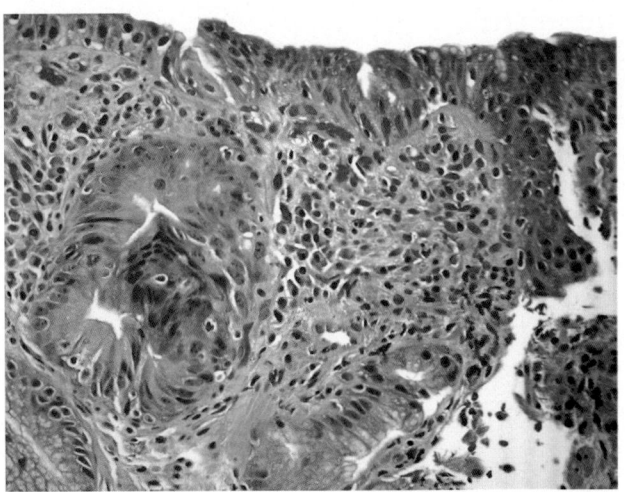

Figure 1-45. Barrett esophagus, indefinite for dysplasia. This is a higher magnification of the field seen in Fig. 1.44. The nucleoli in the glands at the left suggest that the findings are reactive, but the jumbled nuclei on the surface at the left are concerning, but they gradually merge with an area to the right that has the four lines.

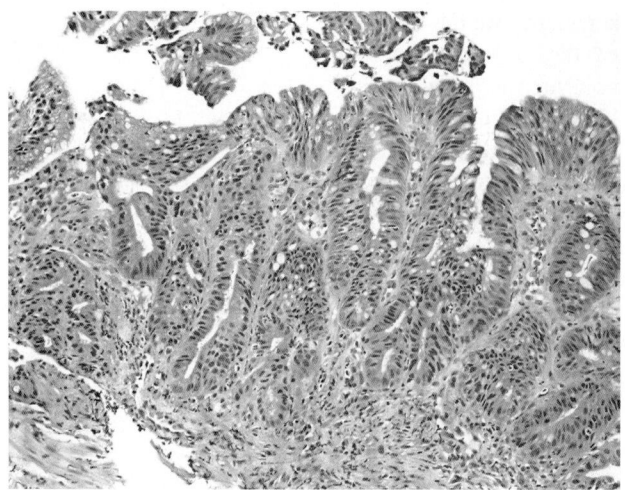

Figure 1-46. Barrett esophagus, indefinite for dysplasia. In this sample, the surface shows prominent nuclear stratification and the lines are obscured. However, the nuclei are smaller than the ones in the deep glands. The features are adenoma-like (low-grade dysplasia), but the key issue is obscuring inflammation. It is no problem to consider high-grade dysplasia in the setting of lots of inflammation, but obscuring inflammation is problematic for diagnosing low-grade dysplasia.

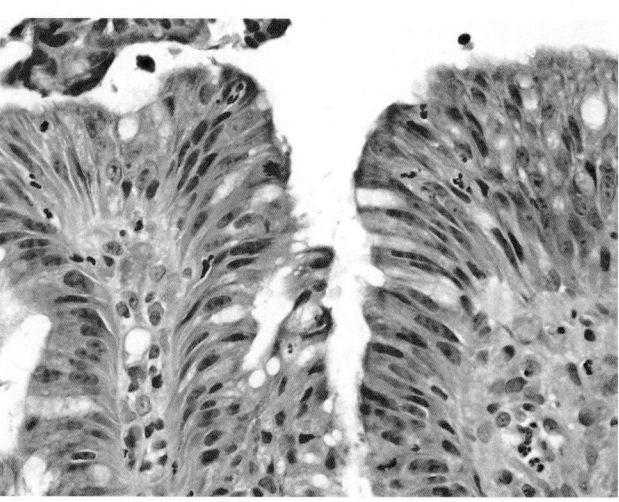

Figure 1-47. Barrett esophagus, indefinite for dysplasia. This is a high-magnification image of the lesion seen in Fig. 1.46. The nucleoli at the surface do suggest that the findings are reactive in the setting of obscuring inflammation, but the features at low magnification are striking such that a "treat and repeat" scenario is not unreasonable.

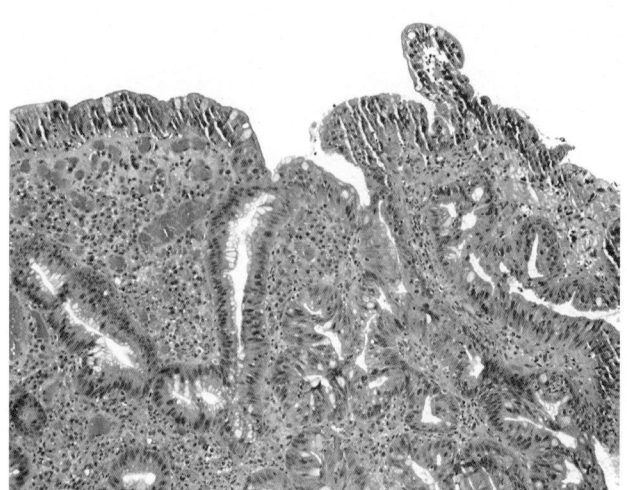

Figure 1-48. Barrett esophagus, indefinite for dysplasia. This image is from a different case from the one seen in Figs. 1.44–1.47. In this example, inflammation is prominent as is "chatter artifact," but there seem to be some surface alterations that are concerning for low-grade dysplasia.

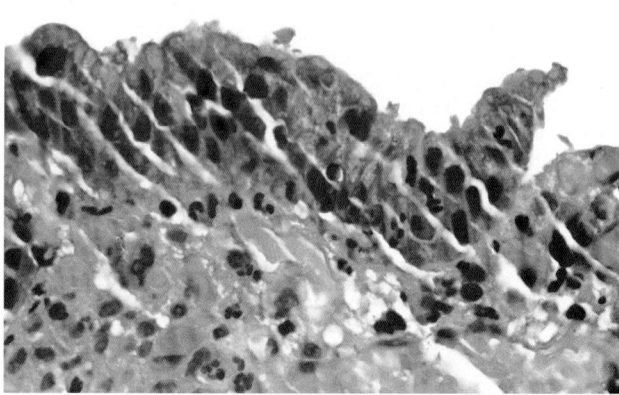

Figure 1-49. Barrett esophagus, indefinite for dysplasia. This image is from the same case as the one in Fig. 1.48. In this area, the surface lines are obscured but there are many neutrophils embedded in the epithelium. The nuclei are dark but not particularly enlarged. Compare their sizes with those of the inflammatory cell nuclei.

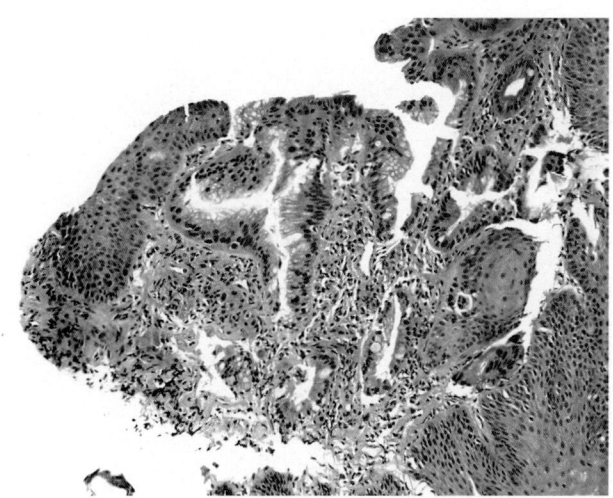

Figure 1-50. Barrett esophagus, indefinite for dysplasia. This is from the same case as that seen in Figs. 1.48 and 1.49. The specimen is tangentially embedded and there are apparent surface hyperchromatic nuclei, but it is not clear if in fact the surface is well represented.

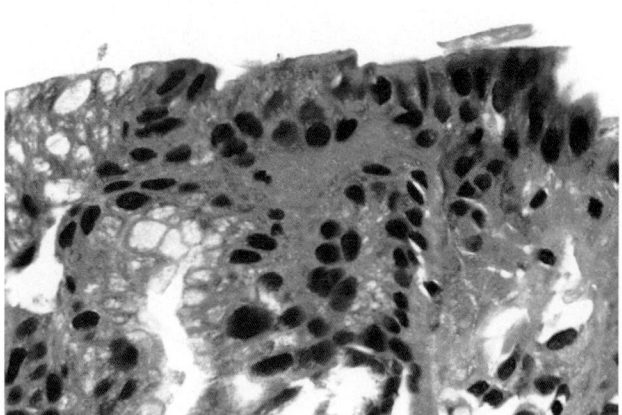

Figure 1-51. Barrett esophagus, indefinite for dysplasia. Although the lines are obscured in this zone, the adjoining areas seem to have preservation of cell polarity. The nuclei are enlarged but not crisply distinct from nuclei that appear unremarkable.

Low-Grade Dysplasia

Low-grade dysplasia should be clearly neoplastic (adenoma-like) and should involve the surface epithelium. It is important not to overdiagnose it because current guidelines endorse mucosal ablation for low-grade dysplasia and mucosal ablation confers a risk for stricture formation even in skilled hands. In prospectively evaluated patients the incidence of low-grade dysplasia should be on the order of 2% to 3% but not more than 5%.[33]

The nuclei in the cells of low-grade dysplasia are larger than those of normal Barrett mucosa, and generally, there is little inflammation in samples confidently diagnosed with low-grade dysplasia. A helpful clue that low-grade dysplasia is present is that one observes an abrupt transition between the dysplastic zone and adjoining zones that are clearly not dysplastic. The surface lines that help to confirm nondysplastic Barrett mucosa are effaced. Classic examples of low-grade dysplasia with intestinal differentiation can resemble colorectal tubular adenomas. When this happens, it is important to consider the possibility of a sample switch with an actual colorectal adenoma before reporting the case. Examples of low-grade dysplasia appear in Figs. 1.52–1.61. In general, low-grade dysplasia should demonstrate loss of the four lines (an overall indication of altered cell architecture and cell polarity) but not loss of nuclear polarity. The long axes of the nuclei should remain more or less perpendicular to the basement membrane. This general concept is further discussed and illustrated in "Colon" chapter with the construct of well aligned rows of nuclei. There is some subjectivity in differentiating low-grade dysplasia from high-grade dysplasia, but this is less important than it was in the past because all dysplasia are currently managed by endoscopic ablation, although gastroenterology societies do suggest peer review of dysplasia cases before mucosal ablation is performed.[10,12]

Staining for TP53 is sometimes useful in confirming an interpretation of low-grade dysplasia—a few darkly stained nuclei on the surface can be identified and the basal glands are labeled. In contrast, alpha-methylacyl-CoA racemase and other markers have not proven useful, at least in our hands.

Most dysplasia cases show intestinal differentiation in that the epithelium is stratified and punctuated by goblet cells in a fashion similar to the appearance of colorectal adenomas, but not all do.[34] On the order of 10% of low-grade dysplasia cases can display gastric-type differentiation, which can manifest either as an appearance similar to that of gastric pyloric gland adenoma (see "Stomach" chapter) or a lesion that resembles a gastric foveolar-type adenoma. In such lesions in Barrett mucosa the background may or may not contain goblet cells but the surface shows dysplastic-appearing nuclei coated by an apical mucin cap akin to that seen in gastric foveolar epithelium, except that the lines are absent. This type of dysplasia is characterized by smaller nuclei than those in

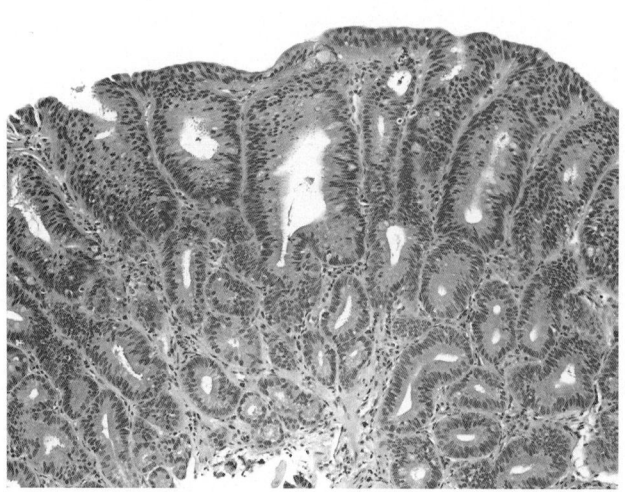

Figure 1-52. Low-grade dysplasia. This case is easy! This lesion is adenoma-like. The surface is involved, and the nuclei at the surface appear similar to those in the glands. The lines are completely obscured throughout the process and most of the nuclei are lined up with their long axes oriented perpendicular to the basement membrane. With a case such as this, some observers might prefer a diagnosis of high-grade dysplasia, but, importantly, presumably all observers would regard this process as dysplastic and endoscopic treatment would be offered.

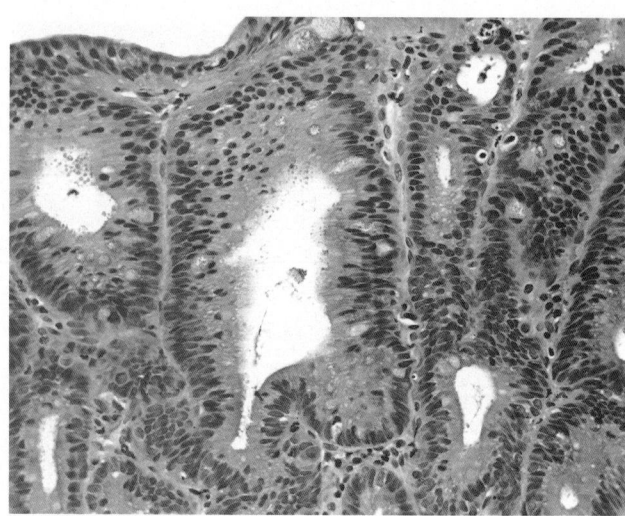

Figure 1-53. Low-grade dysplasia. This is a high-magnification image of the lesion depicted in Fig. 1.52. Overall, the nuclei are oriented perpendicular to the basement membranes.

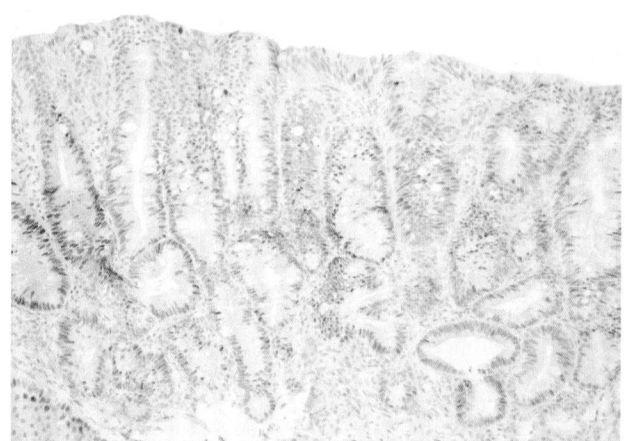

Figure 1-54. Low-grade dysplasia. This is a P53 stain from the lesion depicted in Figs. 1.52 and 1.53. It shows a wild-type pattern and was not particularly helpful in confirming the interpretation.

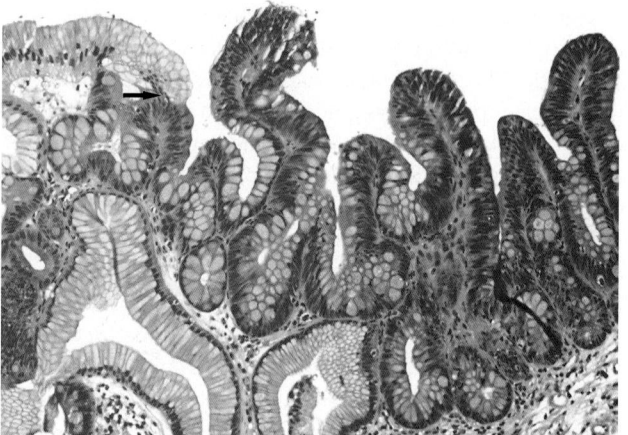

Figure 1-55. Low-grade dysplasia. Note the abrupt demarcation between the low-grade dysplasia and the nondysplastic mucosa. Note also that the lines are obscured and most of the nuclei are oriented in an alignment that is perpendicular to the basement membrane. This latter alignment is lost in high-grade dysplasia.

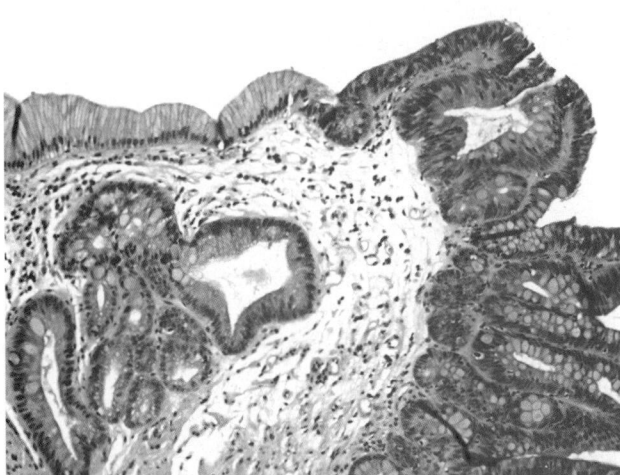

Figure 1-56. Low-grade dysplasia. A sharp demarcation is present between cardiac-type and Barrett mucosa at the left of the image versus the dysplasia at the right.

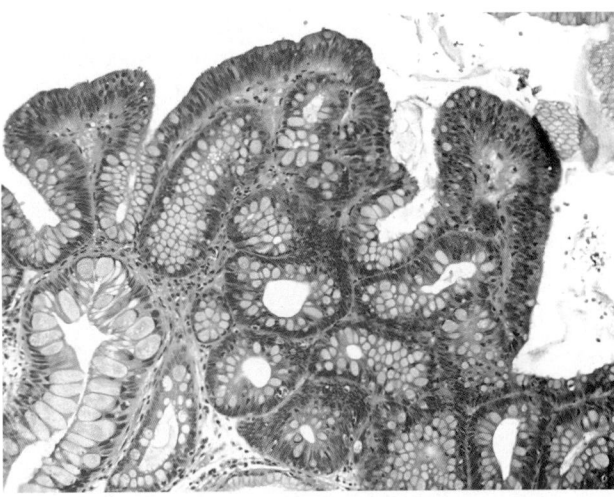

Figure 1-57. Low-grade dysplasia. This field shows that, despite the stratification and loss of the overall cellular polarity (loss of the lines), the nuclear polarity is maintained with the elongated nuclei aligned perpendicularly to the basement membrane.

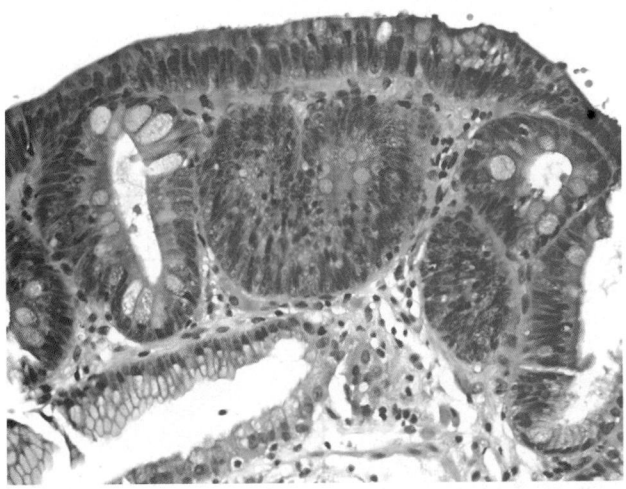

Figure 1-58. Low-grade dysplasia. This high magnification intends to show the alignment of the nuclei with respect to the basement membrane.

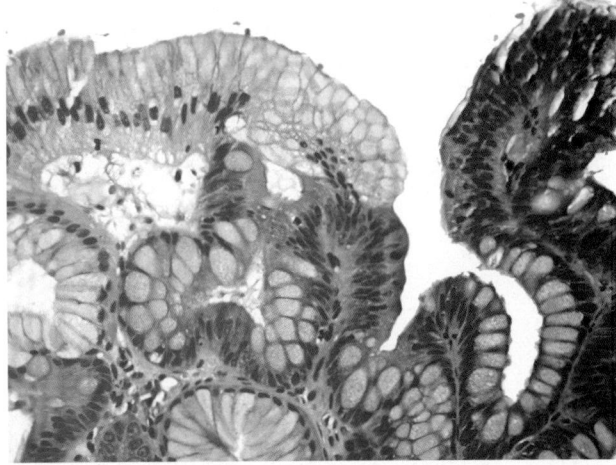

Figure 1-59. Low-grade dysplasia. This image shows areas with sharp demarcations between foci of low-grade dysplasia versus non-dysplastic epithelium.

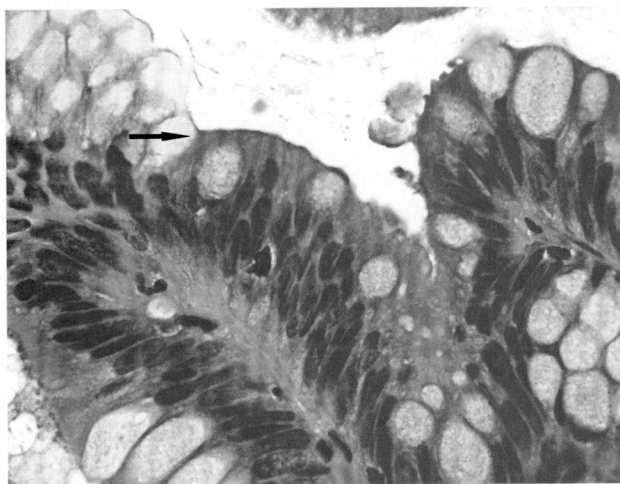

Figure 1-60. Low-grade dysplasia. The *arrow* indicates a zone of demarcation between dysplastic and nondysplastic epithelium. Note that the dysplastic nuclei lack nucleoli in most cells.

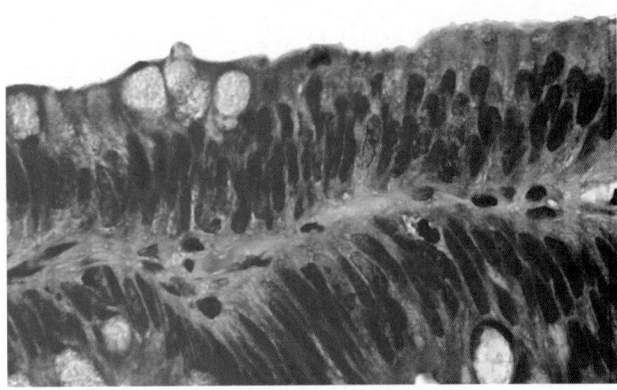

Figure 1-61. Low-grade dysplasia. This very-high-magnification image shows the nuclear features of low-grade dysplasia.

intestinal-type dysplasia, but they are typically slightly hyperchromatic. Examples of this pattern of dysplasia are seen in Figs. 1.62–1.65. Unfortunately, immunolabeling for TP53 is not particularly helpful.

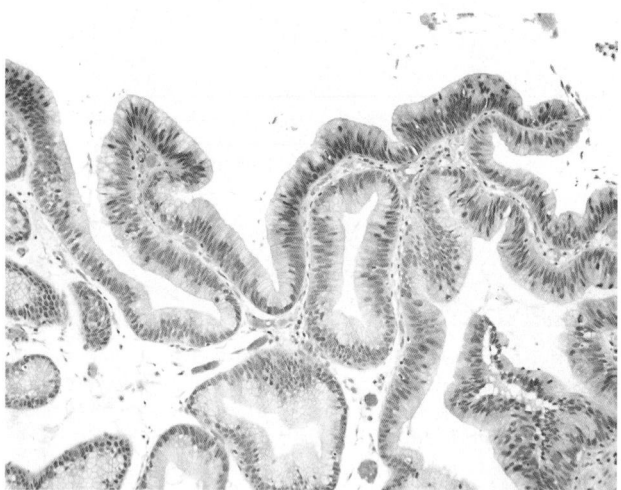

Figure 1-62. Low-grade dysplasia. Rare examples of low-grade dysplasia show gastric foveolar differentiation. The lines are obscured and the nuclei are hyperchromatic, but there are no goblet cells in the area of dysplasia in contrast to the situation in Figs. 1.52–1.61. This pattern of dysplasia can be encountered in a background of Barrett mucosa with goblet cells, but the dysplasia itself shows gastric foveolar differentiation.

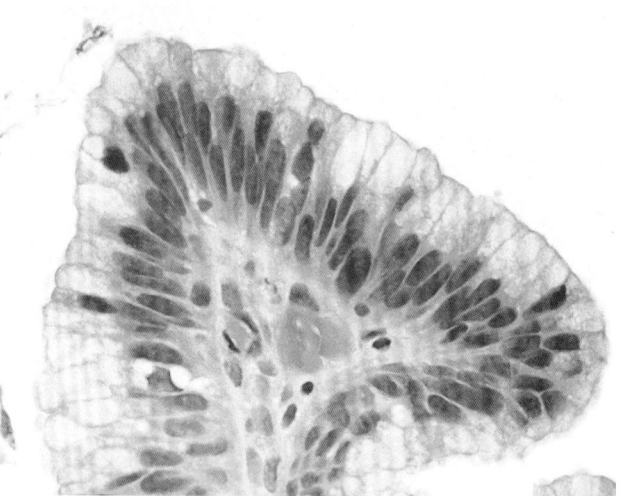

Figure 1-63. Low-grade dysplasia. This is a high-magnification image of the foveolar-type dysplasia seen in Fig. 1.62. Note that the nuclei themselves appear similar to those in the intestinal-type dysplasia seen in Figs. 1.60 and 1.61.

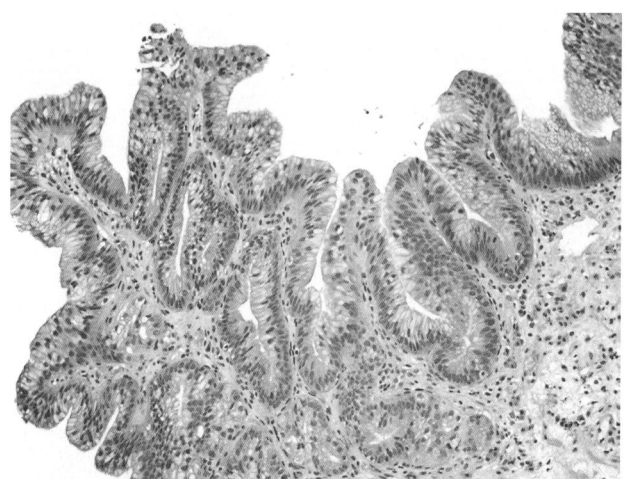

Figure 1-64. Foveolar pattern dysplasia. This case is a bit controversial. It could be interpreted as low-grade dysplasia based on the disorderly alignment of the cells, but some cells have lost their relationship to the membrane (a feature of high-grade dysplasia). This was interpreted as low-grade dysplasia because the nuclei are not particularly enlarged. There are no goblet cells in this area.

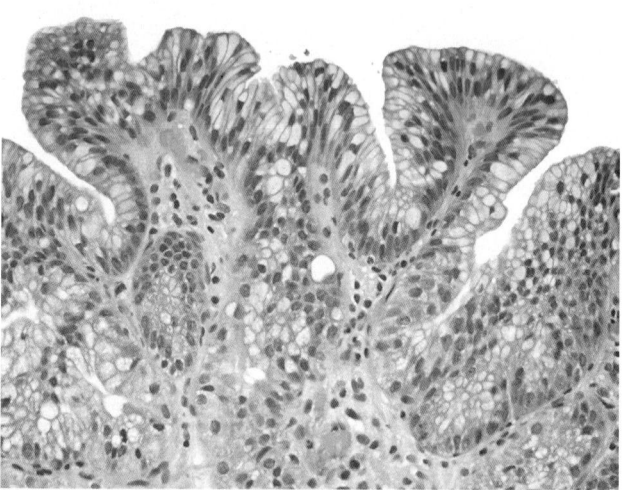

Figure 1-65. Foveolar pattern dysplasia. This is a high-magnification image of the lesion seen in Fig. 1.64.

High-Grade Dysplasia

Generally, high-grade dysplasia is not difficult to recognize and is difficult to overlook. At low magnification the area appears hyperchromatic and stands out from any nondysplastic mucosa in the sample. It is generally not particularly inflamed, but even examples showing inflammation appear extremely hyperchromatic at low magnification. The alterations usually can be detected in the surface epithelium. Prominent nucleoli are not a usual feature of high-grade dysplasia, but there are exceptions. In most cases, there is still plenty of lamina propria between the glands. Figs. 1.66 and 1.67 show a characteristic example of high-grade dysplasia with all the key features. Although there are a few neutrophils (indicated), the nuclear hyperchromasia is in excess of that which can be explained by a reparative process. Furthermore, there are often prominent nucleoli in a reactive process and the nuclei shown are quite dense appearing. Many nuclei both in the pits and at the surface have completely lost their relationship to the basement membrane and have rounded up and are arranged in a jumbled configuration. A similar lesion is shown in Figs. 1.68 and 1.69.

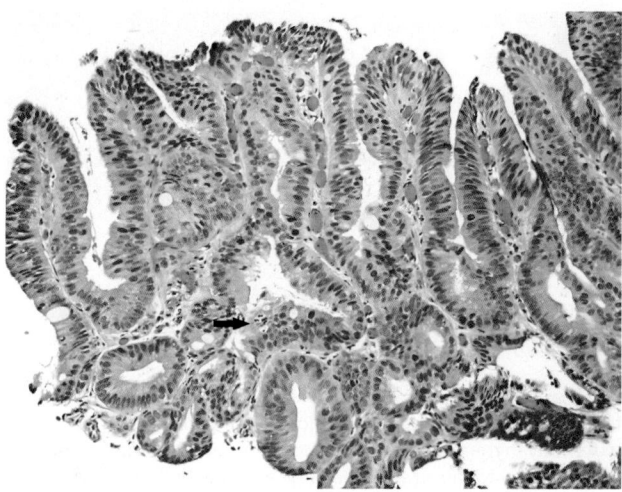

Figure 1-66. High-grade dysplasia. In a case like this, finding acute inflammation (*arrow*) need not detract from the diagnosis. In this case, the degree of nuclear hyperchromasia is in excess of that which can be attributed to inflammation. Note that the nuclei at the surface are hyperchromatic and many have lost their relationship. There are also many nuclei in the glands that are hyperchromatic and have rounded up and lost their alignment with the basement membrane.

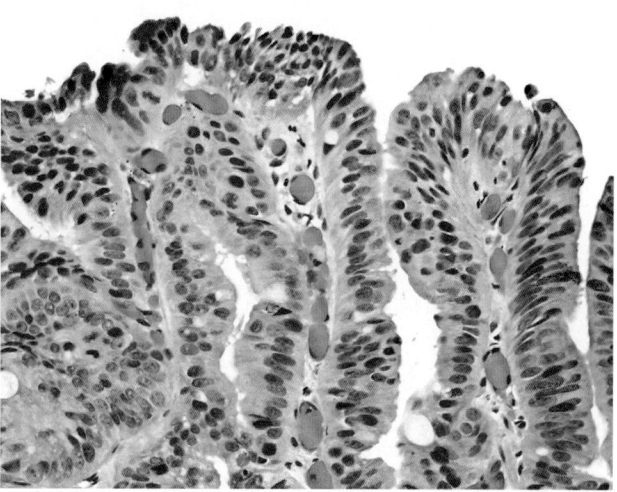

Figure 1-67. High-grade dysplasia. This is a high-magnification image of the lesion seen in Fig. 1.66. The rounded hyperchromatic nuclei are the key feature. Note that nucleoli are not a prominent feature.

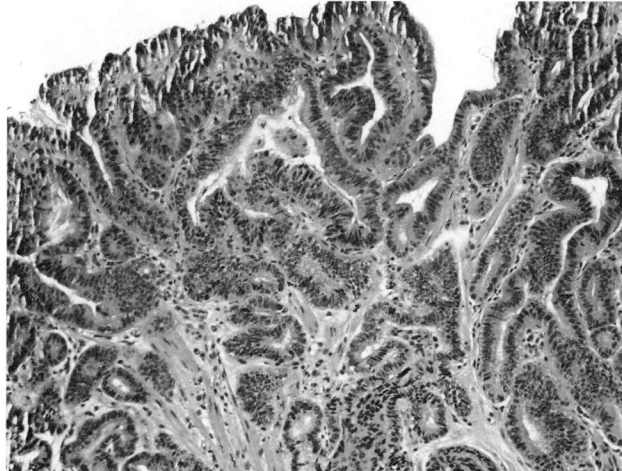

Figure 1-68. High-grade dysplasia. The key finding is striking nuclear hyperchromasia.

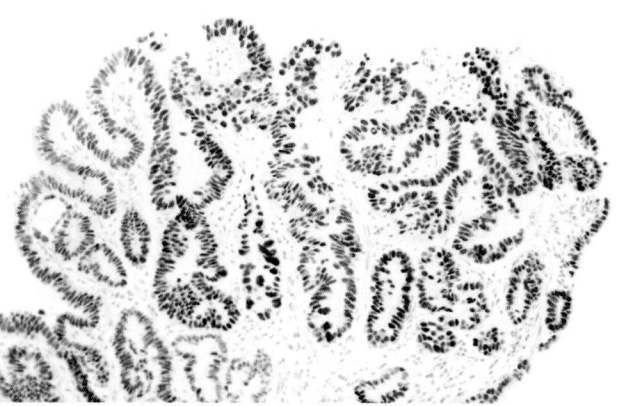

Figure 1-69. High-grade dysplasia. This is a P53 immunostain. This strong diffuse nuclear labeling pattern is characteristic of high-grade dysplasia. Some examples of low-grade dysplasia show strong labeling, but usually just a few surface cells are labeled. In this example, the surface nuclei are strongly reactive.

Nuclear hyperchromasia is the key finding, although the glands are crowded in this example as well. Some examples of high-grade dysplasia feature markedly enlarged nuclei, sometimes in the absence of glandular crowding, such as the case shown in Figs. 1.70 and 1.71.

Most cases of high-grade dysplasia show some degree of nuclear elongation and stratification akin to the features in colorectal adenomas. A subset of cases shows an unusual pattern of small tubules, each lined by a monolayer of hyperchromatic nuclei (Figs. 1.72 and 1.73). Because the monolayer appearance is unusual and lacks nuclear stratification, it has been referred to as a "nonadenomatous" form of high-grade dysplasia by some,[35] but others have considered this pattern as evidence for gastric differentiation in high-grade dysplasia.[36,37] None of this has any effect on management, but such cases are still part of high-grade dysplasia.

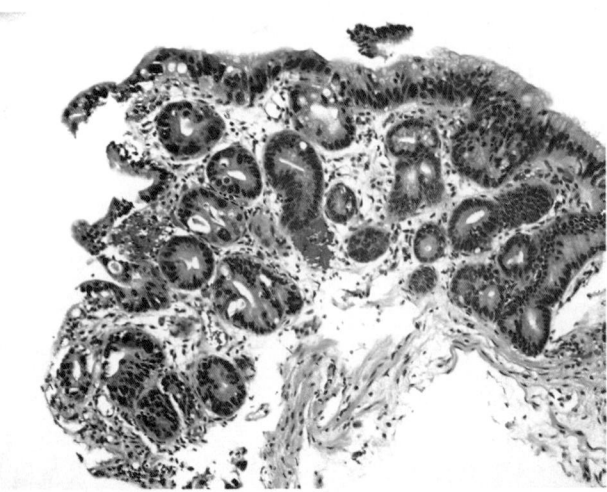

Figure 1-70. High-grade dysplasia. Even though there is no glandular crowding, the giant hyperchromatic nuclei in some of the glands and on the surface at the left part of the image are sufficient for a high-grade dysplasia diagnosis.

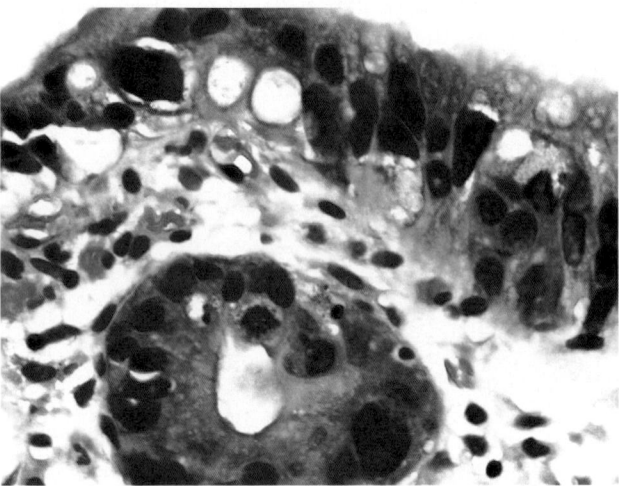

Figure 1-71. High-grade dysplasia. This is a very-high-magnification image of the lesion depicted in Fig. 1.70. The nuclei are extremely hyperchromatic. Compare their sizes (including the smaller ones) to the sizes of the lamina propria inflammatory cells.

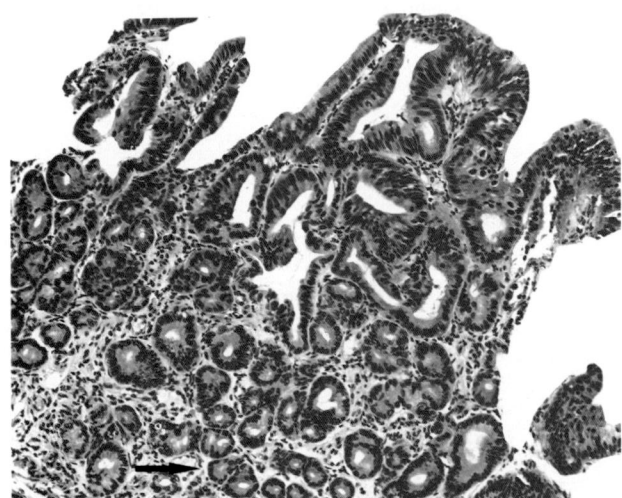

Figure 1-72. High-grade dysplasia. Although the surface shows loss of nuclear polarity and somewhat stratified nuclei, the *arrow* indicates some deep glands that also show high-grade dysplasia in a pattern consisting of small tubules each lined by a monolayer of tiny hyperchromatic nuclei that are not elongated like those of classic dysplasia. Because of the lack of nuclear stratification, some colleagues have referred to this pattern as "nonadenomatous" and others have regarded it as a form of gastric-type differentiation. The main thing is to be aware that some examples of high-grade dysplasia lack nuclear stratification.

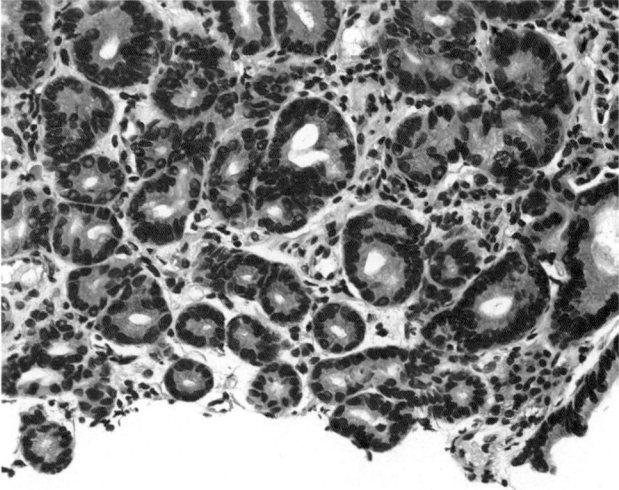

Figure 1-73. High-grade dysplasia. This is a high-magnification image of the deep dysplastic glands seen in Fig. 1.72.

Immunolabeling for TP53 can be helpful in confirming an impression of high-grade dysplasia when there is doubt. If the histologic features are already classic, there is no reason to perform immunolabeling, but about 85% to 90% of the time, if immunolabeling is added, strong labeling like that seen in Fig. 1.69 will confirm the impression. Thankfully, such strong labeling is typically present in the "small cell" pattern depicted in Figs. 1.72 and 1.73. As noted earlier, TP53 is a tumor suppressor protein that is active during cell division as a normal component and has a short half-life. Because TP53 is a molecule put in place to prevent cancer development during the course of normal cell proliferation, some labeling is to be expected in the proliferative compartment of the mucosa. As such, there is always nuclear labeling in the basal layer of the squamous epithelium and in the pits of the stomach. When the *TP53* gene is mutated, this usually results in a TP53 protein with an extra-long half-life, so it accumulates in the nuclei of the cells and can be detected by immunolabeling. However, there is a subset of high-grade dysplasia cases in which there is biallelic loss of the *TP53* gene. In this form of dysplasia, the cells have absolutely no TP53 to depend on and there is complete absence of staining in the dysplastic nuclei. This pattern has been termed the "null pattern" and can be exploited for diagnosis just as well as the strongly reactive pattern. The dysplasia/neoplasia cases shown in Figs. 1.74–1.78 display the null pattern of TP53 labeling that confirms the diagnosis. In addition, Figs. 1.77 and 1.78 show "buried dysplasia." This means that there is a coating of squamous epithelium on top of the dysplasia. There have been articles that express concern that this is a huge issue in patients who have had mucosal ablation procedures but it is not. We would not have this image if our endoscopy colleagues did not find and biopsy this area. Furthermore, there is nearly always separate surface dysplasia in patients with buried dysplasia and exceptions are rare.[38] The "Endoscopic Mucosal Resections" section also features examples of buried dysplasia.

The line between high-grade dysplasia and early carcinoma can be difficult to draw, and some features that are helpful in confirming an interpretation of intramucosal carcinoma are discussed later. We diagnosed the lesion seen in Figs. 1.79–1.81 as high-grade dysplasia rather than early carcinoma, but the irregular growth pattern of the dilated deeper glands could be interpreted as evidence of early invasion.[39]

Lastly, there are cases of high-grade dysplasia that display either gastric foveolar differentiation or differentiation similar to that seen in pyloric gland adenomas of the stomach,

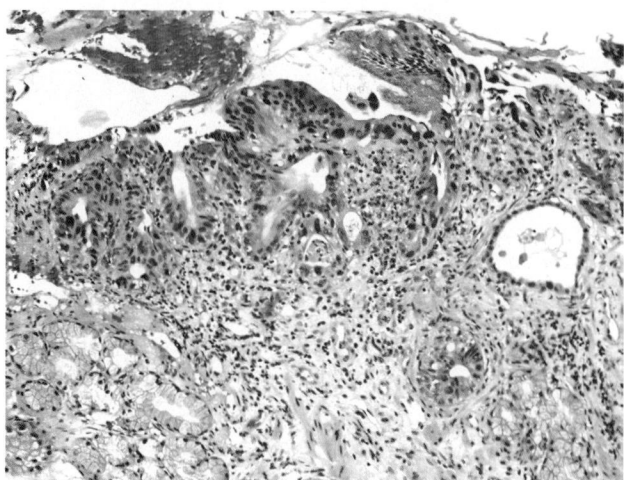

Figure 1-74. Intramucosal carcinoma. Such cases are controversial, and some colleagues might regard this lesion as high-grade dysplasia. The glands in the center seem to be growing parallel to the surface, and the luminal necrosis in the center is a feature of the earliest invasion into the lamina propria. However, this case is shown because it has a special pattern of P53 labeling, as seen in Fig. 1.75.

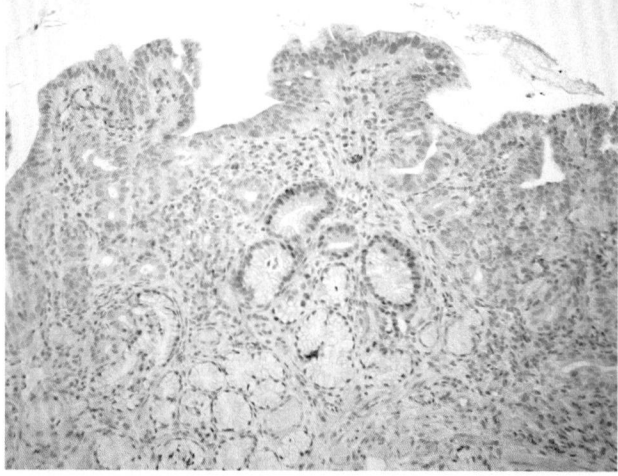

Figure 1-75. Intramucosal carcinoma. This is a P53 stain from the lesion seen in Fig. 1.75. There are cardiac glands in the lower left of both images, but a few additional nondysplastic/nonneoplastic glands have popped into the center of the field. These cardiac glands all show light nuclear wild-type P53 labeling. The dysplasia/early carcinoma, however, shows complete absence of P53 labeling, which is just as useful for confirming a diagnosis as finding strong labeling. This finding indicates that the *TP53* gene and any P53 protein it might have produced to keep neoplasia at bay has been wiped out on both copies of the gene in the neoplastic cells. This can be from deletions/allelic loss. Biallelic inactivation of the gene is at work in the dysplasia.

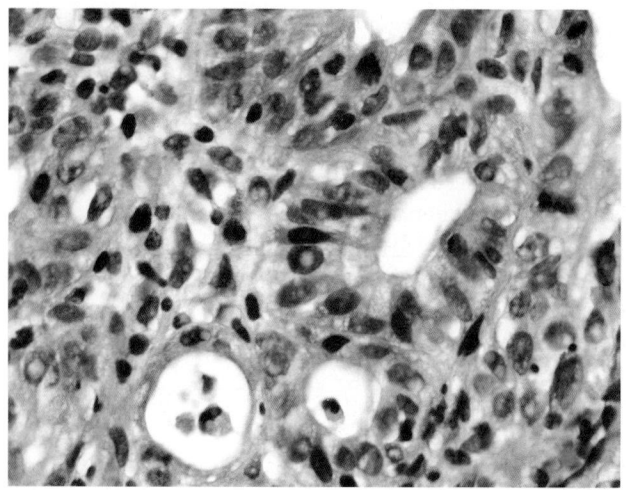

Figure 1-76. Intramucosal carcinoma. This is a very-high-magnification image of the lesion seen in Figs. 1.74 and 1.75. The two glands at the bottom of the image have luminal necrosis.

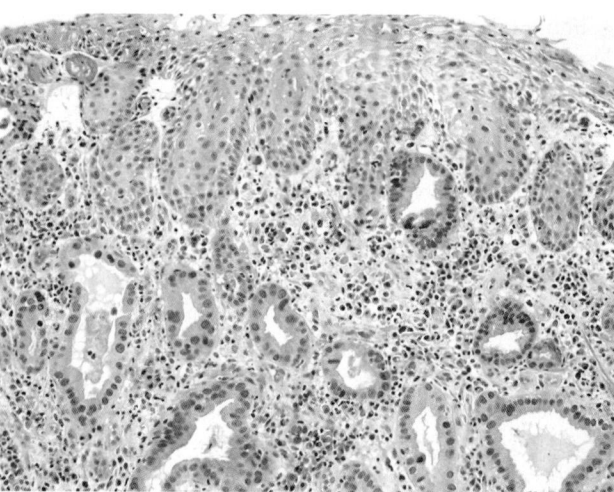

Figure 1-77. Intramucosal carcinoma. This example is seen beneath reactive squamous epithelium with reactive (pseudoepitheliomatous) squamous epithelial changes. The glands contain luminal debris and several of the nuclei contain large nucleoli, a feature of early invasion. This area was detected endoscopically, even though it is coated with squamous epithelium. Case reports of "buried" neoplasia after mucosal ablation raised initial concerns, but this concern is overstated based on accumulated data.

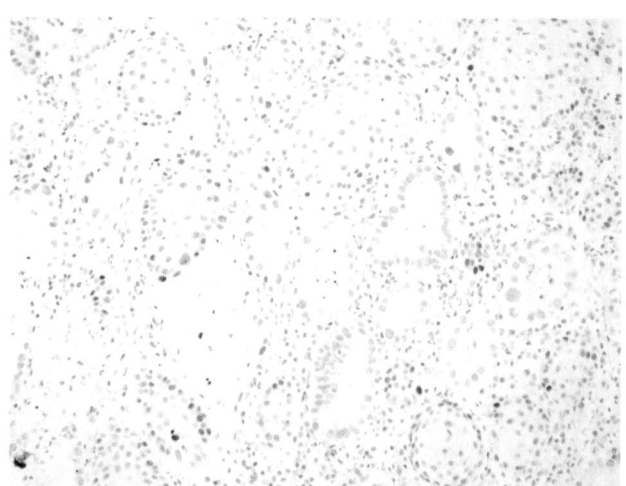

Figure 1-78. Intramucosal carcinoma. This P53 stain shows labeling in reactive squamous epithelium and a few reactive cardiac-type glands but is entirely nonreactive in the large dysplastic/neoplastic nuclei such that it is a helpful stain in confirming the impression of neoplasia.

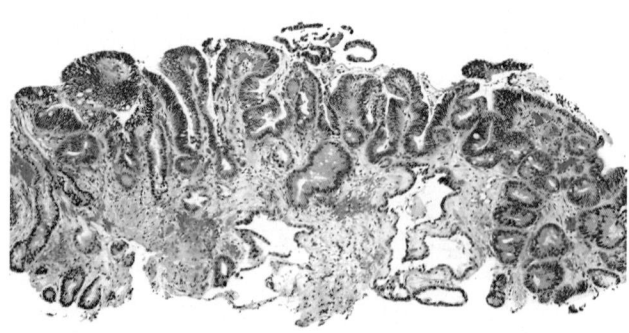

Figure 1-79. High-grade dysplasia versus intramucosal carcinoma. The glands at the right and left and surface of the lesion in this image are composed of cells with hyperchromatic enlarged nuclei. In contrast, there are some dilated glands in the center that grow in an abnormal arrangement and are lined by cells with small hyperchromatic nuclei, a pattern of high-grade dysplasia. Some would regard this pattern as that of intramucosal carcinoma because the glands are convoluted and growing parallel (instead of perpendicular) to the surface. In the modern era of endoscopic treatment of both dysplasia and early carcinoma, this distinction is not critical.

as discussed in "Stomach" chapter. This type of dysplasia can arise in a background of intestinal metaplasia, but it still has gastric-type differentiation.[34] The important point is that the nuclei in this pattern of dysplasia are paler than those seen in conventional-type dysplasia and this form of dysplasia is diagnosed by attention to nuclear multilayering and loss of nuclear polarity (Figs. 1.82–1.85). For this pattern, TP53 immunolabeling often fails to add information.

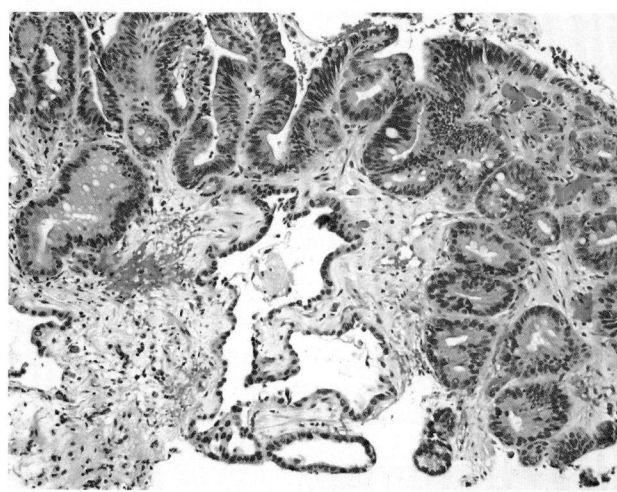

Figure 1-80. High-grade dysplasia versus intramucosal carcinoma. This is a high-magnification image of the area in Fig. 1.79. We report this pattern as intramucosal carcinoma, but it is acceptable to report it as high-grade dysplasia to forestall overtreatment in centers with overzealous surgeons.

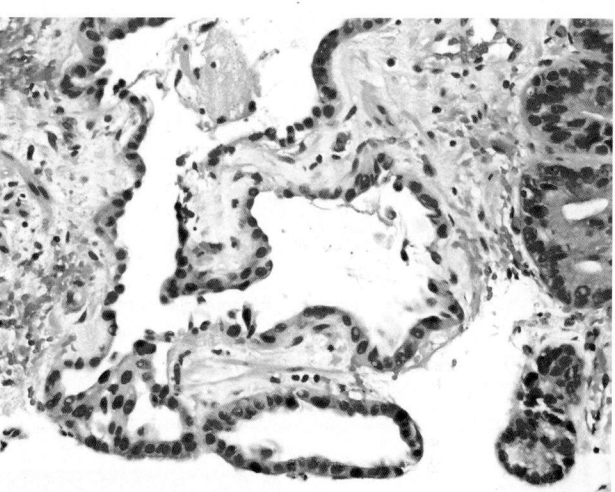

Figure 1-81. High-grade dysplasia versus intramucosal carcinoma. This is a higher-magnification image of the key area seen in Figs. 1.70 and 1.80. The nuclei are abnormal and hyperchromatic in a gland with an abnormal infiltrative growth pattern.

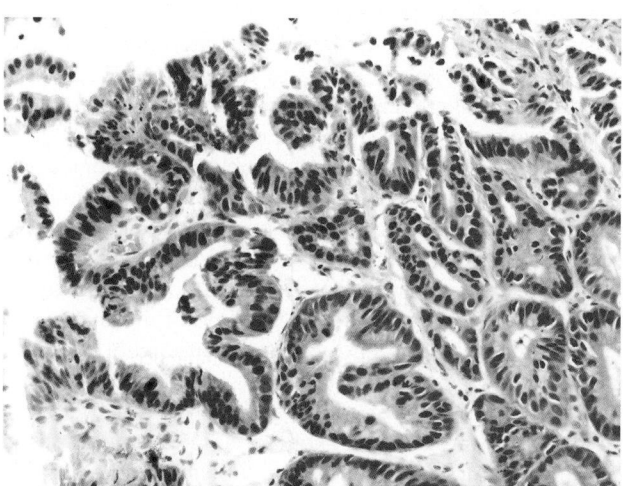

Figure 1-82. High-grade dysplasia, foveolar differentiation. Many of the cells in this image have apical mucin caps in the fashion of gastric foveolar cells. This example is easy to diagnose as high-grade dysplasia because the nuclei are enlarged and hyperchromatic.

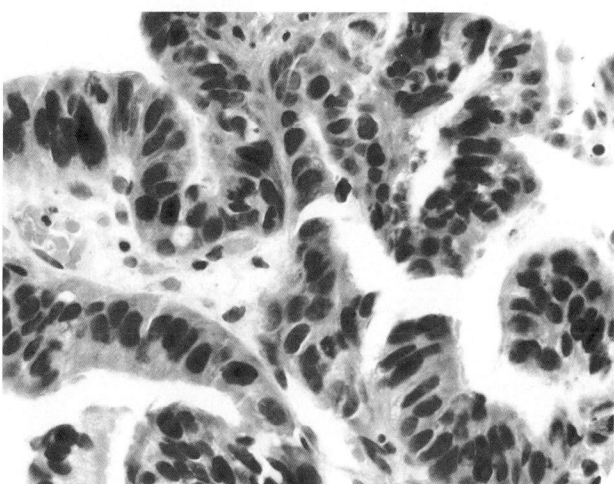

Figure 1-83. High-grade dysplasia, foveolar differentiation. There are no goblet cells, and there are cells with gastric-type mucin at the left.

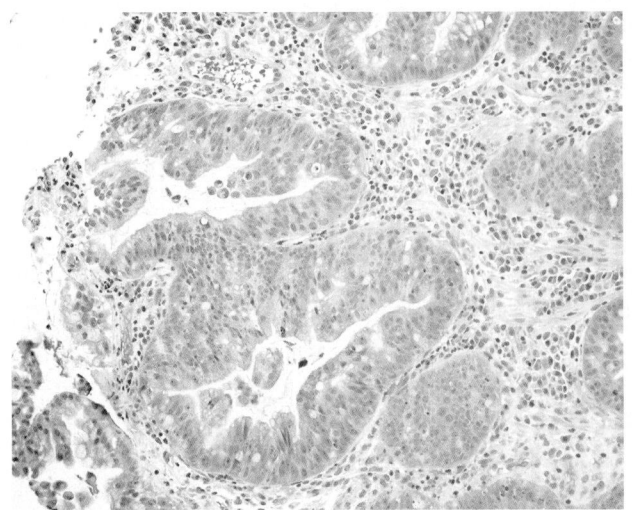

Figure 1-84. High-grade dysplasia, foveolar differentiation. Cases like this are tricky to diagnose because the nuclei are not hyperchromatic. Many cells have gastric-type mucin, but the key to diagnosis is noting the loss of nuclear polarity.

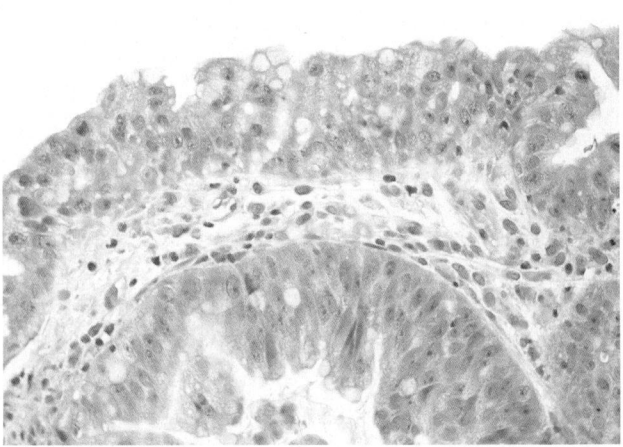

Figure 1-85. High-grade dysplasia, foveolar differentiation. This high-magnification image shows the gastric foveolar-type mucin to advantage. The nuclei are jumbled and some have nucleoli.

PEARLS & PITFALLS: Basal "Crypt" Dysplasia

This is a controversial area. This pattern was described in 2006 using the above mentioned terminology (the glands in the stomach are pits and glands rather than crypts, but because the mucosa is intestinalized the term "crypts" makes sense).[31,40] This pattern of course makes sense. Biology is a continuum such that we would expect that occasional cases of dysplasia would be sampled before the findings have appeared on the surface. The trouble is that it is subjective to differentiate epithelial changes that simply reflect reactive glands (Figs. 1.37–1.40) from cases in which there is dysplasia without a surface component. Often these issues can be resolved by adding a few recuts. We will admit to being inconsistent in how we handle such cases. Using the indefinite category for such lesions will result in follow-up with resampling and using the basal dysplasia category may result in mucosal ablation, so caution is advised. In some cases, the nuclear alterations are striking and akin to those of classic high-grade dysplasia, and these cases can be diagnosed as "high-grade dysplasia, basal pattern" with no qualms concerning whether the patient receives mucosal ablation. However, it is unclear which lesions are low-grade dysplasia, basal pattern. In the initial study, the authors suggested "lumping" these cases in the low-grade category, but at the time of the publication, universal ablation for low-grade dysplasia had yet to be endorsed, so the stakes were low. For this reason, some observers prefer not to use this category.

These are the cases for which P53 immunolabeling can help for a diagnosis of dysplasia. Without strong labeling, we are more likely to classify the findings as indefinite. Some examples of cases are shown in Figs. 1.41, 1.86–1.91. Fortunately this issue is not common. Our advice is to err on the side of indefinite for dysplasia unless the nuclear alterations are really striking, especially in the absence of P53 immunolabeling. The patient will be followed but not ablated. Here are some approaches:

1. Atypical basal glands with surface maturation, slight nuclear alterations—Barrett mucosa, negative for dysplasia
2. Atypical basal glands with surface maturation, prominent atypical nuclei, gradual maturation to surface and gradual transition to glands that are clearly reactive, wild-type P53 labeling—Barrett mucosa, negative for dysplasia

3. Atypical basal glands with surface maturation, prominent atypical nuclei, abrupt transition to more mature nuclei with maturation at surface, wild-type P53 labeling—Safer to regard as indefinite for dysplasia to avoid overtreatment

4. Atypical basal glands with surface maturation, prominent atypical nuclei, abrupt transition to more mature nuclei with maturation at surface, abnormal P53 labeling—basal pattern dysplasia. If there is no loss of nuclear polarity in the glands in question—low grade. If there is loss of nuclear polarity in the glands in question—then high-grade basal pattern dysplasia

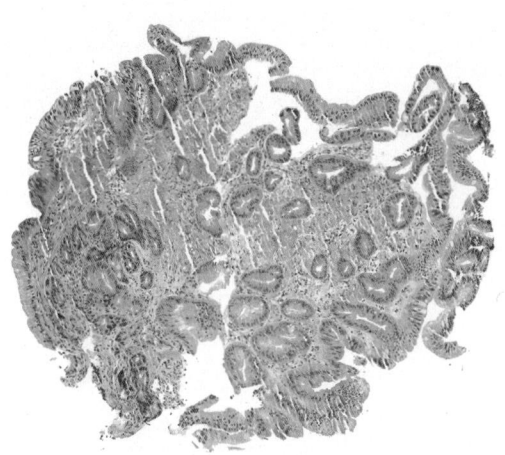

Figure 1-86. Basal pattern dysplasia. Note that this sample is badly embedded and that there is surface epithelium on all sides. Most of the surface epithelium has the characteristic lines of nondysplastic Barrett mucosa, but at the upper right, this is not clear. There is a zone of glands with hyperchromatic nuclei in the lower left, but the surface is not fully evaluable in this zone.

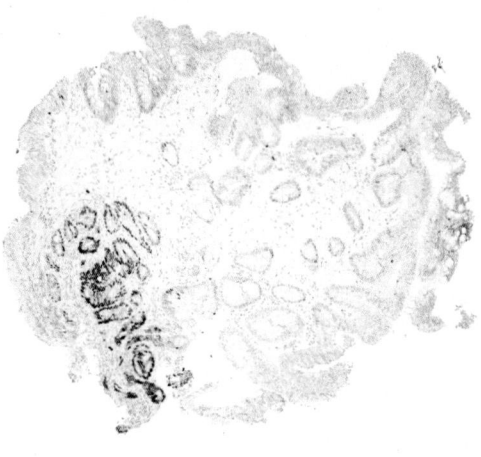

Figure 1-87. Basal pattern dysplasia. This is a P53 stain from the case shown in Fig. 1.86. A zone of strong nuclear labeling conforms to the area in Fig. 1.86. Note that several glands at the right of the field have wild-type staining. This pattern altogether can be diagnosed as basal pattern dysplasia, but it acceptable to diagnose it as indefinite for dysplasia, which will prompt close follow-up and additional sampling.

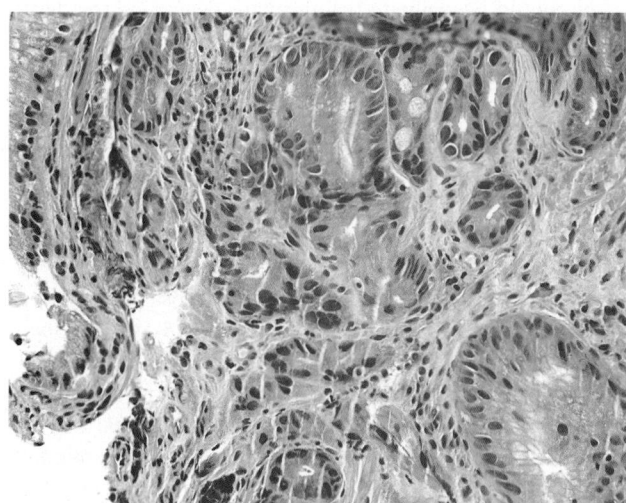

Figure 1-88. Basal pattern dysplasia. This is a high-magnification image of the area seen in Figs. 1.86 and 1.87. The nuclei are enlarged and hyperchromatic compared with the nuclei in the gland to the lower right. This lesion could be interpreted as low-grade dysplasia, basal pattern. Were there striking loss of nuclear polarity and striking nuclear enlargement, this would be high-grade dysplasia, basal pattern. However, if there is any doubt, the indefinite category should be used because a dysplasia diagnosis (low or high grade) often results in mucosal ablation.

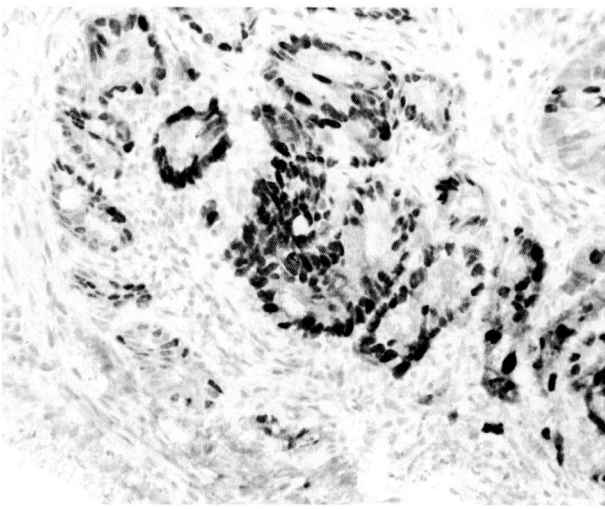

Figure 1-89. Basal pattern dysplasia. This is a high-magnification image of the P53 preparation from the case seen in Figs. 1.86–1.88.

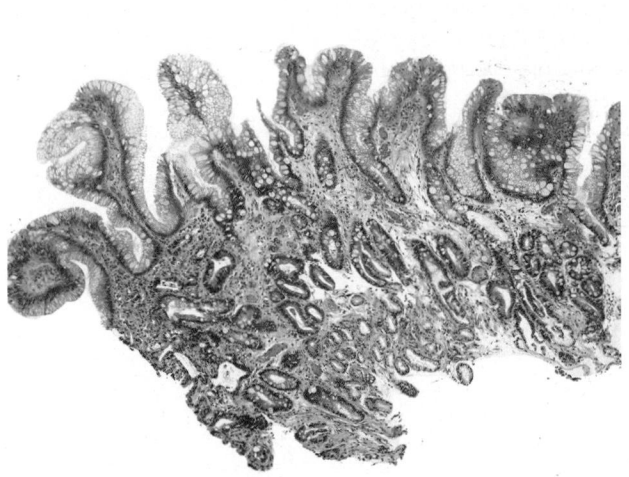

Figure 1-90. Intramucosal carcinoma with apparent surface maturation. There is a carcinoma invading the lamina propria at the left side of the tissue fragment. Seeing a mature surface in this zone may simply mean that the lesion has spread laterally and an involved surface a small distance away was simply not sampled. Recuts of apparent basal pattern lesions sometimes show zones of surface involvement.

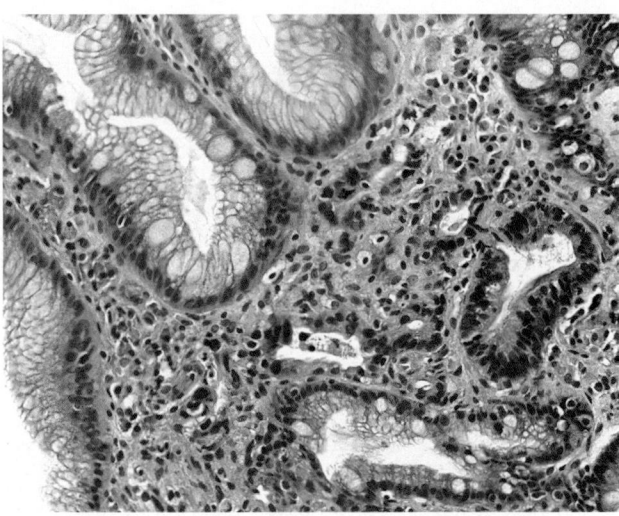

Figure 1-91. Intramucosal carcinoma with apparent surface maturation. This is a high-magnification image of the lesion seen in Fig. 1.90. Atypical glands with angulated contours and luminal necrotic debris are present in the lamina propria beneath a surface of non-dysplastic Barrett mucosa.

Intramucosal Adenocarcinoma and Adenocarcinoma

In theory it is not possible to diagnose intramucosal carcinoma on mucosal biopsy samples because the tissue beneath the mucosa has not been evaluated, but in practical terms, one can have a good idea based on the findings in the mucosal biopsy alone! Because of this, we do render diagnoses of intramucosal carcinoma (invasion into the lamina propria) on mucosal samples, in part because we know that this interpretation will prompt an EMR and if deeper invasion is found at this time, an esophagectomy will follow. It is always nice to give a patient a chance at endoscopic treatment! Some institutions diagnose adenocarcinoma with a note that the patient should be evaluated clinically to determine the depth of invasion and whether the lesion is amenable to endoscopic treatment. Either approach is reasonable depending on who might read the report, but we prefer the first, because it could prevent overtreatment by some surgeons who continue to practice using standards from an era when endoscopic treatments were not widely available and accepted in the United States.

Intramucosal carcinoma indicates invasion into the mucosa and is staged as T1a[1], which differs from the approach in the colon wherein mucosal invasion is staged as Tis because there is negligible lymphatic access in the lamina propria of the colon, as discussed further in "Colon" chapter. Esophageal carcinomas that invade the submucosa are staged as T1b[1]. The problem with intramucosal carcinoma is that desmoplasia is not well developed. Features associated with early invasion include luminal necrosis of the glands, an architecture with back-to-back glands, the presence of nucleoli in atypical glands, and glands that grow parallel to the surface.[41,42] Examples of intramucosal carcinoma appear in Figs. 1.92–1.99, illustrating the criteria noted earlier. After a diagnosis of intramucosal carcinoma is given on mucosal biopsies, the current standard of care is mucosal resection and ablation, which is discussed later. Intramucosal adenocarcinoma is adenocarcinoma, it is simply T1a and thereby usually associated with a good outcome following endoscopic treatment.[43] Even some lesions that invade the superficial submucosa can be managed with endoscopic treatments.[44,45]

There are two hints that deep invasion is present when a mucosal biopsy is reviewed.

The first: If there is prominent desmoplasia (Fig. 1.100), invasion into at least the submucosa is likely. Desmoplasia essentially means scarring and is discussed in more detail in the "Colon" chapter.

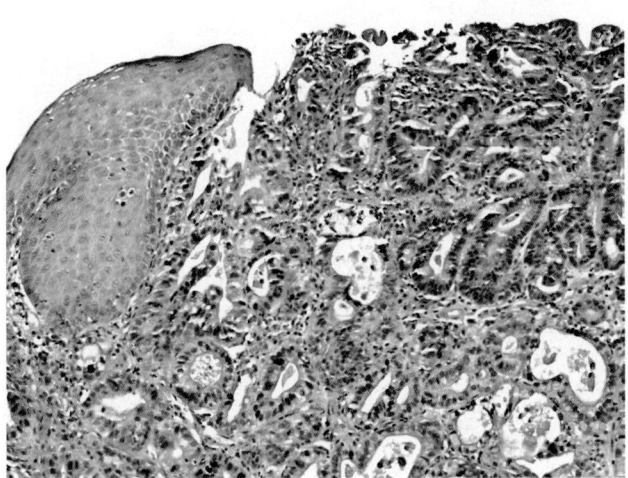

Figure 1-92. Intramucosal carcinoma. The glands are crowded together and have effaced the lamina propria. Many contain luminal debris. Some contain more open nuclei than those encountered in high-grade dysplasia. This open appearance is imparted by nucleoli.

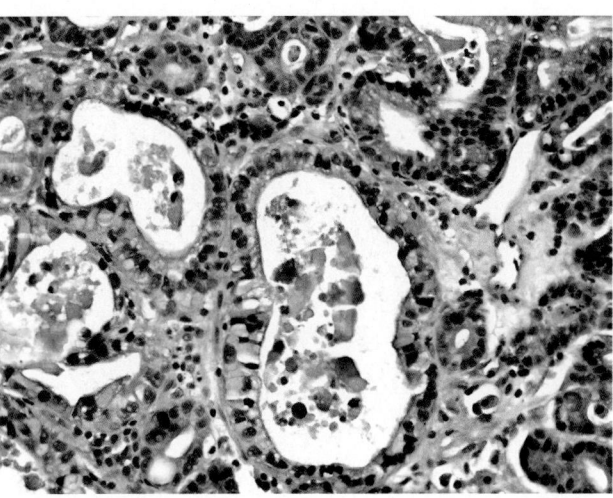

Figure 1-93. Intramucosal carcinoma. Many of the nuclei have prominent nucleoli. This is a high-magnification image of the lesion seen in Fig. 1.92.

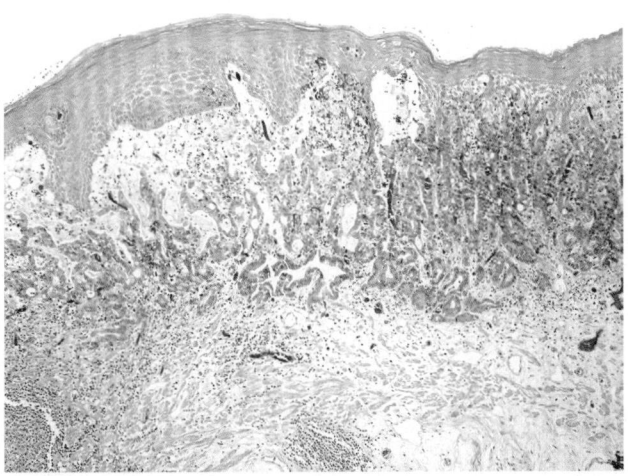

Figure 1-94. Intramucosal carcinoma. This example is coated by squamous epithelium (but the endoscopist still spotted this area and sampled it). Although desmoplasia is not well developed, the glands grow in an angulated manner and several run parallel to the surface. The carcinoma is seen in the lamina propria. The wisps of muscle below it are wisps of muscularis mucosae, probably duplicated muscularis mucosae.

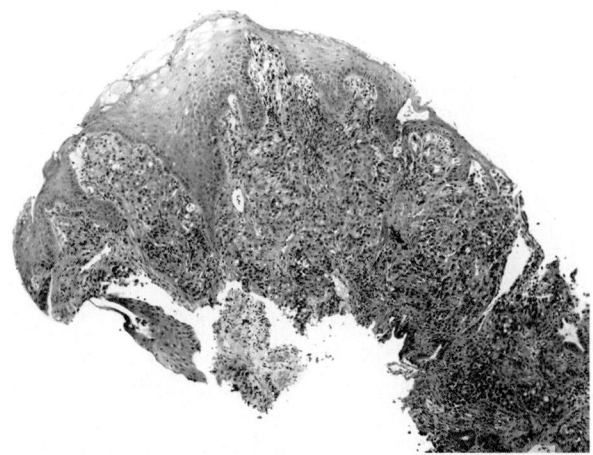

Figure 1-95. Intramucosal carcinoma. It is difficult to determine where one glands starts and another stops in this lesion that effaces the lamina propria.

The second: If there is pagetoid extension of single adenocarcinoma cells into the squamous epithelium (Figs. 1.101 and 1.102), there is invariably an associated deeply invasive underlying carcinoma, but this pattern is uncommon in biopsies.[42,46]

Most adenocarcinomas that have invaded beyond the lamina propria are straightforward to diagnose and not subtle. They can have mucinous and signet cell patterns akin to those in gastric carcinoma, and some are poorly differentiated and can require immunolabeling to be classified (Figs. 1.103–1.105). At present, HER2 testing is added for esophageal adenocarcinomas and the scheme for scoring is the same as that for gastric carcinomas and addressed in detail in "Stomach" chapter.

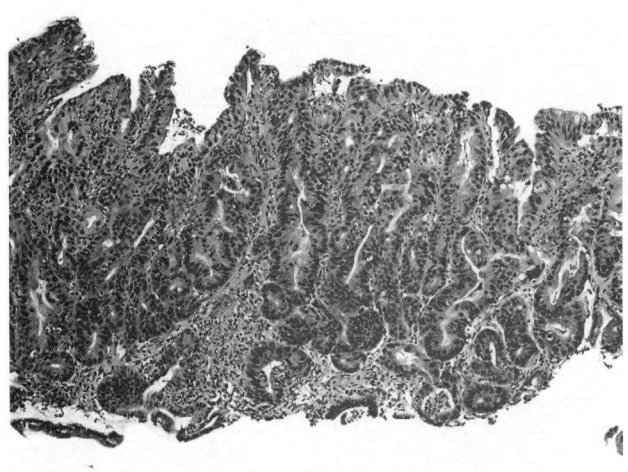

Figure 1-96. Intramucosal carcinoma. This lesion has features of high-grade dysplasia with hyperchromatic nuclei, but some of the glands bud off from larger ones, some have luminal necrosis, and some grow parallel to the surface. Cases such as this are often interpreted as high-grade dysplasia, which is acceptable for the purposes of modern treatments, as lesions such as this are unlikely to metastasize.

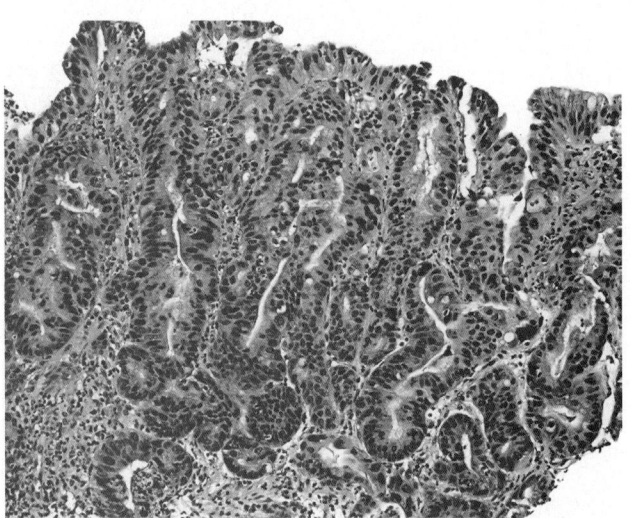

Figure 1-97. Intramucosal carcinoma. This is a high-magnification image of the lesion seen in Fig. 1.96. It is the complex architecture of the process that merits an interpretation of intramucosal carcinoma rather than high-grade dysplasia. The glands do not form individual tubules but instead interanastomose.

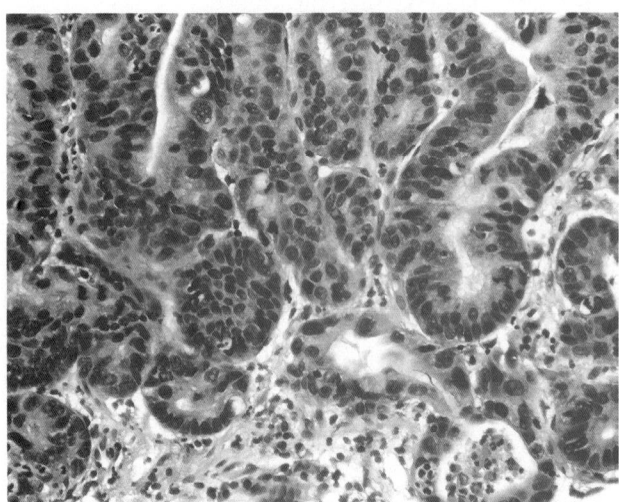

Figure 1-98. Intramucosal carcinoma. This is another high-magnification image of the lesion shown in Figs. 1.96 and 1.97 intended to show the luminal necrosis at the lower right and the abnormal complex architecture of the glands.

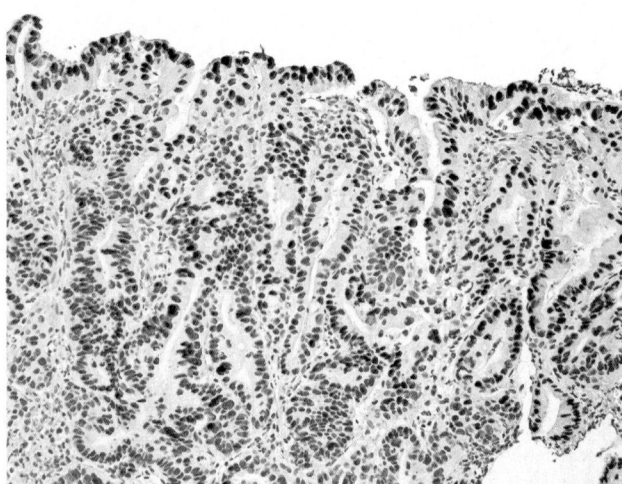

Figure 1-99. Intramucosal carcinoma. This is a CDX2 stain from the case seen in Figs. 1.96–1.98. There was no reason to perform this labeling—the laboratory that handled the sample was in the habit of adding CDX2 labeling to all esophageal biopsies. The strong nuclear labeling certainly supports that the lesion displays intestinal differentiation.

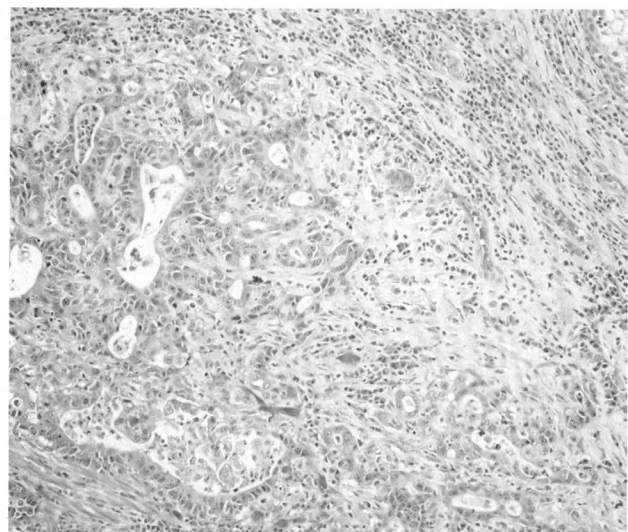

Figure 1-100. Adenocarcinoma. This adenocarcinoma is accompanied by desmoplasia (scarring in response to the lesion). This finding on a biopsy sample suggests that there may be deeper invasion than into the lamina propria.

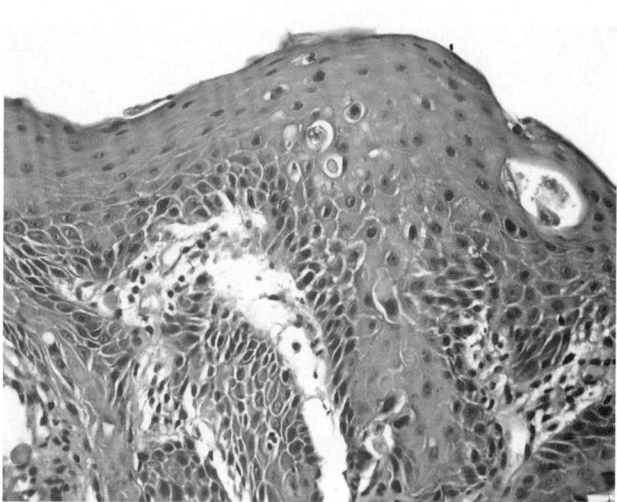

Figure 1-101. Adenocarcinoma. In this case, there is pagetoid extension of single adenocarcinoma cells into accompanying squamous mucosa in the sample. This finding suggests that a deeply invasive carcinoma is present and is an ominous sign.

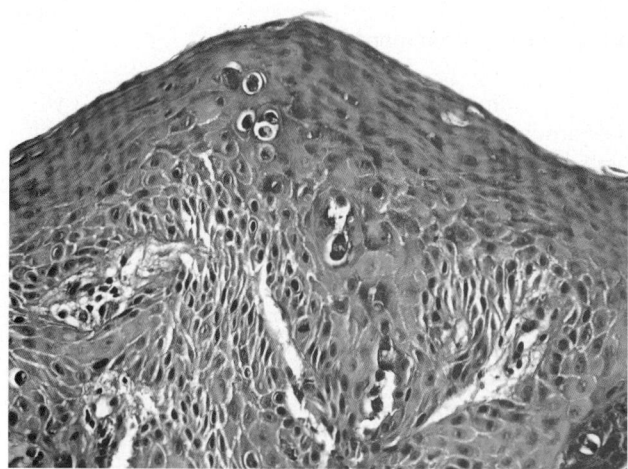

Figure 1-102. Adenocarcinoma. This is PAS/AB stain from the case seen in Fig. 1.101. The PAS highlights glycogen in the superficial squamous epithelium (the basal cells lack glycogen), but the adenocarcinoma cells contain bluish alcian blue–reactive mucin.

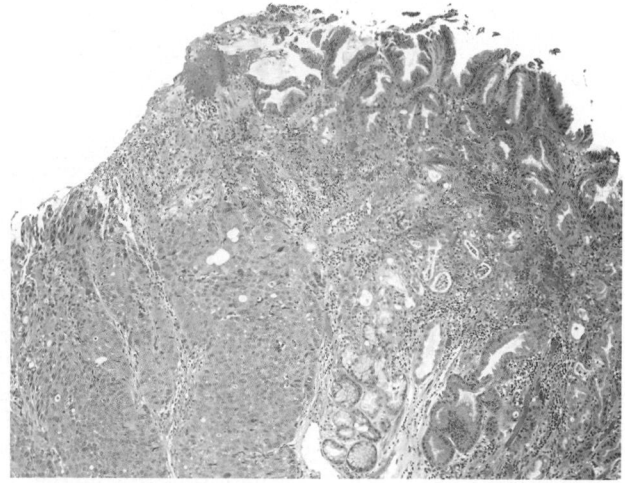

Figure 1-103. Poorly differentiated carcinoma associated with columnar epithelium in the esophagus. This lesion has a suggestion of gland formation (adenocarcinoma), but it is difficult to assure that it is not a squamous cell carcinoma.

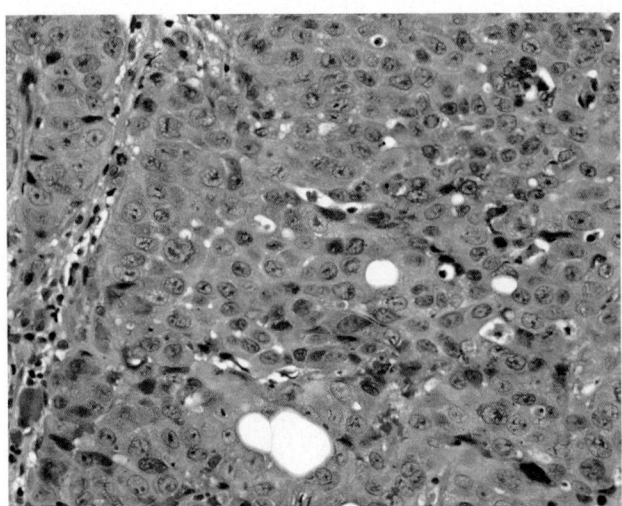

Figure 1-104. Poorly differentiated carcinoma. This is a high-magnification image of the lesion seen in Fig. 1.103. The cells are arranged in sheets and some have prominent nucleoli.

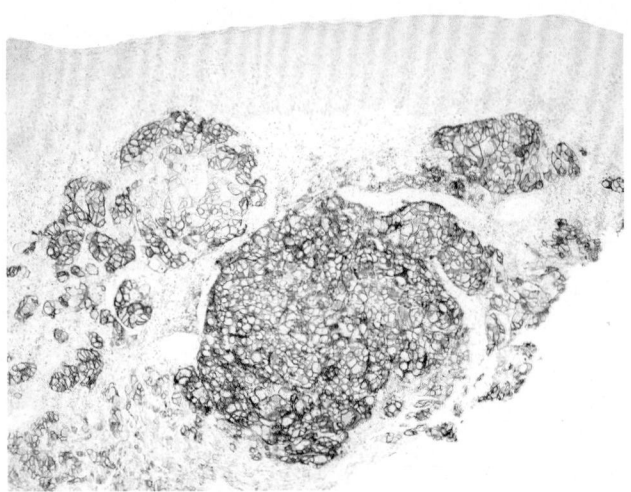

Figure 1-105. Poorly differentiated carcinoma. This strongly reactive BEREP4 stain supports an interpretation of poorly differentiated adenocarcinoma. This staining was performed to determine if HER2 testing should be done. HER2 testing is discussed in the "Stomach" chapter, but the same criteria are used for gastric and esophageal adenocarcinomas.

FAQ: How are dysplasia and early carcinoma managed?

Answer: Before we discuss EMR samples, it is worth considering how dysplasia and early carcinomas are managed. The 2016 American College of Gastroenterologists suggestions for management and follow-up of Barrett mucosa and estimates for likelihood of progression to carcinoma are given in Table 1.1. Essentially, all dysplasia is currently managed by mucosal ablation, **including low-grade dysplasia**, so endoscopy societies have suggested expert pathology review before treatment. Unfortunately, criteria for whom to regard as an expert are not well established,[47] but interobserver variability can be an issue in assessing dysplasia no matter who is reviewing such that it is always a good idea to review cases with colleagues[29]; it is seen as prudent to have peer review as a matter of course before performing mucosal ablation. Generally, flat/invisible dysplasia is ablated using radiofrequency ablation, whereas dysplasia that forms a visible lesion is resected endoscopically either with EMR or endoscopic submucosal dissection. The latter technique provides a better en bloc sample that typically has negative lateral margins, but the former is quicker and several adjoining areas can be removed piecemeal.[48] Most mucosal ablation is performed using radiofrequency ablation,[49] but there are a few other techniques that can be used, including cryotherapy.[50]

TABLE 1.1: American College of Gastroenterology (ACG)

Dysplasia Grade	Further Documentation	Follow-up, ACG/AGA	Estimated Likelihood of Progression
None	None	3–5 y	0.2%–0.5%/year initially, later up to 9%
Indefinite	Repeat after optimization of acid suppression in 3–6 months. If another indefinite, follow up	12 months	Data unclear
Low grade	Expert confirmation, ablation	Every 6 months during the first year, then annually	0.7%/year
High-grade or intramucosal carcinoma	Expert confirmation. EMR recommended if biopsies are taken from an area of mucosal irregularity coupled with RFA	Every 3 months for the first year, every 6 months for the second year, then annually	7%/year (HGD)

EMR, endoscopic mucosal resection; HGD, high-grade dysplasia; RFA, radiofrequency ablation.
Adapted from Shaheen NJ, Falk GW, Iyer PG, Gerson LB; American College of Gastroenterology. ACG clinical guideline: diagnosis and management of Barrett's esophagus. *Am J Gastroenterol.* 2016;111(1):30-50.

Endoscopic Mucosal Resection Specimens

EMR specimens are the more common samples received compared with submucosal dissections and are more prone to interpretation issues because they are often simply tossed into a jar of formalin, which causes them to curl. Ideally, they should be pinned to a corkboard or wax board, but they are often too tiny to pin without ruining them. The main thing is to have a way to orient them before they are sectioned. Ideally, they are breadloafed and embedded so that each slice shows the surface mucosa and some deep submucosa.[44] It can be helpful to ink the deep (submucosal) margin, but if this is not done, diathermy (cautery) is usually apparent to offer a clue about the location of the margins.

There are two forms of artifact that are often encountered in EMRs, and once they are understood, most EMRs can be readily assessed. The first is that the surface is often iatrogenically damaged. This is because, to perform an EMR, often the surface mucosa is sucked into a plastic cap after injecting the submucosa to create a polyplike lesion that is then removed by polypectomy. As such, the surface is rubbed and sometimes the most superficial epithelium is denuded. The second artifact is that, once the sample is removed and tossed into fixative, the sample curls as noted earlier. This gives an appearance that the lateral (mucosal) margin is a deep margin.

It is especially important when evaluating EMRs to be aware that, in patients with Barrett mucosa, the muscularis mucosae becomes disorganized and duplicated or even triplicated in response to cycles of damage and repair.[2,51-53] This can easily result in misinterpretation of lamina propria as submucosa and overstaging of the lesion as T1b when the stage is in fact T1a. Remember that T1a indicates invasion into lamina propria and T1b indicates invasion into submucosa.[1] **The space between the duplicated and original muscularis mucosae is still lamina propria!!!** A number of EMR samples, some annotated to highlight the issue with the muscularis mucosae, are shown in Figs. 1.106–1.120.

For clinical treatment purposes, it does not matter which layer of the mucosa is invaded, but clinical colleagues like to know a depth of invasion because they like a number and a quantitation. They also like to know the status of the sample margins. There are some

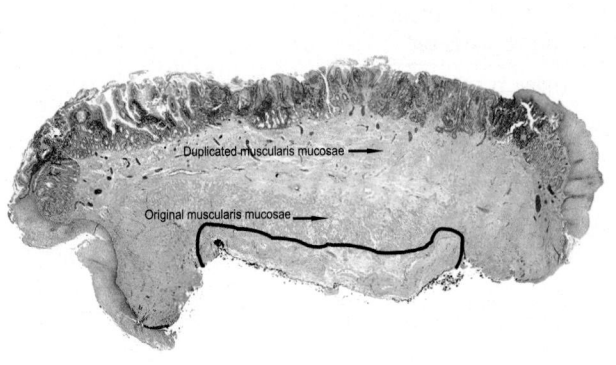

Figure 1-106. Endoscopic mucosal resection (EMR) specimen. This image illustrates some key issues in interpreting these samples. There is a lesion present in the upper right portion of the specimen. Note that the right lesion is covered by squamous epithelium (buried or pseudoregression pattern). The sample was not pinned to a corkboard such that it has curled, but it is well embedded. A *thick black line* separates the muscularis mucosae from the submucosa. The original muscularis mucosae is annotated, as is the duplicated muscularis mucosae. The loose tissue between these two muscle layers in not submucosa, it is part of the lamina propria! Note also that the surface epithelium appears damaged—this is probably from the procedure to perform the EMR, in which a cap is applied to the lesion's surface and suction is applied. In this example, the muscularis mucosae layers are so thick that the endoscopist barely obtained any submucosa.

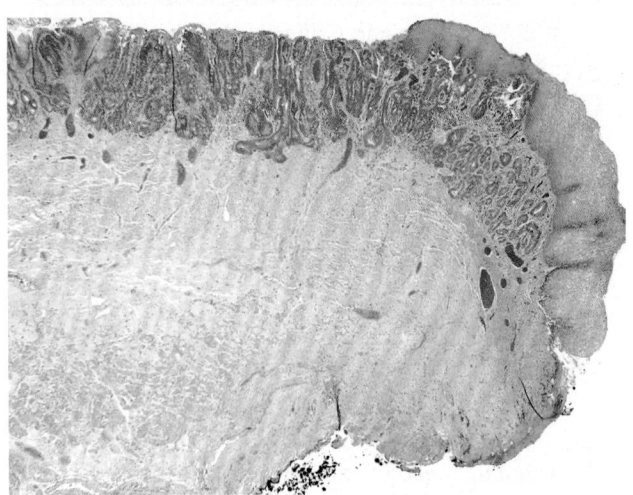

Figure 1-107. Endoscopic mucosal resection (EMR) specimen. This is a higher-magnification image of the right side of the lesion seen in Fig. 1.106. There is an intramucosal carcinoma that invades the lamina propria. The squamous epithelium and the accompanying lamina propria has curled such that the lateral margin masquerades as a deep margin. The actual deep margin does not begin until the middle of the image, where a submucosal vessel is seen; the muscularis mucosae is draped over it!

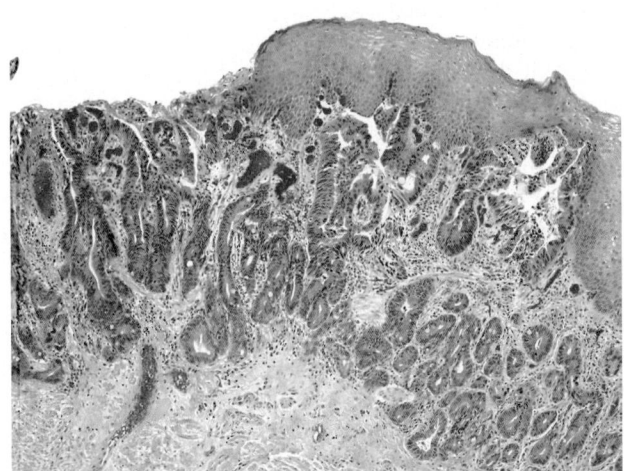

Figure 1-108. Endoscopic mucosal resection (EMR) specimen. This is a higher-magnification image of the lesion seen in Figs. 1.106 and 1.107. The intramucosal carcinoma consists of glands with luminal necrosis and angulated growth. Note that the surface at the left part of the image has been altered during the EMR operation itself.

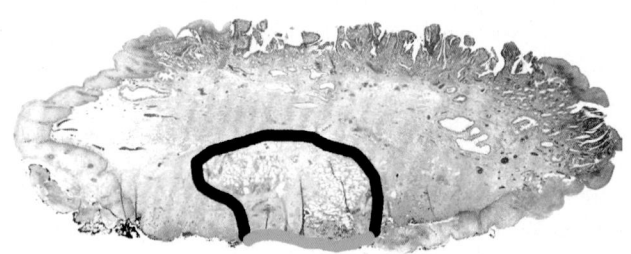

Figure 1-109. Endoscopic mucosal resection (EMR) specimen. In this example, the junction between the mucosa and submucosa is delineated with a *thick black line*. It drapes over some submucosal glands; their presence is proof that the cordoned off area is indeed submucosa! The *thick green line* thus is the true deep (submucosal) margin, and the rest of the apparent "deep" area is in fact lateral margin! The squamous epithelium itself has curled around to the apparent deep margin. This is an artifact of tissue retraction associated with diathermy (cautery) used in the EMR. In the top center, a few glands are arranged parallel to the surface in the lamina propria (not the submucosa).

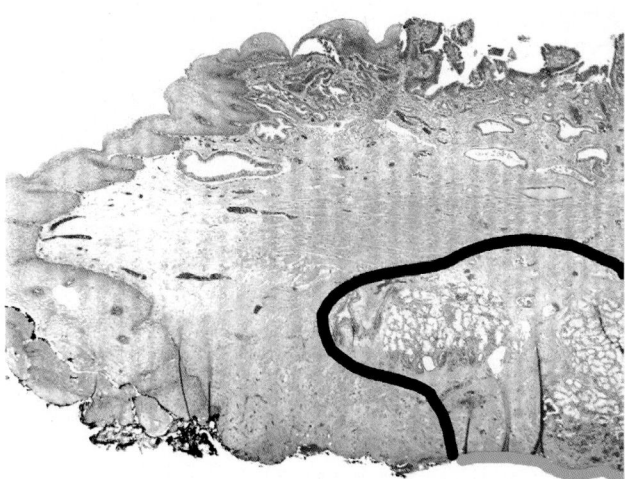

Figure 1-110. Endoscopic mucosal resection (EMR) specimen. This is a higher-magnification image of the left side of the tissue seen in Fig. 1.109. The *thick black line* separates the mucosa and submucosa. The thick muscularis mucosae has draped over the submucosal gland to the left. The deep (submucosal) margin is indicated by the *thick green line*, but the apparent deep tissue inked with *black* India ink is in fact a lateral margin consisting of curled squamous epithelium and muscularis mucosae. There is an intramucosal carcinoma invading into duplicated disorganized muscularis mucosae at the upper right of the field.

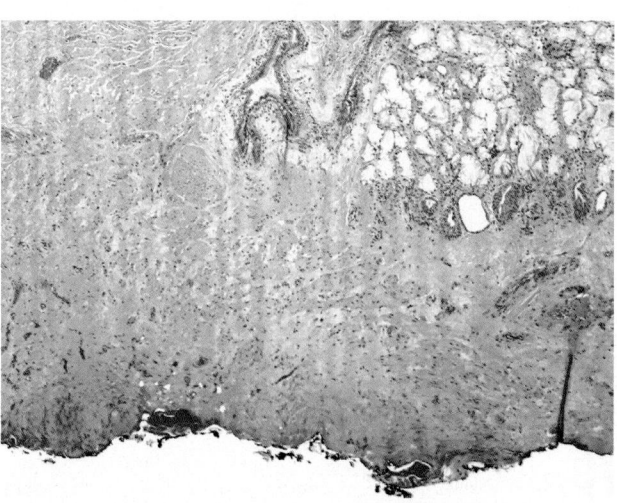

Figure 1-111. Endoscopic mucosal resection (EMR) specimen. This is a high-magnification image of the lateral margin seen at the lower left of Fig. 1.110. Note the muscularis mucosae curling over the submucosal gland at the upper right and painted with India ink at the bottom of the image.

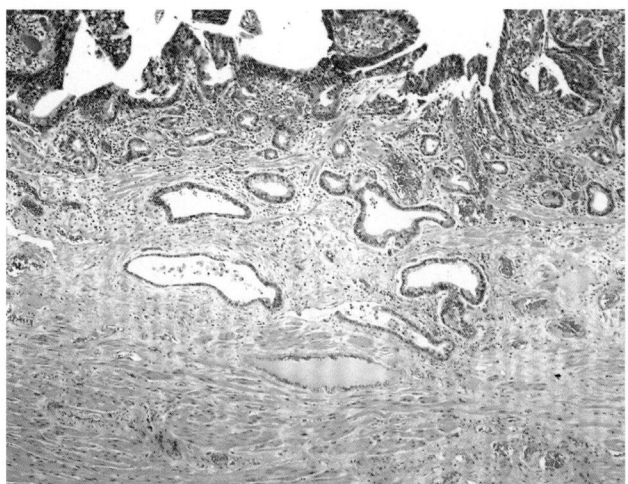

Figure 1-112. Endoscopic mucosal resection (EMR) specimen. This is a high-magnification image of the lesion seen in Figs. 1.109–1.111. The intramucosal carcinoma has invaded into the disorganized muscularis mucosae at the upper right of the image and is in the space between the original muscularis mucosae and the superficial duplicated muscularis mucosae. Note that there is no desmoplastic response to the invasion in this intramucosal carcinoma. In this case, it is easy to see the extent of the lesion because this is an EMR sample but this field should serve as a caution—were this a small biopsy, it would be easy to incorrectly assume that there was submucosal invasion and that the smooth muscle at the bottom was muscularis propria. However, a moment's thought should rectify this idea because the muscularis propria is practically never seen on mucosal biopsies of columnar esophagus.

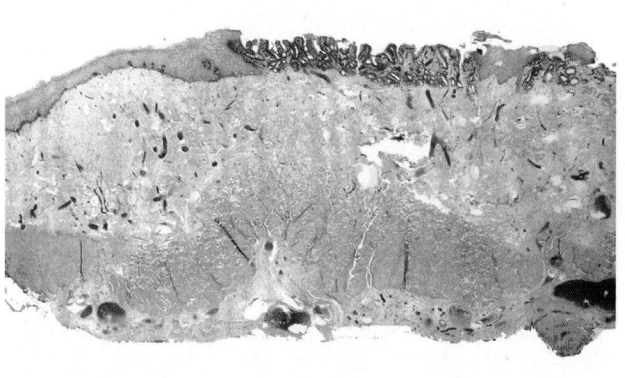

Figure 1-113. Endoscopic mucosal resection (EMR) specimen. This example was pinned well and has not curled much. As such, the bottom of the sample is submucosa and the thick band of smooth muscle near the bottom is the muscularis mucosae. There is additional disorganized smooth muscle above the thick muscularis mucosae.

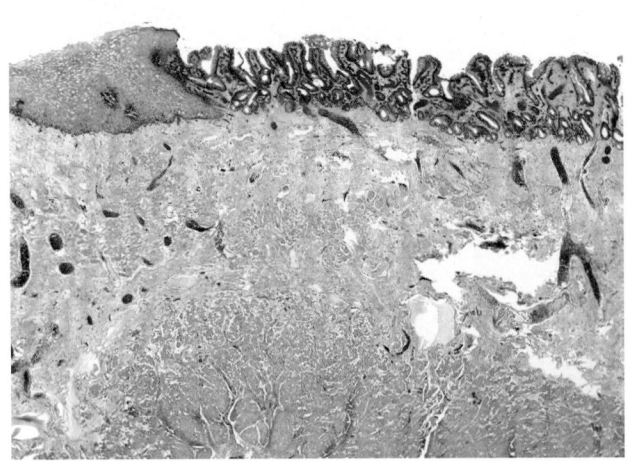

Figure 1-114. Endoscopic mucosal resection (EMR) specimen. This is a higher-magnification image of the EMR seen in Fig. 1.113. This particular EMR lacks dysplasia but shows only reactive Barrett mucosa. However, it gives a good look at the thickened original (lower part of field) muscularis mucosae and disorganized duplicated muscularis mucosae in the center of the image above the original muscularis mucosae.

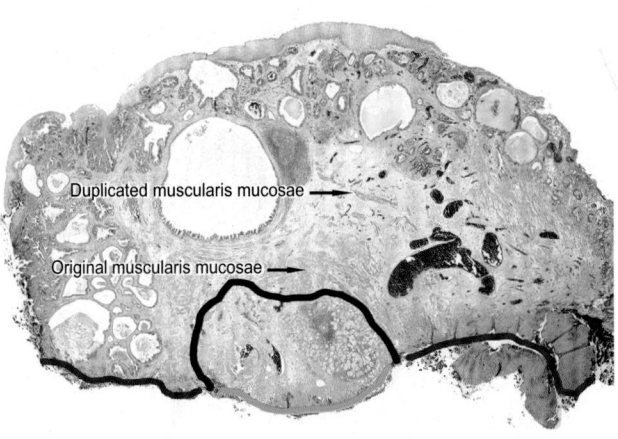

Figure 1-115. Endoscopic mucosal resection (EMR) specimen. This EMR is curled and contains a carcinoma that has invaded the space between the original and duplicated muscularis mucosae (T1a lesion). A *thick black line* separates the mucosa and submucosa. A *thick green line* shows the deep (submucosal) margin, and *thick blue lines* show the lateral margins. There is intramucosal carcinoma at the lateral (mucosal) margin on the left. This is not at the deep margin! This is a common occurrence because endoscopists often resect lesion by means of several side-by-side EMRs. In this case, much of the lesion is buried under squamous epithelium but the endoscopist found it anyway.

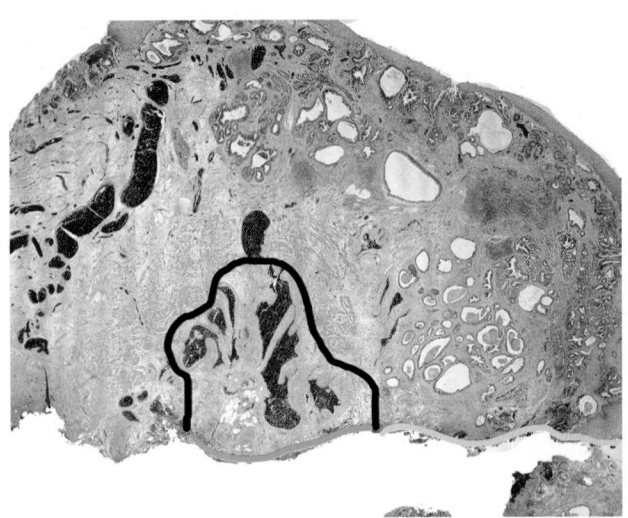

Figure 1-116. Endoscopic mucosal resection (EMR) specimen. This EMR contains an intramucosal carcinoma that has invaded nearly to the submucosa. A *black line* separates the mucosa and submucosa. A *thick green line* shows the deep (submucosal) margin, and a *blue line* shows the lateral margin. This T1a neoplasm is present at the lateral margin.

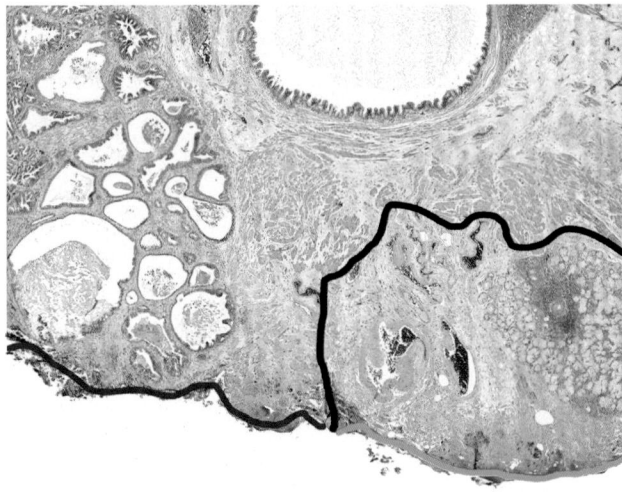

Figure 1-117. Endoscopic mucosal resection (EMR) specimen. This is a high-magnification image of the involved lateral margin from the lesion seen in Fig. 1.115. The *thick black line* shows the demarcation between the mucosa and submucosa. A submucosal gland is present at the right side of the image beneath the *black line*. The *green line* shows the deep (submucosal) margin, and the *blue line* shows the lateral (mucosal) margin. The muscularis mucosae can be seen draping over a large submucosal vessel in the lower central part of the field.

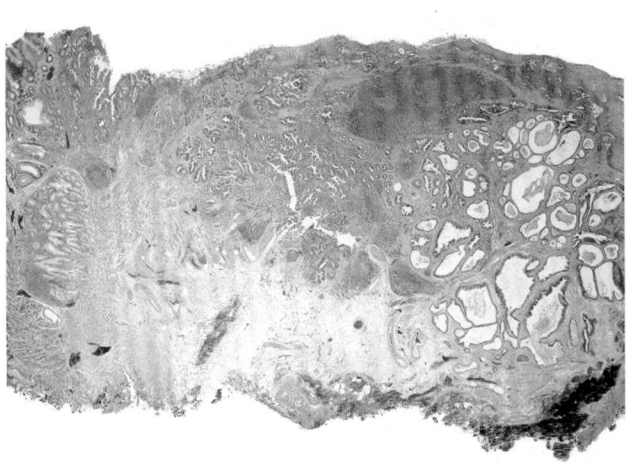

Figure 1-118. Endoscopic mucosal resection (EMR) specimen. This EMR shows a carcinoma that invades the submucosa in the center of the image. In this case, it is worthwhile to measure the depth of invasion starting from the bottom of the original muscularis mucosae.

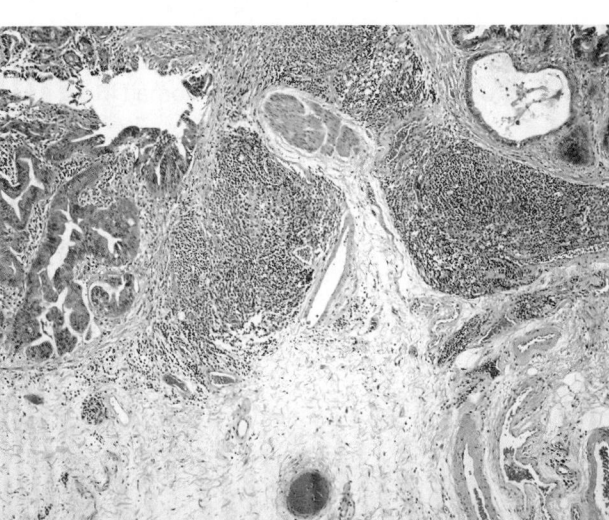

Figure 1-119. Endoscopic mucosal resection (EMR) specimen. This is a higher-magnification image of the lesion seen in Fig. 1.118. A bit of muscularis mucosae is seen in the center of the image, and the carcinoma at the left is invading into the submucosa. Large submucosal vessels are seen at the lower right.

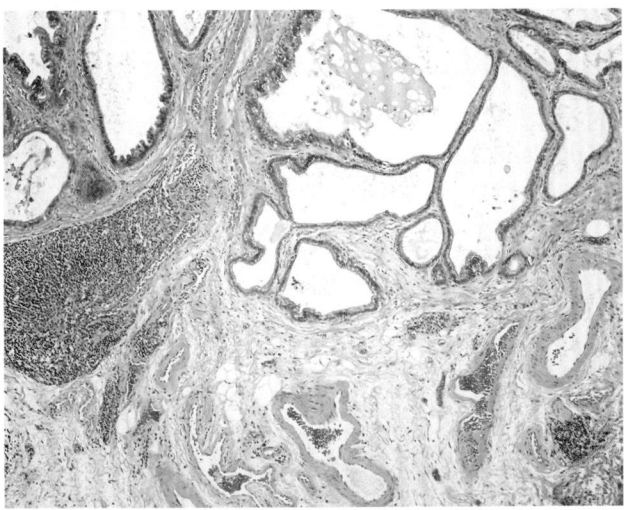

Figure 1-120. Endoscopic mucosal resection (EMR) specimen. A carcinoma has entered the submucosa. Note the large thick vessels in this space!

formalized schemes for reporting this, but in our experience, it is safest to simply describe the depth of invasion in words. For example, "the tumor invades into the space between the initial and duplicated muscularis mucosae." Table 1.2 shows the various schemes that have been developed, and several authors have used "m1-m3" or something similar to account for the various depths that a tumor can invade the mucosa. We usually avoid the classifications with "m1-m3" or "m1-m4" because an oncologist invariably misinterprets the "m" for "mucosal invasion" as the "M" for "metastasis" in the staging manual. Argh.

When tumors invade the submucosa, it is worthwhile to provide a depth of invasion as measured from the base of the muscularis mucosae because these items are in the balance of whether to perform a follow-up esophagectomy. A depth of more than half a millimeter (500 μm) prompts discussion of esophagectomy unless the patient has significant comorbidities.[45] Finding a poorly differentiated component (lots of single cells rather than cells forming glands) or vascular space invasion also prompts this discussion. Such decisions are best made with a clinical team and in light of known comorbidities in the patient.

TABLE 1.2: Reported Subclassification Schemes for Intramucosal Carcinoma (T1a)

Descriptive Designation of Depth of Invasion	Designation, Westerterp Scheme[54]	Designation, Vieth Scheme[55]	Designation, Kaneshiro Scheme[52]
None (Tis, high-grade dysplasia, HGD)	m1	HGD	HGD
Tumor cells invading beyond basement membrane into lamina propria	m2	m1	LP
Tumor cells invading (inner) duplicated muscularis mucosae	m2	m2	IMM
Tumor cells in the space between the duplicated muscularis mucosae and original muscularis mucosae	m2	m3	BMM
Tumor cells into (outer) original muscularis mucosae	m3	m4	OMM

SAMPLE NOTE: Carcinoma Confined to the Lamina Propria

Esophagus, 35 cm (EMR): Intramucosal carcinoma in a background of Barrett mucosa (T1a). The carcinoma invades into the lamina propria. No vascular space invasion seen. No poorly differentiated component seen. The lesion is present at the lateral (mucosal) margin. The deep (submucosal) margin is uninvolved.

SAMPLE NOTE: Carcinoma Invading Into the Submucosa

Esophagus, 37 cm (EMR): Moderately differentiated adenocarcinoma invading into the superficial submucosa (T1b) in a background of Barrett mucosa with extensive high-grade dysplasia. No poorly differentiated component seen. No vascular space invasion. Carcinoma invades to a depth of 0.4 mm measured from the base of the muscularis mucosae and is 1 mm from the deep margin. The deep (submucosal) and lateral (mucosal) margins are uninvolved.

Dysplasia Recapitulation

Composite Fig. 1.121 summarizes the key issues of Barrett dysplasia grading:

Negative for dysplasia—There is surface maturation, preserved overall cell polarity (the four lines), and maintained nuclear polarity (long axes of nuclei are perpendicular to the basement membrane). Lamina propria is plentiful.

Indefinite for dysplasia—There is equivocal surface maturation, equivocally preserved overall cell polarity (the four lines), and maintained nuclear polarity (long axes of nuclei are perpendicular to the basement membrane). Lamina propria is plentiful. Inflammation is often a factor in using the indefinite category.

Low-grade dysplasia—The surface shows areas that lack surface maturation, and there is loss of overall cell polarity (the lines are obscured). Nuclei are hyperchromatic but have overall maintained polarity. Lamina propria is plentiful. Cases with gastric-type differentiation are different and discussed in the earlier text.

Basal pattern dysplasia—There are nuclear features of dysplasia restricted to the pits. Often recut sections will disclose zones of surface alterations.

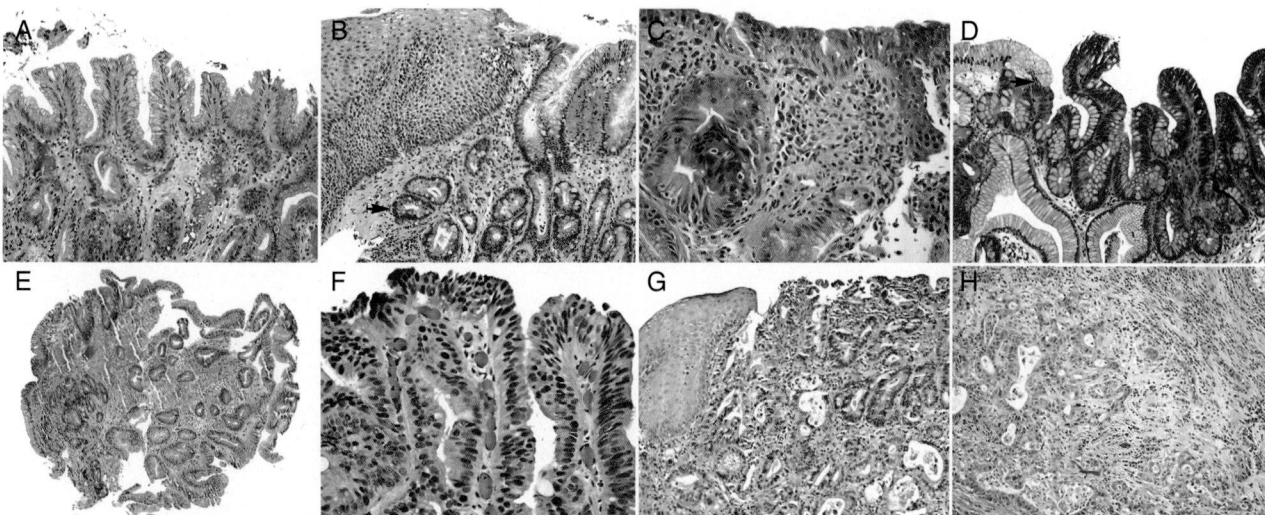

Figure 1-121. Summary of Barrett esophagus and neoplasia. **A:** Negative for dysplasia—there is surface maturation, preserved overall cell polarity (the four lines), and maintained nuclear polarity (long axes of nuclei are perpendicular to the basement membrane). Lamina propria is abundant. **B:** Barrett mucosa with reactive changes. The polarity of the cells is maintained (the four lines), and deeper glands may display mild nuclear alterations. **C:** Indefinite for dysplasia—there is equivocal surface maturation, equivocally preserved overall cell polarity (the four lines), and maintained nuclear polarity (long axes of nuclei are perpendicular to the basement membrane). Lamina propria is plentiful. Inflammation is often a factor in using the indefinite category. **D:** Low-grade dysplasia—the surface shows areas that lack surface maturation, and there is loss of overall cell polarity (the lines are obscured). Nuclei are hyperchromatic but have overall maintained polarity. Lamina propria is plentiful. **E:** Basal pattern dysplasia—there are nuclear features of dysplasia restricted to the glands. Often recut sections will disclose zones of surface alterations. **F:** High-grade dysplasia—the surface shows lack of maturation, and there is loss of overall cell polarity (the lines are obscured). Nuclei are hyperchromatic with loss of polarity. Nucleoli are inconspicuous. Lamina propria is often plentiful (but not always). **G:** Intramucosal carcinoma (lamina propria invasion T1a)—this is the earliest invasive carcinoma and invasion only into the lamina propria can be suggested even on mucosal biopsies because desmoplasia is not yet well developed. The surface shows lack of maturation, and there is loss of overall cell polarity (the lines are obscured). Many nuclei are hyperchromatic with loss of polarity. Large nucleoli are present. Lamina propria is overrun by glands. **H:** Adenocarcinoma invasive into at least the submucosa (at least T1b as seen on mucosal biopsies)—all of the features of intramucosal carcinoma are present as well as angulated glands with desmoplasia. Occasional cases show pagetoid extension of single cells into squamous epithelium.

High-grade dysplasia—The surface shows lack of maturation, and there is loss of overall cell polarity (the lines are obscured). Nuclei are hyperchromatic with loss of polarity. Nucleoli are usually inconspicuous. Lamina propria is often plentiful (but not always). Cases with gastric-type differentiation are different and discussed in the earlier text.

Intramucosal carcinoma (lamina propria invasion T1a)—This is the earliest invasive carcinoma, and invasion only into the lamina propria can be suggested even on mucosal biopsies because desmoplasia is not yet well developed. The surface shows lack of maturation, and there is loss of overall cell polarity (the lines are obscured). Many nuclei are hyperchromatic with loss of polarity. Large nucleoli are present. Lamina propria is overrun by glands.

Adenocarcinoma invasive into at least submucosa (at least T1b as seen on mucosal biopsies)—all of the features of intramucosal carcinoma are present as well as angulated glands with desmoplasia. Occasional cases show pagetoid extension of single cells into squamous epithelium.

FAQ: What is pseudoregression (buried Barrett mucosa)?

Answer: This is a pattern seen after either injury from reflux or injury from mucosal ablation in which squamous mucosa grows on top of columnar mucosa (Barrett mucosa). There were early case reports of carcinomas appearing beneath the squamous mucosa following ablation for dysplasia, but it is currently believed that this concern was overblown and not an issue. In fact, there is virtually always a surface lesion accompanying buried lesions (pseudoregression lesions).[38] In addition, using modern high-resolution endoscopes, many endoscopists are able to see areas that harbor buried lesions. We have already seen examples of these in Figs. 1.94, 1.106, 1.107, 1.109, 1.110, 1.115, 1.116, 1.118, and 1.122. In some of these examples, the endoscopist detected the lesions even though they were buried beneath squamous epithelium and even labeled them "lesion" on the specimen jars. Of course, she is a good endoscopist, but the point is that such lesions can be found by careful gross (endoscopic) examination.

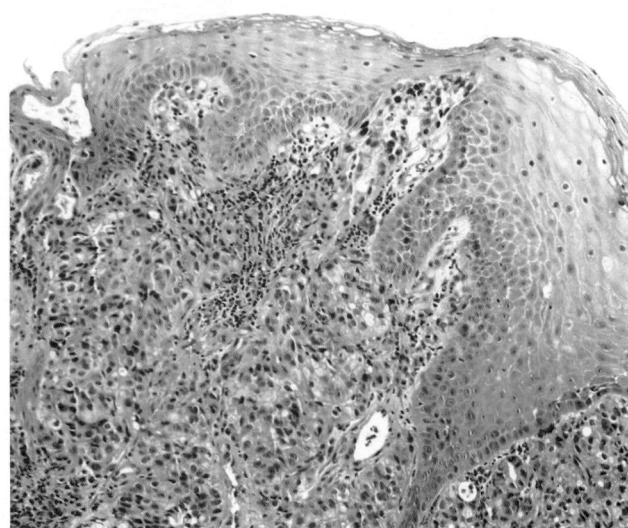

Figure 1-122. "Buried" Barrett-associated neoplasia/pseudoregression. This was once believed to be an issue, but additional data do not support such a concern. In this example, an intramucosal carcinoma, is seen buried under the squamous epithelium.

PEARLS & PITFALLS: Do not Be Fooled by Duplicated Muscularis Mucosae!

Disorganized double and even triple layers of muscularis mucosae are commonly encountered in the injured esophagus with Barrett metaplasia.[2,53] Correctly identifying the layers is easy on resections, but on superficial biopsies, remember that it is unusual to see submucosa, and tissue seen deep to muscularis mucosae on superficial samples is probably not submucosa but instead lamina propria between the duplicated muscularis mucosae and the deeper original muscularis mucosae. Fig. 1.106 shows an EMR sample with a very thick duplicated muscularis mucosae. Imagine a biopsy that is superficial and encompasses the space between the original muscularis mucosae and the duplicated muscularis mucosae. The savvy pathologist knows that that space is not submucosa and reports accordingly.

FAQ: What changes can we expect in samples obtained in patients who have had mucosal ablation?

Answer: The objective of mucosal ablation is to eliminate the dysplasia and, better still, all columnar epithelium. In some patients, follow-up samples show findings indistinguishable from those in undamaged squamous mucosa, but, in many patients, mild fibrosis of the lamina propria, prominent eosinophils, lymphocytosis,[56] and lichenoid changes (prominent intraepithelial lymphocytes and apoptotic squamous epithelial cells) may be encountered. Of course, do not forget to search for candidiasis and viral cytopathic changes.

SQUAMOUS NEOPLASIA

RISK FACTORS

Esophageal squamous neoplasia is uncommon in the United States compared with other regions of the world. Most patients with squamous carcinomas are men, and most are adults at least in their fifties. In contrast to the demographics for adenocarcinomas, which typically affect white men, squamous carcinoma predominates among African-American men.[57] Recent advances in improvement in detecting and treating adenocarcinomas are not mirrored for squamous carcinoma.[58]

The incidence of squamous cell carcinoma is diminishing in comparison with esophageal adenocarcinomas in the United States. In contrast, squamous carcinomas have a high incidence in developing countries, e.g., in southern Africa and China. In Southeast Asians, polymorphisms in *ALDH*, the gene that encodes aldehyde dehydrogenase, are associated with esophageal squamous cell cancer.[59,60] The effects of these polymorphisms are synergistic with alcohol and smoking. *ALDH* polymorphisms also result in accumulation in acetaldehyde, which causes flushing upon ingestion of alcohol in about a third of East Asians (Chinese, Japanese, and Koreans).

Any factor that causes chronic irritation and inflammation of the esophageal mucosa predisposes one to esophageal squamous cell carcinoma. Even skin disease affecting the esophagus can initiate the development of dysplasia/carcinoma of the esophagus. An example of this is lichen planus. However, substantial alcohol intake, especially in combination with smoking, exponentially increases the risk of squamous cell carcinoma (but not adenocarcinoma) and may account for the vast majority of squamous cell carcinoma of the esophagus in the developed world. The combination of smoking and alcohol abuse also results in an increased risk of head and neck cancer. Squamous cell carcinoma of the esophagus is in fact discovered incidentally in 1% to 2% of patients with head and neck cancers.[61]

Chronic esophageal irritation can also result from achalasia and esophageal diverticula such that food is retained and decomposes, releasing various chemical irritants. Frequent consumption of extremely hot beverages seems to increase the incidence of squamous cell carcinoma. Lastly, persons who have ingested lye or other caustic fluids require lifelong surveillance for the development of this cancer.[62]

Nonepidermolytic palmoplantar keratoderma (tylosis) is a rare autosomal dominant disorder defined by *RHBDF2* mutations on chromosome 17q25[63] associated with squamous cell carcinoma of the esophagus.[64] Patients have hyperkeratosis of the palms and soles and thickening of the oral mucosa. Although it confers up to a 95% risk of squamous cell carcinoma of the esophagus by the age of 70 years, it is a rare syndrome.

Squamous cell carcinoma (but not adenocarcinoma) is associated with low socioeconomic status, presumably a reflection of poor nutrition and other lifestyle factors. However, deficiency syndromes associated with this cancer, such as the Plummer-Vinson syndrome (dysphagia, iron-deficiency anemia, and esophageal webs), are becoming uncommon in the developed world as overall nutrition improves. A role for human papillomavirus (HPV) in the development of esophageal squamous cell carcinoma is debatable, even though it is well-established in the anal canal, as discussed in "Anus" chapter. Although HPV DNA detection rates are minimal (0% to 2%) in some studies from low-incidence areas,[65,66] higher rates are reported in high incidence areas, such as China and Iran.[67,68] However, one Mexican study, an area of low tumor incidence, reported the presence of high-risk HPV DNA in 25% of esophageal squamous cell carcinomas.[69] The rate in the United States is about 10%.[70]

SQUAMOUS CARCINOMA PRECURSOR LESIONS
Squamous Dysplasia

Background squamous epithelial dysplasia (intraepithelial neoplasia), low or high grade (including "carcinoma in situ"), can often be encountered at the periphery of invasive squamous cell carcinomas (Figs. 1.123–1.132). As in other sites, the convention is to regard epithelial changes in the bottom half of the epithelium as low-grade dysplasia (the intraepithelial neoplasia terminology is preferred in Europe) and into the top half as high-grade dysplasia. When there is absolutely no maturation at the surface, the term carcinoma in situ can be used, but it really does not matter for treatment purposes. Likewise, it can be difficult to determine when there is very early invasion into the lamina propria because this does not invoke a desmoplastic reaction. However, severe epithelial changes in the bottom half of the epithelium often suggest an adjoining unsampled carcinoma, as noted later. Sometimes reactive conditions can mimic dysplasia, and it is especially important to be cautious in the setting of inflammatory conditions (which themselves predispose to squamous neoplasia). Examples of lichenoid esophagitis[71] and pill-associated esophagitis with prominent epithelial changes are seen in Figs. 1.133–1.136. The reader is also referred to volume 1 of this series.

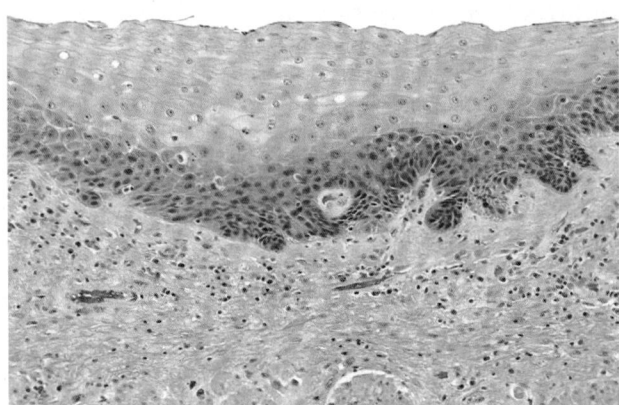

Figure 1-123. Low-grade squamous dysplasia. These lesions are subtle and often difficult to differentiate from reparative changes. The nuclei are hyperchromatic, and there may be mitoses and apoptotic nuclei as seen in the left part of the image. The epithelial changes are restricted to the lower half of the epithelium. In the setting of prominent inflammation, it can be impossible to determine if epithelial changes are reactive or dysplastic. Note that nucleoli are not prominent.

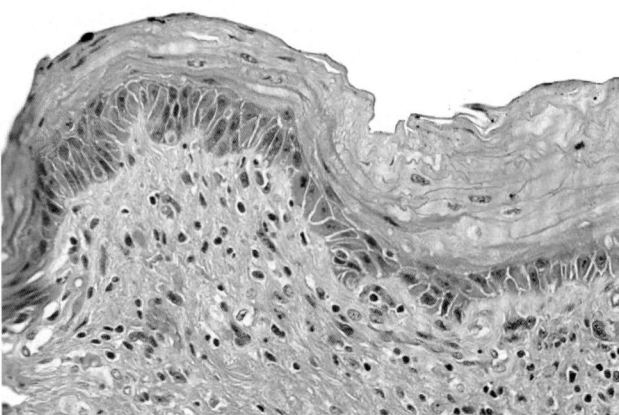

Figure 1-124. Low-grade squamous dysplasia. This case is difficult, but there are no inflammatory features to explain the findings and there are a few apoptotic bodies in the proliferation, which occupies just under half of the epithelial thickness.

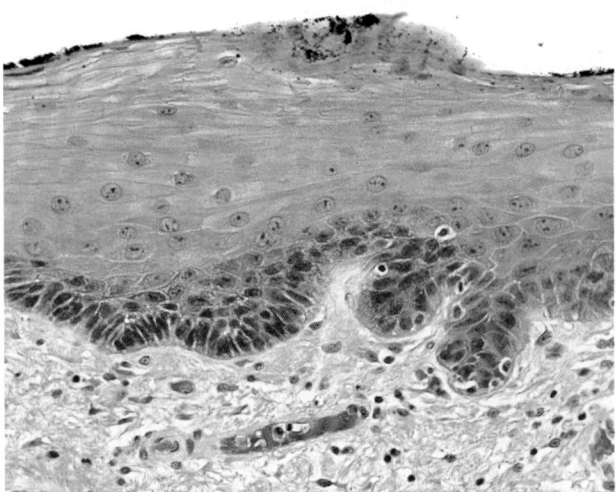

Figure 1-125. Low-grade squamous dysplasia. This is a high-magnification image of the case seen in Fig. 1.123.

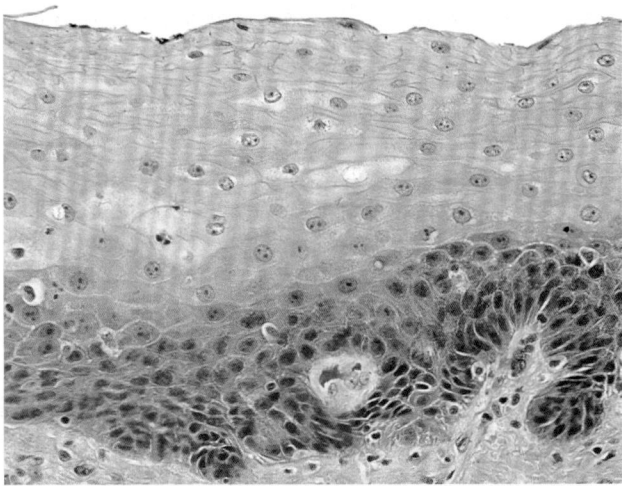

Figure 1-126. Low-grade squamous dysplasia. The nuclei in the basal portion of the epithelium are markedly hyperchromatic.

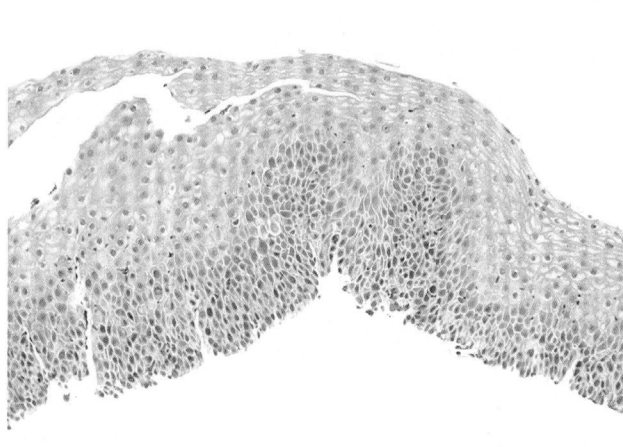

Figure 1-127. Low-grade squamous dysplasia. The basal zone is thickened, and the nuclei are enlarged and hyperchromatic.

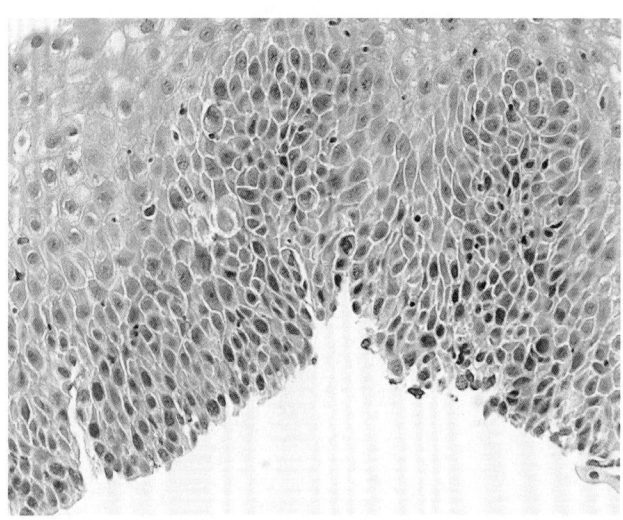

Figure 1-128. Low-grade squamous dysplasia. High magnification shows scattered mitoses and apoptotic bodies.

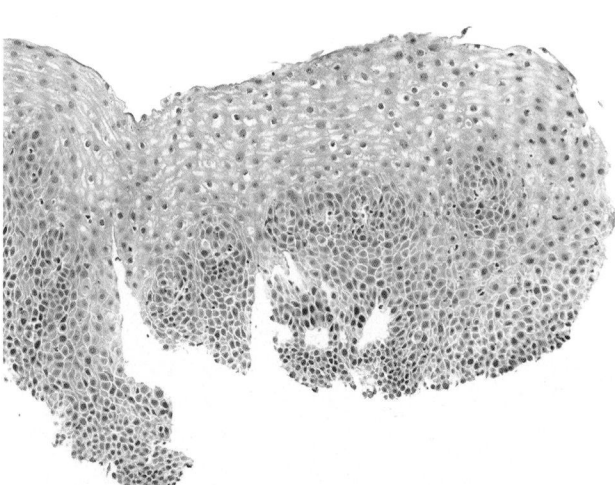

Figure 1-129. Low-grade squamous dysplasia. Note the marked nuclear hyperchromasia in the center of the image. There is no inflammatory process to explain the findings.

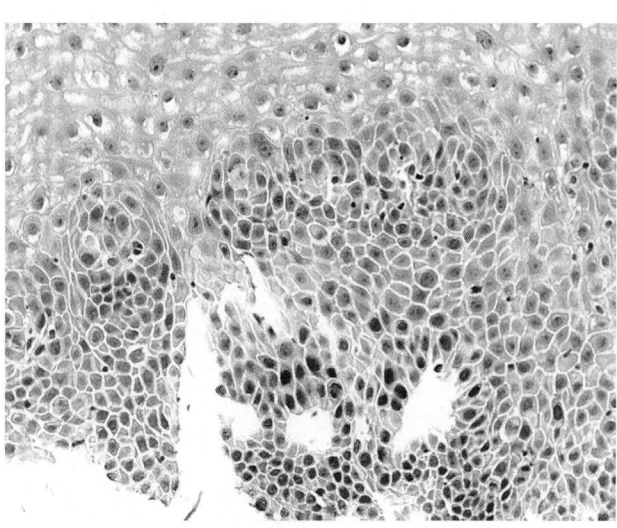

Figure 1-130. Low-grade squamous dysplasia. This is a high-magnification image of the process seen in Fig. 1.129.

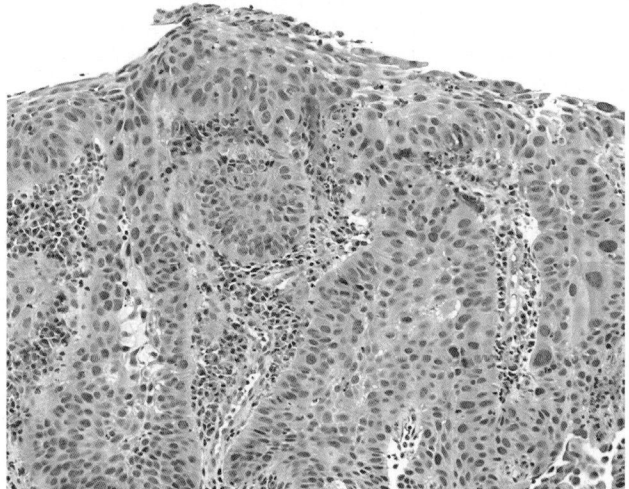

Figure 1-131. High-grade squamous dysplasia. Despite the inflammation, the epithelial changes are in excess of those attributable to inflammation. In Japan, lesions such as this would be regarded as intramucosal carcinomas.

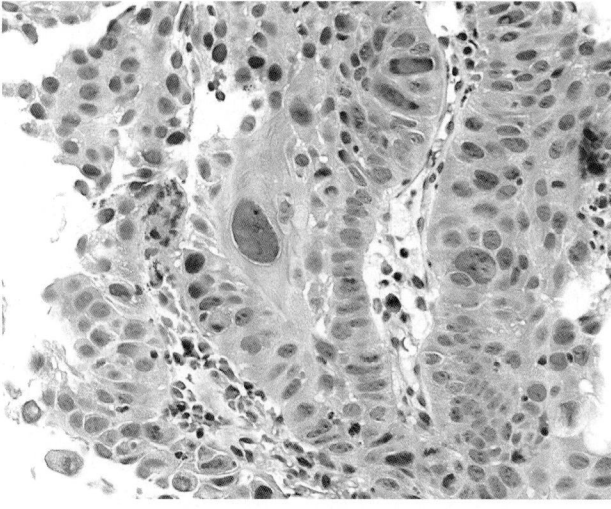

Figure 1-132. High-grade squamous dysplasia. The keratinization is concerning for invasion.

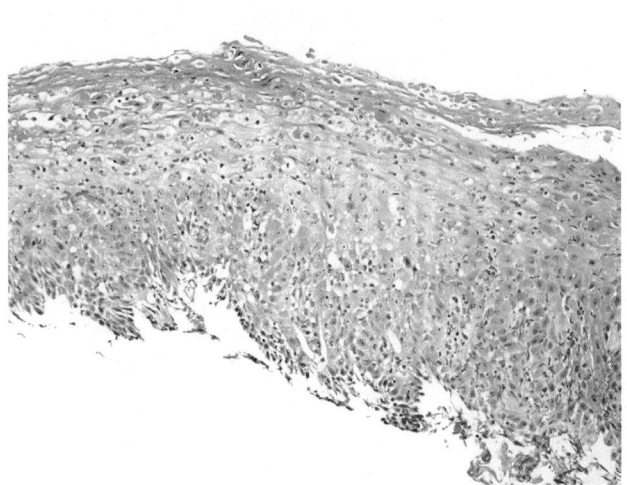

Figure 1-133. Lichenoid esophagitis with marked reactive epithelial changes. The findings are similar to those of low-grade dysplasia, but the striking inflammatory process can explain them. Patients with lichen planus of the esophagus and related lesions are at risk for squamous cell carcinomas and are monitored accordingly, so if these changes are in fact dysplastic and interpreted as reactive, this will not end patient surveillance.

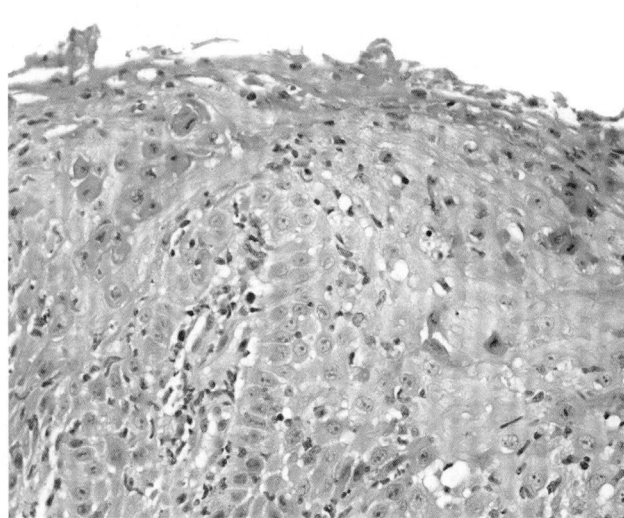

Figure 1-134. Lichenoid esophagitis with marked reactive epithelial changes. The prominent nucleoli suggest a reactive process.

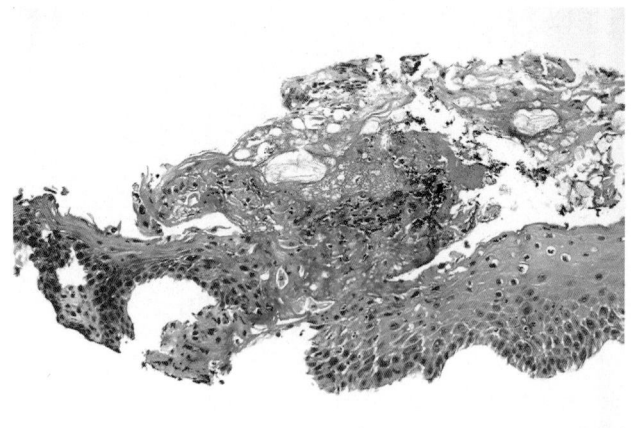

Figure 1-135. Pill esophagitis with striking reactive changes. In the context of the exudate and embedded pill material, these changes are best regarded as reparative.

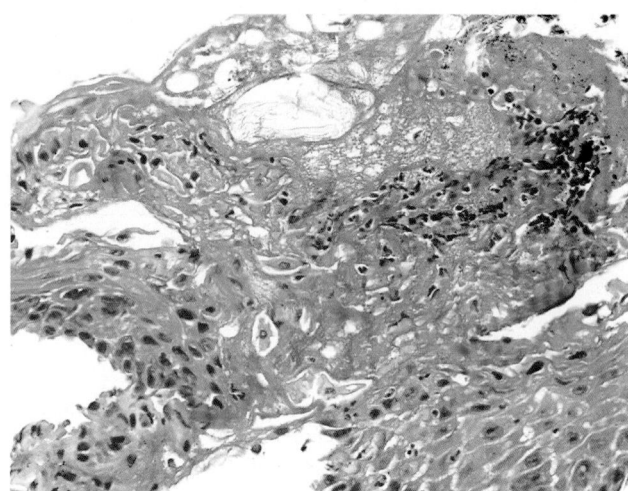

Figure 1-136. Pill esophagitis with striking reactive changes. This is a high-magnification image of the lesion seen in Fig. 1.135. Note the prominent intracellular edema at the lower right. The edema causes the intercellular bridges to appear prominent.

Epidermoid Metaplasia

A peculiar pattern of hyperkeratosis and hypergranulosis, which can be termed "esophageal leukoplakia" (because the endoscopist notes white plaques), but more accurately "epidermoid metaplasia," can be encountered as an isolated finding, but it can also be seen associated with samples showing squamous dysplasia and carcinoma.[72,73] We suspect that this is a precursor lesion. There is also some more scientific rather than histologic evidence that epidermoid metaplasia is a precursor lesion; we have noted that molecular alterations detected by next-generation sequencing mirror those in the associated dysplasias and carcinomas.[74]

Epidermoid metaplasia is easy to overlook unless one is in the know because it appears normal at first glance except that it is metaplastic. Unfortunately, the magnitude of the risk for associated squamous cell dysplasia and carcinoma is not known. The subtle finding to be sought is simply the presence of a granular layer in esophageal squamous epithelium, which is not normal for the esophagus but perfectly normal in skin! Examples of epidermoid metaplasia, one of which is associated with neoplasia, are shown in Figs. 1.137–1.142.

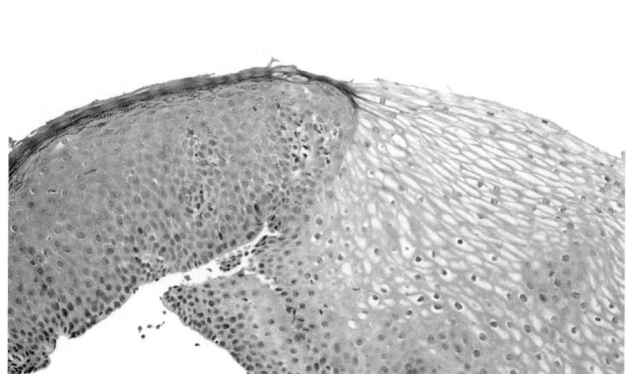

Figure 1-137. Epidermoid metaplasia. This sample appears rather unremarkable at first glance but note the granular layer at the left. Note also that the lesion is sharply demarcated from the uninvolved squamous epithelium.

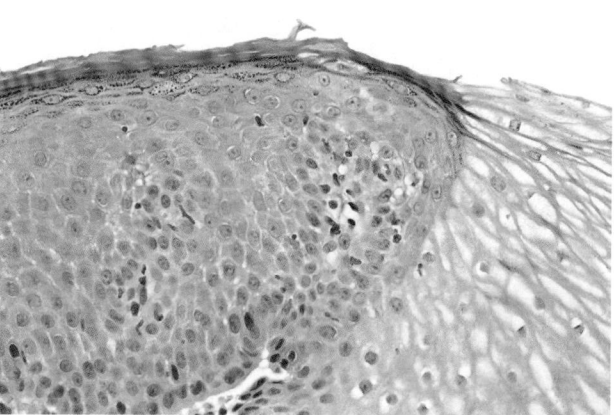

Figure 1-138. Epidermoid metaplasia. This is a high-magnification image of the lesion seen in Fig. 1.137. It shows the sharp demarcation between the normal area and the zone with epidermoid metaplasia.

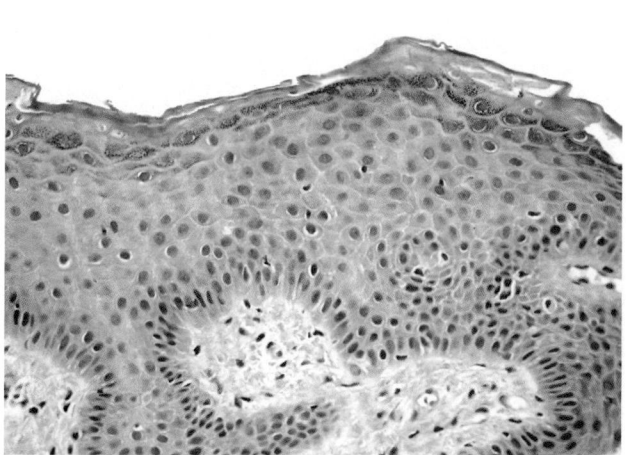

Figure 1-139. Epidermoid metaplasia. Note the granular layer and the surface hyperkeratosis.

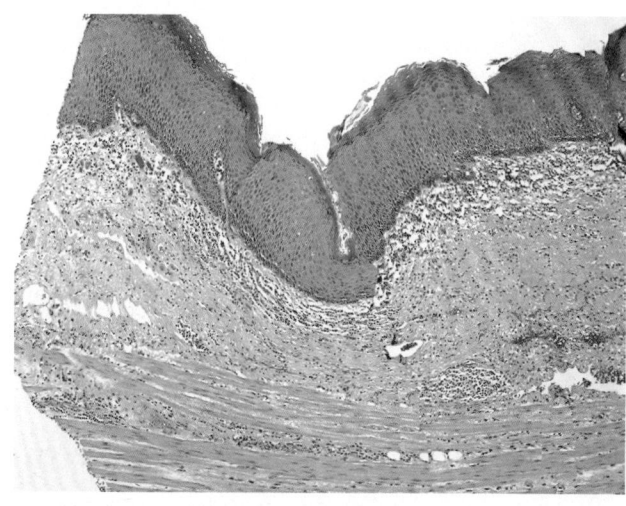

Figure 1-140. Epidermoid metaplasia. This example is from a resection specimen—the indication for resection was squamous cell carcinoma and there was extensive epidermoid metaplasia in the adjoining tissue.

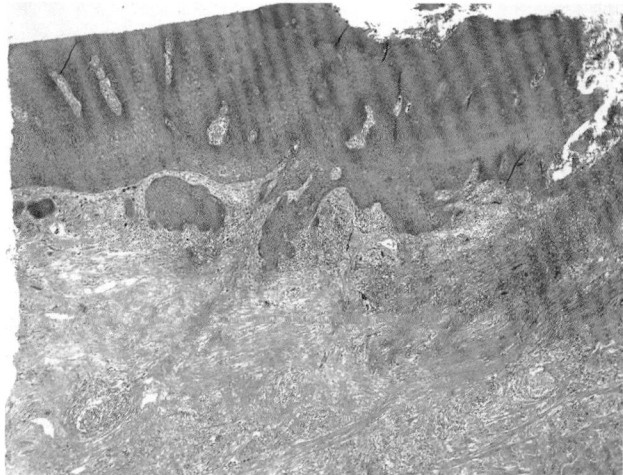

Figure 1-141. Squamous cell carcinoma associated with epidermoid metaplasia. This squamous cell carcinoma was associated with epidermoid metaplasia.

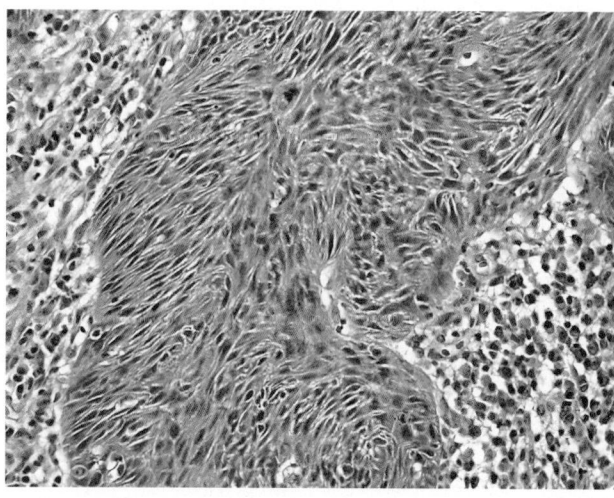

Figure 1-142. Squamous cell carcinoma associated with epidermoid metaplasia. This is a high-magnification image of the carcinoma seen in Fig. 1.141.

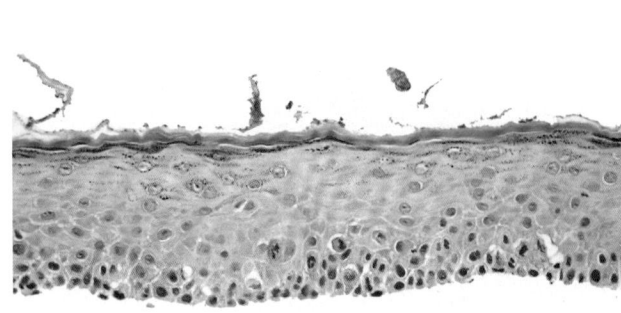

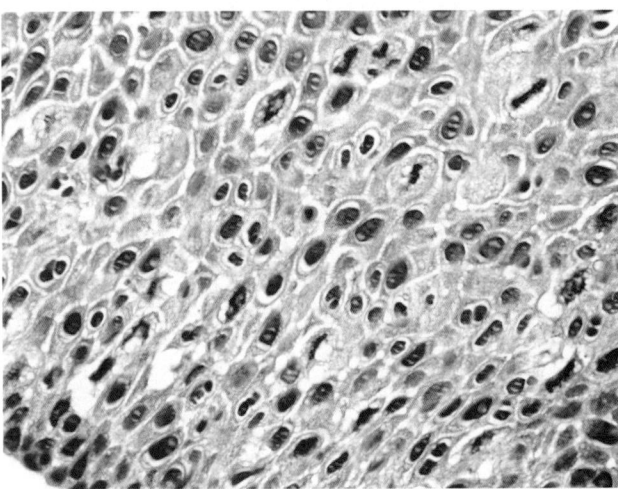

Figure 1-143. Epidermoid metaplasia. This is a tricky case. There is epidermoid metaplasia and apparently dysplasia in the lower half of the mucosa. But, wait, there is more! The patient was taking a taxane medication for a separate carcinoma (breast), and in fact there is taxane effect (note the ring mitoses) in association with epidermoid metaplasia.

Figure 1-144. Taxane effect. In this tangentially embedded focus, it is a real mimicker of dysplasia but note the mitotic arrest.

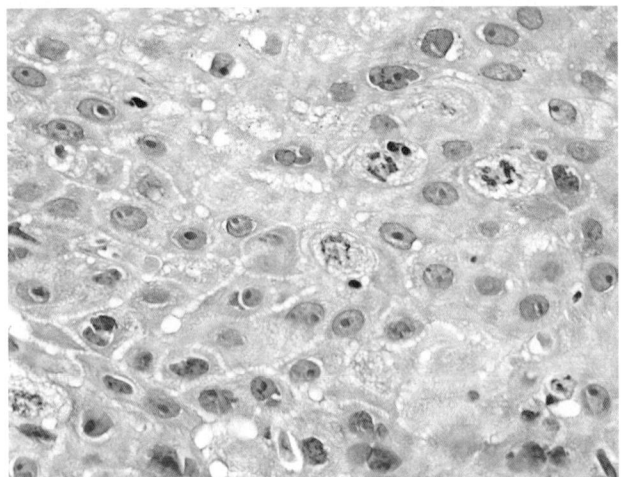

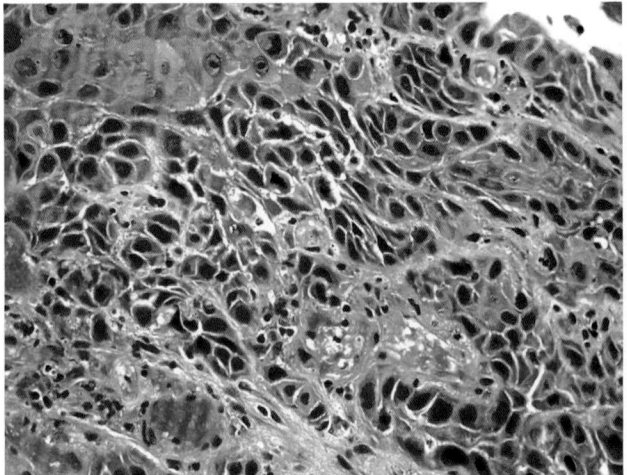

Figure 1-145. Taxane effect. This field is from the same biopsy as the images seen in Figs. 1.143 and 1.144. The mitotic arrest (ring mitoses) is apparent.

Figure 1-146. Esophageal squamous cell carcinoma. Squamous cell carcinoma of the esophagus has the same appearance as it does elsewhere in the body with abnormally keratinized overtly malignant cells.

However, in the spirit of trickery and to introduce the near misses section of this chapter, note that Figs. 1.143–1.145 show a lesion in which a medication effect (taxane effect[75]) mimics dysplasia in a patient with esophageal epidermoid metaplasia! The clue is the ring mitoses.

Squamous Cell Carcinoma

Esophageal squamous cell carcinomas display essentially the same appearance as squamous cell carcinoma in the rest of the body and are usually not a diagnostic problem (Figs. 1.146–1.149). Most are well differentiated with prominent keratinization, but they can be basaloid, spindled, papillary, or verrucous; the latter can be impossible to diagnose on superficial samples but is instead diagnosed in the context of the endoscopic finding—a mass is seen and the pathologist is faced with a bland-appearing thickened mucosa.

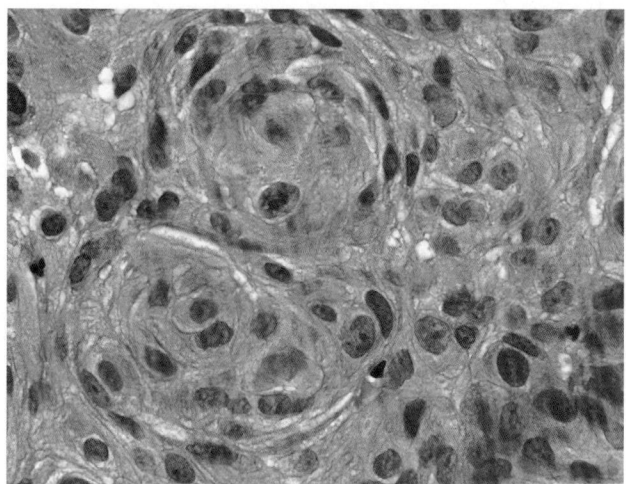

Figure 1-147.   Esophageal squamous cell carcinoma. This example shows whorls of malignant squamous cells.

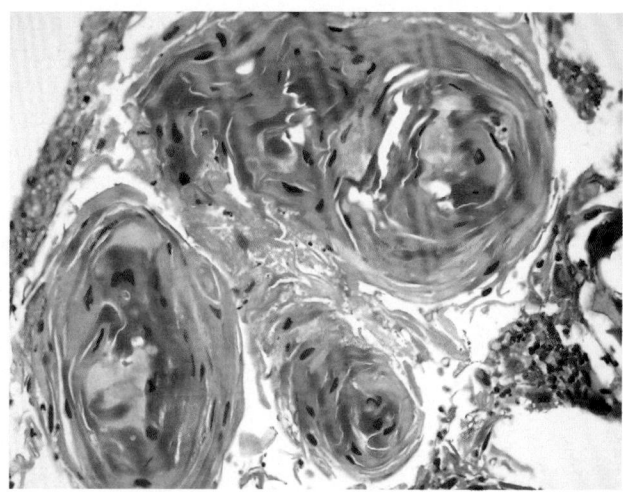

Figure 1-148.   Esophageal squamous cell carcinoma. This biopsy is scant but shows abnormal keratinization in cells arranged in squamous pearls with cytologically malignant nuclei.

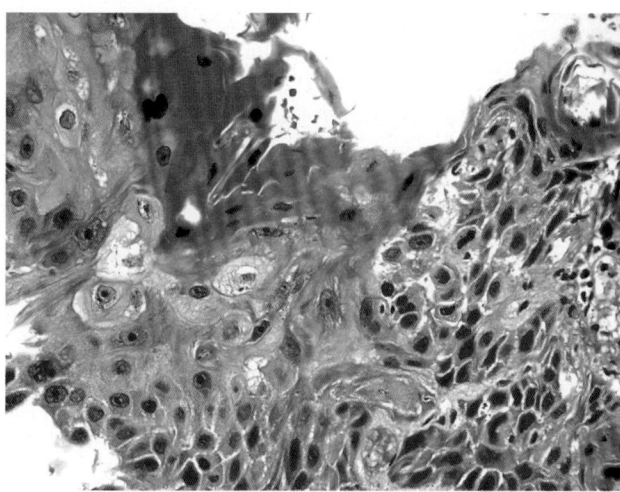

Figure 1-149.   Esophageal squamous cell carcinoma. Even though this sample is superficial, it was from a mass lesion; in this context it can be diagnosed as squamous cell carcinoma.

Squamous carcinomas can assume a prominent spindle cell appearance as well—please remember that a spindle cell malignant neoplasm of the esophagus is almost never a sarcoma.

Like squamous carcinomas elsewhere, esophageal examples express p63, p40, CK5/6, and a host of epithelial markers. Most examples do not pose diagnostic problems, and it is not difficult to obtain repeat samples if an initial biopsy is not fully diagnostic. This is usually a result of superficial sampling. However, when these carcinomas are spindled, melanoma and sarcomas must be excluded. In resection specimens, it is easy to do this by sampling as much of the overlying squamous mucosa as possible to detect an in situ component or a zone of conventional-appearing squamous cell carcinoma. Otherwise, S100 protein (which should be negative) and various keratins are most useful. Do not even think of wasting tissue on a vimentin! **Repeat, never waste tissue on vimentin staining in mucosal biopsies of the gastrointestinal tract.** Rare examples of esophageal squamous carcinoma are associated with Epstein-Barr virus, but such cases are more commonly encountered in the stomach.

Lastly, before moving on to case studies that we regard as "near misses," we would like to point out a pattern that can be seen that superficially mimics low-grade dysplasia that is instead a marker of an unsampled squamous cell carcinoma. Figs. 1.150 and 1.151 are from a case of squamous cell carcinoma of the esophagus. Note that, in one of the fragments, the lower half of the epithelium is replaced by strikingly atypical squamous cells. Were only this fragment sampled, it could be interpreted as low-grade dysplasia because the epithelial changes encompass less than half the thickness of the epithelium. However, the cytologic features are in excess of those expected for low-grade squamous dysplasia. This pattern reflects intraepithelial invasion of the nearby squamous cell carcinoma. It can be termed a lateral spread pattern, but it is important to call attention to it to assure that the endoscopist brings the patient back for additional sampling to search for a subtle unsampled invasive carcinoma.

Table 1.3 outlines some of the demographic and other differences between esophageal adenocarcinoma and squamous cell carcinoma.

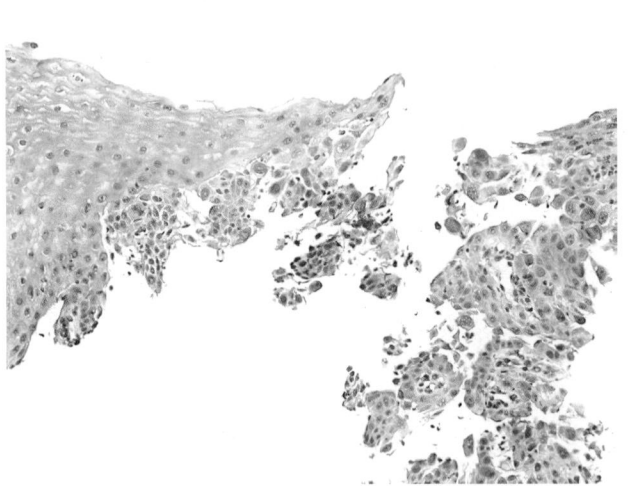

Figure 1-150. Esophageal squamous cell carcinoma. This is a portion of a biopsy of a squamous cell carcinoma that illustrates an important phenomenon. Notice that the carcinoma (not well demonstrated in this field) has spread into the space between the basement membrane and the normal squamous epithelium in the fragment seen at the left and in the center. This results in severely atypical cell being seen in the lower half of the epithelium, a feature of low-grade dysplasia. However, the cytologic changes are far in excess of the subtle ones that form low-grade squamous dysplasia. This pattern has been called a lateral spread pattern.

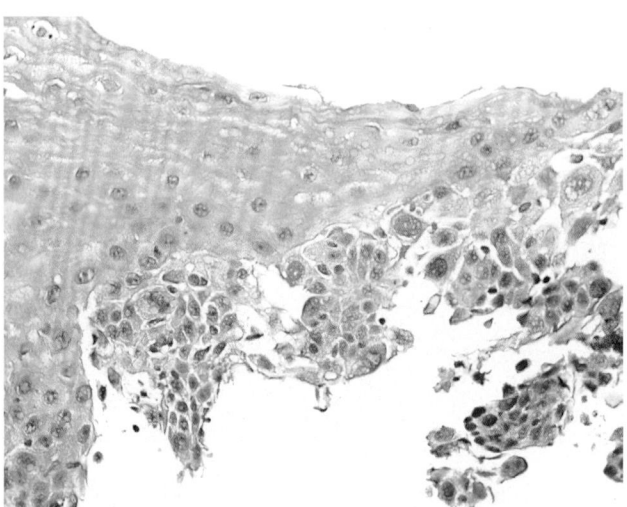

Figure 1-151. Lateral spread pattern. This is a high-magnification image of the fragment seen at the center and at the left in Fig. 1.150. Strikingly atypical cells are seen in the lower half of the epithelium. This finding suggests intraepithelial invasion of an adjoining carcinoma. If only this pattern is seen on a biopsy, the endoscopist should be encouraged to perform extensive resampling with the goal of detecting an occult invasive carcinoma.

TABLE 1.3: Esophageal Adenocarcinoma Versus Squamous Cell Carcinoma (US Population)

Feature	Adenocarcinoma	Squamous Cell Carcinoma
Typical demographics	Older white men	Older black men
Risk factors	Reflux, obesity, smoking	Smoking, alcohol
Precursors	Barrett esophagus; Barrett esophagus with dysplasia	Epidermoid metaplasia (probable), squamous dysplasia

NEAR MISSES

Case 1

Figs. 1.152 and 1.153 were taken from the esophagus and diagnosed as adenocarcinoma arising in association with Barrett mucosa with high-grade dysplasia. As a result, the patient was referred for endoscopic treatment and the biopsies were rereviewed in preparation for this.

WHAT WENT WRONG?

The nuclei are far too hyperchromatic for the usual adenocarcinoma and are arranged in sheets rather than remotely forming glands and have no component of mucin. Some adenocarcinomas and squamous carcinomas are poorly differentiated, but this case is unusual. In Fig. 1.153, where the tumor undermines the squamous epithelium, it shows nuclear molding. Because the carcinoma arises in association with high-grade columnar epithelium (Fig. 1.152), the colleague assumed that it was an adenocarcinoma. It is instead a high-grade neuroendocrine carcinoma, small cell type. Figs. 1.154 and 1.155 show a synaptophysin stain, and Fig. 1.155 highlights the characteristic dotlike staining seen with synaptophysin in small cell carcinomas from all sites. In addition, the extremely high proliferation index using Ki-67 immunolabeling seen in Fig. 1.156 is characteristic of small cell carcinoma. Esophageal high-grade neuroendocrine carcinomas are not common but tend to arise in association with columnar epithelial dysplasia in the US population and in association with high-grade squamous dysplasia in populations in which esophageal squamous lesions are common. This is similar in some ways to high-grade neuroendocrine carcinomas encountered in the colon, which are often associated with an adenomatous (columnar) precursor. In fact, sometimes neuroendocrine differentiation can be seen in Barrett esophagus with high-grade dysplasia (Figs. 1.157 and 1.158)—we would assume that these cells are the precursors to high-grade neuroendocrine carcinomas of the esophagus. An example of an esophageal high-grade neuroendocrine carcinoma of the large cell type is seen in Fig. 1.159.

Neuroendocrine Tumors of the Esophagus

Esophageal neuroendocrine tumors (NETs) are currently classified as differentiated NETs, grade 1 and 2 (carcinoid tumor, atypical carcinoid tumor), and neuroendocrine carcinomas (large and small cell types), grade 3.[76] They are rare (on the order of 100 cases have been reported, and most are high-grade carcinomas/small cell carcinomas). In a large series of carcinoid tumors, <0.1% involved the esophagus.[77] They are only rarely encountered on

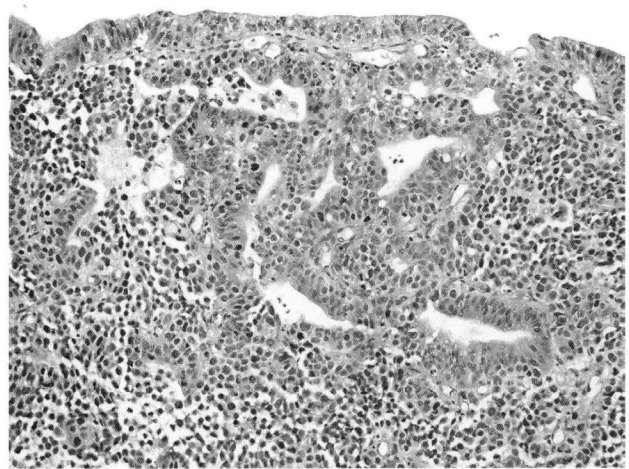

Figure 1-152. High-grade neuroendocrine carcinoma associated with high-grade columnar epithelial dysplasia. A malignant lesion composed of extremely hyperchromatic cells has filled the lamina propria between glands that show high-grade dysplasia features.

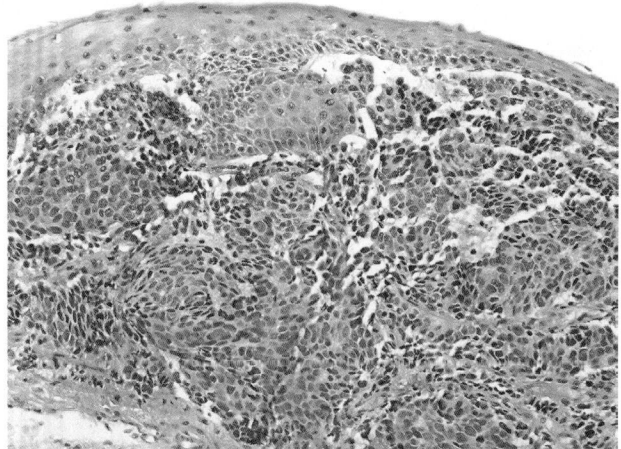

Figure 1-153. High-grade neuroendocrine carcinoma, small cell type. The carcinoma fills the lamina propria beneath the squamous epithelium. The malignant cells show prominent nuclear molding. This is another field from the same lesion as that depicted in Fig. 1.152.

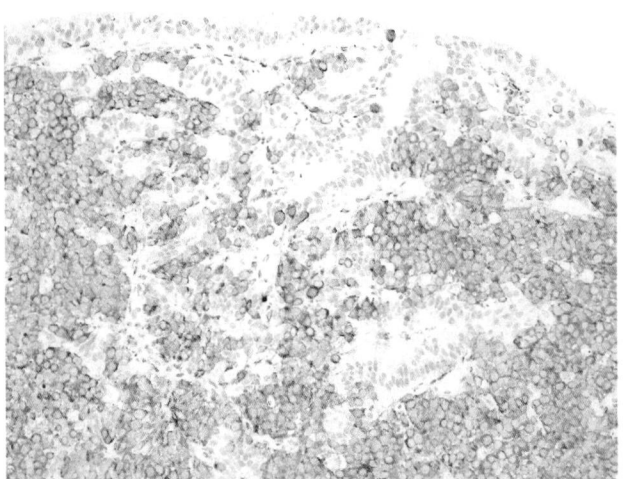

Figure 1-154. High-grade neuroendocrine carcinoma, small cell type. This is a synaptophysin stain, which labels the carcinoma but not many cells in the high-grade columnar epithelial precursor.

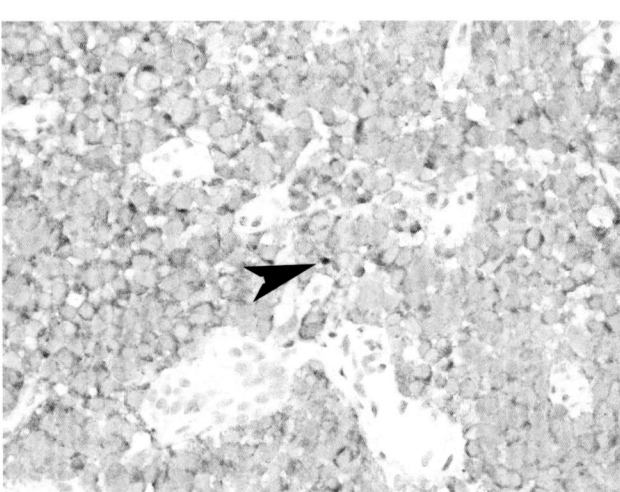

Figure 1-155. High-grade neuroendocrine carcinoma, small cell type. This is a high-magnification image of the lesion seen in Figs. 1.152–1.154. The *arrowhead* indicates dotlike reactivity with the synaptophysin stain, a characteristic feature of small cell carcinoma.

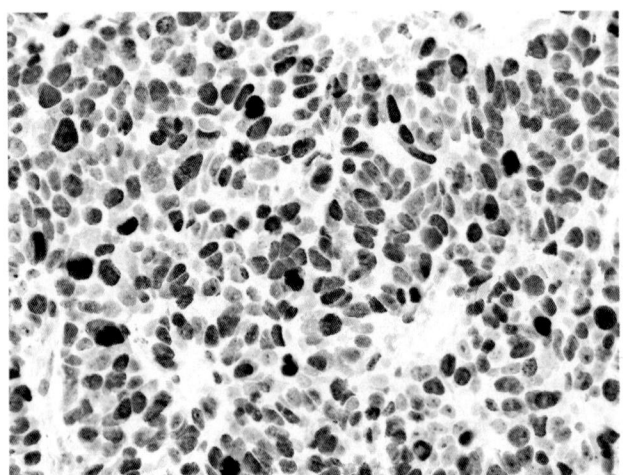

Figure 1-156. High-grade neuroendocrine carcinoma, small cell type. This is a Ki-67 stain of the lesion seen in Figs. 1.152–1.155.

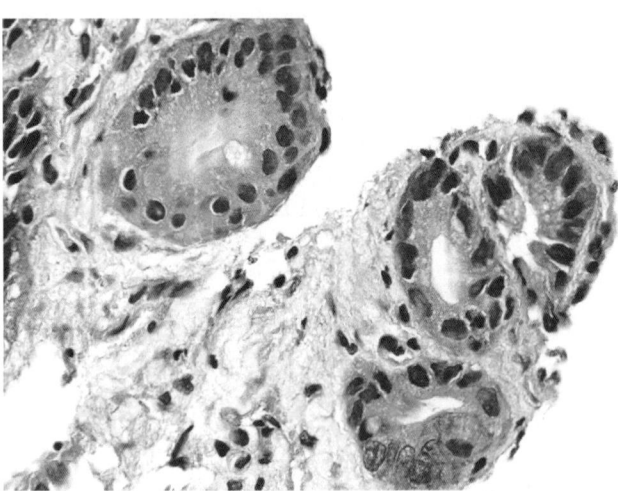

Figure 1-157. High-grade columnar epithelial dysplasia. Note the prominent neuroendocrine cells (Kulchitsky cells) in this example! They are characterized by red granules that point away from the gland lumina.

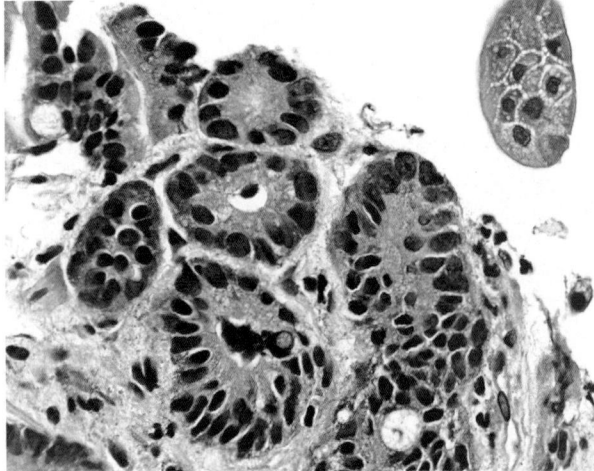

Figure 1-158. High-grade columnar epithelial dysplasia. This example shows cells with neuroendocrine features. It is a different lesion from the one seen in Fig. 1.157.

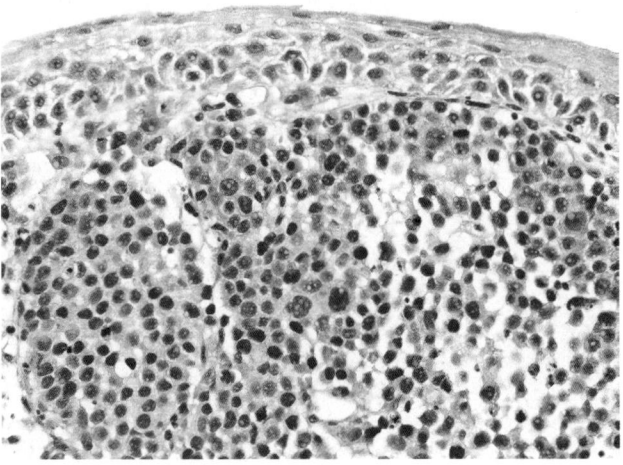

Figure 1-159. High-grade neuroendocrine carcinoma, large cell type. The cells are nested and some are large with large nucleoli.

biopsies. Well-differentiated NETs (carcinoids) of the esophagus resemble those seen in other sites, although in the esophagus most are polypoid and thus appear in the lamina propria on biopsies. They consist of uniform bland tumor cells with an insular pattern and solid to cribriform growth (Figs. 1.160–1.164). On immunolabeling, they express keratin, synaptophysin, and chromogranin. Interestingly, they can be associated with heterotopic oxyntic mucosa.

Like well-differentiated NETs elsewhere, they can be graded by assessing the mitotic activity (to the extent possible in small biopsies, which means that they cannot really be graded) or by performing Ki-67 immunolabeling.[76] As of the 2010 WHO classification of gastrointestinal tumors, well-differentiated NETs were graded as G1 or G2 and the rare lesions with well-differentiated morphology but a high Ki-67 labeling index were included with high-grade neuroendocrine carcinoma, but this has sometimes proved unsatisfactory (because there is different treatment of small cell carcinoma and large cell neuroendocrine carcinoma). As such, the 2017 WHO Classification of Tumours of Endocrine Organs, at least with good data for pancreatic lesions, has added a new category, termed NET G3.[78] This latter category encompasses neoplasms that have an appearance like that of a

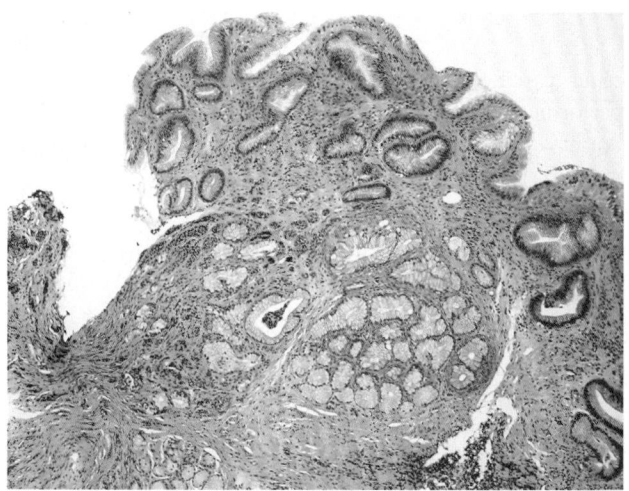

Figure 1-160. Well-differentiated neuroendocrine (carcinoid) tumor of the esophagus. These are rare (rarer than high-grade neuroendocrine carcinomas) in the esophagus. This lesion was found in the tubular esophagus in an area with cardiac-type mucosa.

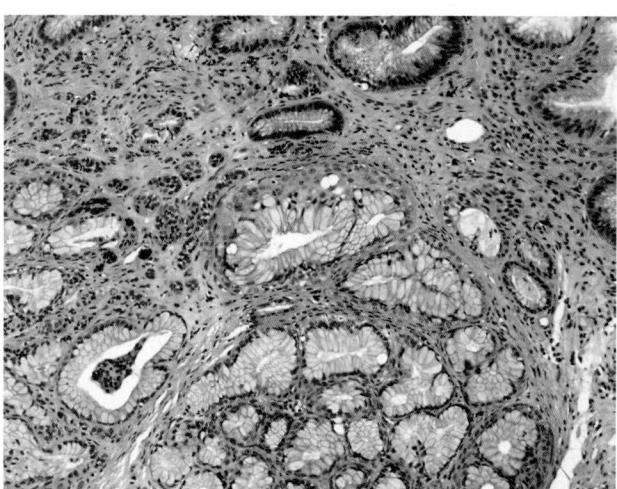

Figure 1-161. Well-differentiated neuroendocrine (carcinoid) tumor of the esophagus. The lesion is to the left. A bit of multilayered epithelium is also present, confirming that the process indeed involved the esophagus rather than the stomach!

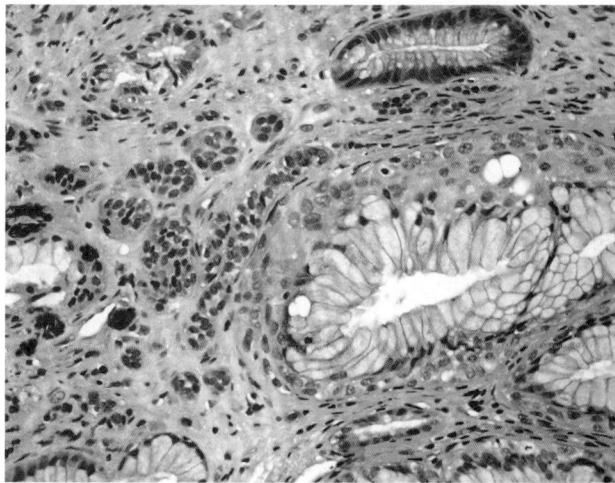

Figure 1-162. Well-differentiated neuroendocrine (carcinoid) tumor of the esophagus. The lesion is bland appearing at high magnification.

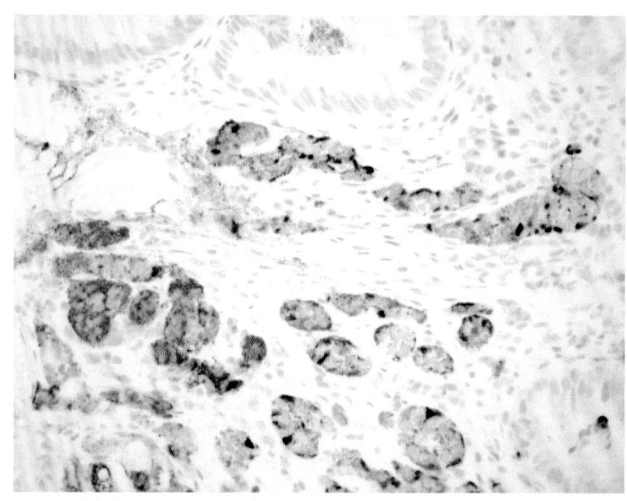

Figure 1-163. Well-differentiated neuroendocrine (carcinoid) tumor of the esophagus. This is a chromogranin stain.

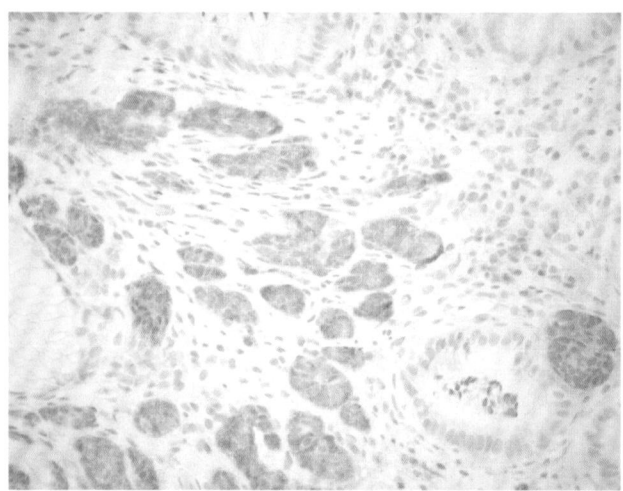

Figure 1-164. Well-differentiated neuroendocrine (carcinoid) tumor of the esophagus. This is a synaptophysin stain.

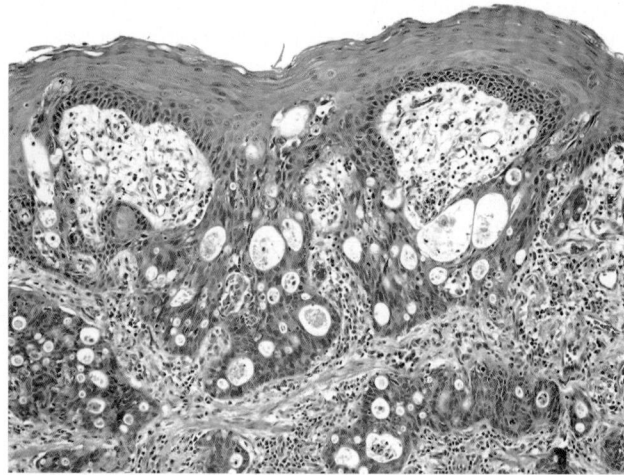

Figure 1-165. Adenosquamous carcinoma of the esophagus. The lesion seems to spill from the base on nondysplastic squamous epithelium.

well-differentiated neuroendocrine (carcinoid) tumor but that have a high proliferation index when Ki-67 labeling is performed. Because this latter category is rare and NET of the esophagus is rare as well, we have not encountered such a lesion. To summarize for neuroendocrine **tumor**[76,78]:

NET G1—<2 mitoses per 10 high-power fields or Ki-67 labeling <3%
NET G2—2 to 20 mitoses per 10 high-power fields or Ki-67 labeling 3% to 20%
NET G3—>20 mitoses per 10 high-power fields or Ki-67 labeling >20.

On the other hand, classic neuroendocrine **carcinoma**s (always grade 3) are high-grade lesions and can be classified as "small cell" or "large cell" types.[76,78] Both types are aggressive lesions. Most arise in men (although they are rare), sometimes in association with Barrett mucosa. These are rare tumors that have not been well studied, but in one Chinese series of patients with resectable disease, the mean age was about 60 years and most patients (about 70%) were men. About 60% were of the small cell rather than of the large cell type. Although nearly 70% were alive after a year, only a third were alive at 3 years, even though the patients had resectable disease.[79] Patients with these carcinomas are often treated with platinum-based chemotherapy. Large cell neuroendocrine carcinomas manifest an organoid pattern with solid nests or acinar structures, whereas small cell carcinomas form solid sheets and nests and are composed of cells with small dark nuclei and minimal cytoplasm or larger cells with more cytoplasm. Adjoining zones of adenocarcinoma or squamous cell carcinoma may be present (the latter may require p63/p40 or CK5/6 staining to detect). They express keratins, synaptophysin, and chromogranin. Some observers also use CD56 immunolabeling, which is hampered by its lack of specificity. Both small cell and large cell neuroendocrine carcinomas are G3 neoplasms:

G3 neuroendocrine carcinoma—mitotic count >20 per 10 high-power field or >20% Ki-67 index.

Case 2

Figs. 1.165 and 1.166 are from an esophageal biopsy. A mass was seen at endoscopy in the middle third of the esophagus. The sample was interpreted as squamous cell carcinoma. Indeed, the lesion does appear to "drip," but there is something amiss for squamous cell carcinoma. Fig. 1.166 gives the clue in that there is mucin in some of the cells. This is an adenosquamous carcinoma. However, it is not horrible to miss this feature—both types (adenocarcinoma and squamous cell carcinoma) are treated the same way, although HER2 testing might be added for adenosquamous carcinoma. This is different from the situation in the prior case—detecting a high-grade neuroendocrine carcinoma results in a different chemotherapy regimen than that for adenocarcinoma.

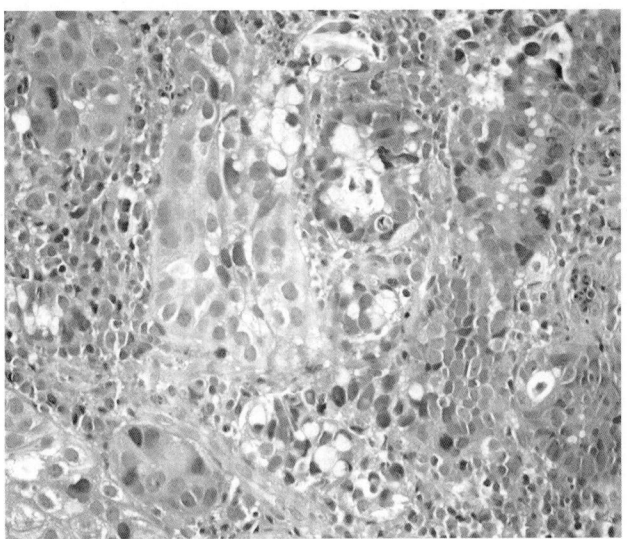

Figure 1-166. Adenosquamous carcinoma of the esophagus. Note the mixture of squamous cells and cells that contain mucin.

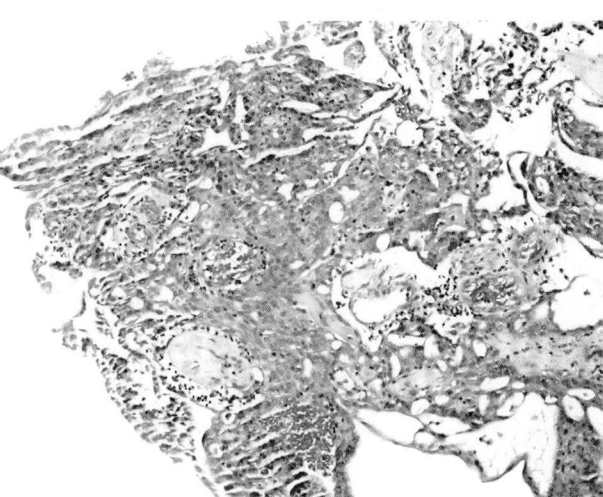

Figure 1-167. Thyroid papillary carcinoma extending directly into the esophagus. The carcinoma has an odd appearance for an esophageal adenocarcinoma.

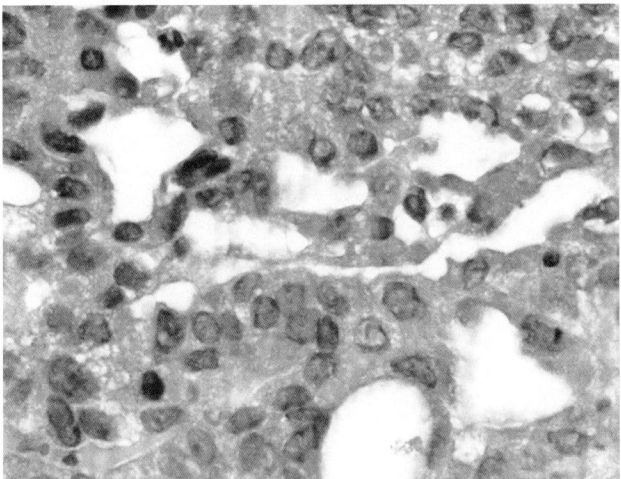

Figure 1-168. Thyroid papillary carcinoma extending directly into the esophagus. A few grooves and intranuclear inclusions are present, but they are easier to see if you know that the patient has a history of a large thyroid carcinoma!

Adenosquamous Carcinoma

Adenosquamous carcinoma arises only rarely in the esophagus. It consists of a mixture of infiltrating squamous cell carcinoma and adenocarcinoma elements. Like squamous cell carcinoma, this variant preferentially affects the middle third of the esophagus. Adenosquamous carcinoma also seems to present at an earlier stage than pure adenocarcinoma or squamous cell carcinoma.[80] The squamous component tends to be more conspicuous than the glandular areas with gradual transitions between the two. Areas of accompanying Barrett mucosa may rarely be identified. The outcome is more favorable than that associated with pure squamous or adenocarcinoma, presumably a result of the smaller size and lower stage at presentation.[80]

Case 3

Figs. 1.167 and 1.168 are images taken from an esophageal biopsy in a 58-year-old woman who complained of dysphagia. The sample was diagnosed as well-differentiated adenocarcinoma, and the patient was referred to one of our institutions for treatment. On review, it was noted that the nuclei appeared rather small compared with those that usually form esophageal adenocarcinomas and also that nucleoli were not a feature. This prompted extensive queries into the clinical history, and we learned that the patient had a history of papillary thyroid carcinoma. Based on this history, we added a thyroglobulin stain, which is seen in Fig. 1.169. In this case, the presence of unusual features in the lesion prompted some digging in the patient's records. Once we considered thyroid carcinoma, the nuclear inclusions and grooves became apparent to us, even though the sample was suboptimal.

Spread of Extraesophageal Carcinoma to the Esophagus

The extraesophageal neoplasms that spread to the esophagus are primarily lung carcinoma (Figs. 1.170 and 1.171) and breast carcinoma, but thyroid carcinoma is known, and rarely, cervix carcinoma can spread to the lung (this requires HPV studies to differentiate from primary esophageal squamous carcinoma), as well as ovary, prostate, and renal carcinoma. Recognition can be impossible without knowledge of pertinent history, but a clue to at least consider an extraesophageal primary is the absence of a precursor component. Immunolabeling can be useful but has limitations. For example, both esophageal and lung adenocarcinoma can express TTF1 and napsin if a polyclonal antibody is used.[81] However, esophageal adenocarcinomas generally lack expression of hormone receptors (estrogen and progesterone receptors) and GATA3, whereas expression of these can suggest metastatic breast carcinoma.

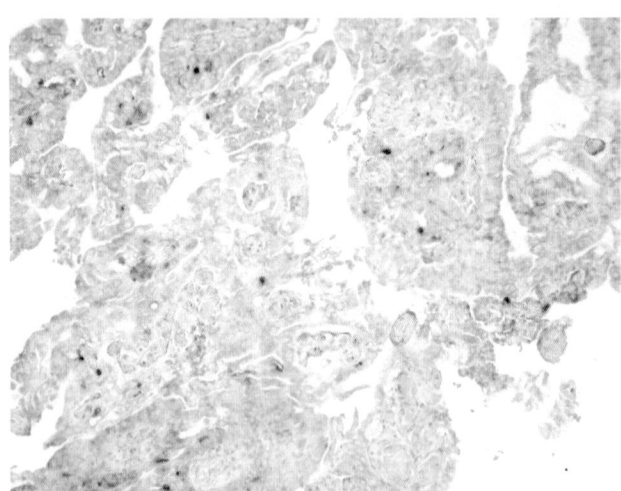

Figure 1-169. Thyroid papillary carcinoma extending directly into the esophagus. The lesion shows expression of thyroglobulin.

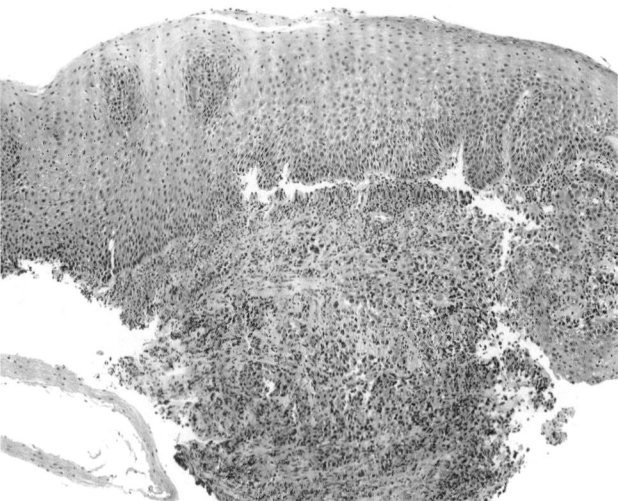

Figure 1-170. Lung carcinoma extending into the lamina propria of the esophagus. This is diagnosed in the context of the history!

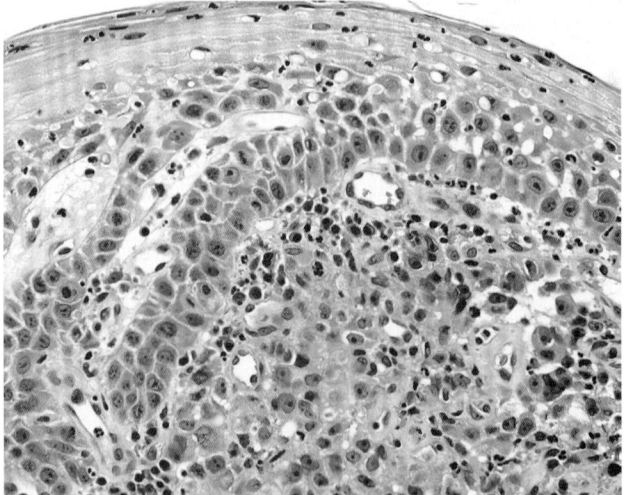

Figure 1-171. Lung carcinoma extending into the lamina propria of the esophagus. Note the reactive changes in the overlying inflamed squamous epithelium.

Case 4

Fig. 1.172 shows a spindle cell lesion that was biopsied from the esophagus. On immunolabeling, it was KIT reactive but CD34 nonreactive. A diagnosis of esophageal GIST was made. The mitotic count was high in keeping with a high-risk lesion, and a resection was performed.

What Went Wrong?

This is a melanoma! Remember that many melanomas show KIT expression and about 20% of mucosal melanomas in fact have *KIT* mutations, the presence of which can be exploited using targeted therapy.[82-85] This is an important pitfall, especially in spindle cell melanomas. Melanoma can masquerade in many forms. It is usually CD34 negative as well. In this particular case, simply looking carefully at the slides gave the correct diagnosis because there was an obvious in situ pigmented component that had been overlooked (Fig. 1.173).

Melanoma

Primary esophageal melanoma is rare, with only about 300 cases reported. It is encountered in adults with a mean age of about 60 years.[86-91] There is a male predominance but no racial predominance. Most esophageal melanomas arise in the distal esophagus. At endoscopy, most are polypoid and pigmented (about 85%). Imaging studies show bulky polypoid masses that bulge intraluminally without associated obstruction. Many examples are pigmented, an obvious diagnostic clue. The rest are whitish and poorly marginated. Primary melanomas may display an in situ component. When present, this finding is extremely useful in establishing the esophagus as the primary site. The malignant cells are spindled to epithelioid with variable pigment and prominent nucleoli, and sometimes prominent intranuclear pseudoinclusions can be found.

The key differential diagnosis is with poorly differentiated carcinoma, which is far more common, and also with high-grade lymphomas. Immunohistochemistry can be critical in establishing the diagnosis of esophageal melanoma, as it is with melanomas elsewhere. Useful antibodies include S100 protein, Sox 10, MART, HMB45, and Melan A. Remember that melanomas are also reactive with CD117/KIT antibodies about 40% of the time, so a panel approach is best; overall, melanomas are usually more pleomorphic than GISTs. The host of masqueraders is usually unmasked using a panel including lymphoid markers (among which is CD30 for anaplastic lymphoma) and pankeratins. Sarcomas are rarely in the differential diagnosis, but, of course, spindled melanomas may lack other melanoma markers aside from S100 protein and Sox 10. Another spindle cell tumor that is strongly S100 protein reactive is cellular (benign) schwannoma. The distinction is on cytologic grounds, with attention to nuclear pleomorphism and large nucleoli, features of melanoma but not of cellular schwannoma. These unusual primary esophageal melanomas have had

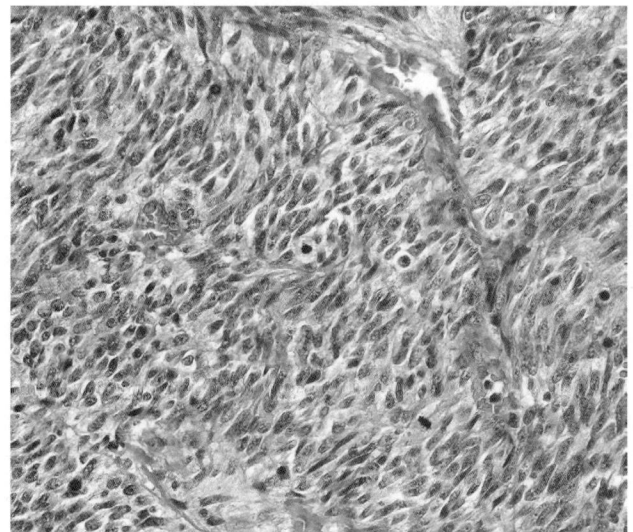

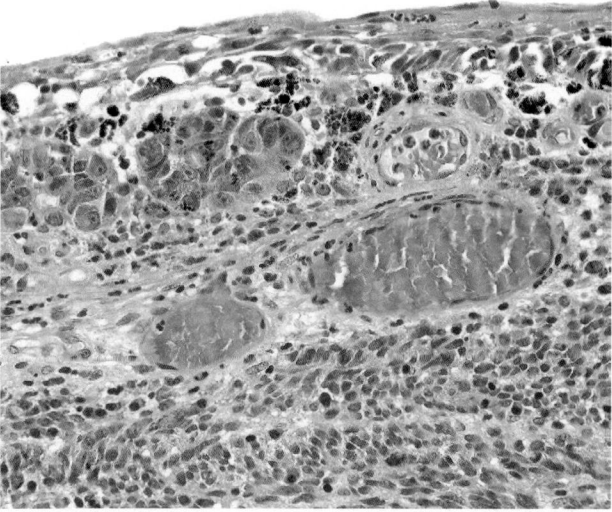

Figure 1-172. Esophageal melanoma with spindle cell features. This lesion displays the monotonous cytologic features that are often seen in gastrointestinal stromal tumors.

Figure 1-173. Melanoma extending into the lamina propria of the esophagus. In this case, a pigmented in situ component gives away the diagnosis.

a dismal prognosis. Based on the literature, only rare patients, whose tumors present early, can be cured. However, newer treatments exploiting PDL1/PD1 blockade may improve the situation, but there are no outcome data available at this point for esophageal melanoma specifically. In one case report a good tumor response was achieved with nivolumab.[92]

Case 5

Fig. 1.174 shows a biopsy from a mass lesion of the distal esophagus. It was submitted on a rush protocol on a Friday night by a surgeon eager to plan an operation for Monday morning and was reported as poorly differentiated carcinoma. The surgeon scheduled the patient for 7 AM the following Monday. The resection resulted in a sinking feeling.

What Went Wrong?

This is a diffuse large B cell lymphoma, which of course is not treated surgically.

On small biopsies of overtly malignant neoplasms for which limited tissue in present in the sample, it can be prudent to begin with a limited immunolabeling panel and an order of unstained sections up front. A panel that can work well consists of S100 protein (to address melanoma), a pankeratin (to address carcinoma), and a CD20 (to address diffuse large B cell lymphoma, the most likely type of lymphoma encountered). If all three of these stains are negative on the first round of immunolabeling, the morphology can be revisited and a second attempt made, which might be directed at GIST (KIT and DOG1). This sequential approach can allow a diagnosis before the tissue is exhausted.

Esophageal Hematopoietic Disorders

Primary esophageal hematopoietic lesions are truly rare, but the majority are extranodal lymphomas. Esophageal lymphoma is defined as an extranodal lymphoma arising in the esophagus itself rather than extending into the esophagus from the mediastinum, stomach, or a contiguous lymph node. The lesion shown in Fig. 1.174 might be regarded as a gastric lymphoma because it is associated with cardiac-type mucosa. However, when lymphomas are found in the esophagus, most are large B cell lymphomas or mucosa-associated lymphoid tissue lymphomas. Any type of lymphoma can be detected in the esophagus, and a discussion of every type is beyond the scope of this section.[93]

Case 6

Fig. 1.175 is from a biopsy taken from a 75-year-old man with dysphagia, and a subtle early lesion was seen by the endoscopist. A diagnosis of intramucosal adenocarcinoma was made. The next day, the endoscopist called and said that she was confused because the patient's symptoms were out of proportion to the histologic diagnosis and to the results of endoscopic ultrasound performed at the time of the endoscopic evaluation.

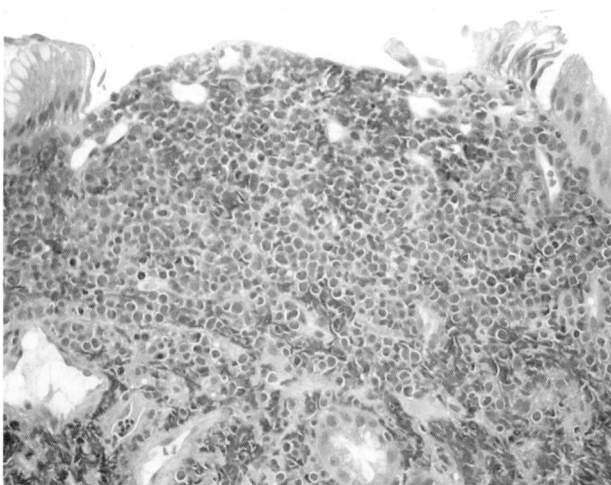

Figure 1-174. Diffuse large B cell lymphoma involving the esophagus. It is easy to consider a poorly differentiated carcinoma in this location.

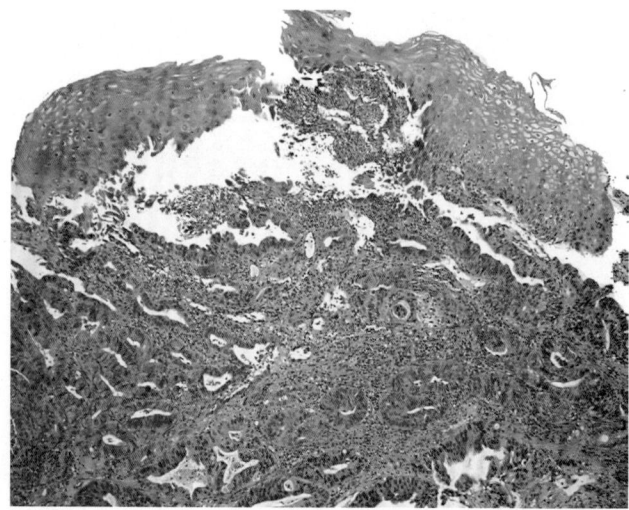

Figure 1-175. Esophageal intramucosal carcinoma with extensive associated inflammation. Be sure to check the areas of exudate!

What Went Wrong?

On rereview, herpes simplex viral cytopathic effect was noted in an eroded area that had been overlooked! The classic viral cytopathic effect is seen in Fig. 1.176 and, just for fun, immunolabeling for herpes simplex virus was performed and is shown in Figs. 1.177 and 1.178.

The message in this case is that we must always remember to look for additional diagnoses once we have made our key diagnosis. It is easy forget to check erosions and ulcers for infectious agents when we diagnose neoplasms, but sometimes treating the infection can make the patient more comfortable while the main issue is dealt with.

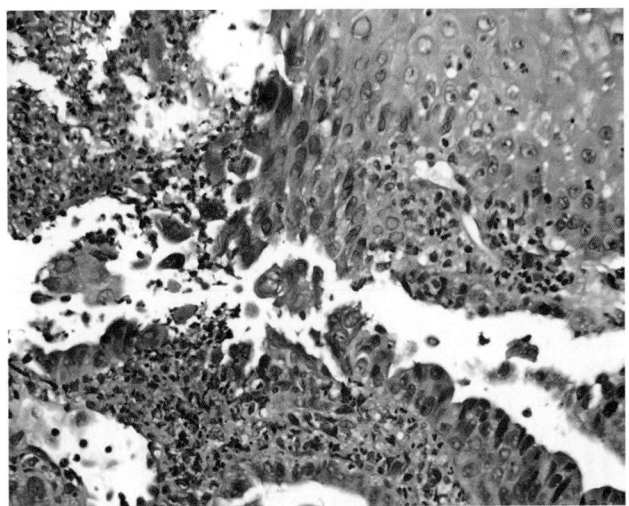

Figure 1-176. Esophageal intramucosal carcinoma with extensive associated inflammation. A careful search in the inflamed zones yielded foci of herpes simplex virus cytopathic effect.

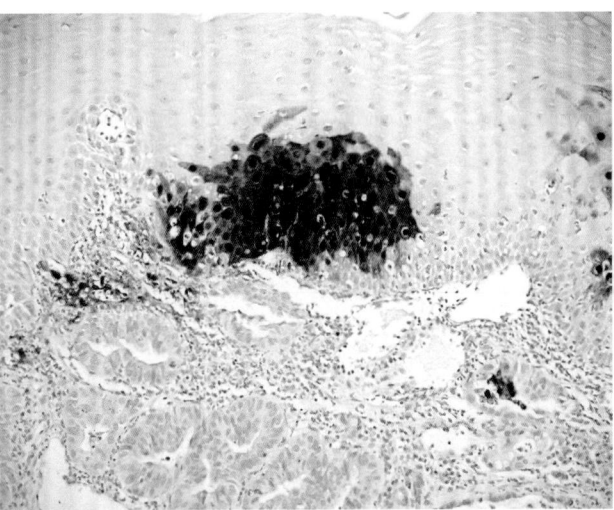

Figure 1-177. Esophageal intramucosal carcinoma with extensive associated inflammation and herpes simplex virus infection. This is a herpes simplex virus immunostain.

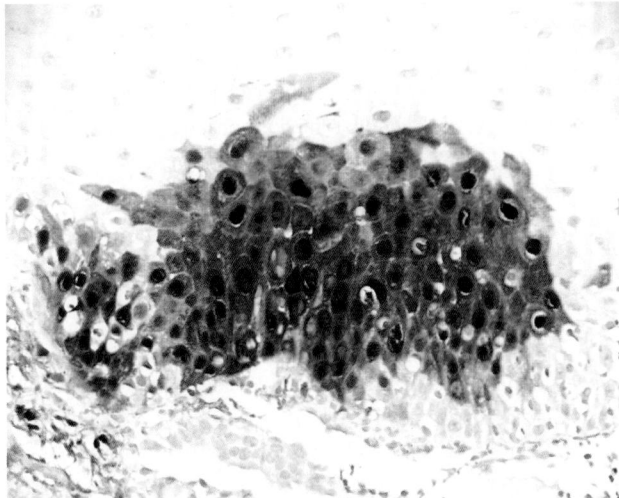

Figure 1-178. Esophageal intramucosal carcinoma with extensive associated inflammation and herpes simplex virus infection. This is a high-magnification image of the preparation shown in Fig. 1.177.

References

1. Amin M, Edge S, Greene F, et al. *AJCC Cancer Staging Manual.* 8th ed. Springer International Publishing AG Switzerland; 2017.

2. Abraham SC, Krasinskas AM, Correa AM, et al. Duplication of the muscularis mucosae in Barrett esophagus: an underrecognized feature and its implication for staging of adenocarcinoma. *Am J Surg Pathol.* 2007;31(11):1719-1725.

3. Glickman JN, Chen YY, Wang HH, Antonioli DA, Odze RD. Phenotypic characteristics of a distinctive multilayered epithelium suggests that it is a precursor in the development of Barrett's esophagus. *Am J Surg Pathol.* 2001;25(5):569-578.

4. Glickman JN, Spechler SJ, Souza RF, Lunsford T, Lee E, Odze RD. Multilayered epithelium in mucosal biopsy specimens from the gastroesophageal junction region is a histologic marker of gastroesophageal reflux disease. *Am J Surg Pathol.* 2009;33(6):818-825.

5. Lack EE, Worsham GF, Callihan MD, et al. Granular cell tumor: a clinicopathologic study of 110 patients. *J Surg Oncol.* 1980;13(4):301-316.

6. Johnston J, Helwig EB. Granular cell tumors of the gastrointestinal tract and perianal region: a study of 74 cases. *Dig Dis Sci.* 1981;26(9):807-816.

7. Ohmori T, Arita N, Uraga N, Tabei R, Tani M, Okamura H. Malignant granular cell tumor of the esophagus. A case report with light and electron microscopic, histochemical, and immunohistochemical study. *Acta Pathol Jpn.* 1987;37(5):775-783.

8. Yoshizawa A, Ota H, Sakaguchi N, et al. Malignant granular cell tumor of the esophagus. *Virchows Arch.* 2004;444(3):304-306.

9. Miettinen M, Sarlomo-Rikala M, Sobin LH, Lasota J. Esophageal stromal tumors: a clinicopathologic, immunohistochemical, and molecular genetic study of 17 cases and comparison with esophageal leiomyomas and leiomyosarcomas. *Am J Surg Pathol.* 2000;24(2):211-222.

10. Fitzgerald RC, di Pietro M, Ragunath K, et al. British Society of Gastroenterology guidelines on the diagnosis and management of Barrett's oesophagus. *Gut.* 2014;63(1):7-42.

11. American Gastroenterological Association, Spechler SJ, Sharma P, Souza RF, Inadomi JM, Shaheen NJ. American Gastroenterological Association medical position statement on the management of Barrett's esophagus. *Gastroenterology.* 2011;140(3):1084-1091.

12. Shaheen NJ, Falk GW, Iyer PG, Gerson LB; American College of Gastroenterology. ACG clinical guideline: diagnosis and management of Barrett's esophagus. *Am J Gastroenterol.* 2016;111(1):30-50; quiz 51.

13. Epstein JA, Cosby H, Falk GW, et al. Columnar islands in Barrett's esophagus: do they impact Prague C&M criteria and dysplasia grade? *J Gastroenterol Hepatol.* 2017;32(9):1598-1603.

14. Aida J, Vieth M, Shepherd NA, et al. Is carcinoma in columnar-lined esophagus always located adjacent to intestinal metaplasia?: a histopathologic assessment. *Am J Surg Pathol.* 2015;39(2):188-196.

15. Chandrasoma P, Wijetunge S, DeMeester S, et al. Columnar-lined esophagus without intestinal metaplasia has no proven risk of adenocarcinoma. *Am J Surg Pathol.* 2012;36(1):1-7.

16. Smith J, Garcia A, Zhang R, DeMeester S, Vallone J, Chandrasoma P. Intestinal metaplasia is present in most if not all patients who have undergone endoscopic mucosal resection for esophageal adenocarcinoma. *Am J Surg Pathol.* 2016;40(4):537-543.

17. Salimian KJ, Waters KM, Eze O, et al. Definition of Barrett esophagus in the United States: support for retention of a requirement for goblet cells. *Am J Surg Pathol.* 2018;42(2):264-268.

18. Bennett C, Moayyedi P, Corley DA, et al. BOB CAT: a large-scale review and Delphi consensus for management of Barrett's esophagus with no dysplasia, indefinite for, or low-grade dysplasia. *Am J Gastroenterol.* 2015;110(5):662-682; quiz 683.

19. Shields HM, Rosenberg SJ, Zwas FR, Ransil BJ, Lembo AJ, Odze R. Prospective evaluation of multilayered epithelium in Barrett's esophagus. *Am J Gastroenterol.* 2001;96(12):3268-3273.

20. Takubo K, Honma N, Arai T. Multilayered epithelium in Barrett's esophagus. *Am J Surg Pathol.* 2001;25(11):1460-1461.

21. Jiang M, Li H, Zhang Y, et al. Transitional basal cells at the squamous-columnar junction generate Barrett's oesophagus. *Nature.* 2017;550(7677):529-533.

22. Sharma P, Dent J, Armstrong D, et al. The development and validation of an endoscopic grading system for Barrett's esophagus: the Prague C & M criteria. *Gastroenterology.* 2006;131(5):1392-1399.

23. Panarelli NC, Yantiss RK. Do ancillary studies aid detection and classification of Barrett esophagus? *Am J Surg Pathol.* 2016;40(8):e83-e93.

24. Ormsby AH, Goldblum JR, Rice TW, et al. Cytokeratin subsets can reliably distinguish Barrett's esophagus from intestinal metaplasia of the stomach. *Hum Pathol*. 1999;30(3):288-294.

25. Ormsby AH, Vaezi MF, Richter JE, et al. Cytokeratin immunoreactivity patterns in the diagnosis of short-segment Barrett's esophagus. *Gastroenterology*. 2000;119(3):683-690.

26. Phillips RW, Frierson HF Jr, Moskaluk CA. Cdx2 as a marker of epithelial intestinal differentiation in the esophagus. *Am J Surg Pathol*. 2003;27(11):1442-1447.

27. Hahn HP, Blount PL, Ayub K, et al. Intestinal differentiation in metaplastic, nongoblet columnar epithelium in the esophagus. *Am J Surg Pathol*. 2009;33(7):1006-1015.

28. Chu PG, Jiang Z, Weiss LM. Hepatocyte antigen as a marker of intestinal metaplasia. *Am J Surg Pathol*. 2003;27(7):952-959.

29. Montgomery E, Bronner MP, Goldblum JR, et al. Reproducibility of the diagnosis of dysplasia in Barrett esophagus: a reaffirmation. *Hum Pathol*. 2001;32(4):368-378.

30. Reid BJ, Haggitt RC, Rubin CE, et al. Observer variation in the diagnosis of dysplasia in Barrett's esophagus. *Hum Pathol*. 1988;19(2):166-178.

31. Lomo LC, Blount PL, Sanchez CA, et al. Crypt dysplasia with surface maturation: a clinical, pathologic, and molecular study of a Barrett's esophagus cohort. *Am J Surg Pathol*. 2006;30(4):423-435.

32. Riddell RH, Goldman H, Ransohoff DF, et al. Dysplasia in inflammatory bowel disease: standardized classification with provisional clinical applications. *Hum Pathol*. 1983;14(11):931-968.

33. Curvers WL, ten Kate FJ, Krishnadath KK, et al. Low-grade dysplasia in Barrett's esophagus: overdiagnosed and underestimated. *Am J Gastroenterol*. 2010;105(7):1523-1530.

34. Vieth M, Montgomery EA, Riddell RH. Observations of different patterns of dysplasia in Barrett's esophagus - a first step to harmonize grading. *Cesk Patol*. 2016;52(3):154-163.

35. Rucker-Schmidt RL, Sanchez CA, Blount PL, et al. Nonadenomatous dysplasia in Barrett esophagus: a clinical, pathologic, and DNA content flow cytometric study. *Am J Surg Pathol*. 2009;33(6):886-893.

36. Mahajan D, Bennett AE, Liu X, Bena J, Bronner MP. Grading of gastric foveolar-type dysplasia in Barrett's esophagus. *Mod Pathol*. 2010;23(1):1-11.

37. Patil DT, Bennett AE, Mahajan D, Bronner MP. Distinguishing Barrett gastric foveolar dysplasia from reactive cardiac mucosa in gastroesophageal reflux disease. *Hum Pathol*. 2013;44(6):1146-1153.

38. Bronner MP, Overholt BF, Taylor SL, et al. Squamous overgrowth is not a safety concern for photodynamic therapy for Barrett's esophagus with high-grade dysplasia. *Gastroenterology*. 2009;136(1):56-64; quiz 351-352.

39. Vieth M, Riddell RH, Montgomery EA. High-grade dysplasia versus carcinoma: east is east and west is west, but does it need to be that way? *Am J Surg Pathol*. 2014;38(11):1453-1456.

40. Coco DP, Goldblum JR, Hornick JL, et al. Interobserver variability in the diagnosis of crypt dysplasia in Barrett esophagus. *Am J Surg Pathol*. 2011;35(1):45-54.

41. Voltaggio L, Montgomery EA. Diagnosis and management of Barrett-related neoplasia in the modern era. *Surgical Pathol Clin*. 2017;10(4):781-800.

42. Zhu W, Appelman HD, Greenson JK, et al. A histologically defined subset of high-grade dysplasia in Barrett mucosa is predictive of associated carcinoma. *Am J Clin Pathol*. 2009;132(1):94-100.

43. Pech O, May A, Manner H, et al. Long-term efficacy and safety of endoscopic resection for patients with mucosal adenocarcinoma of the esophagus. *Gastroenterology*. 2014;146(3):652.e651-660.e651.

44. Greene CL, Worrell SG, Attwood SE, et al. Emerging concepts for the endoscopic management of superficial esophageal adenocarcinoma. *J Gastrointest Surg*. 2016;20(4):851-860.

45. Manner H, Pech O, Heldmann Y, et al. The frequency of lymph node metastasis in early-stage adenocarcinoma of the esophagus with incipient submucosal invasion (pT1b sm1) depending on histological risk patterns. *Surg Endosc*. 2015;29(7):1888-1896.

46. Abraham SC, Wang H, Wang KK, Wu TT. Paget cells in the esophagus: assessment of their histopathologic features and near-universal association with underlying esophageal adenocarcinoma. *Am J Surg Pathol*. 2008;32(7):1068-1074.

47. van der Wel MJ, Jansen M, Vieth M, Meijer SL. What makes an expert Barrett's histopathologist? *Adv Exp Med Biol*. 2016;908:137-159.

48. Terheggen G, Horn EM, Vieth M, et al. A randomised trial of endoscopic submucosal dissection versus endoscopic mucosal resection for early Barrett's neoplasia. *Gut*. 2017;66(5):783-793.

49. Shaheen NJ, Sharma P, Overholt BF, et al. Radiofrequency ablation in Barrett's esophagus with dysplasia. *N Engl J Med*. 2009;360(22):2277-2288.

50. Canto MI, Shin EJ, Khashab MA, et al. Safety and efficacy of carbon dioxide cryotherapy for treatment of neoplastic Barrett's esophagus. *Endoscopy*. 2015;47(7):591.

51. Estrella JS, Hofstetter WL, Correa AM, et al. Duplicated muscularis mucosae invasion has similar risk of lymph node metastasis and recurrence-free survival as intramucosal esophageal adenocarcinoma. *Am J Surg Pathol*. 2011;35(7):1045-1053.

52. Kaneshiro DK, Post JC, Rybicki L, Rice TW, Goldblum JR. Clinical significance of the duplicated muscularis mucosae in Barrett esophagus-related superficial adenocarcinoma. *Am J Surg Pathol*. 2011;35(5):697-700.

53. Lewis JT, Wang KK, Abraham SC. Muscularis mucosae duplication and the musculo-fibrous anomaly in endoscopic mucosal resections for Barrett esophagus: implications for staging of adenocarcinoma. *Am J Surg Pathol*. 2008;32(4):566-571.

54. Westerterp M, Koppert LB, Buskens CJ, et al. Outcome of surgical treatment for early adenocarcinoma of the esophagus or gastro-esophageal junction. *Virchows Arch*. 2005;446(5):497-504.

55. Vieth M, Stolte M. Pathology of early upper GI cancers. *Best Pract Res Clin Gastroenterol*. 2005;19(6):857-869.

56. Kissiedu J, Thota PN, Gohel T, Lopez R, Gordon IO. Post-ablation lymphocytic esophagitis in Barrett esophagus with high grade dysplasia or intramucosal carcinoma. *Mod Pathol*. 2016;29(6):599-606.

57. Brown LM, Hoover R, Silverman D, et al. Excess incidence of squamous cell esophageal cancer among US black men: role of social class and other risk factors. *Am J Epidemiol*. 2001;153(2):114-122.

58. Njei B, McCarty TR, Birk JW. Trends in esophageal cancer survival in United States adults from 1973 to 2009: a SEER database analysis. *J Gastroenterol Hepatol*. 2016;31(6):1141-1146.

59. Brooks PJ, Enoch MA, Goldman D, Li TK, Yokoyama A. The alcohol flushing response: an unrecognized risk factor for esophageal cancer from alcohol consumption. *PLoS Med*. 2009;6(3):e50.

60. Cui R, Kamatani Y, Takahashi A, et al. Functional variants in ADH1B and ALDH2 coupled with alcohol and smoking synergistically enhance esophageal cancer risk. *Gastroenterology*. 2009;137(5):1768-1775.

61. Erkal HS, Mendenhall WM, Amdur RJ, Villaret DB, Stringer SP. Synchronous and metachronous squamous cell carcinomas of the head and neck mucosal sites. *J Clin Oncol*. 2001;19(5):1358-1362.

62. Csikos M, Horvath O, Petri A, Petri I, Imre J. Late malignant transformation of chronic corrosive oesophageal strictures. *Langenbecks Arch Chir*. 1985;365(4):231-238.

63. Blaydon DC, Etheridge SL, Risk JM, et al. RHBDF2 mutations are associated with tylosis, a familial esophageal cancer syndrome. *Am J Hum Genet*. 2012;90(2):340-346.

64. Ellis A, Risk JM, Maruthappu T, Kelsell DP. Tylosis with oesophageal cancer: diagnosis, management and molecular mechanisms. *Orphanet J Rare Dis*. 2015;10:126.

65. Turner JR, Shen LH, Crum CP, Dean PJ, Odze RD. Low prevalence of human papillomavirus infection in esophageal squamous cell carcinomas from North America: analysis by a highly sensitive and specific polymerase chain reaction-based approach. *Hum Pathol*. 1997;28(2):174-178.

66. Poljak M, Cerar A, Seme K. Human papillomavirus infection in esophageal carcinomas: a study of 121 lesions using multiple broad-spectrum polymerase chain reactions and literature review. *Hum Pathol*. 1998;29(3):266-271.

67. Chang F, Syrjanen S, Shen Q, et al. Human papillomavirus involvement in esophageal carcinogenesis in the high-incidence area of China. A study of 700 cases by screening and type-specific in situ hybridization. *Scand J Gastroenterol*. 2000;35(2):123-130.

68. Farhadi M, Tahmasebi Z, Merat S, Kamangar F, Nasrollahzadeh D, Malekzadeh R. Human papillomavirus in squamous cell carcinoma of esophagus in a high-risk population. *World J Gastroenterol*. 2005;11(8):1200-1203.

69. Herrera-Goepfert R, Lizano M, Akiba S, Carrillo-Garcia A, Becker-D'Acosta M. Human papilloma virus and esophageal carcinoma in a Latin-American region. *World J Gastroenterol*. 2009;15(25):3142-3147.

70. Syrjanen K. Geographic origin is a significant determinant of human papillomavirus prevalence in oesophageal squamous cell carcinoma: systematic review and meta-analysis. *Scand J Infect Dis*. 2013;45(1):1-18.

71. Salaria SN, Abu Alfa AK, Cruise MW, Wood LD, Montgomery EA. Lichenoid esophagitis: clinicopathologic overlap with established esophageal lichen planus. *Am J Surg Pathol.* 2013;37(12):1889-1894.

72. Singhi AD, Arnold CA, Crowder CD, Lam-Himlin DM, Voltaggio L, Montgomery EA. Esophageal leukoplakia or epidermoid metaplasia: a clinicopathological study of 18 patients. *Mod Pathol.* 2014;27(1):38-43.

73. Taggart MW, Rashid A, Ross WA, Abraham SC. Oesophageal hyperkeratosis: clinicopathological associations. *Histopathology.* 2013;63(4):463-473.

74. Singhi AD, Arnold CA, Lam-Himlin DM, et al. Targeted next-generation sequencing supports epidermoid metaplasia of the esophagus as a precursor to esophageal squamous neoplasia. *Mod Pathol.* 2017;30(11):1613-1621.

75. Daniels JA, Gibson MK, Xu L, et al. Gastrointestinal tract epithelial changes associated with taxanes: marker of drug toxicity versus effect. *Am J Surg Pathol.* 2008;32(3):473-477.

76. Bosman F, Carneiro F, Hruban R, Theise N, eds. *WHO Classification of Tumours of the Digestive System.* Lyon: IARC; 2010. Bosman F, Jaffee E, Lakhani S, Ohgaki H, eds. *World Health Organization Classification of Tumours.*

77. Modlin IM, Sandor A. An analysis of 8305 cases of carcinoid tumors. *Cancer.* 1997;79(4):813-829.

78. Lloyd R, Osamura R, Kloppel G, Rosai J. *WHO Classification of Tumours of Endocrine Organs.* Lyon: IARC Press; 2017.

79. Deng HY, Ni PZ, Wang YC, Wang WP, Chen LQ. Neuroendocrine carcinoma of the esophagus: clinical characteristics and prognostic evaluation of 49 cases with surgical resection. *J Thorac Dis.* 2016;8(6):1250-1256.

80. Yachida S, Nakanishi Y, Shimoda T, et al. Adenosquamous carcinoma of the esophagus. Clinicopathologic study of 18 cases. *Oncology.* 2004;66(3):218-225.

81. Aulakh K, Chisholm C, Speights V. TTF-1 and napsin-A frequently positive in esophageal and pulmonary adenocarcinomas: dispelling myths and offering new insights. *Mod Pathol.* 2011;24(suppl 1):142A; (Abstract 596).

82. Antonescu CR, Busam KJ, Francone TD, et al. L576P KIT mutation in anal melanomas correlates with KIT protein expression and is sensitive to specific kinase inhibition. *Int J Canc.* 2007;121(2):257-264.

83. Carvajal RD, Antonescu CR, Wolchok JD, et al. KIT as a therapeutic target in metastatic melanoma. *JAMA.* 2011;305(22):2327-2334.

84. Carvajal RD, Hamid O, Antonescu CR. Selecting patients for KIT inhibition in melanoma. *Meth Mol Biol.* 2014;1102:137-162.

85. Carvajal RD, Lawrence DP, Weber JS, et al. Phase II study of nilotinib in melanoma harboring KIT alterations following progression to prior KIT inhibition. *Clin Canc Res.* 2015;21(10):2289-2296.

86. Gollub MJ, Prowda JC. Primary melanoma of the esophagus: radiologic and clinical findings in six patients. *Radiology.* 1999;213(1):97-100.

87. Syrigos KN, Konstadoulakis MM, Ricaniades N, Leandros M, Karakousis CP. Primary malignant melanoma of the esophagus: report of two cases and review of the literature. *In Vivo.* 1999;13(5):421-422.

88. Takubo K, Kanda Y, Ishii M, et al. Primary malignant melanoma of the esophagus. *Hum Pathol.* 1983;14(8):727-730.

89. Volpin E, Sauvanet A, Couvelard A, Belghiti J. Primary malignant melanoma of the esophagus: a case report and review of the literature. *Dis Esophagus.* 2002;15(3):244-249.

90. Wayman J, Irving M, Russell N, Nicoll J, Raimes SA. Intraluminal radiotherapy and Nd:YAG laser photoablation for primary malignant melanoma of the esophagus. *Gastrointest Endosc.* 2004;59(7):927-929.

91. Yoo CC, Levine MS, McLarney JK, Lowry MA. Primary malignant melanoma of the esophagus: radiographic findings in seven patients. *Radiology.* 1998;209(2):455-459.

92. Inadomi K, Kumagai H, Arita S, et al. Bi-cytopenia possibly induced by anti-PD-1 antibody for primary malignant melanoma of the esophagus: a case report. *Medicine.* 2016;95(29):e4283.

93. Swerdlow SH, Campo E, Pileri SA, et al. The 2016 revision of the World Health Organization classification of lymphoid neoplasms. *Blood.* 2016;127(20):2375-2390.

CHAPTER OUTLINE

THE UNREMARKABLE STOMACH

The stomach consists of the cardiac opening, fundus, body, antrum, and pylorus (Fig. 2.1). These sites perform different physiologic functions and accordingly have variable histologic characteristics. Familiarity with these features will aid in both gastric polyp classification and the prognostication of neoplastic processes affected by the presence of background gastritis. For example, the sporadic gastric neuroendocrine tumor (NET) (type III) has a relatively worse prognosis than the NET found in autoimmune gastritis (type I); this important distinction relies upon adequate regional sampling and the information gleaned therein. See also "Well-Differentiated Neuroendocrine Tumors" section.

The gastric wall includes the mucosa, submucosa, muscularis propria, and serosa (Fig. 2.2). The mucosa consists of the epithelium, lamina propria, and muscularis mucosae. Unlike the deep glands, the surface epithelial component is consistent throughout the stomach and is composed of mucus-secreting foveolar cells that line superficial pits (foveolae). Deep to these pits are mucous neck cells and the gastric glands, whose function and cell composition are region dependent (Fig. 2.3). For example, deep glands

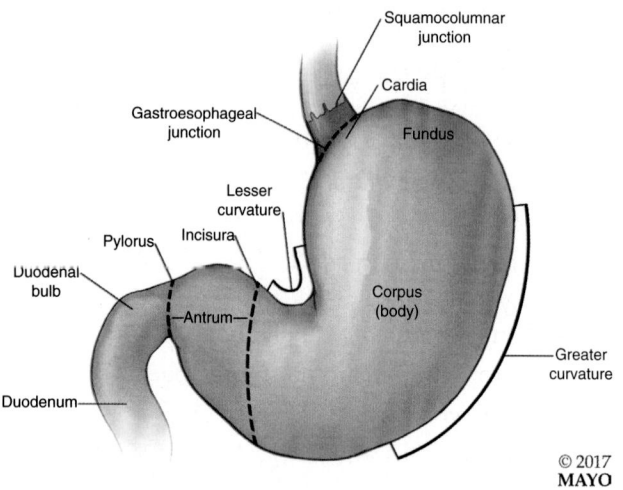

Figure 2-1. The stomach consists of the cardiac opening, fundus, corpus or body, antrum, and pylorus. The fundus and body are the bulk of the stomach, whereas the gastric antrum comprises merely 10%.

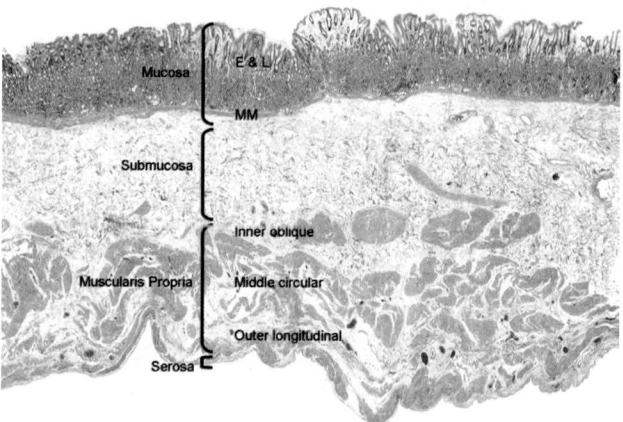

Figure 2-2. A full-thickness section of the stomach wall shows mucosa composed of epithelium and lamina propria (E&L) and muscularis mucosae (MM). Beyond the submucosa is the muscularis propria, which contains three layers of muscle, all of which is covered by serosa (visceral peritoneum).

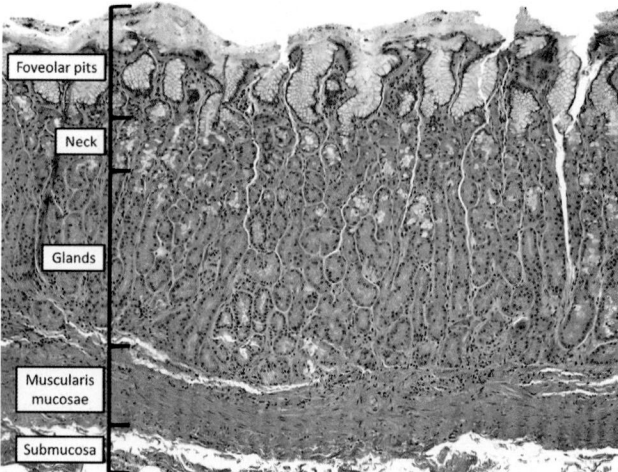

Figure 2-3. The mucosa throughout the stomach is lined by surface foveolar mucin cells, which extend down the gastric pits. Mucous neck cells transition to deep glands, the composition of which varies by gastric subsite. The muscularis mucosae is the deepest layer of the mucosa before reaching submucosa. This section is through the gastric corpus (body and fundus) in which the oxyntic glands comprise approximately 80% of the mucosal thickness, and the foveolar pits are relatively shallow.

found in the gastric cardia are composed of mucus-secreting cells with abundant clear foamy cytoplasm (Fig. 2.4). By comparison, deep glands of the body and fundus contain mixed bluish-purple chief cells, pink parietal cells, and scattered amphophilic enterochromaffinlike (ECL) endocrine cells (Fig. 2.5). In the antrum and pylorus, the deep glands are again mucus secreting and are similar in histology to those in the gastric cardia (Figs. 2.6 and 2.7). Transition zones between these regions may show a variable mixture of gland histology. For a more detailed discussion of the unremarkable stomach, see also "Stomach" chapter, *Atlas of Gastrointestinal Pathology: A Pattern Based Approach to Non-Neoplastic Biopsies.*

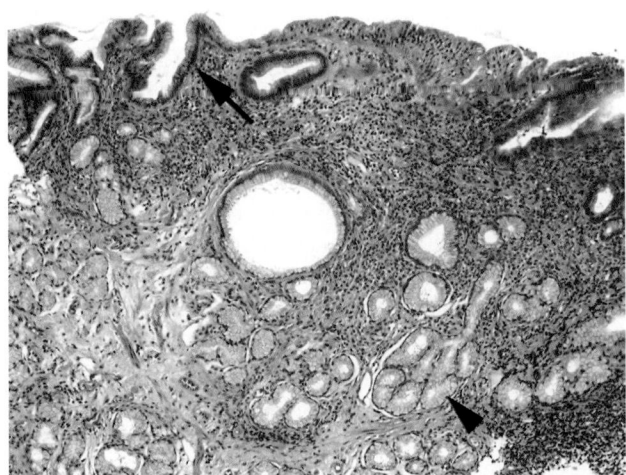

Figure 2-4. The deep glands of the gastric cardia vary between oxyntic type (chief cells and parietal cells, not pictured) and cardiac type, which are lined by cuboidal cells with abundant clear cytoplasm and small flattened nuclei pushed toward the basement membrane (*arrowhead*). These cells are indistinguishable from the pyloric glands found in the gastric antrum. The luminal surface and foveolar pits are lined by foveolar mucin cells (*arrow*), as it is throughout the stomach.

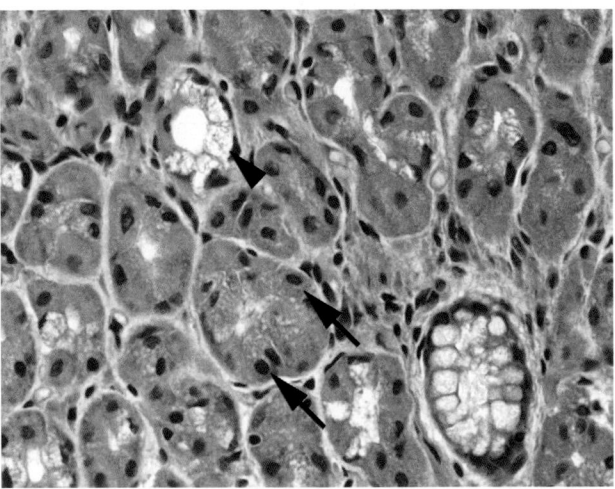

Figure 2-5. The deep glands of the gastric body and fundus are lined by oxyntic glands composed of *pink* parietal cells and *blue* chief cells (*arrows*). Mucous neck cells with clear foamy cytoplasm and eccentric nuclei (*arrowhead*) are normal and should not be mistaken for signet ring cell carcinoma.

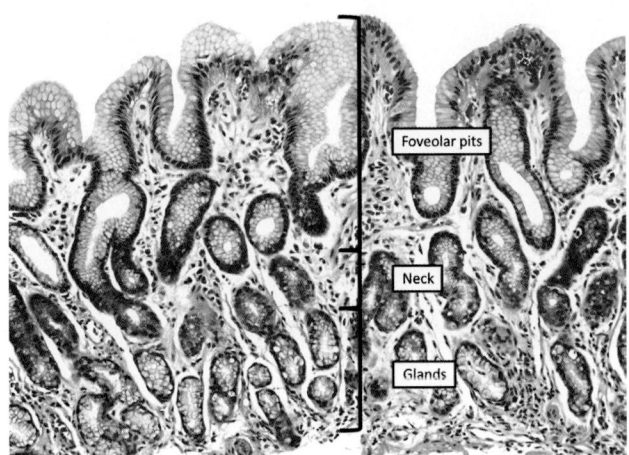

Figure 2-6. The pits of the gastric antrum are lined by foveolar mucin cells and are deeper as compared with the pits in the corpus, extending to 50% of the mucosal thickness. The deep pyloric glands of the antrum are cuboidal with clear cytoplasm.

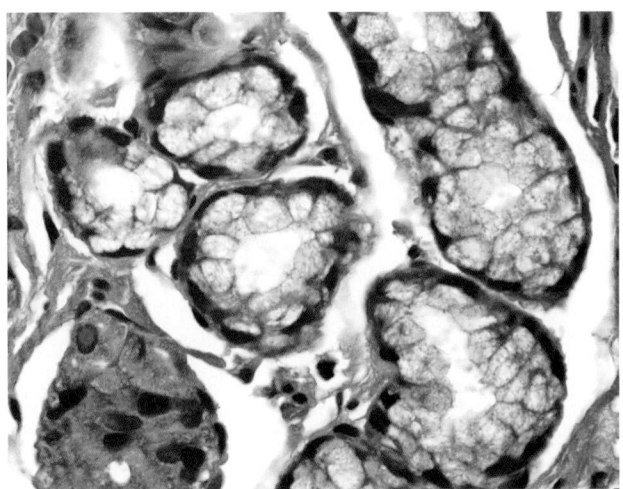

Figure 2-7. The deep glands of the antrum and pylorus contain pyloric-type glands, which are similar in appearance as cardiac-type glands, with cuboidal cells containing abundant clear foamy cytoplasm and small flattened nuclei displaced toward the basement membrane.

The lamina propria between the pits and glands is normally devoid of inflammatory cells and contains inconspicuous lymphovascular channels accessible for metastatic spread of tumor cells. The muscularis mucosae is composed of a thin delicate layer of smooth muscle cells, separating the mucosa from the underlying submucosa, which contains abundant larger lymphatic and vascular structures, also readily able to facilitate metastasis. The muscularis propria of the stomach is composed of three sets of smooth muscle fibers: longitudinal, circular, and oblique. The entire organ is encased by the mesothelial-derived serosa, which forms the boundary to the peritoneal space. Staging of invasive tumors requires accurate identification of each of these layers.

POLYPS

Several features contribute to challenges in gastric polyp classification, even for the skilled pathologist. For example, gastric polyps are far less common than colonic polyps, resulting in a more recent and sparse body of literature; they show significant histologic overlap with one another; and classification is influenced by features of the background flat mucosa. Unlike polyps elsewhere in the tubular gastrointestinal (GI) tract, which are frequently isolated findings, polyps of the stomach often arise in association with an inflammatory backdrop or a polyposis syndrome. Thus, although they may be troublesome to classify, careful attention to the background mucosa with a deliberate effort toward an integrated interpretation will provide important information about prognosis or risk for familial syndromes. Gastric polyps are found in 6% of upper endoscopies and are seen as projections above the adjacent flat mucosa (Fig. 2.8).[1] These proliferative lesions may arise from the epithelium (most common) or from other compartments in the mucosa and submucosa. Table 2.1 lists the most common gastric polyps by chief proliferative compartment and serves as an outline for this segment. This section provides a diagnostic approach for epithelial and hamartomatous polyps; mesenchymal lesions are discussed in a dedicated chapter (see "Mesenchymal Lesions" chapter). An understanding of the normal regions and histologic compartments, reviewed at the beginning of this chapter, will facilitate application of this approach.

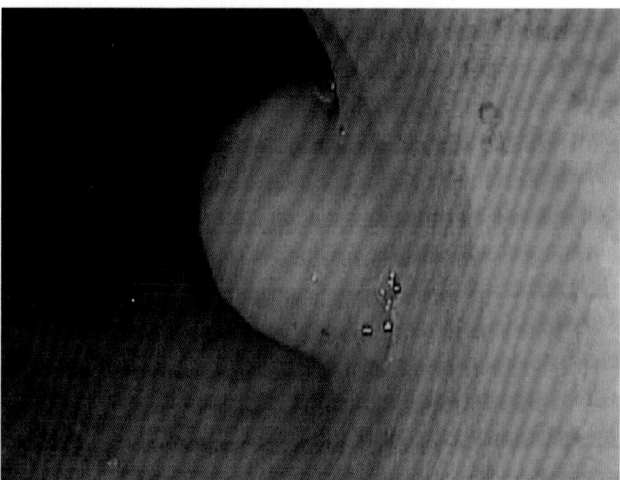

Figure 2-8. Endoscopically, gastric polyps appear exophytic and are mucosal or submucosal based. All gastric polyps require histologic diagnosis.

TABLE 2.1: Gastric Polyps: Categorized by Proliferative Compartment

Heterotopic Polyps

- Pancreatic acinar heterotopia

Hamartomatous Polyps

- Peutz-Jeghers polyp[a]
- Juvenile polyp[a]
- Cronkhite-Canada syndrome–associated polyp[a]
- PTEN hamartoma tumor syndrome and Cowden syndrome–associated polyp[a]

Epithelial Polyps and Hyperplasias

- Hyperplastic polyp, polypoid foveolar hyperplasia, foveolar polyp
- Fundic gland polyp[a]
- Adenomatous polyps
  - Intestinal type
  - Gastric type, foveolar adenoma
  - Gastric type, pyloric gland adenoma
  - Gastric type, oxyntic gland polyp/adenoma
- Carcinomatous polyp, primary or metastatic
- Neuroendocrine tumors

Mesenchymal

- Inflammatory fibroid polyp
- Gastrointestinal stromal tumor
- Leiomyoma
- Vascular lesions
- Granular cell tumor

Other findings that may appear polypoid

- Lymphoid hyperplasia
- Lymphoma
- Xanthoma
- Granuloma
- Amyloidosis
- Hemosiderosis
- Calcium deposit
- Gastritis cystica profunda

[a]Polyps associated with clinical syndromes.
PTEN, phosphatase and tensin homolog.

PANCREATIC HETEROTOPIA

Heterotopic pancreatic tissue is an incidental finding most commonly seen in the wall of the gastric antrum. Endoscopically, it can appear as a submucosal nodule with central umbilication and surface erosion (Fig. 2.9). These are commonly biopsied with clinical concern for a gastrointestinal stromal tumor (GIST), which is endoscopically similar in appearance. However, because the bulk of these lesions are submucosal, superficial biopsies may lack diagnostic material and rebiopsy may be necessary. When well sampled or mucosally resected, these lesions consist of a variable admixture of benign pancreatic acinar cells, islets, and ducts, the latter of which may even connect to the mucosal surface for drainage in larger lesions (Figs. 2.10–2.14). These structures attempt to recapitulate normal pancreatic tissue and maintain a lobular architecture but may appear slightly disorganized. Although the pancreatic acinar cells may be sparse, they are identified by their typical triangular shape, eccentric round nuclei, and abundant eosinophilic to amphophilic granular cytoplasm. Importantly, there is no cytologic atypia, infiltrative border, or desmoplastic stromal reaction. Adjacent or overlying mucosa may show reactive changes or intestinal metaplasia (IM) owing to the digestive secretions of the pancreatic acinar cells.

FAQ: Is there significant difference between pancreatic heterotopia and pancreatic acinar cell metaplasia?

Yes! Pancreatic heterotopia is incidental, and, aside from possible gastric outlet obstruction or ulceration in larger examples, the finding is generally inconsequential and not associated with inflammatory conditions. By comparison, the finding of pancreatic acinar cell metaplasia (PAM) should alert the pathologist to examine the background mucosa more closely for possible autoimmune metaplastic atrophic gastritis (AMAG) as nearly half of AMAG cases contain PAM.[2] Histologic distinction between heterotopia and metaplasia is not always possible, but some clues can favor one over the other. For example, because pancreatic heterotopia is ectopic pancreatic tissue, it often involves the submucosa and contains heterogeneous pancreatic cell types (i.e., some combination of acini, ducts, and islets). In contrast, PAM is the result of single cell transformation (gastric cells to acinar cells) and thus is limited to the mucosa and is homogeneous (composed of acinar cells only) (Fig. 2.15).

PEARLS & PITFALLS

When stumped by a gastric nodule that resembles a well-differentiated NET but fails to stain for neuroendocrine markers such as chromogranin and synaptophysin, consider PAM or pancreatic heterotopia. Often, simply remembering this entity results in an "ah-ha" moment of diagnosis. Pancreatic heterotopia may contain small ducts, a helpful clue. In difficult cases, immunohistochemistry for trypsin or chymotrypsin is positive in pancreatic acinar cells.

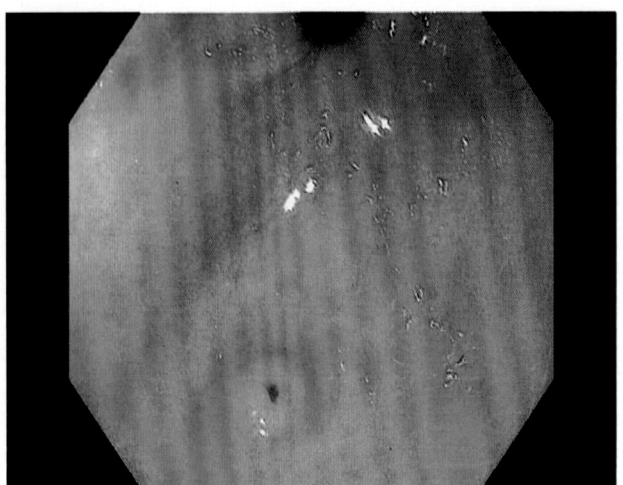

Figure 2-9. Pancreatic heterotopia. A submucosal nodule with a central umbilication is seen in the gastric antrum.

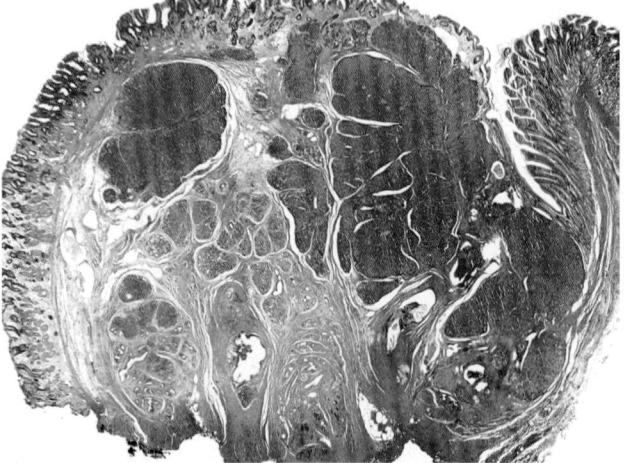

Figure 2-10. Pancreatic heterotopia. Pancreatic heterotopia is found in the wall of the stomach. This EMR specimen shows deep submucosal location as well as mucosal involvement. Note the lobulated appearance of the glands.

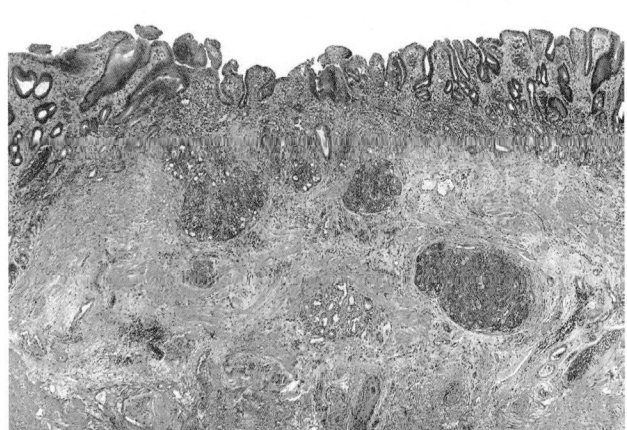

Figure 2-11. Pancreatic heterotopia. This example contains a few lobules of pancreatic acini in the submucosa. The surface epithelium shows mild erosive and reactive changes.

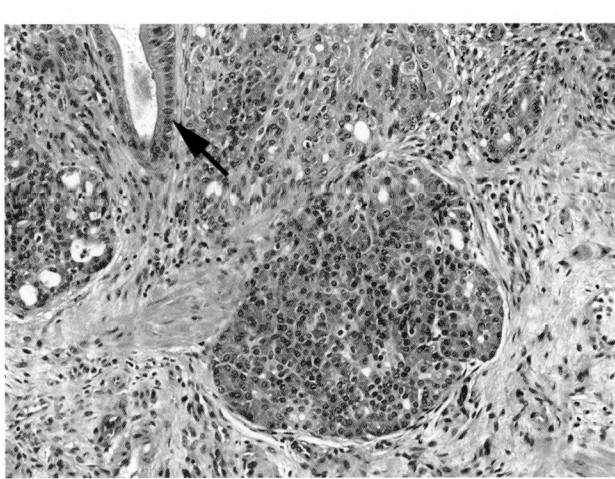

Figure 2-12. Pancreatic heterotopia. Most examples are straightforward with well-developed pancreatic acinar lobules, as seen here. In challenging cases, the presence of a duct (arrow) can be a helpful clue.

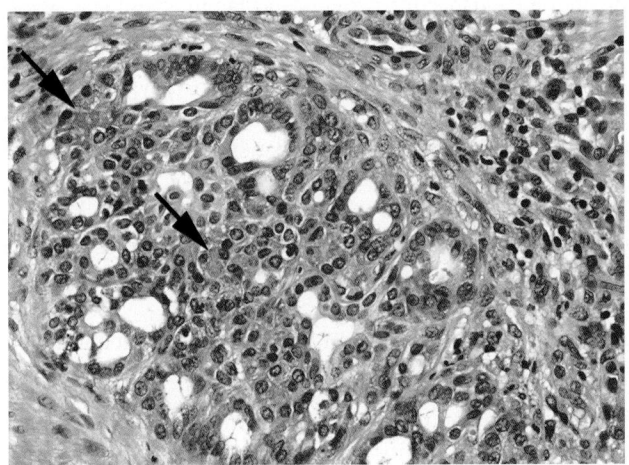

Figure 2-13. Pancreatic heterotopia. Some cases can resemble neuroendocrine tumors, but careful examination for a population of pancreatic acinar cells with eosinophilic granular cytoplasm (arrows) can steer one away from this pitfall. Trypsin or chymotrypsin immunostains would also be reactive in pancreatic acinar cells.

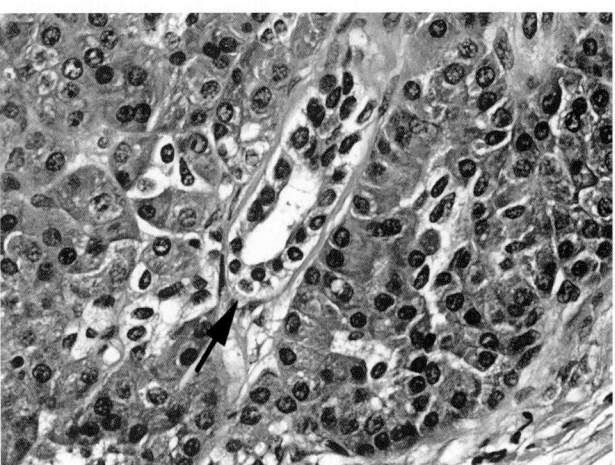

Figure 2-14. Pancreatic heterotopia. A small pancreatic duct (arrow) is a helpful clue in differentiating pancreatic heterotopia from pancreatic metaplasia and neuroendocrine tumor.

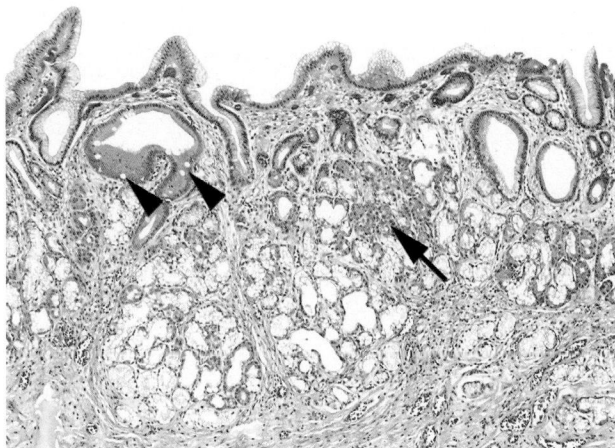

Figure 2-15. Pancreatic acinar metaplasia (PAM). These pancreatic acinar cells (arrow) are admixed with normal antral glands and lack the lobulated organization of pancreatic heterotopia. The acinar cells of either PAM or pancreatic heterotopia may secret enzymes causing adjacent intestinal metaplasia (arrowheads).

HAMARTOMATOUS POLYPS AND SYNDROMIC CONSIDERATIONS

Hamartomatous polyps result from disordered growth of tissues native to the site and can arise from any of the three embryonic layers. These lesions are frequently, but not universally, associated with a clinical syndrome. Compared with their small bowel and colonic counterparts, hamartomatous polyps in the gastric mucosa have nonspecific histology and may be indistinguishable from hyperplastic polyps even in a patient with a known polyposis syndrome.[3] Therefore, this section covers common diagnostic challenges of gastric hamartomatous polyps and some of the syndromic considerations, and additional discussion of polyposis syndromes can be found in the "Small Bowel" chapter.

Peutz-Jeghers Polyp

Peutz-Jeghers syndrome is characterized by hamartomatous polyps of the GI tract and melanocytic mucocutaneous hyperpigmentation.[4] Up to 25% of documented cases are sporadic, but this condition is best known as an autosomal dominant inherited syndrome with 80% of affected families harboring a germline mutation in the *STK11/LKB1* gene.[5,6] Patients with Peutz-Jeghers syndrome have a 93% cumulative lifetime risk for cancer, including carcinomas of the GI tract, breast, ovary, and testis.[7-9] In this context, early recognition of the syndrome allows for appropriate screening and surveillance for patients and family members. World Health Organization (WHO) criteria for the clinical diagnosis of Peutz-Jeghers syndrome are:

1. Detection of three or more histologically confirmed Peutz-Jeghers polyps.

or

2. The presence of *any number* of Peutz-Jeghers polyps in a patient with a family history of the syndrome.

or

3. Detection of characteristic, prominent mucocutaneous pigmentation in the patient with a family history of the syndrome.

or

4. Detection of *any number* of Peutz-Jeghers polyps in a patient with prominent mucocutaneous pigmentation.[10]

1Three of the above four potential methods of diagnosis include histologic identification of Peutz-Jeghers polyps, making pathologic recognition a necessary skill. These hamartomatous polyps have a characteristic appearance, showing compactly spaced glands supported by an arborizing framework of well-developed smooth muscle that is contiguous with the muscularis mucosae (Figs. 2.16–2.23). Gastric polyps, which occur in about 15% to 30% of syndromic patients, are less frequent than small bowel (64%) or colonic polyps (53%).[11] These lesions of the small bowel and colon are not only more common but also highly distinctive; their intact lamina propria with arborizing smooth muscle fibers helps

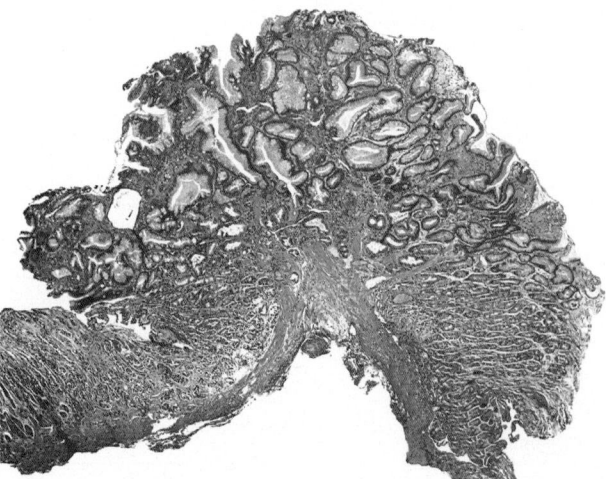

Figure 2-16. Well-developed gastric Peutz-Jeghers polyp. At scanning magnification, an arborizing smooth muscle base is evident along with disorganized, branching, and cystic glands.

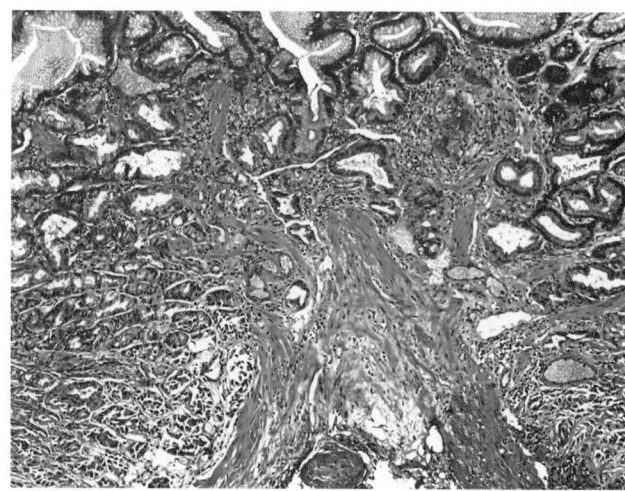

Figure 2-17. Higher magnification of the previous figure. Arborizing bundles of smooth muscle splay out at various angles.

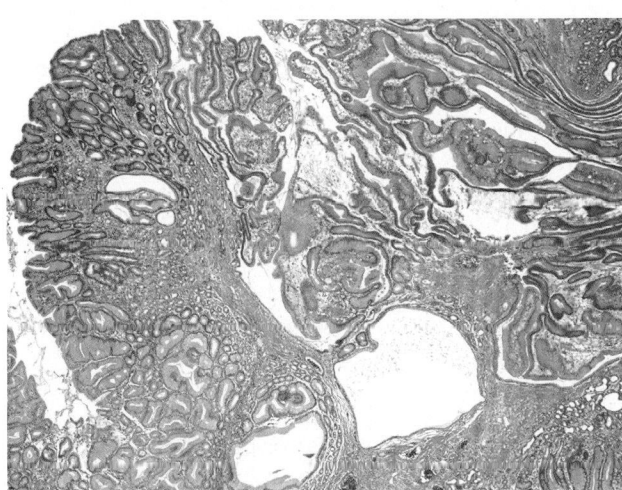

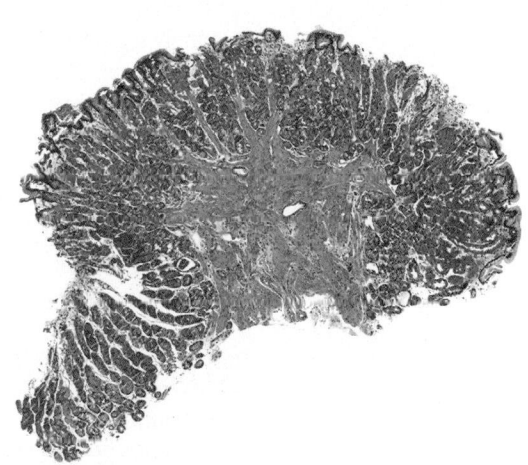

Figure 2-18. Gastric Peutz-Jeghers polyp. This example shows broad areas of foveolar hyperplasia, lamina propria edema, and disorganized gland architecture with dilated glands and abundant admixed smooth muscle.

Figure 2-19. Gastric Peutz-Jeghers polyp. This polyp in the gastric body shows a prominent core of disorganized smooth muscle with branches extending at various angles.

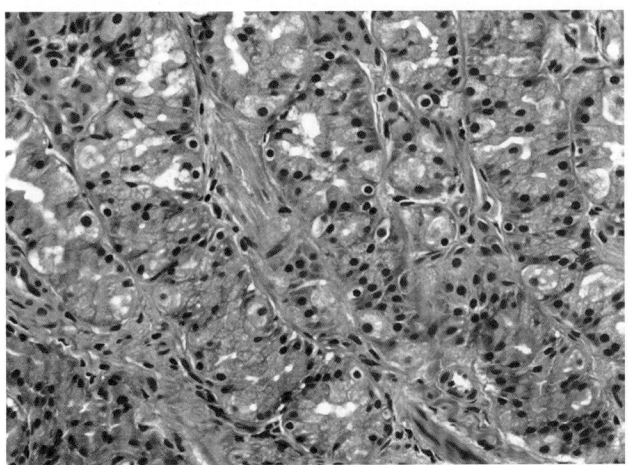

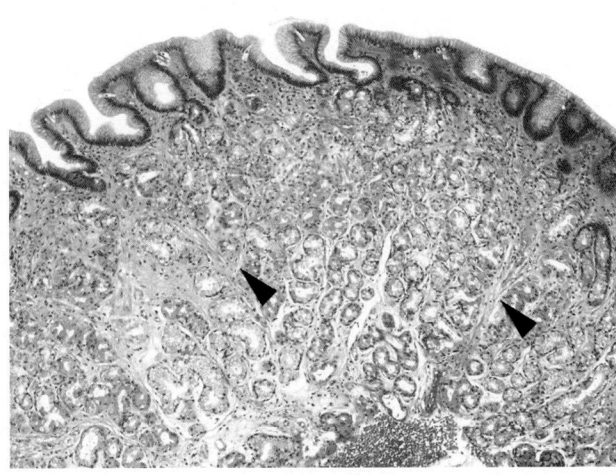

Figure 2-20. Higher magnification of the previous figure. Disorganized small bundles and wisps of smooth muscle are present in the lamina propria and stream at intersecting angles.

Figure 2-21. Gastric Peutz-Jeghers polyp. This polyp is not as well developed as previous examples, but it was retrieved from a patient known to have Peutz-Jeghers syndrome. The glands appear organized and lack dilation or architectural changes, but note the presence of smooth muscle within the lamina propria (*arrowheads*).

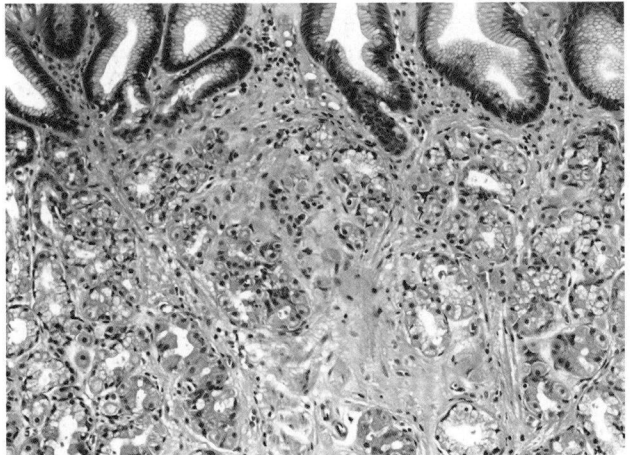

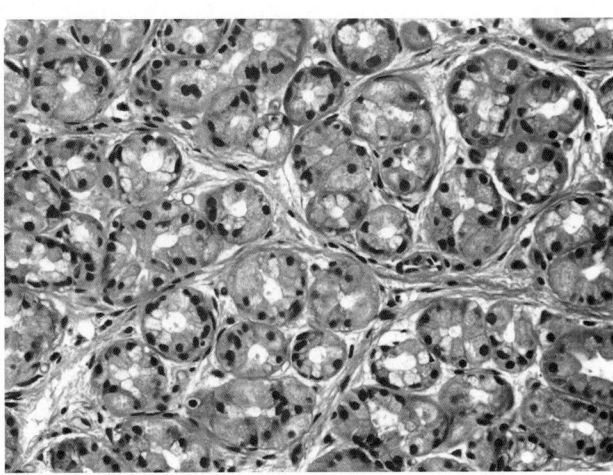

Figure 2-22. Higher magnification of the previous figure. Small disorganized bundles and wisps of smooth muscle expand the lamina propria and branch in different directions.

Figure 2-23. Gastric Peutz-Jeghers polyp. Wisps of intersecting smooth muscle surround glands creating small lobules, a helpful clue in some examples.

differentiate them from juvenile polyps. Gastric Peutz-Jeghers polyps, on the other hand, are routinely indistinguishable from nonspecific gastric hyperplastic polyps or other syndromic gastric polyps. Clues, such as unexplained wisps of smooth muscle in the lamina propria and lobular architecture of the glands (Figs. 2.20–2.23), can improve the sensitivity for hamartomatous polyps of Peutz-Jeghers type.[3,12] Dysplasia is rarely found in these polyps, but patients with the syndrome have significant risk for malignancy elsewhere, including gastric adenocarcinoma outside of the polyp.[13] Given these diagnostic challenges and the clinical implications for both patients and families, a low threshold should be maintained for diagnosis of gastric hamartomatous polyps. Suggesting further bidirectional endoscopy may provide more definitive histologic evidence for Peutz-Jeghers polyps at other sites.

PEARLS & PITFALLS

Although a low threshold for diagnosis of hamartomatous polyps is advocated, caution is advised *against* using gastric polyps to fulfill any of the WHO criteria requiring "histologically confirmed" Peutz-Jeghers polyps. In the stomach, the histologic features are not reliable enough to differentiate syndromic polyps from reactive lesions such as inflammatory/hyperplastic polyps, and the implications are considerable. Instead, compose a descriptive sign out with an explanatory note (see the following note). If the patient has prior GI polyps, it may be worthwhile to review the histology.

SAMPLE NOTE: Gastric Polyp With Features Suggesting Hamartomatous Versus Inflammatory/Hyperplastic Polyp

Stomach, Antrum, Polyp, Biopsy

- Gastric polyp with features suggestive of hamartomatous polyp, see Comment.

Comment

There are no reliable histologic features to distinguish gastric hamartomatous polyps from reactive lesions (i.e., gastric inflammatory/hyperplastic polyps) or to reliably differentiate subtypes of hamartomatous polyps. Nevertheless, the current specimen contains some features that suggest hamartomatous development, such as cystically dilated irregular glands and admixed smooth muscle. Syndromes involving hamartomatous GI polyps (e.g., Peutz-Jeghers syndrome, juvenile polyposis syndrome, Cowden syndrome) should be ruled out clinically. In addition, bidirectional endoscopy is advised, with biopsy of any polypoid lesions in either the upper or lower GI tract, as polyps found outside the stomach are more likely to retain pathognomonic features.

FAQ: I have a patient with single *classic* Peutz-Jeghers polyp, but this patient has no other polyps or family history of Peutz-Jeghers syndrome. What does this mean?

Rare instances of patients with isolated sporadic Peutz-Jeghers polyps have been documented. In nearly all instances, these patients had clinical histories suggesting Peutz-Jeghers syndrome (e.g., concurrent pancreatic cancer, family GI cancer history, metachronous tumors) but failed to meet the WHO criteria. Thus, isolated or sporadic Peutz-Jeghers polyps may occur, but clinicians should be advised that these patients appear to have a cumulative lifetime risk of malignancy similar to those with the syndrome[14] (Figs. 2.24 and 2.25).

Juvenile Polyp

Juvenile polyposis syndrome, the most common of the hamartomatous polyposis syndromes, affects one in 100,000. The syndrome is largely sporadic but can be inherited as autosomal dominant familial syndrome (30%).[15] Both inherited and sporadic forms share similar genetics, with germline mutations in *SMAD4* (also known as *DPC4*) (15%) and the related gene *BMPR1A* (25%), whereas *ENG* is associated with early childhood presentation.[16,17] These

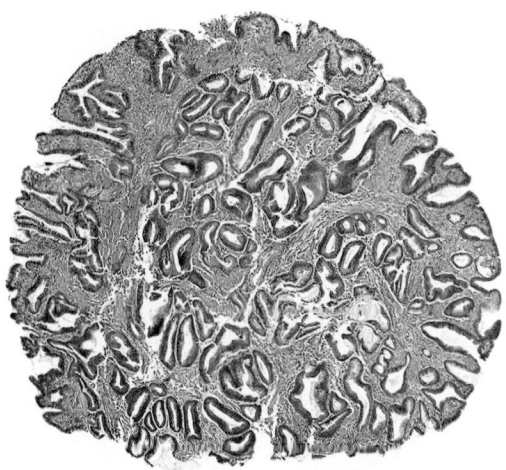

Figure 2-24. Gastric hamartomatous polyp. This gastric polyp was retrieved from a patient without a known syndrome but shows brightly eosinophilic disorganized smooth muscle bundles within the lamina propria suggestive of a hamartomatous polyp.

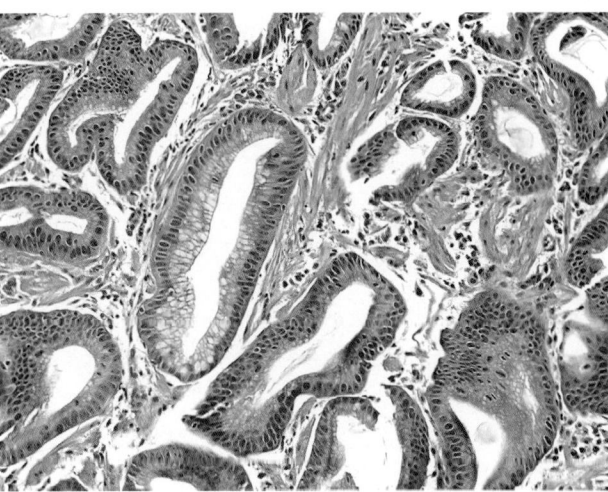

Figure 2-25. Gastric hamartomatous polyp, higher magnification of the previous figure. The foveolar epithelium is separated by disorganized smooth muscle bundles that stream at intersecting angles. Isolated sporadic Peutz-Jeghers polyps are rare but can occur. These patients share the same cumulative lifetime risk of cancer as patients with Peutz-Jeghers syndrome.

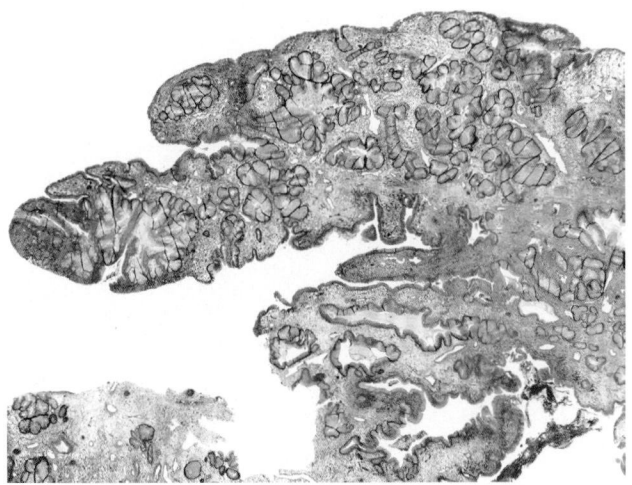

Figure 2-26. Juvenile polyp. This gastric polyp was retrieved from a patient known to have juvenile polyposis syndrome. There are broad fingerlike projections with an excess of lamina propria and inflammation. The glands are abnormally shaped and dilated.

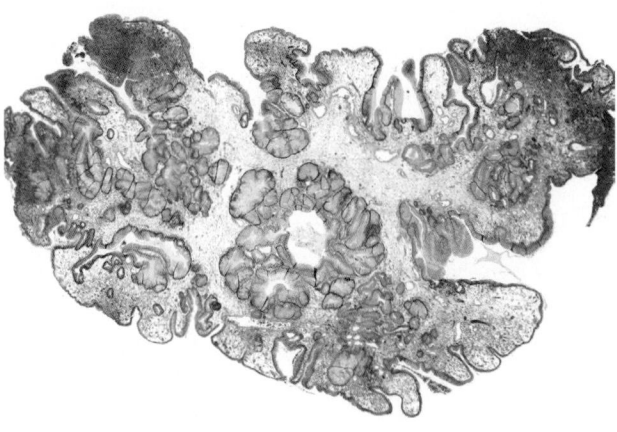

Figure 2-27. Juvenile polyp. These polyps can resemble inflammatory polyps owing to their edematous lamina propria, chronic inflammation, dilated glands, and surface erosion.

genetic changes cause a disruption in the transforming growth factor beta signal transduction pathway and result in an increased risk of malignancy. The overall risk of GI malignancies in these patients is 55%, with colorectal cancer presenting at an average age of 37 years.[18,19]

WHO criteria for the clinical diagnosis of juvenile polyposis syndrome are:

1. More than three to five juvenile polyps of the colorectum
or
2. Juvenile polyps throughout the GI tract
or
3. Any number of juvenile polyps with a family history of juvenile polyposis[20]

In the stomach, juvenile polyps are usually 3- to 20-mm solitary pedunculated lesions with a predilection for the gastric antrum. Like Peutz-Jeghers polyps, juvenile polyps are classified as hamartomatous lesions, but their histologic profiles differ. Juvenile polyps consist primarily of an excess of lamina propria and show abundant distorted and dilated glands (Figs. 2.26–2.30). The combination of lamina propria edema and abundance of distended, mucus-filled glands in combination with inflammatory cells is occasionally mistaken for "inflammatory" or "retention" polyp. This is understandable because solitary

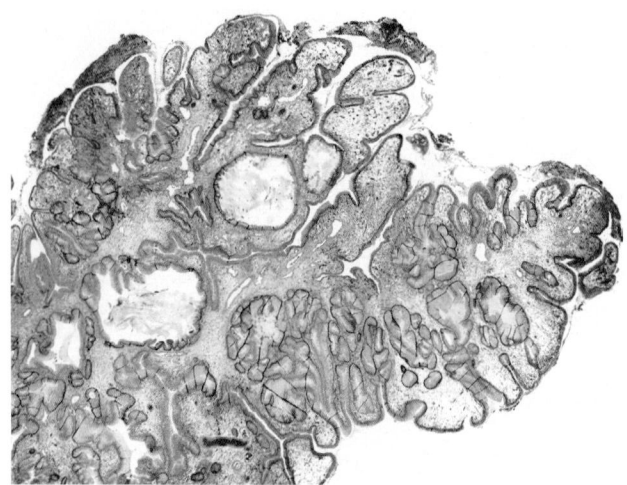

Figure 2-28. Juvenile polyp. Broad and blunt projections characterize this polyp from a patient with known juvenile polyposis syndrome. The lamina propria is edematous and contains inflammatory cells. Surface erosion is present with a fibroinflammatory layer.

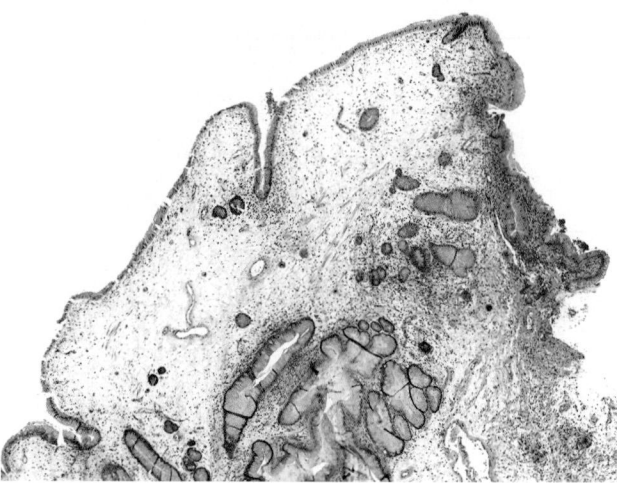

Figure 2-29. Juvenile polyp. Excess lamina propria and disorganized dilated glands are present.

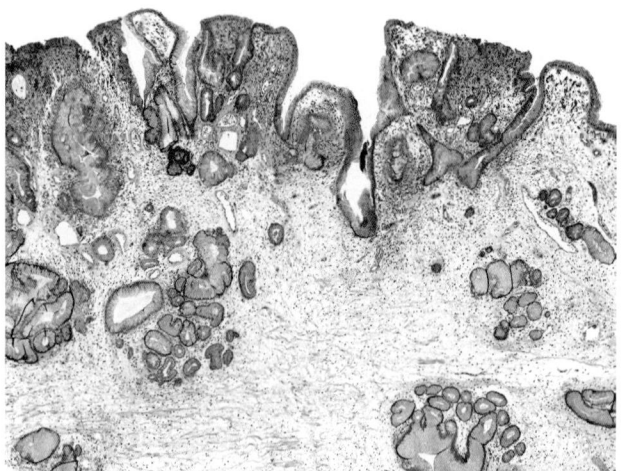

Figure 2-30. Juvenile polyp. Sparse abnormally shaped glands are present with abundant edematous lamina propria, surface erosion, and inflammation. The histologic features are not specific to juvenile polyp, but this example is from a patient known to have the syndrome.

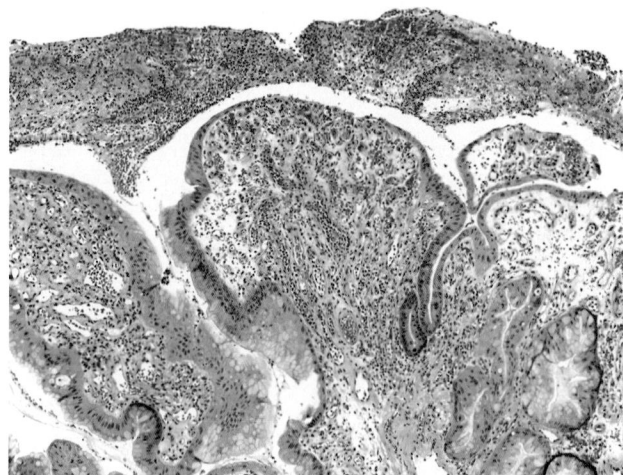

Figure 2-31. Juvenile polyp. Surface erosion, granulation tissue formation, and a fibroinflammatory coating are common nonspecific findings. These changes are also found in inflammatory polyps and large hyperplastic polyps.

or sporadic juvenile polyps may be indistinguishable from inflammatory/retention polyps in either the upper or lower GI tract. Fortunately, and in contrast to sporadic Peutz-Jeghers polyps, there is no documented increased lifetime risk for malignancy reported for sporadic juvenile polyps. Nevertheless, foci of dysplasia are regularly seen in juvenile polyps, underscoring their neoplastic potential and the value of recognition. In the absence of sufficient clinical history, and when the histology precludes definitive classification, patients benefit from a more inclusive diagnosis, such as "juvenile/inflammatory polyp" and a careful note (see the earlier sample note for Peutz-Jeghers syndrome). When multiple similar polyps are encountered, the possibility of a polyposis syndrome should be stated. On the other hand, take care not to label these patients prematurely, as classification of single gastric polyps is often irresolvable. Other syndromes involving hamartomatous GI polyps should be ruled out clinically or by pathologic examination (Figs. 2.31–2.34).

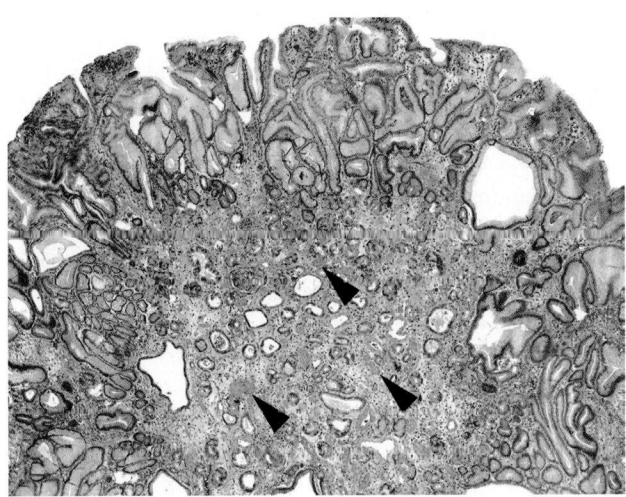

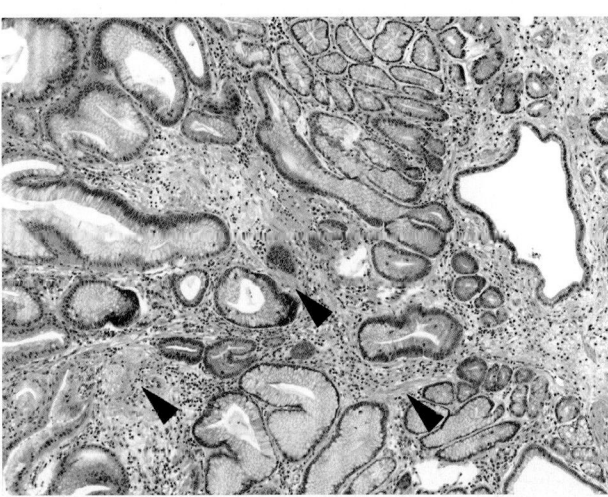

Figure 2-32. Juvenile polyp. This gastric polyp was retrieved from a patient known to have juvenile polyposis syndrome, and it shows features characteristic of juvenile polyps: dilated glands, surface foveolar hyperplasia, and lamina propria edema with inflammation. However, it also contains bundles of smooth muscle scattered in the lamina propria (*arrowheads*), a feature that overlaps with Peutz-Jeghers polyps.

Figure 2-33. Juvenile polyp, higher magnification of the previous figure. The lamina propria contains smooth muscle bundles (*arrowheads*) streaming at various angles. One might consider a diagnosis of Peutz-Jeghers polyps based on this finding; the patient, however, was known to have juvenile polyposis syndrome.

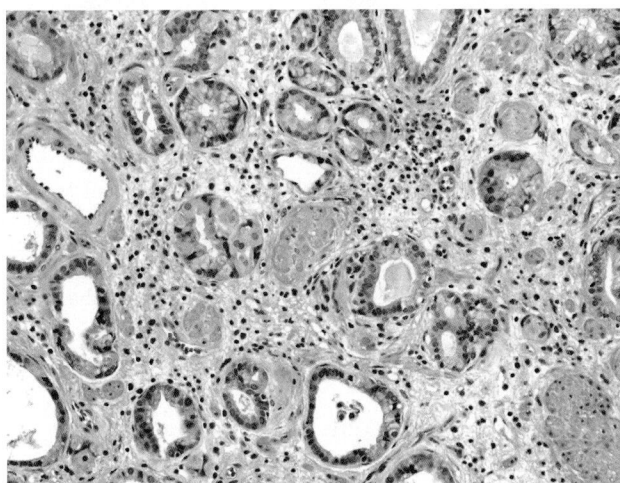

Figure 2-34. Juvenile polyp, separate high-magnification area of the previous figure. Small disorganized bundles of smooth muscle within gastric polyps, such as seen here, are a red flag for hamartomatous polyps, particularly the Peutz-Jeghers type. This example, however, is from a patient with juvenile polyposis syndrome, emphasizing the histologic overlap among gastric syndromic polyps.

PEARLS & PITFALLS: An Approach to Unusual or Potentially Syndromic Gastric Polyps

Akin to gastric Peutz-Jeghers polyps, the gastric juvenile polyp can defy classification and may be indistinguishable from the polyps of other syndromes (e.g., Peutz-Jeghers and Cronkhite-Canada syndrome) and common hyperplastic polyps. When confronted with an unusual gastric polyp the following approach is recommended: (1) use a low threshold to report juvenile polyps (or any hamartomatous polyp); (2) investigate into the patient's medical record for family history, clinical presentation, and endoscopic findings; (3) review any prior pathology specimens, such as previous GI polyps; and (4) communicate with the clinician for a multidisciplinary approach to follow-up or surveillance.

Cronkhite-Canada Syndrome Polyp

Cronkhite-Canada syndrome is a rare, noninherited clinical condition characterized by GI hamartomatous polyposis and the dermatologic triad of alopecia, onychodystrophy, and hyperpigmentation.[21,22] Consider this syndrome when numerous biopsies show juvenile polyp–like features: cystically dilated and tortuous glands containing proteinaceous fluid or inspissated mucus with a background lamina propria showing marked edema and chronic inflammation (Figs. 2.35–2.41).[23] At first glance, the changes resemble inflammatory-type polyps and are nonspecific in the absence of clinical information, but the tip-off will be the diffuse nature of the changes and the lack of intervening normal mucosa. Given the 55% 5-year mortality rate, consideration for and recognition of this condition is critical such that patients receive appropriate treatment.

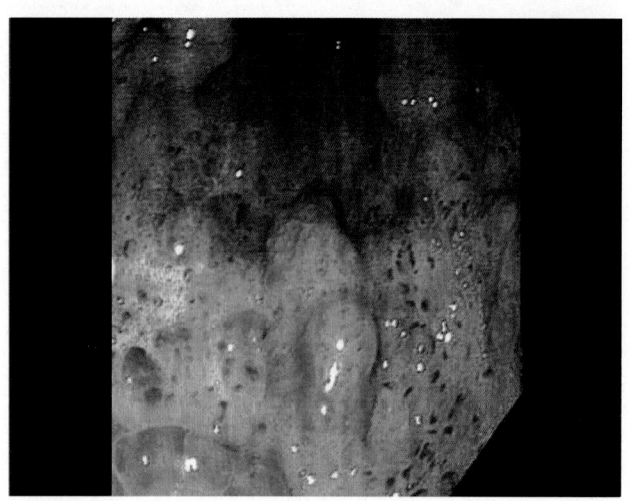

Figure 2-35. Cronkhite-Canada syndrome. Diffuse polyposis is seen in the stomach (pictured) and throughout the upper and lower gastrointestinal tract.

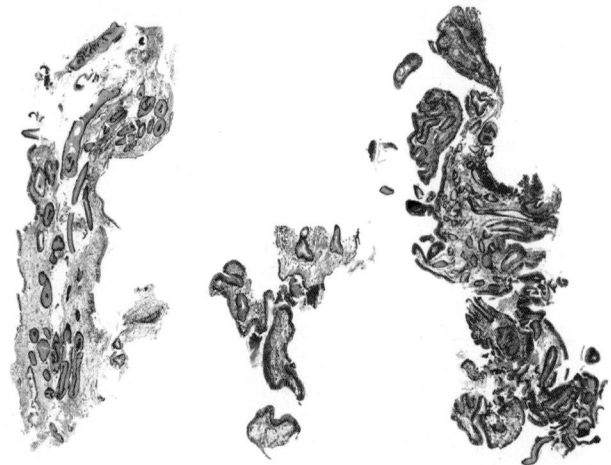

Figure 2-36. Cronkhite-Canada syndrome, gastric antrum. Multiple biopsies of the stomach show the diffuse nature of this disease. The mucosa is atrophic with abundant edematous lamina propria, similar to that seen in juvenile polyps. The similarities between the antrum, body, and fundus (see the next two figures) emphasize the diffuse process.

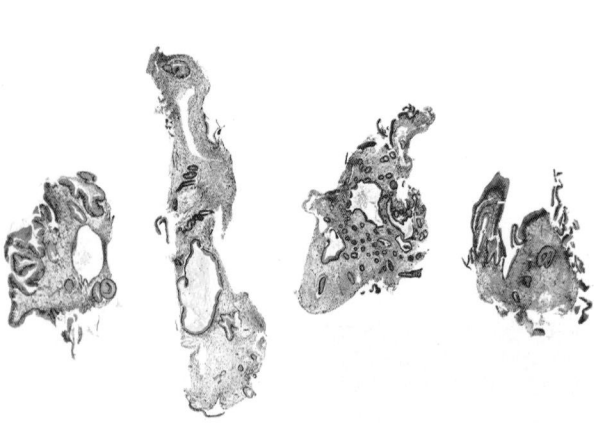

Figure 2-37. Cronkhite-Canada syndrome, gastric body. These biopsies from the gastric body show cystically dilated glands and marked lamina propria edema. At first glance, they resemble juvenile polyps. However, these changes are found in random samples of nonpolypoid mucosa. One of the key diagnostic clues to Cronkhite-Canada syndrome is the involvement of nonpolypoid mucosa.

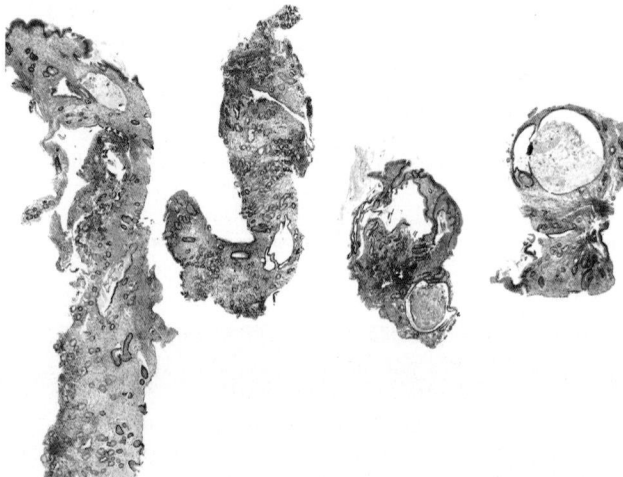

Figure 2-38. Cronkhite-Canada syndrome, gastric fundus. As in the previous two figures, multiple biopsies of the gastric fundus show diffuse changes involving all tissue fragments. There is atrophy of the oxyntic glands, abundant lamina propria edema, and cystically dilated glands with inspissated proteinaceous material.

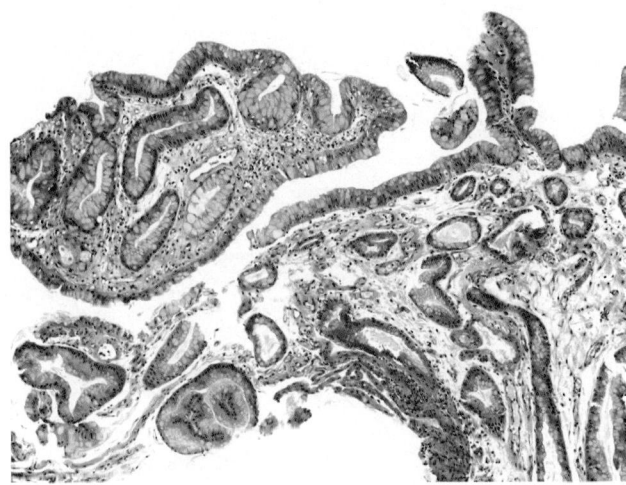

Figure 2-39. Cronkhite-Canada syndrome. Polypoid and nonpolypoid mucosa is histologically similar to juvenile polyps. The edematous lamina propria contains variable inflammation, and focal areas may show erosion and reactive epithelial changes.

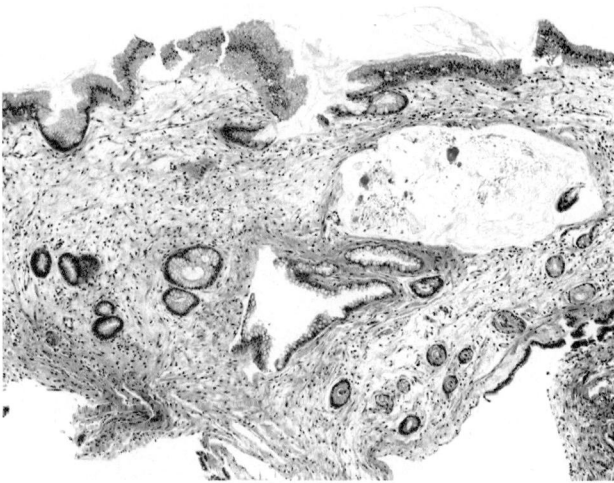

Figure 2-40. Cronkhite-Canada syndrome. There is an excess of edematous lamina propria and dilated irregular glands. In isolation, the findings suggest a juvenile polyp or inflammatory polyp. When these changes are found diffusely in both polypoid and nonpolypoid mucosa, consider Cronkhite-Canada syndrome and look for the clinical triad of alopecia, onychodystrophy (changes in nail color or quality), and hyperpigmentation.

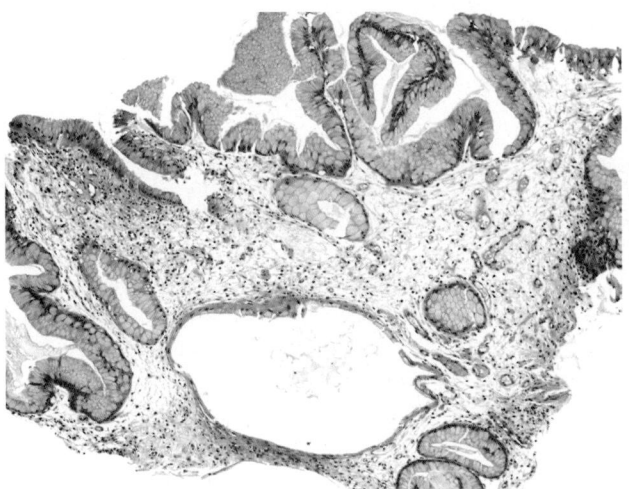

Figure 2-41. Cronkhite-Canada syndrome. The mucosa contains cystically dilated glands and edematous lamina propria with sparse inflammatory cells, similar in appearance to juvenile polyps.

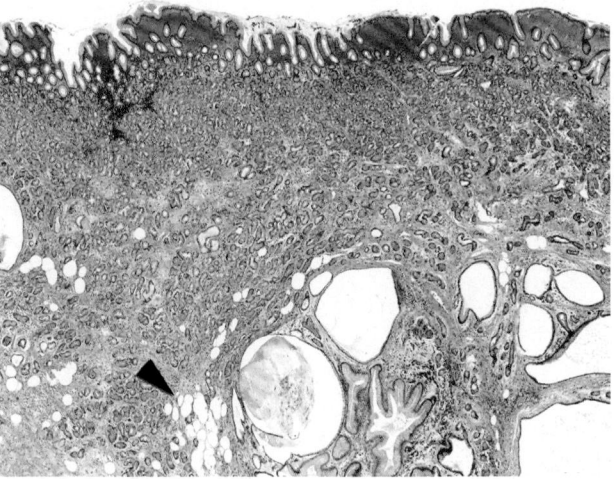

Figure 2-42. Cowden syndrome gastric polyp. Gastrointestinal lesions in PTEN hamartoma tumor syndrome or Cowden syndrome include hamartomatous polyps, lipomas, ganglioneuromas, and inflammatory polyps. This gastric hamartomatous polyp from a patient with Cowden syndrome contains mucosal adipocytes (*arrowhead*) and dilated, distorted glands.

PTEN Hamartoma Tumor Syndrome and Cowden Syndrome Polyp

Cowden syndrome is inherited in an autosomal dominant fashion and is the best described phosphatase and tensin homolog (PTEN) hamartoma syndrome with 66% to 100% of affected individuals reported to have gastric or duodenal polyps.[24-26] The range of clinical manifestations of Cowden syndrome includes mucocutaneous and extracutaneous hamartomatous tumors in multiple organ systems and characteristic dermatologic manifestations, such as trichilemmomas, oral fibromas, and punctate palmoplantar keratoses. This syndrome is highly associated with an increased risk of carcinomas of the breast (cumulative risk as high as 85%), endometrium (13% to 28%), thyroid (3% to 35%), kidney (13% to 34%), and colorectum (66% to 93%).[25-27] This increased risk of malignancy underscores the importance of reporting any hamartomatous polyp within the gastric mucosa and thus alerting clinicians to screen for a polyposis syndrome. Gastrointestinal lesions include hamartomatous polyps, lipomas, ganglioneuromas, and inflammatory polyps (Figs. 2.42–2.44). These lesions may

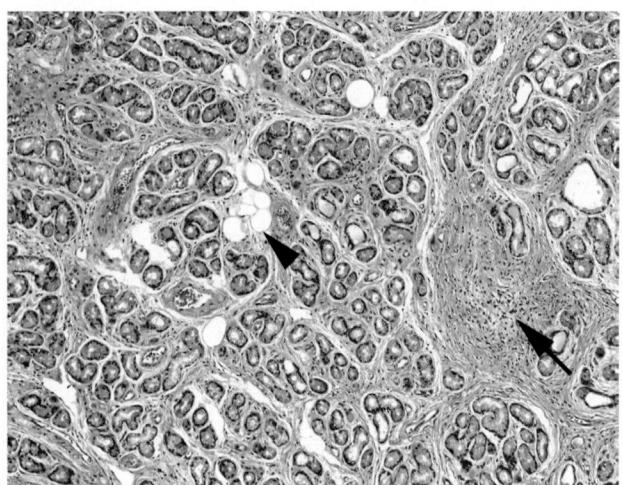

Figure 2-43. Cowden syndrome gastric polyp. This polyp shows lobules of glands, similar to that of Peutz-Jeghers polyps, but the presence of adipocytes (*arrowhead*) and neural tissue (*arrow*) argue against this diagnosis. This mixed hamartomatous polyp is from a patient with Cowden syndrome.

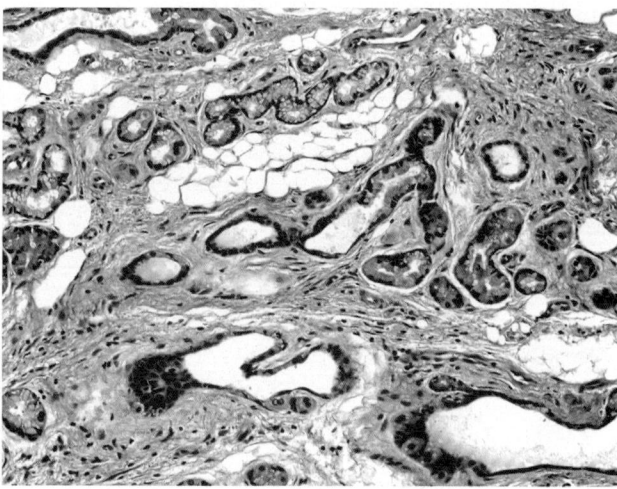

Figure 2-44. Cowden syndrome gastric polyp. The lamina propria between these distorted gastric glands is myxoid and contains hamartomatous elements, such as adipose tissue.

also be found in Bannayan-Riley Ruvalcaba syndrome and adult Lhermitte-Duclos disease, both rare disorders characterized by *PTEN* mutations. Proteus and proteus-like syndromes, although also belonging to the *PTEN* mutation family, do not feature GI hamartomas as a prominent finding.

> **PEARLS & PITFALLS: An Algorithm for Separating Gastric Hyperplastic and Hamartomatous Polyps**
>
> When encountering an unusual hyperplasticlike gastric polyp (e.g., containing foveolar hyperplasia, dilated and distorted glands, lamina propria edema, and chronic inflammation), always consider the possibility of a hamartomatous polyp or syndrome, even in the absence of any obvious hamartomatous element. An algorithmic approach is provided in Fig. 2.45.

EPITHELIAL POLYPS

Epithelial polyps are the most commonly encountered gastric polyps. These include gastric hyperplastic polyps, fundic gland polyps (FGPs), and adenomatous polyps, all of which are associated with distinctly different clinical contexts, as discussed later. Less common epithelial lesions manifesting as polyps include NETs, discussed separately in this chapter.

Hyperplastic Polyp

These benign epithelial proliferations are the second most common type of gastric polyp, and, in contrast to the incidental colonic hyperplastic polyp, gastric hyperplastic polyps are highly associated with background mucosal injury (85%), including *Helicobacter* infection (25%), reactive/chemical gastropathy (21%), AMAG (12%), and environmental metaplastic atrophic gastritis (8%).[28] Other associated conditions include mucosal ulcerations and erosions, ostomy sites, and gastroesophageal reflux disease, which, notably, are also forms of mucosal injury. Although they may be found at any age, gastric hyperplastic polyps occur more frequently with increasing age (mean age 65 to 75 years) and are female predominant. The lesions are solitary in 75% of cases and, owing to their foveolar origin, are found in all regions of the stomach with fairly even distribution. When large, these lesions may cause gastric outlet obstruction (Fig. 2.46); recurrence following polypectomy or endoscopic resection is common (up to 50%).[29,30]

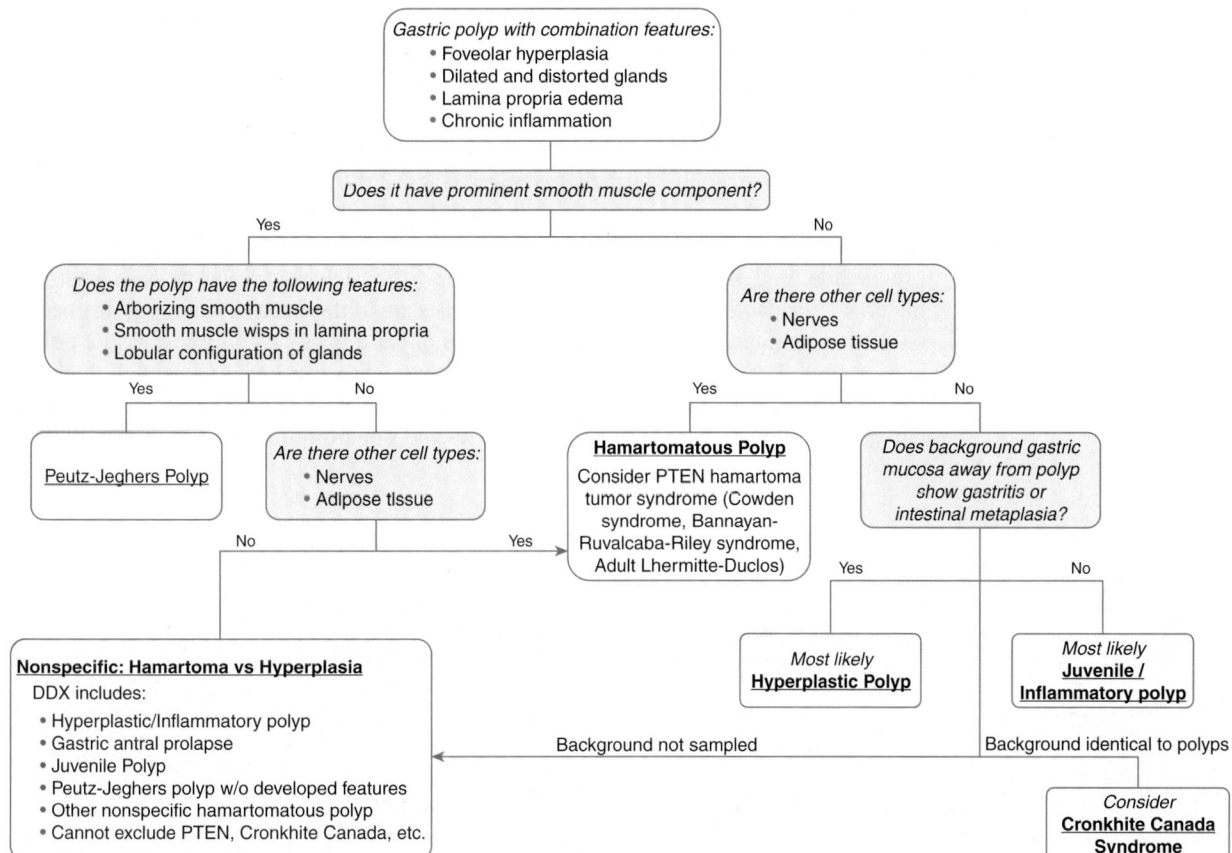

Gastric polyp with combination features:
- Foveolar hyperplasia
- Dilated and distorted glands
- Lamina propria edema
- Chronic inflammation

Does it have prominent smooth muscle component?

Yes → *Does the polyp have the following features:*
- Arborizing smooth muscle
- Smooth muscle wisps in lamina propria
- Lobular configuration of glands

Yes → Peutz-Jeghers Polyp

No → *Are there other cell types:*
- Nerves
- Adipose tissue

No → **Nonspecific: Hamartoma vs Hyperplasia**
DDX includes:
- Hyperplastic/Inflammatory polyp
- Gastric antral prolapse
- Juvenile Polyp
- Peutz-Jeghers polyp w/o developed features
- Other nonspecific hamartomatous polyp
- Cannot exclude PTEN, Cronkhite Canada, etc.

Yes → **Hamartomatous Polyp**

No → *Are there other cell types:*
- Nerves
- Adipose tissue

Yes → **Hamartomatous Polyp**
Consider PTEN hamartoma tumor syndrome (Cowden syndrome, Bannayan-Ruvalcaba-Riley syndrome, Adult Lhermitte-Duclos)

No → *Does background gastric mucosa away from polyp show gastritis or intestinal metaplasia?*

Yes → *Most likely* **Hyperplastic Polyp**

No → *Most likely* **Juvenile / Inflammatory polyp**

Background not sampled → **Nonspecific: Hamartoma vs Hyperplasia**

Background identical to polyps → *Consider* **Cronkhite Canada Syndrome**

Figure 2-45. A flow diagram for interpreting unusual gastric polyps. The histologic overlap of hyperplastic and syndromic gastric polyps can be a challenge during routine signout, but most can be handled by applying the simple algorithmic approach illustrated in this figure.

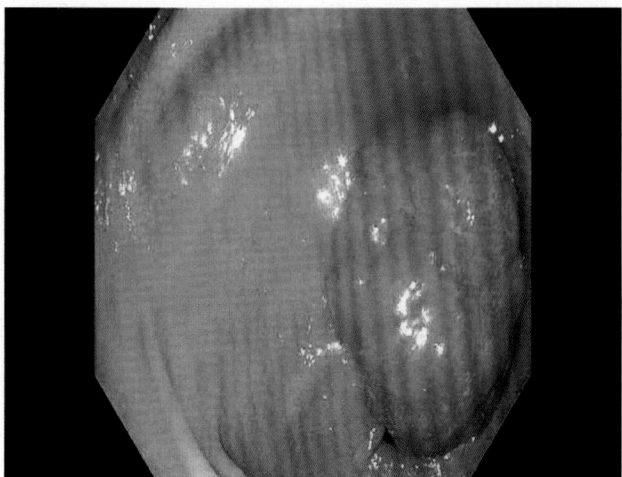

Figure 2-46. Gastric hyperplastic polyp. This antral-based gastric polyp protrudes into the lumen with a lobulated appearance. The entire lesion should be resected for histologic evaluation, and a separate jar containing tandem biopsies of the surrounding flat mucosa should also be submitted by the endoscopist to evaluate for background etiologic factors (e.g., *H. pylori*, AMAG).

Histologically, the polypoid mucosa often has a broad pedicle and shows elongated and distorted pits lined by a single layer of foveolar epithelial cells. There is wide histologic variability: the gastric pits and glands may show cystic dilation separated by edematous lamina propria with mixed inflammatory cells (Fig. 2.47), or there may be glandular crowding with gastric foveolar hyperplasia (Fig. 2.48). Surface erosion is common and may be accompanied by reactive epithelial changes (Figs. 2.49 and 2.50). Always ensure that a quick search for IM and dysplasia is performed (Figs. 2.51 and 2.52). Given the high association with surrounding mucosal inflammation and damage, and the potential for neoplastic progression, pathologists should carefully review the background flat mucosa when such material is available. Because not all endoscopists are in the habit of doing so, this necessitates advising them to submit separate samples of flat mucosa every time a gastric polyp is encountered. Recommended biopsy protocols exist, the most widely accepted of which is the Sydney protocol, which includes five mucosal samples: two each from greater and lesser curvatures (to include both antrum and body) and one from incisura (transition zone).

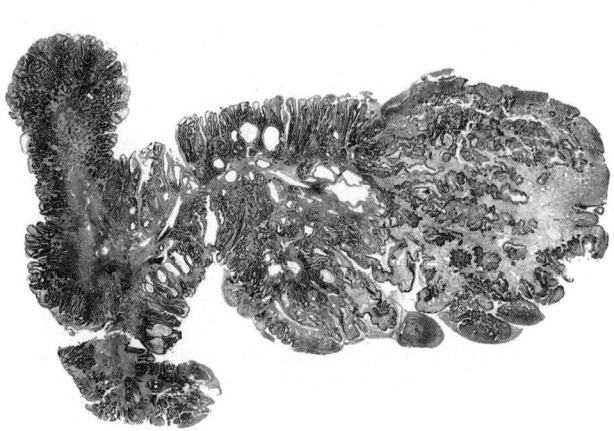

Figure 2-47. Gastric hyperplastic polyp. Gastric hyperplastic polyps have a wide range of appearances. This example shows a broad, rounded fingerlike projection at low magnification, with tortuous distorted and dilated glands, abundant lamina propria, and surface erosion. The features are similar to the juvenile polyp in Fig. 2.25, but this patient does not have a history of juvenile polyposis syndrome.

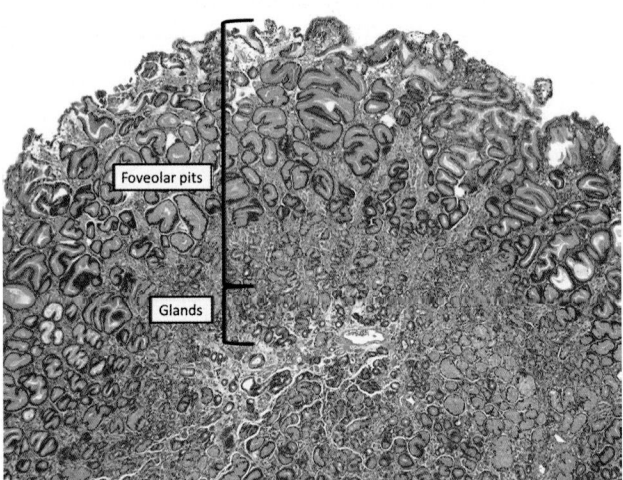

Figure 2-48. Gastric hyperplastic polyp. The histologic spectrum ranges from stroma-rich, like the previous example, to gland-rich, as seen here. This polyp contains tightly packed glands and marked foveolar hyperplasia with elongated tortuous foveolar pits, similar to chemical/reactive gastropathy. In this case, the gastric pits comprise about 80% of the mucosal thickness (normal is up to 25% in the body/fundus and up to 50% in the antrum).

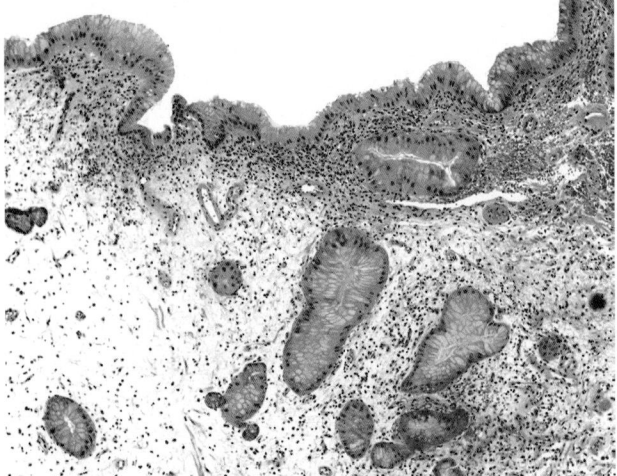

Figure 2-49. Reactive atypia in a gastric hyperplastic polyp. Epithelial cells may show reactive changes, such as mild nuclear hyperchromasia and enlargement due to inflammation or erosion.

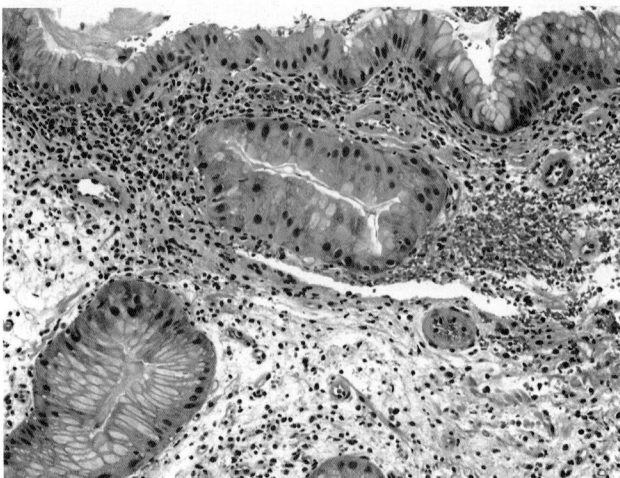

Figure 2-50. Reactive atypia in a gastric hyperplastic polyp, higher magnification of the previous figure. Reassuring features for reactive atypia are the presence of preserved nuclear to cytoplasmic ratio, indistinct nucleoli, lack of nuclear crowding, and absence of an abrupt transition from normal.

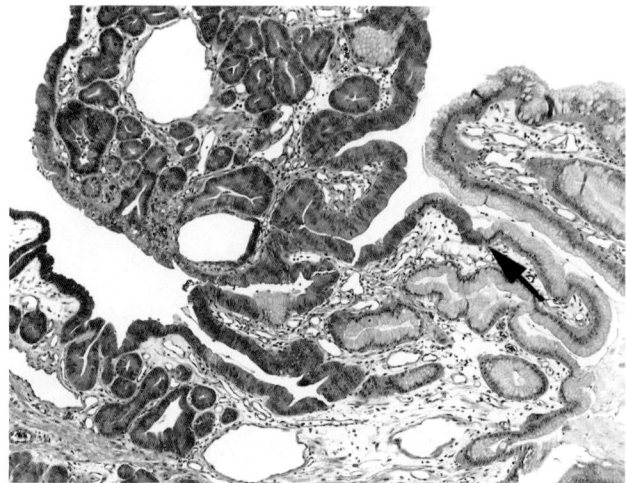

Figure 2-51. Low-grade dysplasia arising in a hyperplastic polyp. Most dysplasia can be identified at low magnification by the presence of stark hyperchromasia and nuclear crowding. An abrupt transition from normal to dysplastic (*arrow*) is a helpful clue. The nuclei in this example remain elongated, and the glandular architecture is simple, supporting classification as low-grade dysplasia.

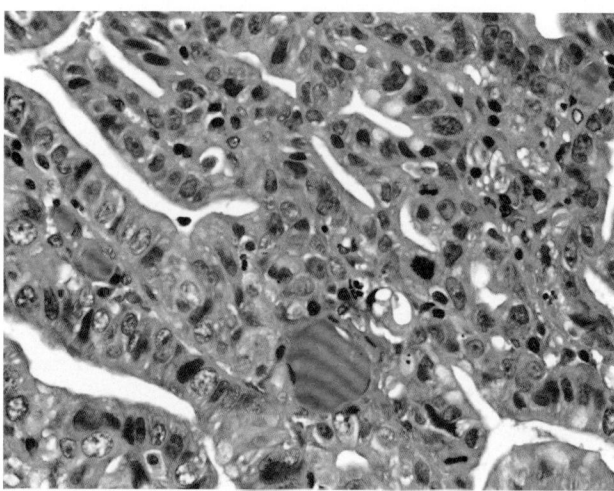

Figure 2-52. High-grade dysplasia. Both glands and cells are crowded in this example. The glands are back to back and architecturally complex. The cells are no longer elongated and show loss of nuclear polarity. Prominent nucleoli and irregular nuclear contours are present. Frequent mitoses and apoptoses are evident.

> **PEARLS & PITFALLS: The Background Flat Mucosa May Reveal the Etiology of the Hyperplastic Polyp**
>
> Always search for an etiologic factor when encountering these reactive lesions. Treatment of an underlying condition, such as eradication of *Helicobacter* infection, can prevent further polyp formation and recurrence.

SAMPLE NOTE: Gastric Hyperplastic Polyp Submitted Without Background Flat Mucosa

Stomach, Antrum, Polyp, Biopsy

- Gastric hyperplastic polyp, see Comment.

Comment
Gastric hyperplastic polyps are reactive lesions highly associated with mucosal injury and inflammation. Should repeat endoscopy be performed, separately submitted biopsies of the background flat mucosa to evaluate the gastric environment would be of interest.

Despite their classification as a regenerative growth, large (>2 cm) polyps may harbor IM or dysplasia and subsequent risk of malignant transformation (2% to 20%).[28,31-33] Similar to other areas of the GI tract, gastric dysplasia is categorized as negative for dysplasia, low-grade dysplasia (LGD), high-grade dysplasia (HGD), or indefinite for dysplasia. The microscopic features also parallel those seen in other areas of the GI tract with LGD showing epithelial changes of hyperchromasia, nuclear elongation, and pseudostratification extending to the mucosal surface (Fig. 2.51). Other features include nuclear atypia, prominent nucleoli, and increased mitoses and apoptoses. High-grade epithelial dysplasia is characterized by greater nuclear pleomorphism, anisonucleosis, loss of cell polarity, and architectural complexity with back-to-back or cribriform gland formation (Fig. 2.52). These descriptive terms sound quite similar to the words used to describe the conventional tubular adenoma, yet gastric dysplasia remains slightly more challenging to interpret. Contributors to this struggle include the array of gastric dysplastic lesions (e.g., gastric adenomas include foveolar, intestinal, pyloric gland, and oxyntic gland types; see later discussion) and the frequency of background gastric inflammatory changes, from which one must differentiate reactive and dysplastic lesions. The abrupt histologic transition of dysplasia remains the best practical tool in dysplasia assessment and is evident even at low magnification.

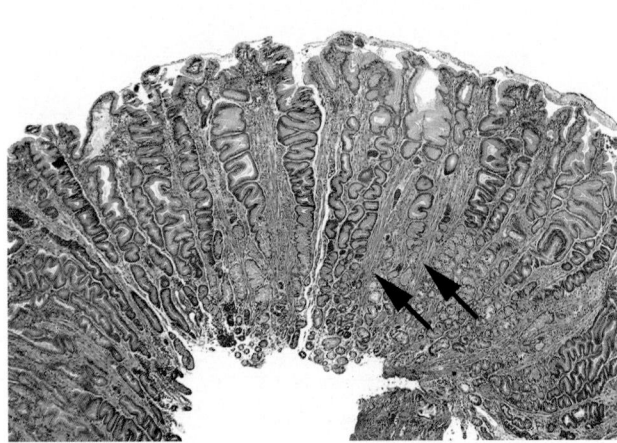

Figure 2-53. Gastric antral prolapse. Gastric antral prolapse can produce polypoid areas, not to be mistaken for hyperplastic polyps. The presence of tortuous gastric pits and exuberant smooth muscle (*arrows*) streaming perpendicular to the luminal surface are features of antral prolapse.

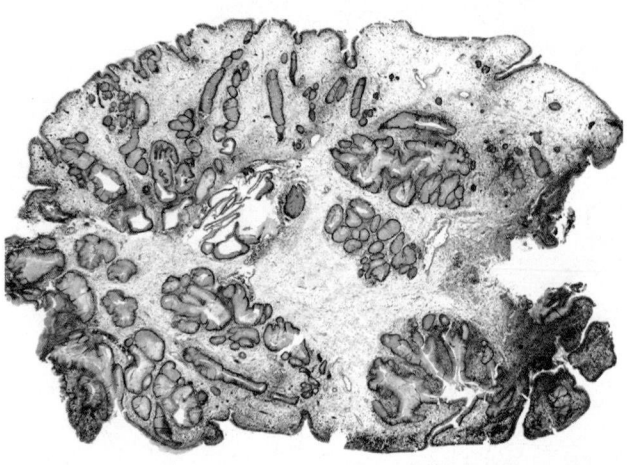

Figure 2-54. Gastric hyperplastic polyp. This example is small, rounded and contains an excess of pale edematous lamina propria, variably distorted glands, and inflammation. Compare this example with the juvenile polyp from Fig. 2.26. There are no reliable histologic features to differentiate the two entities aside from the presence of background mucosal damage (e.g., *H. pylori*, AMAG, gastritis), which favors a gastric hyperplastic/inflammatory polyp.

The gastric hyperplastic polyp is plagued with challenges in differential diagnoses. Gastric mucosal prolapse may form polypoid areas, but this finding is usually limited to the gastric antrum. Histologically, mucosal prolapse lacks the highly edematous stroma and cystic dilated glands/pits of hyperplastic polyps. Instead, the lamina propria contains streaming strands of smooth muscle arranged perpendicular to the gastric surface, and pits show corkscrew tortuosity such as that seen in chemical gastropathy (Fig. 2.53). Several other conditions enter into the differential diagnosis, most of which show so much histologic overlap as to be indistinguishable from one another. The most common of these is the inflammatory polyp, which contains variable degrees of inflammation in combination with features also seen in hyperplastic polyps, such as foveolar hyperplasia, cystic and distorted glands, lamina propria edema, and surface ulceration/erosion. In some instances, these features show so much histologic overlap with the hyperplastic polyp that the inflammatory polyp probably represents the same process at different temporal intervals. That is to say, inflamed hyperplastic polyps may be indistinguishable from inflammatory polyps, and when the inflammation of an inflammatory polyp subsides, it may resemble a hyperplastic polyp or juvenile polyp (Figs. 2.47 and 2.54). Interpretation and sign out of these overlapping gastric lesions can be handled in a fashion similar to that for the gastric hamartomatous polyps (see later discussion). Some observers prefer to lump these lesions together, signing them as "inflammatory/hyperplastic polyps."

Other differential diagnoses include hamartomatous polyps such as juvenile polyps and Peutz-Jeghers polyps (Fig. 2.55), which also can be histologically indistinguishable in the stomach despite having highly characteristic morphology in the colon and small bowel.[3] Thus, if there is suspicion for a hamartomatous polyposis syndrome after the review of gastric biopsies, include a diagnosis comment suggesting that bidirectional endoscopy could identify other sites of involvement and more characteristic histology. Other hamartomatous tumor syndromes, such as the PTEN hamartomatous tumor syndromes (i.e., Cowden syndrome, Bannayan-Riley-Ruvalcaba syndrome, and adult Lhermitte-Duclos disease) and Cronkhite-Canada syndrome also display polyps that overlap histologically with gastric hyperplastic polyps. However, attention to clues such as nonepithelial components, such as adipocytes or neural proliferations within the polyps, should alert one to the possibility of a PTEN syndrome (Figs. 2.42–2.44). Cronkhite-Canada syndrome, although often referred to as a hamartomatous polyposis syndrome, actually represents diffuse mucosal changes that endoscopically appear nodular and/or polypoid owing to intervening areas of mucosal atrophy. These submitted "polyps" are similar to hyperplastic polyps as they contain dilated and cystic glands, lamina propria edema, and variable inflammation. Clues to diagnosis

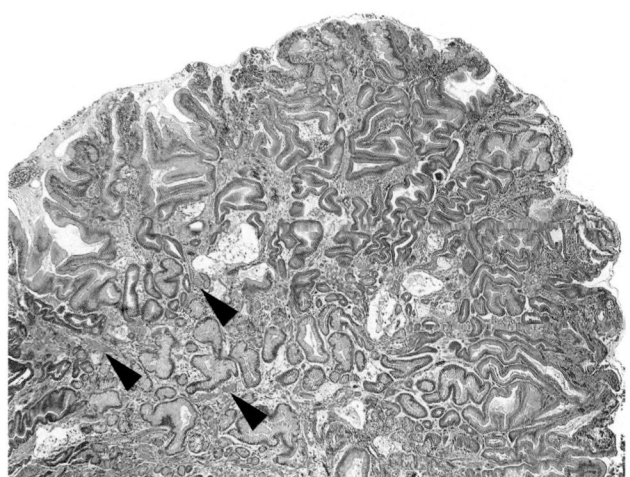

Figure 2-55. Gastric hyperplastic polyp. This hyperplastic polyp features crowded glands with architectural distortion and foveolar hyperplasia, in contrast to the previous example, which was more edematous and less cellular. The small disorganized bundles of smooth muscle (*arrowheads*) in the lamina propria raise the possibility of a hamartomatous polyp, but the background mucosa in this case showed erosive iron pill gastritis (not pictured), supporting this as a reactive lesion over a hamartomatous polyp.

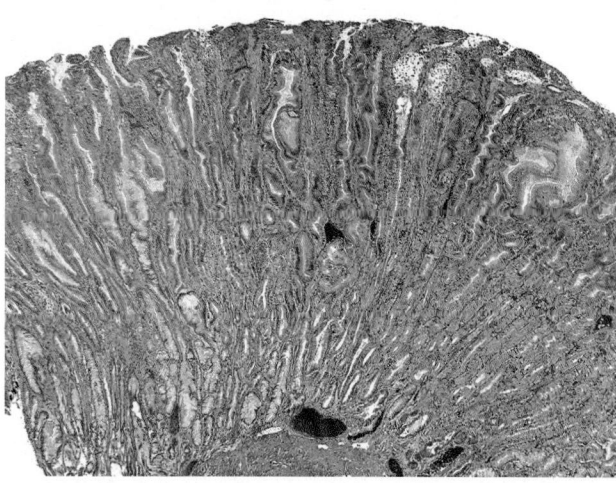

Figure 2-56. Menetrier disease. Compared with the foveolar hyperplasia seen in the previous figure, the marked foveolar hyperplasia in Menetrier disease is diffuse, giving rise to giant gastric folds throughout the stomach.

include diffuse changes throughout the upper and lower GI tract in both the polypoid and *nonpolypoid* mucosa and the finding of other ectodermal features (e.g., onychodystrophy and alopecia) (Figs. 2.35–2.41). Changes found in Menetrier disease are limited to the gastric body and fundus but are diffuse with striking foveolar hyperplasia and an absence of intervening normal mucosa (Fig. 2.56). The provided algorithmic approach (Fig. 2.45) can help differentiate these challenging cases (Fig. 2.57).

CHECKLIST: Diagnostic Considerations for Gastric Hyperplastic Polyps

□ Always check background flat mucosa for inflammatory causes, such as *Helicobacter pylori* or autoimmune gastritis
□ Gastric hyperplastic polyp
□ Inflammatory polyp
□ Gastric antral prolapse
□ Gastric Peutz-Jeghers polyp
□ Gastric juvenile polyp
□ PTEN syndromes (Cowden syndrome, Bannayan-Riley-Ruvalcaba syndrome, adult Lhermitte-Duclos disease)
□ Cronkhite-Canada syndrome
□ Menetrier disease

Fundic Gland Polyp

Fundic gland polyps (FGPs) comprise 77% of all gastric polyps,[1] are found exclusively in areas where fundic glands reside (i.e., body and fundus only), and are typically sessile and small (<2 mm, and rarely >1 cm). They may arise either sporadically or associated with a syndrome, the best known of which is familial adenomatous polyposis (FAP) syndrome, and this results in unique clinicopathologic characteristics for each group (see Table 2.2). Sporadic FGPs are usually single or few in number (Fig. 2.58) and are asymptomatic incidental findings that, in contrast to hyperplastic polyps, are not associated with an inflammatory or atrophic mucosal backdrop. In fact, their presence is inversely correlated with *Helicobacter* infection

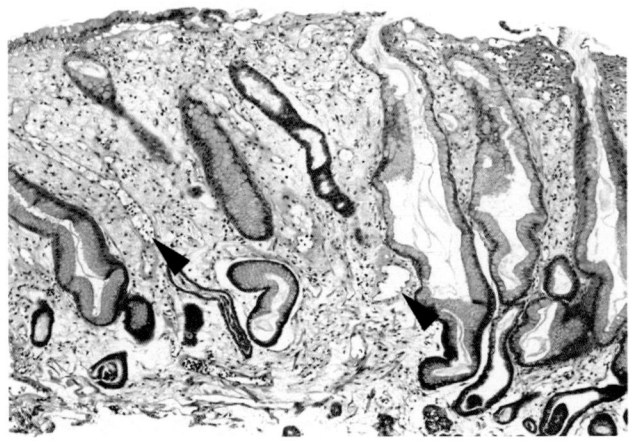

Figure 2-57. Gastric hyperplastic polyp. Lamina propria edema, mild foveolar hyperplasia, and scattered chronic inflammatory cells can be seen in both hyperplastic and inflammatory polyps. This small polyp arose in a backdrop of portal hypertensive gastropathy (not pictured) and contains ectatic vessels in the lamina propria (*arrowheads*). Findings in the background flat mucosa aid in classifying gastric polyps.

TABLE 2.2: Fundic Gland Polyps: Sporadic Versus FAP Associated

Features	Sporadic	FAP-Associated
Number	Single; few when multiple (40%)	Multiple (90%); carpet of hundreds to thousands
Male to female ratio	F > M	F = M
Age	5th–6th decade; no children	3rd decade; can occur in children
Mutations	β-catenin	APC gene mutation; CTNNB1/β-catenin
Frequency of LGD	Low (<1%)	High (nearly half)
Progression to carcinoma	None reported	Case reports only
Surveillance	None, even when dysplasia detected	Upper endoscopy every 1–3 years for detection of duodenal and periampullary lesions; no specific surveillance for FGPs, even when dysplasia detected

F, female; FAP, familial adenomatous polyposis; FGP, fundic gland polyp; LGD, low-grade dysplasia; M, male.

and active gastritis.[34] In the sporadic setting, it is widely accepted that proton pump inhibitor (PPI) use is associated with FGPs,[35] and although these lesions reportedly regress with medication cessation, no proven causal pathogenetic relationship between PPIs and FGPs exists.[36] Other clinical associations include gastroesophageal reflux disease, gastric heterotopia, and colonic polyps (hyperplastic in men and adenomas in women).

Histologically, these polyps consist of dilated cystic oxyntic glands with distorted glandular architecture admixed with normal-appearing glands (Figs. 2.59 and 2.60). Parietal cells balloon into the lumen with snoutlike protuberances, sometimes resulting in exfoliated anucleate blebs with eosinophilic granules that clog the gland outlets

(Figs. 2.61 and 2.62). Some cystic spaces may be lined by columnar epithelium as a result of adjacent gastric pit dilation (Fig. 2.63), but most are lined by chief cells and parietal cells. The findings, for practical purposes, are identical to that of PPI effect, and distinction requires correlation with an endoscopic lesion (Fig. 2.64). Likewise, there are no differentiating histologic features between syndromic and sporadic FGPs, but the clinicopathologic features are distinct. For example, nearly all patients with FAP have FGPs (12.5% to 88% of patients with FAP, depending on age at time of endoscopy) and these polyps are more numerous than sporadic FGPs, often with hundreds or thousands in a carpet-like distribution.[37] FAP-associated FGPs also occur earlier than in the sporadic setting (third decade vs. fifth to sixth decade) and can be found among the pediatric population, which is exceptionally rare for sporadic FGPs. A key distinction of FAP-associated FGPs is their association with low-grade epithelial dysplasia, which is reported in up to half of cases (Figs. 2.65–2.69). Despite the high prevalence of dysplasia in these lesions, the risk of malignant transformation is exceptionally low, with only case reports in the literature.[38,39] By comparison, dysplasia develops in less than 1% of sporadic FGPs and has never been associated with progression to carcinoma.[34,40] Given the rarity of both HGD and carcinoma in either sporadic or FAP settings, surveillance is unnecessary for LGD in an FGP and surgical resection is never advised. Patients with FAP do require continued surveillance for other risk factors, however, such as duodenal polyposis and periampullary adenomas and adenocarcinomas.[41] Upper endoscopy and biopsy of selected polyps is recommended every 1 to 3 years, with closer screening warranted when a gastric adenoma is detected.

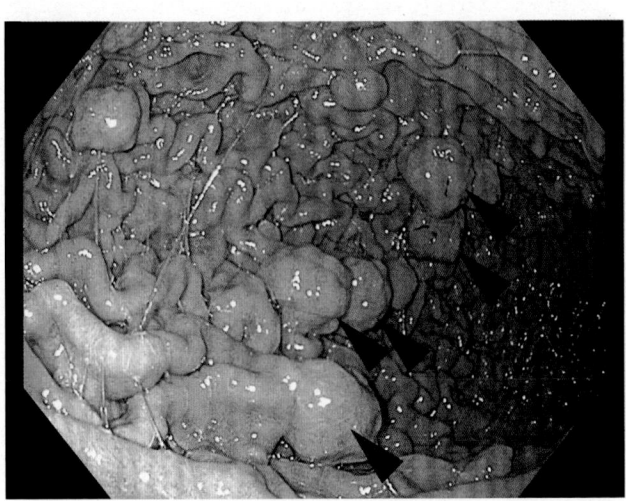

Figure 2-58. Fundic gland polyps (FGP). Multiple small sessile lesions (*arrowheads*) are seen in the gastric body. Sporadic FGPs may be multiple but usually few in number. When innumerable FGPs carpet the gastric corpus, consider a syndromic cause, such as familial adenomatous polyposis syndrome, *MutYH*-associated polyposis, or gastric adenocarcinoma and proximal polyposis syndrome.

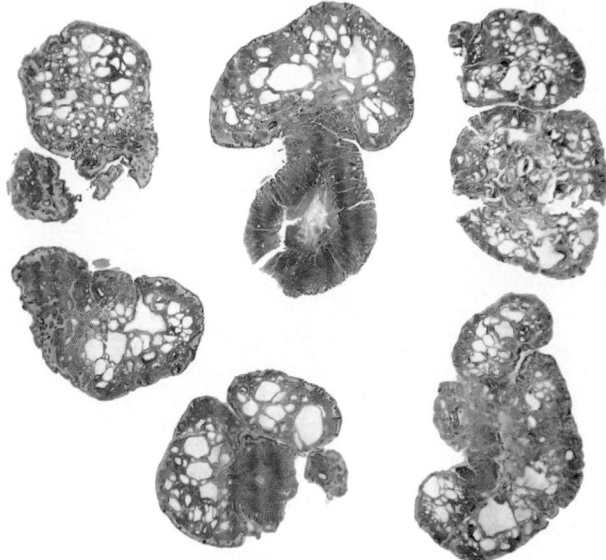

Figure 2-59. Fundic gland polyps, scanning magnification. These polypoid tissue fragments show dilated cystic glands with distorted architecture. Multiple polyps are frequently found, although endoscopists typically only sample one or two.

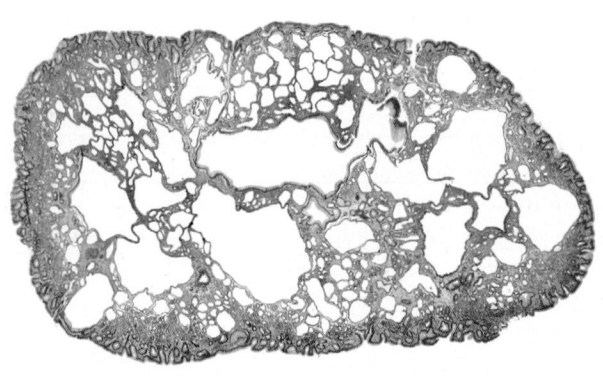

Figure 2-60. Fundic gland polyp. These small round polyps are expanded by cystically dilated oxyntic glands, and there is no significant increase in stroma. The surface epithelium is foveolar and unremarkable.

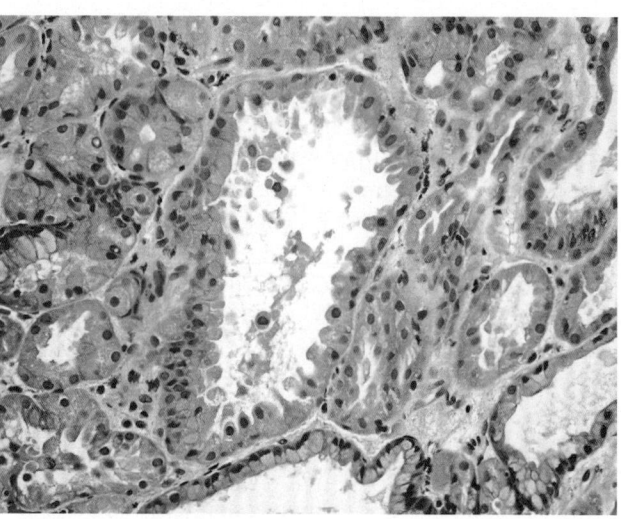

Figure 2-61. Fundic gland polyp. The cystic spaces are dilated oxyntic glands and are lined by *pink* parietal cells and *blue* chief cells. The parietal cells balloon into the lumen with snoutlike protuberances, and the lumen contains exfoliated cells.

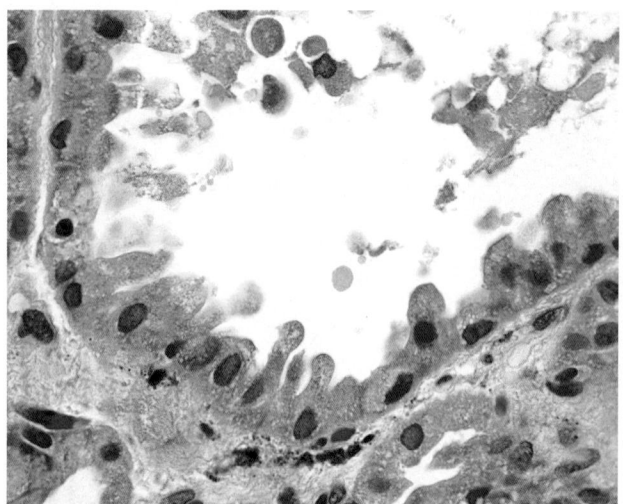

Figure 2-62. Fundic gland polyp. At high magnification, the parietal cells have brightly eosinophilic granular cytoplasm that protrudes toward the lumen, similar to apocrine metaplasia in the breast. The apical snouts produce anucleate granular blebs within the cystic space.

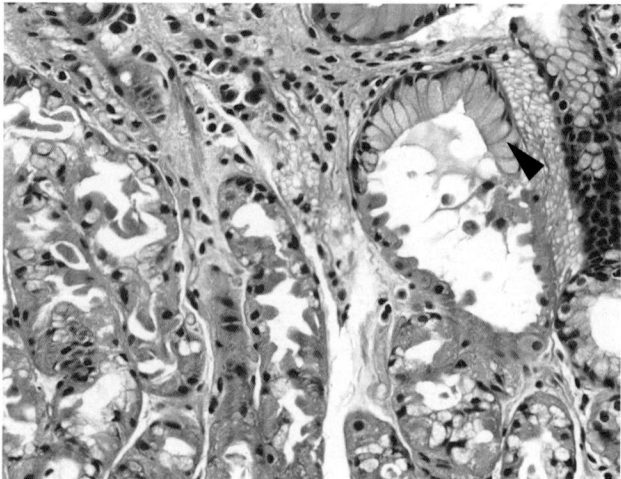

Figure 2-63. Fundic gland polyp. Some cystic spaces are partially lined by foveolar mucous cells (*arrowhead*), but this variation does not indicate a mixed polyp. The background dilated oxyntic glands and apical snouting of parietal cells are characteristic for fundic gland polyp.

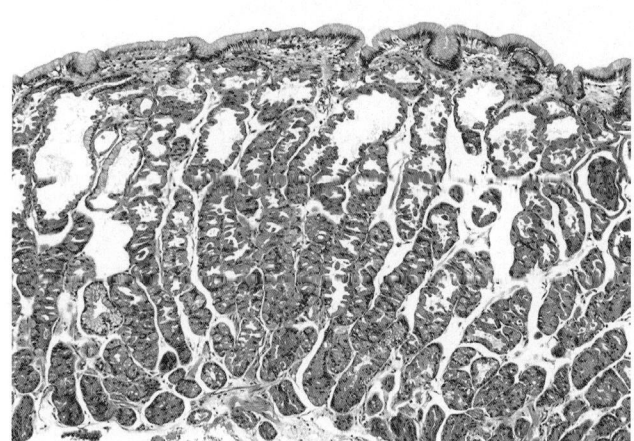

Figure 2-64. Proton pump inhibitor (PPI) effect. PPIs are associated with diffuse oxyntic gland dilation and apical snouting of parietal cells, similar to that seen in fundic gland polyps. Distinction between the two requires endoscopic correlation with a polypoid lesion or with medication history.

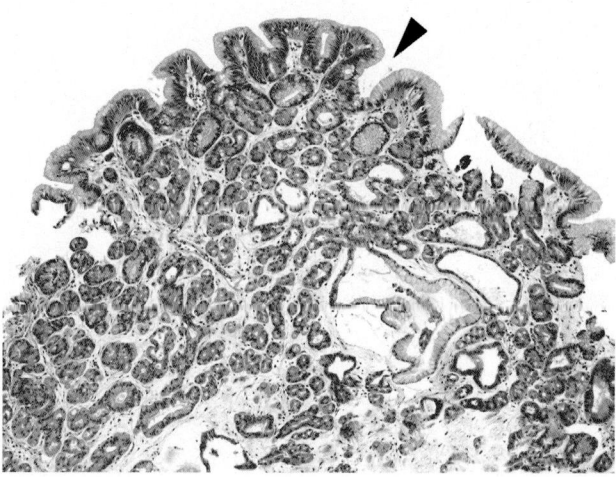

Figure 2-65. Low-grade dysplasia in a fundic gland polyp. Low-grade dysplasia is best identified as an area of eye-catching hyperchromasia at low magnification. An abrupt transition (*arrowhead*) between normal foveolar epithelium and an area of hyperchromasia is a helpful clue.

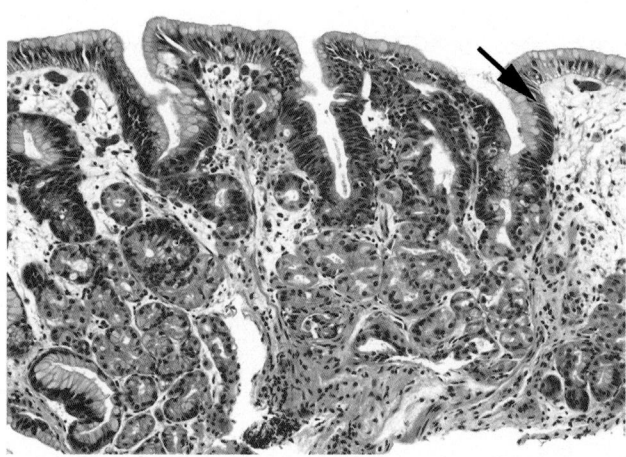

Figure 2-66. Low-grade dysplasia in a fundic gland polyp. Dysplasia in FGPs occurs in half of patients with FAP syndrome. Dysplasia can also be found in sporadic FGPs but is seen in <1%. An abrupt transition (*arrow*) from nondysplastic to dysplastic epithelium can usually be identified. The dysplastic foveolar epithelial cells show pseudostratification and nuclear crowding, imparting an area of distinct hyperchromasia.

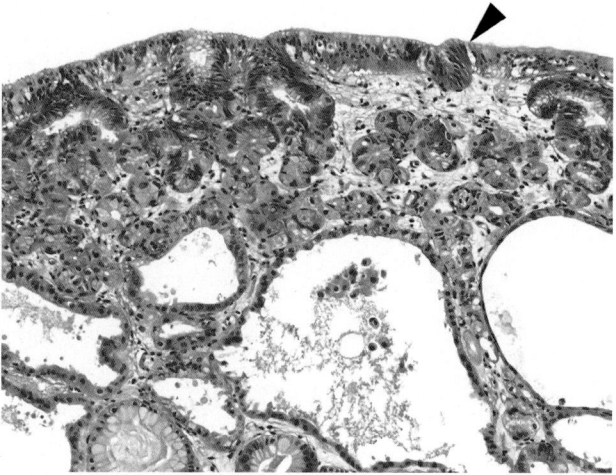

Figure 2-67. Low-grade dysplasia in a fundic gland polyp. Dysplasia affects the surface foveolar cells overlying the dilated oxyntic glands and extends down the foveolar-lined gastric pits. An abrupt surface transition (*arrowhead*) from nondysplastic cells is present.

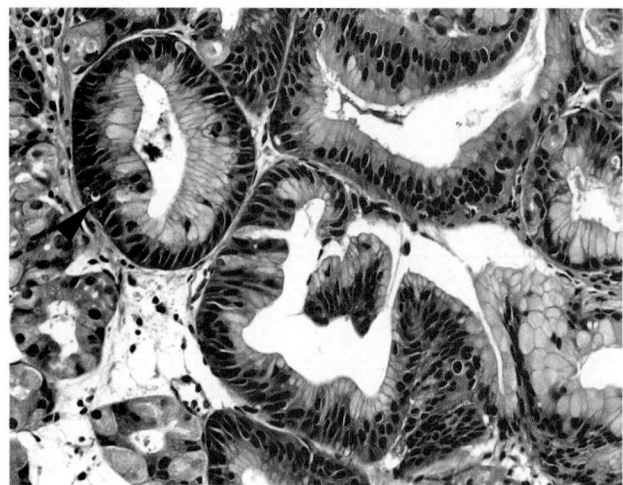

Figure 2-68. Low-grade dysplasia in a fundic gland polyp. Dysplasia affects the foveolar epithelium overlying the fundic glands and shows cytologic features of pseudostratification, nuclear crowding, increased mitotic activity, and apoptotic activity (*arrowhead*).

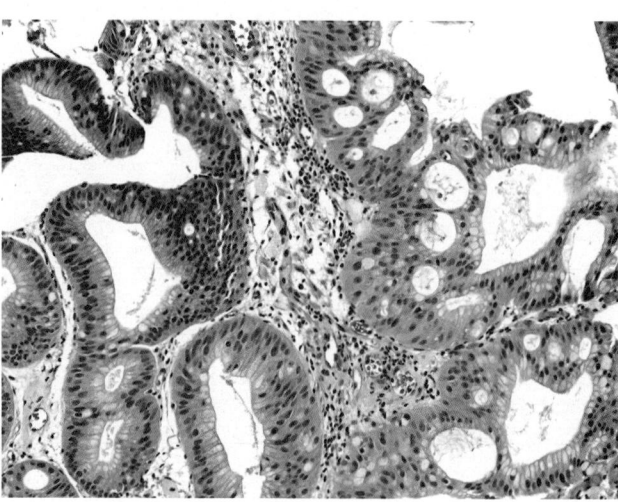

Figure 2-69. Low- and high-grade dysplasia in a fundic gland polyp. A distinct change in architecture and cytology is seen in the right side of the figure and can be arguably interpreted as high-grade dysplasia, in contrast to the characteristic low-grade dysplasia seen on the left. Dysplasia in fundic gland polyps, whether low or high grade, has negligible risk for malignant transformation.

An exception in FAP that is discussed later in this chapter is the syndrome termed gastric adenocarcinoma and proximal polyposis syndrome (GAPPS). GAPPS is a rare subvariant of FAP characterized by many FGPs and gastric adenocarcinoma.

FAQ: What is the surveillance protocol for LGD in an FGP? Are there differences in follow-up for LGD in sporadic versus FAP-associated FGPs?

Clinicians may be advised that *no surveillance is necessary* for LGD arising in FGPs, *whether FAP associated or sporadic*. This is a frequent finding, occurring in nearly half of patients with FAP, but progression to HGD or carcinoma is so rare as to be case report material. Carcinoma arising in a sporadic FGP has never been reported. Thus, specific follow-up for LGD arising in FGPs is unnecessary. However, other than the special situation of GAPPS noted earlier and later in the chapter, patients with FAP should continue their scheduled interval surveillance for duodenal polyposis and periampullary lesions, as these lesions carry risk for malignant progression.

PEARLS & PITFALLS

Diffuse fundic gland hyperplasia is commonly ascribed to PPI usage, but do not overlook the possibility of Zollinger-Ellison (ZE) syndrome when massive oxyntic gland hyperplasia is seen. This tumor-mediated syndrome is the result of a gastrinoma of the small bowel or pancreas causing elevated serum gastrin, which stimulates oxyntic gland hyperplasia and excessive gastric acid secretion, resulting in subsequent ulcers of the stomach or small bowel. This same gastrin stimulation can also give rise to gastric NETs (type 2), as a result of ECL-cell hyperplasia, discussed later in this chapter. Although most ZE syndrome cases are sporadic, 30% are the result of a defect in the *MEN1* tumor suppressor gene associated with the autosomal dominant syndrome multiple endocrine neoplasia type 1 (MEN1). As the name implies, it is important to identify these patients because they are at risk for neoplasia in multiple endocrine organs. Neoplasms of the pituitary, parathyroid, and pancreas (and small bowel) have conferred the moniker the "3P syndrome." Clinical testing for serum gastrin levels ≥10 times normal can suggest ZE syndrome, but more than half of patients with ZE have nondiagnostic serum gastrin results. In these cases, consider other studies such as gastric pH, imaging studies of the small bowel and pancreas, somatostatin receptor scintigraphy, and *MEN1* genotyping.

FAQ: What causes innumerable carpetlike FGPs?

When FGPs are innumerable, consider syndromic etiologies such as FAP, attenuated FAP, GAPPS, *MutYH*-associated polyposis, and sporadic FGPosis.[42,43] Differentiating these requires correlation with family history, physical examination, endoscopic findings, and genetic testing. Mutations of the *APC* gene are at the root of FAP and attenuated FAP. Point mutations of this same *APC* gene have also been identified in the more recently described GAPPS, which is now regarded as an FAP variant.[43] Mutations in *MutYH* characterize *MutYH*-associated polyposis, and mutations of *CTNNB1* (the gene that encodes for β-catenin) are seen in sporadic fundic gland polyposis (as well as nonsyndromic sporadic FGPs).[42,44]

KEY FEATURES: FGPs

- FGPs are the **most common type of gastric polyp**.
- Endoscopic finding of a discreet lesion separates FGPs from oxyntic gland hyperplasia such as seen in PPI use and ZE syndrome.
- Histologically, they are composed of **dilated cystic oxyntic glands** with hypertrophic parietal cells, some of which have **apocrine-like snouts**.
- Sporadic FGPs are typically single, **whereas innumerable polyps may be seen in the syndromic setting**.
- Syndromic associations include FAP syndrome, attenuated FAP, GAPPS, *MutYH*-associated polyposis, and sporadic fundic gland polyposis syndrome.
- **LGD** is common in FAP-associated FGPs (~50%) and uncommon in sporadic FGPs (<1%), but all have **negligible risk for malignant transformation and do not require surveillance**.

ADENOMATOUS POLYPS

By convention, polypoid dysplasia in the stomach is designated "gastric adenoma," and the degree of dysplasia is graded similar to other parts of the GI tract: low grade, high grade, or indefinite for dysplasia (Figs. 2.70–2.77). Similar to colon tubular adenomas, a diagnosis of gastric adenoma implies at least LGD. Gastric adenomas come in several varieties, including the intestinal type, foveolar type, pyloric gland adenoma (PGA), and oxyntic gland polyp/adenoma (see Table 2.3). Our understanding of this area continues to evolve, and much of the previous literature is difficult to interpret owing to several factors: (1) Divergent histologic criteria between Japanese and Western practices; Japanese pathologists, who contributed a significant bulk of the 20th century literature on this subject, did not require invasion to diagnose "carcinoma," whereas invasion is an explicit criterion of Western practice.[45] (2) Revision of nomenclature as a result of this discrepancy; definitions of gastric epithelial neoplasia were harmonized in the Vienna classification published in 2000, resulting in a system congruent with Western understanding.[46] (3) Subsequent ongoing revisions of polyp classification and nomenclature; oxyntic gland polyp/adenoma was previously classified as "gastric adenocarcinoma with chief cell differentiation."[47] (4) Lack of recognition or underreporting of certain gastric adenomas; for example, in one study, PGA was the third most common gastric polyp, yet only rare case reports were published on this entity previously.[48] (5) Histologic blends of "hybrid" polyps; these defy specific classification and continue to muddle the literature. Ongoing study in this area will most certainly yield new updates before a revised edition of this text. In the meantime, the following section depicts our current understanding for each of the gastric adenomas. Some bear risk for malignant progression, but each is remarkably different in prognosis and clinicopathologic associations, discussed later. As with gastric hyperplastic polyps, sampling the background flat mucosa is important to identify other risk factors (e.g., *H. pylori*, IM) and associated conditions such as AMAG.

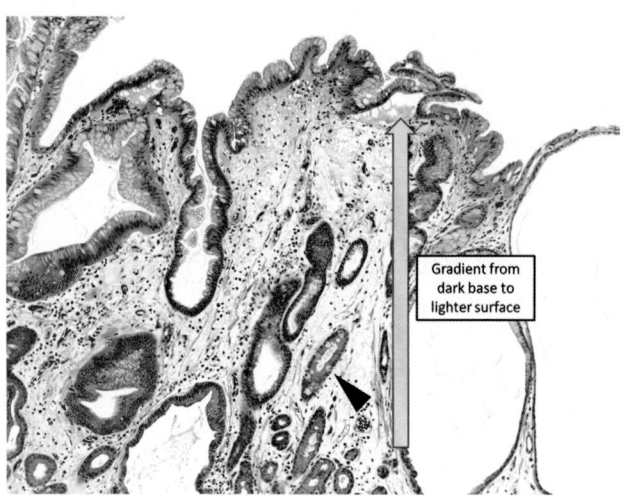

Figure 2-70. Reactive changes, negative for dysplasia. Areas of intestinal metaplasia (*arrowhead*) may be hyperchromatic at low power. However, this polyp shows a gradual gradient toward the lighter mature surface. Surface maturation is a reassuring feature for nondysplastic reactive changes.

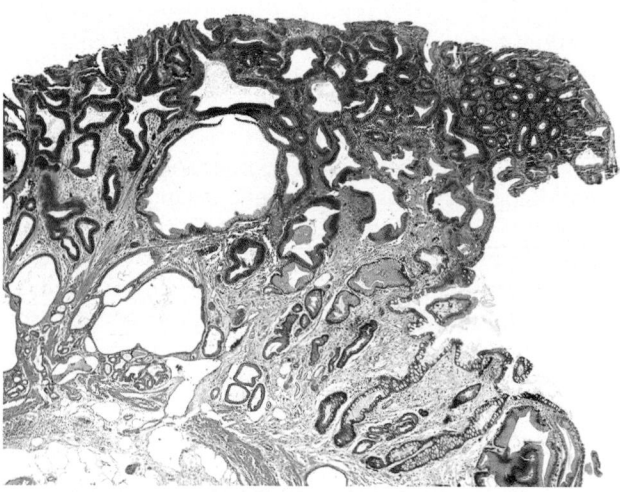

Figure 2-71. Gastric adenoma, intestinal type (low-grade dysplasia implied). The designation as "gastric adenoma" implies at least low-grade dysplasia. The hyperchromasia is striking at low magnification and extends to the mucosal surface. Note the abrupt transition from nondysplastic adjacent mucosa.

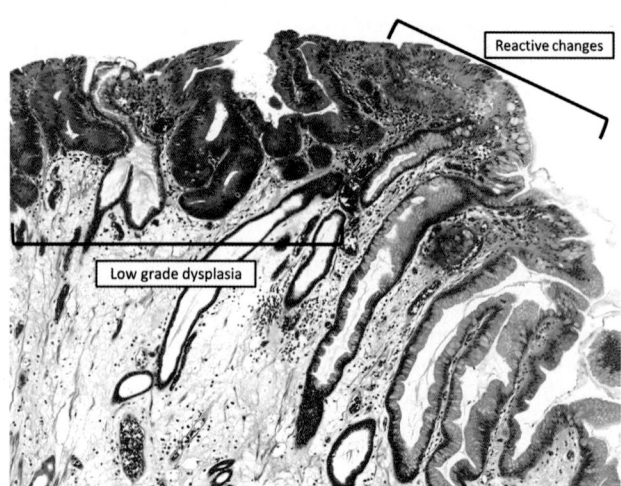

Figure 2-72. Gastric adenoma, intestinal type. LGD is dramatically hyperchromatic at low magnification. The crowded cells extend to the mucosal surface, and there is an abrupt transition from non-dysplastic epithelium. Reactive changes can mimic LGD, and this juxtaposition is a nice contrast, showing slight hyperchromasia but no nuclear crowding. Also note the gradual color gradient in the reactive area versus the abrupt change in LGD.

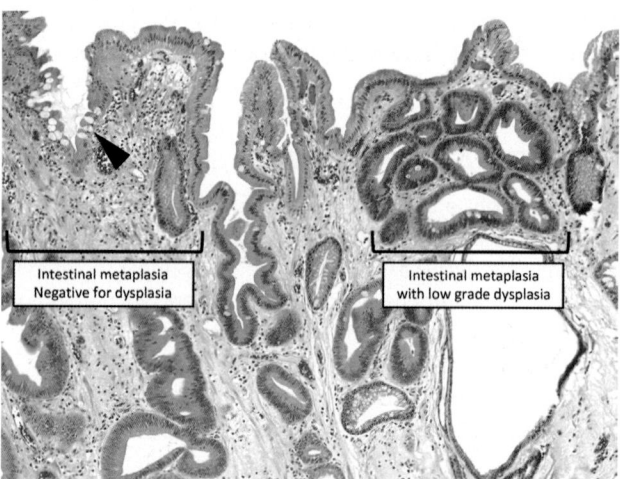

Figure 2-73. Gastric adenoma, intestinal type. Involvement of the surface epithelium is a helpful clue to dysplasia, but beware of tangential embedding. In this example, the area of LGD is hyperchromatic and eye-catching but does not involve the overlying surface epithelium. Search out areas of background intestinal metaplasia (*arrowhead*) for comparison. The marked contrast in hyperchromasia between the two areas supports LGD.

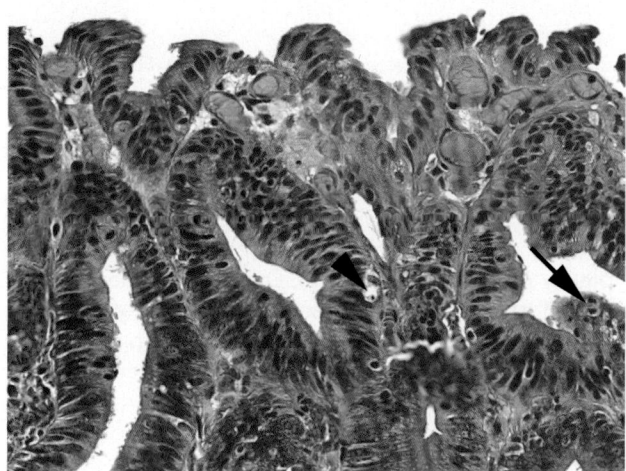

Figure 2-74. Low-grade dysplasia. Gastric adenoma, intestinal type (goblet cells not seen in this field). Dysplasia in this example is conventional, similar to that seen in a colonic tubular adenoma. The architecture is simple with well-formed glands, and the nuclei are elongated, pseudostratified, and crowded. Mitotic activity (*arrow*) and apoptoses (*arrowhead*) are increased.

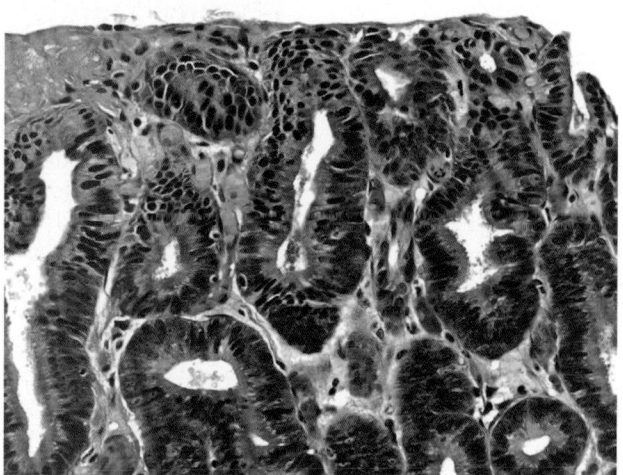

Figure 2-75. Gastric adenoma, intestinal type (goblet cells not seen in this field). The cells at the top of this photo are starting to show more rounded nuclei (loss of nuclear polarity) instead of elongated nuclei. The combination of architectural complexity, loss of nuclear polarity, and increased cytologic atypia are criteria for high-grade dysplasia.

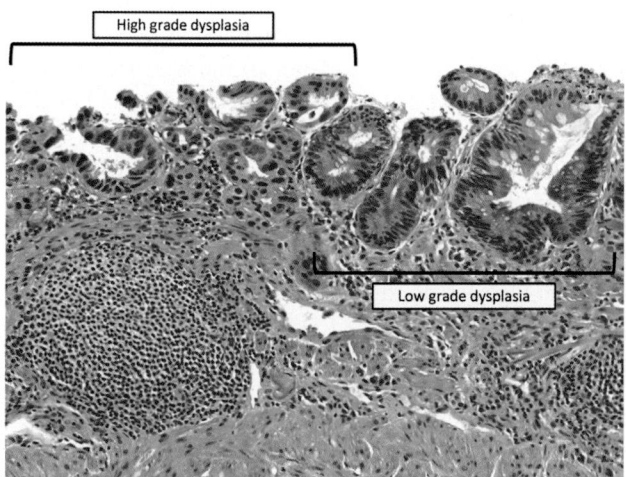

Figure 2-76. High-grade dysplasia and low-grade dysplasia in gastric adenoma, intestinal type. A diagnosis of gastric adenoma implies low-grade dysplasia. When high-grade dysplasia is seen, it is listed first. The cells in high-grade dysplasia show disorganization with loss of nuclear polarity and marked nuclear atypia characterized by variability in both size and shape as compared with neighboring cells. In contrast, the cells of low-grade dysplasia retain nuclear polarity and appear organized and relatively uniform, despite the hyperchromasia and nuclear crowding.

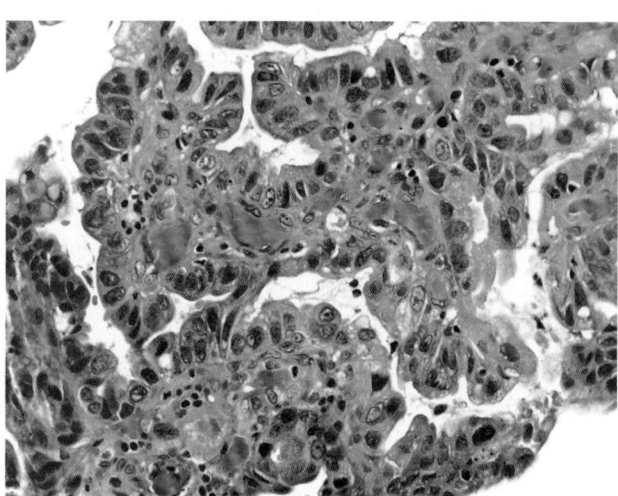

Figure 2-77. High-grade dysplasia in gastric adenoma, intestinal type (goblet cells not seen in this field). These cells have an increased nuclear to cytoplasmic ratio, appear disorganized owing to loss of nuclear polarity, and show marked nuclear variability in size and shape.

PEARLS & PITFALLS: A Diagnosis of "Gastric Adenoma" Implies Low-Grade Dysplasia, Similar to Colon Tubular Adenomas

By convention, a designation of "gastric adenoma" implies the presence of at least LGD, similar to colon tubular adenomas. Unlike HGD in colon tubular adenomas, which requires both cytologic and architectural complexity, these features are not required for HGD in gastric adenomas. In this way, dysplasia grading of gastric adenomas is more similar to dysplasia grading in Barrett mucosa, whereby loss of nuclear polarity, glandular crowding, and pleomorphism are sufficient for HGD; architectural complexity is not required for HGD in gastric adenomas. Furthermore, because "adenoma" and "low-grade dysplasia" are synonymous, it is unnecessary to use the redundant nomenclature of "low-grade dysplasia arising in a gastric adenoma." Rather, a simplified diagnosis of "gastric adenoma" is sufficient and conveys the presence of LGD. When HGD is identified, however, it is worthwhile to list the HGD first: "high-grade dysplasia in a gastric adenoma, foveolar type."

See also "Esophagus" chapter and "Colon" chapter.

Gastric Adenoma, Intestinal Type

Intestinal-type gastric adenomas comprise the bulk of all gastric adenomas, the others being relatively rare. They are single, well circumscribed, sessile, or pedunculated and are typically <2 cm. Although they can arise in any area of the stomach, they have a predilection for the gastric antrum/pylorus (61%) and are found more commonly in men than women (3:1), occurring in the sixth and seventh decades.[49] Histologically, the epithelial lining of this adenoma contains goblet cells and/or Paneth cells and by definition is dysplastic. The dysplasia is conventional (similar to that seen in a tubular adenoma) and is characterized by the presence of hyperchromatic mucin-depleted elongated cells with crowding and nuclear pseudostratification extending to involve the surface (Figs. 2.70–2.75). LGD has simple architecture with small glands, whereas HGD shows architectural complexity (cribriforming, budding, branching, or crowding) in addition to other cytological changes such as ovoid nuclei with loss of nuclear polarity, increased nuclear to cytoplasmic ratio (N:C), prominent nucleoli, clumped chromatin, and irregular nuclear contours (Figs. 2.76 and 2.77). Approximately 40% of intestinal-type gastric adenomas harbor HGD and nearly one-fourth progress to adenocarcinoma.[49] This is in contrast to the gastric foveolar-type adenoma, discussed next, which rarely harbors HGD or carcinoma. Nearly all intestinal-type adenomas arise in association with background IM, gastric atrophy, and gastritis, again emphasizing the importance of separately sampling the background gastric mucosa (Figs. 2.78–2.88).

FAQ: We do not see gastric adenomas often. What should I advise my clinician?

Clinicians should be aware that gastric adenomas with intestinal subtype confer a high rate of synchronous HGD (40%) and invasive adenocarcinoma (24%). Accordingly, complete endoscopic excision should be assured, and the lesion should be processed entirely to examine for areas of invasive carcinoma. Furthermore, additional biopsies of the background flat mucosa should be submitted separately, as these lesions are associated with *separate foci* of adenocarcinoma (16%), flat dysplasia (6%), and IM (97%). These background gastric biopsies also serve to identify other highly associated conditions, such as *H. pylori* (42%) and background gastritis (71%; environmental metaplastic atrophic gastritis [EMAG] 52% and AMAG 19%).[49]

TABLE 2.3: Gastric Adenomatous Polyps

Features		Intestinal Type	Foveolar Type	Pyloric Gland Adenoma	Oxyntic Gland Polyp/ Adenoma
Morphology low power		Fig. 2.77	Fig. 2.93	Fig. 2.99	Fig. 2.119
Morphology high power		Fig. 2.83	Fig. 2.96	Fig. 2.110	Fig. 2.122
Size		<2 cm	<1 cm	1–2 cm	0.2–0.8 cm
Location		Antrum > body/fundus	Body/fundus ≫ antrum	Body	Fundus and cardia
Mean age		60s	40s	70s	60s
Male to female ratio		M ≫ F (3:1)	F = M	F ≫ M (3:1)	F = M
HGD		++ (44%)	-	++ (51%)	-
Adenocarcinoma		+ (24%)	-	+ (12%–30%)	-
Background IM		Yes (virtually 100%)	No	Yes (60%)	No
Associated conditions		*H. pylori* (42%) EMAG (52%) AMAG (19%) Flat dysplasia (6%)	FAP (70%)	AMAG (40%)	GERD (100%)
IHC staining characteristics	MUC5AC (Foveolar) MUC6 (Pyloric) MUC 2 & CDX2 (Intestinal)	-	+	+	-
		-	-	+	+
		+	-	- (Background IM will stain)	-

AMAG, autoimmune metaplastic atrophic gastritis; EMAG, environmental metaplastic atrophic gastritis; F, female; FAP, familial adenomatous polyposis; GERD, gastroesophageal reflux disease; HGD, high-grade dysplasia; IHC, immunohistochemistry; IM, intestinal metaplasia; LGD, low-grade dysplasia; M, male.

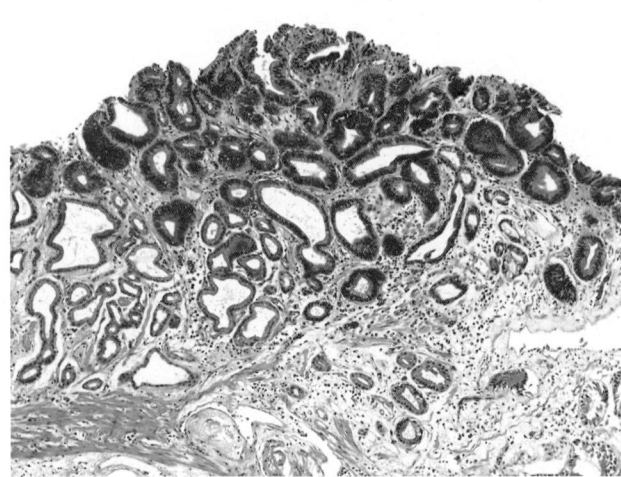

Figure 2-78. Gastric adenoma, intestinal type. The most common gastric adenoma subtype is the intestinal type. It is fairly easy to identify owing to the marked hyperchromasia at low magnification and presence of goblet cells.

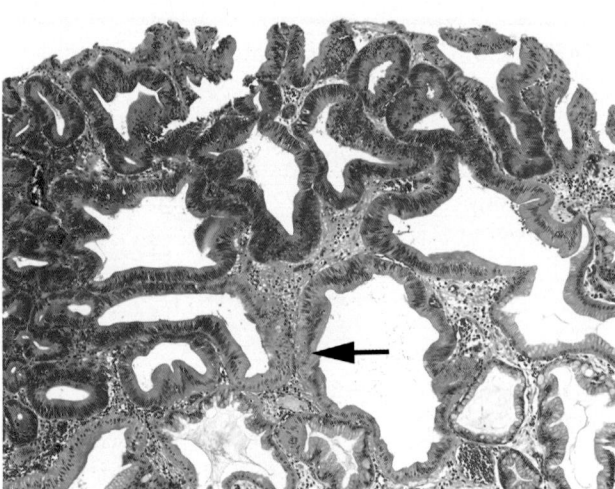

Figure 2-79. Gastric adenoma, intestinal type. There is an abrupt transition (*arrow*) from nondysplastic to dysplastic epithelium.

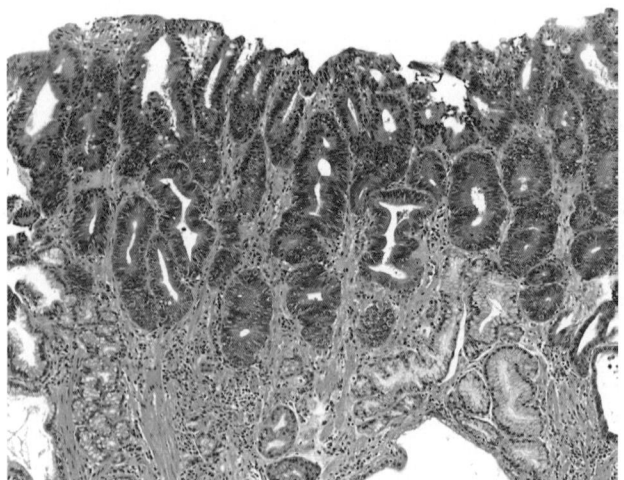

Figure 2-80. Gastric adenoma, intestinal type. The marked hyperchromasia and presence of goblet cells make intestinal-type adenomas easy to classify as compared with other subtypes.

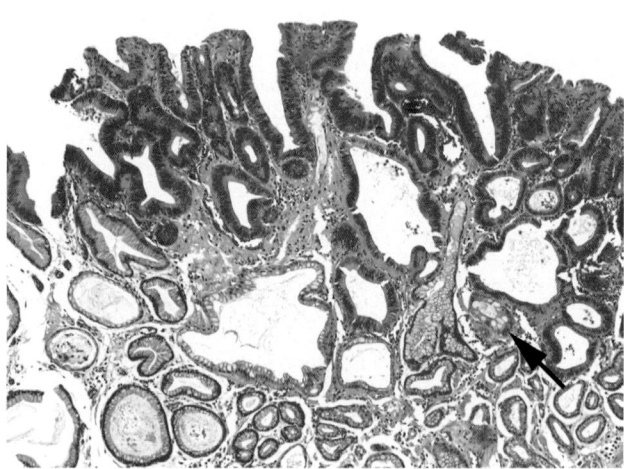

Figure 2-81. Gastric adenoma, intestinal type. Goblet cells may be sparse in some intestinal type adenomas, but the adjacent mucosa may provide clues, such as foci of intestinal metaplasia (*arrow*).

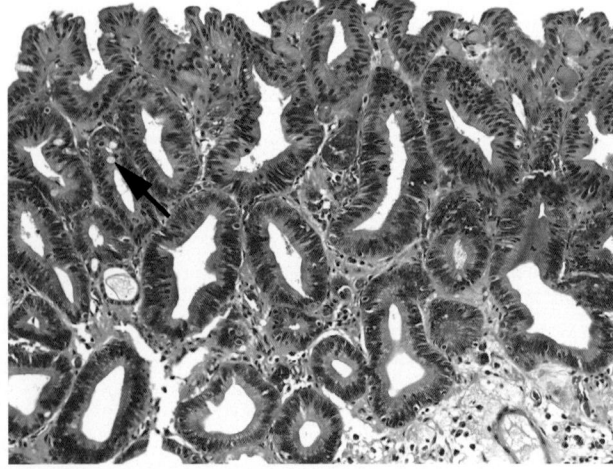

Figure 2-82. Gastric adenoma, intestinal type. The cytologic features of intestinal-type gastric adenomas are similar to the conventional colonic tubular adenoma, with elongated and crowded pseudostratified nuclei. Goblet cells (*arrow*) are usually present.

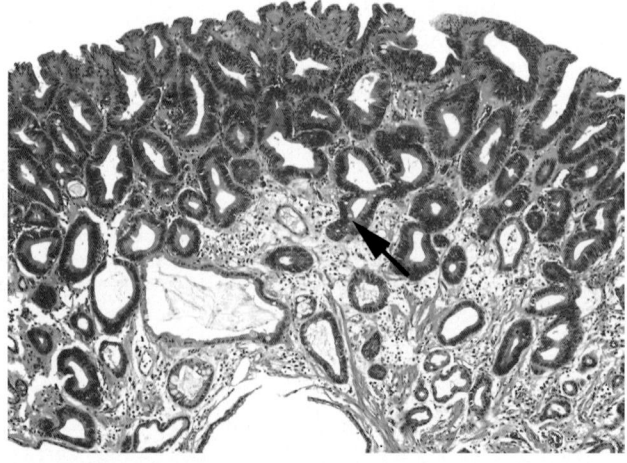

Figure 2-83. Gastric adenoma, intestinal type. These lesions are readily diagnosed at low magnification, with strong resemblance to the colonic tubular adenoma. The presence of goblet cells (*arrow*) are also a helpful clue to classification.

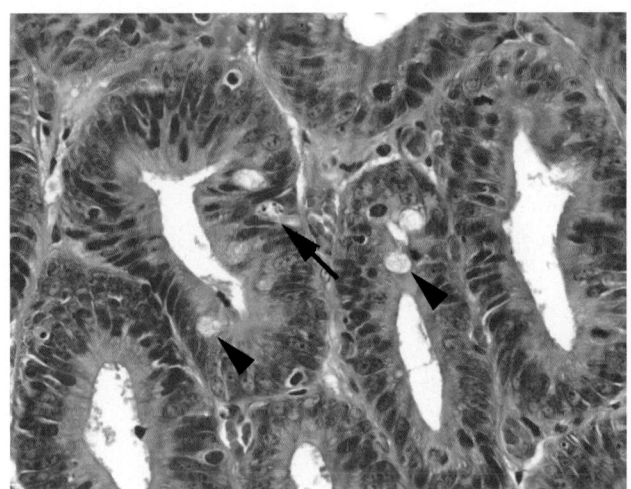

Figure 2-84. Gastric adenoma, intestinal type. By definition, gastric adenomas are at least low-grade dysplasia. Although crowded and pseudostratified, the nuclei remain polarized and organized. There may be increased mitoses and apoptoses (*arrow*). The presence of goblet cells (*arrowheads*) classifies this gastric adenoma as intestinal type.

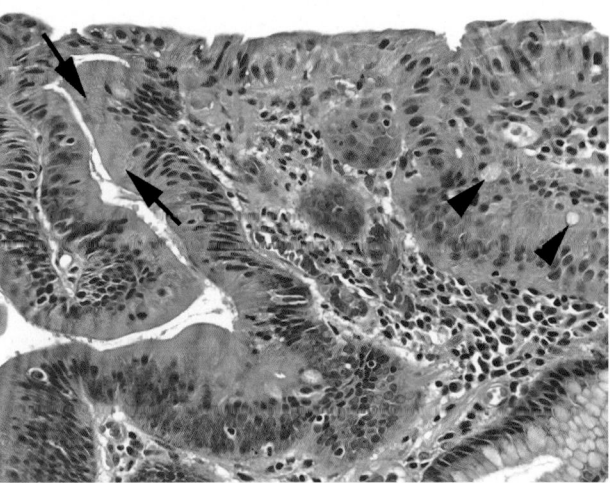

Figure 2-85. Gastric adenoma, intestinal type. Cytoplasmic features are key to differentiating the gastric adenoma subtypes. For intestinal-type gastric adenomas, the presence of goblet cells (*arrowheads*) is the easiest clue to spot. However, also note the smooth pale eosinophilic cytoplasm (*arrows*) in the intervening cells. The luminal surface has a stiff eosinophilic border, and the cytoplasm lacks clearing, foaminess, or a mucin cap.

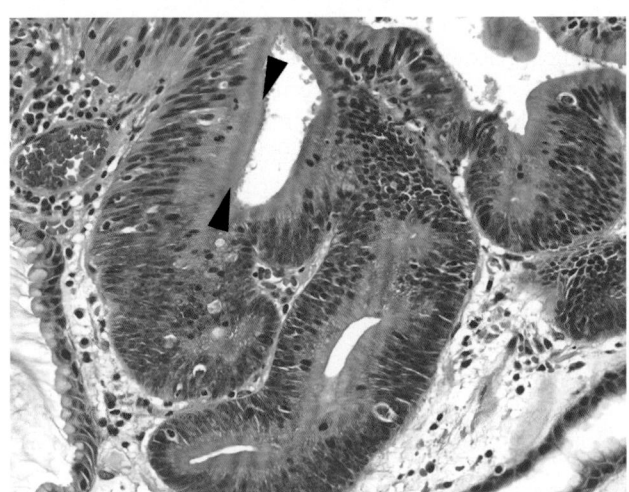

Figure 2-86. Gastric adenoma, intestinal type. These cells share a stiff eosinophilic border at the luminal surface, and a microvillous brush border can sometimes be seen (*arrowheads*). The cytoplasm is smooth, pale, and eosinophilic. The absence of clearing, foaminess, and mucin distinguish this from other gastric adenoma subtypes, especially when goblet cells are absent.

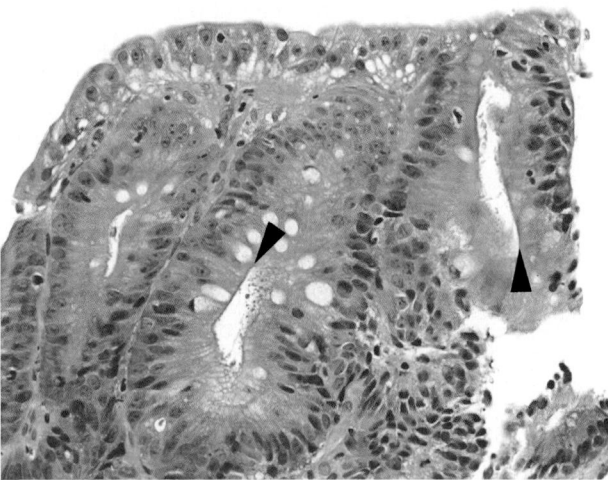

Figure 2-87. Gastric adenoma, intestinal type. When goblet cells are abundant, classification of the intestinal-type gastric adenoma is straightforward. Take a moment to note the cytoplasmic qualities of the intervening cells, which appear pale and smooth. The stiff luminal border (*arrowheads*) is distinctly eosinophilic.

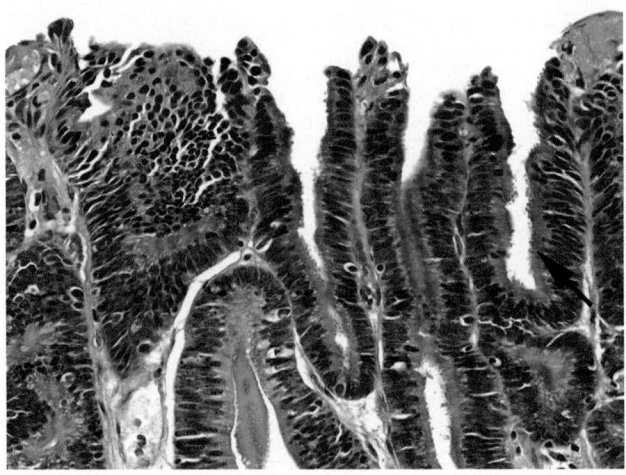

Figure 2-88. Gastric adenoma, intestinal type. A microvillous brush border (*arrow*) is present in this intestinal-type gastric adenoma. In the absence of goblet cells, the smooth *pink* cytoplasm and lack of a mucin cap or cytoplasmic clearing are helpful features.

Gastric Adenoma, Foveolar Type

Adenomas composed entirely of dysplastic foveolar-type epithelium are rare. They are typically solitary, arise more commonly in the body/fundus, and show equal gender distribution with a mean age of 44 years.[49,50] These lesions usually contain no more than LGD and are lined by gastric epithelial mucin cells with a neutral mucin cap (Figs. 2.88–2.99). Immunohistochemistry for MUC5AC (gastric mucin marker) can confirm gastric differentiation, whereas negative markers include MUC6 (pyloric mucin marker), MUC2, and CDX2 (intestinal markers). In contrast to intestinal type, foveolar-type adenomas tend to occur in otherwise normal, nonatrophic gastric mucosa and rarely harbor HGD or carcinoma.[49,50] Furthermore, background IM is the exception (found in <3% of cases) and no flat epithelial dysplasia is found in the nonpolypoid areas.[49] This stark dissimilarity between the intestinal and foveolar adenomas have led investigators to postulate divergent genetic pathways for each, but although most harbor some detectable genetic alteration, no statistically significant differences in any particular genetic alteration (*APC*, *CTNNB1*, *KRAS* mutations, and MSI) were found between the intestinal and foveolar types.[51]

FAQ: Are there any known associations for foveolar-type gastric adenomas?

A genetic background of FAP syndrome can be found in 68% of foveolar-type gastric adenomas. These syndrome-associated gastric foveolar adenomas are found more commonly in the gastric antrum and herald severe duodenal adenomatosis.[52]

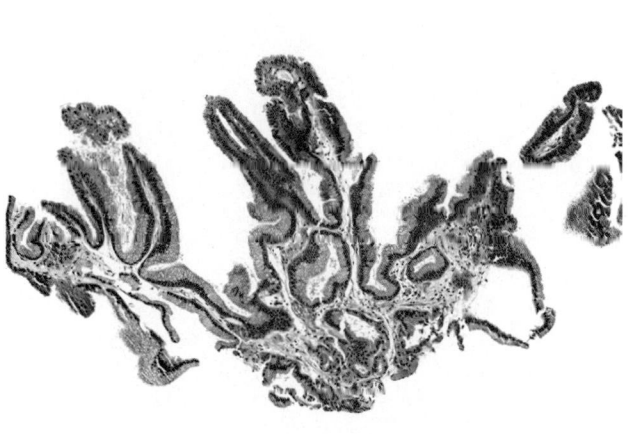

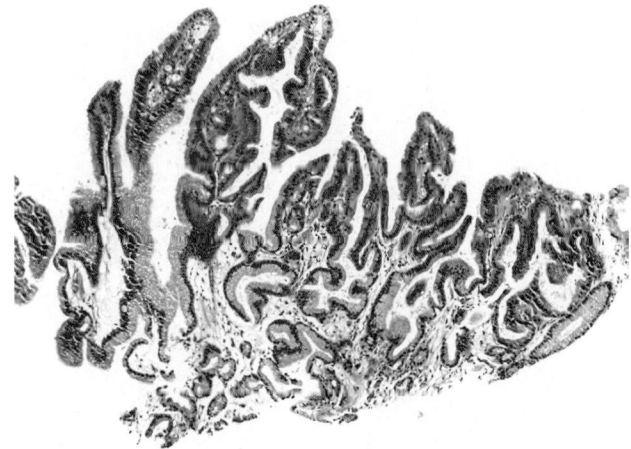

Figure 2-89. Gastric adenoma, foveolar type (low-grade dysplasia implied). By definition, gastric adenomas are at least low-grade dysplastic. At low magnification, this gastric polyp is distinctly hyperchromatic and easy to spot as a dysplastic lesion.

Figure 2-90. Gastric adenoma, foveolar type. This gastric polyp is hyperchromatic a low magnification due to the presence of low grade dysplasia.

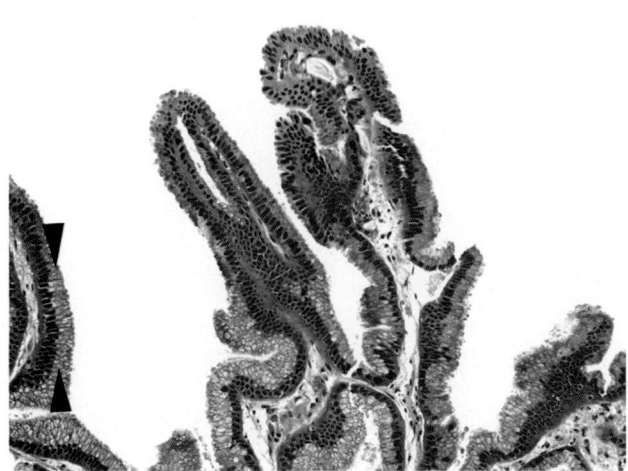

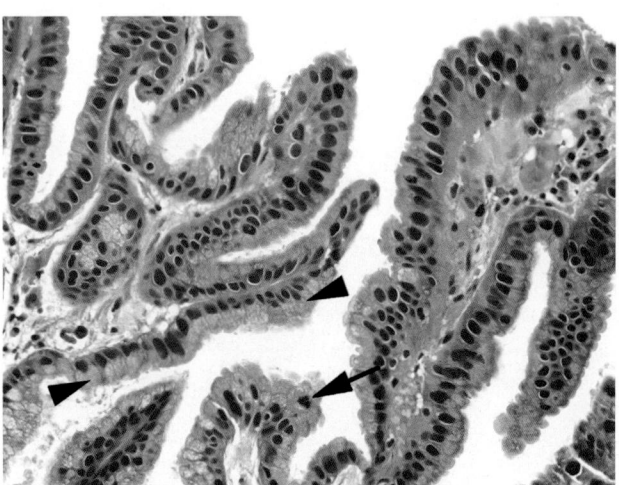

Figure 2-91. Gastric adenoma, foveolar type. The cells of the foveolar type gastric adenoma recapitulate normal foveolar cells, which have a clear mucin cap (*arrowheads*). This cytoplasmic feature distinguishes foveolar adenomas from other gastric adenomas.

Figure 2-92. Gastric adenoma, foveolar type. The nuclei of this foveolar-type adenoma are slightly crowded and disorganized, but they remain basally located, without the degree of pseudostratification seen in intestinal-type gastric adenomas. The key to classification, however, is the presence of a pale pink to clear apical mucin cap along the luminal surface (*arrowheads*). Mitotic activity is present (*arrow*).

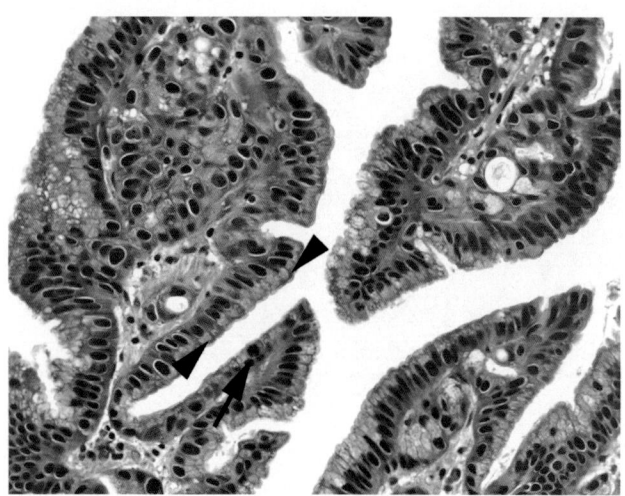

Figure 2-93. Gastric adenoma, foveolar type. The nuclei of this foveolar-type adenoma are slightly elongated and crowded but basally located and lack the degree of elongation and pseudostratification seen in intestinal-type gastric adenomas. The presence of pale pink to clear cytoplasmic mucin at the apical border (*arrowheads*) is key to classification. Mitotic activity is present (*arrow*).

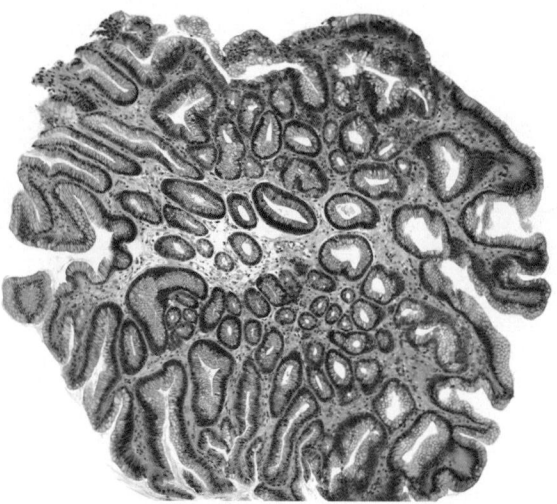

Figure 2-94. Gastric adenoma, foveolar type. At low magnification, this polyp is distinctly hyperchromatic, indicating that it contains at least low-grade dysplasia and should be categorized as a gastric adenoma. The clear mucinous cap along the surface epithelial cells, evident even at low magnification, indicates foveolar subtype.

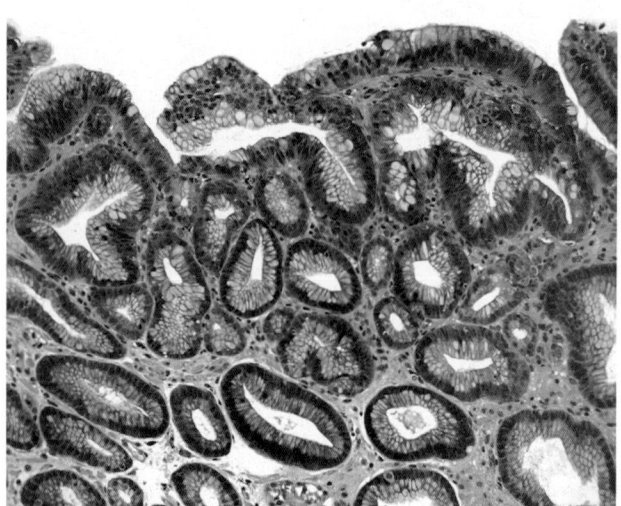

Figure 2-95. Gastric adenoma, foveolar type, higher magnification of the previous figure. The cells are columnar with crowded and basally located nuclei. The presence of an apical mucin cap indicates foveolar differentiation.

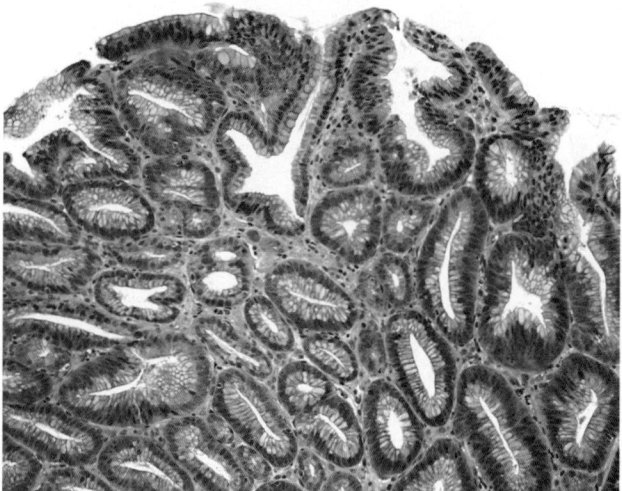

Figure 2-96. Gastric adenoma, foveolar type. These columnar cells have crowded nuclei and some pseudostratification but not to the degree seen in intestinal-type gastric adenomas. The absence of goblet cells and the presence of a pale pink to clear apical mucin cap identify this gastric adenoma as foveolar subtype.

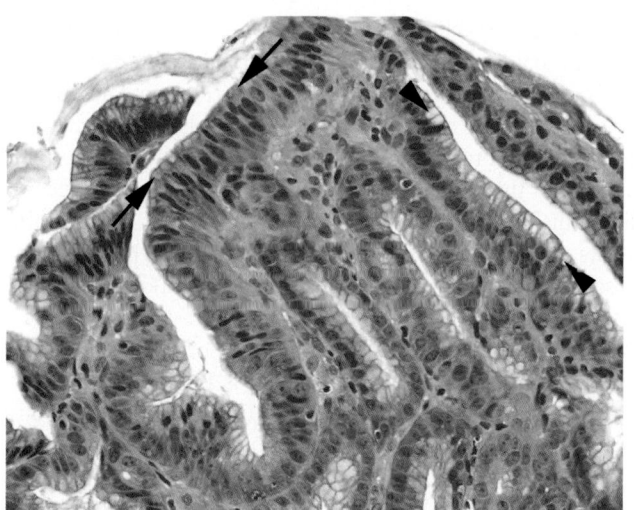

Figure 2-97. Gastric adenoma, foveolar type. Compare these epithelial cells to those found in intestinal-type gastric adenomas. These nuclei are crowded and pseudostratified, but the key differentiating feature is the cytoplasmic quality. Foveolar-type gastric adenomas have a pale pink to clear apical mucin cap (*arrows and arrowheads*) not found in intestinal-type gastric adenomas.

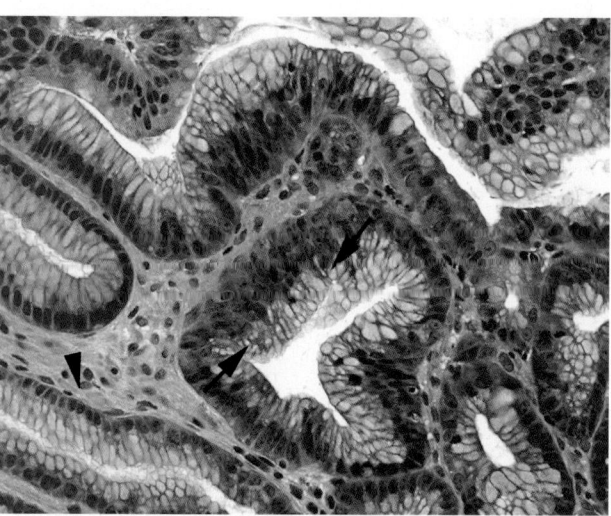

Figure 2-98. Gastric adenoma, foveolar type. This low-grade dysplastic gland is lined by cells with crowded pseudostratified nuclei and apical mucin caps (*arrows*). Adjacent nondysplastic foveolar epithelium (*arrowhead*) is in the field for comparison.

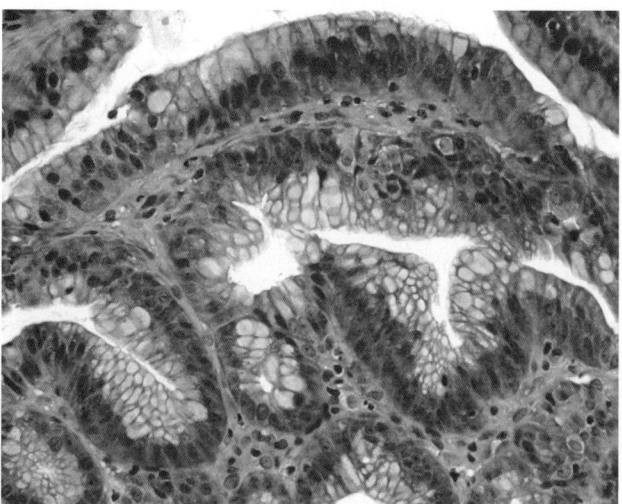

Figure 2-99. Gastric adenoma, foveolar type. The apical mucin cap on these dysplastic cells identifies this polyp as a foveolar-type gastric adenoma. Unlike intestinal-type and pyloric-type gastric adenomas, these lesions rarely harbor high-grade dysplasia or carcinoma, and the background mucosa is usually normal and nonatrophic.

Pyloric Gland Adenoma

PGAs are neoplastic lesions with malignant potential and can be found in a variety of GI sites, with the stomach being the most common, followed by the duodenal bulb, bile duct, gallbladder, duodenum, and main pancreatic duct.[48,53] In the stomach, they are 1 to 2 cm, have a marked female predominance (75%), and arise in older individuals (mean age, 73 years).[48,50] Histologically, they are composed of closely packed pyloric gland–like tubules with a single layer of cuboidal to low columnar epithelial cells containing round nuclei and pale to eosinophilic cytoplasm with ground glass appearance. These lesions can be histologically heterogenous (Figs. 2.100–2.117), and this variability, in combination with the overall infrequency of these lesions (2.7% of all gastric polyps), causes challenges in recognition.[48,50] Application of immunohistochemical stains is helpful in problematic cases: pyloric gland adenomas (PGAs) demonstrate coexpression of MUC5AC (foveolar mucin marker) and MUC6 (pyloric mucin marker) (Figs. 2.118 and 2.119), and are nonreactive for MUC2 or CDX2 (both intestinal mucin markers).[50] By comparison, gastric foveolar-type adenomas are reactive for MUC5AC only, and gastric intestinal-type adenomas show reactivity for MUC2 and/or CDX2. Most centers, however, do not have these helpful MUC stains readily available, and so a good number of pathologists will rely upon routine hematoxylin and eosin (H&E) stains for this diagnosis. Helpful histologic clues include the lack of an apical mucin cap, distinguishing it from gastric foveolar-type adenoma, and the absence of intralesional goblet cells, distinguishing it from gastric intestinal-type adenoma. Based on morphologic features, some observers suggest that PGAs and oxyntic gland polyp/adenomas are closely related lesions.[54,55]

Although PGAs lack intralesional goblet cells, 60% of PGAs show associated background IM and 40% are associated with AMAG,[50] a key feature of which is IM. Thus, adequate mucosal sampling is important to identify the gastric environment in which these lesions arise. These lesions are composed of a bland monolayer of pyloric-type cells (Fig. 2.110), well described in early papers, and conventional LGD (similar to that seen in tubular adenomas) is found in slightly more than half of PGAs (63%) (Fig. 2.111).[50] Note that all PGAs, whether they contain conventional dysplasia or not, are considered at least low-grade dysplastic, a view that has developed over time since the original descriptions.[56] This notion is further supported by the frequent association with HGD (51%) (Figs. 2.113–2.115) and adjacent adenocarcinoma (12% to 30%) (Figs. 2.116 and 2.117), a feature that also underscores the importance of adequate sampling[50]; complete excision is the treatment of choice. PGAs have been reported to occur in FAP syndrome (6% of patients), but these lesions show similar genetic background as sporadic PGAs (i.e., *KRAS* and *GNAS* mutations).[54,55,57]

PEARLS & PITFALLS

IM is seen in association with 60% of PGAs. This is important to note for several reasons.

First, the presence of background IM can mislead one to a diagnosis of gastric intestinal-type adenoma; avoid this misstep by carefully scrutinizing the lesional tissue, which, in a PGA, will contain predominantly cuboidal and low columnar cells with pale to eosinophilic ground glass cytoplasm and lack intralesional goblet cells.

Second, 40% of PGAs arise in the setting of AMAG,[48,50] a key feature of which is IM. Thus, the finding of IM in association with a PGA should trigger a workup for AMAG (i.e., gastrin and chromogranin immunohistochemical stains) when sufficient background gastric mucosa is available. A diagnosis of AMAG may be rendered when a *constellation of features is found limited to the gastric* **body and fundus** (the gastrin immunohistochemistry confirms this location by the *absence* of staining for G-cells):

- Intestinal metaplasia
- "Antralization" (atrophy of oxyntic glands and pyloric metaplasia)
- Linear or nodular ECL-cell hyperplasia, confirmed by chromogranin
- Inactive chronic gastritis, characterized by a low-lying lymphocytic infiltrate

By comparison, the gastric antrum (confirmed by gastrin immunohistochemistry highlighting abundant G-cells), will be near normal (at most, reactive/chemical gastropathy) (see "Gastric Well-Differentiated Neuroendocrine Tumors, Type 1" section for more details).

Finally, for those fortunate enough to have access to MUC2, MUC5AC, and MUC6 immunohistochemistry, areas of transition from PGA to background IM can demonstrate MUC2 reactivity. Take care to interpret the stain results in areas of lesional tissue. PGA should be reactive for MUC5AC and MUC6 and nonreactive for MUC2 (Figs. 2.118 and 2.119).

FAQ: What is the recommended surveillance for PGA?

No specific surveillance recommendations exist for gastric PGA, but clinicians should be advised that PGAs are neoplastic lesions with malignant potential (12% to 30% are associated with adjacent adenocarcinoma). As such, complete excision is recommended, along with sampling of the background flat mucosa to evaluate for AMAG, which is found in 40% of cases.

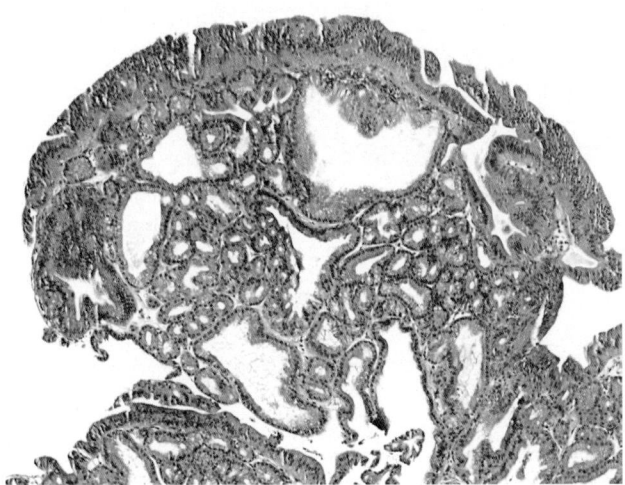

Figure 2-100. Pyloric gland adenoma (low-grade dysplasia is implied). The morphologic heterogeneity of PGAs contributes to lack of recognition, but several key unifying features can aid in diagnosis. For example, at low magnification, this polyp is predominantly composed of closely packed pyloric gland–like tubules. As with colon tubular adenomas, the diagnosis of PGA implies at least low-grade dysplasia.

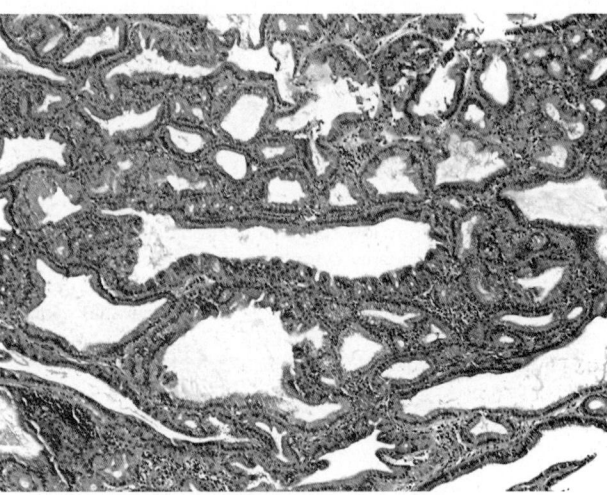

Figure 2-101. Pyloric gland adenoma. Some areas may show back-to-back well-formed tubules, whereas other areas may have dilated and distorted glands, but the cells lining these areas are the same. Despite the bland appearance, these lesions are all considered at least low-grade dysplasia.

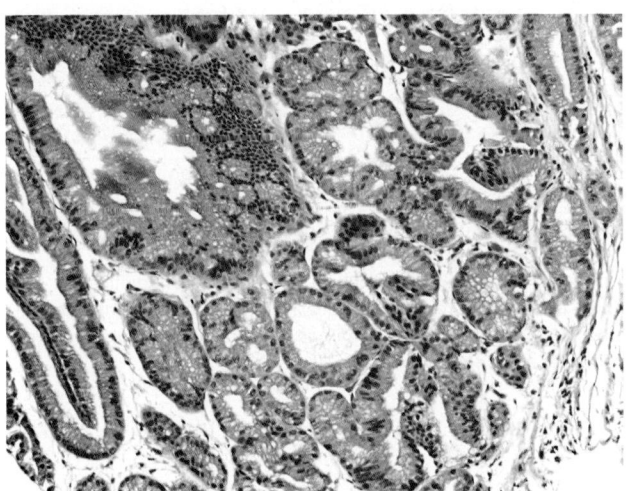

Figure 2-102. Pyloric gland adenoma. PGAs are a composed of a monolayer of low columnar or cuboidal cells with abundant clear to foamy cytoplasm and basally located nuclei. These polyps are considered low grade dysplasia despite the lack of conventional dysplasia (such as that seen in colon tubular adenomas).

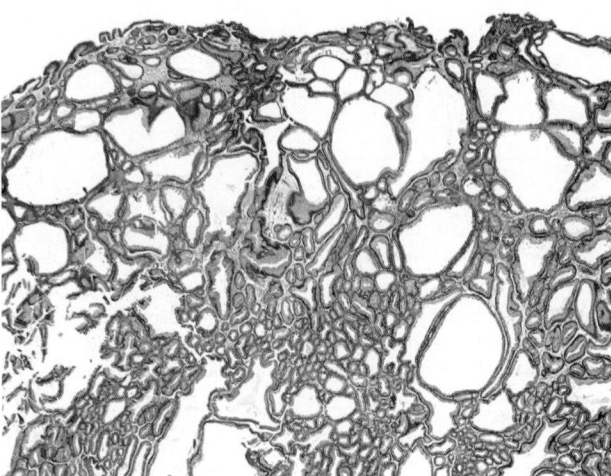

Figure 2-103. Pyloric gland adenoma. At low magnification, this PGA shows closely packed pyloric gland–like tubules, some of which are cystically dilated and distorted. The lesion lacks stroma-rich or edematous areas, and the presence of back-to-back glands indicates an epithelial proliferative process. PGA, by definition, has at least low-grade dysplasia.

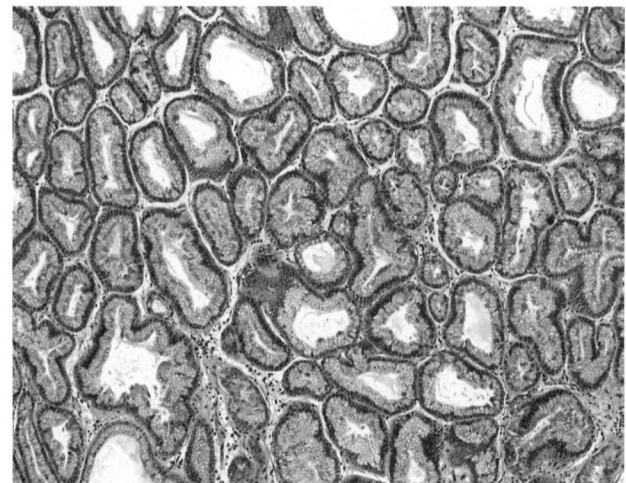

Figure 2-104. Pyloric gland adenoma. These back-to-back glands are composed of uniform low columnar to cuboidal cells with abundant ground glass or foamy cytoplasm. The nuclei are small and basally located. Original descriptions did not consider areas containing a monolayer of bland cells dysplastic, but this view has evolved over time, and all PGAs are now considered at least low-grade dysplasia regardless of whether conventional dysplasia is present.

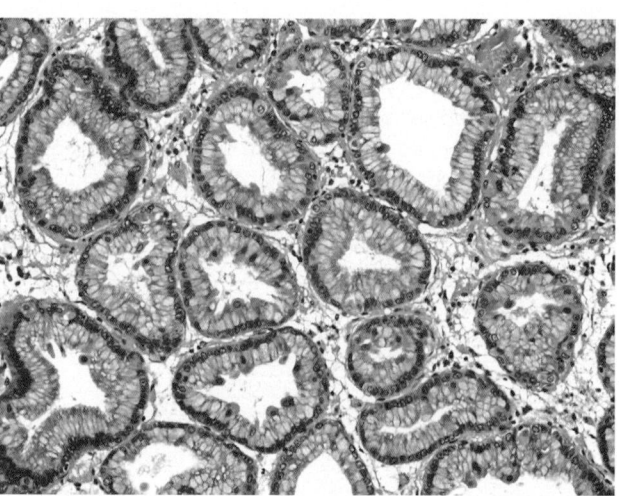

Figure 2-105. Pyloric gland adenoma. The proliferative tubules are pyloric gland–like, with uniform basally located small nuclei and abundant clear foamy cytoplasm.

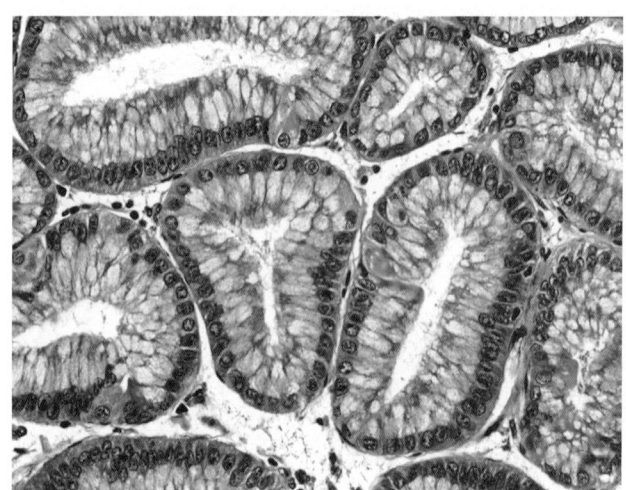

Figure 2-106. Pyloric gland adenoma. These cells are low columnar with round basally located nuclei. The cytoplasmic quality helps subclassify gastric adenomas, and PGAs have eosinophilic to clear cytoplasm with ground glass or foamy appearance.

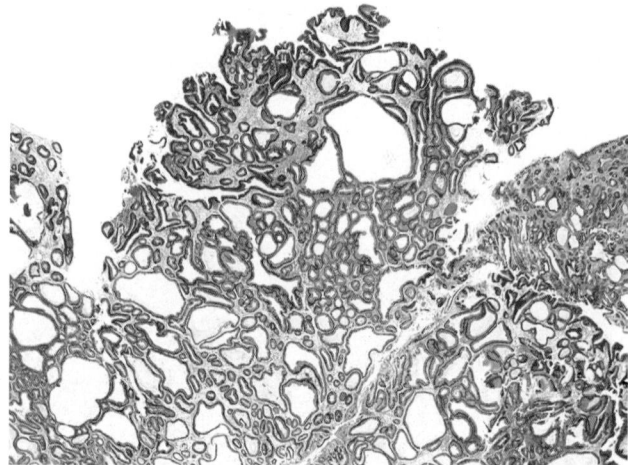

Figure 2-107. Pyloric gland adenoma. At low magnification, this polyp contains more cystically dilated glands than previous examples. There is absence of stroma-rich areas or lamina propria edema, and focal areas show closely packed smaller tubules.

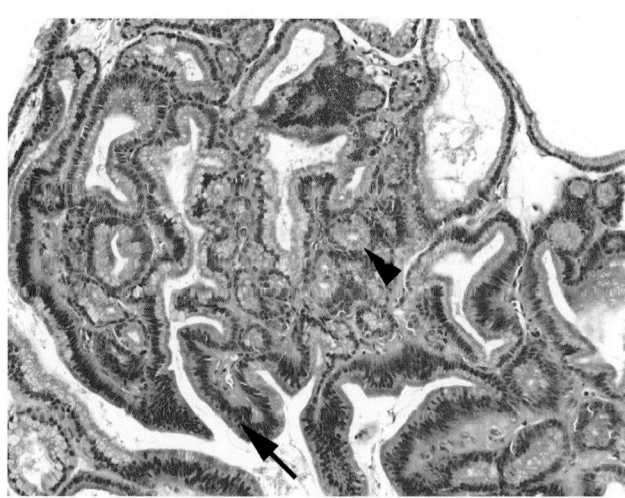

Figure 2-108. Pyloric gland adenoma. PGAs can be morphologically heterogeneous, and this example shows a PGA lined by both columnar cells with eosinophilic cytoplasm (*arrow*) and cuboidal cells with clear foamy cytoplasm (*arrowhead*).

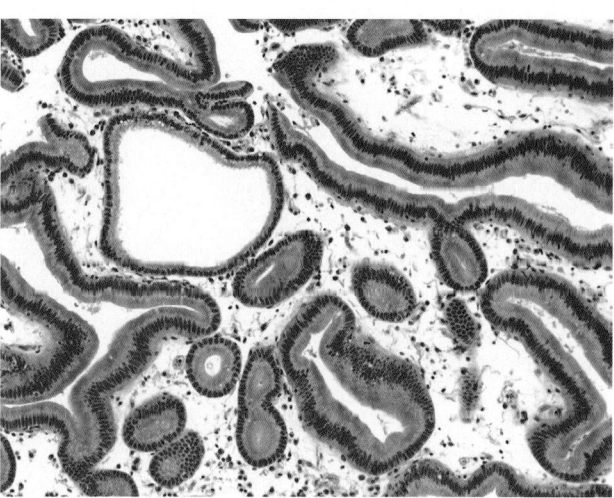

Figure 2-109. Pyloric gland adenoma. Another area in the previous polyp shows more of the columnar cells with eosinophilic ground glass cytoplasm. This morphologic heterogeneity contributes to difficulty in diagnostic recognition. These polyps are considered low-grade dysplasia despite the lack of conventional dysplasia (such as seen in tubular adenomas).

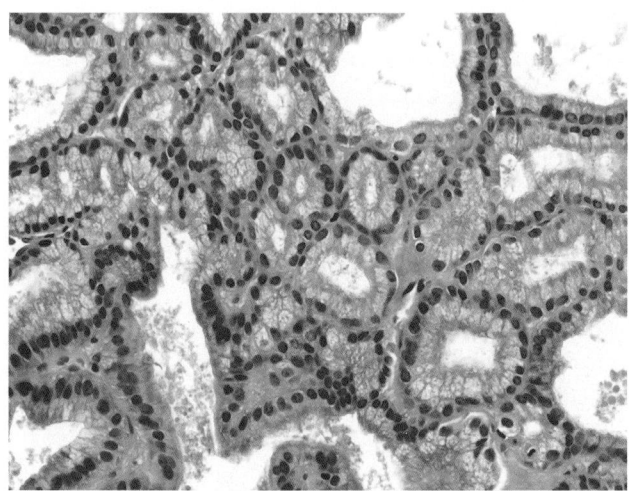

Figure 2-110. Pyloric gland adenoma. Yet a different area of the same polyp shows the more characteristic cuboidal cells with round basally located nuclei and abundant foamy clear cytoplasm. One can appreciate the similarity between these areas and the normal pyloric glands found in the gastric antrum and pylorus. Original descriptions did not consider areas containing a monolayer of bland cells dysplastic, but this view has evolved over time, and all PGAs are now considered at least low-grade dysplasia regardless of whether conventional dysplasia is present.

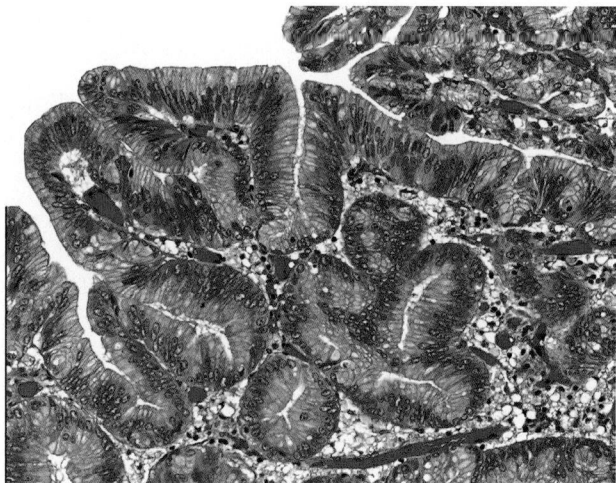

Figure 2-111. Pyloric gland adenoma with conventional low-grade dysplasia. This example shows more cytologic atypia, especially along the surface epithelium where the cells are overlapping and show pseudostratification. There is some disorganization in glandular architecture, but the nuclei maintain polarity and there is abundant cytoplasm. Although all PGAs are considered low-grade dysplasia, this example shows conventional dysplasia like that seen in a typical colonic tubular adenoma.

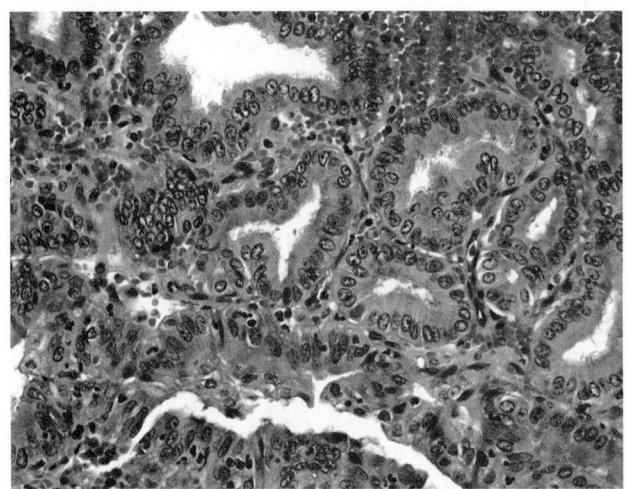

Figure 2-112. Pyloric gland adenoma. This is another example of the variability in cytoplasmic quality found in PGAs. Rather than clear and foamy, this example shows eosinophilic ground glass cytoplasm.

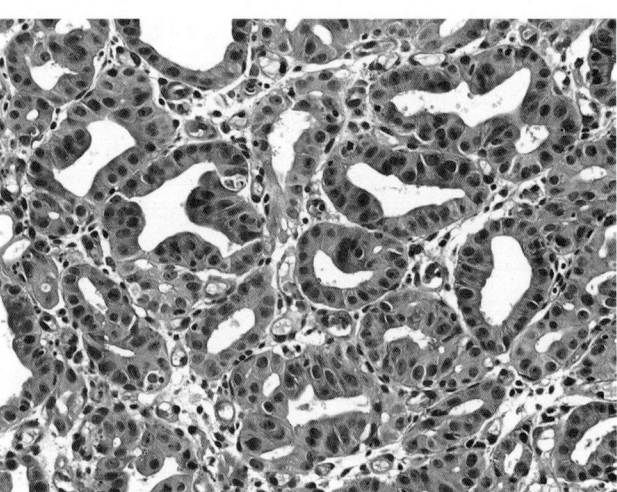

Figure 2-113. High-grade dysplasia in a pyloric gland adenoma. The nuclei in this example are highly atypical with variation in size and shape. The nuclei are no longer situated in an orderly fashion along the basement membrane but instead are haphazardly arranged.

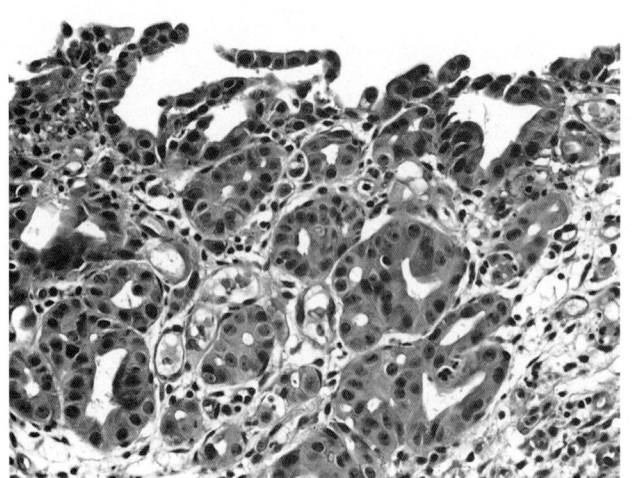

Figure 2-114. High-grade dysplasia in a pyloric gland adenoma. High-grade dysplasia is found in half of PGAs. These glands are cribriforming, and the cells show marked nuclear atypia. There is loss of nuclear polarity, variation in size and shape, and prominent nucleoli.

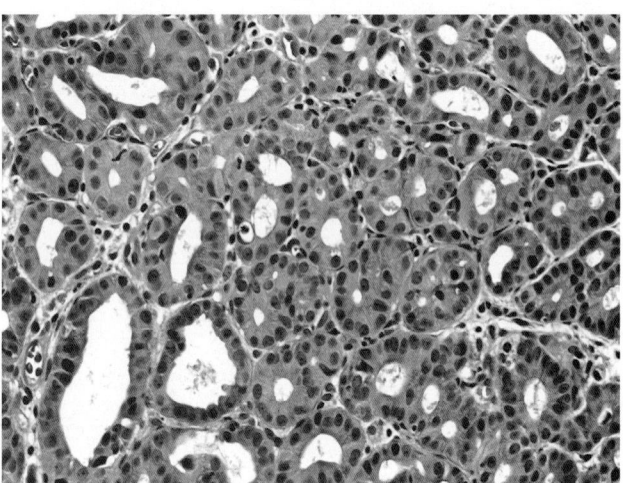

Figure 2-115. High-grade dysplasia in a pyloric gland adenoma. The glandular architecture is complex with crowding and cribriforming. The nuclei show variation in size and shape, have irregular nuclear borders, and contain prominent nucleoli.

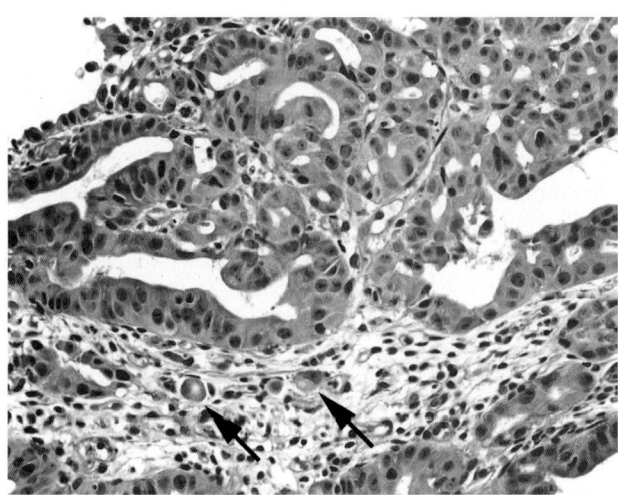

Figure 2-116. Adenocarcinoma in a pyloric gland adenoma. Associated or adjacent adenocarcinoma is reported in up to one-third of PGAs. Look carefully in busy areas with complex architecture. Single infiltrating cells (*arrows*) are diagnostic for adenocarcinoma invasive into the lamina propria (pT1).

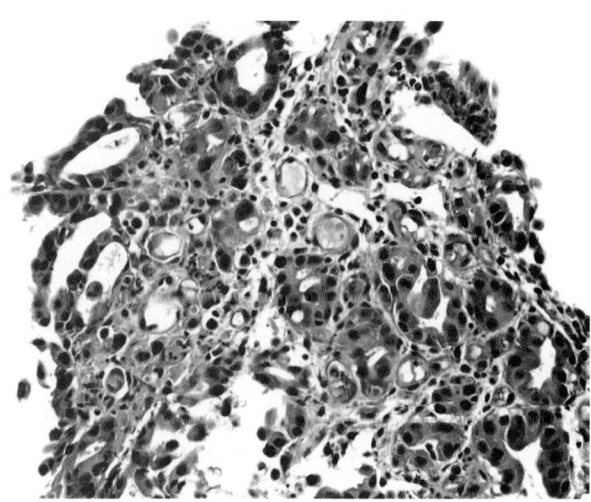

Figure 2-117. Adenocarcinoma in a pyloric gland adenoma. This adenocarcinoma is poorly differentiated and arising from a PGA.

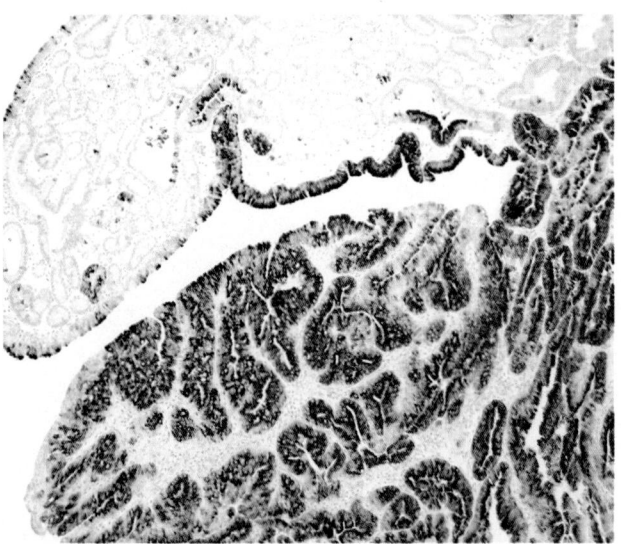

Figure 2-118. Pyloric gland adenoma, MUC5AC expression. MUC5AC is a marker for foveolar differentiation and is expressed in PGAs along with MUC6, which indicates pyloric differentiation. These immunostains may be helpful in challenging cases, but most PGAs can be distinguished by H&E.

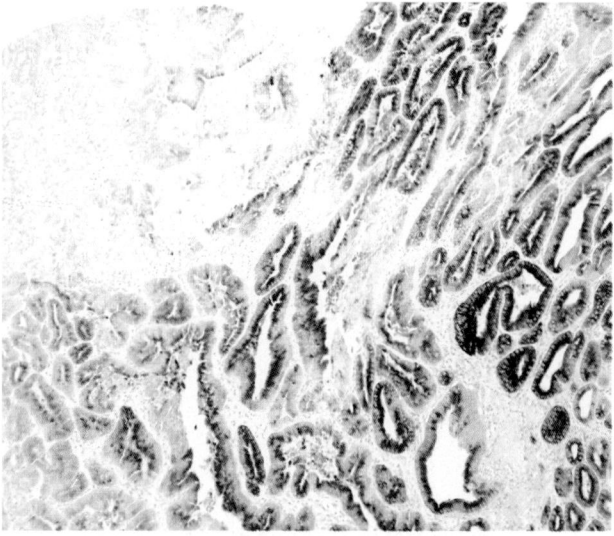

Figure 2-119. Pyloric gland adenoma, MUC6 expression. PGAs coexpress foveolar (MUC5AC) and pyloric (MUC6) immunohisto-chemistry. They are negative for intestinal markers MUC2 and CDX2. These immunostains may be applied in challenging cases, but they are not readily available in most laboratories, making H&E recognition essential.

Oxyntic Gland Polyp/Adenoma

The oxyntic gland polyp/adenoma is one example of the challenges in the nomenclature of gastric neoplasia. This uncommon gastric lesion was previously classified as both an adenocarcinoma (the so-called gastric adenocarcinoma of fundic gland type/chief cell predominant type or gastric adenocarcinoma with chief cell differentiation) and a benign "chief cell hyperplasia" or FGP variant by several authors.[58-60] However, the bland cytologic features of the lesion and low Ki-67 proliferation rate (<2%) in combination with the benign clinical course prompted a proposal for reclassification as "oxyntic gland polyp/adenoma."[47] These rare lesions are encountered as small (0.2 to 0.8 cm) single polypoid growths in the gastric fundus (70%) or cardia (30%), with equal distribution among men and women, and are found uniformly in the setting of gastroesophageal reflux disease.[47] Histologically, they are characterized by a deep proliferation of oxyntic glands arranged in cords and clusters (Figs. 2.120–2.125). Thin wisps of smooth muscle separate the glands (Figs. 2.123 and 2.124), but there is no desmoplastic stromal response to suggest invasion. The predominant cells are monotonous pale gray-blue (basophilic or amphophilic) columnar cells resembling chief cells; interspersed are smaller numbers of eosinophilic parietal cells and clear mucous cells. The cells lack overt cytologic atypia, mitotic activity, or necrosis. Assessment for dysplasia in these lesions and whether they are best classified as polyps or adenomas remains unclear until further studies clarify the pathogenesis. However, in their series, Singhi and colleagues point out that no reported cases have shown true recurrence or progression of disease. Similar to PGAs, these lesions are associated with *GNAS* mutations[61] and are reactive for MUC6 (a pyloric marker) by immunohistochemistry (Fig. 2.126). They can be differentiated from PGAs by their negative MUC5AC (a foveolar marker) immunoreactivity (Fig. 2.127).

FAQ: What is the appropriate follow-up for this lesion?

The nomenclature ranges from benign (oxyntic gland polyp, chief cell hyperplasia, chief cell hamartoma) to benign neoplasia (oxyntic gland polyp/adenoma) to malignant (gastric adenocarcinoma of fundic gland/chief cell predominant type and gastric adenocarcinoma with chief cell differentiation), but clinicians may be assured that despite the evolving nomenclature, the data are quite clear that these lesions are biologically benign. These lesions have been reported to persist when incompletely resected, but no reported cases have shown true recurrence or progression of disease. Thus, complete endoscopic excision of these lesions is sensible, whereas surgical intervention is overkill.

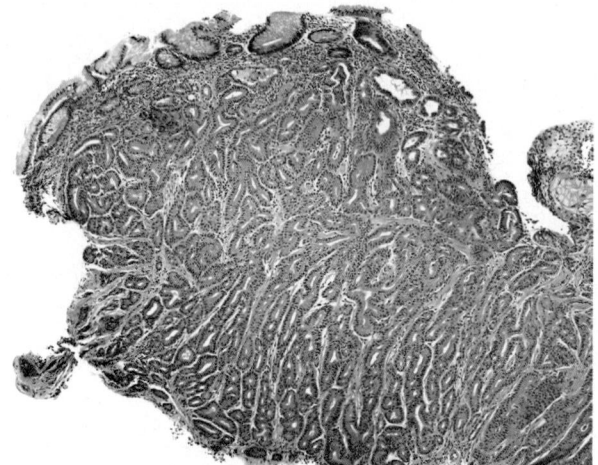

Figure 2-120. Oxyntic gland polyp/adenoma. These are typically small subcentimeter lesions found in the gastric fundus with a proliferation of cords and clusters of oxyntic glands. The surface foveolar epithelium is unchanged.

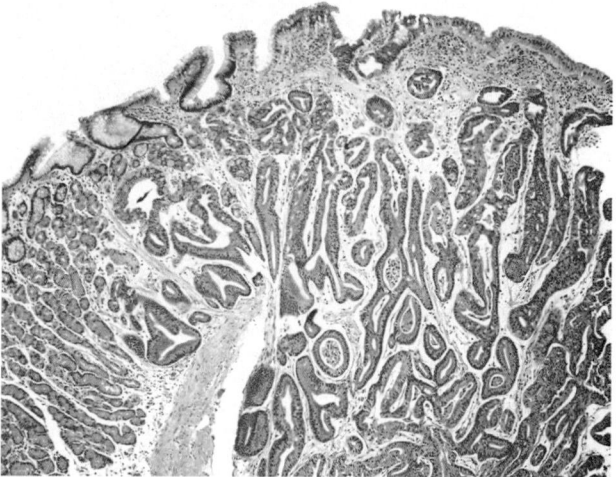

Figure 2-121. Oxyntic gland polyp/adenoma. This example shows an abrupt change from normal oxyntic gland architecture at the left to distorted cords of oxyntic cells at the right. The surface foveolar epithelium is normal.

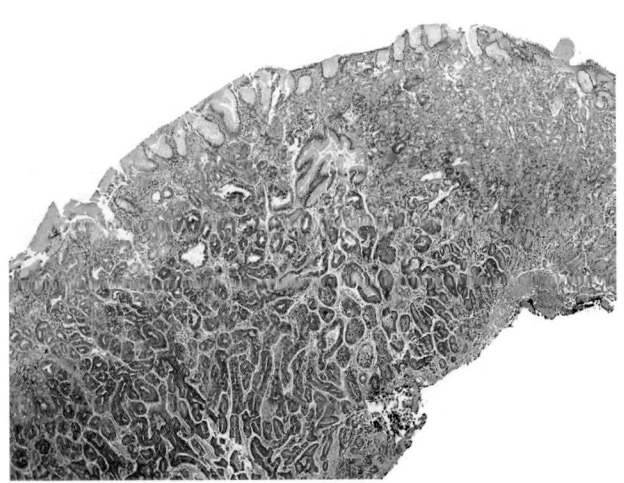

Figure 2-122. Oxyntic gland polyp/adenoma. There is a deep proliferation of oxyntic glands arranged in cords and clusters, whereas the overlying foveolar epithelium is unchanged. The far right of this biopsy shows normal oxyntic mucosa for comparison.

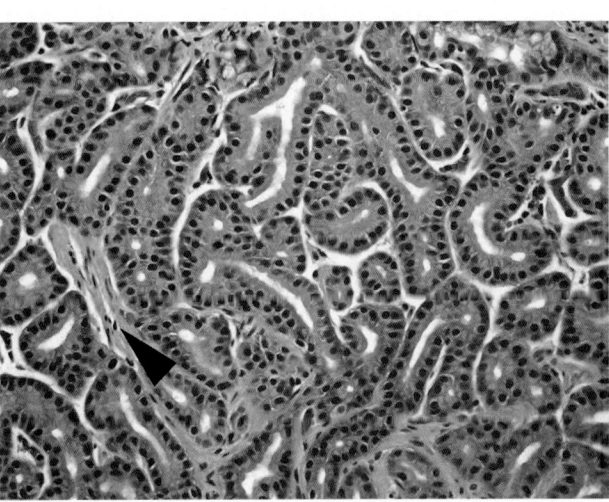

Figure 2-123. Oxyntic gland polyp/adenoma. The cells in this example are bland and exquisitely uniform. They are arranged in long tubules or cords separated by smooth muscle strands in the lamina propria (*arrowhead*).

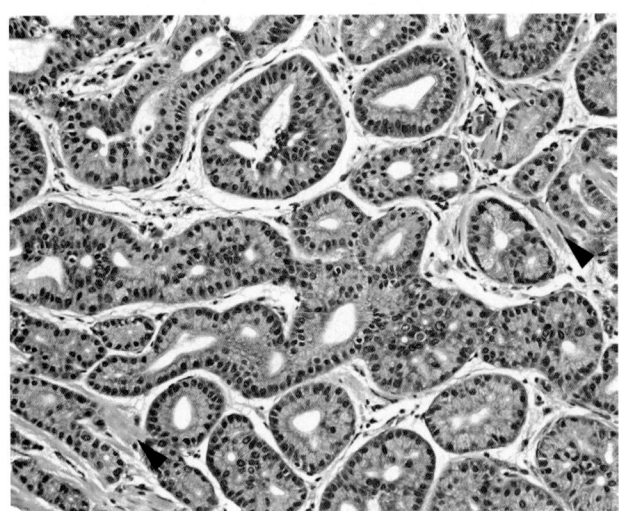

Figure 2-124. Oxyntic gland polyp/adenoma. Another example demonstrates some heterogeneity in the cells of this lesion. Although the cells are oxyntic in origin, this may not be evident at high-power views. The arrangement of the cells in cords separated by smooth muscle strands (*arrowheads*) and the deep location within oxyntic mucosa are clues to the diagnosis.

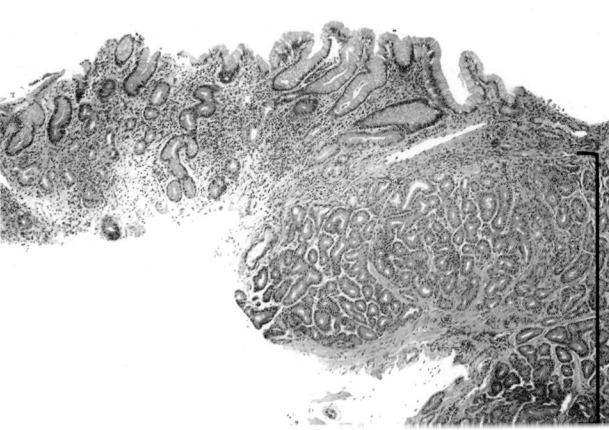

Figure 2-125. Oxyntic gland polyp/adenoma. Note the deep proliferation of glands (*bracket*) that has embedded smooth muscle between the cords of cells. This example arises in a backdrop of autoimmune metaplastic atrophic gastritis.

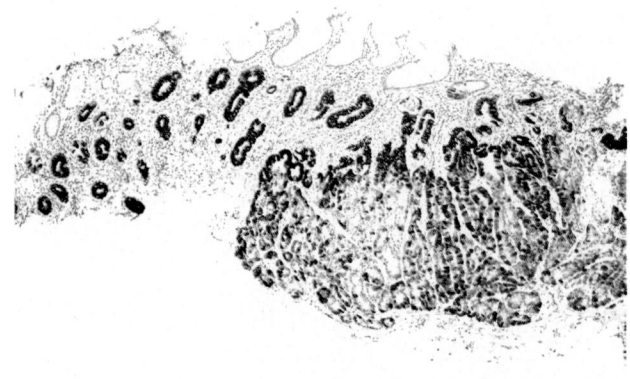

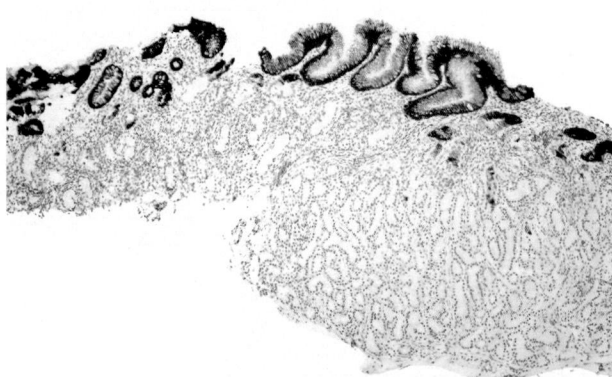

Figure 2-126. Oxyntic gland polyp/adenoma, MUC6 immunohistochemistry. These lesions demonstrate MUC6 (pyloric differentiation) immunoreactivity and are negative for MUC5AC (foveolar).

Figure 2-127. Oxyntic gland polyp/adenoma, MUC5AC immuno-histochemistry. There is no expression of MUC5AC foveolar differentiation in the tumor cells. Note the reactivity of the normal overlying foveolar epithelial cells, which serve as internal control.

KEY FEATURES: Gastric Adenomas (See Table 2.3)

- **Polypoid dysplasia** is designated as gastric adenoma and is classified as **low-grade** or **high-grade** dysplasia.
- Varieties include **intestinal type**, **foveolar type**, PGA, and **oxyntic gland polyp/adenoma**.
- **Intestinal-type gastric adenoma:**
  - Contains **goblet cells** with or without Paneth cells
  - Frequently associated with **HGD** (44%) and **adenocarcinoma** (24%)
  - High frequency of background **gastritis (e.g. *H. pylori*, AMAG, EMAG)**
  - Immunohistochemistry (IHC) profile: **MUC2+, CDX2+,** MUC5AC−, MUC6−
- **Foveolar-type gastric adenoma:**
  - Lined by foveolar epithelial cells, identified by its **mucin cap**
  - Associated with **FAP (70%)**
  - **Low risk of adenocarcinoma** (<1%)
  - IHC profile: **MUC5AC+,** MUC6−, MUC2−
- Pyloric gland adenoma:
  - Closely packed tubules lined by cuboidal **pyloric gland cells with ground glass cytoplasm**
  - Frequently associated with **HGD** (51%) and **adenocarcinoma** (30%)
  - Strong association with **AMAG** (40%) and **background IM** (60%)
  - IHC profile: **MUC5AC+, MUC6+,** MUC2−, CDX2−
- **Oxyntic gland polyp/adenoma:**
  - **Deep cords and clusters of oxyntic glands** without cytologic atypia or desmoplasia
  - Biologically **benign**
  - Associated with gastroesophageal reflux disease (100%)
  - IHC profile: **MUC6+,** MUC5AC− MUC2−, CDX2−
- Regardless of subtype, polyps should be managed by **complete excision**; additional **biopsies should be taken of mucosa away from the polyp** to evaluate for gastritis, IM, flat dysplasia, and other synchronous lesions.

ADENOCARCINOMA

Globally, gastric cancer is among the top five leading causes of cancer and a leading cause of cancer death. The highest incidence worldwide is in Asia, central Europe, and South America.[62,63] In the United States, the overall incidence rates are modest but remain greater than those of esophageal cancer, and when compared with Caucasians, the incidence is increased in all non-Caucasian ethnic and racial groups including Hispanics, Asian, and African-Americans.[64] Although gastric cancer remains a deadly disease, the incidence and mortality rates have fallen dramatically over the past 80 years.[63] Advances in endoscopic techniques have improved detection of early gastric cancer (defined as pT1), and adjuvant chemotherapy contributes to improved overall mortality and 5-year survival rates.[65,66] Stage remains the most important prognostic indicator, but a number of considerations affect biopsy interpretation, such as tumor location and stage, Lauren classification, morphologic variants, background mucosa characteristics, genetic considerations, and biomarker profile, as discussed later.

APPROACH TO THE BIOPSY

Tumor Location and Staging: Esophageal Versus Gastric

Organ subsite remains an important prognostic indicator, and treatment indications differ if the carcinoma involves the gastric cardia or gastroesophageal junction (GEJ). For example, for proximal tumors involving the GEJ or gastric cardia, radiation therapy may be added to adjuvant chemotherapy before resection. These proximal tumors are on the rise in developed countries and are associated with risk factors for gastroesophageal reflux.[66] By comparison, distal gastric cancers, which are associated with diet and *H. pylori* infection, have been decreasing worldwide as a result of improved diet and health care. For staging purposes, the esophagus and stomach are differentiated by the American Joint Committee on Cancer staging manual (eighth edition) based on involvement of and proximity to the GEJ.[67] Carcinomas entirely on either side of the GEJ are easily classified as either esophageal or gastric cancers, respectively. For tumors involving the GEJ, these are considered gastric when the tumor midpoint is greater than 2 cm into the stomach, whereas those with tumor midpoints 2 cm or less into the stomach are staged as esophageal cancers (Fig. 2.128).

Staging of gastric cancers is based on depth of invasion and is independent of tumor size. Any invasion into the lamina propria, muscularis mucosae, or submucosa is considered pT1. Recall, these intramucosal carcinomas have access to the rich lymphatics within the gastric lamina propria, allowing for lymphatic spread and lymph node metastases. The T1 category is further divided into pT1a (invasion into the lamina propria or muscularis mucosae) and pT1b (invasion into the submucosa). pT2 tumors invade the muscularis propria, pT3 penetrate the subserosal connective tissue, and tumors that involve the visceral peritoneum are considered pT4. This last category is further subdivided as pT4a (involvement of visceral peritoneum only) and pT4b (involvement of adjacent organs or structures) (Fig. 2.129). Early gastric cancers are tumors with invasion limited to the lamina propria, muscularis mucosae, or submucosa (pT1) and may be amenable to conservative endoscopic mucosal resection (EMR) if they meet specific criteria. Early studies were limited to small lesions with specific endoscopic features (e.g., exophytic vs depressed), whereas recent studies cite more liberal criteria that include early submucosal invasion. Examples of tumors amenable to EMR include (1) intramucosal nonulcerated differentiated tumors >2 cm, (2) intramucosal ulcerated differentiated tumors ≤3 cm, (3) intramucosal nonulcerated undifferentiated tumors ≤2 cm, and (4) submucosal invasion <500 μm (sm1) differentiated tumor ≤3 cm.[68] Thus, tumor differentiation, as well as depth of invasion, is an important feature to include in the pathology report.

FAQ: What anatomic landmark distinguishes esophageal from gastric tumors?

Tumors entirely proximal or entirely distal to the GEJ are simply classified as esophageal or gastric, respectively. For tumors that involve the GEJ, the distance of the tumor's midpoint is taken into account. A somewhat arbitrary distance of 2 cm is the cutoff: the tumor is considered esophageal if its midpoint is ≤2 cm into the stomach, and gastric if >2 cm (see Fig. 2.128).

PEARLS & PITFALLS: GEJ Is Not Interchangeable With Squamocolumnar Junction

Determining whether a tumor is gastric versus esophageal relies upon its positional relationship with the GEJ and not the squamocolumnar junction (SCJ); these two are *not* synonymous (see Fig. 2.128). The GEJ is defined anatomically, whereas the SCJ is defined histologically, and these two do not always coincide. Take, for example, in Barrett esophagus, where the SCJ has moved caudally into the tubular esophagus as the result of columnar metaplasia. This distinction is important because the American Joint Committee on Cancer definition of gastric cancer utilizes the GEJ and not the SCJ. These landmarks can be identified endoscopically or at the grossing bench by the following distinctive features:

GEJ: Proximal end of gastric folds, or the notch where the pouched stomach meets the tubular esophagus.

SCJ: The line where squamous mucosa (which has a pale glossy appearance) meets the columnar mucosa (which appears reddish and has a coarse texture).

PEARLS & PITFALLS: Staging Challenges in pT3 and pT4 Tumors

It is possible for a tumor to invade through the muscularis propria (pT3) of the stomach and directly extend into the gastrocolic or gastrohepatic ligament, or the greater or lesser omentum, without perforating the visceral peritoneum. In these cases, the lesion should be classified as pT3. Note these structures and organs are covered in visceral peritoneum, and pT4 designation is reserved for tumors with invasion into this visceral peritoneum.

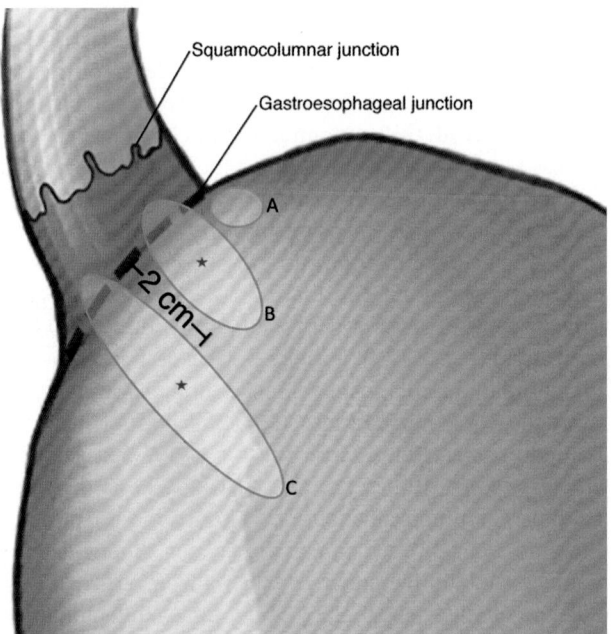

Figure 2-128. Criteria for gastric versus esophageal classification. The gastroesophageal junction (GEJ), not the squamocolumnar junction, serves as a reference point for tumor classification as gastric or esophageal. Any tumor entirely distal to the GEJ (not involving the GEJ) is classified as a gastric tumor (A) regardless of midpoint location. For tumors involving the GEJ, do not classify the tumor based on the location of the bulk of the tumor. Instead, the tumor midpoint (*stars*) is the important reference point. Those with a tumor midpoint ≤2 cm into the stomach (B) are esophageal, and those with tumor midpoint >2 cm into the stomach (C) are gastric.

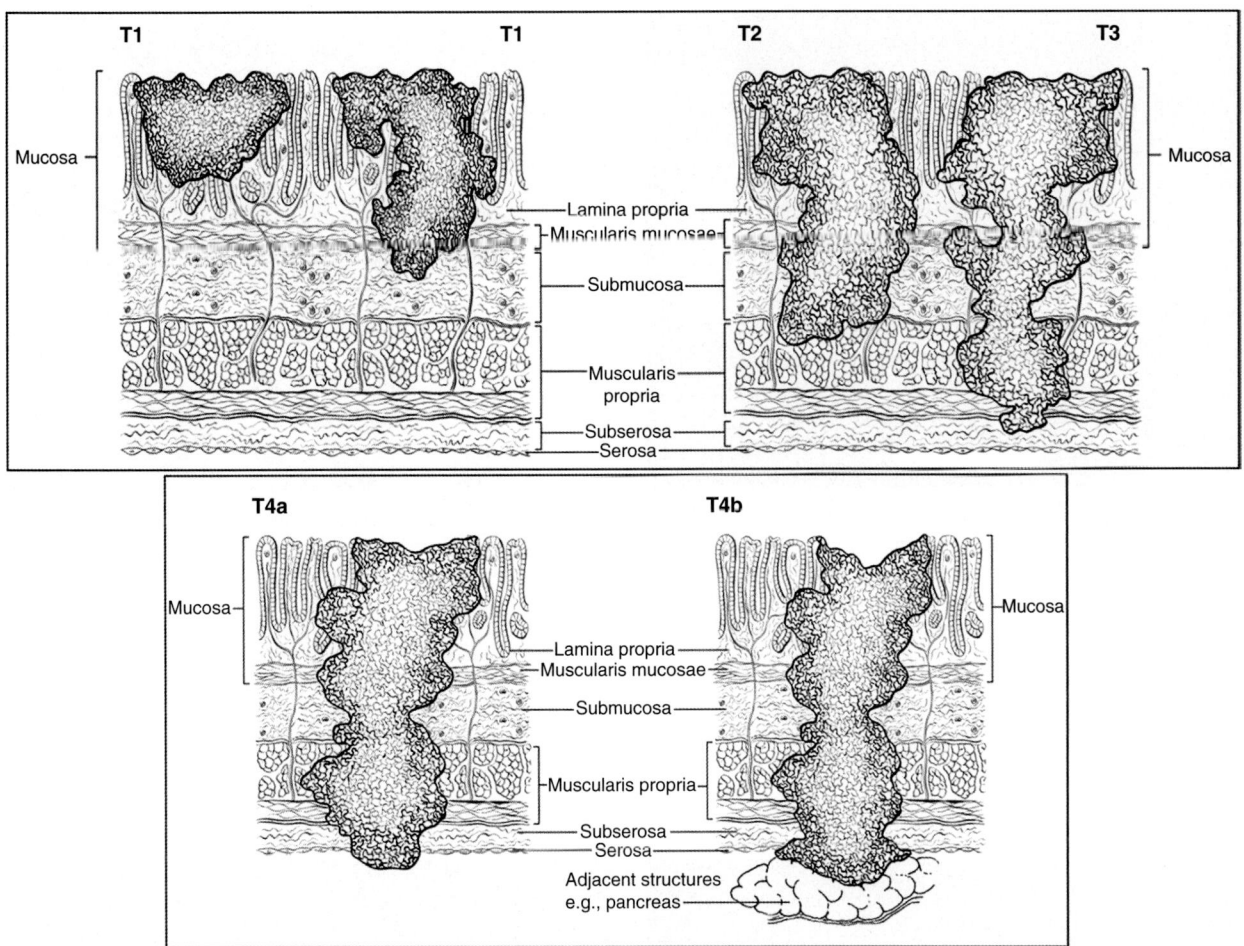

Figure 2-129. Pathologic T staging of gastric cancer, AJCC eighth edition. T1 is divided into lamina propria invasion (pT1a) and invasion into submucosa (pT1b). Involvement of muscularis propria is pT2, whereas invasion beyond the muscularis propria into the subserosal tissue is pT3. Penetration of the serosa (visceral peritoneum) is pT4a, and when adjacent structures are involved the stage is designated pT4b. (Used with permission of the American Joint Committee on Cancer [AJCC], Chicago, IL. The original source for this material is the *AJCC Cancer Staging Atlas*. [2006]. Greene FL, Compton CC, Fritz AG, et al. [eds.]. Springer Science and Business Media, LLC. www.springerlink.com.)

TUMOR CLASSIFICATION: LAUREN, MING, AND WHO MORPHOLOGIC VARIANTS

In addition to providing basic histologic typing, the Lauren tumor type offers significant prognostic information and is simple to apply.[69] The Lauren tumor type is divided into two chief categories: intestinal-type and diffuse-type gastric adenocarcinomas; tumors that do not fit into these two categories are considered indeterminate unclassified types. Mass-forming and expansile gastric adenocarcinomas that arise in a backdrop of IM are classified as intestinal type (Figs. 2.130 and 2.131). By comparison, adenocarcinomas that have an infiltrative growth pattern and arise without the backdrop of IM are classified as diffuse type. The classic example for diffuse type is the signet ring cell carcinoma with endoscopic characteristics of poor insufflation (linitis plastica) and the absence of an endoscopically visible mass lesion (Figs. 2.132–2.134), features that contribute to the worse prognosis as compared with the intestinal type. The relative frequencies are 50% to 67% for intestinal type, 29% to 35% for diffuse type, and 3% to 21% for indeterminate type.[70] A similar two-tiered Ming grading system is used by some pathologists, in which the categories "expanding type" and "infiltrative type" correlate with Lauren's intestinal and diffuse types, respectively.

The Lauren classification is used most widely by pathologists but does not specify the morphologic variants. The WHO 2010 classification of gastric carcinomas includes seven major tumor varieties, including adenocarcinoma, adenosquamous carcinoma, carcinoma with lymphoid stroma (medullary carcinoma), hepatoid adenocarcinoma, squamous cell

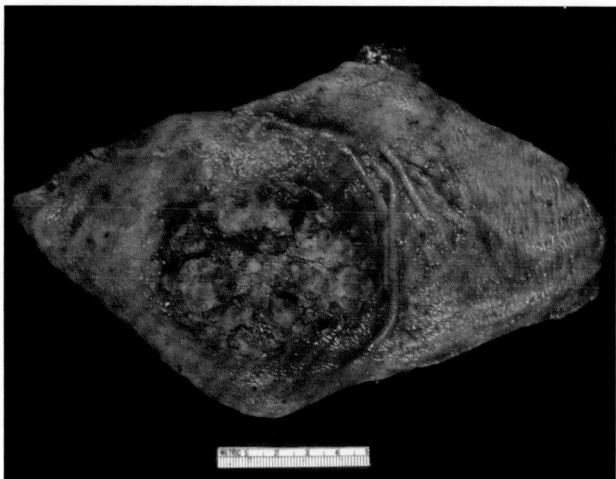

Figure 2-130. Gastric adenocarcinoma, intestinal type, gross specimen. The gross pathology of gastric cancer correlates closely with histologic classification in the Lauren and Ming systems. This large, mass-forming exophytic growth represents an intestinal type (Lauren) or expanding type (Ming) even without histologic review.

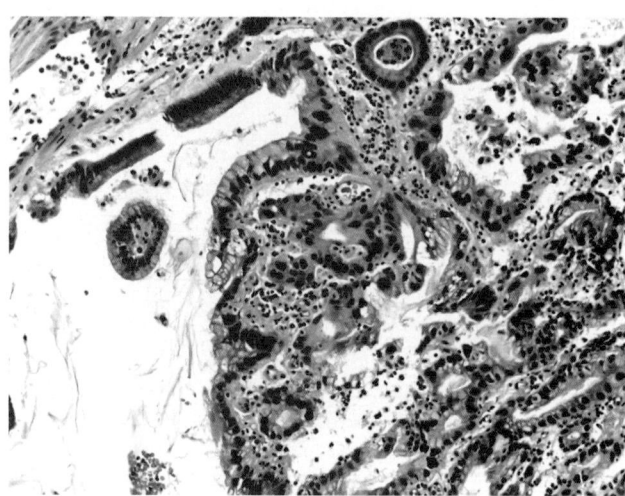

Figure 2-131. Gastric adenocarcinoma, representative histology of the previous figure. Histologic features show the mass lesion is composed of malignant glands with an expansile growth pattern.

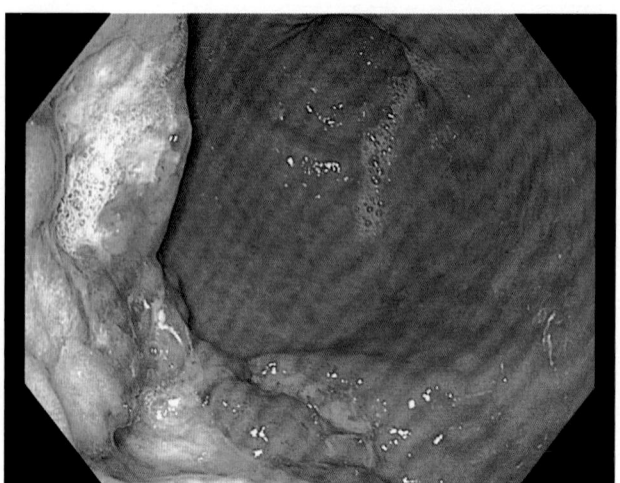

Figure 2-132. Stomach linitis plastica, endoscopic view. The stomach shows loss of rugal folds and has a stiff "leather bottle" quality that results in poor insufflation and distensibility. No mass lesion is visible, but this endoscopic feature is synonymous with gastric adenocarcinoma, diffuse type (Lauren) or infiltrating type (Ming).

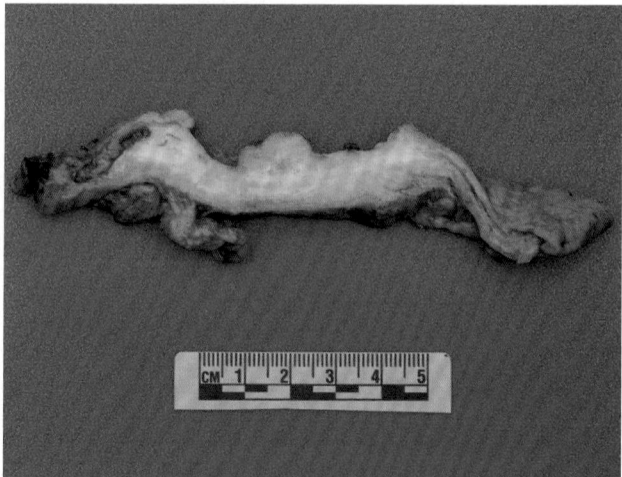

Figure 2-133. Stomach linitis plastica, gross specimen cross section. The gastric wall is thickened and stiff without an obvious mass lesion. Histologic sections reveal diffuse infiltration of the gastric wall by sheets of discohesive malignant cells.

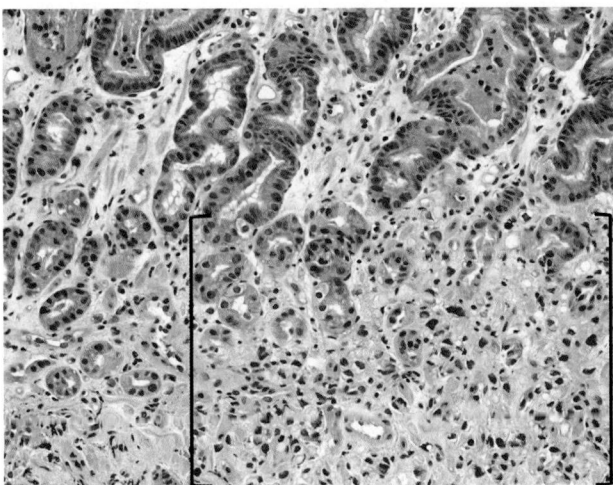

Figure 2-134. Gastric adenocarcinoma, representative histology of the previous figure. Histologic features show architecturally intact superficial mucosa without an expansile mass lesion. Instead, single discohesive malignant cells (*brackets*) infiltrate the mucosa without much disruption of the glands. This pattern is classified as diffuse type by Lauren or infiltrating type by Ming, both simple bimodal classification systems. By WHO classification, this tumor is a poorly cohesive carcinoma variant.

carcinoma, undifferentiated carcinoma, and neuroendocrine carcinoma (NEC).[71] The WHO adenocarcinoma group is further divided into additional morphologic subtypes, including papillary, tubular, mucinous, poorly cohesive carcinomas, and mixed carcinoma; the differentiating histologic features are summarized in Table 2.4. Although most multivariate analyses show no effect of these tumor types (aside from the poorly performing small cell carcinoma) on prognosis independent of grade or stage,[72] this morphologic classification is useful to include in a biopsy report to assist pathologist colleagues who will review surgical margin frozen sections or work up metastatic deposits. Of the adenocarcinoma variants, two WHO morphologic subtypes correlate with the Lauren diffuse type: (1) mucinous adenocarcinoma, defined as having at least 50% extracellular mucin pools (with or without signet ring cells), and (2) poorly cohesive adenocarcinoma, which includes the signet ring cell variant as well as other variants. In general, these WHO, Lauren, and Ming groups correlate closely.[73]

Signet ring cell carcinoma is a specific subset of poorly cohesive carcinomas that is composed predominantly of discohesive single cells with distended cytoplasmic mucin that displaces and eccentrically compresses the nucleus. This designation should be restricted to tumors composed predominantly of the signet ring cell type, as other variants of poorly cohesive carcinomas may also infiltrate in a diffuse or single cell pattern, but are mucin poor (Figs. 2.135–2.163). In either case, these are the carcinomas that provide the most challenge on endoscopic biopsies because they lack the helpful red flag of an endoscopic mass, and stromal desmoplasia is frequently absent. Examine gastric biopsies with careful attention to areas of pallor, crush artifact, or slightly increased cellularity. Make sure to account for every cell in the tissue and call out any possible mimickers before moving on (e.g., crushed oxyntic glands, mucous neck cells, xanthoma cells). If there is any uncertainty, a pancytokeratin immunostain can aid in highlighting the architecture of epithelial cells (Figs. 2.142 and 2.152), and consultation with a fellow surgical pathologist may clarify matters. Squamous cell carcinomas may be either keratinizing or nonkeratinizing, and adenosquamous carcinomas should have at least 25% squamous component by volume mixed with a glandular component. Biopsy material may not be wholly representative, and final morphologic classification can be either reserved for or revised following review of the resection specimen. The carcinoma with lymphoid stroma (also referred to as medullary carcinoma or lymphoepithelioma-like carcinoma) may resemble well differentiated tubular adenocarcinomas or undifferentiated carcinomas with poorly formed sheets of tumor cells, but in all instances it contains a prominent stromal lymphoid infiltrate, sometimes nearly obscuring the carcinoma itself (Figs. 2.164–2.171). This tumor has reactivity

TABLE 2.4: WHO 2010 Classification of Gastric Carcinomas

Tumor Type	Histologic Features	
Adenocarcinoma		
Papillary	Exophytic tumor with finger-like or frond-like projections containing fibrovascular cores Usually low grade	
Tubular	Branching and anastomosing tubules with dilated or slit-like lumen Usually low grade	
Mucinous	>50% extracellular mucin pools May contain signet ring cells Lauren classification = diffuse type	
Poorly cohesive carcinomas (signet ring cell and other variants)	Infiltrating single cells or small aggregates Signet ring cell type is a specific subset composed predominantly of signet ring cells containing a clear droplet of cytoplasmic mucin displacing the nucleus Lauren classification = diffuse type	
Mixed	Mixture of morphologically identifiable components (e.g., tubular, papillary, poorly cohesive)	
Adenosquamous carcinoma	≥25% squamous component mixed with glandular	
Carcinoma with lymphoid stroma	Poorly differentiated carcinoma with prominent lymphoid infiltrate Associated with Epstein-Barr virus Better prognosis	
Hepatoid adenocarcinoma	Resembles hepatocellular carcinoma with large polygonal cells containing abundant eosinophilic cytoplasm May express alpha-fetoprotein	
Squamous cell carcinoma	Either keratinizing or nonkeratinizing	
Undifferentiated carcinoma	High-grade carcinoma not classifiable among other categories	
Neuroendocrine carcinoma (NEC)		
Large cell NEC	Poorly differentiated High grade Marked nuclear atypia Synaptophysin+ or chromogranin+ May have: Focal necrosis Ki-67 >20% >20 mitoses per 10 HPF	Cells are large and pleomorphic Moderate amount of cytoplasm Prominent nucleoli
Small cell NEC		Cells are small Finely granular chromatin ("salt and pepper") Indistinct nucleoli
Mixed adenoneuroendocrine carcinoma (MANEC)		>30% each of gland-forming and neuroendocrine areas (Adenocarcinomas showing immunoreactivity for neuroendocrine markers is not sufficient for diagnosis.)

for Epstein-Barr virus–encoded RNA by in situ hybridization (EBER ISH) and is more commonly seen in the proximal stomach, among men and in a younger age group. Some observers have reported significantly better prognosis via longer disease-free survival and overall cancer survival attributed to the younger age at presentation and less lymph node metastasis.[74,75] Another interesting variant, hepatoid adenocarcinoma, morphologically resembles hepatocellular carcinoma with large polygonal cells containing abundant eosinophilic granular cytoplasm (Figs. 2.172–2.175). These hepatoid gastric adenocarcinomas can raise concern for metastatic hepatocellular carcinoma and may even express immunoreactivity for alpha-fetoprotein (AFP) and glypican-3, which are also reactive in hepatocellular carcinomas.[76] SALL4 immunohistochemistry may help differentiate these tumors, as it is expressed in 89% of AFP-positive hepatoid gastric adenocarcinomas and negative in most hepatocellular carcinoma.[76] However, we would caution that a subset of primary liver hepatocellular carcinomas are SALL4 reactive; these latter tumors tend to be aggressive but, thankfully, targetable.[77] Tumors demonstrating features that are not classifiable into one of the other WHO categories are considered undifferentiated carcinomas.

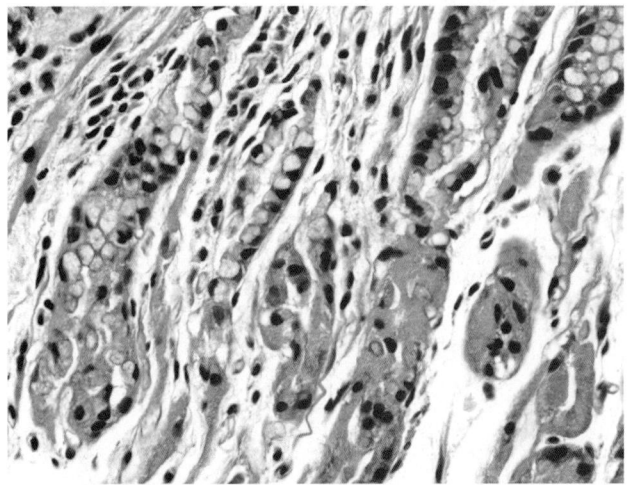

Figure 2-135. Benign gastric mucous neck cells. Do not overcall carcinoma when benign gastric mucous neck cells are seen. These mucous filled cells found in the neck of gastric pits/glands are inconspicuous in normal tissues but can appear concerning when tissue is crushed, fragmented, or reactive. Do not make a diagnosis of signet ring carcinoma unless there is 100% certainty; suggest rebiopsy if the diagnosis is unclear.

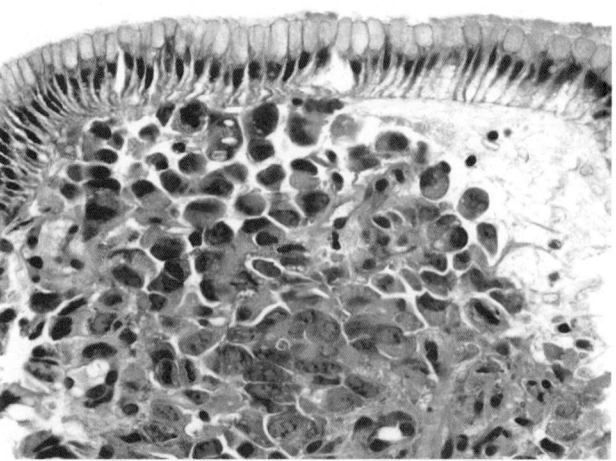

Figure 2-136. Gastric adenocarcinoma, diffuse type. These discohesive cells are infiltrating beneath an intact and benign surface epithelium.

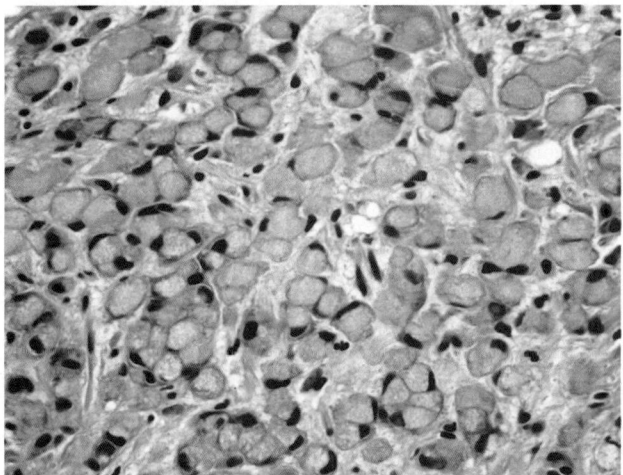

Figure 2-137. Gastric adenocarcinoma, diffuse type. Single discohesive and non-gland-forming cells infiltrate the wall of the stomach. The cytoplasm is filled with mucin and pushes the nucleus off to one side, similar in profile to a signet ring.

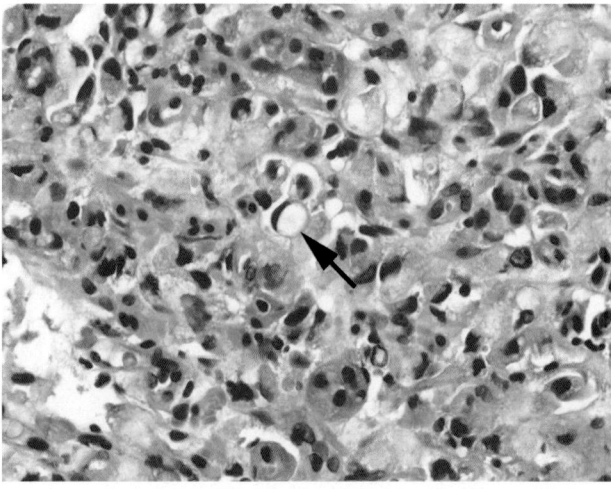

Figure 2-138. Gastric adenocarcinoma, diffuse type, with signet ring cells. True signet ring cells (arrow) have cytoplasm distended with a clear vacuole of mucin that displaces and compresses the nucleus.

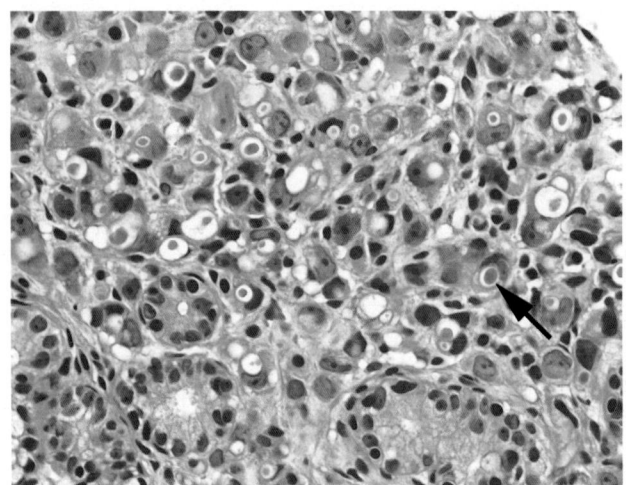

Figure 2-139. Metastatic lobular breast carcinoma. These tumor cells appear similar to signet ring cells, but lobular breast carcinoma cells do not contain mucin. Instead, there is a single round cytoplasmic vacuole with a sharply demarcated border, which sometimes contains a dense hyaline eosinophilic body (*arrow*) imparting a targetoid appearance.

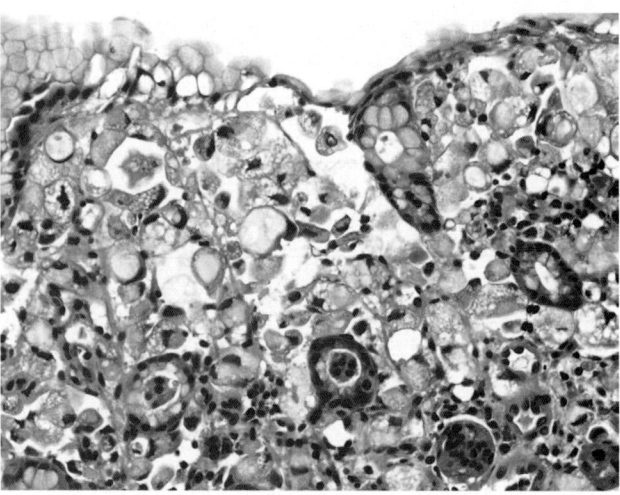

Figure 2-140. Gastric adenocarcinoma, diffuse type, with signet ring cells. Signet ring cells have distended clear cytoplasm filled with mucin that displaces the nucleus to the periphery. This example shows marked variation in size and shape among the signet ring cells.

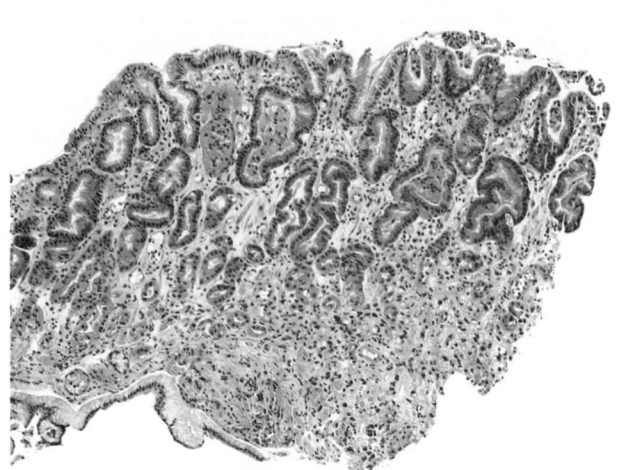

Figure 2-141. Gastric adenocarcinoma, diffuse type. At low magnification, one can appreciate how the malignant cells diffusely infiltrate the gastric mucosa without forming an obvious mass lesion. The surface epithelium is intact, and the gastric pits remain relatively evenly spaced. The absence of significant architectural disturbance makes the diffuse type of gastric adenocarcinoma more difficult to spot than the intestinal mass-forming type.

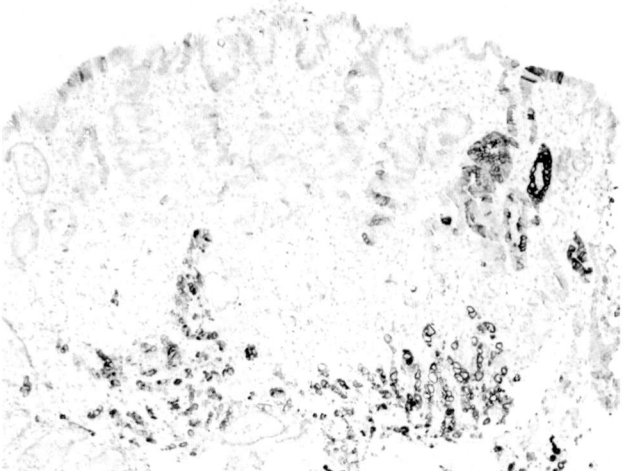

Figure 2-142. Gastric adenocarcinoma, diffuse type, cytokeratin 7 immunohistochemistry of the previous figure. A cytokeratin immunostain can be helpful to assess the architecture in difficult cases. In this example, CK7 highlights a lack of normal gland formation and single infiltrating cells at the base of the biopsy.

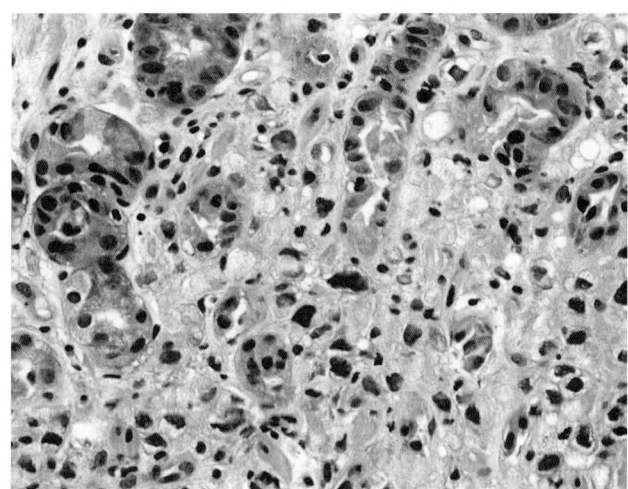

Figure 2-143. Gastric adenocarcinoma, diffuse type, higher magnification of the previous figure. The cells in this example are markedly atypical with large, irregularly shaped nuclei that vary in size.

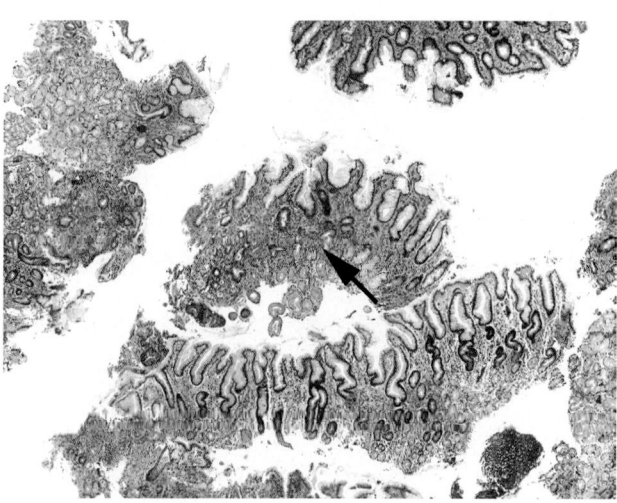

Figure 2-144. Gastric adenocarcinoma, diffuse type. Take care to look closely at "busy" gastric biopsies. At low magnification, the inflammatory cells and reactive gastropathy changes obscure a focus of gastric adenocarcinoma (*arrow*). One good rule of thumb is to always review gastric biopsies at high magnification and mentally account for all cells present.

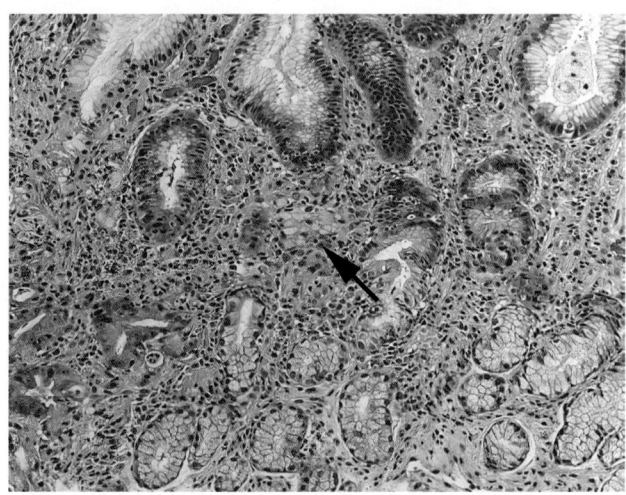

Figure 2-145. Gastric adenocarcinoma, diffuse type, higher magnification of the previous figure. Amid a background of acute and chronic inflammation, this cluster of signet ring cells (*arrow*) could be easily overlooked. Do not forget to always look beyond the first (obvious) diagnosis.

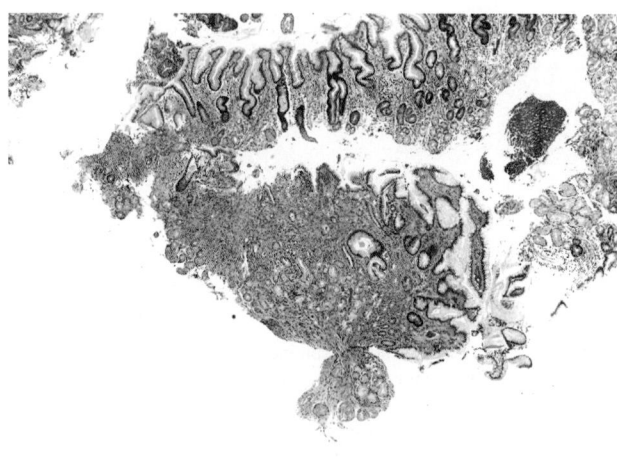

Figure 2-146. Gastric adenocarcinoma, diffuse type. This low-power view shows a "busy" gastric biopsy with surface erosion and abundant inflammation. Always look closer at areas that appear abnormal at low magnification.

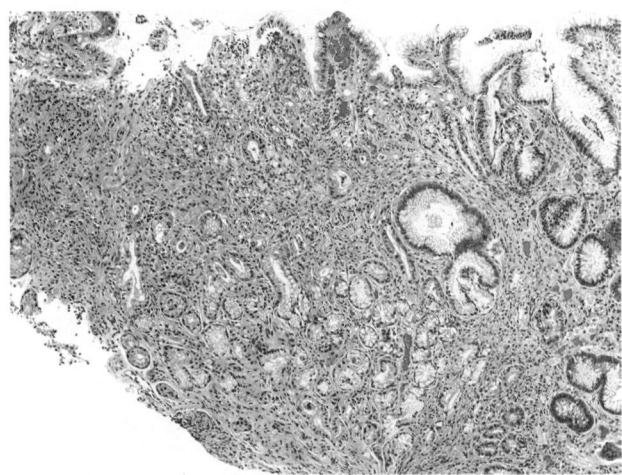

Figure 2-147. Gastric adenocarcinoma, diffuse type, higher magnification of the previous figure. Even at midpower magnification, the adenocarcinoma hiding in this busy tissue fragment is not clear. The malignant cells blend into the background of inflammation which is distracting one's eye.

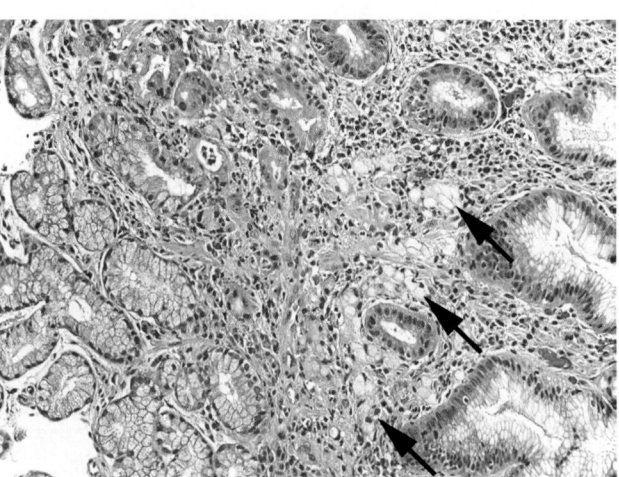

Figure 2-148. Gastric adenocarcinoma, diffuse type, higher magnification of the previous figure. These sneaky signet ring cell clusters (*arrows*) are only visible at high magnification, underscoring the importance of reviewing each gastric biopsy at high power and mentally registering each and every cell.

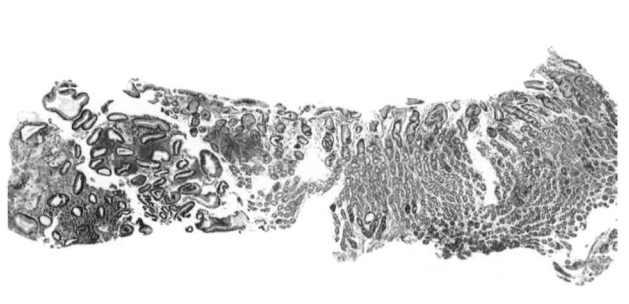

Figure 2-149. Gastric adenocarcinoma, diffuse type. This low-power view shows gastric mucosa with an area of edema and lamina propria hemorrhage. It looks harmless at this power, but any area of abnormality should always trigger a higher-power perusal.

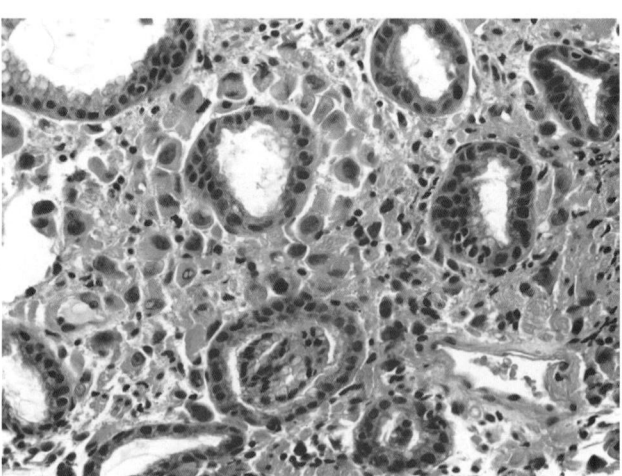

Figure 2-150. Gastric adenocarcinoma, diffuse type, higher magnification of the previous figure. Impossible to see at low magnification, these small malignant cells infiltrate between the benign glands, leaving the architecture relatively intact.

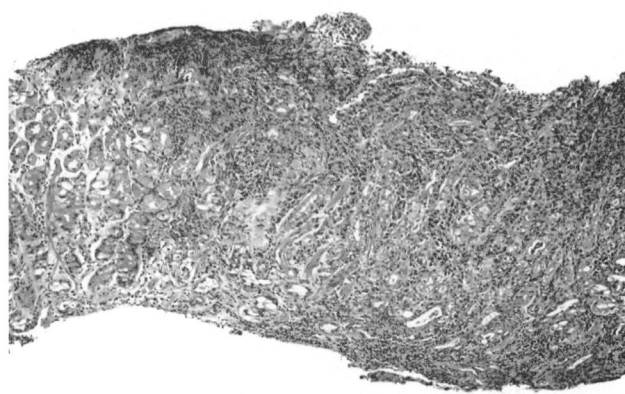

Figure 2-151. Gastric adenocarcinoma, diffuse type. Areas of gastric erosion and chronic inflammation should always trigger a closer examination. Inflammation can be particularly devious in hiding gastric cancer.

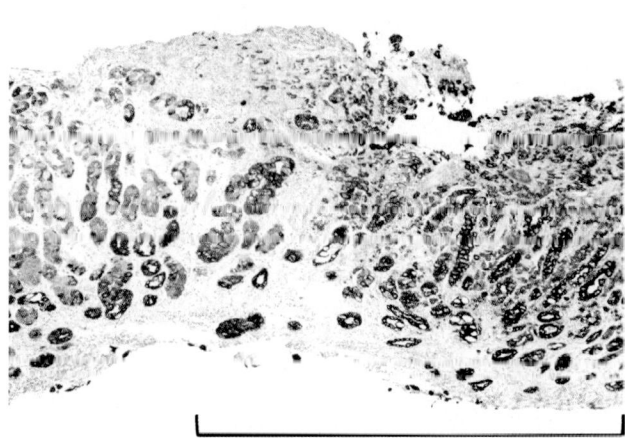

Figure 2-152. Gastric adenocarcinoma, diffuse type, pancyto-keratin immunostain of the previous figure. A pancytokeratin stain highlights a broad area containing single infiltrating cells (*bracket*). The extent of invasive carcinoma is frequently surprising when highlighted in this manner and demonstrates how challenging it is to discern these cells on H&E. Contrast the malignant area against the normal glandular architecture to the left.

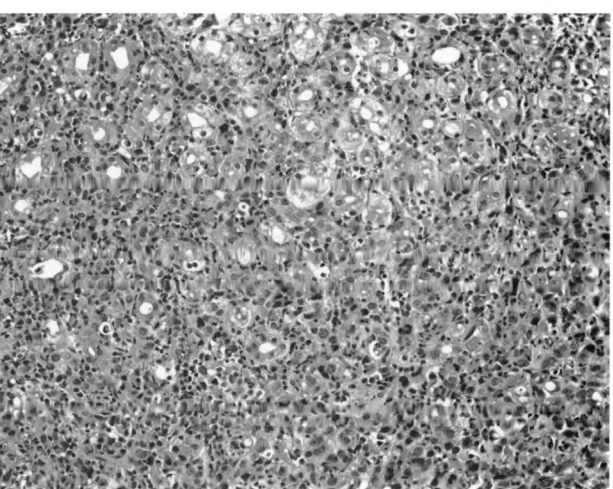

Figure 2-153. Gastric adenocarcinoma, diffuse type, higher magnification of the previous figure. The malignant cells are obscured by the inflammatory backdrop. Some remnant benign glands add to the difficulty in diagnosis. Even at this magnification, it can be challenging to point out the malignant cells. Always take a moment to go to high magnification and mentally account for each cell.

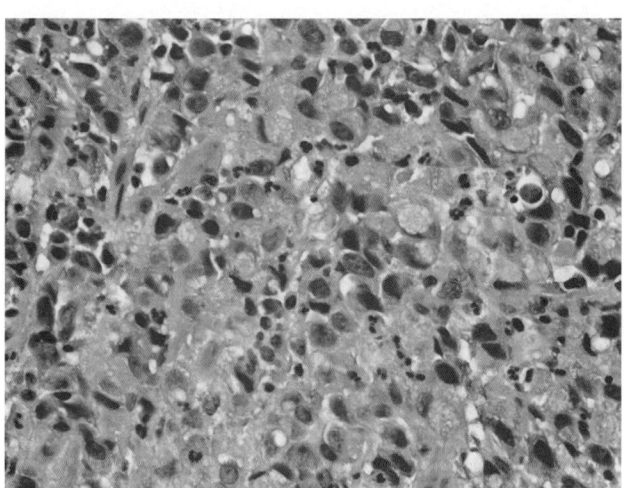

Figure 2-154. Gastric adenocarcinoma, diffuse type, higher magnification of the previous figure . High magnification reveals many malignant cells admixed with acute and chronic inflammatory cells. At this magnification, it is possible to name each cell present as benign or malignant.

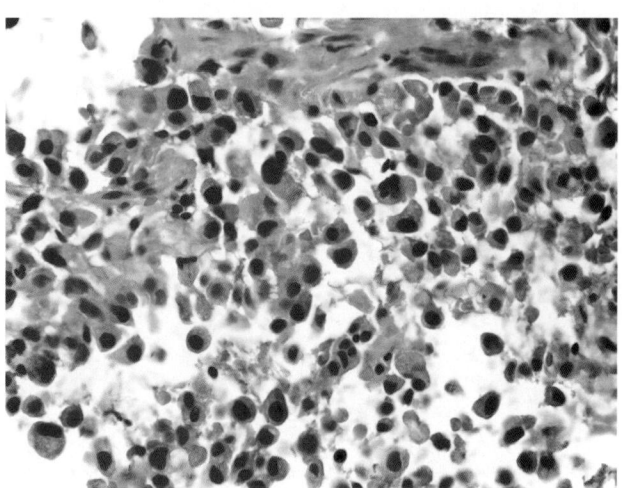

Figure 2-155. Gastric adenocarcinoma, diffuse type. These discohesive tumor cells are characteristic of diffuse-type adenocarcinoma by Lauren classification, infiltrative type by Ming classification, and poorly cohesive carcinoma by WHO classification. The cells lack clear cytoplasmic mucin vacuoles and thus are not true signet ring cells.

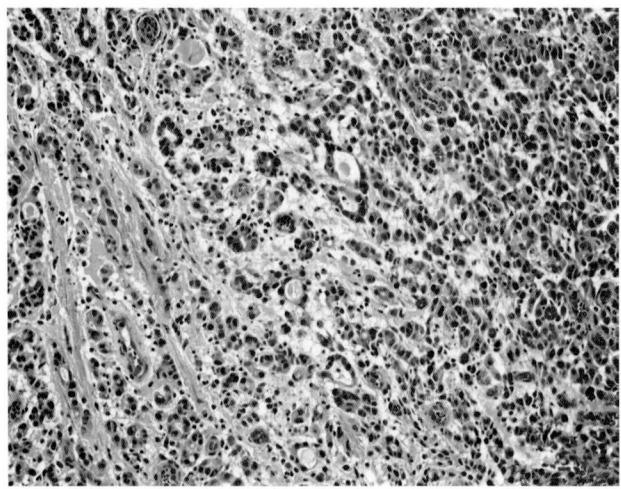

Figure 2-156. Gastric adenocarcinoma, diffuse type. Another example of the infiltrative discohesive tumor cells found in diffuse-type adenocarcinoma. These cells permeate the gastric wall without forming a mass lesion and frequently have no background gastritis or other gastric pathology.

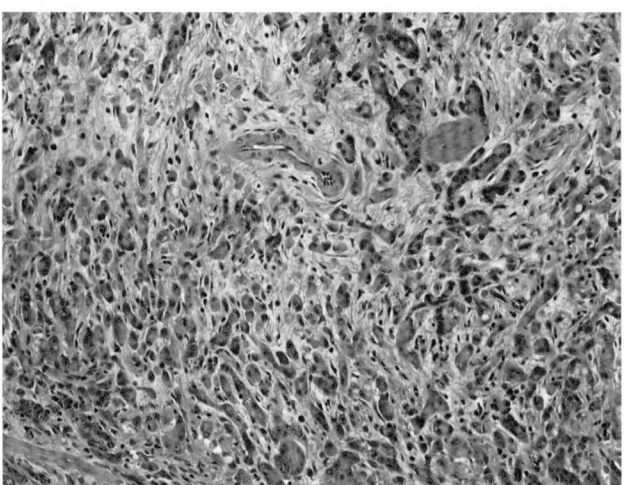

Figure 2-157. Gastric adenocarcinoma, diffuse type, eosinophilic variant. The cells in this unusual example of diffuse-type adenocarcinoma are deeply eosinophilic and lack intracytoplasmic mucin. This is classified as a poorly cohesive carcinoma by the WHO classification, which includes signet ring cell and other variants. The tumor contains <50% glands and is therefore poorly differentiated.

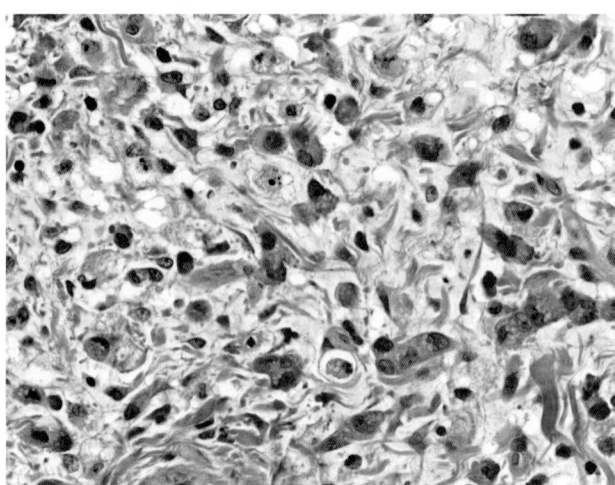

Figure 2-158. Gastric adenocarcinoma, diffuse type, eosinophilic variant. The cells are markedly atypical with eosinophilic cytoplasm and a myxoid backdrop. These are not signet ring cells because they lack the characteristic clear vacuole of intracytoplasmic mucin.

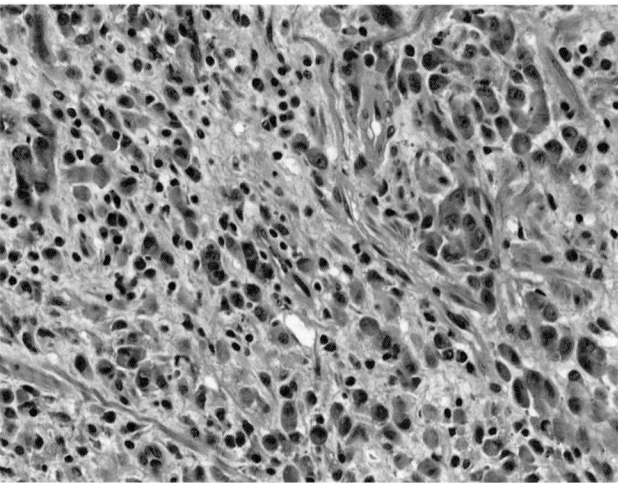

Figure 2-159. Gastric adenocarcinoma, diffuse type, eosinophilic variant. This unusual variant contains cells that have abundant eosinophilic cytoplasm without mucin. Some areas show cohesive malignant cells arranged in cords.

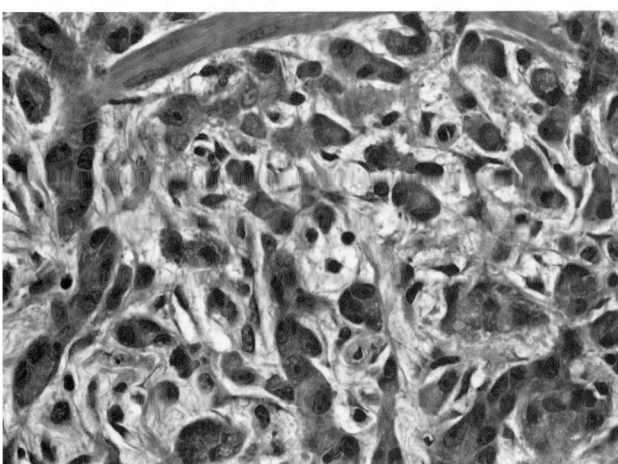

Figure 2-160. Gastric adenocarcinoma, diffuse type, eosinophilic variant. The tumor cells appear plasmacytoid with irregular nuclei containing conspicuous nucleoli. These should not be mistaken for signet ring cells, as they lack the characteristic compressed nucleus and cytoplasmic mucin vacuole.

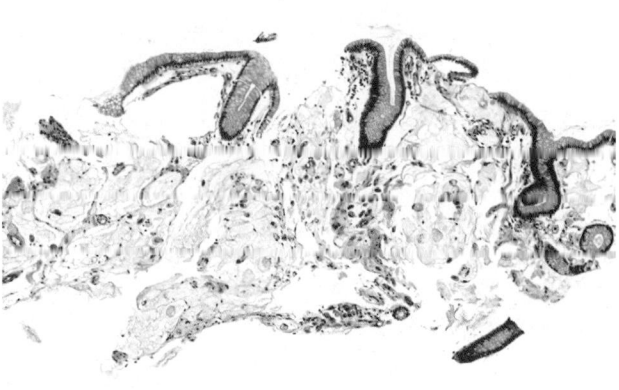

Figure 2-161. Gastric adenocarcinoma, WHO mucinous type. These tumors contain >50% extracellular mucin pools and are considered a diffuse type by Lauren classification and are poorly differentiated by definition.

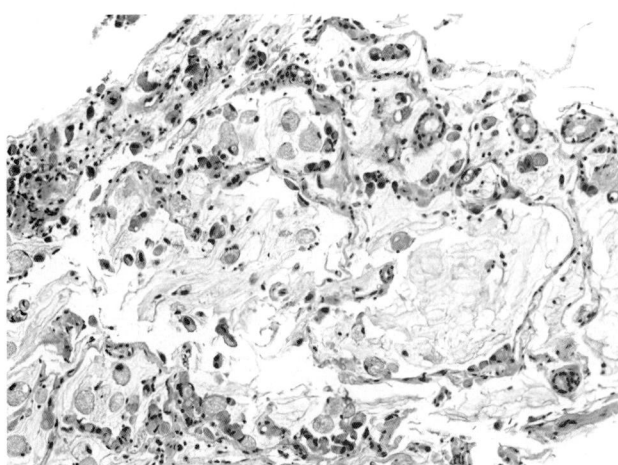

Figure 2-162. Gastric adenocarcinoma, WHO mucinous type, Lauren diffuse type. There is abundant intracellular and extracellular mucin, the latter of which comprises >50% of the tumor.

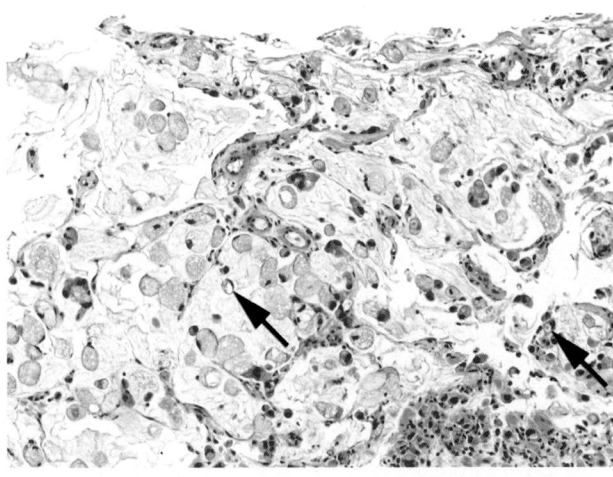

Figure 2-163. Gastric adenocarcinoma, WHO mucinous type, Lauren diffuse type. Mucinous adenocarcinoma may or may not contain signet ring cells (*arrows*).

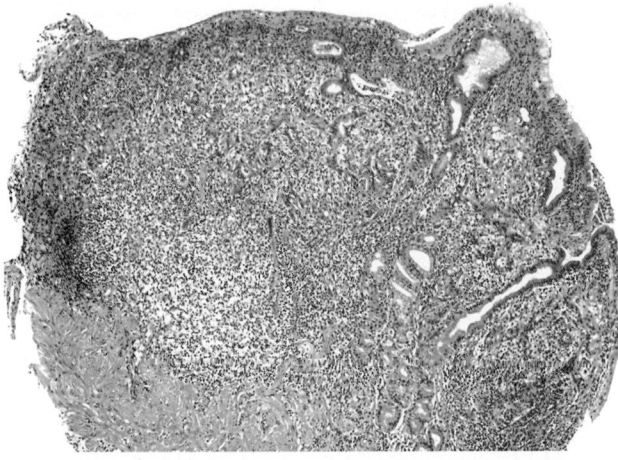

Figure 2-164. Gastric adenocarcinoma with lymphoid stroma (EBV-associated gastric adenocarcinoma). At low magnification, this mass-forming lesion shows a prominent lymphoid infiltrate that obscures the glands. At first glance, one might consider a lymphoid neoplasm such as MALT lymphoma.

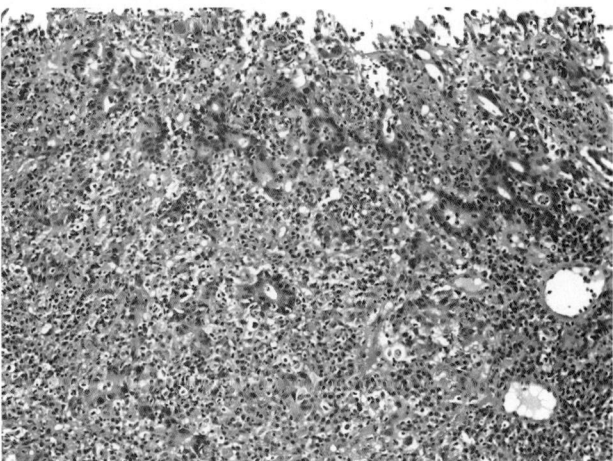

Figure 2-165. Gastric adenocarcinoma with lymphoid stroma (EBV-associated gastric adenocarcinoma). Higher magnification of the previous figure shows abnormal distorted and abortive glands with prominent intraepithelial lymphocytes. These features are reminiscent of lymphoepithelial lesions found in MALT lymphoma, but do not be fooled, and take a closer look at higher power.

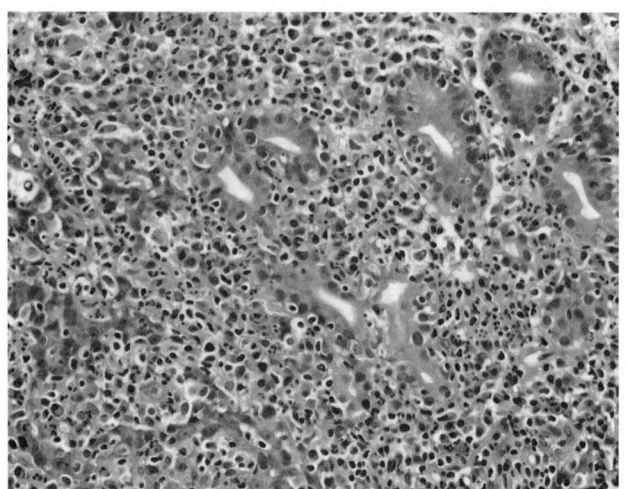

Figure 2-166. Gastric adenocarcinoma with lymphoid stroma (EBV-associated gastric adenocarcinoma). The intact glands show abundant intraepithelial lymphocytes, but the abnormal glands are composed of malignant cells, indicating this is in fact a carcinoma and not a lymphoma.

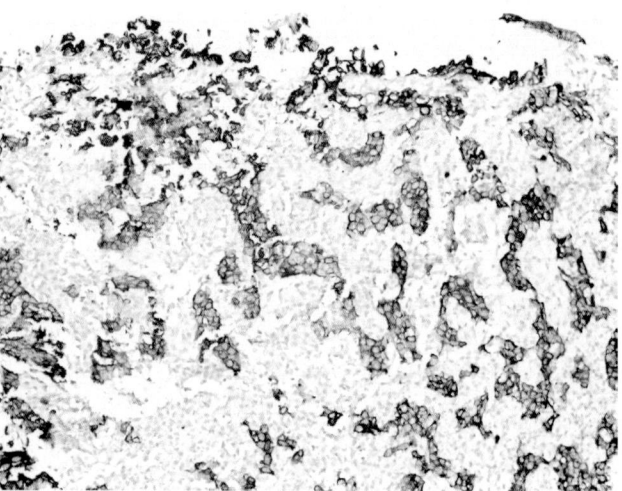

Figure 2-167. Gastric adenocarcinoma with lymphoid stroma (EBV-associated gastric adenocarcinoma), pancytokeratin immunostain. Immunohistochemistry highlights the poorly formed glands, which are more abundant than visualized on H&E and infiltrative in architecture.

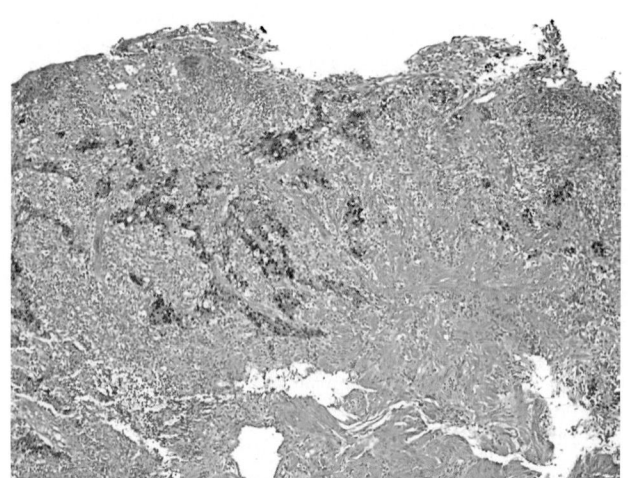

Figure 2-168. Gastric adenocarcinoma with lymphoid stroma (EBV-associated gastric adenocarcinoma), in situ hybridization for Epstein-Barr virus encoded RNA (EBER ISH). A subset of adenocarcinomas with lymphoid stroma will show positivity for EBER ISH localized to the tumor nuclei, as in this example.

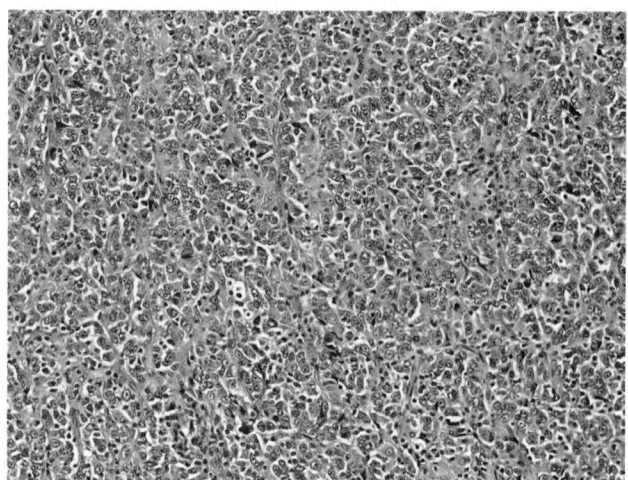

Figure 2-169. Gastric adenocarcinoma with lymphoid stroma (EBV-associated gastric adenocarcinoma). Another example of a poorly differentiated gastric carcinoma with abundant lymphoid cells. The lymphocytes in close association with these sheets of malignant cells are a clue to the diagnosis of EBV-associated gastric cancer and a relatively better prognosis.

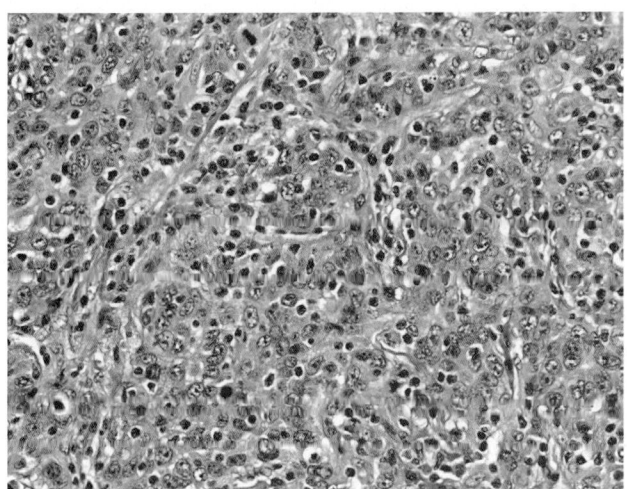

Figure 2-170. Gastric adenocarcinoma with lymphoid stroma (EBV-associated gastric adenocarcinoma). Higher magnification of the previous figure shows syncytial sheets of tumor cells with indistinct cell borders and numerous intratumoral lymphocytes. Previous names for this tumor include medullary carcinoma or lymphoepitheliallike carcinoma. The tumor is considered poorly differentiated because it has <50% gland formation.

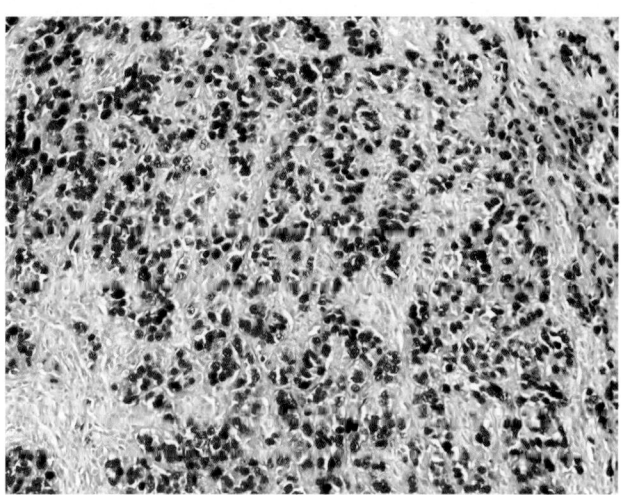

Figure 2-171. Gastric adenocarcinoma with lymphoid stroma (EBV-associated gastric adenocarcinoma). In situ hybridization for Epstein-Barr encoded RNA shows the tumor nuclei contain EBV RNA. This finding is associated with a better prognosis.

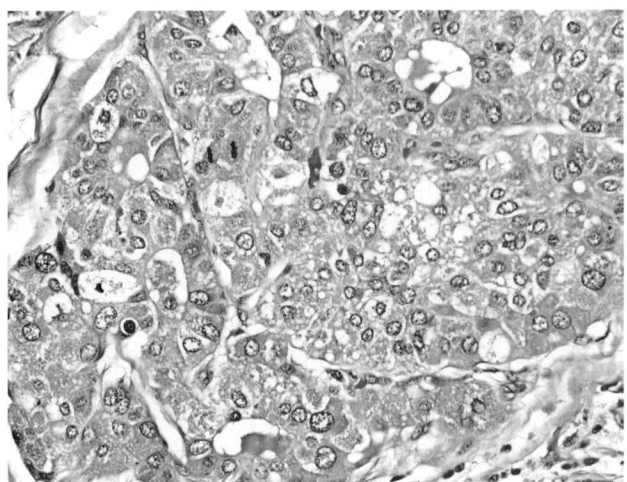

Figure 2-172. Gastric adenocarcinoma, WHO hepatoid variant. This tumor resembles hepatocellular carcinoma with large polygonal cells containing abundant granular cytoplasm. Pseudoacini may be present, and this example even shows bile formation.

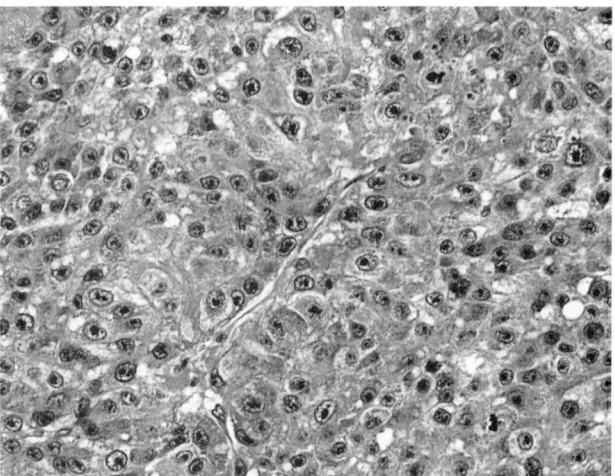

Figure 2-173. Gastric adenocarcinoma, WHO hepatoid variant. This gastric cancer shows sheets of malignant cells with abundant eosinophilic granular cytoplasm and prominent nucleoli arranged in sheets or wide trabeculae with fine endothelial spaces simulating hepatic sinusoids. The cytology and architecture are hepatoid. Exclusion of metastatic hepatocellular carcinoma to the stomach may require correlation with radiologic findings.

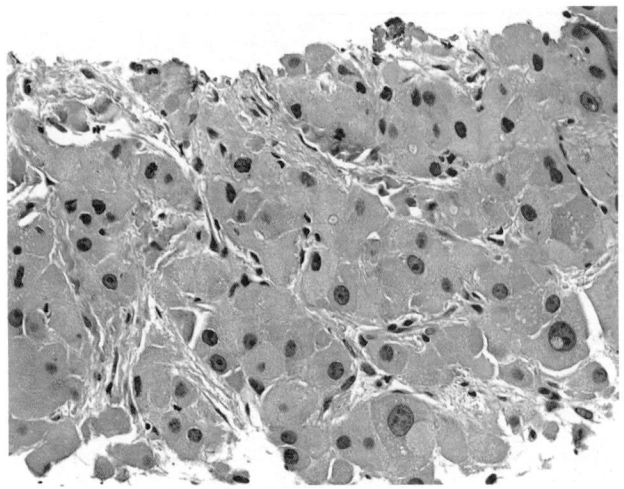

Figure 2-174. Gastric adenocarcinoma, WHO hepatoid variant. The tumor is composed of large cells with abundant eosinophilic cytoplasm and round nuclei with prominent nucleoli arranged in vague trabeculae. The delicate vasculature reinforces the similarity to widened hepatic plates and sinusoids.

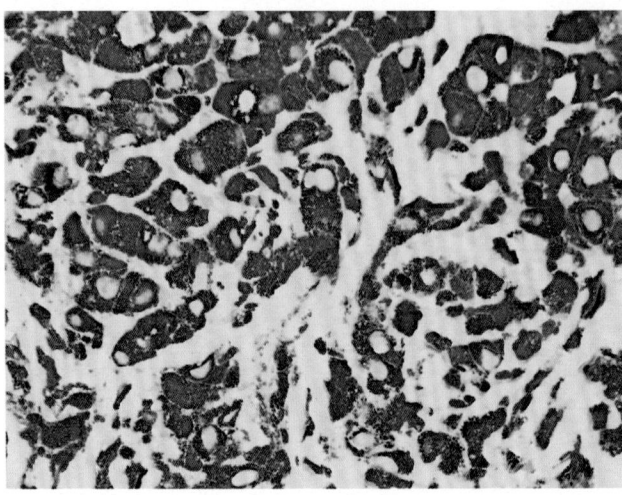

Figure 2-175. Gastric adenocarcinoma, WHO hepatoid variant, hepatocyte-specific antigen (HSA). Hepatoid variant of primary gastric carcinoma may be reactive for HSA (pictured), AFP, and glypican-3, all of which are also reactive in hepatocellular carcinoma. SALL-4 can help differentiate these tumors, as it is positive in most gastric hepatoid carcinomas and negative in hepatocellular carcinoma.

NECs are classified as such by their poorly differentiated high-grade cytology and marked nuclear atypia, although this was not always the case. The now outdated WHO 2010 classification of neuroendocrine neoplasms defined three grades based purely on mitotic rate and Ki-67 index, with the high grade (G3) category defined as >20 mitoses per 10 HPF or Ki-67 proliferation index >20% without regard to histologic atypia.[71] This older WHO 2010 classification regarded G3 neoplasms as synonymous with poorly differentiated NECs. However, when investigators divided the G3 group into morphologically well- and poorly differentiated tumors, the poorly differentiated tumors had different etiologies, genetic alterations, and response to treatment with worse survival outcomes.[78-82] For these reasons, the updated classification of endocrine tumors (WHO 2017) now relies first on morphologic features; a tumor should be identified as well differentiated or poorly differentiated before further stratification by mitotic count and Ki-67 proliferative index. In the case of poorly differentiated morphology, these should always be classified as NECs and staged as carcinomas.[83] This group can be further divided into (1) small cell type, in which the cells are small with finely granular "salt and pepper" chromatin and inconspicuous nucleoli (Figs. 2.176–2.179); (2) large cell type, in which the cells are large with a moderate amount of cytoplasm and prominent nucleoli (Figs. 2.180–2.181); and (3) mixed neuroendocrine-nonneuroendocrine neoplasm (MiNEN; previously "mixed adenoneuroendocrine carcinoma" or MANEC), in which the tumor is composed of at least 30% both NET and adenocarcinoma or other high-grade carcinoma. Immunoreactivity for neuroendocrine markers within an adenocarcinoma does not indicate MiNEN.

FAQ: What is the preferred classification system: Lauren, Ming, or WHO subtypes?

The Lauren system is the most commonly used classification system, dividing tumors into either "intestinal type" (mass-forming lesions with a backdrop of IM, such as seen in Figs. 2.130 and 2.131) or "diffuse type" (non–mass forming infiltrative tumors without an identifiable precursor lesion, such as seen in Figs. 2.132–2.134). The Ming classification is similar with "expanding" and "infiltrating" types that correlate with the Lauren's intestinal and diffuse types, respectively. All three (Lauren, Ming, and WHO) correlate closely, as described in the earlier text, and morphologic classification is helpful for frozen section interpretation and metastatic workups. Aside from the poorly performing small cell carcinoma, multivariate analyses show no effect of tumor type on prognosis, independent of grade or stage.

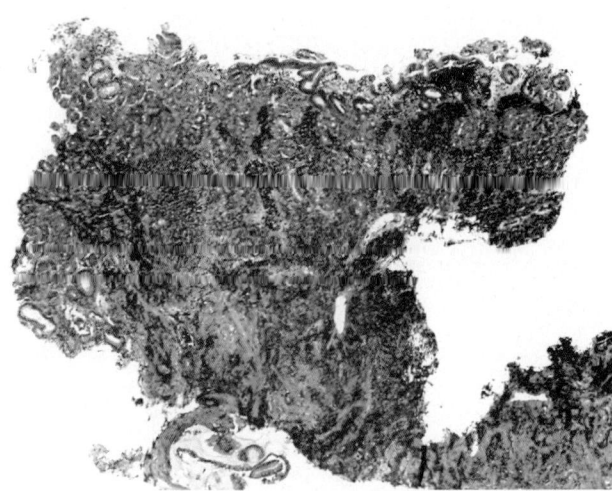

Figure 2-176. Gastric neuroendocrine carcinoma, small cell type. At low magnification, this gastric biopsy is markedly abnormal with a deeply basophilic infiltrate and considerations include lymphoma and poorly differentiated carcinoma.

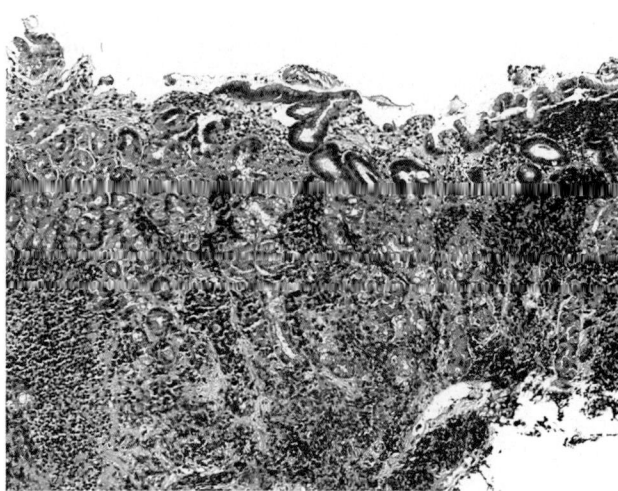

Figure 2-177. Gastric neuroendocrine carcinoma, small cell type. Higher magnification of the previous figure shows infiltrative highly atypical cells with prominent crush artifact.

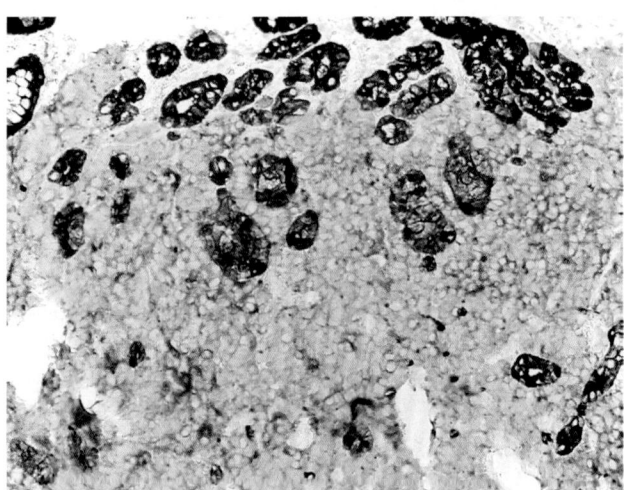

Figure 2-178. Gastric neuroendocrine carcinoma, small cell type, CAM 5.2 immunohistochemistry. Immunohistochemical stains show the tumor cells are positive for epithelial differentiation, thus ruling out lymphoma. Chromogranin (not pictured) was also positive, supporting neuroendocrine differentiation. Based on the high-grade morphology, this tumor qualifies as a poorly differentiated neuroendocrine carcinoma, G3, and is classified as small cell type because of the typical small cell features of high nuclear to cytoplasmic ratio, scant cytoplasm, absence of nucleoli, prominent nuclear molding, and crush artifact.

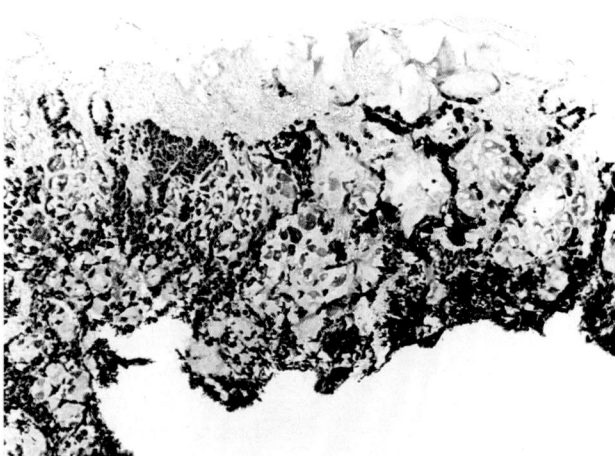

Figure 2-179. Gastric neuroendocrine carcinoma, small cell type, KI-67 immunohistochemistry. The proliferation index of the previous figures shows near 100% Ki-67 labeling in the tumor cells. This further supports a diagnosis of NEC.

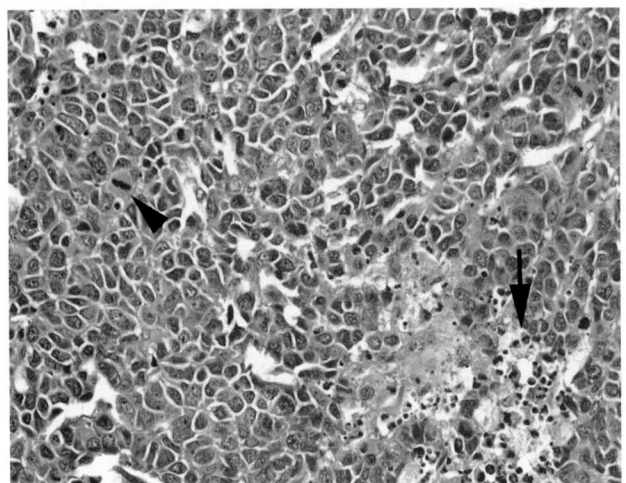

Figure 2-180. Gastric neuroendocrine carcinoma, large cell type. The high-grade cytologic features of this neuroendocrine neoplasm (confirmed by chromogranin and synaptophysin, not pictured) classify it as a poorly differentiated neuroendocrine carcinoma (G3) and not a well-differentiated neuroendocrine tumor. These cells are large with variation in size and shape, angulated nuclei, prominent nucleoli, and visible cytoplasm, differentiating it from small cell type. Frequent mitoses (*arrowhead*) and areas of necrosis (*arrow*) are present.

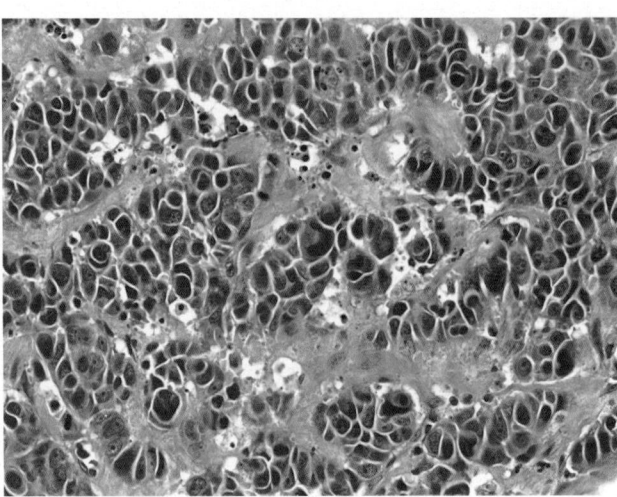

Figure 2-181. Gastric neuroendocrine carcinoma, large cell type. Another example shows large pleomorphic cells with variable amounts of cytoplasm and prominent nucleoli. A chromogranin immunostain (not pictured) confirms neuroendocrine differentiation, and the cytologic features classify this as a poorly differentiated neuroendocrine carcinoma, G3, large cell type. Note the frequent mitotic activity and areas of punctate necrosis.

FAQ: What does it mean when a signet ring cell carcinoma is not staining for mucin?

Not all tumors with single infiltrating cells are signet ring cell carcinomas. True signet ring cells have cytoplasm distended with a clear vacuole of mucin that displaces and compresses the nucleus (Fig. 2.138). Other poorly cohesive or diffuse type variants without intracytoplasmic mucin may have eosinophilic cytoplasm instead (Figs. 2.157–2.160) and should be classified as diffuse type gastric adenocarcinoma *without* the "signet ring" designation. Do not forget to consider metastatic lobular breast carcinoma, which may also mimic signet ring cells. Lobular breast carcinoma cells contain intracytoplasmic lumina, which can mimic the mucin vacuole of signet ring cells. However, the single round vacuole found in lobular breast carcinoma cells have thick sharply demarcated edges, sometimes contain a dense hyaline eosinophilic body imparting a "targetoid" appearance (Fig. 2.139), and are not mucicarminophilic. They can be differentiated from gastric cancer with immunohistochemistry for breast markers such as GCDFP or GATA3.

FAQ: How does one differentiate NET from NEC?

Based on WHO 2017 classification, NECs are identified by their poorly differentiated high-grade morphology (Figs. 2.180 and 2.181), independent of mitotic count or Ki-67 proliferative index. This is a departure from previous WHO 2010 classification for neuroendocrine neoplasms, which stratified tumors based purely on mitoses and Ki-67. The updated system not only indicates prognosis and response to therapy more reliably but is also more intuitive to pathologists. Tumors that are morphologically well differentiated are classified as well-differentiated NETs and can be further graded based on mitotic and Ki-67 cutoffs. See later in this chapter for a discussion on well-differentiated NETs.

PEARLS & PITFALLS: Histologic Grading of Gastric Adenocarcinomas

The histologic grading of adenocarcinomas is a three-tiered system and is based on the extent of glandular differentiation. Tumors with >95% gland formation are G1 (well differentiated), 50% to 95% are G2 (moderately differentiated), and <50% G3 (poorly differentiated or undifferentiated) (Figs. 2.182–2.185). The following tumor subtypes are automatically G3: Lauren diffuse type, WHO mucinous (Figs. 2.161–2.163), WHO poorly cohesive (including signet ring and other variants), and WHO undifferentiated.

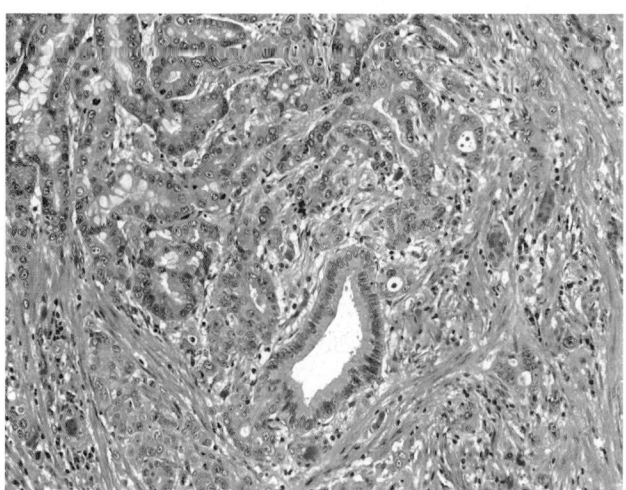

Figure 2-182. Gastric adenocarcinoma, intestinal type, G1 well differentiated. Gastric adenocarcinomas are graded histologically by the degree of gland formation. Tumors with >95% gland formation are G1 (well differentiated).

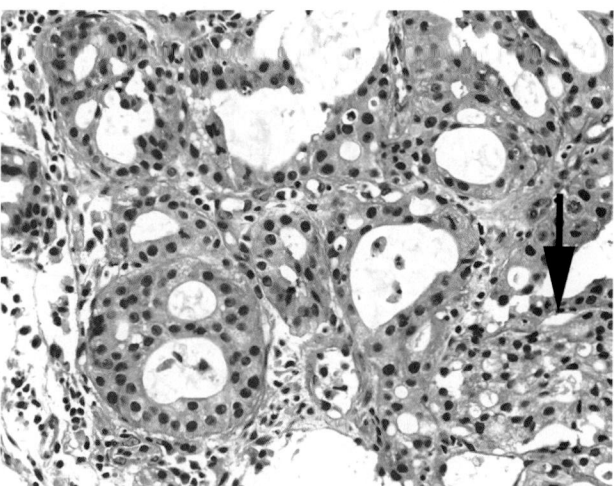

Figure 2-183. Gastric adenocarcinoma, intestinal type, G2 moderately differentiated. Tumors with 50%–95% gland formation are graded as G2 (moderately differentiated). Some areas of this carcinoma show poor gland formation and sheets of tumor cells (*arrow*).

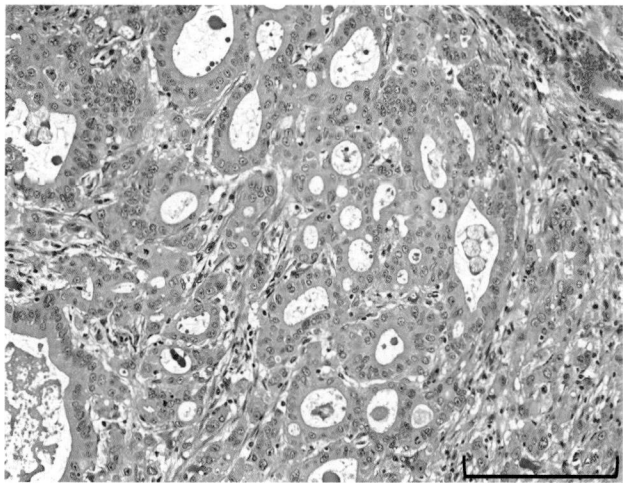

Figure 2-184. Gastric adenocarcinoma, intestinal type, G2 moderately differentiated. Glands make up most of this tumor (in the 50%–95% range), whereas some areas show no gland formation (*bracket*). This tumor is best graded as G2, moderately differentiated.

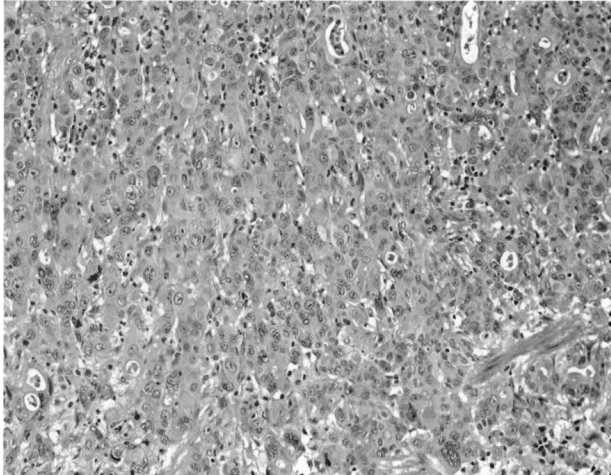

Figure 2-185. Gastric adenocarcinoma, intestinal type, G3 poorly differentiated. Tumors with <50% gland formation are graded as G3, poorly differentiated. This example shows only rare glandular lumina.

RISK FACTORS AND GENETIC CONSIDERATIONS
Background Mucosa

One cannot overstate the importance of examining the background gastric mucosa whenever a gastric lesion is encountered. This background mucosa can reveal additional information about a patient's risk factors for gastric adenocarcinoma and it should be sampled routinely, either by the endoscopist at the time of biopsy or, in the case of a gastrectomy, by the prosector at the grossing bench. Features to look for include background IM, *Helicobacter* infection, AMAG, and precursor polyps or areas of flat dysplasia.

Analogous to the adenoma-carcinoma sequence in colorectal cancer, gastric carcinogenesis is a multistep and multifactorial process, with a sequence of precursor histologic findings that progress from IM to LGD, HGD, and carcinoma. Although IM is a known risk factor for gastric cancer, the overall risk of gastric cancer in a patient with IM is extremely low compared with the risk of adenocarcinoma in a patient with Barrett esophagus.[84] Known risk factors for IM can be divided into two categories: (1) EMAG, which encompasses both *H. pylori* gastritis (typically an active chronic superficial plasmacytic inflammation) and chemical/reactive gastropathy (characterized by tortuous "corkscrew" hyperplasia of the antral foveolae and pits, lamina propria smooth muscle streaming toward the surface, and attenuation of foveolar mucin) related to high salt intake, smoking, alcohol consumption, and chronic bile reflux; and (2) AMAG. Recall, the IM (and other histologic abnormalities) found in EMAG is antral predominant, which is in direct contrast to the body-predominant IM (and other histologic abnormalities) found in AMAG. For more detailed discussion on EMAG and AMAG, see *Atlas of Gastrointestinal Pathology: A Pattern-Based Approach to Non-Neoplastic Biopsies*.

In 1994, based on epidemiologic evidence, the International Agency for Research on Cancer recognized *H. pylori* as a class 1 carcinogen and primary cause of gastric adenocarcinoma. Only a small minority of infected individuals develop gastric cancer (three cases per year for every 10,000 infected persons), which is predominantly intestinal type, and progression is multifactorial owing to influences such as host susceptibility, environmental forces, and bacterial strain (e.g., CagA strains are associated with a higher frequency of precancerous lesions and gastric cancer). Left untreated, *H. pylori* infection results in a long latency period (four or more decades) and progresses from chronic active nonatrophic gastritis to multifocal atrophic gastritis, and then to IM, dysplasia, and intestinal type invasive carcinoma.[85,86] Patients with AMAG are also at risk for gastric neoplasia, including both NETs and adenocarcinoma. The incidence of adenocarcinoma in these patients is seven times more frequent than in the general population, with an overall prevalence of 2%.[87] Do not forget to check the background mucosa for other associated precursor lesions, such as gastric adenomas, hyperplastic polyps, or syndromic hamartomatous polyps. Flat dysplasia is an uncommon finding in the stomach usually associated with chronic atrophy (*H. pylori* or AMAG) and can be graded in a two-tiered system similar to gastric adenomas (LGD and HGD).

CHECKLIST: Before Signing Out a Gastric Adenocarcinoma, Examine the Background Mucosa Away From the Lesion for the Following

- ☐ Intestinal metaplasia
  - ○ Environmental metaplastic atrophic gastritis (antral predominant)
    - ■ *H. pylori* (active and chronic superficial plasmacytic gastritis)
    - ■ Chemical/reactive gastropathy (e.g., high-salt diet, smoking, alcohol, bile reflux)
  - ○ AMAG (body/fundus predominant)
- ☐ Precursor polyps
  - ○ Gastric adenomas
  - ○ Hyperplastic polyps
  - ○ Syndromic hamartomatous polyps
- ☐ Flat dysplasia

FAQ: What is *H. pylori* CagA and how does it relate to gastric cancer?

Bacteria have developed several mechanisms to secrete proteins or to inject toxins into target cells. *H. pylori* injects the oncoprotein cytotoxin-associated antigen A (CagA) into host cells. Once inside the cell, CagA is phosphorylated and acts as a scaffold or hub protein that disrupts multiple host signaling pathways and targets the apical junctional complex of the epithelial cell. Different domains of the CagA protein interfere with signaling cascades, which results in cytoskeleton rearrangements and degradation of signal transduction pathways that maintain normal epithelial differentiation, including cell adhesion, cell polarity, and the inhibition of cell migration. CagA is also a highly antigenic protein that elicits interleukin-8 production resulting in a pronounced inflammatory response. These factors all play into the development of gastric adenocarcinoma and mucosa-associated lymphoid tissue (MALT) extranodal marginal zone lymphoma.

Environmental Risk Factors

There are distinctive differences in the geographic and ethnic incidence of gastric cancer. Emigrants acquire risk similar to that of their destination population, and such findings strongly suggest that exposure to environmental factors plays an important role in gastric cancer development. A number of dietary factors also play a significant role, including salt and salt-preserved foods, such as salted fish, cured meat, and salted-pickled vegetables. Modern refrigeration has reduced the need for this kind of food preservation and is cited as a reason for the decreasing incidence of gastric cancers.[88,89] However, regional and ethnic consumption patterns persist and continue to correlate with gastric cancer incidence. Another contributor is N-nitroso compounds, which are formed endogenously and following ingestion of dietary nitrates (found in some cheeses and cured meats but largely in natural foods, such as vegetables and potatoes). Diets high in fried food, processed meat and fish, and alcohol are associated with an increased risk of gastric carcinoma, whereas fruits, vegetables, and fiber appear protective. Obesity, smoking, occupational exposures, previous history of stomach surgery, and blood group A all contribute, but the most important environmental risk factor is *H. pylori*. Epstein-Barr virus also contributes to 5% to 10% of gastric cancers, as discussed earlier.

FAQ: What is the link between nitrates, nitrites, and nitrosamines and gastric cancer? Which of these ingredients do I need to avoid, exactly?

Do not quit your hot dog habit just yet. High consumption of processed meats, such as ham, bacon, sausages, and hot dogs, is linked to an increased gastric cancer risk, and many attribute this to the food additives nitrates and nitrites that retard microbial spoilage, preserve meat's recognizable appearance, and enhance flavor. As a group, these compounds containing an –NO group are referred to as N-nitroso compounds, which *all become the same end product when consumed*. Nitrates (NO_3) are inert until they are reduced to nitrites (NO_2) by oral bacteria, are swallowed, and, upon hitting the acidic gastric juices, are converted to nitrous acid (HNO_2), which then binds to amines, amides, and amino acids to form nitrosamines. Major sources of human exposure to *N*-nitroso compounds include diet, occupational exposure, and smoking, but in vivo formation accounts for up to 75% (that is right, your body is making most of it!).[90] Several studies have investigated the potential association between dietary consumption of nitrates, nitrites, and nitrosamines with gastric cancer. Increased consumption of nitrites and *N*-nitrosodimethylamine are linked to an increased risk for gastric cancer,[91] whereas several studies have demonstrated a *protective effect of nitrates*,[91-93] and this was found related to the high levels of nitrates found in green leafy vegetables. Researchers conclude that higher intake of antioxidants relative to nitrates offers protective effects. So, although the hype surrounding nitrate-free products is not entirely a load of bologna, a few bites of broccoli may be kinder to your GI tract.

Familial Predisposition

Most gastric cancers are sporadic, but about 10% of cases occur with aggregation within families. Truly hereditary familial gastric cancer accounts for 1% to 3% of the global burden of gastric cancer and comprises at least two major syndromes: hereditary diffuse gastric cancer (HDGC) and GAPPS of the stomach (essentially a variant of FAP).

Hereditary Diffuse Gastric Cancer

HDGC is inherited in an autosomal dominant pattern with high penetrance. Nearly 50% of HDGC is associated with germline truncating mutations of the *CDH1* gene, located on chromosome 16q22.1, which was first identified in three Maori families from New Zealand that were predisposed to diffuse gastric cancer. More than 75 families with nearly 4,000 probands have since been identified, and we now know these mutations are not concentrated in a single hotspot but are evenly distributed along the CDH1 gene in several different exons and, to date, more than 155 different germline CDH1 mutations have been identified.[94,95]

Quick Fact: *CDH1* is a tumor suppressor gene that requires a second hit for tumor formation. The *CDH1* gene provides instructions for making the E-cadherin protein, which is a membrane-bound cell-adhesion molecule that also acts as a tumor suppressor protein, preventing cells from growing or dividing too rapidly. Simply put, *CDH1* and E-cadherin are important in controlling cellular cohesion (cells sticking together) and division. The mechanism by which the second allele of E-cadherin is inactivated is diverse and includes promoter hypermethylation, mutation, and loss of heterozygosity, any of which results in loss of E-cadherin expression. Functionally, the resulting loss of cellular cohesion leads to an increased ability for tumor cells to invade and migrate, a feature seen in diffuse gastric cancers and invasive lobular breast carcinomas.

The lifetime risk of gastric cancer in individuals from these families is 70% for men and 56% for women, and the average age of onset is 38 years (range 14 to 82 years).[94,95] Asymptomatic carriers of the mutation are recommended prophylactic total gastrectomy generally between ages 20 and 30 years, during which the risk of gastric cancer rises from <1% to 4%.[95] Women in these affected families also have a 42% cumulative risk of lobular breast carcinoma, with increased risk before age 30.[94] Cases of signet ring cell appendiceal and colorectal cancers have also been reported, but these do not appear increased as compared with those in non-*CDH1*-mutated populations.[94]

Histologically, the tumors in these patients are identical to sporadic diffuse gastric cancers and are similarly challenging to identify (Figs. 2.186–2.195). In situ lesions or pagetoid spread of signet ring cells are described commonly in the literature with *CDH1*-mutated diffuse gastric cancer, but identifying these nearly invisible lesions requires skillful experience and, in most cases, prior knowledge of the patient's history.

FAQ: When should I raise the possibility of HDGC in my report?

Consensus guidelines for *CDH1* mutation testing include the following criteria:
1. Two gastric cancer cases in a family regardless of age (at least on confirmed diffuse type)
2. Diffuse gastric cancer in an individual <40 years
3. Personal or family history (first- or second-degree relative) of diffuse gastric cancer and lobular breast cancer, one diagnosed <50 years.[95]

Other patients in whom testing should be considered include:
1. Bilateral lobular breast cancer or family history (first- or second-degree relative) of ≥2 cases of lobular breast cancer <50 years
2. Personal or family history (first- or second-degree relative) of cleft lip/palate in a patient with diffuse gastric cancer
3. Any individual with in situ signet ring cells and/or pagetoid spread of signet ring cell on a gastric biopsy

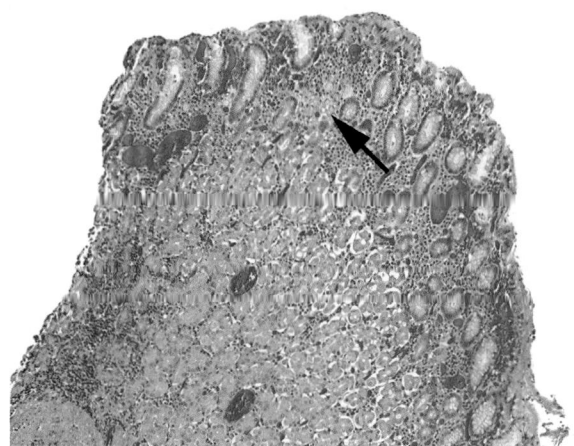

Figure 2-186. Hereditary diffuse gastric cancer, *CDH1* mutated. A nearly invisible focus of early gastric cancer (*arrow*) is found in this prophylactic gastrectomy specimen from a patient known to carry a CDH1 germline mutation. Without prior knowledge of the patient's history, such a small focus could easily be missed.

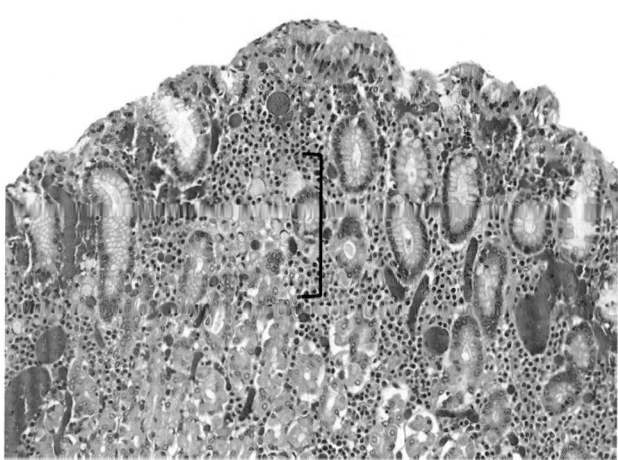

Figure 2-187. Hereditary diffuse gastric cancer, *CDH1* mutated, higher power of the previous figure. The small cluster of signet ring cells (*bracket*) invade into the lamina propria without disturbing the overall architecture or surface epithelium, making it extremely difficult to detect.

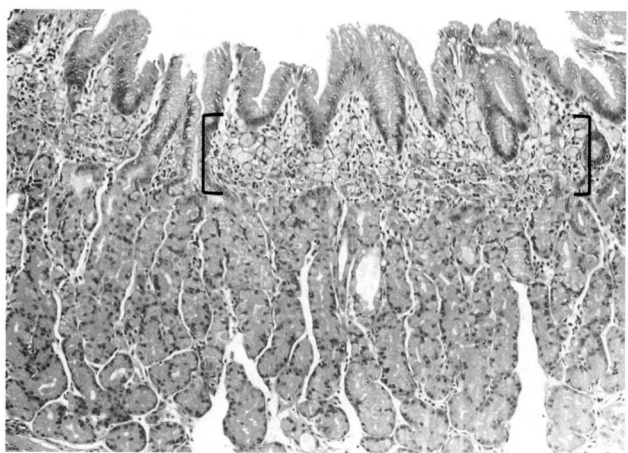

Figure 2-188. Hereditary diffuse gastric cancer, *CDH1* mutated. Another example of early gastric cancer in a patient with CDH1 gene mutation shows subepithelial signet ring cells (*brackets*) infiltrating the lamina propria without disturbing the overall architecture or surface mucosa, features that would normally alert the pathologist to take a closer look.

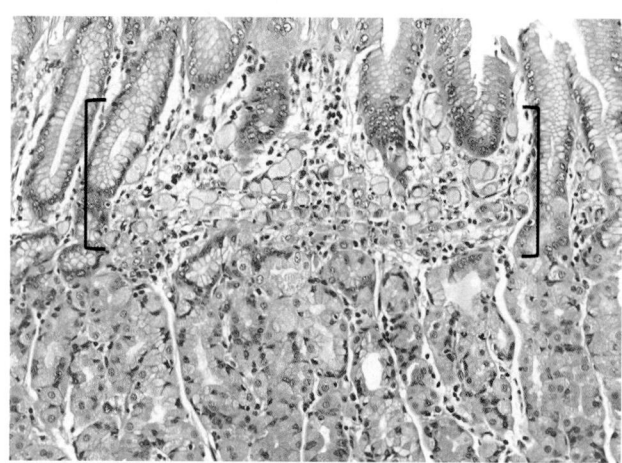

Figure 2-189. Hereditary diffuse gastric cancer, *CDH1* mutated, higher magnification of the previous figure. These pale signet ring cells (*brackets*) infiltrate the lamina propria and cause no epithelial or stromal reaction. Note the absence of background gastritis or intestinal metaplasia.

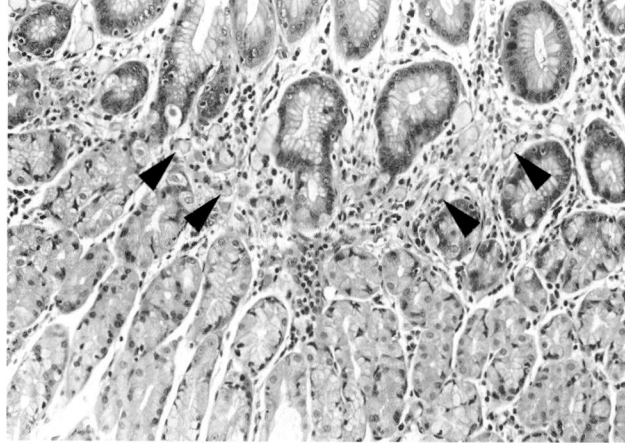

Figure 2-190. Hereditary diffuse gastric cancer, *CDH1* mutated. Single cells (*arrowheads*) are so subtle as to be nearly invisible. Even with knowledge of the patient's clinical history, finding these foci on a prophylactic gastrectomy can be extremely challenging.

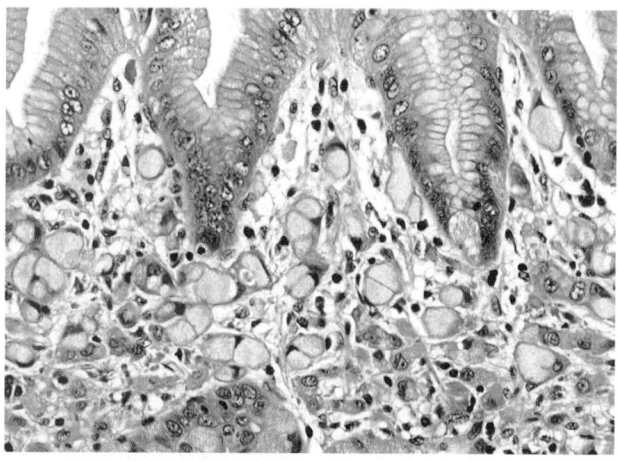

Figure 2-191. Hereditary diffuse gastric cancer, *CDH1* mutated. Signet ring cells are easier to identify when sufficient numbers cluster together. The absence of an expansile lesion, surface change, or stromal changes is highly characteristic.

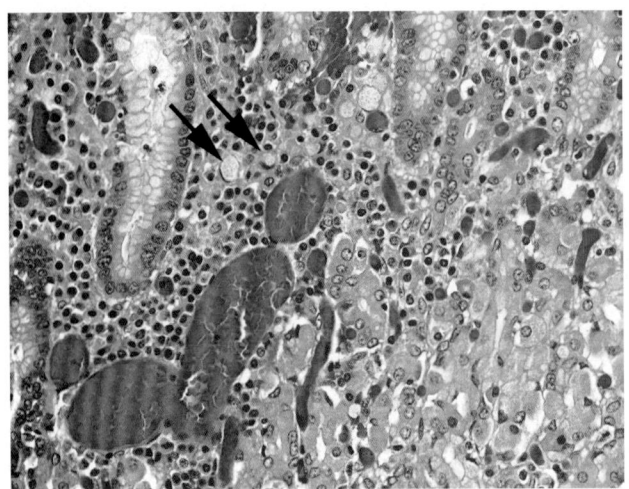

Figure 2-192. Hereditary diffuse gastric cancer, *CDH1* mutated. This example has a backdrop of inactive chronic gastritis that obscures an already difficult diagnosis. Single malignant signet ring cells (*arrows*) are surrounded by chronic inflammatory cells.

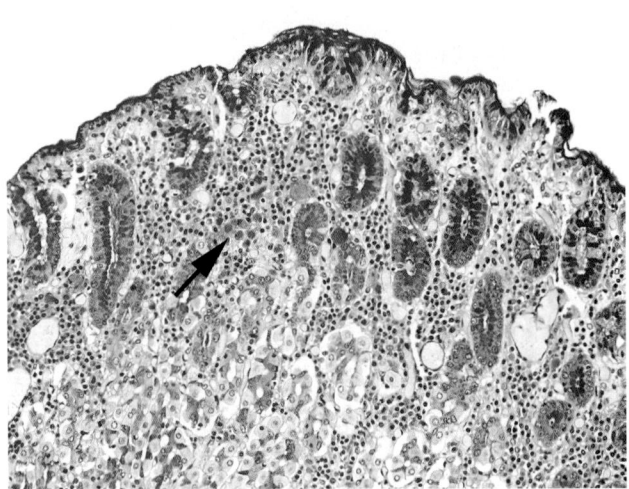

Figure 2-193. Hereditary diffuse gastric cancer, *CDH1* mutated, PAS stain. Some experts suggest performing PAS stain in lieu of H&E to screen prophylactic gastrectomy specimens. The PAS stain highlights tumor cells (*arrow*), providing a better contrast as compared with H&E. This technique can also be helpful in biopsy material.

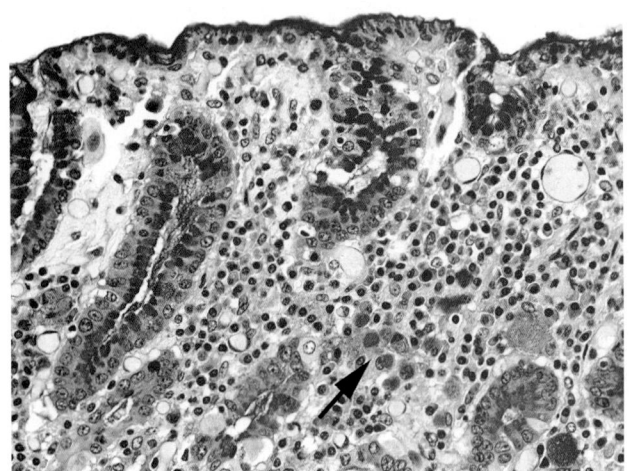

Figure 2-194. Hereditary diffuse gastric cancer, *CDH1* mutated, PAS stain, higher magnification of the previous figure. The mucin within the signet ring cells (*arrow*) are PAS positive.

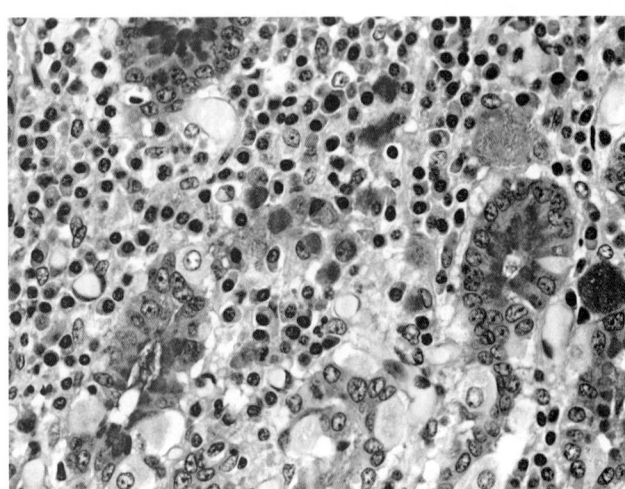

Figure 2-195. Hereditary diffuse gastric cancer, *CDH1* mutated, PAS stain, higher magnification of the previous figure. Individual signet ring cells are highlighted by PAS. Although many cells contain intracytoplasmic mucin, benign cells maintain normal architecture and gland formation. By comparison, the signet ring cells are single, discohesive, and disorganized.

FAQ: How do I process the prophylactic gastrectomy specimen?

Prophylactic gastrectomy is performed for cancer risk reduction, typically between 20 and 30 years of age in patients with known CDH1 mutations. Examination of the entire mucosa is essential, and one study showed at least five occult tumor foci in all cases.[96] Systematic submission of the entire mucosa can be performed by cutting transverse strips and submitting the stomach sequentially from proximal to distal. When multiple sections are embedded in each block, the average case may yield 200 to 300 blocks. Coupled with a gross photograph, these blocks can be mapped to assist in pinpointing the exact tumor location at the time of signout. Mapping also allows for concentrated screening in high-risk areas, such as the proximal stomach, where nearly two-thirds of tumors are found (37% anterior proximal fundus and 27% cardia/proximal fundus).[96] Histologically, early and in situ lesions are difficult to detect because the surface epithelium remains undisturbed. Some observers recommend periodic acid–Schiff (PAS) stain in lieu of H&E (Figs. 2.193–2.195), to improve detection of lesions and reduce the time required to screen cases.[97]

PEARLS & PITFALLS: Complete Submission of a Prophylactic Total Gastrectomy May Yield Several Hundred Blocks!

Examination of the entire mucosa is important to identify areas of occult diffuse gastric cancer. The typical prophylactic gastrectomy results in about 500 sections, and even when multiple sections are embedded within a single block, the average case may yield 200 to 300 blocks. Undoubtedly, for most centers, this will be a significant increase in block/slide production, and strategic planning with the histology laboratory is critical to prevent bottlenecking of other urgent clinical work. For these gastrectomies, completing the slide production over several days while also prioritizing other patient material can ease the burden on the laboratory and provide a more humane signout for the pathologist of record. Although this increases the turnaround time for final reporting, the delay is inconsequential, as prophylactic cases have little clinical urgency.

FAQ: Can E-cadherin immunohistochemistry be used to identify *CDH1*-related HDGC?

Germline mutations in the *CDH1* gene encoding E-cadherin are detected in nearly half of patients with HDGC. Among these patients, E-cadherin immunohistochemistry shows reduced or absent expression in the tumor foci and retained expression in the intervening nonneoplastic mucosa.[98] However, sporadic tumors may also show decreased or absent E-cadherin immunoreactivity, making this stain ineffective as a diagnostic marker for *CDH1*-related HDGC.

FAQ: Is there a role for endoscopic surveillance for patients with HDGC?

There are no reliable screening tests that allow for early detection of diffuse gastric cancer. Prophylactic gastrectomy is the treatment of choice for *CDH1* mutation carriers after age 20 years, but annual endoscopic surveillance may be considered for patients under the age of 20 years, patients who refuse or postpone gastrectomy (e.g., fertility concerns), and individuals who have genetic variants of undetermined significance. Note, however, that because diffuse gastric carcinomas do not form endoscopically visible lesions, endoscopic surveillance is likely to have extremely low detection rates for cancers in these patients. Random mapping biopsies may be sent to pathology, but the estimated number of biopsies necessary to capture a single focus of cancer (90% detection rate) is theoretically projected at 1768![96]

KEY FEATURES: Hereditary Diffuse Gastric Cancer

- **Autosomal dominant** with high penetrance
- **Nearly 50% attributed to mutations in the *CDH1* gene encoding E-cadherin**
- Lifetime risk of gastric cancer is 70% for men and 56% for women, with mean age 38 years (range 14 to 82 years)
- Endoscopic surveillance is not endorsed owing to ineffective detection of cancer
- Prophylactic total gastrectomy is recommended between ages 20 and 30 years
- The **entire specimen should be mapped** and submitted for histologic evaluation
- **Nearly 70% of tumors are found in the proximal stomach**
- PAS may be more helpful than H&E in the detection of early and small lesions (e.g., in situ or pagetoid spread)

Gastric Adenocarcinoma and Proximal Polyposis of the Stomach

GAPPS was initially identified in 2012 and is characterized by the autosomal dominant transmission of fundic gland polyposis with dysplasia and intestinal-type gastric adenocarcinoma that are restricted to the proximal stomach, with no evidence of duodenal or colorectal polyposis or other hereditary GI cancer syndrome.[99,100] The defining point mutations in exon 1B of the *APC* gene may also be found in some patients with FAP,[43] suggesting that GAPPS may represent a variant of FAP.[101] Fewer than a dozen families have been identified in the literature, and GAPPS is characterized by incomplete penetrance, with polyposis presenting in patients as young as 10 years and the median age for adenocarcinoma arising at 50 years (range 33 to 75 years), making it important for pathologists to consider this entity.[99,100,102] Proposed diagnostic criteria include (1) gastric polyps limited to the body/fundus without colorectal or duodenal polyposis; (2) >100 gastric polyps (or >30 polyps if known first-degree relative with GAPPS); (3) polyps are primarily FGPs, some of which have dysplasia (or any family member with dysplastic FGP or gastric carcinoma); and (4) autosomal dominant pattern of inheritance.[99]

KEY FEATURES: GAPPS

- Gastric adenocarcinoma and proximal polyposis of the stomach is a **variant of FAP**
- Point mutation in **exon 1B of *APC* gene**
- **Autosomal dominant** inheritance with **incomplete penetrance**
- **Carpet of >100 FGPs, some dysplastic,** in body/fundus, as early as age 10 years
- **Gastric adenocarcinoma,** usually intestinal type, presents at **median age 50 years (33 to 75 years)**
- **Absence of colorectal or duodenal polyps** is required
- **Absence of other inherited polyposis syndromes** is also required (Figs. 2.196–2.202)

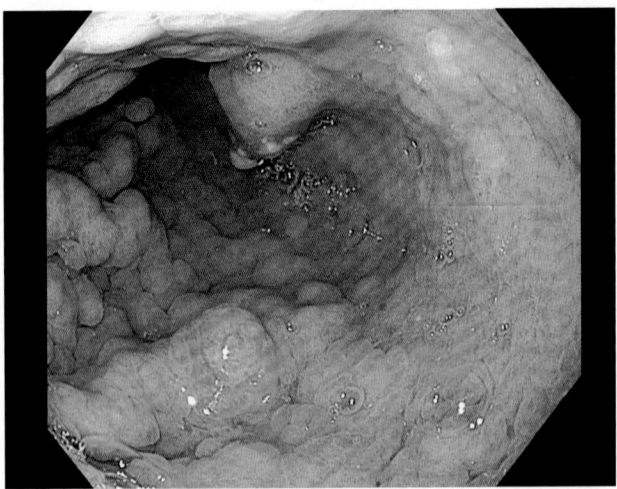

Figure 2-196. Gastric adenocarcinoma and proximal polyposis syndrome, endoscopic view. Diagnostic criteria include >100 gastric polyps limited to the gastric body/fundus (endoscopic view pictured) *without* colorectal or duodenal polyposis and autosomal dominant inheritance.

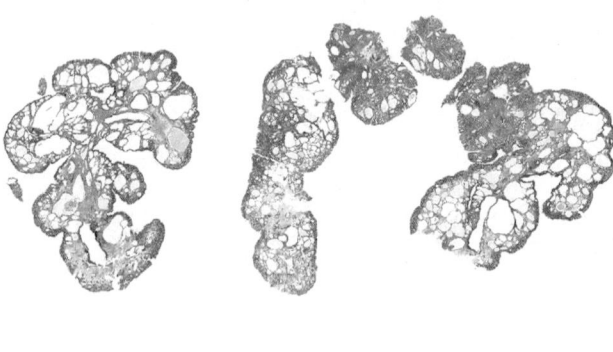

Figure 2-197. Fundic gland polyps in a patient with GAPPS. The polyps in GAPPS are primarily fundic gland polyps (pictured).

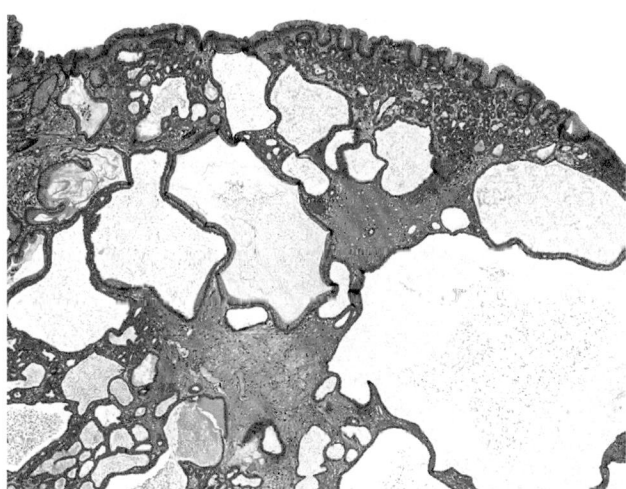

Figure 2-198. Fundic gland polyp in a patient with GAPPS. Most of the polyps found in GAPPS are fundic gland polyps. This example shows cystically dilated glands amid oxyntic glands and overlying normal foveolar epithelium.

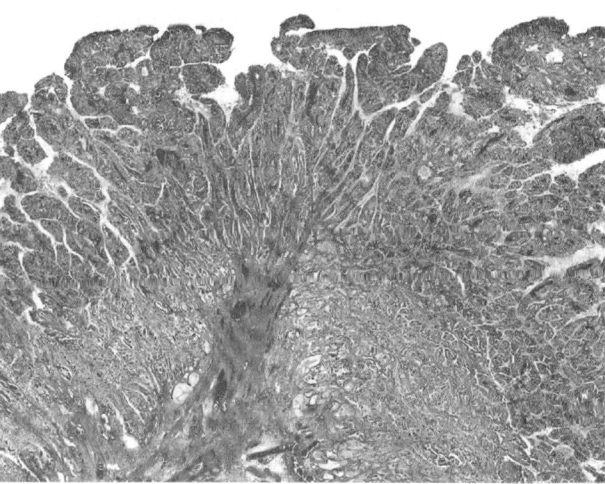

Figure 2-199. Pyloric gland adenoma in a patient with GAPPS. This patient had a large gastric pyloric gland adenoma (pictured) giving rise to adenocarcinoma, in addition to hundreds of fundic gland polyps.

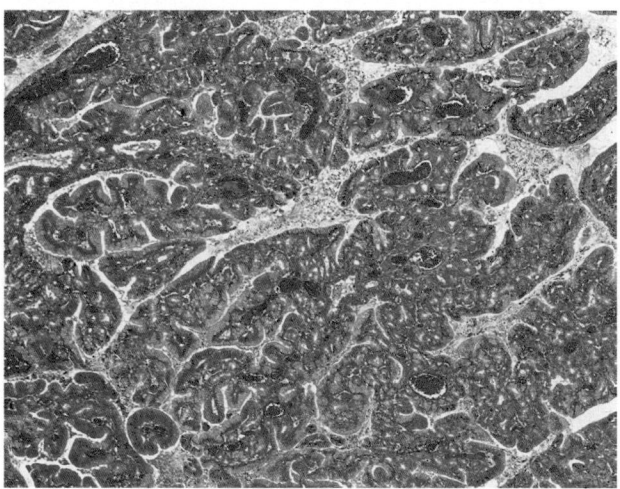

Figure 2-200. Pyloric gland adenoma (PGA) in a patient with GAPPS, higher magnification of the previous figure. Architecturally, PGAs are composed of back-to-back tubules, which when large can form papillary or frondlike extensions.

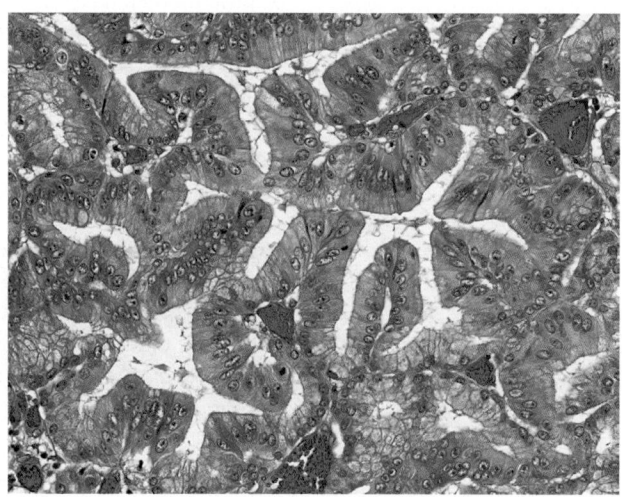

Figure 2-201. Pyloric gland adenoma (PGA) in a patient with GAPPS, higher magnification of the previous figure. The cells of PGA can be columnar to cuboidal and have abundant clear to eosinophilic cytoplasm with a ground glass or foamy appearance.

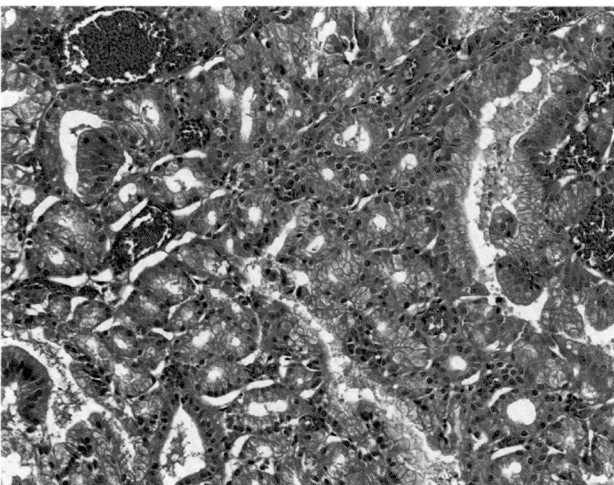

Figure 2-202. Pyloric gland adenoma in a patient with GAPPS. Other areas closely resemble pyloric glands, with closely packed small glands composed of cuboidal cells with clear foamy cytoplasm and nuclei pushed toward the basement membrane.

Other Hereditary Cancer Syndromes

Gastric cancer has also been described in association with certain other inherited cancer syndromes, including Lynch syndrome (hereditary nonpolyposis colorectal cancer), FAP, Li-Fraumeni syndrome, Peutz-Jeghers syndrome, juvenile polyposis, hereditary breast and ovarian cancer syndrome, and possibly PTEN hamartoma tumor (Cowden) syndrome, but these frequently present with benign gastric polyps, when present, and are all fairly rare causes of gastric cancer.

BIOMARKER TESTING 101

Programed Death Receptor-1/Programed Death Ligand-1 (PD-1/PD-L1)

The PD-1/PD-L1 pathway is involved in immune checkpoint surveillance that regulates T-lymphocyte activation. By suppressing T-cell activation, tumors that express PD-1/PD-L1 are able to hide from the immune system. This PD-L1 protein expression has changed the way we think about tumor biology, and it has been identified in lymphoma, non–small cell lung cancer, glioblastoma, melanoma, and malignancies in the kidney, breast, and GI tract, among others.[103] By targeting PD-1 or PD-L1 protein on these tumor cells, a growing number of monoclonal antibody therapies allow restoration of the body's T-cell antitumor function. This therapy has been so effective that in late 2017 the US Food and Drug Administration (FDA) granted accelerated approval to pembrolizumab (KEYTRUDA®, Merck & Co., Inc.) for patients with recurrent locally advanced or metastatic gastric or GEJ adenocarcinoma whose tumors express PD-L1 as determined by FDA-approved testing. At the time of this publication, only PD-L1 IHC 22C3 pharmDx (Dako) is approved, but this information is rapidly evolving, and up-to-date information can be found at http://www.fda.gov/CompanionDiagnostics. For more information about PD-1/PD-L1 function and immunohistochemical testing and interpretation, see "Colon" chapter.

> **PEARLS & PITFALLS: PD-1 and PD-L1 Negative Results on Archived Material**
>
> If PD-L1 expression is not detected in an older archived gastric cancer specimen, the FDA recommends assessing the feasibility of a fresh tumor biopsy for repeat testing.

Human Epidermal Growth Factor Receptor 2 (HER2)

Human epidermal growth factor receptor 2 (*HER2*), also known as CerB-2 and *ERBB2*, is a proto-oncogene located on chromosome 17q21 that encodes a transmembrane protein with tyrosine kinase activity, is a member of the HER receptor family, and is involved in signal transduction pathways leading to cell growth and differentiation.[104]

Quick fact: Proto-oncogenes are the normal inactive precursors of oncogenes. Recall, tumors may arise owing to oncogene activation (turning on) or tumor suppressor gene inactivation (turning off).

Amplification of the *HER2* gene and overexpression of its product were first discovered in breast cancer, in which it is significantly associated with worse outcomes.[105] Other carcinomas also demonstrate HER2 overexpression, including colorectal, ovarian, prostatic, lung, gastroesophageal, and gastric, although a direct link to outcomes is not as clear in these sites.[106] In 2010, a landmark study demonstrating the efficacy of trastuzumab in gastric and gastroesophageal carcinoma was published: "Trastuzumab in combination with chemotherapy versus chemotherapy alone for treatment of HER2-positive advanced gastric or gastro-oesophageal junction cancer (ToGA): a phase 3, open-label, randomized controlled trial."

Quick fact: *Open-label or open trial* is when both researchers and participants know which treatment is being administered. In a *randomized controlled trial*, patients are randomly assigned to either an intervention (in this case trastuzumab in combination with standard chemotherapy) or control group (in this case, chemotherapy alone). Clinical trials are conducted in "phases," and each phase has a different purpose:

Phase I: Experimental treatment is tested on a small group of people (20 to 80) for the first time. The purpose is to evaluate safety and identify side effects.

Phase II: Experimental treatment is tested on a larger group of people (100 to 300) to determine effectiveness and further evaluate safety.

Phase III: Experimental treatment is administered to large groups of people (1000 to 3000) and compared against standard treatment. Effectiveness, side effects, and safety are further assessed.

Phase IV: This phase follows FDA approval and availability of the treatment for the public. Researchers continue to track safety and monitor information about risks, benefits, and optimal use.

Trastuzumab is a monoclonal antibody directed against HER2 (for more information about monoclonal antibodies, see "Colon", chapter). It was one of the first molecular-targeted drugs developed and was introduced for treatment of HER2-positive advanced breast cancer. As stated in the study's title, the ToGA trial demonstrated that the addition of trastuzumab to standard chemotherapy results in increased overall survival among patients with HER2-expressing unresectable gastric and gastroesophageal tumors.[107] The benefit was modest (2.1 months improvement in progression-free survival and 2.7 months improvement in median overall survival) but was statistically significant and resulted in early termination of the study. As a result of the ToGA trial, trastuzumab is the first molecular-targeted agent approved by the FDA for treatment in gastric cancer and other molecular HER2 agents continue to be tested (e.g., pertuzumab, lapatinib).

Combined guidelines from the College of American Pathologists (CAP), American Society of Clinical Pathology (ASCP), and American Society of Clinical Oncology (ASCO) recommend that patients with HER2-positive tumors be offered combination chemotherapy and HER2-targeted therapy as the initial treatment of either primary or metastatic disease.[108] Thus, it is imperative to determine the HER2 status in advanced gastric or gastroesophageal adenocarcinoma to select patients who may benefit from treatment. These CAP/ASCP/ASCO guidelines endorse immunohistochemistry for HER2 as the initial test of choice. However, it is not as simple as applying one's knowledge of breast cancer HER2 testing to these gastric/gastroesophageal cancers (Figs. 2.203–2.212). Interpretation of HER2 IHC relies on three fundamental factors: stain location, extent, and intensity, and there are

---

PEARLS & PITFALLS: Beware False-Positive Staining Patterns!

IM and dysplastic epithelium commonly stain with partial membranous reactivity (Fig. 2.209). Stay alert to this pitfall and *inspect well-preserved areas of invasive tumor only* (Fig. 2.210). Recall, positive staining is linear *membranous* reactivity, either *complete or incomplete* lateral/basolateral, in 10% of tumor cells for resections or a single cancer cell cluster (≥5 cells) in biopsy specimens. Avoid calling *false-positive* results in the following scenarios:

- Cytoplasmic or nuclear reactivity only (Fig. 2.212)
- Isolated luminal membrane staining (Fig. 2.211)
- Granular or pericellular pattern
- Metaplasia or regenerative changes (e.g., near ulceration)
- Edge or crush artifact
- IM or dysplasia (Figs. 2.209 and 2.210)
- Signet ring cells with marginated cytoplasmic staining

PEARLS & PITFALLS: Select the Tissue Block With the Lowest-Grade Tumor Morphology!

As mentioned earlier, HER2 overexpression is seen more frequently in the intestinal phenotype (24%) and mixed tumors (20%) as compared with diffuse signet ring cell type (0% to 6%).[109,110] Low-grade tumors show greater frequency of HER2 positivity compared with high grade,[111] and so *block selection should target the lowest-grade tumor and areas showing intestinal differentiation* to have the highest prospect of positive HER2 result. Other rare morphologic variants of gastric adenocarcinoma (e.g., adenosquamous, papillary, hepatoid) lack sufficient data for comment. *More than one tissue block may be tested if the tumor is morphologically heterogeneous.*

Figure 2-203. HER2 negative, score 1+. A sufficient number of tumor cells are staining in this biopsy specimen (one cancer cell cluster of ≥5 cells), and membranous staining is present. However, the intensity of the stain is 1+, as it is barely perceptible, even at high magnification (40x). A score of 1+ is considered negative, and there is no need to reflex to FISH testing.

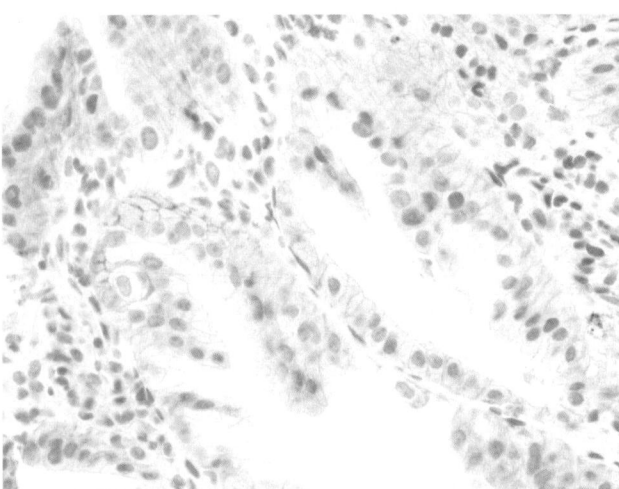

Figure 2-204. HER2 negative, score 1+. In this biopsy example, the staining criteria are met, with basal, lateral, and basolateral staining present in at least ≥5 cells of this tumor cell cluster. However, the stain is faint and requires 40x magnification to be perceptible. This 1+ staining intensity is considered negative, and there is no need to reflex to FISH testing.

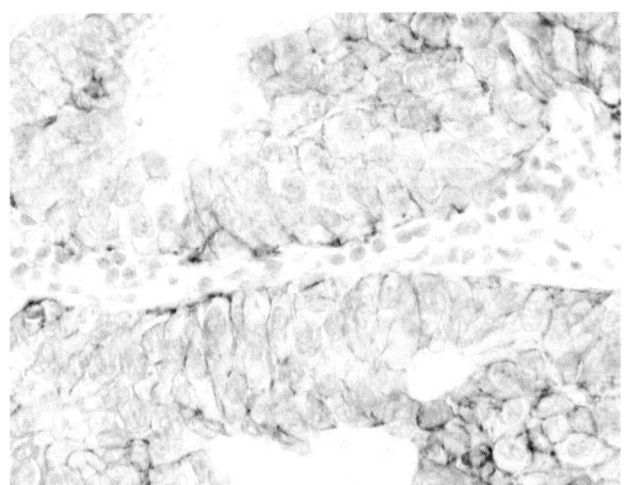

Figure 2-205. HER2 equivocal, score 2+. Sufficient tumor cells are staining (at least one cancer cell cluster defined as ≥5 cells in a biopsy) in a basolateral membranous pattern. However, the staining intensity is weak to moderate and is best seen at 10–20x. This is scored as 2+ and requires follow-up with FISH studies.

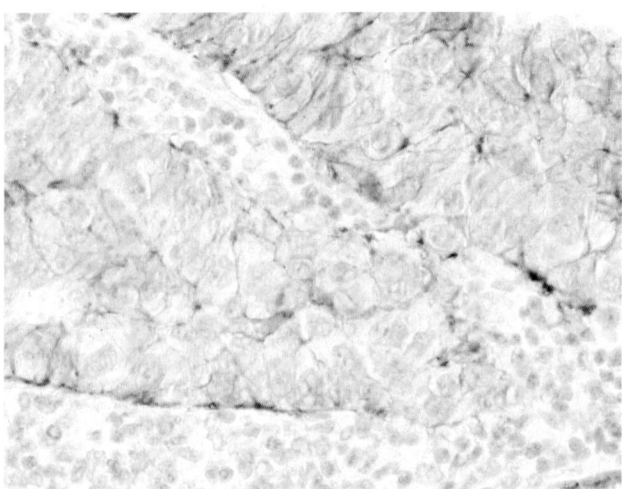

Figure 2-206. HER2 equivocal, score 2+. Complete or incomplete basolateral staining is present in a sufficient number of tumor cells (at least one cancer cell cluster defined as ≥5 cells in a biopsy). Compared with breast carcinoma, which requires circumferential membranous staining, discontinuous basal/lateral membranous staining is acceptable with gastric cancers. However, the staining intensity is weak to moderate and is best seen at 10–20x. This is scored as 2+ and requires follow-up with FISH studies to determine whether the patient can benefit from trastuzumab therapy.

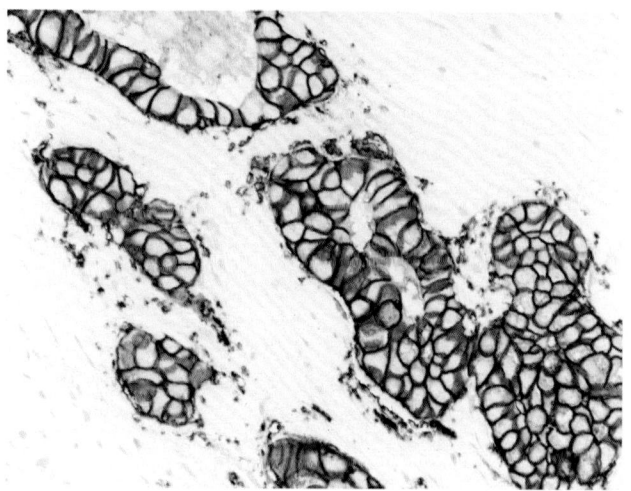

Figure 2-207. HER2 positive, score 3+. Sufficient tumor cells are staining (at least one cancer cell cluster defined as ≥5 cells in a biopsy) in a complete membranous pattern with strong reactivity visible at low magnification (2–4x). A 3+ interpretation is positive and requires no additional FISH testing. Although this example shows complete membranous reactivity, gastric HER2 interpretation requires only basal, lateral, or basolateral staining.

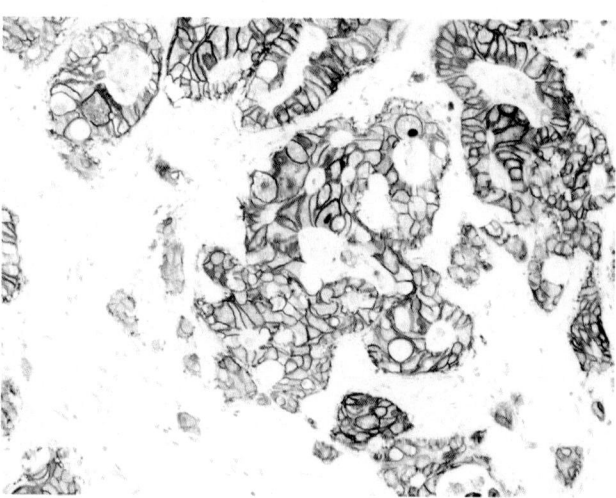

Figure 2-208. HER2 positive, score 3+. At least 10% of tumor cells in a resection specimen must show reactivity to be properly graded. This example shows strong and complete membranous reactivity in the tumor cells visible at low magnification (2–4x). A score of 3+ is considered positive, and patients may benefit from trastuzumab therapy.

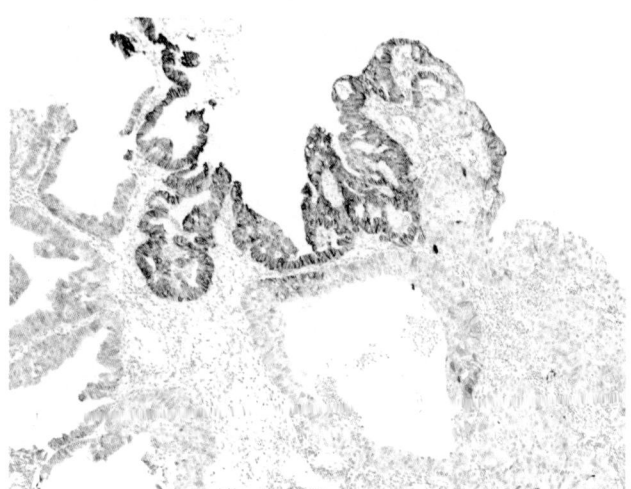

Figure 2-209. HER2 negative, score 0. Beware of strong staining in areas of overlying dysplasia (pictured) or intestinal metaplasia. Areas of metaplasia or regenerative changes near ulcers may also show false-positive reactivity. Interpretation of HER2 should be limited to the invasive carcinoma only, and it is helpful to have the H&E handy for correlation.

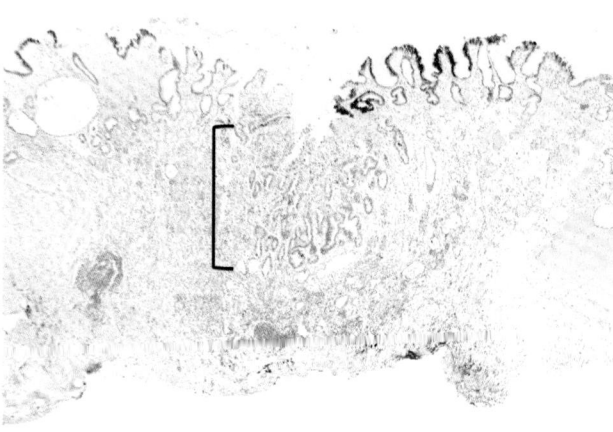

Figure 2-210. HER2 negative, score 0. The invasive cancer (*bracket*) is negative for HER2, but the overlying dysplastic epithelium shows strong reactivity. This is a common false-positive pitfall to avoid; always inspect well-preserved areas of invasive tumor only.

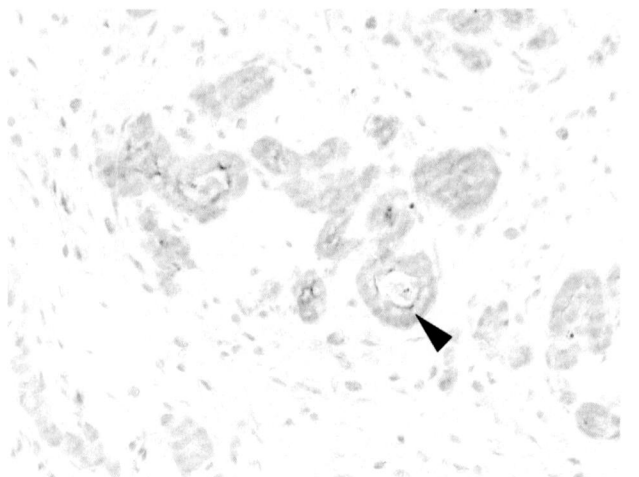

Figure 2-211. HER2 negative, score 0. Although there appears to be linear membranous reactivity in at least five tumor cells, this shows an isolated luminal staining pattern (*arrowhead*). True positive staining requires basal, lateral, or basolateral membranous reactivity.

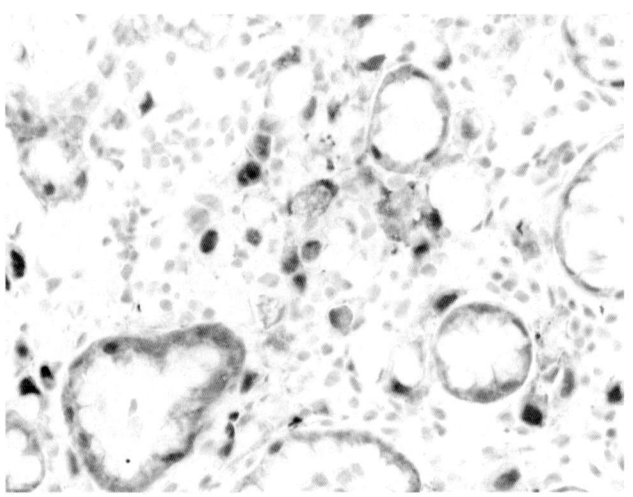

Figure 2-212. HER2 negative, score 0. There is moderate to strong reactivity in at least five tumor cells, but the staining patterns are nuclear, cytoplasmic, granular, and extracellular. True linear membranous reactivity in a lateral/basolateral distribution is absent. This HER2 should be interpreted as negative.

TABLE 2.5: Evaluation of HER2 Immunohistochemistry in Gastric Adenocarcinoma

Membranous Complete or Basolateral Staining	Objective With Visible Staining	Surgical Specimen Criteria	Biopsy Specimen Criteria	Score	Interpretation by IHC	Next Step
None or any membranous		<10% of cancer cells	No cells staining	0	Negative	None
Faint or barely perceptible	40x	≥10% of cancer cells	1 cancer cell cluster (≥5 cells)	1+	Negative	None
Weak to moderate	10–20x			2+	Equivocal	HER2 FISH or other ISH study
Strong	2–4x			3+	Positive	None

FISH, fluorescence in situ hybridization; IHC, immunohistochemistry; ISH, in situ hybridization.

several key differences in the interpretation as compared with breast carcinoma (see Table 2.5). First, and perhaps most importantly, *stain location* does not require complete circumferential membranous staining. Instead, basal, basolateral, or lateral staining is adequate (Figs. 2.205 and 2.206). The exception is isolated luminal membrane staining, which is considered negative (Fig. 2.211). Second, *stain extent* requires a minimum amount of tumor cell reactivity: ≥10% in resection specimens or at least 1 cancer cell cluster, defined as ≥5 cells, in biopsy specimens. Finally, if these two previous criteria are met, a score may be applied based on stain intensity: 1+ for faint or barely perceptible (seen only on 40x objective, Figs. 2.203 and2.204), 2+ for weak to moderate (visible at 10 to 20x, Figs. 2.205 and 2.206), or 3+ for strong (seen at 2 to 4x, Figs. 2.207 and 2.208). If the tumor fails to meet minimum thresholds for location or extent, it is scored as 0. Scores of 0 and 1+ are considered negative results, and no additional testing is required, as these patients will not benefit

TABLE 2.6: Comparison of HER2 Scoring Between Gastroesophageal and Breast Carcinomas

		Gastroesophageal Adenocarcinoma	Breast Carcinoma
IHC criteria	Extent	Biopsy: 1 tumor cluster (≥5 cells) Resection: ≥10% tumor cells	>10% tumor cells
	Circumferential membrane staining required	No. Basal, basolateral, lateral, or complete acceptable.	Yes
	Fixation requirements	None	6–72 hours; 10% neutral buffered formalin
ISH criteria	Single probe HER2 copy number	≥6.0 signals per cell	Same
	Dual probe HER2/CEP17 ratio and HER2 copy number	Ratio ≥2.0 with ≥4.0 signals/cell Ratio ≥2.0 with <4.0 signals/cell Ratio <2.0 with ≥6.0 signals/cell	Same
Positive HER2 Features	Tumor types	25% Intestinal 10% Mixed 5% Diffuse (signet ring cell)	25% Ductal
	Tumor location	30% GE junction 15% Gastric	Not applicable

GE, gastroesophageal; IHC, immunohistochemistry; ISH, in situ hybridization.

from trastuzumab therapy. A score of 2+ is equivocal and requires additional testing by fluorescence in situ hybridization (FISH) analysis or other in situ hybridization method (e.g., silver in situ hybridization, chromogenic in situ hybridization, and dual-color dual-hapten in situ hybridization). Criteria for in situ hybridization results are listed in Table 2.6.

FAQ: Should HER2 testing be performed on biopsy or resection specimens? What about metastases?

Any tumor tissue may be tested, but preferably treatment-naive tumor. Biopsy or resection specimens are both acceptable, and either primary or metastatic tumor is suitable. HER2 rates in the ToGA trial were similar between biopsy and surgical specimens (23.2% and 19.7%, respectively).[107,112] Other studies confirm that HER2 amplification is similar between paired resection and biopsy specimens, as well as their metastatic samples (>90% concordance).[112-116] Given the overall high degree of concordance, HER2 testing on neoplastic tissue from *primary or metastatic* tumor in either *biopsy or resections* specimens is appropriate. Selection of tumor tissue acquired *before the initiation of trastuzumab therapy* is preferred if such specimens are available and adequate.

FAQ: Are there requirements for tissue fixation?

No. Unlike breast carcinoma, there are no specific fixation requirements for HER2 testing of gastric/gastroesophageal adenocarcinoma (see Table 2.6).

PEARLS & PITFALLS: Scoring of HER2 IHC in Gastric Cancer Is Different From Scoring in Breast Cancer

The Ruschoff/Hofmann scoring method for gastric cancer, adapted from the ToGA trial, has a lower threshold as compared with that of breast cancer. Complete membranous staining is *not* required. *Any* linear membranous (not cytoplasmic) basolateral, lateral, or complete staining is considered sufficient for further scoring, *except* in the case of isolated luminal membrane staining. The scoring method then takes into account two additional factors: intensity of staining and minimum amount of tumor cells positive. Intensity of staining is scored as 1+ faint or barely perceptible, visible only on 40x objective; 2+ weak to moderate, visible at 10 to 20x; and 3+ strong, visible at 2 to 4x. This staining must be seen in at least *10% of tumor cells in resections*, or in a *single cancer cell cluster (≥5 cells) in a biopsy specimen.*[117] See Table 2.5 and Figs. 2.203–2.208.

FAQ: How many biopsy fragments are required?

At minimum, five biopsies should be taken at the time of endoscopy. However, clinicians should be advised that six to eight biopsy fragments are optimal owing to tumor heterogeneity.[118] Make sure to communicate any concerns for adequacy, in particular if the HER2 result is negative or uninterpretable.

It is never a bad idea to have a generous sample at first pass. If subsequent genomic testing is requested (there is currently not sufficient evidence to recommend for or against), this archived tissue expedites the process and obviates the need for rebiopsy.

FAQ: Are HER2 results reliable on fine needle aspiration (FNA) specimens? Is it appropriate to use an FNA specimen if it is the only material available?

HER2 testing on FNA specimens (cell blocks) is an acceptable alternative *if it is the only material available*, as per CAP/ASCP/ASCO guidelines. However, this recommendation is extrapolated primarily from breast carcinoma data, and limited conclusive data are available for gastric/gastroesophageal cancers. Given the wide variations in tissue handling and processing of cytologic samples (e.g., use of decalcification and fixative selection: proprietary vs. alcohol based vs. direct formalin vs. alternative), laboratories should *confirm test performance* of HER2 assays on these types of specimens *before reporting patient results*. There are no set regulations guiding this practice, and testing paradigms may be determined by the local laboratory director.

FAQ: Should clinicians wait for HER2 results before initiating therapy?

No. Many centers send out testing to reference laboratories, which may increase turnaround time for HER2 results. Although most oncologists will be anxious to receive these results, there is no need to know HER2 status before starting chemotherapy. If HER2 results are subsequently positive, clinicians may later add trastuzumab to the treatment plan. In addition, most patients with gastric cancer are symptomatic at the time of diagnosis and will benefit from immediate oncologic management. For pathologists, the turnaround time benchmark is 90% of reports within 10 working days from the date of procedure. For send outs, 90% of specimens should be sent within 3 days of tissue processing.

FAQ: Why do scoring criteria for HER2 IHC differ between gastric and breast cancers?

Interpretation of gastric HER2 IHC is based on criteria used in the ToGA trial. Recall, this trial demonstrated survival benefit among patients with HER2-positive tumors when trastuzumab was added to their chemotherapy regimens. The HER2 scoring system used in this study differed from breast scoring, hence the variation in criteria. For gastric/gastroesophageal cancers, complete circumferential membranous staining is *not* required. Instead, any basal, basolateral, lateral, or complete membranous staining may be scored (Figs. 2.203–2.208). Note, however, that isolated luminal membrane staining is negative (Fig. 2.211), as is isolated nuclear or cytoplasmic staining (Fig. 2.212). Scoring then relies on additional factors, such as extent of tumor cells staining and intensity of staining, as detailed in Table 2.6.

FAQ: Why not just perform FISH on all patients?

In gastric cancers, HER2 testing by FISH and IHC show only moderate fidelity, as up to 20% of gastric cancers with negative IHC interpretation (0 or 1+) show positive amplification by FISH. However, *no significant survival benefit* from trastuzumab is seen in these patients and, as a result, IHC is the first-line test for HER2 overexpression.[119] This is in contrast to the experience with breast carcinoma whereby an extremely low threshold to perform FISH is maintained and every attempt is sought to achieve a positive HER2 result. Partially driving this practice is the high efficacy of trastuzumab in HER2+ breast carcinoma along with the low toxicity profile of the drug. This makes trastuzumab low risk and potentially high yield for clinicians to include in their arsenal against breast cancer. However, this does not hold true for gastric cancers, and thus the testing algorithms diverge. Unlike in breast cancer, there is *no significant survival benefit for trastuzumab if IHC is 0 or 1+ even when FISH shows HER2 amplification*. On the other hand, if there is uncertainty over IHC scoring of 1+ versus 2+, the best approach is to simply reflex to FISH.

FAQ: Should I ever repeat HER2 testing?

No. There are no data to support repeat HER2 testing if initial testing is negative, although some clinical colleagues may request this.

PEARLS & PITFALLS: The Path Report Should Specify the Antibodies and Probes Used

Several HER2 antibodies are offered through various vendors, and there is *no specific recommended antibody*. The ToGA trial used HercepTest, whereas other studies have applied Ventana 4B5 or Thermo Fischer Scientific CB11, and even more variations are available on the market. Although concordance among antibodies is moderate to good, the ASCO/CAP/ASCP guidelines strongly recommend laboratories *specify the antibodies and probes used for the test*.[120] An example of this standard verbiage is included later. The guidelines also emphasize that assays should be appropriately validated for HER2 IHC and ISH on gastroesophageal adenocarcinoma specimens, although this is standard practice for any laboratory test. As with any other test, 20 positive and 20 negative gastroesophageal adenocarcinomas should be verified for FDA-approved tests, and 40 samples for laboratory-developed tests.

Example verbiage for inclusion in report:

Method: Testing is performed using FDA-approved Ventana Pathway HER2 (4B5) rabbit monoclonal primary antibody and a proprietary detection system. No expression (HER2 score of 0), low expression (HER2 score of 1+), and high expression (HER2 score of 3+) controls are used. All controls show appropriate reactivity.

Scoring: Scoring is performed according to the following article: Ruschoff J, Dietel M, Baretton G, et al. HER2 diagnostics in gastric cancer-guideline validation and development of standardized immunohistochemical testing. *Virchows Arch.* 2010; 457(3):299-307.

CHECKLIST: Steps to Reporting HER2 in Gastric/Esophageal Carcinoma

☐ Advise clinicians to begin other chemotherapy while waiting for HER2 results; trastuzumab may be added later if HER2 results are positive

☐ IHC is the first test of choice; reflex to ISH only if results are 2+ equivocal

☐ No special fixation constraints required

☐ Use biopsy, resection, or metastatic sample from treatment-naive tumor

☐ Cytology cell block is appropriate if no other tissue is available

☐ Select the tissue block with lowest-grade or intestinal-type carcinoma

☐ Score with three factors:

    ○ Stain location: Complete or basolateral membranous

    ○ Stain extent: >10% in resection; 1 cluster of ≥5 cells in biopsy

    ○ Stain intensity: 1+ weak (40x); 2+ moderate (10 to 20x); 3+ strong (2 to 4x)

☐ Report:

    ○ Negative: 0 or 1+

    ○ Equivocal: 2+

    ○ Positive: 3+

☐ Take action:

    ○ Negative: 0 or 1+ → None

    ○ Equivocal: 2+ → Send for ISH HER2

    ○ Positive: 3+ → None

☐ Specify antibodies and probes used in path report

WELL-DIFFERENTIATED NEUROENDOCRINE TUMORS (FORMERLY "CARCINOID")

Based on WHO 2017 classification, well-differentiated neuroendocrine tumors (WD-NETs) are distinguished from NECs by their morphologic features, independent of mitotic count or Ki-67 proliferative index. This is a departure from previous WHO 2010 classification for neuroendocrine neoplasms, in which tumors were stratified based solely on mitoses and Ki-67. The updated system not only more reliably indicates prognosis and response to therapy but is also more intuitive to pathologists. For example, tumors that are morphologically uniform are classified as WD-NETs, whereas NECs are classified by their poorly differentiated high-grade cytology and marked nuclear atypia. NEC is discussed separately in the gastric adenocarcinoma section "Tumor Classification", as its prognosis and staging more closely reflect those of gastric adenocarcinoma.

Most gastric WD-NETs are composed of ECL cells, typically in the corpus and fundus (90%),[121] which express chromogranin A or synaptophysin by immunohistochemistry. Endoscopically they appear as submucosal nodules or polyps (Fig. 2.213), sometimes with ulcerations. Gastric WD-NETs are classified into three groups, each arising in different clinical contexts (see Table 2.7), and each with divergent prognoses and treatment protocols. In isolation, the tumors are histologically indistinguishable and are composed of nests or trabeculae of small, uniform, polygonal, or cuboidal cells with lightly eosinophilic and finely granular cytoplasm. The nuclei are round or oval with smooth nuclear borders and stippled chromatin with indistinct nucleoli. The key to differentiating the three types of gastric WD-NETs from one another requires examination of the nonpolypoid background mucosa, yet again underscoring the importance of background gastric biopsies with all gastric lesions.

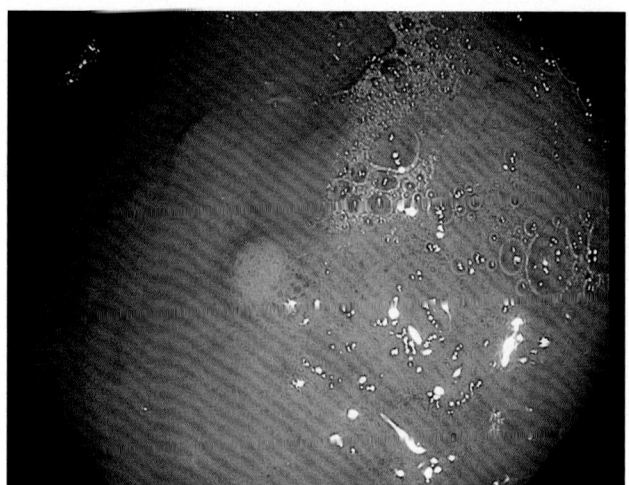

Figure 2-213. Gastric well-differentiated neuroendocrine tumor. This pale endoscopic nodule appears submucosal. The background gastric mucosa also shows a mosaic pattern and patchy atrophy.

TABLE 2.7: Comparison of Gastric Well-Differentiated Neuroendocrine Tumors

	Type 1	Type 2	Type 3
Frequency	70%–80% of gastric NETs	Rare	10%–15% of gastric NETs
Focality	Multifocal	Multifocal	Solitary lesion
Size	0.5–1.0 cm	≤1.5 cm	Variable; one third >2 cm
Location	Body/Fundus	Body/Fundus	Anywhere in stomach
Associated with	Hypergastrinemia Hypochlorhydria/ achlorhydria AMAG ECL-cell hyperplasia Pernicious anemia	Hypergastrinemia MEN1 Zollinger-Ellison syndrome	Sporadic No clinical associations
Clinical behavior	Usually benign Rare metastases	30% metastasize	Dependent on size and depth of invasion
Demographics	F ≫ M 70%-80% of patients are 50's–60's	M = F Mean age 50	M > F Mean age 65

GASTRIC WELL-DIFFERENTIATED NEUROENDOCRINE TUMOR, TYPE I

Type I gastric WD-NETs are the most common and arise in the setting of AMAG. These occur in middle-aged women (70% to 80%) and are the result of ECL-cell hyperplasia. In AMAG, the autoimmune destruction of parietal cells leads to reduced gastric acid production and loss of feedback inhibition of gastrin secretion in the antral G cells (i.e., the G cells cannot turn off gastrin secretion). The resulting hypergastrinemia stimulates ECL cells to proliferate, which appear as multiple small nodules in the body/fundus of the stomach. Technically, this early change represents a *reversible* hyperplasia, but may progress to malignancy, especially as tumors enlarge. As compared with type II and type III gastric WD-NETs, type I lesions have an excellent prognosis with exceedingly low rates of metastatic disease.[122] EMR of any visible lesions and close endoscopic follow-up is prudent, but there are no existing guidelines for surveillance. Antrectomy to remove the stimulatory G cells has also proven useful as long-term therapy, and treatment of underlying pernicious anemia is required because the absence of parietal cells also results in a deficit of intrinsic factor, the transporter for vitamin B12.[123] Differentiating this well-performing tumor from other gastric WD-NETs requires examination of the background flat mucosa (Figs. 2.214–2.229). Look for the constellation body/fundus-predominant characteristics of AMAG: (1) IM, (2) atrophy of oxyntic glands, (3) inactive chronic gastritis (typically low-lying and lymphocytic, in contrast to the superficial plasmacytic inflammation of *H. pylori*), (4) linear or nodular ECL-cell hyperplasia (≥5 cells in a row or cluster as highlighted by chromogranin or other neuroendocrine immunohistochemistry), and (5) pyloric metaplasia (and sometimes pancreatic acinar cell metaplasia).

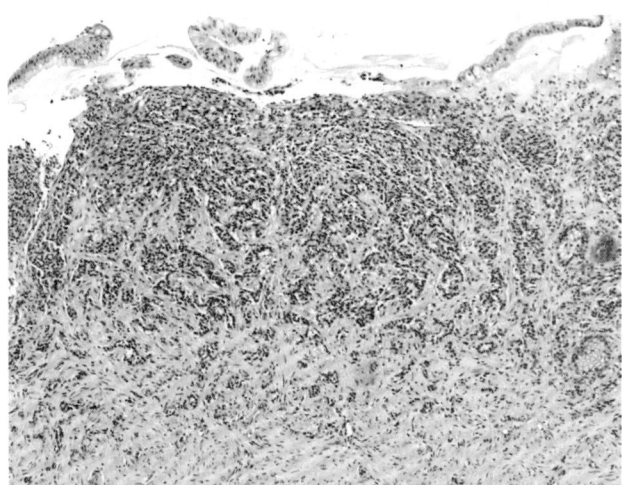

Figure 2-214. Gastric WD-NET, histology of the previous figure. At low magnification, this is an expansile lesion composed of sheets of uniform cells with a slightly trabecular architecture. The base of the lesion is invading into the muscularis mucosae. The prognosis of this lesion depends upon the etiopathogenesis, which can be deduced from the changes found in the background nonlesional sample.

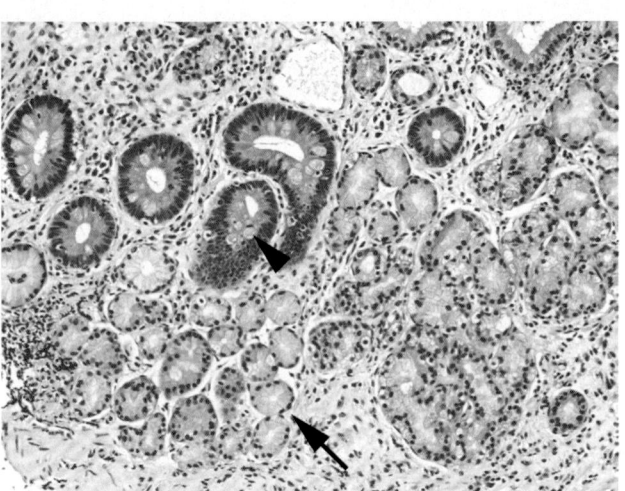

Figure 2-215. Autoimmune metaplastic atrophic gastritis, background mucosa of the previous figure. Background nonlesional gastric tissue is important when encountering a WD-NET in the stomach. Type 1 WD-NETs have an excellent prognosis and arise in the setting of AMAG, which shows a constellation of features. The oxyntic glands are absent in this image because of complete oxyntic gland atrophy, and this is accompanied by background chronic inflammation, intestinal metaplasia (*arrowhead*), and pyloric metaplasia (*arrow*).

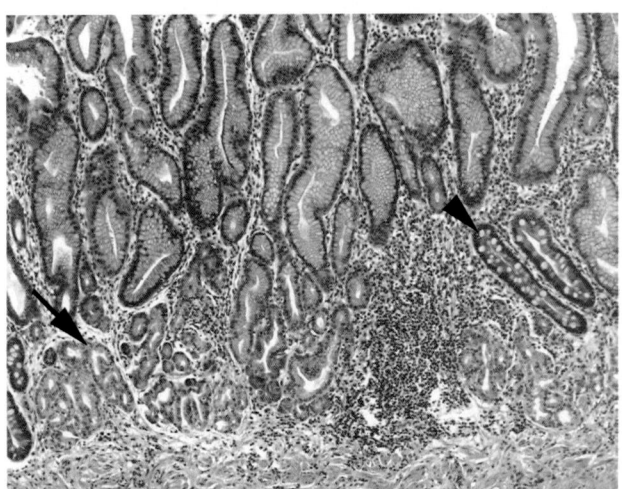

Figure 2-216. Autoimmune metaplastic atrophic gastritis. At lower magnification, one can appreciate the complete absence of oxyntic glands, the presence of a low-lying lymphocytic infiltrate, intestinal metaplasia (*arrowhead*), and pyloric gland metaplasia (*arrow*). These features, in conjunction with ECL-cell hyperplasia (not pictured), indicate AMAG.

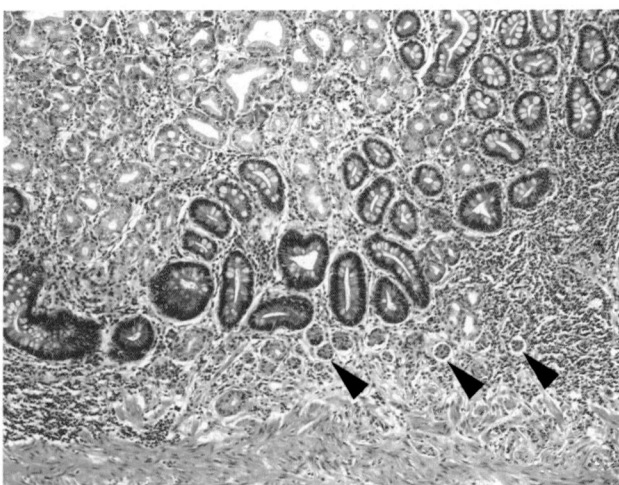

Figure 2-217. Autoimmune metaplastic atrophic gastritis, nodular ECL-cell hyperplasia. ECL-cell hyperplasia is not always visible on H&E stain, but these small nodular aggregates (*arrowheads*) stain with chromogranin. To diagnose AMAG, one must find linear or nodular ECL-cell hyperplasia (defined as at least five adjacent cells) in combination with oxyntic gland atrophy (note the absence of the typical *pink* parietal cell and *blue* chief cells), low-lying lymphocytic inflammation, intestinal metaplasia, and pyloric gland metaplasia.

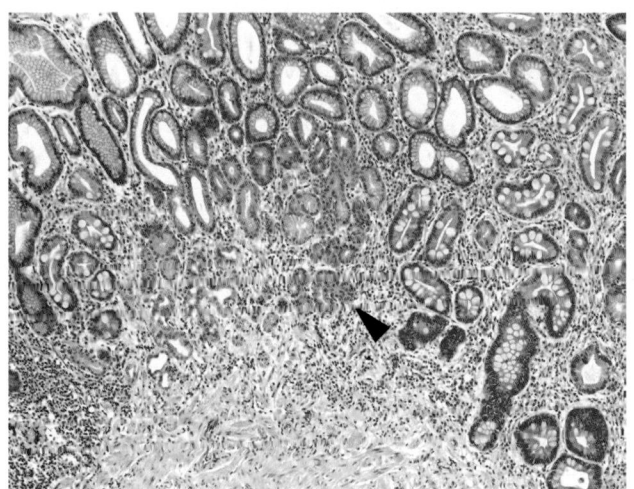

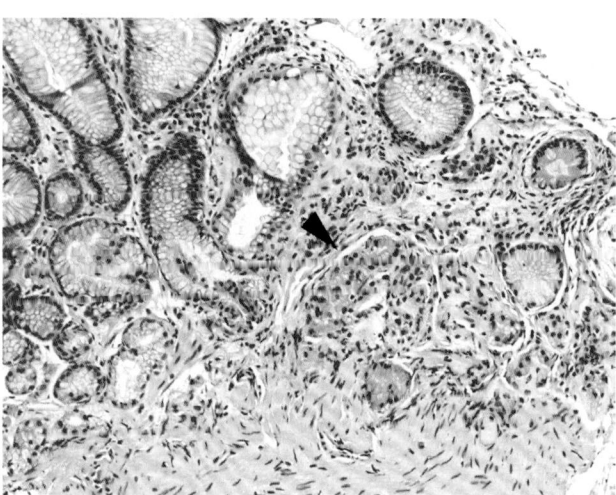

Figure 2-218. Autoimmune metaplastic atrophic gastritis, nodular ECL-cell hyperplasia. Nodular ECL-cell hyperplasia (*arrowhead*) can be confirmed by chromogranin immunostain (not pictured). The mucosa additionally shows a combination of complete atrophy of oxyntic glands, low-lying lymphocytic inflammation, intestinal metaplasia, and pyloric metaplasia. The absence of oxyntic glands leads to loss of acid secretion, which normally inhibits gastrin secretion. In the absence of acid, gastrin levels increase and lead to ECL-cell hyperplasia, seen here.

Figure 2-219. Autoimmune metaplastic atrophic gastritis, nodular ECL-cell hyperplasia. Uninhibited gastrin secretion results in nodular hyperplasia of ECL cells (*arrowhead*), which can become neuroendocrine tumors. The size cutoff varies by publication (0.5 vs. 0.5 cm). However, because the metastatic rate of small lesions is negligible, one practical approach is to report all small ECL-cell nodules as nodular hyperplasia and reserve the term WD-NET for endoscopically visible lesions submitted as nodules or polyps.

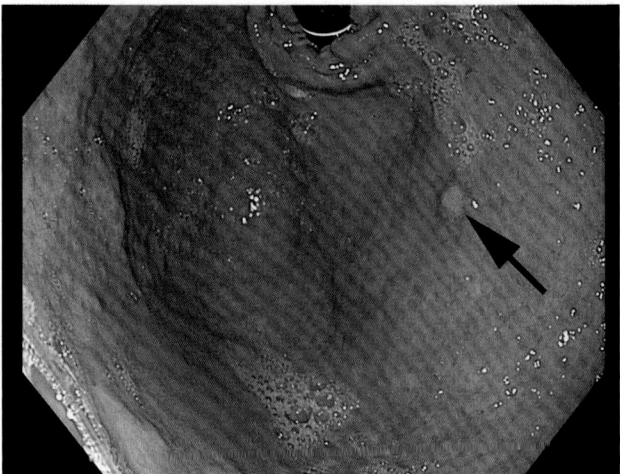

Figure 2-220. WD-NET arising in AMAG, endoscopy. This endoscopically visible lesion is a WD-NET, and the background gastric mucosa is nodular with atrophy. Biopsy samples of the background mucosa (previous figures) show histologic features of AMAG, including numerous areas containing nodular ECL-cell hyperplasia. Size cutoffs for differentiating hyperplasias from NETs are arbitrary, and the authors take a practical approach in calling lesions WD-NETs only if they correlate with an endoscopically visible lesion (*arrow*).

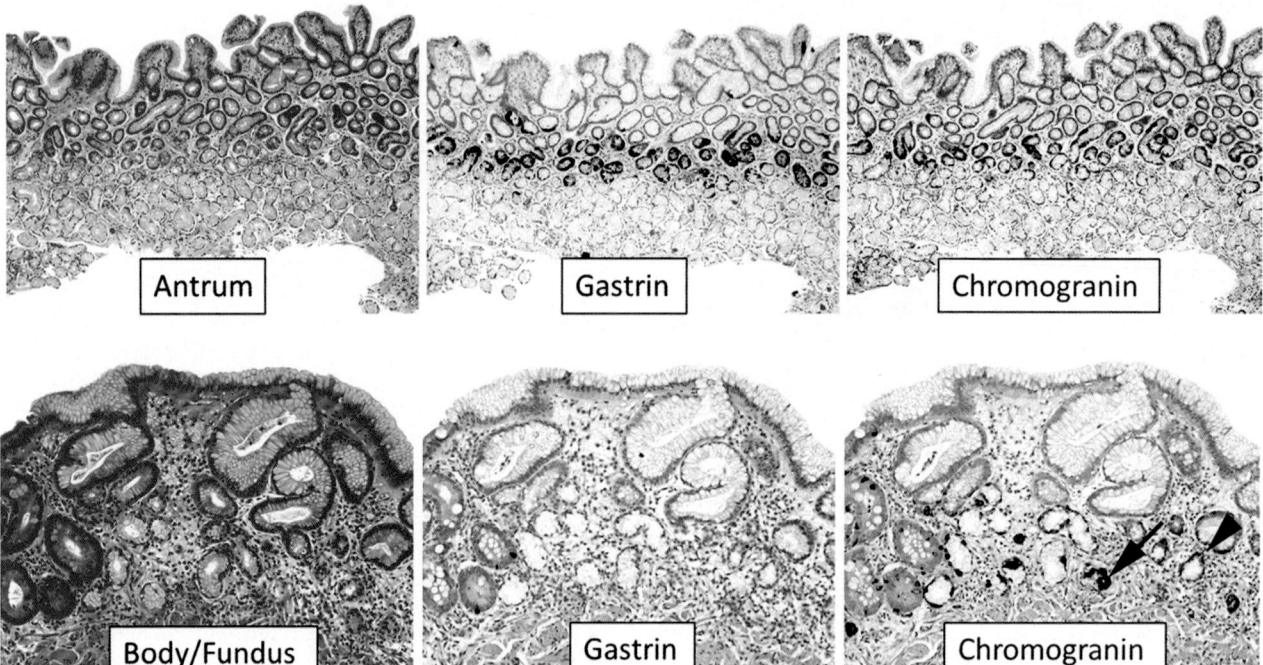

Figure 2-221. Quick tutorial on the interpretation of AMAG. AMAG is a body-predominant disease. Biopsies of the gastric antrum (*top row*) are essentially unremarkable or may show changes of chemical/reactive gastropathy. Gastrin and chromogranin stains in the antrum highlight the normal band of stimulatory "G" cells that secrete gastrin. By comparison, the gastric body and fundus (*bottom row*) show a constellation of features that can be identified by H&E, including (1) partial or complete atrophy of oxyntic glands; (2) lymphocytic inflammation, often low lying; (3) intestinal metaplasia; and (4) pyloric gland metaplasia. The features are almost indistinguishable from gastric antral tissue containing intestinal metaplasia. Therefore, a gastrin stain can be performed to confirm the *absence* of G cells (which reside *only* in the true antrum), thus identifying the tissue as true body/fundus with atrophy. A chromogranin stain highlights the final diagnostic feature of ECL-cell hyperplasia, either linear (*arrowhead*) or nodular (*arrow*).

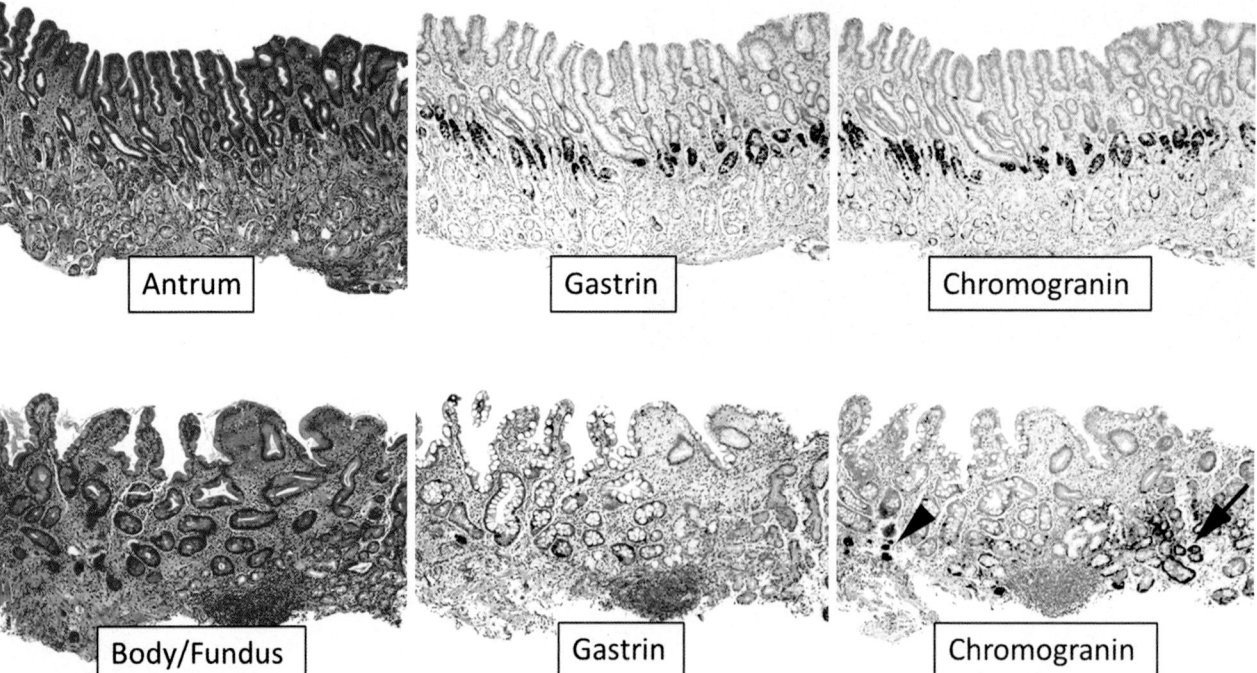

Figure 2-222. Quick tutorial on the interpretation of AMAG. By H&E, the gastric antrum (*top row*) is unremarkable or has chemical/reactive gastropathy, as seen here. The gastric body (*bottom row*) contains red flags to further pursue an AMAG workup. The easiest red flag to spot is *intestinal metaplasia in a biopsy labeled as body/fundus*. Other features include the absence of normal oxyntic glands, a low-lying lymphocytic infiltrate, and pyloric gland metaplasia. Any combination of these should prompt a basic AMAG workup, which includes gastrin and chromogranin immunostains. In the antrum, gastrin and chromogranin both highlight the horizontal band of gastrin-secreting G cells. In the body/fundus, the widespread absence of G cells is expected and confirms the tissue source. Chromogranin highlights linear (*arrow*) and nodular (*arrowhead*) ECL-cell hyperplasia.

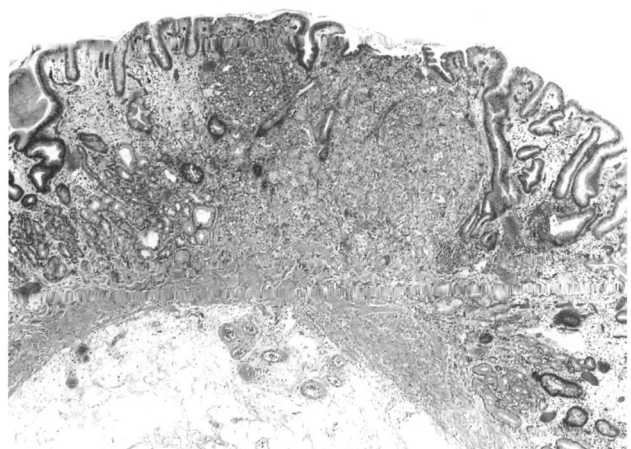

Figure 2-223. WD-NET arising in AMAG. At low magnification, this tumor is expansile and composed of small nests of cells. The background mucosa appears atrophic with intestinal metaplasia and pyloric-type glands.

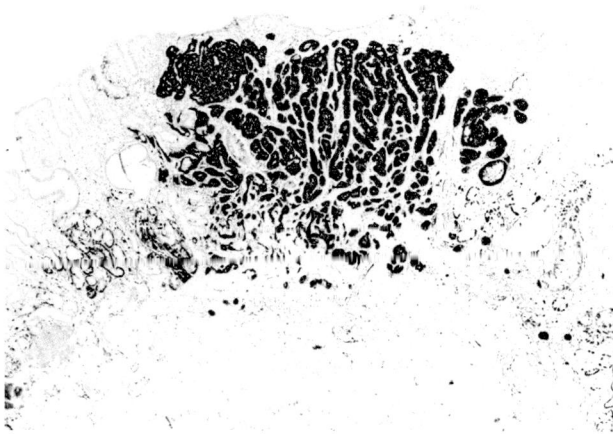

Figure 2-224. WD-NET arising in AMAG. A chromogranin immunostain of the previous case highlights the tumor cells, confirming neuroendocrine differentiation.

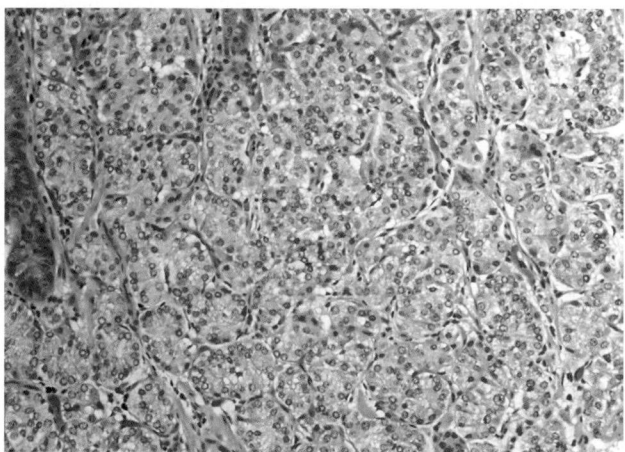

Figure 2-225. WD-NET arising in AMAG, higher magnification of the previous figure. The tumor cells are uniform and arranged in small nests and cords.

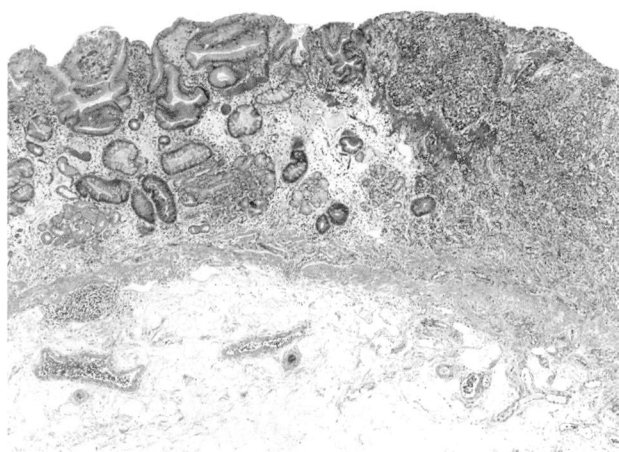

Figure 2-226. WD-NET arising in AMAG. The mucosa adjacent to the tumor (right) provides clues to the pathogenesis and prognosis. A specific combination of features offers a telltale story of AMAG: complete atrophy of oxyntic glands, chronic inflammation, intestinal metaplasia, and pyloric metaplasia. ECL-cell hyperplasia can be found on the chromogranin stain.

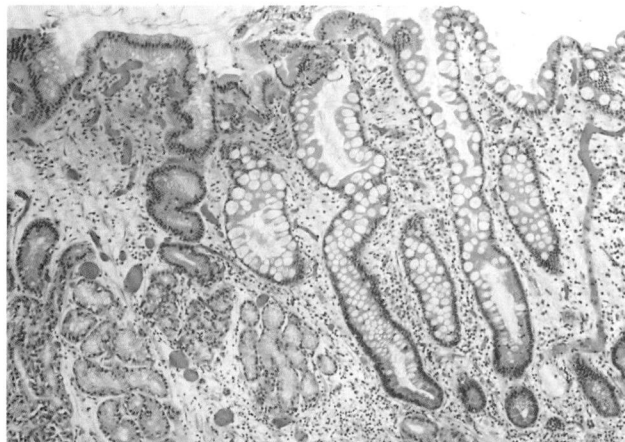

Figure 2-227. AMAG, background mucosa of the previous figure. The H&E features show a complete absence of oxyntic glands (no chief cells or parietal cells), chronic inflammation, intestinal metaplasia, and pyloric metaplasia. The last feature of AMAG (ECL-cell hyperplasia) can be confirmed by chromogranin immunostain.

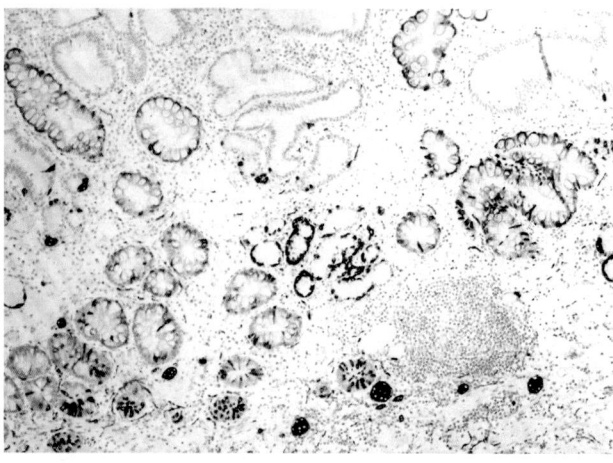

Figure 2-228. AMAG, linear and nodular ECL-cell hyperplasia, chromogranin stain. Linear and nodular ECL-cell hyperplasia is defined as five or more adjacent chromogranin reactive cells.

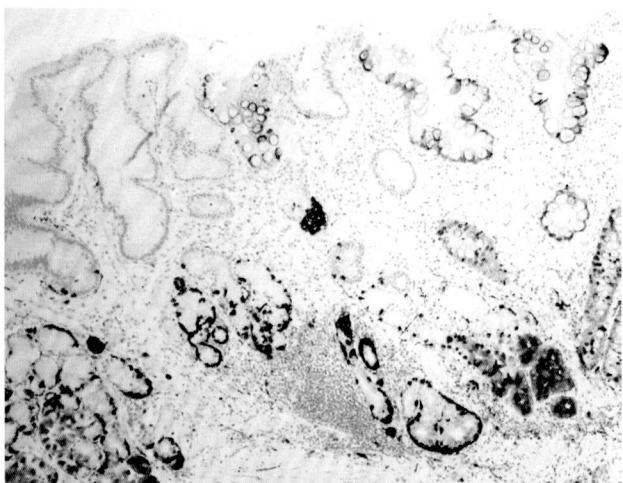

Figure 2-229. AMAG, linear and nodular ECL-cell hyperplasia, chromogranin stain. Linear and nodular ECL-cell hyperplasia is defined as five or more adjacent chromogranin reactive cells.

GASTRIC WELL-DIFFERENTIATED NEUROENDOCRINE TUMOR, TYPE II

Type II NETs (Fig. 2.230) are rare and arise in the setting of ZE syndrome due to MEN1 syndrome or a gastrin-secreting tumor elsewhere in the GI tract. Similar to the mechanism in AMAG, the uninhibited gastrin secretion stimulates ECL cells to proliferate, resulting in WD-NETs (often multiple). These type II tumors have worse prognosis than type I, with metastasis in about 30% of cases.[122] However, type II tumors behave distinctly better than type III tumors, again underscoring the importance of differentiating WD-NETs, which can be achieved by reviewing tandem biopsies of the nonpolypoid mucosa (Figs. 2.230–2.237). Biopsies of the background mucosa in ZE syndrome show oxyntic gland hyperplasia (Fig. 2.231) (as compared with atrophy in AMAG), and diffuse endocrine cell hyperplasia can be identified by immunohistochemistry. Local resection of the NET, evaluation for metastatic disease, and resection of the stimulatory gastrin-secreting tumor (usually found in the small bowel) is the mainstay of therapy.[122]

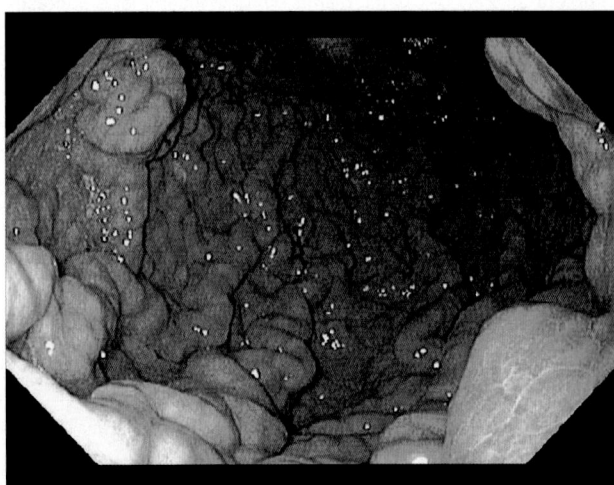

Figure 2-230. Zollinger-Ellison syndrome in a patient with MEN1, endoscopic view. The gastric folds are hypertrophic.

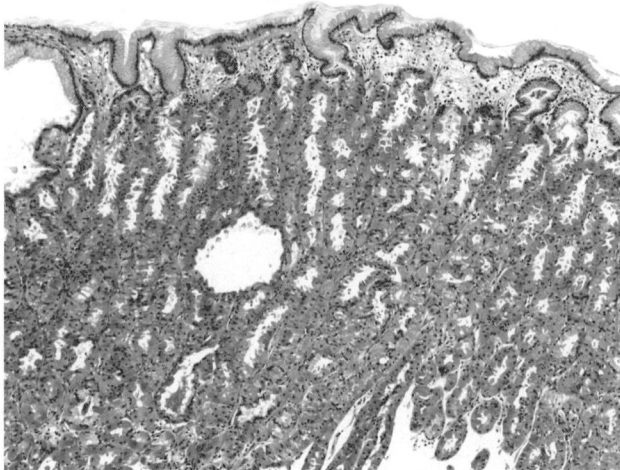

Figure 2-231. Gastric oxyntic mucosa of a patient with Zollinger-Ellison syndrome. These patients have a gastrin-secreting tumor (gastrinoma), often found in the small bowel, and the resulting hypergastrinemia causes direct stimulation of oxyntic mucosa to secrete copious amounts of acid. Biopsies show hyperplastic oxyntic mucosa with proton pump inhibitor effect (pictured); PPIs are prescribed to suppress acid secretion. Curative treatment relies on identification and resection of the gastrinoma.

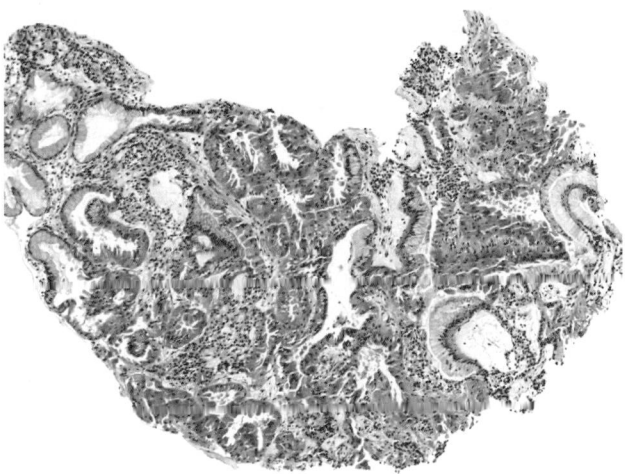

Figure 2-232. WD-NET arising in gastric oxyntic mucosa of a patient with Zollinger-Ellison syndrome. Multiple nests of uniform cells are present between the oxyntic glands.

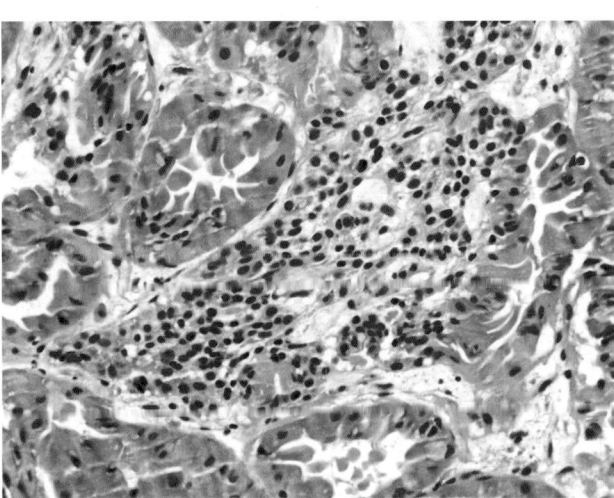

Figure 2-233. WD-NET arising in gastric oxyntic mucosa of a patient with Zollinger-Ellison syndrome. Higher magnification of the previous figure shows uniform tumor cells without prominent nucleoli.

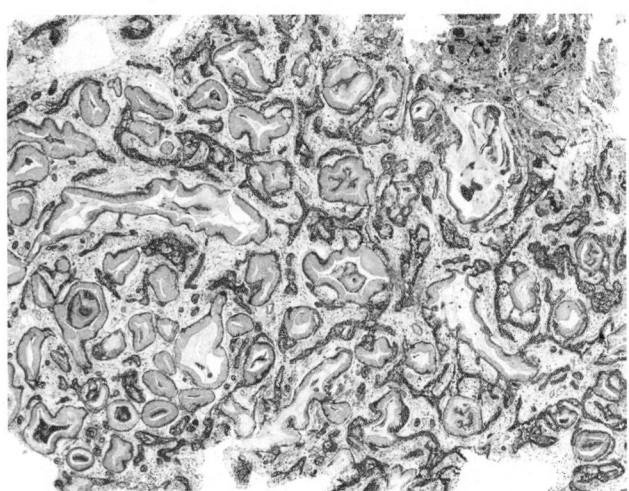

Figure 2-234. WD-NET arising in gastric oxyntic mucosa of a patient with Zollinger-Ellison syndrome. Biopsies submitted as gastric "nodules" show extensive involvement of the gastric mucosa by WD-NET.

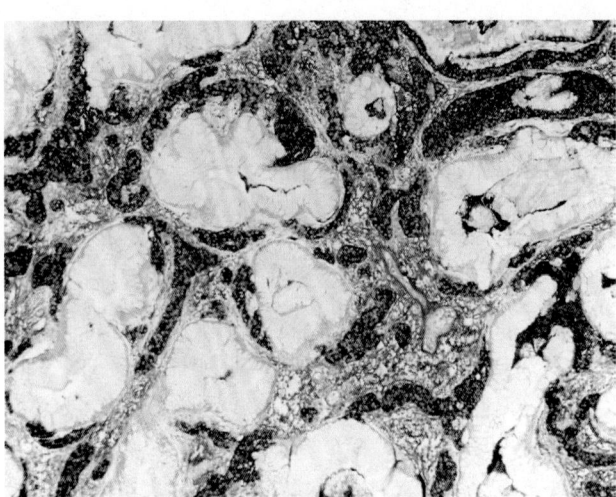

Figure 2-235. WD-NET arising in gastric oxyntic mucosa of a patient with Zollinger-Ellison syndrome, chromogranin immunostain. The tumor cells are reactive for chromogranin.

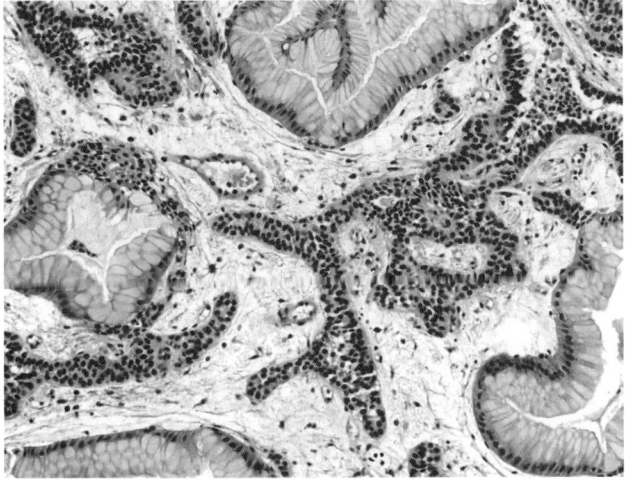

Figure 2-236. WD-NET arising in gastric oxyntic mucosa of a patient with Zollinger-Ellison syndrome. Another look at the tumor cells, which appear remarkably uniform.

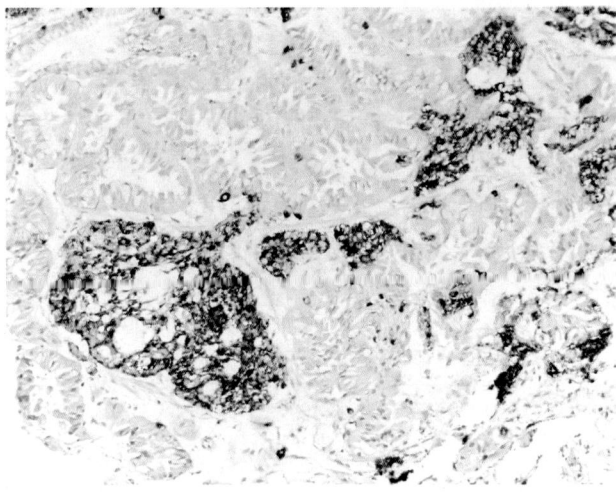

Figure 2-237. WD-NET arising in gastric oxyntic mucosa of a patient with Zollinger-Ellison syndrome, chromogranin immunostain.

GASTRIC WELL-DIFFERENTIATED NEUROENDOCRINE TUMOR, TYPE III

Type III gastric WD-NET (Figs. 2.238–2.241), the second most frequent type, has no associated clinical syndrome or context; rather, these lesions are sporadic. Type I and type II tumors arise predominantly in the gastric body and are multiple, whereas type III tumors can arise anywhere in the stomach and are typically solitary. In contrast to the excellent prognosis of type I and type II tumors, lymph node metastasis is found in 71% of type III tumors measuring >2 cm.[124] Small <1 cm tumors rarely metastasize, but in all cases of type III tumors, surgical resection is advised. Type III WD-NETs are not associated with any specific background mucosal changes.

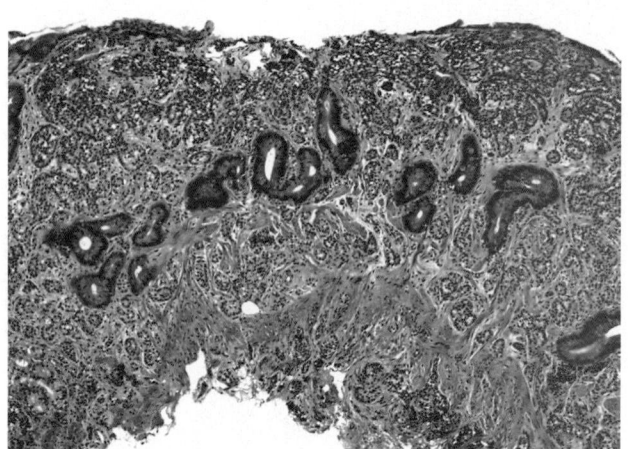

Figure 2-238. Gastric WD-NET. These tumors are staged by both size and depth of invasion. For example, this tumor, which invades into the submucosa would be staged as pT1, but only if the tumor is ≤1 cm. Anything >1 cm is automatically pT2 even if only superficially invasive.

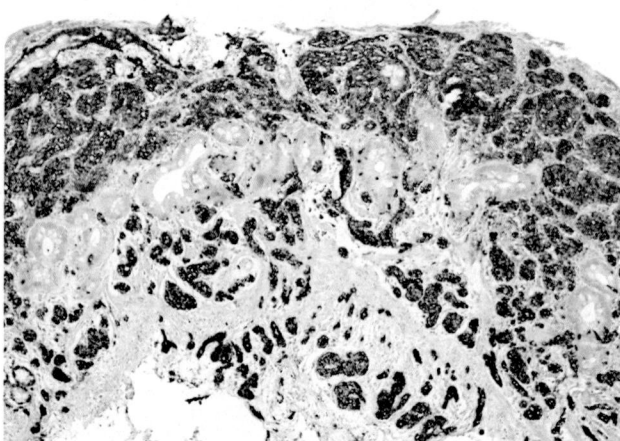

Figure 2-239. Gastric WD-NET chromogranin stain of the previous figure. A chromogranin stain highlights the tumor cells, confirming their neuroendocrine differentiation.

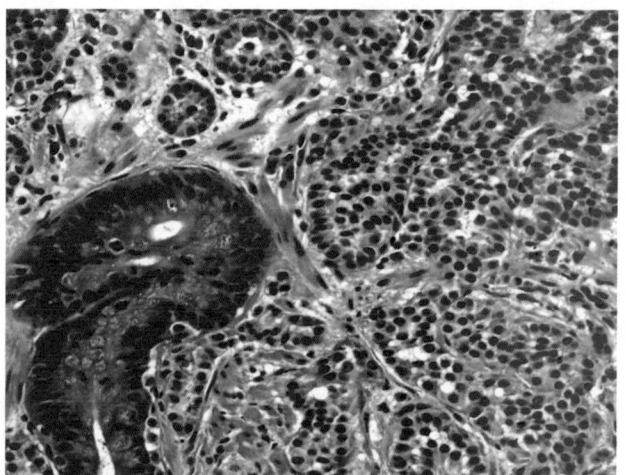

Figure 2-240. Gastric WD-NET. Differentiation (well differentiated vs poorly differentiated) is determined by morphology. Uniform cells such as seen here define this tumor as a well-differentiated NET. Grading, by comparison, is determined by mitotic count and Ki-67 proliferation.

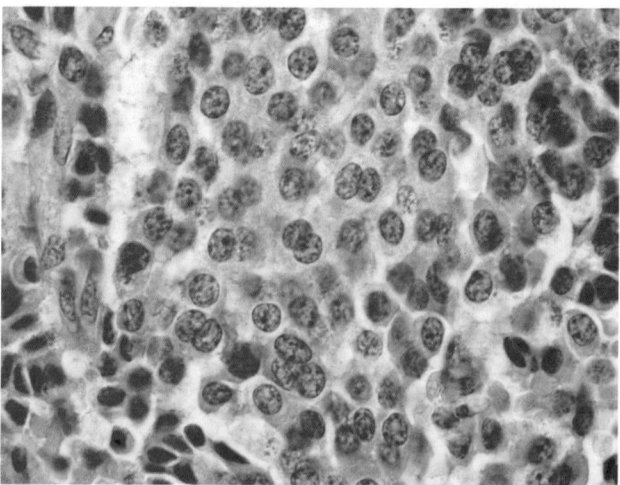

Figure 2-241. Gastric WD-NET. Well-differentiated NETs have uniform round nuclei that are similar in size and shape (pictured). The chromatin is "salt and pepper" with indistinct nucleoli. If there is significant pleomorphism (variation in shape) and anisonucleosis (variation in nuclear size), consider a diagnosis of poorly differentiated neuroendocrine carcinoma, instead.

SAMPLE NOTE: Well-Differentiated NET Arising in AMAG

Stomach, Body, Nodule, Biopsy

- Well-differentiated NET (G1), type I, arising in a backdrop of AMAG, see Comment.

Comment

Type I gastric WD-NETs arise in the setting of hypergastrinemia owing to AMAG and are well-performing tumors. The rate of metastatic disease to lymph nodes or distant sites is negligible and, if the lesion is amenable, conservative EMR is adequate treatment. Patients with AMAG are at risk for pernicious anemia, dysplasia, and gastric adenocarcinoma. Continued endoscopic surveillance is suggested, if clinically appropriate.

FAQ: What is the size cutoff for a NET versus hyperplasia, and what is the significance?

Size cutoffs for NETs vary based on published sources. For example:

College of American Pathologists

≥0.5 mm	Neuroendocrine tumor
<0.5 mm	In situ, neuroendocrine dysplasia or hyperplasia

World Health Organization

≥0.5 cm	Neuroendocrine tumor
>0.5 mm–<0.5 cm	Microcarcinoid
≤0.5 mm	Endocrine cell hyperplasia

The discrepancy in size criteria is a nonissue for type III WD-NETs, which are typically bulky masses at presentation, but it can cause some confusion for type I and II lesions, which are stimulated by excess gastrin and can range from minute endocrine cell aggregates (technically reversible hyperplasias) to larger neoplasms that persist even following removal of the gastrin stimulus. Because the metastatic rate of small lesions is negligible, the authors exercise a more practical approach over measuring endocrine cell aggregates: the term WD-NET is reserved for *endoscopically visible nodules or polyps* (Figs. 2.213 and 2.220), whereas endocrine aggregates found on random samples are described as hyperplasia (Figs. 2.221, 2.222, 2.228, and 2.229). Far more important than splitting hairs over this nomenclature, identifying the features in the background mucosa (AMAG vs. ZE vs normal/nonspecific) provides information for subtyping, prognostication, and treatment.

PEARLS & PITFALLS: Grading of WD-NET Requires Both Mitotic Count and Ki-67 Proliferative Index

WD-NETs are graded by both mitotic index and Ki-67 proliferation index (Figs. 2.242–2.244). The Ki-67 index frequently results in a higher grade than mitotic count, and studies have shown these grade-discordant tumors more likely to have metastases to lymph nodes and distant sites, perineural invasion, small vessel invasion, and overall survival.[125] In cases for which grade results are discordant, *assign the higher grade.*

WHO 2017 Classification of Neuroendocrine Neoplasms

WD-NET G1	<3% Ki-67	<2 mitoses/10 HPF
WD-NET G2	3% to 20% Ki-67	2–20 mitoses/10 HPF
WD-NET G3	>20% Ki-67	>20 mitoses/10 HPF

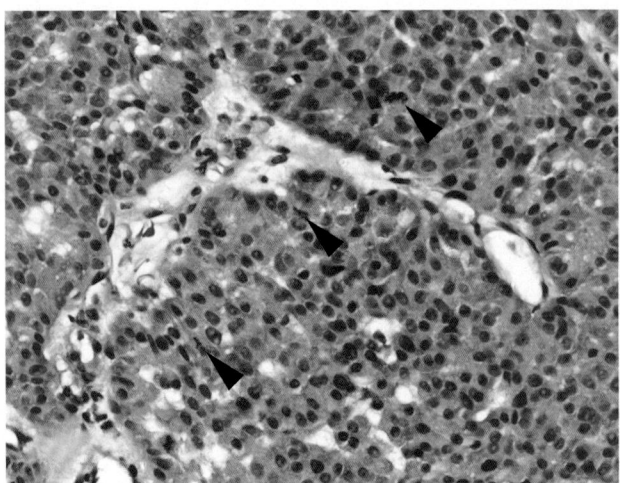

Figure 2-242. Gastric WD-NET, grade 3. Tumor differentiation and tumor grade are independent assessments and a well differentiated tumor can be high grade, even if that sounds counterintuitive. Differentiation is dependent on cell morphology; this case is well differentiated because the tumor cells are uniform. Grading, however, is based on mitotic activity and Ki-67 proliferation index. Any tumor with >20 mitoses in 10 HPF is G3, even if well differentiated. This example shows three mitoses (*arrowheads*) within a single HPF.

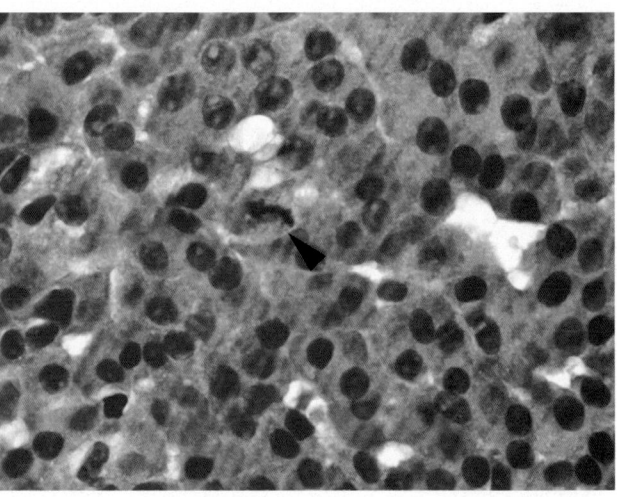

Figure 2-243. Gastric WD-NET, grade 3, higher magnification of the previous figure. This mitotically active (*arrowhead*) tumor reaches the threshold for >20 mitoses in 10 HPF and is considered high grade (G3). However, the tumor is well differentiated because the cells are uniform, have smooth nuclear borders, and nucleoli are absent. Differentiation is morphologic, whereas tumor grade is based on mitoses and Ki-67.

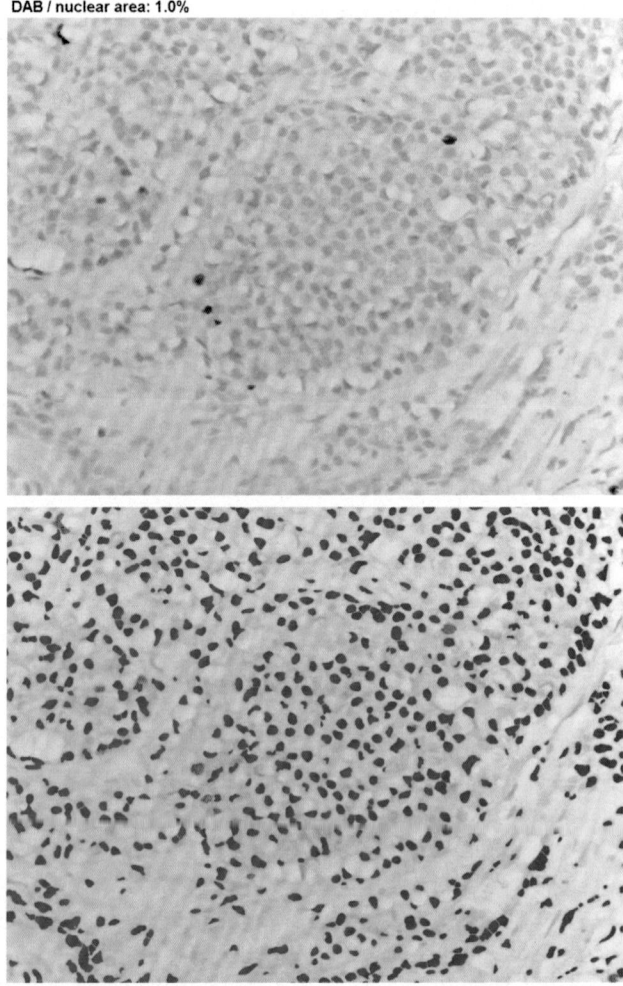

Figure 2-244. Digital image analysis for Ki-67 proliferation index. Digital image analysis software can automate the counting of cells, reducing burden on pathologists. The top image is a photomicrograph of Ki-67 immunohistochemistry in a WD-NET submitted to the software program. The bottom image displays what the program identifies as tumor cells (*marked blue*) and Ki-67 positive cells (*marked gold*) with an automated 1% count in this example.

Note of Caution

Performing Ki-67 labeling on type 1 WD-NETs can be misleading because a sizable minority of them (up to about a third) have the proliferation of a G2 tumor but behave like grade 1 lesions.[126] If this testing is performed (some do not add it), the results may benefit from a disclaimer.

FAQ: Can I eyeball the Ki 67 or does this require a manual count?

A minimum of 500 cells (suggested range 500 to 2000) is counted to determine the Ki-67 index, which is reported as the percent of positive tumor cells. Manual counting is time consuming, and a number of studies have examined different techniques for Ki-67 index, including digitized automatic counting and eyeballing. Digital image analysis software is not widely available and requires software modification to prevent inaccurate counting, for example, intratumoral or peritumoral lymphocytes (Fig. 2.244). Eyeballing in areas of highest density "hot spots" is accurate in higher-grade lesions, but when tumors are close to grade cutoffs, *it is best to perform manual count*. Then again, anyone who has attempted to tally up 500 to 2000 cells under the microscope knows how quickly one can lose track of which cells have been counted. A simple and economical approach is to print out a photo or screenshot of a hot spot area and manually cross off each cell as it is counted (Fig. 2.245). Take care to exclude lymphocytes, which will skew the Ki-67 count higher.

PEARLS & PITFALLS: Grading by Mitotic Rate Requires Counting 50 HPF But Is Reported as per 10 HPF

The mitoses in 50 HPF should be counted to accurately grade the tumor. This number is divided by five to report mitoses per 10 HPF. These minimum requirements for grading (50 HPF for mitotic count and 5000 to 2000 cells for Ki-67 index) presume there is enough tissue for accurate grading, but small biopsy material may be insufficient in many cases. See the following sample note.

SAMPLE NOTE: When Small Biopsies Contain Insufficient WD-NET for Mitotic Count or Ki-67 Index Grading

Stomach, Antrum, Polyp, Biopsy

- Well-differentiated neuroendocrine tumor, see Comment.

Comment

There is insufficient tumor cell quantity to accurately grade this WD-NET (minimum requirement 50 HPF for mitotic count and 500 cells for Ki-67 proliferation index). Based on the available material, this tumor appears to be (G1, G2, G3). Final grading will be revised following review of a larger sample (e.g., excision specimen).

PEARLS & PITFALLS: Both Size and Depth of Invasion Are Considered in Staging of Gastric WD-NETs

Although the depth of invasion defines most staging criteria, gastric WD-NETs are among the few that also take into account tumor size at the lower stages. For example, staging criteria by depth is fairly typical, with invasion into the lamina propria and submucosa staged as pT1, *but only if the tumor is ≤1 cm*. Any tumor >1 cm is automatically pT2 or higher, even if superficially invasive. Once tumors invade at least into the muscularis propria, the tumors are staged by depth regardless of size: pT2, involvement of muscularis propria, pT3, involvement of subserosa, pT4, invasion of serosa or adjacent tissue/organs.

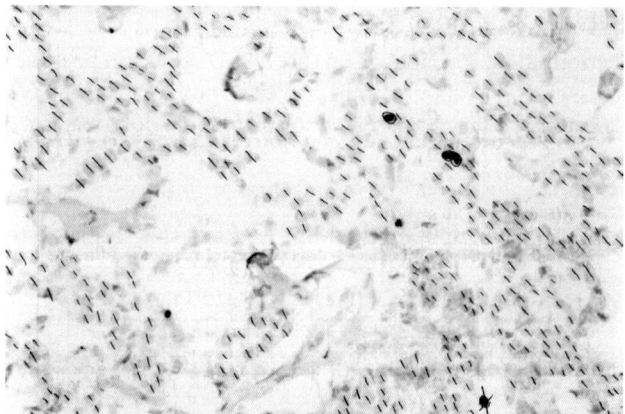

Figure 2-245. Manual count for Ki-67 proliferation index. A simple computer printout is quick and economical if digital image analysis software is not available. Each cell can be marked off during the 500–2000 cell count to avoid duplicate counts. To facilitate turn-around time, ancillary staff can be trained in this method for reporting Ki-67 proliferation index.

MALT LYMPHOMA

GI lymphomas are challenging to recognize because the GI tract serves many immunologic functions, and there is considerable histologic overlap between benign inflammatory conditions and malignant lymphomas. In-depth coverage of lymphomas is beyond the scope of this text and is left to our subspecialty hematopathology colleagues. We encourage a low threshold to liberally share cases with such experts, but any pathologist reviewing GI biopsies will be faced with gastric MALT extranodal marginal zone lymphoma. The tools given in the following text are intended to ensure readers are comfortable triaging these cases and are confident in recognizing features requiring additional workup and consultation with hematopathology colleagues.

Gastric MALT lymphoma is driven by *H. pylori* infection, and eradication of the organism is the first-line treatment of MALT lymphoma, resulting in remission in nearly 80% of cases.[127] At low magnification, a robust and expansile deep chronic inflammatory infiltrate is the first red flag to evaluate further for MALT lymphoma (Figs. 2.246–2.250). At higher magnification, the infiltrate is typically composed of monomorphic small lymphocytes with pericellular clearing or "halos" (Figs. 2.251–2.254). Features that serve as red flags to differentiate a malignant infiltrate from benign gastritis include glandular destruction, in which lymphocytes (usually three or more) invade the glandular epithelium and disrupt normal architecture (i.e., lymphoepithelial lesions) (Figs. 2.251–2.257) and the presence of dense lymphoid infiltrates involving the muscularis mucosae (Figs. 2.246–2.248).[128] These features should trigger immunohistochemical workup, including, at minimum, CD3, CD20, and CD43. This limited and economical panel can identify about half of MALT lymphomas, which will show aberrant coexpression of CD43+ in the predominantly CD20+ B-cell infiltrate (Fig. 2.258). The CD3 immunostain will provide a contrast by highlighting any T cells, which normally express CD43. If this panel is insufficient to make a diagnosis, expansion to a more comprehensive immunohistochemical panel will show the following pattern in MALT lymphoma: CD20+, CD79a+, BCL2+, CD5–, CD10–, cyclin D1–, CD23– CD43± (Figs. 2.259–2.264). This fundamental panel will also differentiate other mature B-cell neoplasms, such as chronic lymphocytic leukemia/small lymphocytic lymphoma (CD5+), follicular lymphoma (CD10+), and mantle cell lymphoma (cyclin D1/BCL1+).

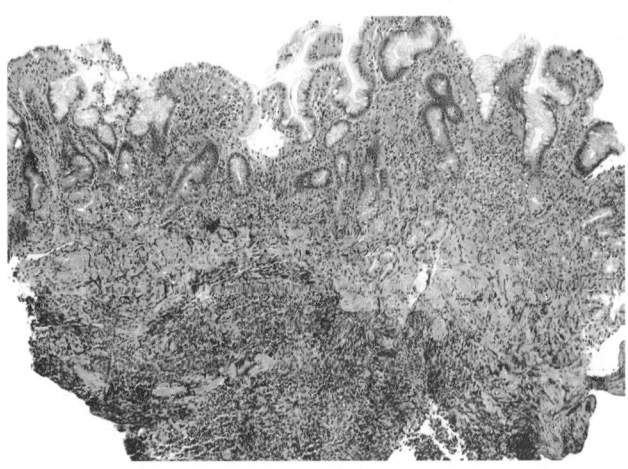

Figure 2-246. Gastric MALT lymphoma. Features that should trigger a MALT lymphoma workup are seen here, including a deep monotonous lymphoid infiltrate that is gland destructive and splaying out the muscularis mucosae.

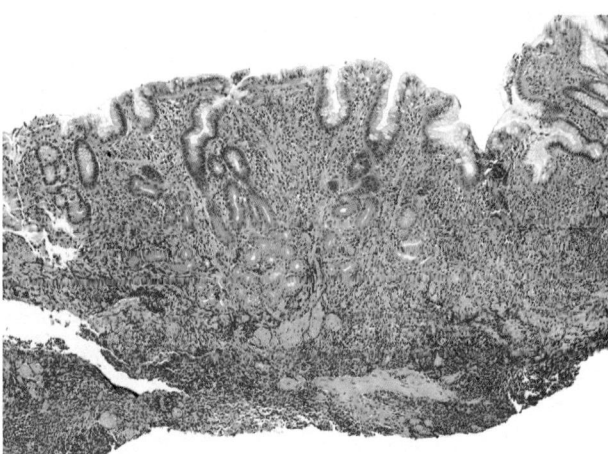

Figure 2-247. Gastric MALT lymphoma. The infiltrate at low power is far more robust than expected for a simple chronic gastritis. The lymphoid infiltrate is densely packed, gland destructive, deep, and expanding the muscularis mucosae.

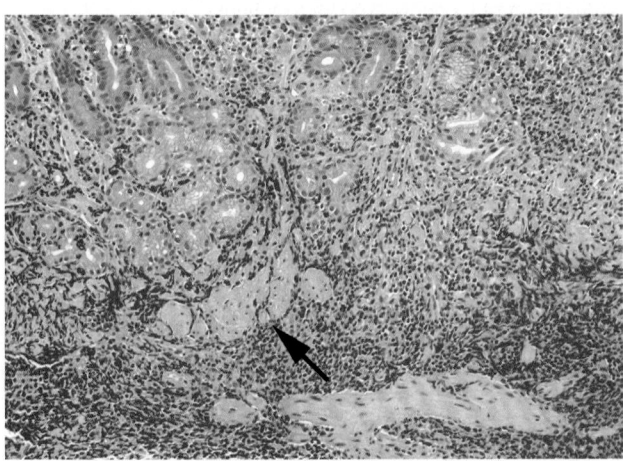

Figure 2-248. Gastric MALT lymphoma, higher magnification of the previous figure. The infiltrate is deep, dense, and composed of a monotonous population of lymphocytes. The lymphoid cells not only cross the muscularis mucosae but also spread the muscle bundles (*arrow*) apart.

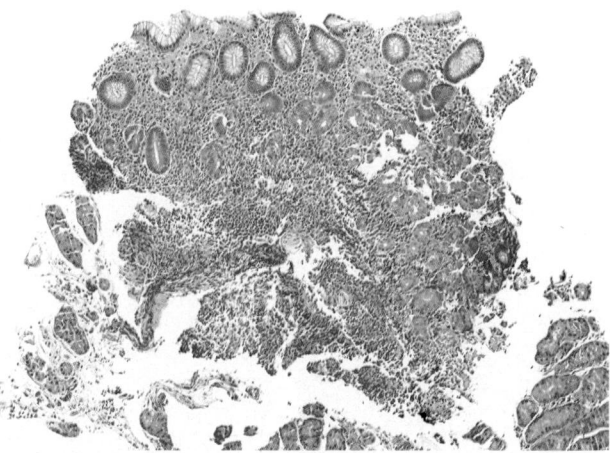

Figure 2-249. Gastric MALT lymphoma. The infiltrate is more dense and monotonous than the usual chronic gastritis. At low magnification, the expansile and gland-destructive quality should trigger further workup for lymphoma.

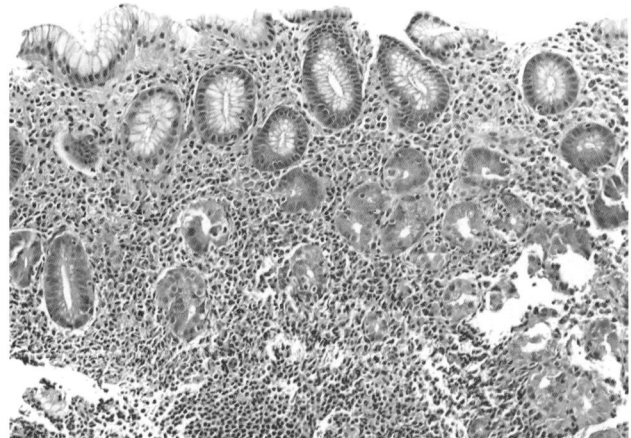

Figure 2-250. Gastric MALT lymphoma, higher magnification of the previous figure. Gland destruction is seen in the center of the field, as lymphocytes invade the glandular epithelium.

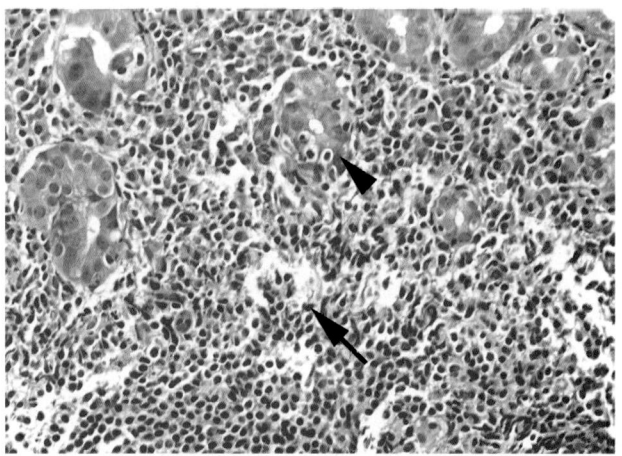

Figure 2-251. Gastric MALT lymphoma, higher magnification of the previous figure. Lymphoepithelial lesions are characterized by lymphocytes (usually ≥3) invading the glandular epithelium and disrupting the normal architecture (*arrowhead*). Destroyed glands (*arrow*) leave areas of drop-out which are filled in by the monotonous lymphocytes.

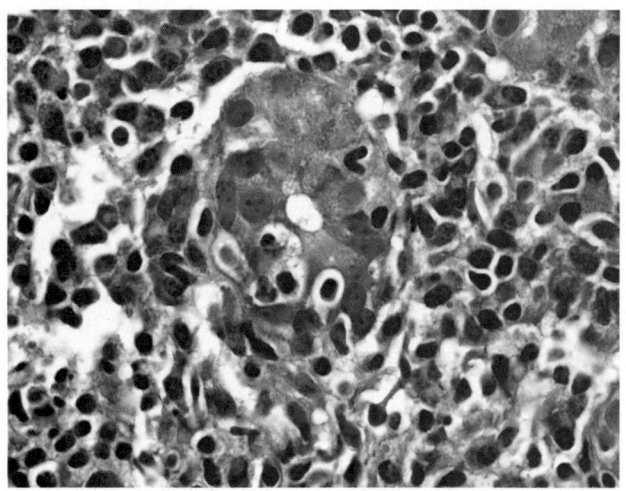

Figure 2-252. Lymphoepithelial lesion of gastric MALT lymphoma. The malignant lymphoid cells invade the glandular epithelium and disrupt the normal architecture. A feature of the malignant cells is the pericellular clearing or halo around each cell.

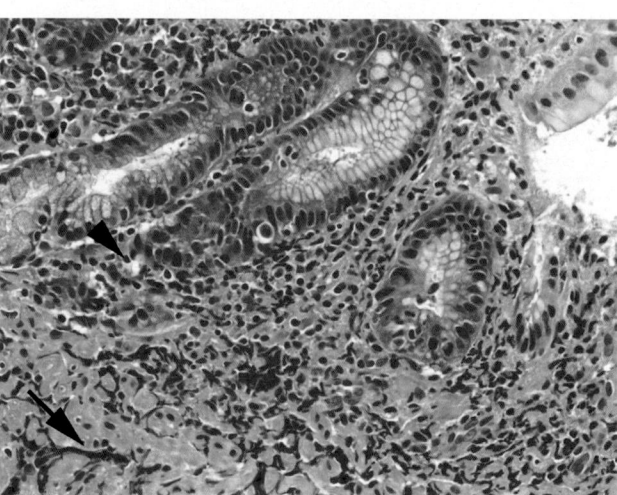

Figure 2-253. Gastric MALT lymphoma. These malignant lymphocytes are destroying areas of glandular epithelium (*arrowhead*) and muscularis mucosae (*arrow*). Features of glandular destruction and muscularis mucosae abnormality are not seen in benign gastritis and should prompt further workup for lymphoma.

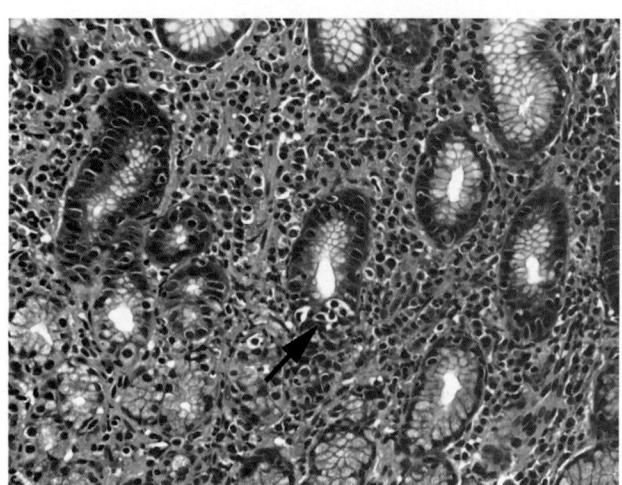

Figure 2-254. Lymphoepithelial lesion of gastric MALT lymphoma. These lymphocytes have a characteristic pericellular halo seen in MALT lymphoma cells. The presence of three or more lymphocytes invading the glandular epithelium (*arrow*) is called a lymphoepithelial lesion (LEL). Compared with benign intraepithelial lymphocytosis, which are T cells, these LELs are composed of malignant B cells.

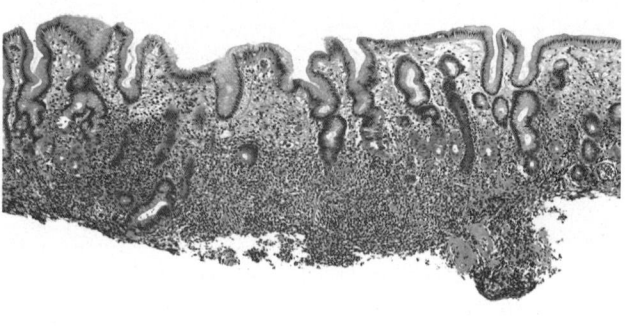

Figure 2-255. Gastric MALT lymphoma. At low magnification, this infiltrate differs from a benign chronic gastritis because it is deep, dense, and monotonous with gland destruction.

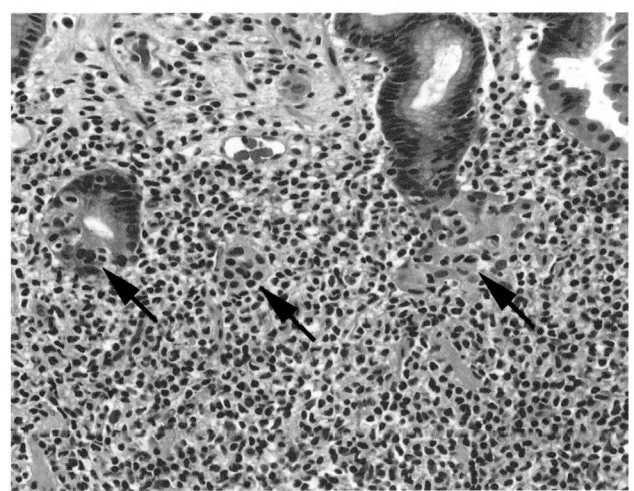

Figure 2-256. Lymphoepithelial lesions in gastric MALT lymphoma, higher magnification of the previous figure. Lymphoepithelial lesions are seen in various stages (*arrows*). On the far left, the gland structure is still visible. The far right shows marked disruption of the glandular architecture, but remnant epithelial cells are still visible. The center lesion is a nearly destroyed gland and is barely visible.

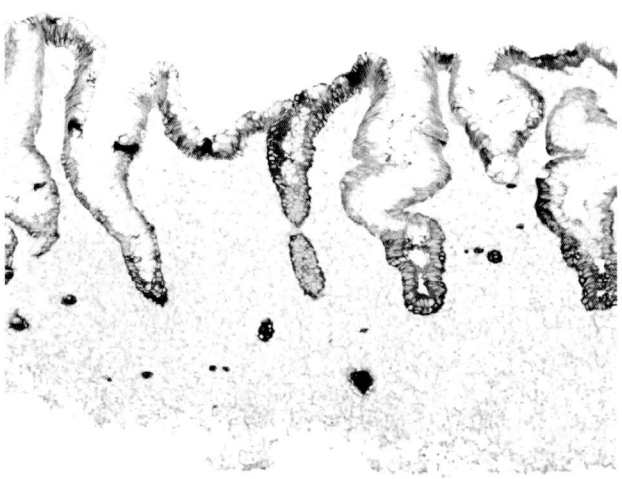

Figure 2-257. Gastric MALT lymphoma, pancytokeratin stain. A pancytokeratin stain can be helpful in highlighting residual glands and areas of lymphoepithelial lesions, which may be obscured by the dense lymphocytic infiltrate on H&E.

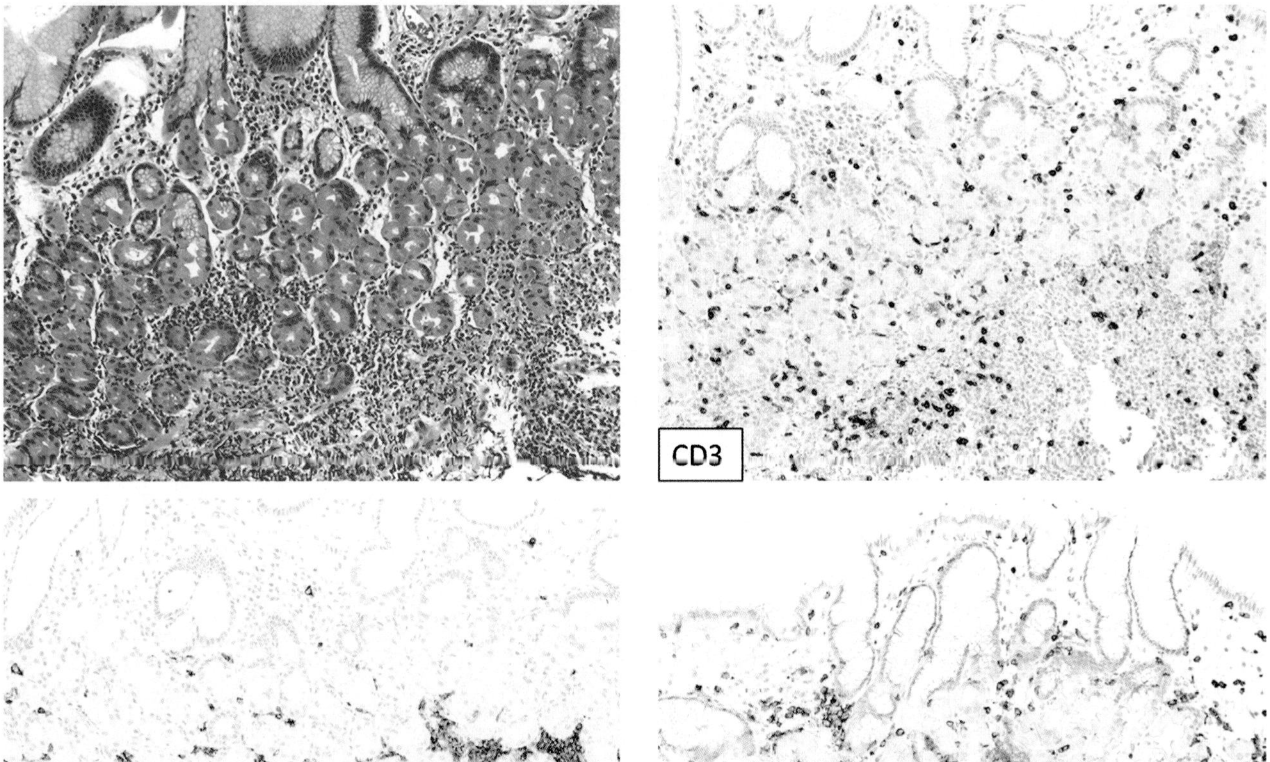

Figure 2-258. Gastric MALT lymphoma, CD20+ with coexpression of CD43+. About half of gastric MALT lymphomas can be identified by a limited immunopanel of CD3, CD20, and CD43. These tumors show aberrant coexpression of CD43+ (normally found in T cells) in the predominantly CD20+ B-cell infiltrate. The CD3 immunostain provides a contrast by highlighting the T cells. Should this panel fail to solidify a diagnosis, an extended immunopanel can be performed.

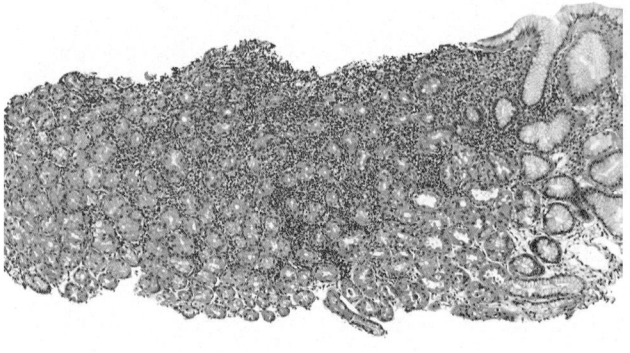

Figure 2-259. Gastric MALT lymphoma. This infiltrate is just a little too dense and too monotonous to consider chronic gastritis. Some areas appear expansile, whereas others appear gland destructive. In these instances, it is best to rule out lymphoma.

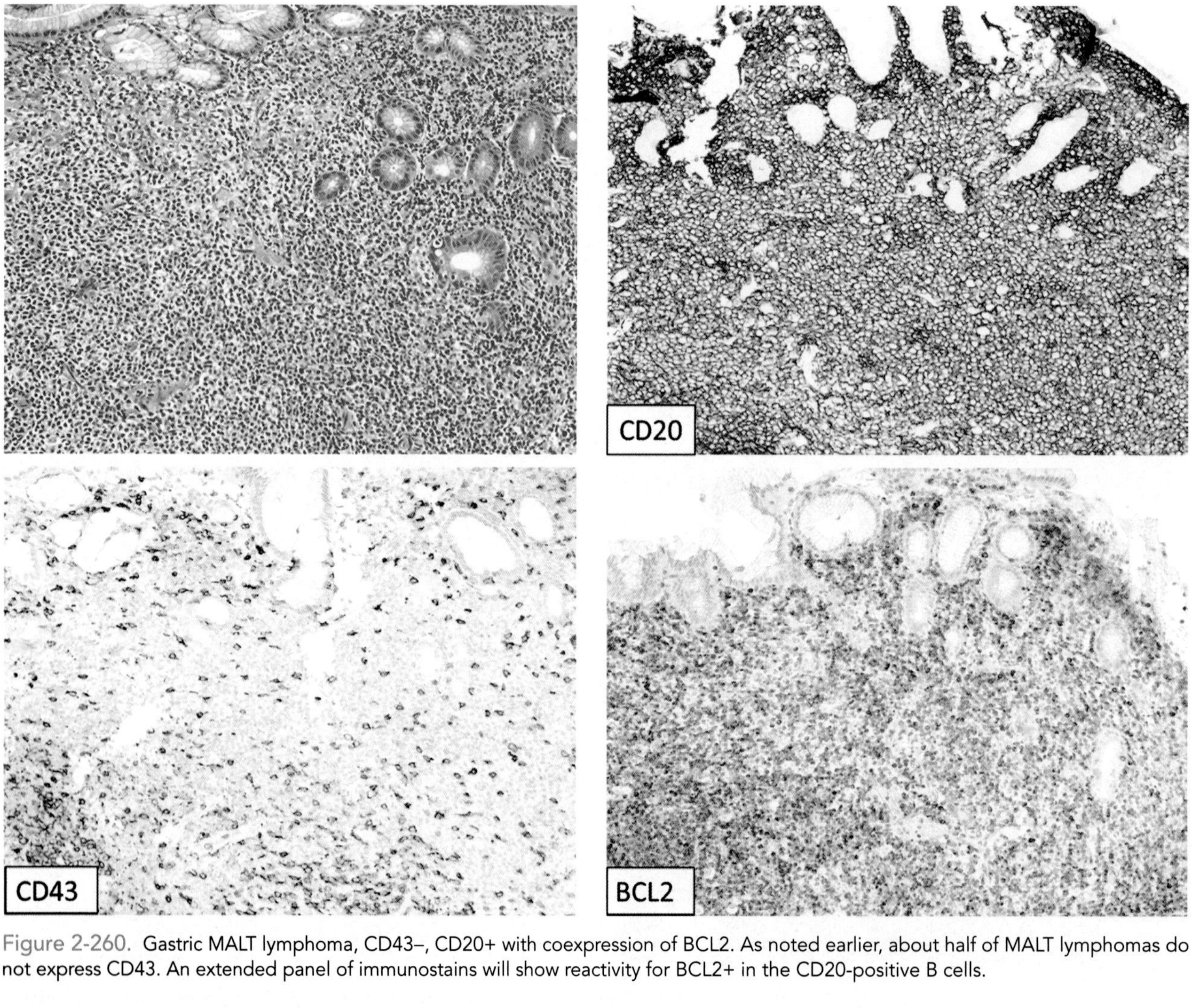

CD20

CD43

BCL2

Figure 2-260. Gastric MALT lymphoma, CD43–, CD20+ with coexpression of BCL2. As noted earlier, about half of MALT lymphomas do not express CD43. An extended panel of immunostains will show reactivity for BCL2+ in the CD20-positive B cells.

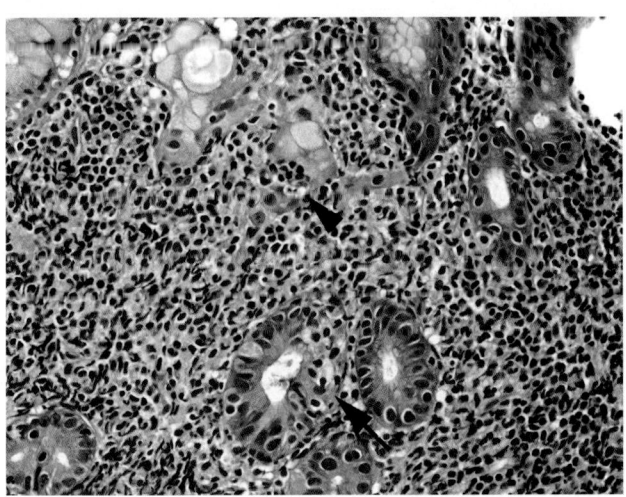

Figure 2-261. Lymphoepithelial lesions in gastric MALT lymphoma. Lymphoepithelial lesions can be found in various stages. Early lesions show ≥3 tumor lymphocytes invading the glandular epithelium (*arrow*). More mature lesions show disruption of glandular architecture with degenerating epithelial cells (*arrowhead*).

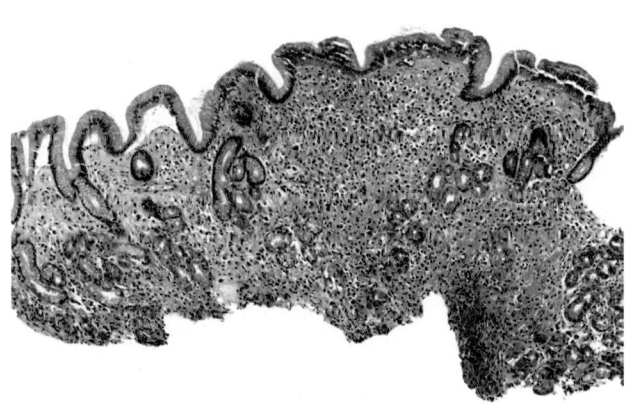

Figure 2-262. Plasmacytoid variant of gastric MALT lymphoma. At low power, the architecture of this gastric biopsy is abnormal. The lamina propria appears expanded and cellular, whereas the glands are irregularly distributed. The pigment is incidental hemosiderin.

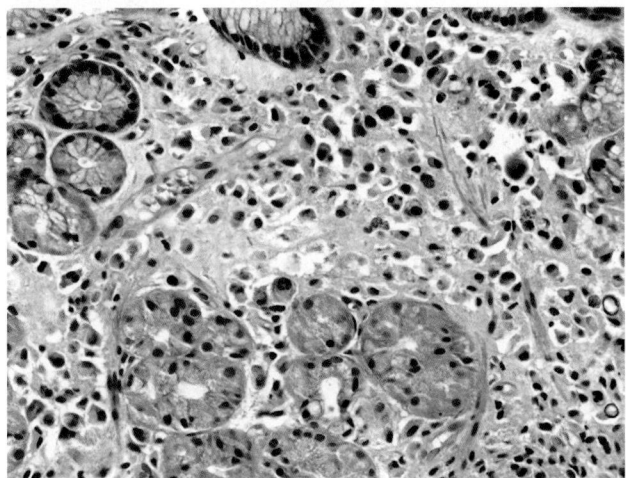

Figure 2-263. Plasmacytoid variant of gastric MALT lymphoma, higher magnification of the previous figure. Do not be falsely reassured by the presence of a plasmacytic infiltrate in this case. The plasma cells in the lamina propria are atypical with binucleate forms and marked variation in size. A plasmacytic clone is found in 30% of MALT lymphomas. The pigment is incidental hemosiderin.

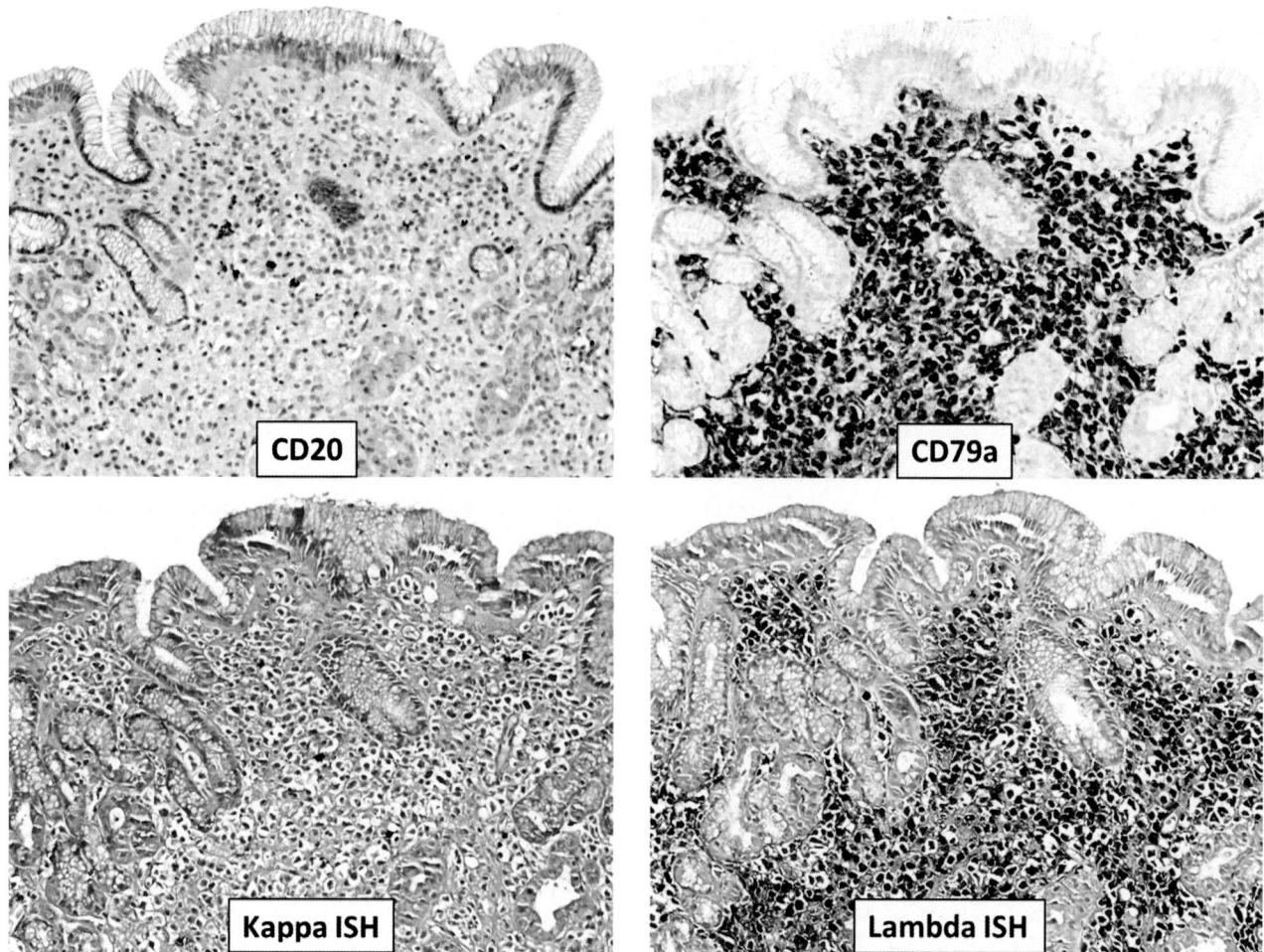

Figure 2-264. Plasmacytoid variant of gastric MALT lymphoma, higher magnification of the previous figure. These subtle MALT lymphomas can be CD20 negative but should express CD79a and show kappa or lambda restriction. This example shows CD20−, CD79a+, and lambda restriction.

PEARLS & PITFALLS: Always Report *H. pylori* Status

H. pylori treatment and eradication is effective and results in remission in up to 80% of gastric MALT lymphomas. However, a subset of tumors contains molecular genetic changes of t(11;18)(q21;q21) that have been associated with the failure of MALT lymphoma to regress after *H. pylori* eradication therapy and may arise in the absence of *H. pylori* infection.[129] Reporting of *H. pylori* status stratifies patients into prognostic groups and directs treatment (e.g., the addition of radiotherapy or chemotherapy).

PEARLS & PITFALLS: Plasmacytoid MALT Lymphoma Variant as a Pitfall

Do not be falsely reassured by the presence of a plasmacytic infiltrate and assume it represents *H. pylori* gastritis. Although *H. pylori* gastritis is associated with a plasmacytic infiltrate compared with the typical lymphoid infiltrate of MALT lymphoma, a plasmacytic clone is present in about 30% of MALT lymphomas, and the plasmacytoid variant of MALT lymphoma can be subtle and tricky (Figs. 2.262 and 2.263).[130] Do not forget to always assess for a deep, expansile, or destructive pattern, even if the cells appear predominantly plasmacytic. Immunostains for CD20 can also be negative in the plasmacytoid variant, another pitfall to diagnosis, but the variant will stain for CD79a and show either kappa or lambda restriction (Figs. 2.264 and 2.265).

FAQ: How does one handle biopsies for posttreatment assessment of MALT lymphoma?

Biopsies from treated patients largely show regression of lymphoma, with sparse residual lymphoid cells that are insufficient for further workup, and yet cannot be cleared as complete remission (Figs. 2.266 and 2.267). In these cases, the first step is immunohistochemistry for *H. pylori* to ensure eradication. Following this, should sufficient lymphoid cells be available, a limited immunohistochemical panel mirroring the original immunoprofile of the tumor cells (e.g., if the tumor was CD43+, then the limited panel of CD20/CD43/CD3 is sufficient) may be useful in confirming residual disease. However, immunohistochemistry is not necessary, and a histological grading system for posttreatment evaluation of gastric MALT lymphoma includes the following categories[131]:

Complete remission: absent or scattered lymphoid/plasma cells

Probable Minimal Residual Disease (pMRD): aggregates of lymphoid cells or lymphoid nodules with empty lamina propria

Responding Residual Disease: Dense, diffuse, nodular lymphoid infiltrate with or without lymphoepithelial lesions, with partially empty lamina propria

No Change: Dense, diffuse, nodular lymphoid infiltrate with lymphoepithelial lesions and no change in lamina propria

The differentiation of complete remission from pMRD is not always histologically clear-cut, but this distinction is not too important because a diagnosis of pMRD is not an indication for further treatment and clinicians manage this as a state of remission.

SAMPLE NOTE: Probable Minimal Residual Disease of MALT Lymphoma

Although the presence of patchy basal lymphoid aggregates is consistent with pMRD, this finding is not necessarily an indication for further treatment and could be managed as a state of remission with appropriate follow-up.

Reference:
Copie-Bergman C, Gaulard P, Lavergne-Slove A, et al. Proposal for a new histological grading system for post-treatment evaluation of gastric MALT lymphoma. *Gut.* 2003;52(11):1656. PMID:14570741; PMCID:PMC1773845.

CHECKLIST: Features that Trigger MALT Lymphoma Workup or Consult

- ☐ Predominantly lymphocytic infiltrate
- ☐ Deep monotonous lymphoid infiltrates
- ☐ Expansile lymphoid infiltrate
- ☐ Lymphocytes with pericellular clearing or halos
- ☐ Lymphoid infiltrate correlating with endoscopic nodule or mass
- ☐ Destructive lymphoid infiltrates invading glands ("lymphoepithelial lesions")
- ☐ Dense lymphoid infiltrates traversing the muscularis mucosae

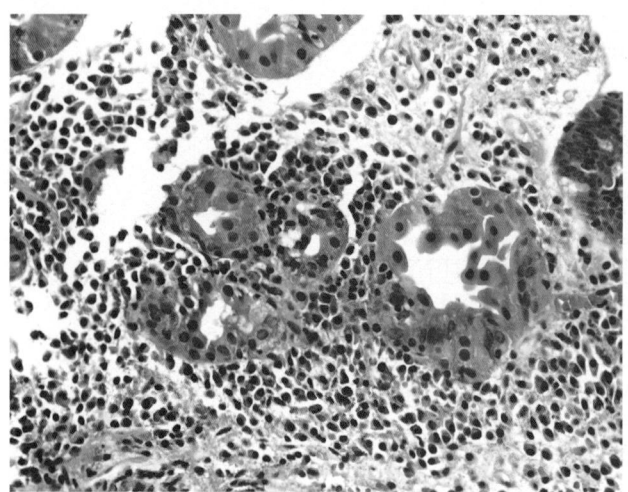

Figure 2-265. Lymphoepithelial lesion in plasmacytoid variant of gastric MALT lymphoma. These malignant plasma cells are invading the glandular epithelium and destroying the normal architecture.

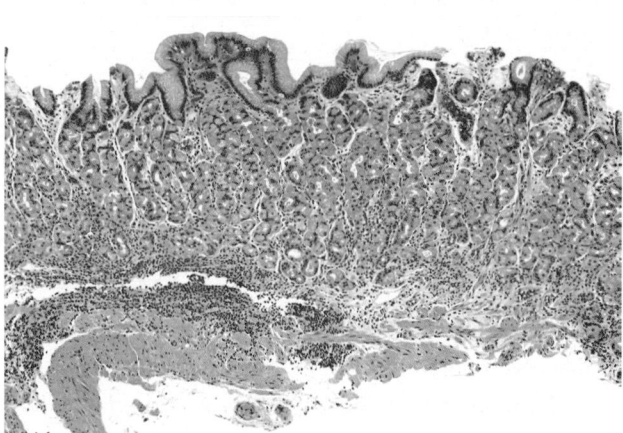

Figure 2-266. Probable minimal residual disease. Some residual lymphoid cells are common following treatment of MALT lymphoma. So long as they are not dense, diffuse, nodular, or accompanied by lymphoepithelial lesions, these are considered probable minimal residual disease. This designation is not an indication for further treatment but should be managed as a state of remission.

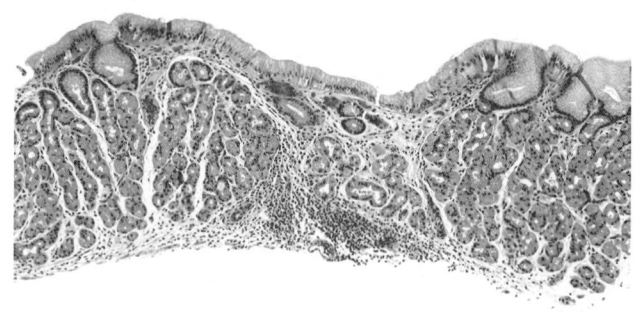

Figure 2-267. Probable minimal residual disease. Sometimes residual lymphoid cells are present in posttreatment biopsies yet are insufficient in size to immunophenotype. These can simply be reported as probable minimal residual disease, which is managed clinically as a state of remission.

MESENCHYMAL LESIONS

Mesenchymal lesions cover a broad spectrum of mesodermally derived tumors, which are covered more completely in "Mesenchymal Tumors" chapter. Select mesenchymal polyps common to the stomach are briefly covered herein, including the inflammatory fibroid polyp (IFP), gastrointestinal stromal tumor (GIST), leiomyoma, and granular cell tumor (GCT).

INFLAMMATORY FIBROID POLYP

IFP was first described in 1949 by Vanek as "gastric submucosal granulomas with eosinophilic infiltration."[132] IFPs can occur in all ages but are most common in age 50 to 60 years and have a slightly higher incidence in women.[121] They are rare lesions with an estimated relative prevalence of 0.09%.[133,134] IFPs present most often as a solitary polyp or submucosal nodule in the gastric pylorus or distal antrum (Fig. 2.268) and are typically small (<1.5 cm) and sessile.[135] They are characterized by CD34 immunoreactive spindle and stellate stromal cells mixed with inflammatory cells (predominantly eosinophils) in a myxoid or edematous stroma and thin-walled vessels (Figs. 2.269–2.274). The spindle cells are sometimes seen swirling or forming an "onion skin" pattern around vessels (Figs. 2.271–2.273). Although this was once believed a reactive lesion, activating mutations have been identified in the platelet-derived growth factor receptor alpha (*PDGFRα*) gene. This mutation is also found in a subset of GISTs, typically the gastric benign epithelioid variant that does not have a *KIT* mutation. IFPs are now viewed as *PDGFRα*-driven benign neoplasms.[135] These tumors rarely cause clinical symptoms; however, a few cases of large gastric IFPs causing gastric outlet obstruction have been reported.[136] They are believed to have no malignant potential, thus no endoscopic follow-up is recommended after initial histologic confirmation, unless symptomatic, in which case complete resection is recommended.[137]

KEY FEATURES: IFP

- *PDGFRα*-mutation-driven **benign neoplasms**
- Mean age **50 to 60 years with female predominance**
- Solitary, sessile **submucosal** nodule in the **antrum/pylorus**
- **Stellate and spindle cells** mixed with inflammatory cells, predominantly **eosinophils**
- Myxoid or edematous stroma with thin-walled vessels
- Spindle cells are sometimes seen swirling or forming an **onion skin pattern around vessels**
- **CD34+** immunohistochemistry highlights spindle/stellate cells
- Excision required only if symptomatic

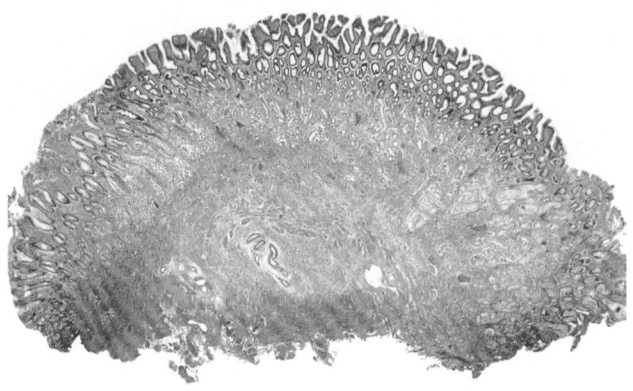

Figure 2-268. Inflammatory fibroid polyp. The most common location for IFP is the gastric antrum, as seen here. The epicenter of these lesions is submucosal, and they appear endoscopically as a nodule.

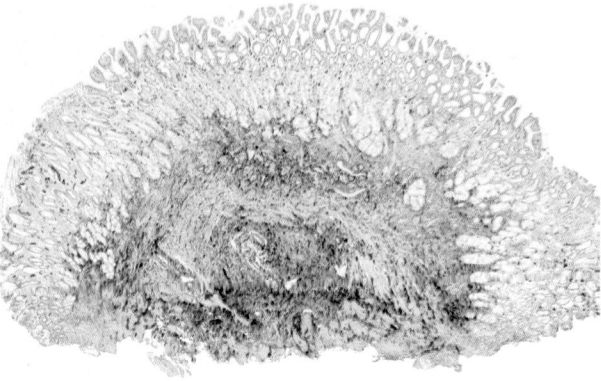

Figure 2-269. Inflammatory fibroid polyp, CD34 immunohistochemistry of the previous figure. A CD34 highlights the scope of this benign lesion, which is surprisingly more extensive than appreciated on H&E.

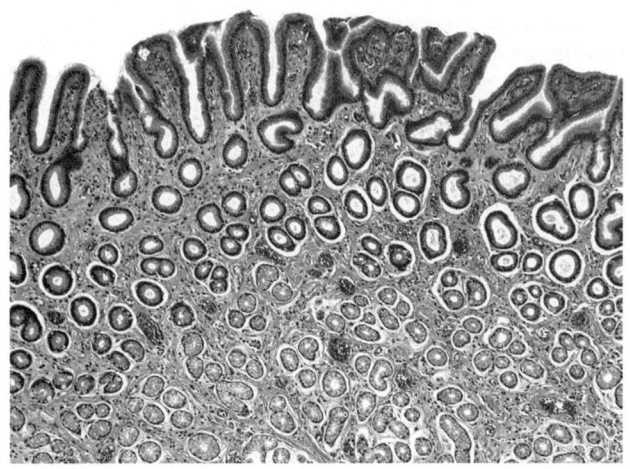

Figure 2-270. Inflammatory fibroid polyp. The spindle cells extend from the submucosa and percolate through the lamina propria toward the surface. However, the findings are subtle and one can appreciate how a superficial biopsy might be challenging to interpret. Diagnostic clues include unexplained bland spindle cells and the presence of eosinophils.

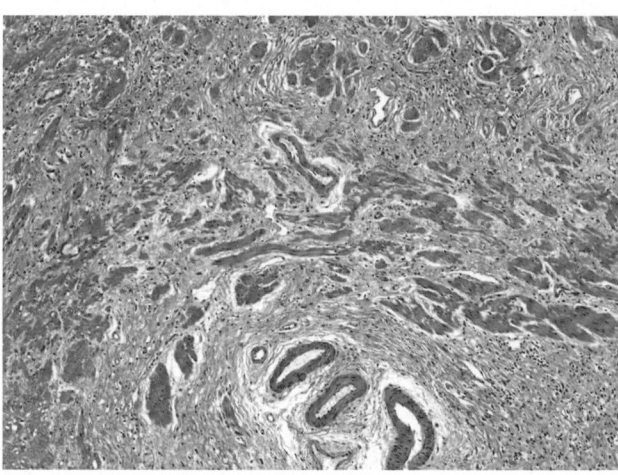

Figure 2-271. Inflammatory fibroid polyp. The spindle cells may swirl concentrically around vessels in an onion skin pattern, as seen here. As the spindle cells extend upward, they traverse the muscularis mucosae and splay the muscle fibers.

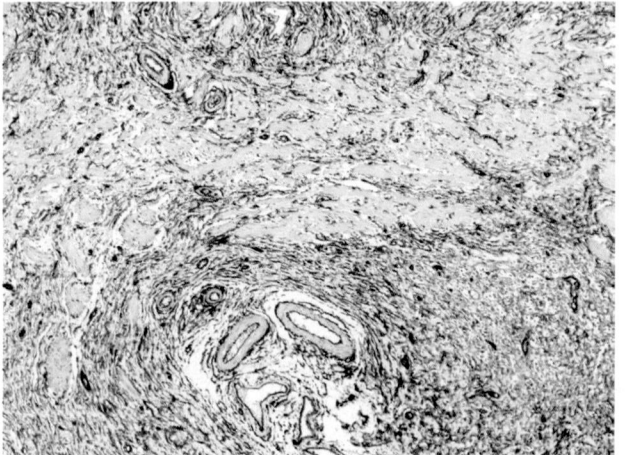

Figure 2-272. Inflammatory fibroid polyp, CD34 immunohistochemistry of the previous figure. CD34 highlights the spindle cells of the IFP, which are more abundant than appreciated by H&E.

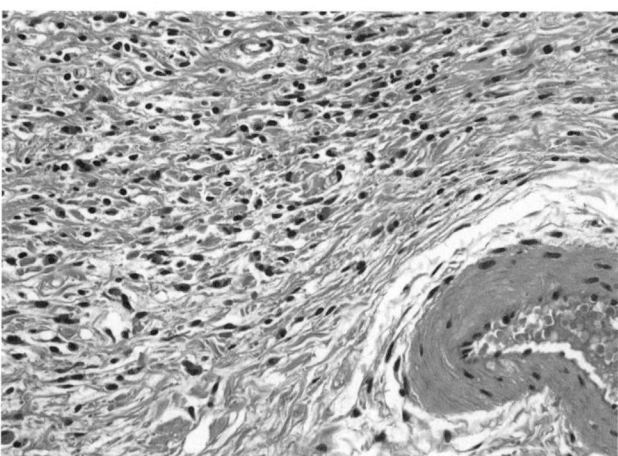

Figure 2-273. Inflammatory fibroid polyp. Higher magnification shows the bland spindle cells forming a concentric pattern around the artery. Intimately admixed are frequent eosinophils, an extremely helpful diagnostic clue to this entity.

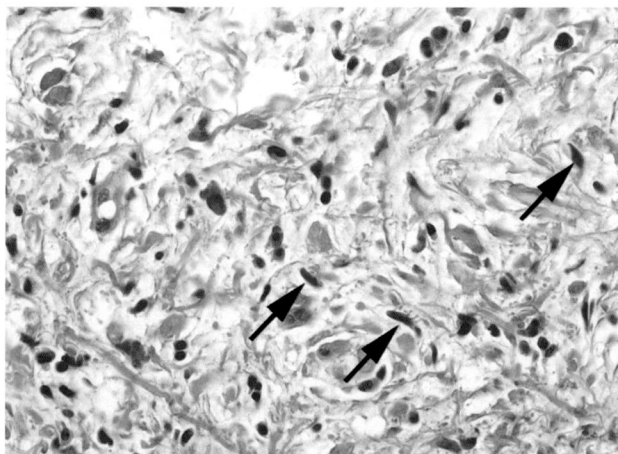

Figure 2-274. Inflammatory fibroid polyp. Some IFPs appear more edematous or myxoid. In these areas, the spindle cells (arrows) may be sparse. Often the first clue to diagnosis is the eye-catching eosinophils.

GASTROINTESTINAL STROMAL TUMOR

GISTs are rare mesenchymal tumors derived from the interstitial cells of Cajal (the pacemaker cells of the GI tract), which reside between the inner circular and outer longitudinal layers of the muscularis propria (Figs. 2.275–2.276). GISTs account for 1% to 3% of all malignant GI tumors,[138] or about 5,000 new cases per year in the United States.[139,140] Although these tumors may arise anywhere along the luminal GI tract, the most common site is the stomach, and they are often found incidentally during upper endoscopy for indications unrelated to the tumor.[141] Most GISTs contain a mutation of the protooncogenes *KIT* (75%) or *PDGFRA* (5%) with known positivity for CD117 (c-KIT) in 95% of the tumors.[142] GISTs lacking cytoplasmic immunoreactivity for CD117 show reactivity for DOG-1 immunohistochemistry (overall 97%), an equally sensitive and specific marker.[140,143,144] The majority of GISTs exhibit stereotypical features of monotonous bland spindled or epithelioid cells with pale eosinophilic cytoplasm and oval nuclei with vesicular chromatin (Figs. 2.277–2.280). The most reliable prognostic factors are site, size of primary tumor, and mitotic index. Endoscopic ultrasound and CT scans are important to determine local and metastatic spread.[145-147] If the tumor is metastatic or unresectable, imatinib (a tyrosine-kinase inhibitor) is the first-line chemotherapeutic agent of choice in tumors expressing c-kit mutation.[148-150] Be attentive to any epithelioid GISTs with multinodular or plexiform growth, or lymphovascular invasion, as these features are red flags for the imatinib-resistant GISTs found in Carney-Stratakis syndrome, an autosomal dominant familial syndrome characterized by paraganglioma and GIST with germline mutations in succinate dehydrogenase genes *SDHB*, *SDHC*, or *SDHD*.[151] These GISTs are found almost exclusively in the stomach, have absent SDHB immunohistochemistry, and have higher risk of metastatic disease irrespective of the usual GIST prognostic predictors.[151-153] Other SDHB-negative GISTs can be found in Carney triad and sporadic pediatric SDHB-deficient tumors.

KEY FEATURES: GIST

- Arise from **interstitial cells of Cajal** found in the **muscularis propria**
- **Stomach is the most common site**, although can arise anywhere along GI tract
- Small fascicles of monotonous pale eosinophilic cells, **spindled (70%)**, **epithelioid (20%)**, or mixed (10%)
- Immunohistochemistry: **CD117+ (95%), DOG-1+ (97%), CD-34+ (60%)**
- Prognosis of most GISTs rely on site, size, and mitotic activity
- Most GISTs have **mutation-specific response to tyrosine kinase** inhibitors, such as imatinib
- **Red flags: Multinodular or plexiform** growth, **lymphovascular invasion** indicate **SDH-deficient** GISTs, a feature of **Carney-Stratakis syndrome**
- **SDH-deficient** GISTs are found almost **exclusively in the stomach**, are more likely to **metastasize**, and are **resistant to imatinib** therapy

LEIOMYOMA

Leiomyomas are benign smooth muscle tumors, typically asymptomatic and found incidentally.[154-156] Endoscopically they appear as rounded submucosal lesions with intact overlying mucosa (Fig. 2.281) and range in size from 0.5 to 20 cm.[157] Both leiomyomas and GISTs can grow inwardly and outwardly to form a dumbbell shape, although leiomyomas are more likely to grow intraluminally (vs. GIST, which expands predominantly in an extramural fashion). Histologically, the tumor is composed of intersecting bundles of smooth muscle without atypia, frequent mitotic activity, or necrosis (Figs. 2.282–2.284). The tumor can be differentiated from GIST, which is CD117 or DOG-1 positive, whereas leiomyoma is smooth muscle actin and desmin positive and negative for CD117/DOG-1.

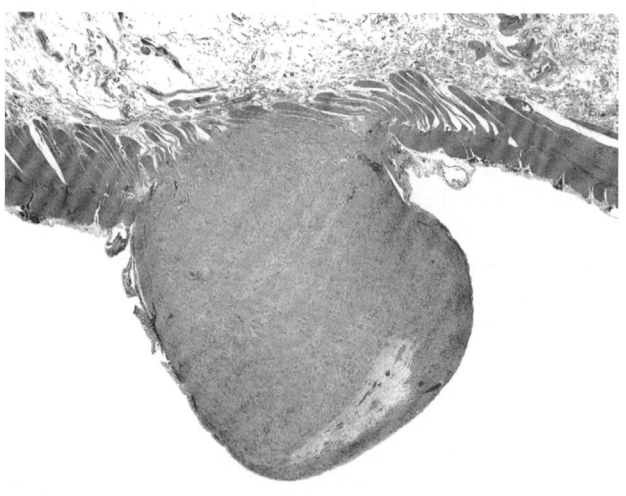

Figure 2-275. Gastrointestinal stromal tumor (GIST). These lesions derive from the interstitial cells of Cajal and arise almost exclusively from the myenteric (Auerbach) plexus, which is located between the inner circular and outer longitudinal layers of the muscularis propria (pictured). For this reason, a spindle cell lesion arising from the muscularis mucosae cannot be a GIST.

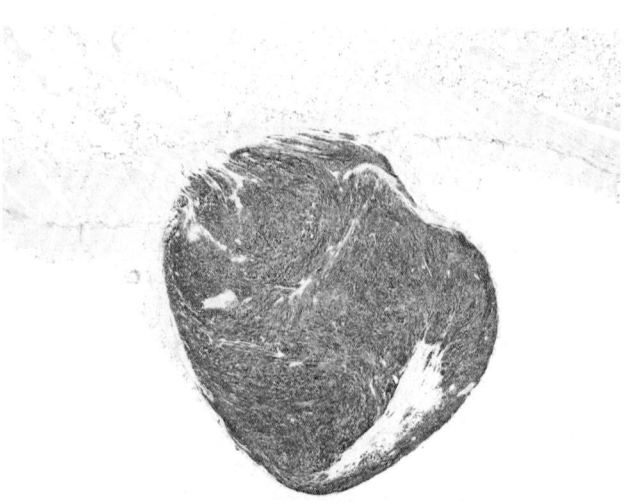

Figure 2-276. Gastrointestinal stromal tumor (GIST), CD117 immunohistochemistry of the previous figure. CD117 immunoreactivity confirms the diagnosis in 95% of cases. CD117-negative GISTs can be stained for DOG1.

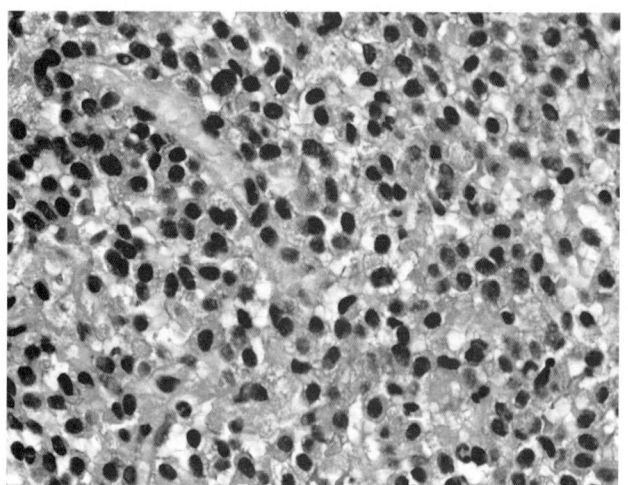

Figure 2-277. GIST, epithelioid type. The cells are round and fairly uniform. There is no prognostic significance to the morphologic variant.

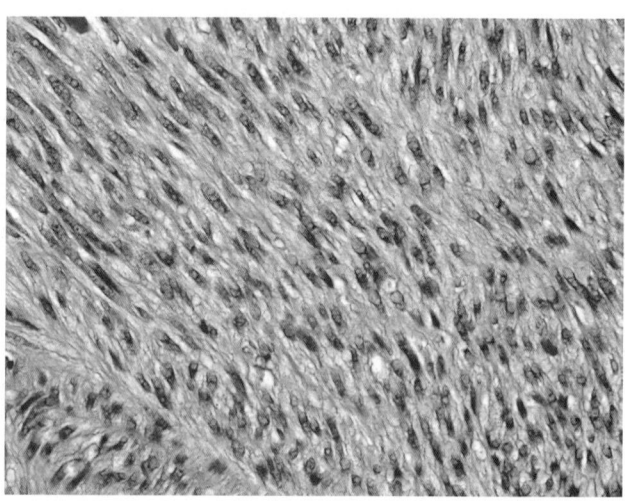

Figure 2-278. GIST, spindled type. These cells are elongated with cigar-shaped nuclei.

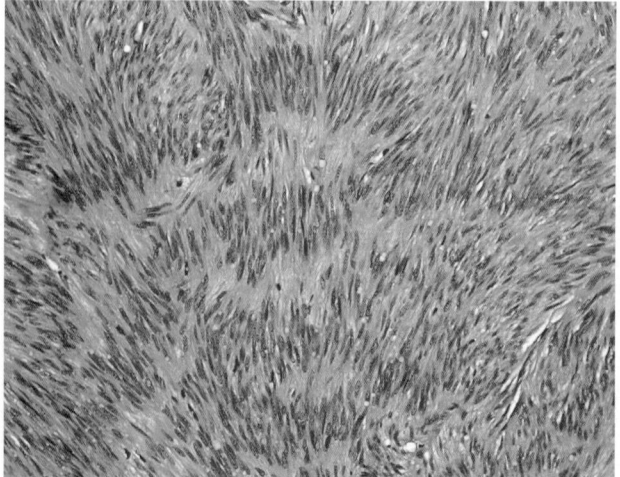

Figure 2-279. GIST. These tumors can take on many morphologic variations and are wonderful mimickers of other tumors. This region shows features similar to Verocay bodies found in schwannomas.

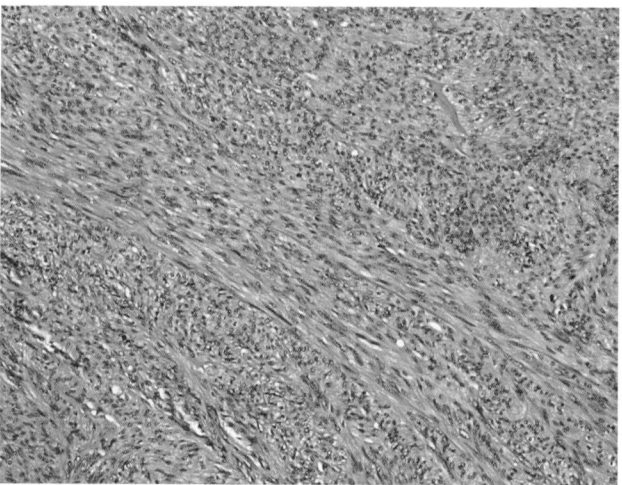

Figure 2-280. GIST. Perpendicular fascicles of spindle cells raise the differential for leiomyoma. GISTs are excellent mimickers of other tumors.

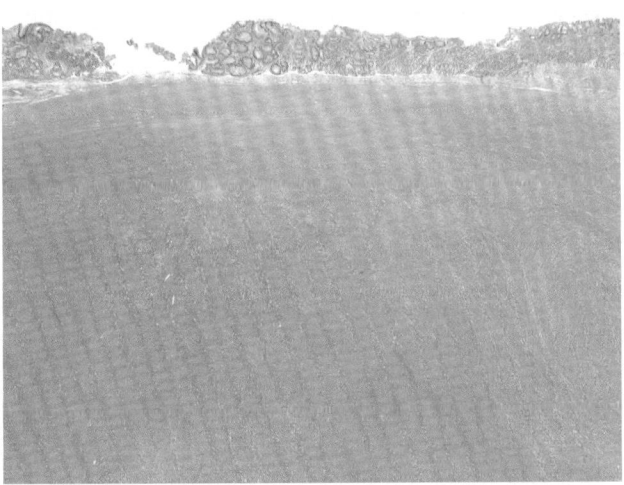

Figure 2-281. Leiomyoma. This spindle cell neoplasm arises from the muscularis mucosae. Because of this location, the diagnosis cannot be GIST.

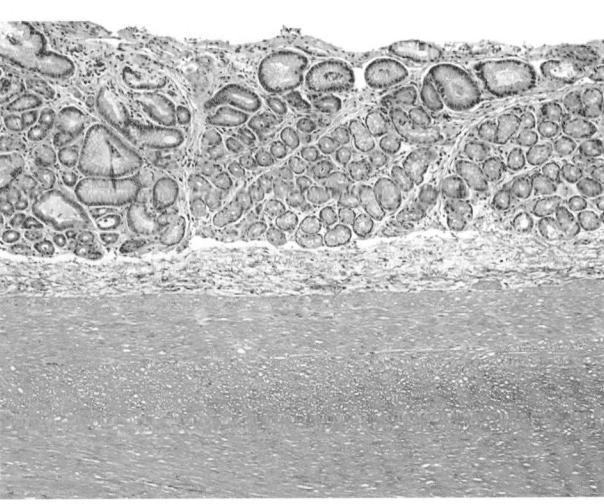

Figure 2-282. Leiomyoma, higher magnification of the previous figure. The tumor arises from the muscularis mucosae, and the cells are bland and spindled.

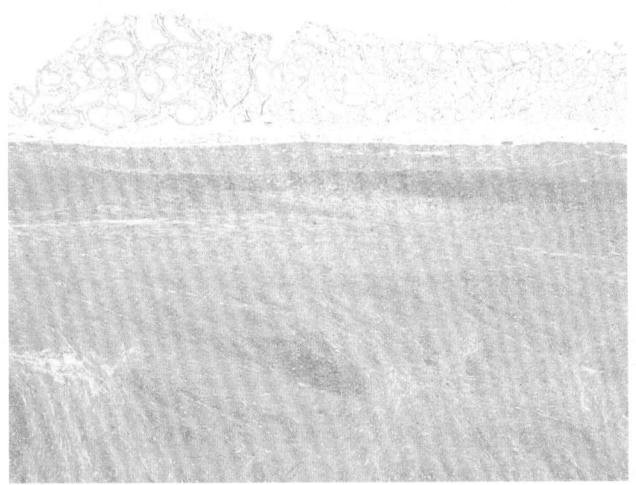

Figure 2-283. Leiomyoma, smooth muscle actin (SMA) immunohistochemistry. SMA confirms the smooth muscle differentiation of this tumor.

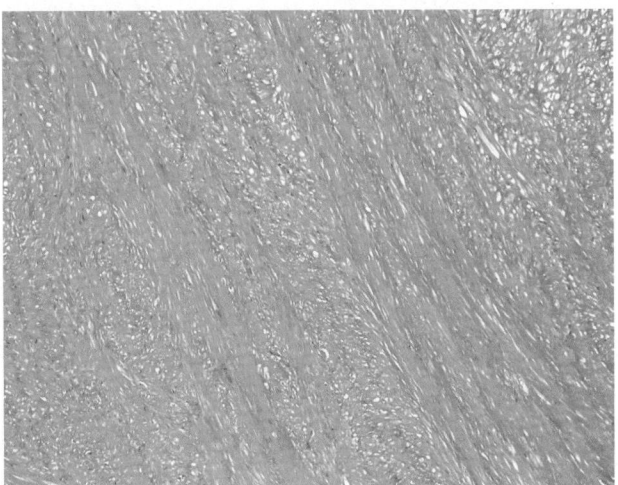

Figure 2-284. Leiomyoma. The smooth muscle bundles characteristically intersect at perpendicular angles.

GRANULAR CELL TUMOR

For unknown reasons, about half of gastric GCTs occur synchronously with esophageal GCTs.[158] These lesions tend to occur equally in both sexes, most frequently in the fourth to sixth decade of life.[158] Endoscopically, they are found incidentally in the proximal stomach, range from a few millimeters in size up to 7 cm, and appear as a yellow subepithelial mass or nodule that resembles a lipoma.[158] Histologically, the submucosal tumor is composed of sheets of uniform polygonal tumor cells with abundant eosinophilic granular cytoplasm and small hyperchromatic nuclei (Figs. 2.285 and 2.286). The cytoplasmic accumulation of secondary lysosomes is PAS positive and diastase resistant, whereas immunohistochemistry shows the tumors are positive for S100 and NSE and negative for HMB45, keratins, and desmin. The vast majority of GCTs are benign, but malignant and metastatic cases have been reported.[159]

KEY FEATURES: GCT

- About 50% of gastric GCTs will have accompanying esophageal GCT
- Mean age 50 years, M = F

- **Submucosal** epicenter, with **sheets of polygonal cells** containing **abundant granular eosinophilic cytoplasm**
- Cytoplasmic accumulation of **PAS-D+ secondary lysosomes**
- Immunohistochemistry positive: **S100+**, NSE+
- Immunohistochemistry negative: HMB45–, cytokeratin–, desmin–

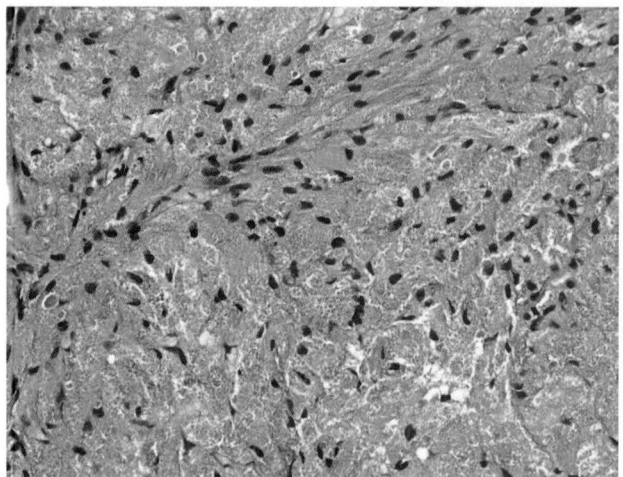

Figure 2-285. Granular cell tumor. The tumor cells have indistinct cell borders and slightly atypical angulated nuclei. There is abundant eosinophilic and granular cytoplasm.

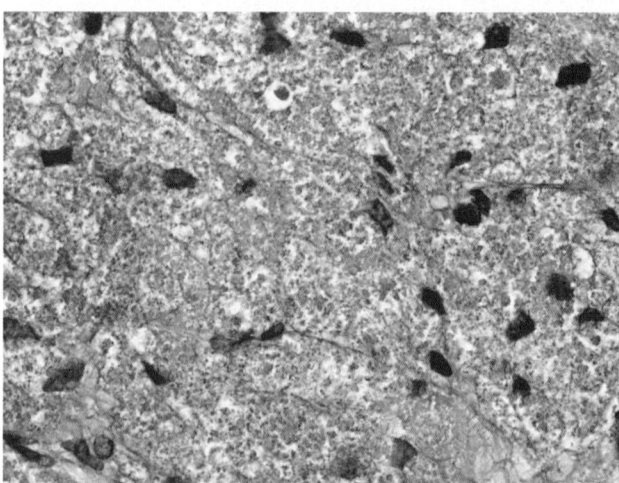

Figure 2-286. Granular cell tumor. Oil immersion shows the granular quality of the cytoplasm, which by electron microscopy is filled with lysosomes (not pictured).

NEAR MISS

METASTATIC LOBULAR BREAST CARCINOMA

New diagnoses of diffuse-type gastric cancer in women should include at least one immunohistochemical marker to exclude metastatic lobular breast carcinoma, such as GATA3. Although breast cancer metastasis to the GI tract is a rare occurrence, the stomach is the most common location aside from the liver, and the discohesive infiltrating cells of lobular breast carcinoma can be easily mistaken for a primary diffuse-type gastric cancer (Figs. 2.287–2.294). Differentiation of these tumors relies almost entirely upon immunohistochemical confirmation, an important step because the treatment of these tumors diverge. A diagnosis of primary gastric cancer leads to surgical management, whereas metastatic breast cancer may benefit from chemotherapeutic options depending on the hormone receptor status. Histologically, metastatic lobular breast cancer cells infiltrate the lamina propria individually or in single-file cords (Fig. 2.288). These uniform small discohesive cells characteristically lack E-cadherin (Fig. 2.289), a surface cohesion molecule. Because diffuse-type gastric cancer lacks a precursor lesion, this metastatic pattern is nearly indistinguishable from a primary gastric tumor. A PAS stain is negative for cytoplasmic PAS staining or intracytoplasmic mucin (Fig. 2.290), whereas most gastric signet ring cell carcinomas will show PAS staining. One helpful clue to metastatic lobular breast carcinoma is the presence of intracytoplasmic lumina, which have a sharply demarcated edge and may contain a hyaline globule imparting a targetoid appearance (Fig. 2.294).

PEARLS & PITFALLS: Metastatic Lobular Breast Carcinoma

- **Metastatic lobular breast carcinoma and primary diffuse-type gastric cancer can be indistinguishable by H&E**
- Both lesions are unassociated with background gastritis or precursor lesion
- Make it a habit to perform a GATA3 on all new diagnoses of diffuse-type gastric adenocarcinoma; GATA3 should be negative in primary gastric cancer
- Clear intracytoplasmic lumina with hyaline globules imparting a targetoid appearance is a clue to lobular breast cancer

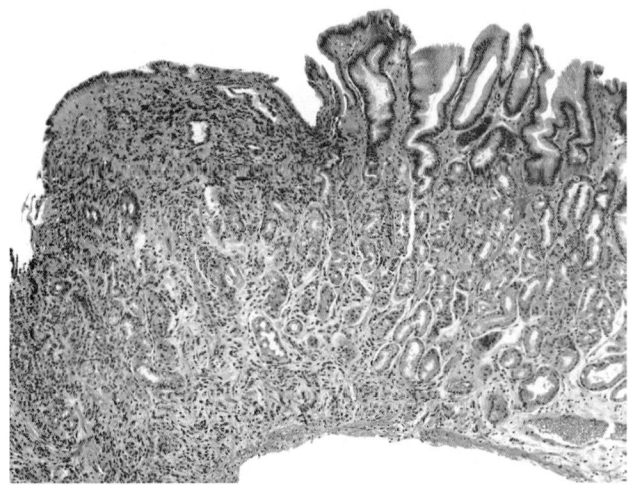

Figure 2-287. Metastatic lobular breast carcinoma. Single infiltrating hyperchromatic cells invade through the lamina propria. At low magnification, one might consider inactive chronic gastritis or diffuse-type gastric adenocarcinoma.

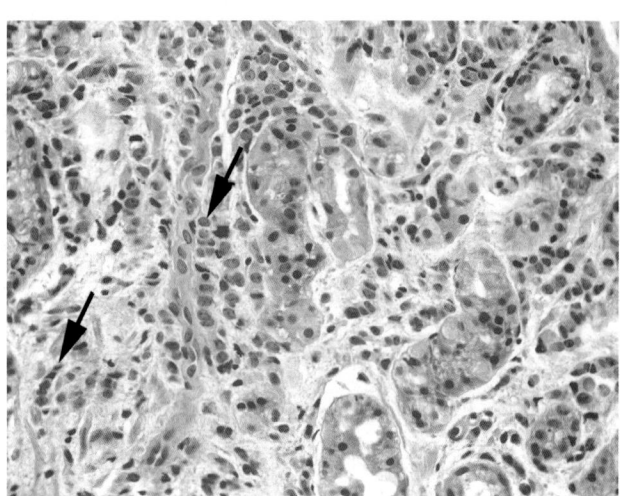

Figure 2-288. Metastatic lobular breast carcinoma, higher magnification of the previous figure. Single-file cords (arrows) are highly characteristic of invasive lobular carcinoma of the breast.

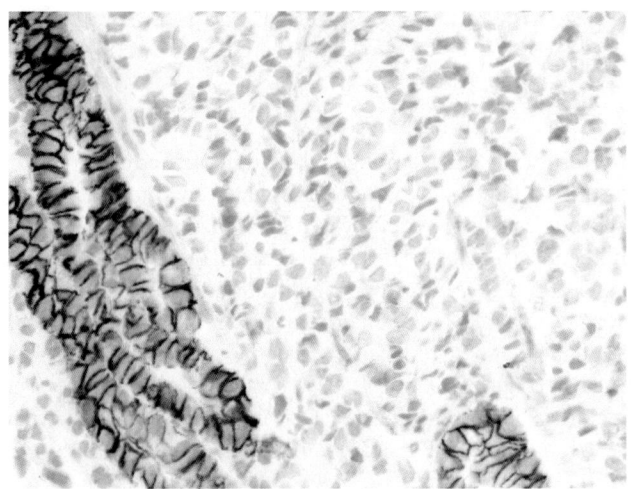

Figure 2-289. Metastatic lobular breast carcinoma, E-cadherin immunostain. Lobular carcinoma of the breast has a characteristic loss of cell adhesion molecule E-cadherin. This feature can also be seen in primary gastric carcinomas of diffuse type and therefore should not be considered a reliable marker for breast origin.

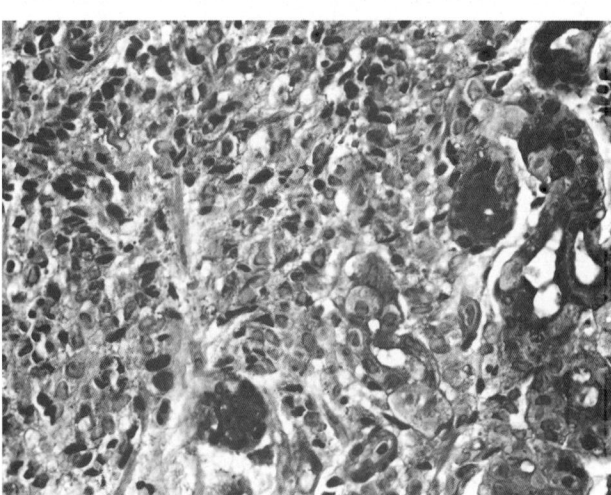

Figure 2-290. Metastatic lobular breast carcinoma, PAS stain. The tumor cells of lobular breast carcinoma do not show cytoplasmic reactivity for PAS or contain mucin.

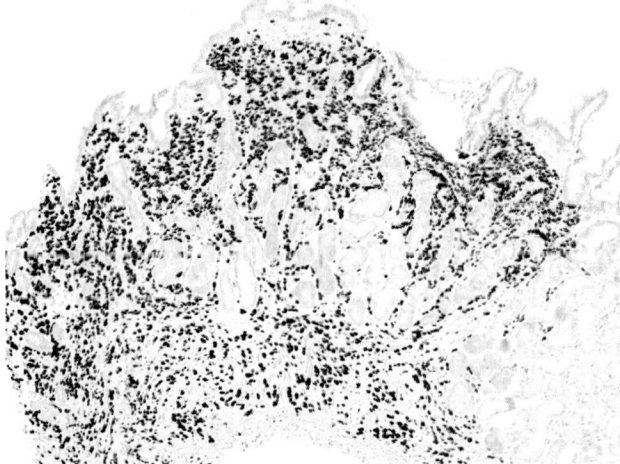

Figure 2-291. Metastatic lobular breast carcinoma, GATA3 immunostain. GATA3 is a reliable marker that highlights tumors of breast origin and is negative in gastric cancer.

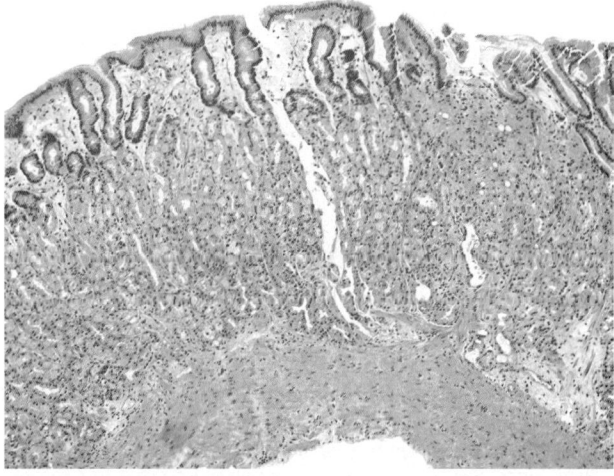

Figure 2-292. Metastatic lobular breast carcinoma. This example is extremely subtle, underscoring the importance of always reviewing gastric biopsies at high magnification and accounting for each cell.

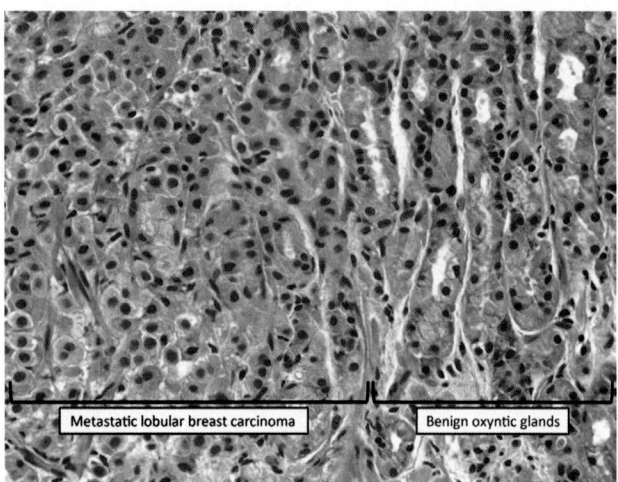

Figure 2-293. Metastatic lobular breast carcinoma, higher magnification of the previous figure. The metastatic cells are uniform and bland with slightly eosinophilic cytoplasm that blends in with the benign oxyntic glands. In all gastric biopsies, take a moment to point out individual cells and try to place a name to them, rather than grouping them together in one's mind.

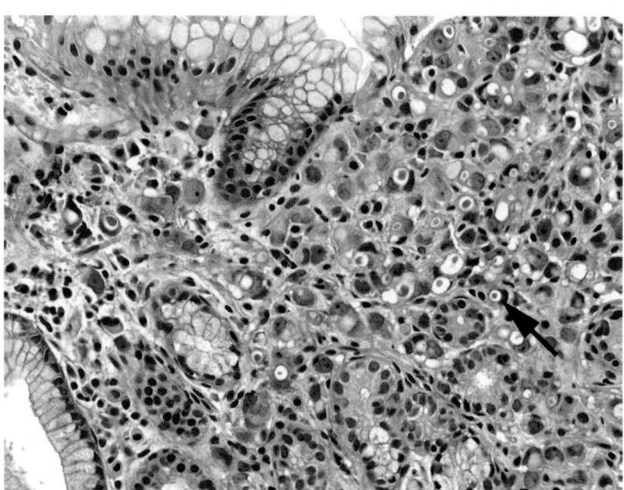

Figure 2-294. Metastatic lobular breast carcinoma. Although at first glance the tumor cells resemble signet ring cells, note the intracytoplasmic lumina with distinct borders and the single hyaline inclusion. These targetoid cells (*arrow*) are characteristic of lobular breast carcinoma.

GASTRIC XANTHOMA

These subepithelial aggregates of histiocytes are submitted as endoscopic nodules, polyps, or plaques and cause no diagnostic difficulty for pathologists when encountered in the gallbladder (i.e., cholesterolosis) but can prove tricky when seen in the stomach (Figs. 2.295–2.302). The most common concern among extramural consultations is exclusion of diffuse-type gastric cancer (Figs. 2.295–2.297). At low magnification, an area of pallor is eye-catching as the foamy histiocytes expand the lamina propria (Fig. 2.298). Collections of bland macrophages with abundant foamy cytoplasm are usually subepithelial but can be found anywhere within the tissue (Fig. 2.299 and 2.301). Small and crushed biopsies provide the most challenging material, but application of CD68 immunohistochemistry is almost always helpful (Figs. 2.297 and 2.302). PAS stain is negative for intracytoplasmic mucin (Fig. 2.300).

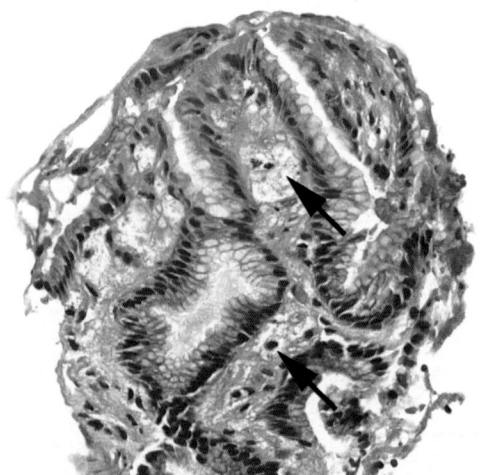

Figure 2-295. Gastric xanthoma in a crushed and suboptimal biopsy. By H&E, several cells in this biopsy are hard to name (*arrows*). They are subepithelial in the lamina propria and contain clear cytoplasm. Small and crushed biopsies are always difficult to interpret, and diffuse-type gastric cancer raises the stakes even further. Do not hesitate to request repeat biopsy if the diagnosis is unclear.

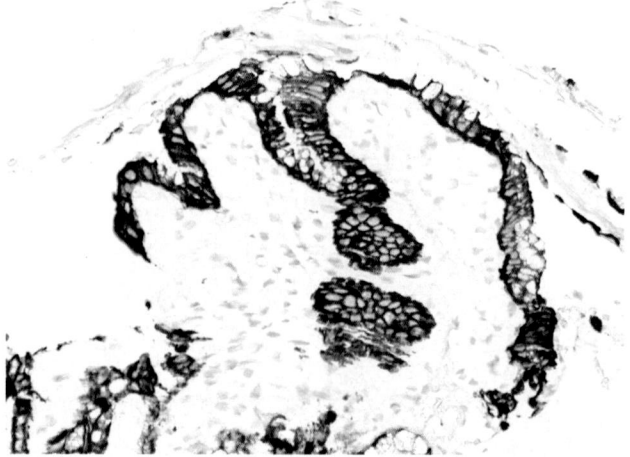

Figure 2-296. Gastric xanthoma, pancytokeratin immunostain of the previous figure. A pancytokeratin stain can highlight the gastric foveolar and glandular architecture and provide reassurance that the cells are not invasive carcinoma cells.

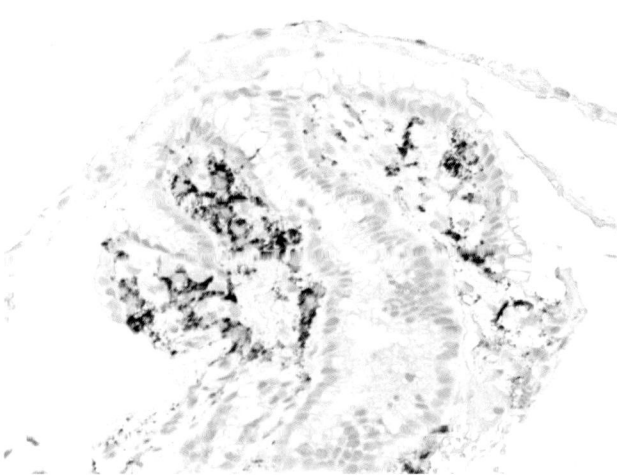

Figure 2-297. Gastric xanthoma, CD68 immunostain. A CD68 immunostain in this example highlights the scant crushed cells, confirming they are foamy macrophages and not signet ring cells.

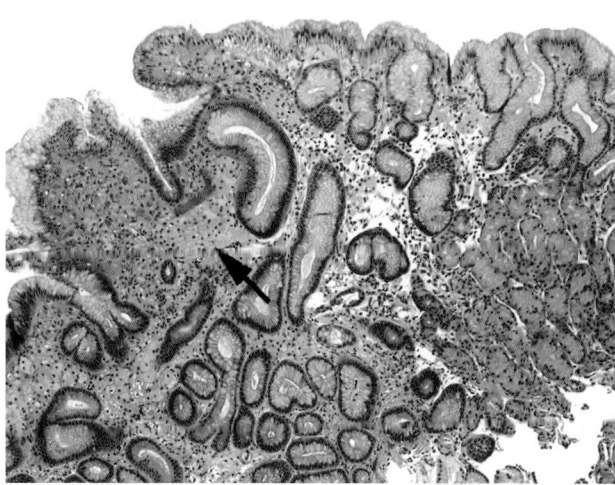

Figure 2-298. Gastric xanthoma. Gastric xanthoma cells can mimic a diffuse-type gastric cancer at low magnification. All areas of increased cellularity or pallor (*arrow*) should be reviewed more closely to exclude a sneaky diffuse-type gastric cancer.

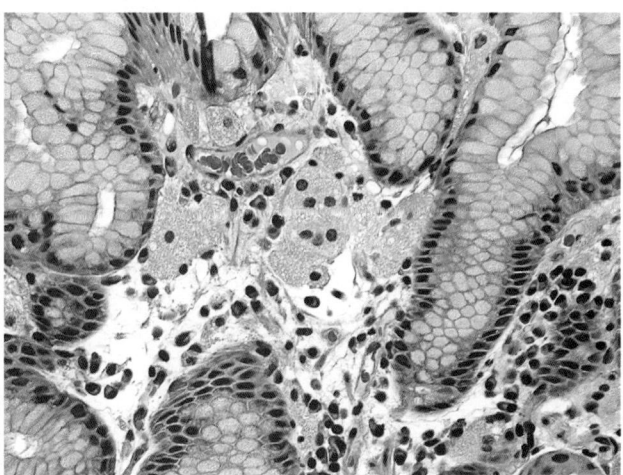

Figure 2-299. Gastric xanthoma, higher magnification of the previous figure. Gastric xanthomas are composed of collections of foamy macrophages. At high magnification, they have bland uniform nuclei and abundant foamy cytoplasm that makes them, in most cases, easy to distinguish from diffuse gastric cancer by H&E alone.

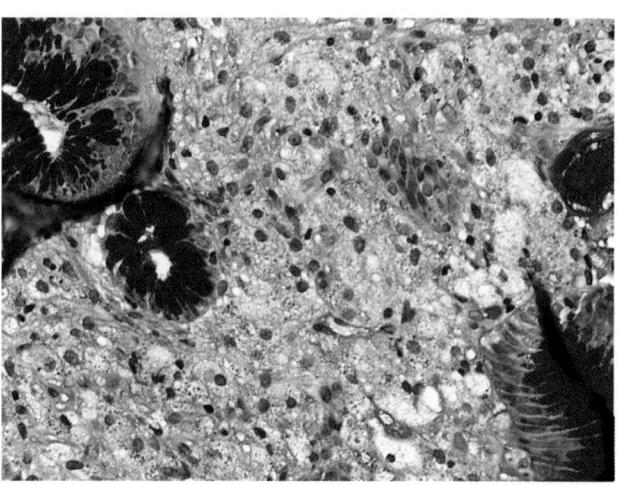

Figure 2-300. Gastric xanthoma, PAS stain. The cytoplasm of foamy macrophages is not PAS positive and does not contain mucin.

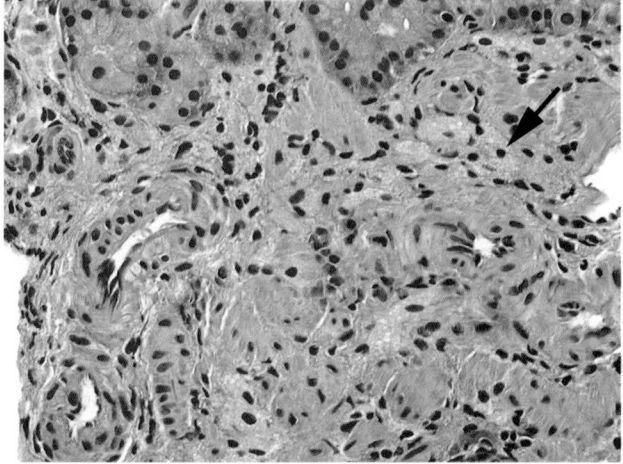

Figure 2-301. Gastric xanthoma. This example is more challenging, as the foamy macrophages (*arrow*) are embedded within the muscularis mucosa and raise concern for a sneaky invasive diffuse-type gastric cancer.

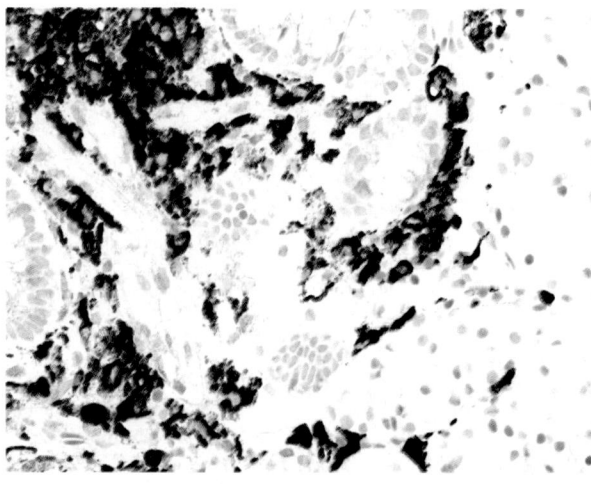

Figure 2-302. Gastric xanthoma, CD68 immunostain of the previous figure. Immunohistochemistry confirms histiocytic differentiation and reassures that these are benign cells.

GASTRITIS CYSTICA PROFUNDA

Do not mistake this rare benign lesion for adenocarcinoma. Gastritis cystica profunda (GCP) is characterized by downgrowth of cystically dilated gastric glands through the muscularis mucosae into the submucosa (Figs. 2.303–2.308), with or without polypoid hyperplasia (gastritis cystica polyposa), and typically has a backdrop of chronic inflammation.[160] The proliferation of these benign displaced glands should not be interpreted as malignant. Some have postulated that inflammation causes mucosal erosion and migration of epithelial cells into the submucosa, followed by cystic dilation. Mucosal prolapse and herniation of glands into the submucosa is thought to be the pathogenesis in cases of prior instrumentation (65%), but this lesion can also be found in unoperated stomachs.[161-163] These lesions are associated with older age, male gender, and proximal location, and rare examples are found in combination with true gastric cancer (0.7% of gastric cancers).[164] A helpful history of prior surgery and prior biopsy can be key to avoiding overdiagnosis, and histologically these submucosal glands are lined by bland nonneoplastic epithelial cells (Figs. 2.304, 2.306, and 2.308).

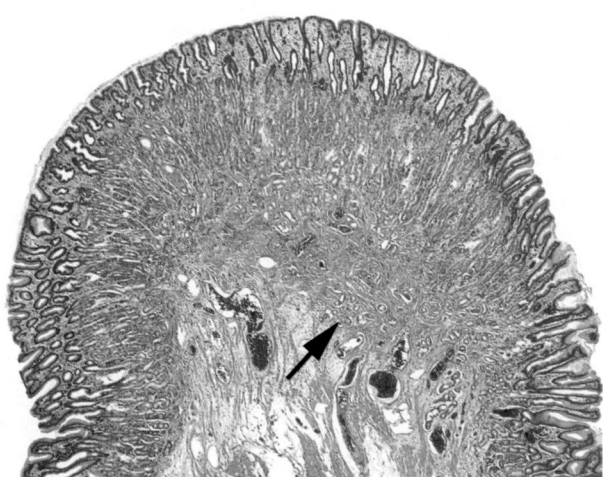

Figure 2-303. Gastritis cystica profunda. Herniating into the submucosa are collections of gastric glands (*arrow*). At scanning magnification, these submucosal glands appear disorganized and raise concern for an invasive adenocarcinoma.

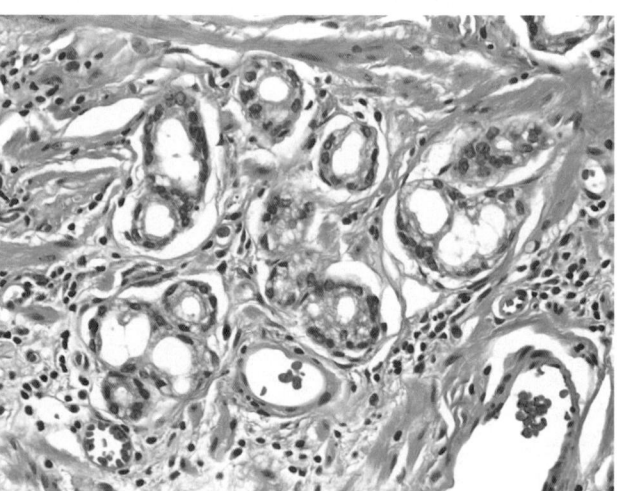

Figure 2-304. Gastritis cystica profunda, higher magnification of the previous figure. Upon closer review, these submucosal glands are bland and lined by benign epithelial cells.

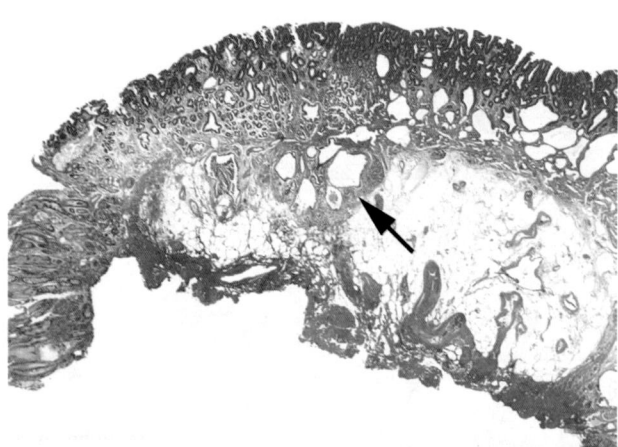

Figure 2-305. Gastritis cystica profunda. An endoscopic mucosal resection shows a gastric adenoma with surface epithelial hyperchromasia. Deep to this are glands that extend into the submucosa (*arrow*). The association with overlying dysplasia certainly raises concern for an invasive adenocarcinoma.

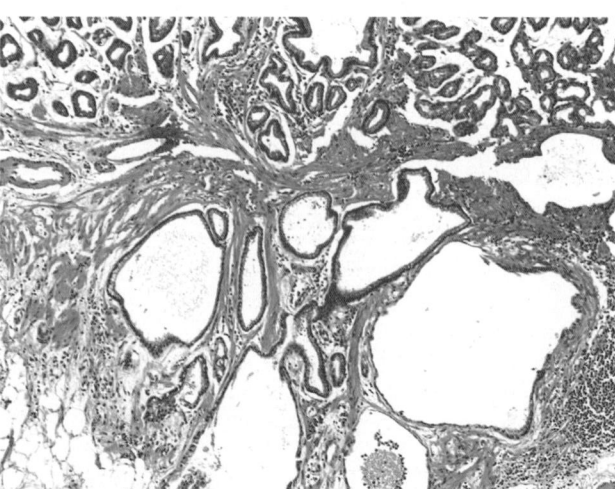

Figure 2-306. Gastritis cystica profunda, higher magnification of the previous figure. A closer examination of the submucosal glands shows they are lined by bland, benign epithelial cells and are cystically dilated. A dive into the electronic medical record reveals that this lesion was previously biopsied. The submucosal glands are likely herniated owing to prior instrumentation, a characteristic history for GCP.

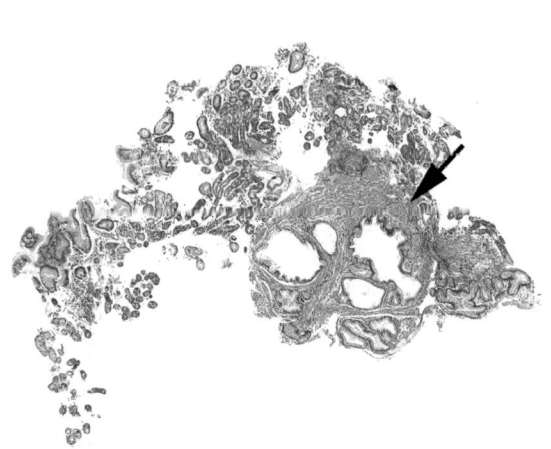

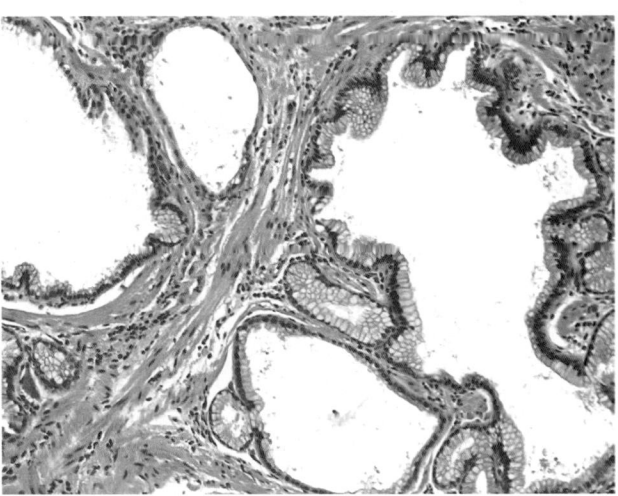

Figure 2-307. Gastritis cystica profunda. Cystically dilated glands are present in the submucosa of this gastric biopsy (*arrow*). A background of inactive chronic gastritis is present, which is characteristic for GCP. Even at this magnification, the glands appear benign and misplaced.

Figure 2-308. Gastritis cystica profunda, higher magnification of the previous figure. The epithelial cells lining the herniated glands are uniform and show no pleomorphism, stratification, or atypia.

INACTIVE CHRONIC GASTRITIS HIDES TUMORS

A theme throughout this chapter has been the emphasis on not diagnosing a chronic gastritis and moving on too quickly. Lymphoid aggregates and dense collections of chronic inflammatory cells can appear hyperchromatic and busy, masking other important findings. To avoid overlooking sneaky tumor cells, always take a moment to review gastric biopsies at higher magnification and make sure each cell in the biopsy is acknowledged. Avoid mentally grouping cells together as inactive chronic gastritis or lymphoid aggregates; instead, pause and put a name to each cell. Once this becomes a habit, it happens automatically and swiftly. This attention to each cell prevents overlooking sneaky signet ring cells, gastric MALT lymphomas, metastatic lobular breast carcinomas, and other subtle tumors, as well as nonneoplastic findings, such as viral cytopathic effect (Figs. 2.309 and 2.310).

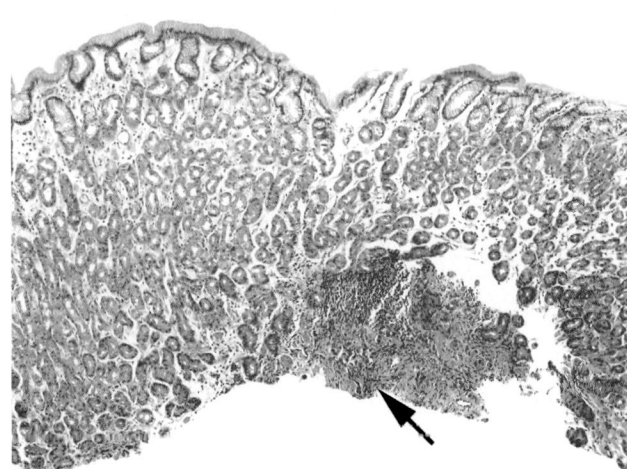

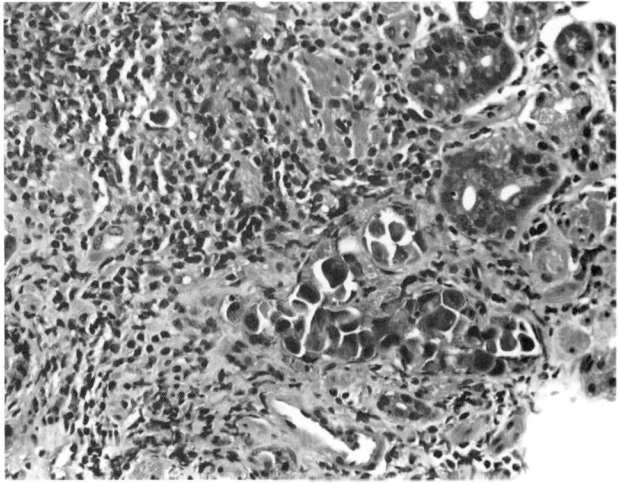

Figure 2-309. Tumor hiding in a lymphoid aggregate. Pattern recognition is key in pathology, and pathologists quickly group together like findings, such as clusters of lymphocytes in inactive chronic gastritis. However, always take a moment to look at higher magnification and acknowledge each cell in case there is tumor hiding there (*arrow*).

Figure 2-310. Tumor hiding in a lymphoid aggregate, higher magnification of the previous figure. These intralymphatic tumor cells were nearly obscured by the surrounding lymphoid infiltrate but are clearly visible at high magnification.

References

1. Carmack SW, Genta RM, Schuler CM, Saboorian MH. The current spectrum of gastric polyps: a 1-year national study of over 120,000 patients. *Am J Gastroenterol.* 2009;104(6):1524-1532.

2. Jhala NC, Montemor M, Jhala D, et al. Pancreatic acinar cell metaplasia in autoimmune gastritis. *Arch Pathol Lab Med.* 2003;127(7):854-857.

3. Lam-Himlin D, Park JY, Cornish TC, Shi C, Montgomery E. Morphologic characterization of syndromic gastric polyps. *Am J Surg Pathol.* 2010;34(11):1656-1662.

4. Beggs AD, Latchford AR, Vasen HF, et al. Peutz-Jeghers syndrome: a systematic review and recommendations for management. *Gut.* 2010;59(7):975-986.

5. Hemminki A, Markie D, Tomlinson I, et al. A serine/threonine kinase gene defective in Peutz-Jeghers syndrome. *Nature.* 1998;391(6663):184-187.

6. Volikos E, Robinson J, Aittomaki K, et al. LKB1 exonic and whole gene deletions are a common cause of Peutz-Jeghers syndrome. *J Med Genet.* 2006;43(5):e18.

7. Giardiello FM, Welsh SB, Hamilton SR, et al. Increased risk of cancer in the Peutz-Jeghers syndrome. *N Engl J Med.* 1987;316(24):1511-1514.

8. Hearle N, Schumacher V, Menko FH, et al. Frequency and spectrum of cancers in the Peutz-Jeghers syndrome. *Clin Cancer Res.* 2006;12(10):3209-3215.

9. Jeghers H, Mc KV, Katz KH. Generalized intestinal polyposis and melanin spots of the oral mucosa, lips and digits; a syndrome of diagnostic significance. *N Engl J Med.* 1949;241(26):1031-1036.

10. Offerhaus GJA BM, Gruber SB. Peutz-Jeghers syndrome. In: Bosman FT, Carneiro F, Hruban RH, et al, eds. *Tumors of the Digestive System.* Lyon, France: IACR; 2010:160-170.

11. Latchford AR, Phillips RK. Gastrointestinal polyps and cancer in Peutz-Jeghers syndrome: clinical aspects. *Fam Cancer.* 2011;10(3):455-461.

12. Tse JY, Wu S, Shinagare SA, et al. Peutz-Jeghers syndrome: a critical look at colonic Peutz-Jeghers polyps. *Mod Pathol.* 2013;26(9):1235-1240.

13. Giardiello FM, Brensinger JD, Tersmette AC, et al. Very high risk of cancer in familial Peutz-Jeghers syndrome. *Gastroenterology.* 2000;119(6):1447-1453.

14. Burkart AL, Sheridan T, Lewin M, Fenton H, Ali NJ, Montgomery E. Do sporadic Peutz-Jeghers polyps exist? Experience of a large teaching hospital. *Am J Surg Pathol.* 2007;31(8):1209-1214.

15. Burt RW, Bishop DT, Lynch HT, Rozen P, Winawer SJ. Risk and surveillance of individuals with heritable factors for colorectal cancer. WHO Collaborating Centre for the Prevention of Colorectal Cancer. *Bull World Health Organ.* 1990;68(5):655-665.

16. Howe JR, Roth S, Ringold JC, et al. Mutations in the SMAD4/DPC4 gene in juvenile polyposis. *Science.* 1998;280(5366):1086-1088.

17. Sweet K, Willis J, Zhou XP, et al. Molecular classification of patients with unexplained hamartomatous and hyperplastic polyposis. *JAMA.* 2005;294(19):2465-2473.

18. Howe JR, Mitros FA, Summers RW. The risk of gastrointestinal carcinoma in familial juvenile polyposis. *Ann Surg Oncol.* 1998;5(8):751-756.

19. Giardiello FM, Hamilton SR, Kern SE, et al. Colorectal neoplasia in juvenile polyposis or juvenile polyps. *Arch Dis Child.* 1991;66(8):971-975.

20. Offerhaus GJA HJ. Juvenile polyposis. In: Bosman FT, Carneiro F, Hruban RH, et al, eds. *WHO Classification of Tumors of the Digestive System.* Lyon, France: IARC; 2010:166-167.

21. Cronkhite LW Jr, Canada WJ. Generalized gastrointestinal polyposis; an unusual syndrome of polyposis, pigmentation, alopecia and onychotrophia. *N Engl J Med.* 1955;252(24):1011-1015.

22. Nakamura M, Kobashikawa K, Tamura J, et al. Cronkhite-Canada syndrome. *Intern Med.* 2009;48(17):1561-1562.

23. Daniel ES, Ludwig SL, Lewin KJ, Ruprecht RM, Rajacich GM, Schwabe AD. The Cronkhite-Canada syndrome. An analysis of clinical and pathologic features and therapy in 55 patients. *Medicine (Baltim).* 1982;61(5):293-309.

24. Heald B, Mester J, Rybicki L, Orloff MS, Burke CA, Eng C. Frequent gastrointestinal polyps and colorectal adenocarcinomas in a prospective series of PTEN mutation carriers. *Gastroenterology.* 2010;139(6):1927-1933.

25. Kato M, Mizuki A, Hayashi T, et al. Cowden's disease diagnosed through mucocutaneous lesions and gastrointestinal polyposis with recurrent hematochezia, unrevealed by initial diagnosis. *Intern Med.* 2000;39(7):559-563.

26. Levi Z, Baris HN, Kedar I, et al. Upper and lower gastrointestinal findings in PTEN mutation-positive Cowden syndrome patients participating in an active surveillance program. *Clin Transl Gastroenterol.* 2011;2:e5.

27. Tan MH, Mester JL, Ngeow J, Rybicki LA, Orloff MS, Eng C. Lifetime cancer risks in individuals with germline PTEN mutations. *Clin Canc Res.* 2012,18(2):400-407.

28. Abraham SC, Singh VK, Yardley JH, Wu TT. Hyperplastic polyps of the stomach: associations with histologic patterns of gastritis and gastric atrophy. *Am J Surg Pathol.* 2001;25(4):500-507.

29. Koch HK, Lesch R, Cremer M, Oehlert W. Polyps and polypoid foveolar hyperplasia in gastric biopsy specimens and their precancerous prevalence. *Front Gastrointest Res.* 1979;4:183-191.

30. Koga S, Watanabe H, Enjoji M. Stomal polypoid hypertrophic gastritis: a polypoid gastric lesion at gastroenterostomy site. *Cancer.* 1979;43(2):647-657.

31. Zea-Iriarte WL, Sekine I, Itsuno M, et al. Carcinoma in gastric hyperplastic polyps. A phenotypic study. *Dig Dis Sci.* 1996;41(2):377-386.

32. Ginsberg GG, Al-Kawas FH, Fleischer DE, Reilly HF, Benjamin SB. Gastric polyps: relationship of size and histology to cancer risk. *Am J Gastroenterol.* 1996;91(4):714-717.

33. Orlowska J, Jarosz D, Pachlewski J, Butruk E. Malignant transformation of benign epithelial gastric polyps. *Am J Gastroenterol.* 1995;90(12):2152-2159.

34. Genta RM, Schuler CM, Robiou CI, Lash RH. No association between gastric fundic gland polyps and gastrointestinal neoplasia in a study of over 100,000 patients. *Clin Gastroenterol Hepatol.* 2009;7(8):849-854.

35. Zelter A, Fernandez JL, Bilder C, et al. Fundic gland polyps and association with proton pump inhibitor intake: a prospective study in 1,780 endoscopies. *Dig Dis Sci.* 2011;56(6):1743-1748.

36. Vieth M, Stolte M. Fundic gland polyps are not induced by proton pump inhibitor therapy. *Am J Clin Pathol.* 2001;116(5):716-720.

37. Bianchi LK, Burke CA, Bennett AE, Lopez R, Hasson H, Church JM. Fundic gland polyp dysplasia is common in familial adenomatous polyposis. *Clin Gastroenterol Hepatol.* 2008;6(2):180-185.

38. Garrean S, Hering J, Saied A, Jani J, Espat NJ. Gastric adenocarcinoma arising from fundic gland polyps in a patient with familial adenomatous polyposis syndrome. *Am Surg.* 2008;74(1):79-83.

39. Zwick A, Munir M, Ryan CK, et al. Gastric adenocarcinoma and dysplasia in fundic gland polyps of a patient with attenuated adenomatous polyposis coli. *Gastroenterology.* 1997;113(2):659-663.

40. Wu TT, Kornacki S, Rashid A, Yardley JH, Hamilton SR. Dysplasia and dysregulation of proliferation in foveolar and surface epithelia of fundic gland polyps from patients with familial adenomatous polyposis. *Am J Surg Pathol.* 1998;22(3):293-298.

41. Offerhaus GJ, Giardiello FM, Krush AJ, et al. The risk of upper gastrointestinal cancer in familial adenomatous polyposis. *Gastroenterology.* 1992;102(6):1980-1982.

42. Torbenson M, Lee JH, Cruz-Correa M, et al. Sporadic fundic gland polyposis: a clinical, histological, and molecular analysis. *Mod Pathol.* 2002;15(7):718-723.

43. Li J, Woods SL, Healey S, et al. Point mutations in exon 1B of APC reveal gastric adenocarcinoma and proximal polyposis of the stomach as a familial adenomatous polyposis variant. *Am J Hum Genet.* 2016;98(5):830-842.

44. Abraham SC, Nobukawa B, Giardiello FM, Hamilton SR, Wu TT. Sporadic fundic gland polyps: common gastric polyps arising through activating mutations in the beta-catenin gene. *Am J Pathol.* 2001;158(3):1005-1010.

45. Lauwers GY, Shimizu M, Correa P, et al. Evaluation of gastric biopsies for neoplasia: differences between Japanese and Western pathologists. *Am J Surg Pathol.* 1999;23(5):511-518.

46. Schlemper RJ, Riddell RH, Kato Y, et al. The Vienna classification of gastrointestinal epithelial neoplasia. *Gut.* 2000;47(2):251-255.

47. Singhi AD, Lazenby AJ, Montgomery EA. Gastric adenocarcinoma with chief cell differentiation: a proposal for reclassification as oxyntic gland polyp/adenoma. *Am J Surg Pathol.* 2012;36(7):1030-1035.

48. Vieth M, Kushima R, Borchard F, Stolte M. Pyloric gland adenoma: a clinico-pathological analysis of 90 cases. *Virchows Arch.* 2003;442(4):317-321.

49. Abraham SC, Montgomery EA, Singh VK, Yardley JH, Wu TT. Gastric adenomas: intestinal-type and gastric-type adenomas differ in the risk of adenocarcinoma and presence of background mucosal pathology. *Am J Surg Pathol.* 2002;26(10):1276-1285.

50. Chen ZM, Scudiere JR, Abraham SC, Montgomery E. Pyloric gland adenoma: an entity distinct from gastric foveolar type adenoma. *Am J Surg Pathol.* 2009;33(2):186-193.

51. Abraham SC, Park SJ, Lee JH, Mugartegui L, Wu TT. Genetic alterations in gastric adenomas of intestinal and foveolar phenotypes. *Mod Pathol.* 2003;16(8):786-795.

52. Spigelman AD, Williams CB, Talbot IC, Domizio P, Phillips RK. Upper gastrointestinal cancer in patients with familial adenomatous polyposis. *Lancet.* 1989;2(8666):783-785.

53. Bakotic BW, Robinson MJ, Sturm PD, Hruban RH, Offerhaus GJ, Albores-Saavedra J. Pyloric gland adenoma of the main pancreatic duct. *Am J Surg Pathol.* 1999;23(2):227-231.

54. Hackeng WM, Montgomery EA, Giardiello FM, et al. Morphology and genetics of pyloric gland adenomas in familial adenomatous polyposis. *Histopathology.* 2017;70(4):549-557.

55. Hashimoto T, Ogawa R, Matsubara A, et al. Familial adenomatous polyposis-associated and sporadic pyloric gland adenomas of the upper gastrointestinal tract share common genetic features. *Histopathology.* 2015;67(5):689-698.

56. Choi WT, Brown I, Ushiku T, et al. Gastric pyloric gland adenoma: a multicentre clinicopathological study of 67 cases. *Histopathology.* 2018;72(6):1007-1014.

57. Wood LD, Salaria SN, Cruise MW, Giardiello FM, Montgomery EA. Upper GI tract lesions in familial adenomatous polyposis (FAP): enrichment of pyloric gland adenomas and other gastric and duodenal neoplasms. *Am J Surg Pathol.* 2014;38(3):389-393.

58. Ueyama H, Yao T, Nakashima Y, et al. Gastric adenocarcinoma of fundic gland type (chief cell predominant type): proposal for a new entity of gastric adenocarcinoma. *Am J Surg Pathol.* 2010;34(5):609-619.

59. Matsukawa A, Kurano R, Takemoto T, Kagayama M, Ito T. Chief cell hyperplasia with structural and nuclear atypia: a variant of fundic gland polyp. *Pathol Res Pract.* 2005;200(11-12):817-821.

60. Muller-Hocker J, Rellecke P. Chief cell proliferation of the gastric mucosa mimicking early gastric cancer: an unusual variant of fundic gland polyp. *Virchows Arch.* 2003;442(5):496-500.

61. Kushima R, Sekine S, Matsubara A, Taniguchi H, Ikegami M, Tsuda H. Gastric adenocarcinoma of the fundic gland type shares common genetic and phenotypic features with pyloric gland adenoma. *Pathol Int.* 2013;63(6):318-325.

62. Parkin DM, Bray F, Ferlay J, Pisani P. Global cancer statistics, 2002. *CA Cancer J Clin.* 2005;55(2):74-108.

63. Jemal A, Bray F, Center MM, Ferlay J, Ward E, Forman D. Global cancer statistics. *CA Cancer J Clin.* 2011;61(2):69-90.

64. Siegel RL, Miller KD, Jemal A. Cancer statistics, 2017. *CA Cancer J Clin.* 2017;67(1):7-30.

65. Ahn HS, Lee HJ, Yoo MW, et al. Changes in clinicopathological features and survival after gastrectomy for gastric cancer over a 20-year period. *Br J Surg.* 2011;98(2):255-260.

66. Brown LM, Devesa SS. Epidemiologic trends in esophageal and gastric cancer in the United States. *Surg Oncol Clin N Am.* 2002;11(2):235-256.

67. Amin MB, Greene FL, Edge SB, et al. The Eighth Edition AJCC Cancer Staging Manual: continuing to build a bridge from a population-based to a more "personalized" approach to cancer staging. *CA Cancer J Clin.* 2017;67(2):93-99.

68. Park JC, Lee YK, Kim SY, et al. Long-term outcomes of endoscopic submucosal dissection in comparison to surgery in undifferentiated-type intramucosal gastric cancer using propensity score analysis. *Surg Endosc.* 2018;32(4):2046-2057.

69. Lauren P. The two histological main types of gastric carcinoma: diffuse and so-called intestinal-type carcinoma. An attempt at a histo-clinical classification. *Acta Pathol Microbiol Scand.* 1965;64:31-49.

70. Cimerman M, Repse S, Jelenc F, Omejc M, Bitenc M, Lamovec J. Comparison of Lauren's, Ming's and WHO histological classifications of gastric cancer as a prognostic factor for operated patients. *Int Surg.* 1994;79(1):27-32.

71. Bosman FT, Carneiro F, Hruban RH, et al., ed *WHO Classification of Tumours of the Digestive System.* 4th ed. Lyon: WHO Press; 2010.

72. Talamonti MS, Kim SP, Yao KA, et al. Surgical outcomes of patients with gastric carcinoma: the importance of primary tumor location and microvessel invasion. *Surgery.* 2003;134(4):720-727; discussion 727-729.

73. Luebke T, Baldus SE, Grass G, et al. Histological grading in gastric cancer by Ming classification: correlation with histopathological subtypes, metastasis, and prognosis. *World J Surg.* 2005;29(11):1422-1427; discussion 1428.

74. van Beek J, zur Hausen A, Klein Kranenbarg E, et al. EBV-positive gastric adenocarcinomas: a distinct clinicopathologic entity with a low frequency of lymph node involvement. *J Clin Oncol.* 2004;22(4):664-670.

75. Zur Hausen A, van Rees BP, van Beek J, et al. Epstein-Barr virus in gastric carcinomas and gastric stump carcinomas: a late event in gastric carcinogenesis. *J Clin Pathol.* 2004;57(5):487-491.

76. Ushiku T, Shinozaki A, Shibahara J, et al. SALL4 represents fetal gut differentiation of gastric cancer, and is diagnostically useful in distinguishing hepatoid gastric carcinoma from hepatocellular carcinoma. *Am J Surg Pathol.* 2010;34(4):533-540

77. Yong KJ, Gao C, Lim JS, et al. Oncofetal gene SALL4 in aggressive hepatocellular carcinoma. *N Engl J Med.* 2013;368(24):2266-2276.

78. Tang LH, Untch BR, Reidy DL, et al. Well-differentiated neuroendocrine tumors with a morphologically apparent high-grade component: a pathway distinct from poorly differentiated neuroendocrine carcinomas. *Clin Cancer Res.* 2016;22(4):1011-1017.

79. Yachida S, Vakiani E, White CM, et al. Small cell and large cell neuroendocrine carcinomas of the pancreas are genetically similar and distinct from well-differentiated pancreatic neuroendocrine tumors. *Am J Surg Pathol.* 2012;36(2):173-184.

80. Basturk O, Yang Z, Tang LH, et al. The high-grade (WHO G3) pancreatic neuroendocrine tumor category is morphologically and biologically heterogenous and includes both well differentiated and poorly differentiated neoplasms. *Am J Surg Pathol.* 2015;39(5):683-690.

81. Raj N, Valentino E, Capanu M, et al. Treatment response and outcomes of grade 3 pancreatic neuroendocrine neoplasms based on morphology: well differentiated versus poorly differentiated. *Pancreas.* 2017;46(3):296-301.

82. Sorbye H, Welin S, Langer SW, et al. Predictive and prognostic factors for treatment and survival in 305 patients with advanced gastrointestinal neuroendocrine carcinoma (WHO G3): the NORDIC NEC study. *Ann Oncol.* 2013;24(1):152-160.

83. Lloyd RV OR, Kloppel G, Rosai J. *WHO Classification of Tumours of Endocrine Organs.* Vol 10. 4th ed. Lyon: IARC; 2017.

84. Fennerty MB. Gastric intestinal metaplasia on routine endoscopic biopsy. *Gastroenterology.* 2003;125(2):586-590.

85. Correa P. Human gastric carcinogenesis: a multistep and multifactorial process—first American Cancer Society Award Lecture on cancer epidemiology and prevention. *Cancer Res.* 1992;52(24):6735-6740.

86. Correa P, Haenszel W, Cuello C, Tannenbaum S, Archer M. A model for gastric cancer epidemiology. *Lancet.* 1975;2(7924):58-60.

87. Park JY, Cornish TC, Lam-Himlin D, Shi C, Montgomery E. Gastric lesions in patients with autoimmune metaplastic atrophic gastritis (AMAG) in a tertiary care setting. *Am J Surg Pathol.* 2010;34(11):1591-1598.

88. Coggon D, Barker DJ, Cole RB, Nelson M. Stomach cancer and food storage. *J Natl Cancer Inst.* 1989;81(15):1170-1182.

89. La Vecchia C, Negri E, D'Avanzo B, Franceschi S. Electric refrigerator use and gastric cancer risk. *Br J Cancer.* 1990;62(1):136-137.

90. Tricker AR. N-nitroso compounds and man: sources of exposure, endogenous formation and occurrence in body fluids. *Eur J Cancer Prev.* 1997;6(3):226-268.

91. Song P, Wu L, Guan W. Dietary nitrates, nitrites, and nitrosamines intake and the risk of gastric cancer: a meta-analysis. *Nutrients.* 2015;7(12):9872-9895.

92. La Vecchia C, Ferraroni M, D'Avanzo B, Decarli A, Franceschi S. Selected micronutrient intake and the risk of gastric cancer. *Cancer Epidemiol Biomarkers Prev.* 1994;3(5):393-398.

93. Palli D, Russo A, Decarli A. Dietary patterns, nutrient intake and gastric cancer in a high-risk area of Italy. *Cancer Causes Control.* 2001;12(2):163-172.

94. Hansford S, Kaurah P, Li-Chang H, et al. Hereditary diffuse gastric cancer syndrome: CDH1 mutations and beyond. *JAMA Oncol.* 2015;1(1):23-32.

95. van der Post RS, Vogelaar IP, Carneiro F, et al. Hereditary diffuse gastric cancer: updated clinical guidelines with an emphasis on germline CDH1 mutation carriers. *J Med Genet.* 2015;52(6):361-374.

96. Fujita H, Lennerz JK, Chung DC, et al. Endoscopic surveillance of patients with hereditary diffuse gastric cancer: biopsy recommendations after topographic distribution of cancer foci in a series of 10 CDH1-mutated gastrectomies. *Am J Surg Pathol.* 2012;36(11):1709-1717.

97. Lee AF, Rees H, Owen DA, Huntsman DG. Periodic acid-schiff is superior to hematoxylin and eosin for screening prophylactic gastrectomies from CDH1 mutation carriers. *Am J Surg Pathol.* 2010;34(7):1007-1013.

98. Barber ME, Save V, Carneiro F, et al. Histopathological and molecular analysis of gastrectomy specimens from hereditary diffuse gastric cancer patients has implications for endoscopic surveillance of individuals at risk. *J Pathol.* 2008;216(3):286-294.

99. Worthley DL, Phillips KD, Wayte N, et al. Gastric adenocarcinoma and proximal polyposis of the stomach (GAPPS): a new autosomal dominant syndrome. *Gut.* 2012;61(5):774-779.

100. Yanaru-Fujisawa R, Nakamura S, Moriyama T, et al. Familial fundic gland polyposis with gastric cancer. *Gut.* 2012;61(7):1103-1104.

101. McDuffie LA, Sabesan A, Allgaeuer M, et al. beta-Catenin activation in fundic gland polyps, gastric cancer and colonic polyps in families afflicted by 'gastric adenocarcinoma and proximal polyposis of the stomach' (GAPPS). *J Clin Pathol.* 2016;69(9):826-833.

102. Repak R, Kohoutova D, Podhola M, et al. The first European family with gastric adenocarcinoma and proximal polyposis of the stomach: case report and review of the literature. *Gastrointest Endosc.* 2016;84(4):718-725.

103. Guan J, Lim KS, Mekhail T, Chang CC. Programmed death Ligand-1 (PD-L1) expression in the programmed death receptor-1 (PD-1)/PD-L1 blockade: a key player against various cancers. *Arch Pathol Lab Med.* 2017;141(6):851-861.

104. Akiyama T, Sudo C, Ogawara H, Toyoshima K, Yamamoto T. The product of the human c-erbB-2 gene: a 185-kilodalton glycoprotein with tyrosine kinase activity. *Science.* 1986;232(4758):1644-1646.

105. Slamon DJ, Clark GM, Wong SG, Levin WJ, Ullrich A, McGuire WL. Human breast cancer: correlation of relapse and survival with amplification of the HER-2/neu oncogene. *Science.* 1987;235(4785):177-182.

106. Yan M, Schwaederle M, Arguello D, Millis SZ, Gatalica Z, Kurzrock R. HER2 expression status in diverse cancers: review of results from 37,992 patients. *Cancer Metastasis Rev.* 2015;34(1):157-164.

107. Bang YJ, Van Cutsem E, Feyereislova A, et al. Trastuzumab in combination with chemotherapy versus chemotherapy alone for treatment of HER2-positive advanced gastric or gastro-oesophageal junction cancer (ToGA): a phase 3, open-label, randomised controlled trial. *Lancet.* 2010;376(9742):687-697.

108. Bartley AN, Washington MK, Ventura CB, et al. HER2 testing and clinical decision making in gastroesophageal adenocarcinoma: guideline from the College of American Pathologists, American Society for Clinical Pathology, and American Society of Clinical Oncology. *Arch Pathol Lab Med.* 2016;140(12):1345-1363.

109. Cruz-Reyes C, Gamboa-Dominguez A. HER2 amplification in gastric cancer is a rare event restricted to the intestinal phenotype. *Int J Surg Pathol.* 2013;21(3):240-246.

110. Kunz PL, Mojtahed A, Fisher GA, et al. HER2 expression in gastric and gastroesophageal junction adenocarcinoma in a US population: clinicopathologic analysis with proposed approach to HER2 assessment. *Appl Immunohistochem Mol Morphol.* 2012;20(1):13-24.

111. Park JS, Rha SY, Chung HC, et al. Clinicopathological features and prognostic significance of HER2 expression in gastric cancer. *Oncology.* 2015;88(3):147-156.

112. Okines AF, Thompson LC, Cunningham D, et al. Effect of HER2 on prognosis and benefit from peri-operative chemotherapy in early oesophago-gastric adenocarcinoma in the MAGIC trial. *Ann Oncol.* 2013;24(5):1253-1261.

113. Janjigian YY, Werner D, Pauligk C, et al. Prognosis of metastatic gastric and gastroesophageal junction cancer by HER2 status: a European and USA International collaborative analysis. *Ann Oncol.* 2012;23(10):2656-2662.

114. Pirrelli M, Caruso ML, Di Maggio M, Armentano R, Valentini AM. Are biopsy specimens predictive of HER2 status in gastric cancer patients? *Dig Dis Sci.* 2013;58(2):397-404.

115. Qiu Z, Sun W, Zhou C, Zhang J. HER2 expression variability between primary gastric cancers and corresponding lymph node metastases. *Hepatogastroenterology.* 2015;62(137):231-233.

116. Bozzetti C, Negri FV, Lagrasta CA, et al. Comparison of HER2 status in primary and paired metastatic sites of gastric carcinoma. *Br J Cancer.* 2011;104(9):1372-1376.

117. Ruschoff J, Dietel M, Baretton G, et al. HER2 diagnostics in gastric cancer-guideline validation and development of standardized immunohistochemical testing. *Virchows Arch.* 2010;457(3):299-307.

118. Gullo I, Grillo F, Molinaro L, et al. Minimum biopsy set for HER2 evaluation in gastric and gastro-esophageal junction cancer. *Endosc Int Open*. 2015;3(2):E165-E170.

119. Bang YJ. Advances in the management of HER2-positive advanced gastric and gastroesophageal junction cancer. *J Clin Gastroenterol*. 2012;46(8):637-648.

120. Abrahao-Machado LF, Jacome AA, Wohnrath DR, et al. HER2 in gastric cancer: comparative analysis of three different antibodies using whole-tissue sections and tissue microarrays. *World J Gastroenterol*. 2013;19(38):6438-6446.

121. Stolte M, Sticht T, Eidt S, Ebert D, Finkenzeller G. Frequency, location, and age and sex distribution of various types of gastric polyp. *Endoscopy*. 1994;26(8):659-665.

122. Borch K, Ahren B, Ahlman H, Falkmer S, Granerus G, Grimelius L. Gastric carcinoids: biologic behavior and prognosis after differentiated treatment in relation to type. *Ann Surg*. 2005;242(1):64-73.

123. Burkitt MD, Pritchard DM. Review article: pathogenesis and management of gastric carcinoid tumours. *Aliment Pharmacol Ther*. 2006;24(9):1305-1320.

124. Rorstad O. Prognostic indicators for carcinoid neuroendocrine tumors of the gastrointestinal tract. *J Surg Oncol*. 2005;89(3):151-160.

125. McCall CM, Shi C, Cornish TC, et al. Grading of well-differentiated pancreatic neuroendocrine tumors is improved by the inclusion of both Ki67 proliferative index and mitotic rate. *Am J Surg Pathol*. 2013;37(11):1671-1677.

126. Chen WC, Warner RR, Ward SC, et al. Management and disease outcome of type I gastric neuroendocrine tumors: the Mount Sinai experience. *Dig Dis Sci*. 2015;60(4):996-1003.

127. Raderer M, Kiesewetter B, Ferreri AJ. Clinicopathologic characteristics and treatment of marginal zone lymphoma of mucosa-associated lymphoid tissue (MALT lymphoma). *CA Cancer J Clin*. 2016;66(2):153-171.

128. Isaacson PG, Spencer J. Malignant lymphoma of mucosa-associated lymphoid tissue. *Histopathology*. 1987;11(5):445-462.

129. Ye H, Liu H, Raderer M, et al. High incidence of t(11;18)(q21;q21) in *Helicobacter pylori*-negative gastric MALT lymphoma. *Blood*. 2003;101(7):2547-2550.

130. Bacon CM, Du MQ, Dogan A. Mucosa-associated lymphoid tissue (MALT) lymphoma: a practical guide for pathologists. *J Clin Pathol*. 2007;60(4):361-372.

131. Copie-Bergman C, Gaulard P, Lavergne-Slove A, et al. Proposal for a new histological grading system for post-treatment evaluation of gastric MALT lymphoma. *Gut*. 2003;52(11):1656.

132. Vanek J. Gastric submucosal granuloma with eosinophilic infiltration. *Am J Pathol*. 1949;25(3):397-411.

133. Carmack SW, Vemulapalli R, Spechler SJ, Genta RM. Esophagitis dissecans superficialis ("sloughing esophagitis"): a clinicopathologic study of 12 cases. *Am J Surg Pathol*. 2009;33(12):1789-1794.

134. Rossi P, Montuori M, Balassone V, et al. Inflammatory fibroid polyp. A case report and review of the literature. *Ann Ital Chir*. 2012;83(4):347-351.

135. Rittershaus AC, Appelman HD. Benign gastrointestinal mesenchymal BUMPS: a brief review of some spindle cell polyps with published names. *Arch Pathol Lab Med*. 2011;135(10):1311-1319.

136. Morandi E, Pisoni L, Castoldi M, Tavani E, Trabucchi E. Gastric outlet obstruction due to inflammatory fibroid polyp. *Ann Ital Chir*. 2006;77(1):59-61.

137. Stolte M. Clinical consequences of the endoscopic diagnosis of gastric polyps. *Endoscopy*. 1995;27(1):32-37; discussion 59-60.

138. Cassier PA, Ducimetiere F, Lurkin A, et al. A prospective epidemiological study of new incident GISTs during two consecutive years in Rhone Alpes region: incidence and molecular distribution of GIST in a European region. *Br J Cancer*. 2010;103(2):165-170.

139. Fletcher CD, Berman JJ, Corless C, et al. Diagnosis of gastrointestinal stromal tumors: a consensus approach. *Hum Pathol*. 2002;33(5):459-465.

140. Miettinen M, El-Rifai W, H L Sobin L, Lasota J. Evaluation of malignancy and prognosis of gastrointestinal stromal tumors: a review. *Hum Pathol*. 2002;33(5):478-483.

141. Miettinen M, Sarlomo-Rikala M, Lasota J. Gastrointestinal stromal tumors: recent advances in understanding of their biology. *Hum Pathol*. 1999;30(10):1213-1220.

142. Goddard AF, Badreldin R, Pritchard DM, Walker MM, Warren B. The management of gastric polyps. *Gut*. 2010;59(9):1270-1276.

143. Dei Tos AP, Laurino L, Bearzi I, Messerini L, Farinati F. Gastrointestinal stromal tumors: the histology report. *Dig Liver Dis.* 2011;43 Suppl 4:S304-S309.

144. Liegl-Atzwanger B, Fletcher JA, Fletcher CD. Gastrointestinal stromal tumors. *Virchows Arch.* 2010;456(2):111-127.

145. Caletti G, Deviere J, Fockens P, et al. Guidelines of the European Society of Gastrointestinal Endoscopy (ESGE) Part II: retroperitoneum and large bowel, training. The European Endosonography Club working party. *Endoscopy.* 1996;28(7):626-628.

146. Van Dam J, Brady PG, Freeman M, et al. Guidelines for training in electronic ultrasound: guidelines for clinical application. From the ASGE. American Society for Gastrointestinal Endoscopy. *Gastrointest Endosc.* 1999;49(6):829-833.

147. Nesje LB, Laerum OD, Svanes K, Odegaard S. Subepithelial masses of the gastrointestinal tract evaluated by endoscopic ultrasonography. *Eur J Ultrasound.* 2002;15(1-2):45-54.

148. Casali PG, Jost L, Reichardt P, Schlemmer M, Blay JY. Gastrointestinal stromal tumours: ESMO clinical recommendations for diagnosis, treatment and follow-up. *Ann Oncol.* 2009;20 Suppl 4:64-67.

149. Casali PG VJ, Kotasek D, LeCesne A, Reichardt P, Blay JY. Imatinib mesylate in advanced gastrointestinal stromal tumors (GIST): survival analysis of the intergroup EORTC/ISG/AGITG randomized trial in 946 patients. *Eur J Cancer.* 2005;3:201; abstract 711.

150. Debiec-Rychter M, Sciot R, Le Cesne A, et al. KIT mutations and dose selection for imatinib in patients with advanced gastrointestinal stromal tumours. *Eur J Cancer.* 2006;42(8):1093-1103.

151. Carney JA, Stratakis CA. Familial paraganglioma and gastric stromal sarcoma: a new syndrome distinct from the Carney triad. *Am J Med Genet.* 2002;108(2):132-139.

152. Pasini B, McWhinney SR, Bei T, et al. Clinical and molecular genetics of patients with the Carney-Stratakis syndrome and germline mutations of the genes coding for the succinate dehydrogenase subunits SDHB, SDHC, and SDHD. *Eur J Hum Genet.* 2008;16(1):79-88.

153. Gaal J, Stratakis CA, Carney JA, et al. SDHB immunohistochemistry: a useful tool in the diagnosis of Carney-Stratakis and Carney triad gastrointestinal stromal tumors. *Mod Pathol.* 2011;24(1):147-151.

154. Miettinen M, Sarlomo-Rikala M, Sobin LH, Lasota J. Esophageal stromal tumors: a clinicopathologic, immunohistochemical, and molecular genetic study of 17 cases and comparison with esophageal leiomyomas and leiomyosarcomas. *Am J Surg Pathol.* 2000;24(2):211-222.

155. Hyun JH, Jeen YT, Chun HJ, et al. Endoscopic resection of submucosal tumor of the esophagus: results in 62 patients. *Endoscopy.* 1997;29(3):165-170.

156. Pidhorecky I, Cheney RT, Kraybill WG, Gibbs JF. Gastrointestinal stromal tumors: current diagnosis, biologic behavior, and management. *Ann Surg Oncol.* 2000;7(9):705-712.

157. Davis GB, Blanchard DK, Hatch GF III, et al. Tumors of the stomach. *World J Surg.* 2000;24(4):412-420.

158. Wang LM, Chetty R. Selected unusual tumors of the stomach: a review. *Int J Surg Pathol.* 2012;20(1):5-14.

159. Matsumoto H, Kojima Y, Inoue T, et al. A malignant granular cell tumor of the stomach: report of a case. *Surg Today.* 1996;26(2):119-122.

160. Franzin G, Novelli P. Gastritis cystica profunda. *Histopathology.* 1981;5(5):535-547.

161. Okada M, Iizuka Y, Oh K, Murayama H, Maekawa T. Gastritis cystica profunda presenting as giant gastric mucosal folds: the role of endoscopic ultrasonography and mucosectomy in the diagnostic work-up. *Gastrointest Endosc.* 1994;40(5):640-644.

162. Park JS, Myung SJ, Jung HY, et al. Endoscopic treatment of gastritis cystica polyposa found in an unoperated stomach. *Gastrointest Endosc.* 2001;54(1):101-103.

163. Yu XF, Guo LW, Chen ST, Teng LS. Gastritis cystica profunda in a previously unoperated stomach: a case report. *World J Gastroenterol.* 2015;21(12):3759-3762.

164. Choi MG, Jeong JY, Kim KM, et al. Clinical significance of gastritis cystica profunda and its association with Epstein-Barr virus in gastric cancer. *Cancer.* 2012;118(21):5227-5233.

CHAPTER OUTLINE

THE UNREMARKABLE SMALL BOWEL

Endoscopically, the small bowel is composed of homogeneous pink mucosa with permanent circumferential folds (plicae circulares) and a dense carpet of villi (Fig. 3.1). These plicae are an architectural adaptation to augment the absorptive surface area in the small bowel and correspond histologically to reduplication of the mucosa, which is held together by a submucosa core (Fig. 3.2).

Most neoplastic lesions of the small bowel arise in specific anatomic compartments and, thus, understanding the layers of the small bowel assists in classification and staging of primary small bowel tumors. The small bowel layers are divided into the mucosa, submucosa, muscularis propria, and serosa. Designed for absorption of ingested nutrients, the mucosa is composed of an epithelial component, lamina propria, and muscularis mucosae. The surface epithelium and lamina propria form intraluminal projections called villi; these microscopic fingerlike and leaflike projections cover the entire luminal surface of the small bowel and further enhance surface area for absorption.[1] Each villus is covered by a single layer of epithelial cells of varying types (see later discussion), under which sits the epithelial basement membrane and lamina propria. This lamina propria core contains migratory inflammatory cells as well as a blind-ended lymphatic channel (lacteal) and capillary network, which are accessible for metastatic spread of tumor cells.[2] Although the villi are extensions above the surface architecture, the crypts (of Lieberkühn) are depressions below that extend from the lumen to the muscularis mucosae. The ratio of crypt height to villous length in the normal small bowel varies from 1:3 to 1:5 (Figs. 3.3–3.5).[3]

The villous and crypt epithelium are the source of small bowel carcinomas, which are rare tumors. The villi are lined by tall columnar absorptive epithelial cells, each of which contains an apical brush border composed of microvilli (Figs. 3.6–3.8), and interspersed between the absorptive cells are goblet cells. Scattered endocrine cells are present within the villous epithelium, but they are more abundant within the crypts and give rise to the more common small bowel neuroendocrine tumor. Intraepithelial lymphocytes are normally present as one per five epithelial cells, often reported as 20 per 100 enterocytes when discussing nonneoplastic malabsorptive diseases. The deep crypts additionally contain abundant Paneth cells (Fig. 3.9). The lamina propria rests on the muscularis mucosae, surrounds the crypts, and extends upward into the core of the intestinal villi. It serves as an immunologic organ and contains plasma cells, lymphocytes, eosinophils, histiocytes,

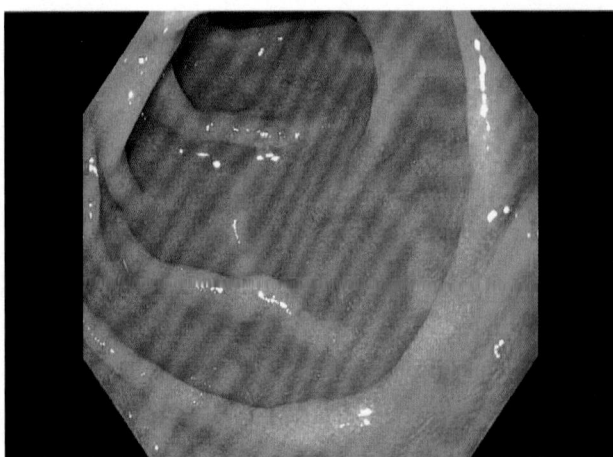

Figure 3-1. Normal small bowel, endoscopic findings in the normal duodenum. A fine carpet of villi lines the duodenal lumen. The circular folds (plicae) of the small bowel have smooth borders.

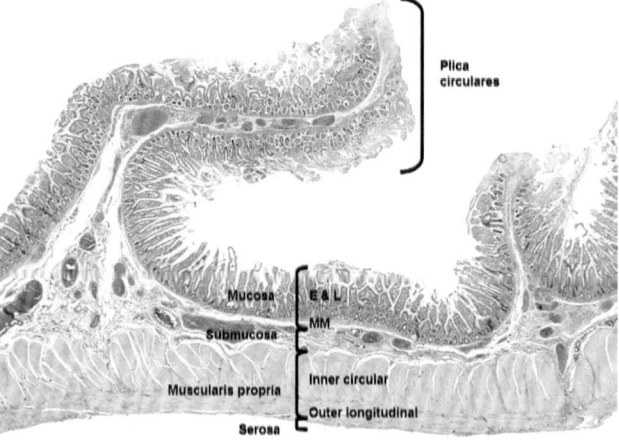

Figure 3-2. Normal small bowel, layers of the small intestine. This resection specimen illustrates the four main layers of the small bowel: mucosa, submucosa, muscularis propria, and serosa. The mucosa consists of epithelium (E), lamina propria (L), and muscularis mucosae (MM). The submucosa sits between the muscularis mucosae and the muscularis propria (MP) and consists of loose fibroconnective tissue and lymphovascular channels. The MP consists of two muscle layers: an inner circular and outer longitudinal. The outermost layer is the serosa. Note the plicae circulares are composed of a reduplication of mucosa held together by a submucosa core.

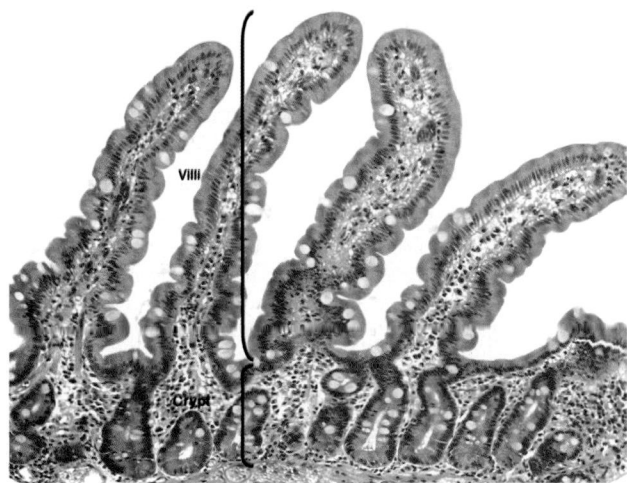

Figure 3-3. Normal small bowel. The crypt to villous ratio in the normal small bowel ranges from 1:3 to 1:5. The epithelial cells lining the villi are tall columnar absorptive cells and are intermittently punctuated by goblet cells. The base of the crypts contains visible bright pink Paneth cells with scattered endocrine cells (unperceivable at this magnification).

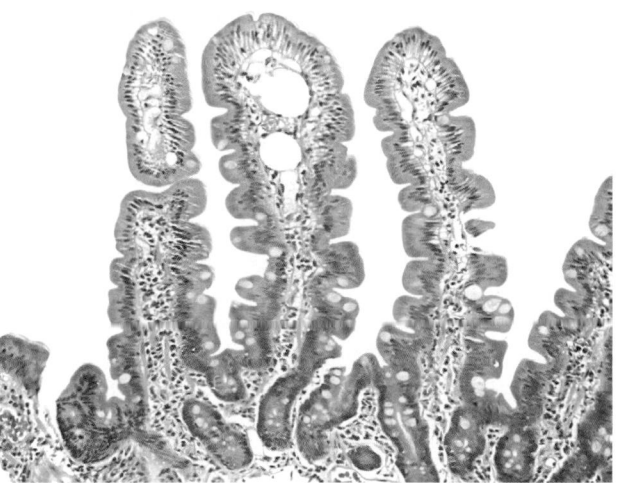

Figure 3-4. Normal small bowel, lacteals. The core of the villi are composed of lamina propria containing migratory chronic inflammatory cells, blood vessels, lymphatic channels, and smooth muscle cells. This example shows dilated lacteals in the tips of the villi, a finding that indicates lymphatic blockage of lymphatic flow of unclear significance.

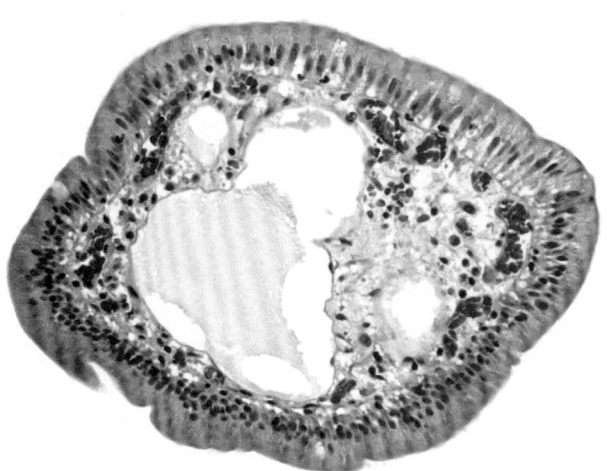

Figure 3-5. Normal small bowel, cross section of villous projection. Higher magnification of a villous core highlights a dilated lymphatic space containing pale eosinophilic serum. Separate capillary vessels contain red blood cells, and scattered chronic inflammatory cells are present in the supporting substance.

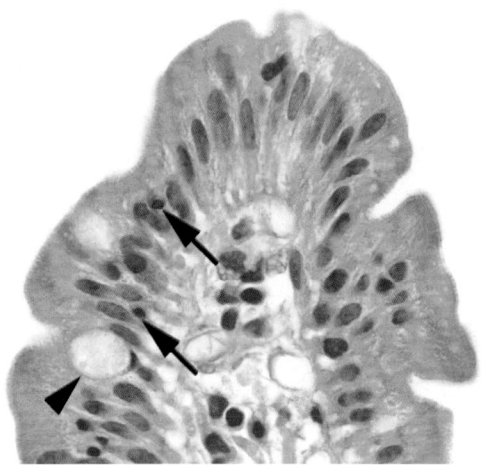

Figure 3-6. Normal small bowel, villous tip. The villous tip is lined by columnar cells with an absorptive brush border composed of microvilli. On H&E stain, this can be visualized as an eosinophilic "fuzzy" border. These absorptive columnar cells are punctuated by goblet cells (*arrowhead*), and small numbers of lymphocytes (*arrows*) may be seen traversing between them.

and mast cells. Like any other immunologic site, the small bowel is susceptible to hematolymphoid disorders and understanding the normal constituents can aid in differentiating benign reactive inflammation from neoplasia (see "Near Miss" section at the end of this chapter for more differentiating clues). Plasma cells are the most abundant cellular lamina propria constituent. Most contain IgA but some contain IgM; in contrast to their abundance in extraintestinal sites, IgG-secreting plasma cells are scarce. Lymphocytes of both B and T lineage are common. The only granulocytes normally found in the lamina propria are eosinophils and mast cells. Like other areas of the gastrointestinal (GI) tract, the muscularis mucosae is composed of a thin layer of smooth muscle cells separating the mucosa from the underlying submucosa. Unique to the small bowel, tufts of smooth muscle radiate from the muscularis mucosae into the lamina propria and extend into the villi (Fig. 3.10).

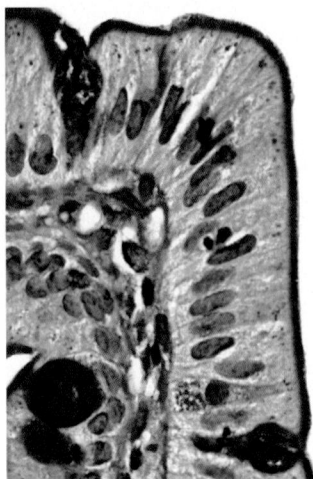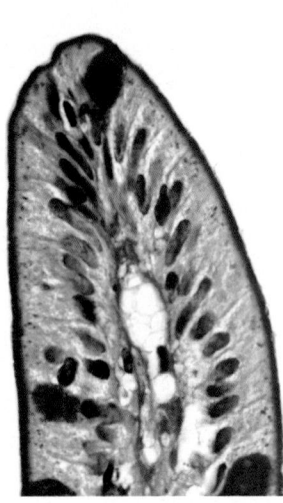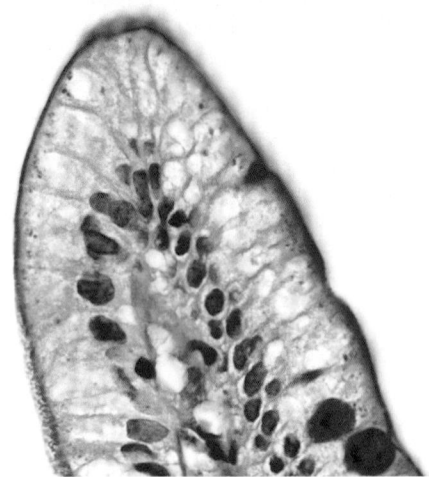

Figure 3-7. Normal small bowel, villous tips (PAS special stain). The microvillous brush border is crisp and deeply eosinophilic on a PAS special stain, which also highlights the goblet cells. Defective, broken, or smudgy brush borders should prompt consideration of microvillous inclusion disease, especially in infants. The cytoplasm of the columnar cells appears pale and homogeneous.

Figure 3-8. Normal small bowel, lipid "hang-up" (PAS special stain). This PAS stain of a villous tip reveals vacuolated cytoplasm of the absorptive columnar cells (compare with the previous figure). This finding indicates lipid within the cytoplasm of the epithelial cells and is commonly seen among patients who have ingested food or drink before endoscopy. When severe, diffuse, or present in the pediatric population, it is worthwhile to consider a lipid transport disorder.

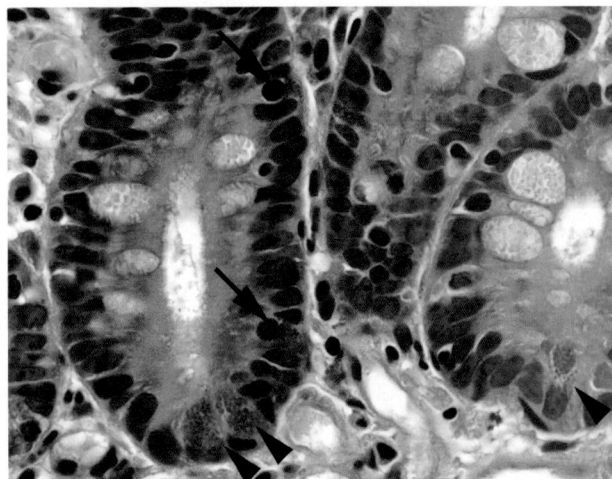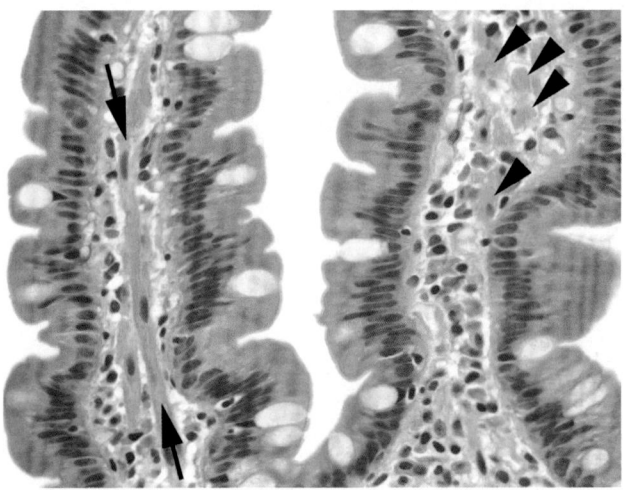

Figure 3-9. Normal small bowel, crypt base. Paneth cells (*arrowheads*) contain abundant brightly eosinophilic coarse granules that face the gland lumen. By comparison, enteroendocrine cells (*arrows*) have deeper red and smaller granules that face the basement membrane.

Figure 3-10. Normal small bowel, smooth muscle within villous core. Delicate tufts of smooth muscle (*arrows*) extend from the muscularis mucosae along the core of the villi. When cut in cross section (*arrowheads*), these can be mistaken for histiocytes, signet ring cell carcinoma, or infectious diseases (such as *Mycobacterium avium intracellulare*).

The submucosa of the duodenum is a source of mesenchymal neoplasms, and it contains ganglion cells of Meissner plexus and lymphatic and vascular structures and is one of only two sites in the GI tract that contains submucosal glands (the other being the esophagus). These Brunner glands are lobular collections of tubuloalveolar glands that are limited to the submucosa of the duodenum. However, up to one-third of them can reside within the deep mucosa in the absence of pathology (Fig. 3.11).[4] These glands are most concentrated at the gastroduodenal junction and gradually decrease in number distally. The glands are lined by cells (Figs. 3.12 and 3.13) that contain periodic acid–Schiff (PAS)-positive and diastase-resistant neutral mucins and scattered endocrine cells that secrete somatostatin, gastrin, and peptide YY. Secretions empty into the luminal crypt spaces by way of small ducts. Distally, the jejunum and ileum lack Brunner glands.

The muscularis propria surrounds the submucosa and is composed of an inner circular and outer longitudinal layer of smooth muscle. Between these layers lies the myenteric plexus of Auerbach, a major neural plexus of the enteric nervous system. Externally, the bowel is enveloped by subserosal connective tissue and the mesothelial-derived serosa.

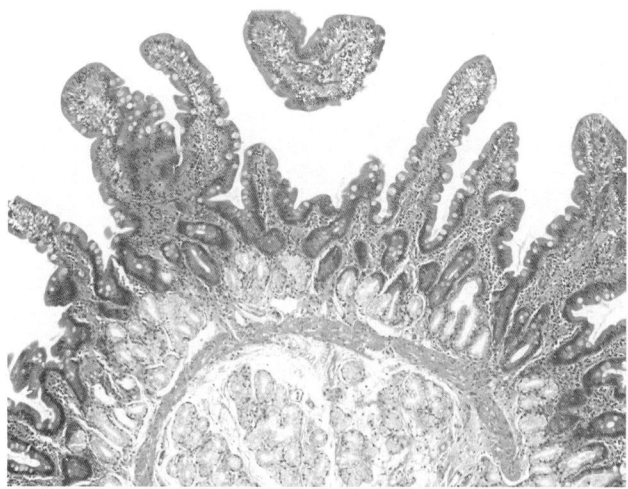

Figure 3-11. Normal small bowel, proximal duodenum with Brunner glands. Brunner glands are found exclusively in the proximal duodenum. Although their bulk lies in the submucosa, extension above the muscularis mucosae is not uncommon, even under normal conditions, as seen here.

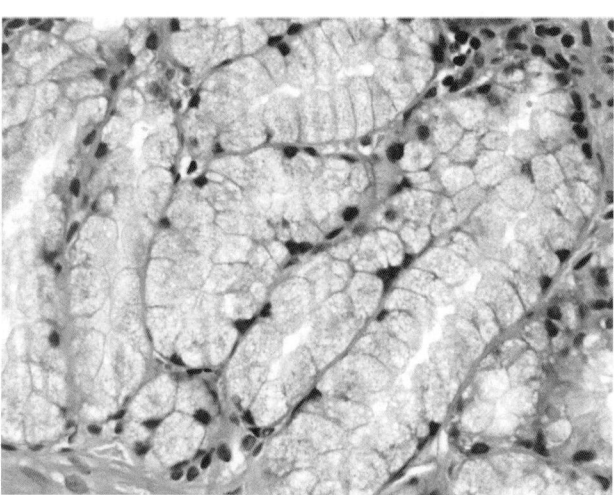

Figure 3-12. Normal small bowel, Brunner glands. Brunner glands are lined by cuboidal to columnar cells with pale, uniform cytoplasm and oval, basally located nuclei.

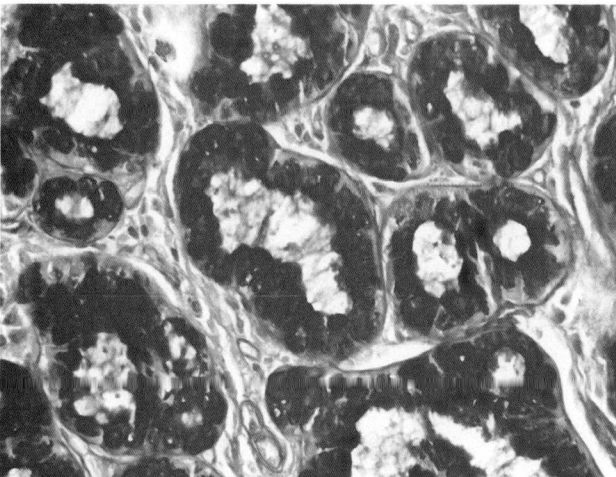

Figure 3-13. Normal small bowel, Brunner glands (PAS special stain). Brunner glands contain PAS-positive and diastase-resistant cytoplasmic mucin. This staining pattern can be helpful in differentiating crushed Brunner glands from a neural tumor.

PEARLS & PITFALLS: Distinctive Differences Among Regions of Small Bowel

Duodenum:

    Contains submucosal Brunner glands, more abundant proximally

    Villi range from slender and fingerlike to broad and leaflike

Jejunum:

    Prominent, tall plicae circulares

    Villi are uniformly slender and fingerlike (Fig. 3.14)

Ileum:

    Submucosal adipose tissue may be present, especially near the ileocecal valve

    Shorter and fewer plicae circulares

    Increased proportion of goblet cells (Fig. 3.15)

    Presence of Peyer patches (abundance of lymphoid aggregates) (Fig. 3.16)

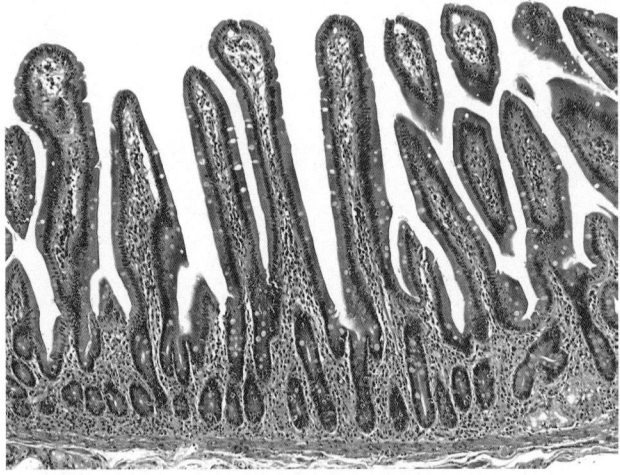

Figure 3-14. Normal small bowel, jejunum. Regional variations exist in the small bowel. For example, the jejunum contains no Brunner glands and has tall slender villi.

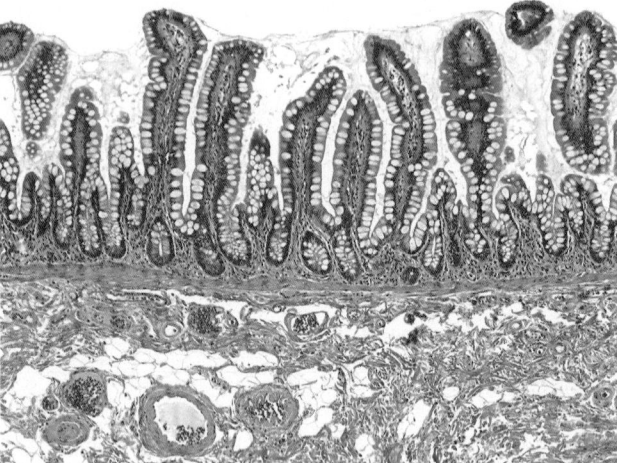

Figure 3-15. Normal small bowel, ileum. The ileum exhibits regional variation with an increased proportion of goblet cells (compare with the previous figure), absence of Brunner glands, and submucosal adipose tissue.

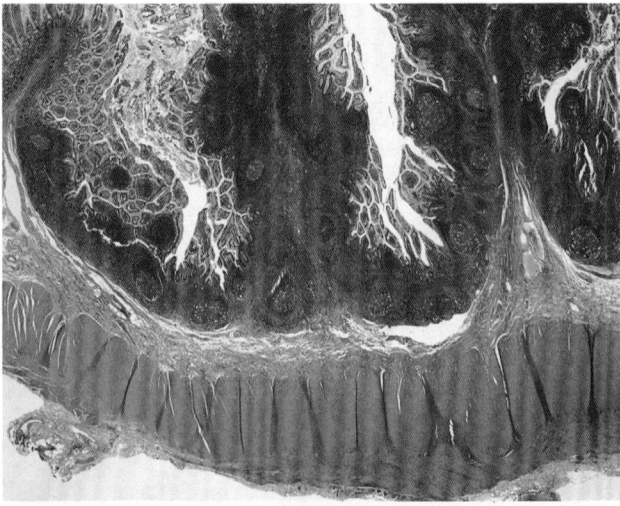

Figure 3-16. Normal small bowel, terminal ileum. Unencapsulated organized lymphoid nodules are found within the mucosa and submucosa of the terminal ileum. These Peyer patches are found exclusively in the terminal ileum, which functions as an immunologic organ (see also Figs. 3.245–3.252).

POLYPS

HETEROTOPIC POLYPS

Heterotopic tissue refers to histologically normal tissue found in abnormal anatomic sites. In the small bowel, heterotopic tissues, such as pancreatic and gastric glands, can produce polypoid lesions that are endoscopically concerning.

Pancreatic Heterotopia

Heterotopic pancreas, sometimes called accessory pancreas, is the presence of normal pancreatic tissue at an abnormal anatomical site. The small intestine is the second most common site (26% of cases) following the stomach (53%), and other frequent locations include the omentum, spleen and hilar region, porta hepatis, gallbladder, distal periesophageal tissue, and mesentery.[5] Presenting symptoms are nonspecific and may include abdominal pain, distension, nausea and vomiting, malaise, anorexia, anemia, weight loss, melena, jaundice, or upper GI bleeding. Most cases are identified incidentally on upper endoscopy and are seen as well-circumscribed, broad-based submucosal nodules with a characteristic central umbilication or dimple seen in most, but not all, cases. Histologically, pancreatic heterotopia is well circumscribed, is predominately submucosal, and comprises three components: (1) characteristic pancreatic acini composed of a single row of pyramidal exocrine epithelial cells featuring granular cytoplasm with an ombré quality, ranging from dense dark purple at the base to bright orange-red at the apex (Fig. 3.17); (2) ducts lined by flat columnar cells; and (3) endocrine cells formed by islets of Langerhans (Fig. 3.18). In the largest study of pancreatic heterotopia (n = 184), all three components were found only in a minority of cases (12.5%) (Fig. 3.19).[5] Thus, diagnosis may be challenging on small biopsy specimens, in particular when lesions are primarily submucosal (Fig. 3.20). Although this ectopia is benign, periampullary lesions are more likely to require resection owing to obstructive jaundice (64%), biliary tract dilatation (41%), and clinically significant abdominal pain (55%). Among lesions in the ampulla of Vater region, retrospective review shows that pancreaticoduodenectomy (Whipple resection) was performed in 64% of patients.[5] With improving endoscopic techniques, more conservative endoscopic resection is the therapy of choice.

KEY FEATURES: Pancreatic Heterotopia

- Pancreatic heterotopia is found most commonly in the **stomach (53%) and small bowel (26%)** but may be found widely in the upper abdomen.
- Endoscopically, lesions are broad-based nodules, and a **characteristic central umbilication** is seen in most, but not all, cases.
- Histologically, the lesion is composed of **benign pancreatic elements**: (1) pancreatic acini with exocrine cells, (2) pancreatic ducts, and (3) islets of Langerhans with endocrine cells.
- Only a **minority of cases (12.5%) contain all three components**.
- Diagnosis can be challenging on biopsy samples, especially in the periampullary region, owing to the submucosal location.
- **Endoscopic resection is the therapy of choice**, but Whipple resection is an alternative if clinically necessary.

Gastric Heterotopia

Gastric heterotopia describes the presence of gastric foveolar epithelium and oxyntic glands in the small bowel mucosa. Some experts view this as an embryologic remnant, whereas others suggest it is a metaplastic response to small bowel injury.[6-10] The largest study identifies gastric heterotopia in 1.9% of more than 28,000 duodenal biopsies, with the duodenal bulb being the most common site (66% of cases). Among patients with gastric heterotopia, *Helicobacter* gastritis was less frequent by a magnitude of fivefold, suggesting that metaplasia is an unlikely cause. The finding is also associated with three times the number of fundic gland polyps, suggesting that these presumed congenital patches may be influenced by proton pump inhibitors. Although most cases are small incidental findings, these lesions can be nodular or polypoid endoscopically. In rare instances, patients may present with iron

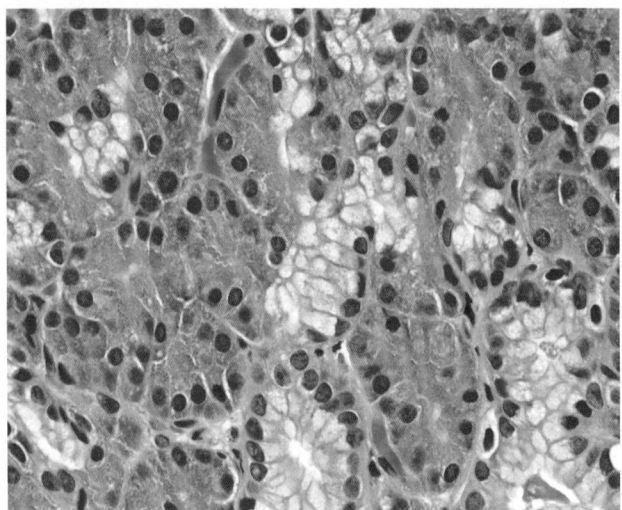

Figure 3-17. Pancreatic heterotopia. Characteristic pancreatic acini are composed of a single row of pyramidal exocrine epithelial cells arranged in acini and featuring finely granular cytoplasm with a tinctorial gradient ranging from dense dark purple at the base to bright orange-red at the apex.

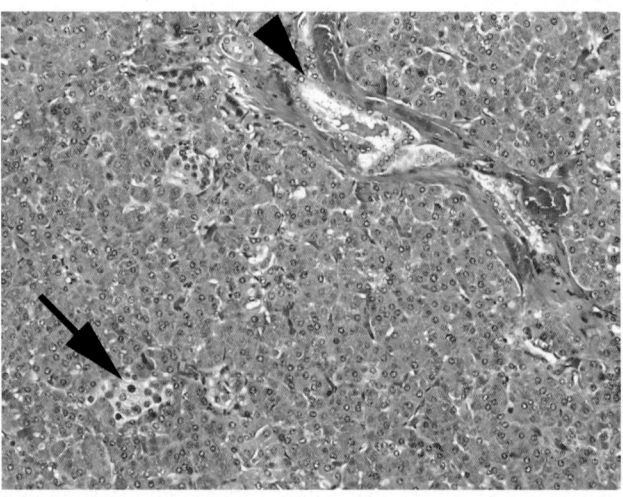

Figure 3-18. Pancreatic heterotopia. A combination of normal pancreatic elements is often present, including ducts lined by flat columnar cells (*arrowhead*), endocrine cells formed by islets of Langerhans (*arrow*), and a backdrop of exocrine epithelial cells.

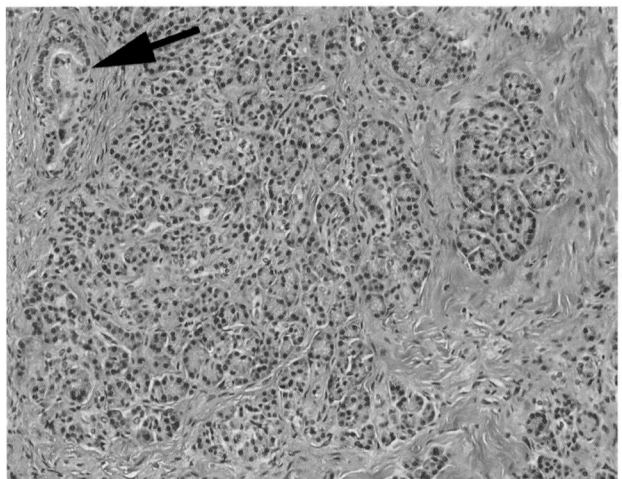

Figure 3-19. Pancreatic heterotopia. Most cases lack all three elements (ducts, endocrine cells, and exocrine cells), such as this case, which shows only ducts (*arrow*) and acini. The pyramidal shape of the exocrine epithelial cells and their acinar arrangement are a clue to pancreatic origin.

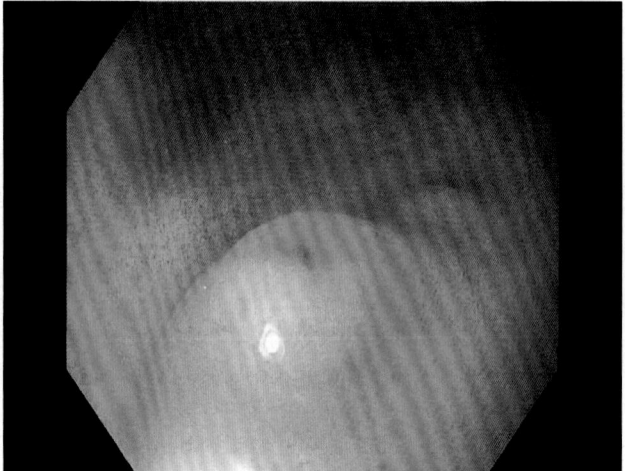

Figure 3-20. Pancreatic heterotopia, endoscopic photo. Lesions may appear polypoid or as a single nodule, and a central umbilication is characteristic, often correlating histologically with a functional pancreatic duct.

deficiency anemia or abdominal pain, and lesions up to 6 cm have been reported.[11] These larger lesions may contain bundles of smooth muscle owing to prolapse resulting from the peristaltic action of the bowel, but this finding should not be mistaken for the hamartomatous Peutz-Jeghers polyp, which has significant familial and screening implications. The diagnostic clue is identification of specialized gastric oxyntic glands among the small bowel crypts. These oxyntic glands are composed of parietal (pink) and chief (blue) cells, and when admixed with pyloric-type or Brunner glands, they may be easy to overlook. Surface foveolar mucin cells are almost always present and can serve as an additional clue to the presence of gastric oxyntic gland heterotopia (Figs. 3.21Figs. 3.21–3.26). If symptomatic, resection is curative.

FAQ: What is the difference between gastric hotorotopia and "nodular chronic peptic duodenitis"?

When gastric foveolar-type epithelium is found in the proximal small bowel, its presence indicates either gastric *heterotopia* or gastric foveolar (mucin cell) *metaplasia*. The distinction is made by the presence of acid-secreting oxyntic glands, which confirm gastric heterotopia. Although their acid secretion contributes to altered pH locally with subsequent foveolar metaplasia, the underlying cause remains gastric heterotopia (Figs. 3.23 and 3.24). In contrast, when gastric foveolar epithelium is found in isolation, without oxyntic glands, this is considered a metaplastic condition and a component of chronic peptic duodenitis (CPD) (Figs. 3.27 and 3.28). The metaplasia is a consequence of chronic acid exposure from upstream pathology (e.g., *H. pylori*) rather than local. Be aware that CPD may be endoscopically nodular or even polypoid. In these cases, a diagnosis of "nodular chronic peptic duodenitis" or "polypoid chronic peptic duodenitis" gives appropriate pathologic correlation to the endoscopist.

KEY FEATURES: Gastric Heterotopia

- Gastric heterotopia is found in **1.9% of duodenal biopsies, two-thirds of which are in the bulb**.
- Histologically, lesions are composed of **specialized gastric parietal cells, chief cells, and surface foveolar epithelium**.
- Lesions are most commonly incidental **small islands**, but can be large nodular or polypoid **masses up to 6 cm**.
- Rarely, patients may present with iron deficiency anemia and resection is curative.

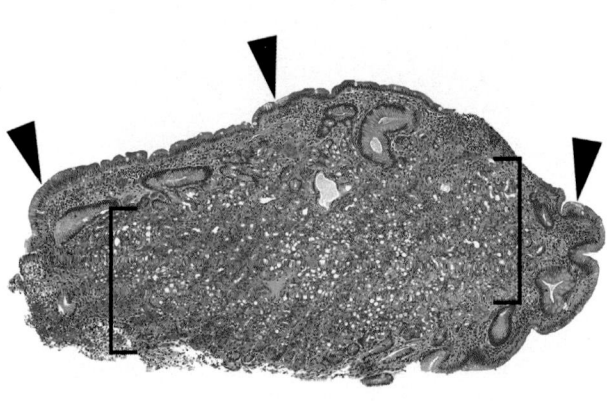
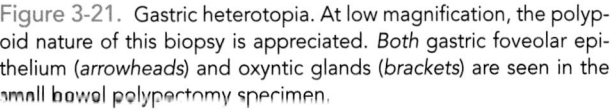

Figure 3-21. Gastric heterotopia. At low magnification, the polypoid nature of this biopsy is appreciated. *Both* gastric foveolar epithelium (*arrowheads*) and oxyntic glands (*brackets*) are seen in the small bowel polypectomy specimen.

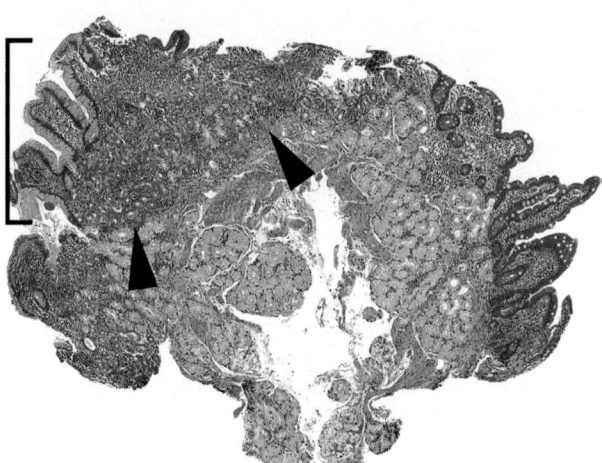

Figure 3-22. Gastric heterotopia. This polypoid duodenal biopsy shows surface foveolar epithelium (*bracket*) that appears pale as compared with normal small bowel surface epithelium (far right). In the deeper lamina propria, gastric oxyntic glands (*arrowheads*) are present and contrast against the pale Brunner glands (far right) normally found in this anatomic site.

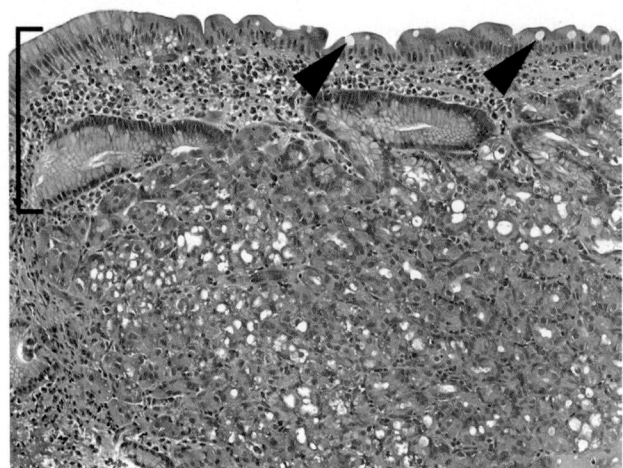

Figure 3-23. Gastric heterotopia. The normal small bowel surface epithelium contains interspersed goblet cells (*arrowheads*) that punctuate a row of columnar enterocytes. By comparison, gastric foveolar epithelium (*bracket*) contains pale apical mucin vacuoles. This appearance has been likened to piano keys or a French tip manicure. Deep in this biopsy, gastric oxyntic glands are present.

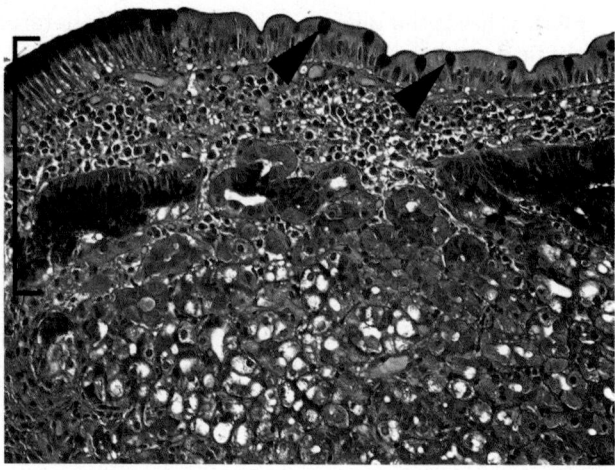

Figure 3-24. Gastric heterotopia, PAS stain of the previous figure. Although gastric heterotopia is an H&E diagnosis, this stain can accentuate the contrast between normal and heterotopic areas in challenging cases. The PAS stain is picked up by both goblet cells (*arrowheads*) and gastric foveolar mucin (*bracket*).

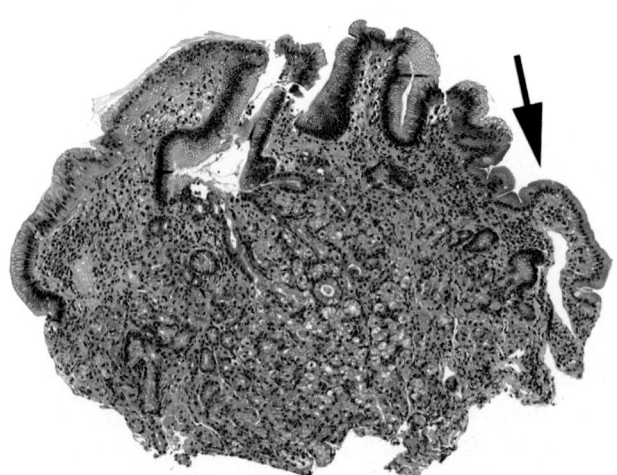

Figure 3-25. Gastric heterotopia. This low-power biopsy shows surface gastric foveolar cells with pale apical mucin caps and deep gastric oxyntic glands. At the far right, normal small bowel surface epithelium (*arrow*) is present for comparison.

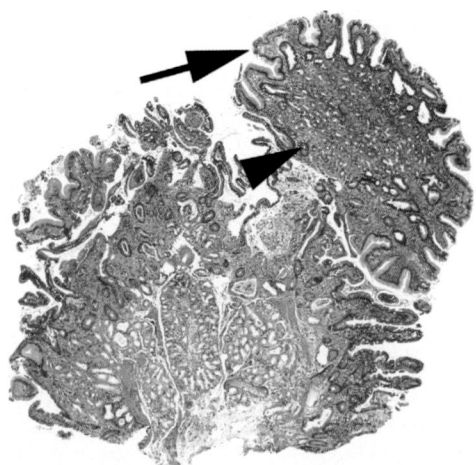

Figure 3-26. Gastric heterotopia. Lesions can be flat, nodular, or polypoid, as in this case. This example is a low-power H&E diagnosis, with pale surface gastric foveolar epithelium (*arrow*) contrasting against the eosinophilic appearance of the background normal small bowel surface and the presence of gastric oxyntic glands in the lamina propria (*arrowhead*) contrasting against deep pale Brunner glands.

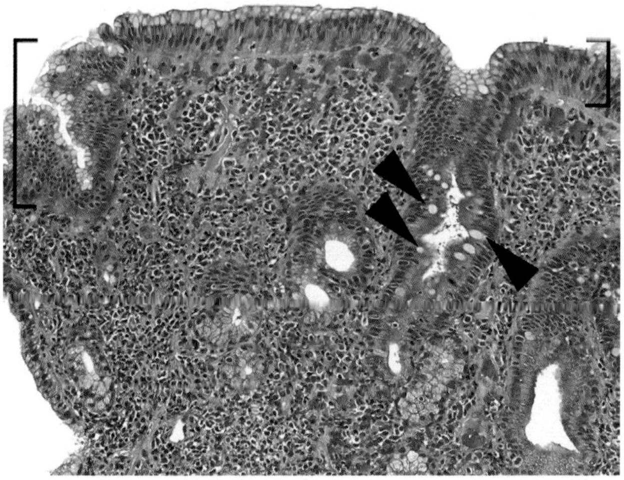

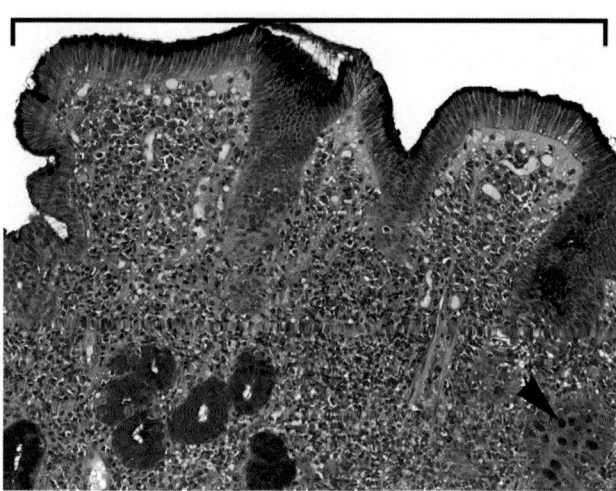

Figure 3-27. Chronic peptic duodenitis. When surface foveo-lar epithelium (*bracket*) is found in the absence of gastric oxyntic glands, consider chronic peptic duodenitis, which is a *metaplastic* condition caused by chronic acid exposure from upstream pathol-ogy (e.g., *H. pylori*). Normal small bowel epithelium with goblet cells (*arrowheads*) is adjacent.

Figure 3-28. Chronic peptic duodenitis, PAS stain of the previ-ous figure. The surface mucin cell metaplasia (*bracket*) picks up the PAS stain diffusely compared with the single scattered goblet cells (*arrowhead*) found in normal small bowel mucosa.

HYPERPLASTIC

Brunner Gland Proliferative Lesion (Hyperplasia, Hamartoma, or Adenoma)

Polyps or nodules composed predominantly of Brunner glands fall into several catego-ries that are frequently indistinguishable histologically. These Brunner gland polyps are found most commonly in the duodenum (recall, the jejunum and ileum lack Brunner glands entirely), although they have been reported in other parts of the small bowel.[12] Brunner gland polyps comprise 5% to 10% of lesions found in the proximal small bowel.[13] Endoscopically, these lesions are polypoid (Fig. 3.29), pedunculated, or submucosal; are found equally among men and women most commonly in the fifth or sixth decades; and vary in size up to 6 cm.[13] Patients with larger lesions may present with GI bleed, obstruc-tion, and jaundice, but in the largest study, 25% were incidental.[13] Under normal con-ditions, Brunner glands are found in the submucosa of the duodenum, are composed of cuboidal cells with abundant foamy clear cytoplasm, and contain basally located nuclei, which may be round or slightly flattened; the appearance is similar to pyloric glands (Figs. 3.11–3.13). By comparison, Brunner gland hyperplasia shows increased submucosal Brunner glands with extension into the lamina propria (Figs. 3.30–3.32), Brunner gland hamartomas are nodular aggregates of submucosal Brunner glands with abundant smooth muscle bands (and sometimes other elements such as fat) and are frequently well circum-scribed (Figs. 3.33–3.38), whereas Brunner gland adenomas show cytologic atypia (Figs. 3.39–3.41). Although this categorization seems fairly straightforward and the literature on this subject has similarly divided Brunner gland proliferations into hyperplasia, hamartoma, and adenoma groupings, there is considerable histologic overlap resulting in difficulty at the scope. For example, Brunner gland hyperplasia is primarily found in CPD, in which repeat cycles of peptic injury and reparative changes result in Brunner glands extending from their normal submucosal location to involve the lamina propria. Yet, large areas of Brunner gland hyperplasia may be encountered independently of CPD, indicating it is not always a reparative process. In addition, when hyperplastic lesions are large, prolapse changes can result in streaming thickened smooth muscle bundles (Fig. 3.32), a feature that overlaps with Brunner gland hamartomas. Finally, Brunner gland adenomas are described to have nuclear atypia, a challenging and sometimes contentious subjective criterion, and examples found in the literature are limited to single case reports or small case series and are morphologically heterogeneous.[12,14-16] These areas of histologic overlap and diagnostic difficulty make definitive classification unfeasible in most cases. To address this problem,

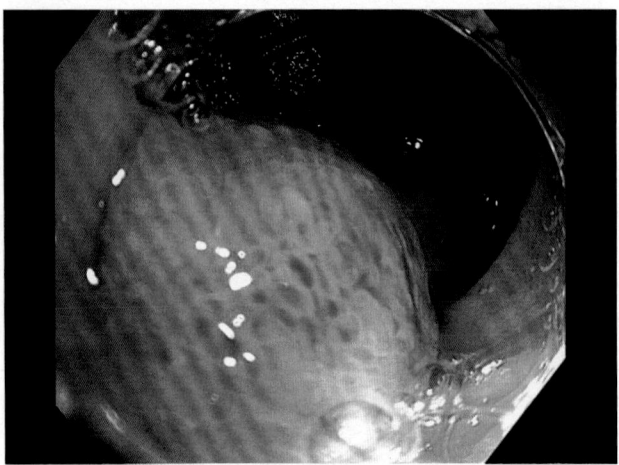

Figure 3-29. Brunner gland proliferative lesion, endoscopic photo. These lesions are found most commonly in the duodenum and are polypoid, as seen here, pedunculated, or submucosal.

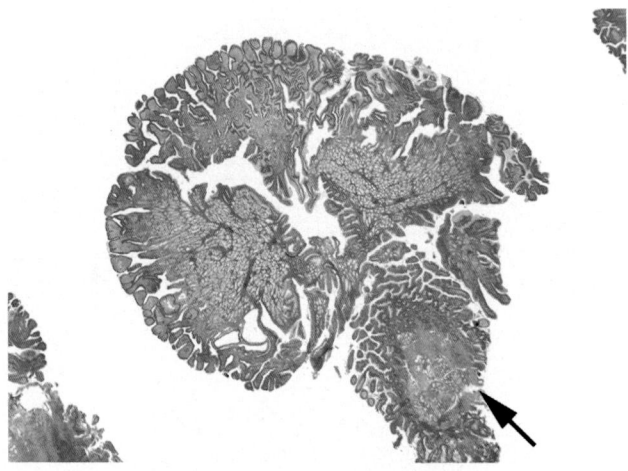

Figure 3-30. Brunner gland hyperplasia. At low magnification, this mucosal-based proliferation of Brunner glands is a pedunculated lesion, with a polyp stalk (*arrow*). Note the expansion of the lamina propria by tightly clustered glands with pale clear cytoplasm.

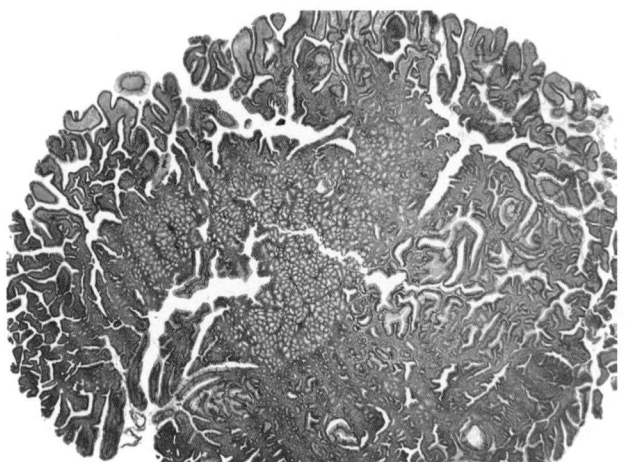

Figure 3-31. Brunner gland hyperplasia, higher magnification of the previous figure. The tightly clustered Brunner glands are fairly uniform is size and shape and have abundant pale clear cytoplasm, evident even at low magnification.

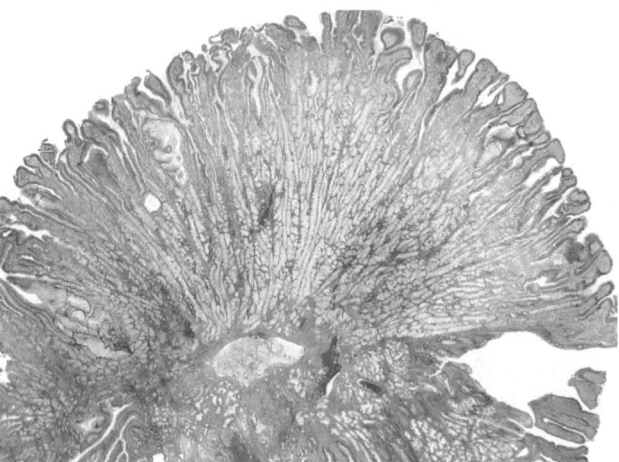

Figure 3-32. Brunner gland hyperplasia. The abundant pale Brunner glands in this example are tightly packed within the mucosa. The streaming appearance is likely due to prolapse of the lesion into the small bowel lumen.

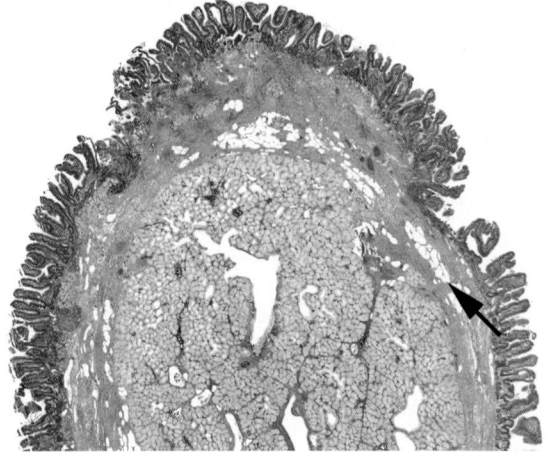

Figure 3-33. Brunner gland hamartoma. The low-power image shows a submucosal nodule of tightly packed pale Brunner glands. Adipose tissue (*arrow*) is also admixed with this lesion, suggesting it is most likely a hamartoma rather than hyperplasia or adenoma.

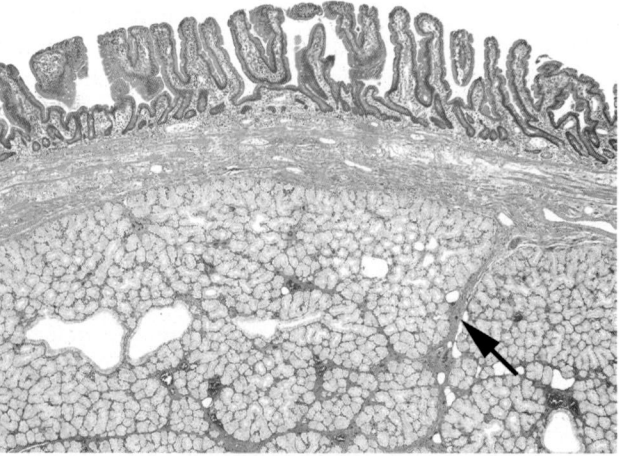

Figure 3-34. Brunner gland hamartoma. Another field of the previous lesion shows the submucosal lesion also contains bands of smooth muscle (*arrow*).

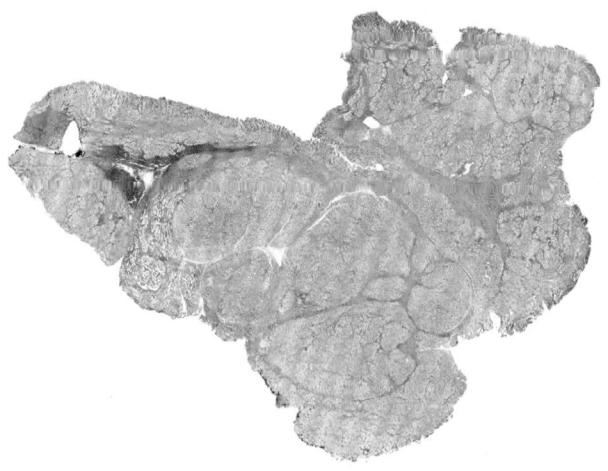

Figure 3-35. Brunner gland hamartoma. These proliferative lesions can achieve sizes up to 6 cm and extend deep when submucosal-based. At low magnification, the pale clusters of Brunner glands are separated into lobules by bands of smooth muscle.

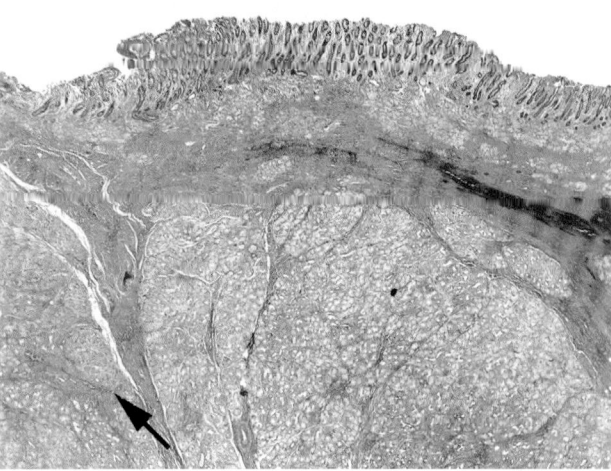

Figure 3-36. Brunner gland hamartoma. Higher magnification of the previous lesion shows sheets and clusters of pale Brunner glands. The individual glands are uniform in size and shape, and ducts are present (*arrow*).

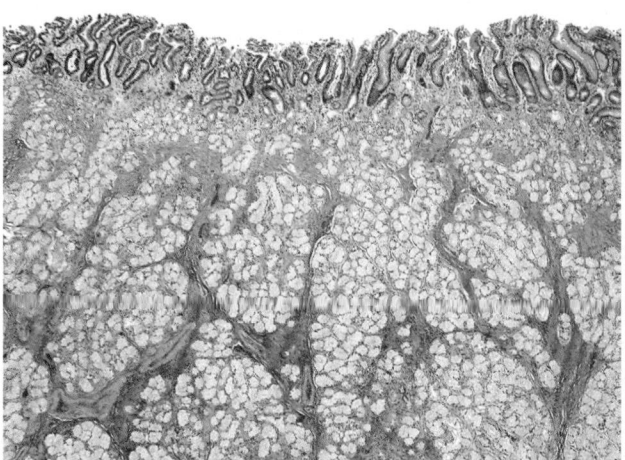

Figure 3-37. Brunner gland hamartoma. This Brunner gland proliferation involves both the mucosa and submucosa and contains bands of smooth muscle.

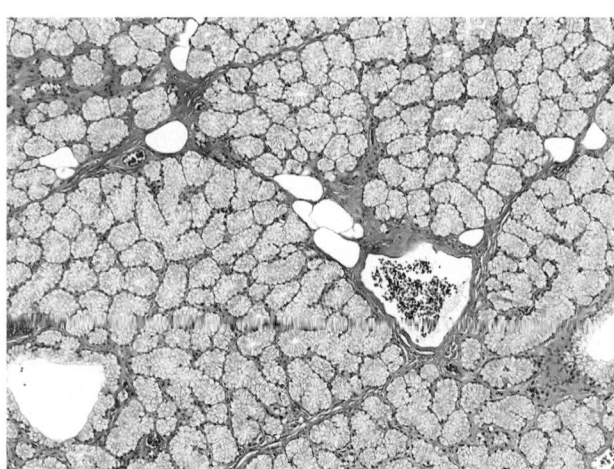

Figure 3-38. Brunner gland hamartoma. In all Brunner gland proliferative lesions, the characteristic feature is an excess of Brunner glands, which are composed of bland cells with abundant clear-to-foamy cytoplasm and small round or flattened nuclei at the periphery.

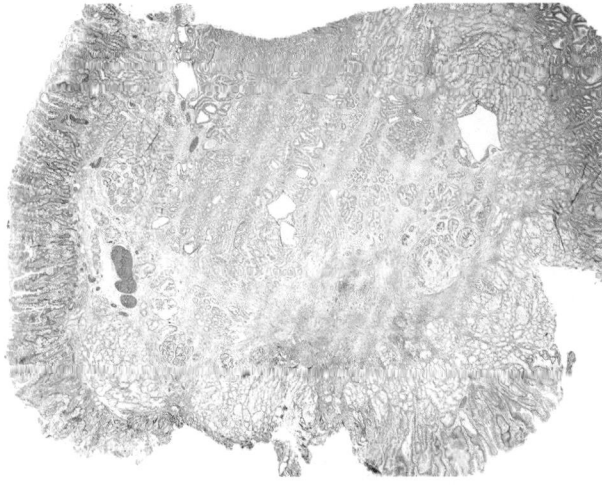

Figure 3-39. Brunner gland adenoma. Brunner gland adenomas show nuclear atypia, but this feature can be subjective, at best. For this reason, and because follow-up studies show no recurrence after local excision, a more general term such as "Brunner gland polyp" or "Brunner gland proliferative lesion" is sufficient at signout.

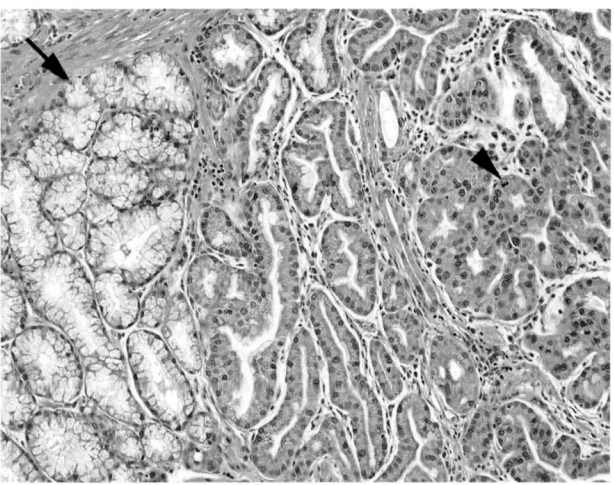

Figure 3-40. Brunner gland adenoma, higher magnification of the previous figure. This area contrasts the atypical Brunner glands (an *arrowhead* highlights a mitotic figure) adjacent to normal Brunner glands (*arrow*).

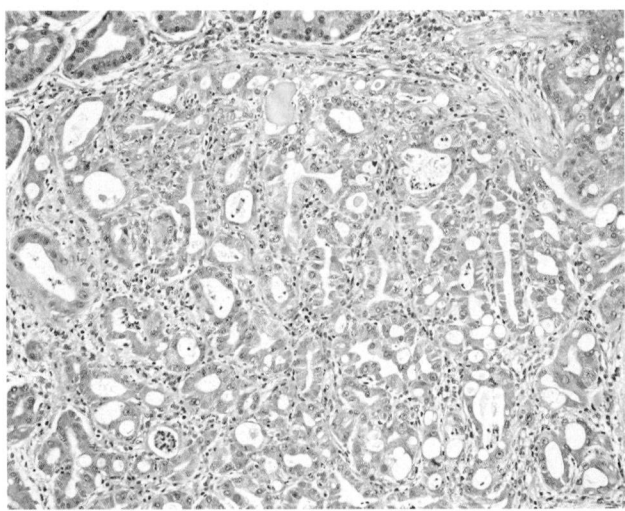

Figure 3-41. Brunner gland adenoma, another area of the previous figure. This area shows glandular disarray and crowding in addition to enlarged nuclei. This Brunner gland proliferative lesion shows unequivocal atypia.

some authors use an encompassing term "Brunner gland proliferating lesion," whereas others simply state "Brunner gland polyp."[13] This sensible approach eases signout aggravation and is supported by follow-up studies showing no recurrence after local excision among lesions without overt high-grade dysplasia or malignancy.[13] Malignancy arising from Brunner gland lesions are exceedingly rare and found only as single case reports.[17-21] One case report details transformation to carcinoma following 17 years of observation, again supporting conservative diagnosis and management owing to long latency.[20] Overlapping morphologic, immunohistochemical, and genetic features (GNAS mutations) with pyloric gland adenomas have been observed among carcinomas and adenomas arising adjacent to Brunner glands[22,23] (see "Pyloric Gland Adenoma" section).

FAQ: What is the difference between Brunner gland hyperplasia and CPD?

A distinction is made between Brunner gland hyperplasia and CPD when other features of peptic change are identifiable. In the proximal small bowel, repeat cycles of peptic injury and repair result in several features, including Brunner glands extending from their normal submucosal location to involve the lamina propria, gastric foveolar (mucin cell) metaplasia of the surface epithelium, increased chronic inflammation with or without intraepithelial lymphocytosis, and mild villous blunting. Neutrophils and erosions may also be present in acute cases. In CPD, the function of Brunner gland hyperplasia is to increase the number of alkaline-secreting glands for neutralization of abnormally high acid levels due to some upstream pathologic process (e.g., *H. pylori*). Thus, *CPD is a clinically important clue to upstream pathology*, whereas the term *Brunner gland hyperplasia is a nonspecific descriptor*. Take note that CPD can result in a nodular or polypoid appearance of the small bowel, similar to Brunner gland proliferative lesions; these may be designated as nodular or polypoid CPD when appropriate.

SAMPLE NOTE: Brunner Gland Proliferative Lesion (Hyperplasia, Hamartoma, or Adenoma)

Duodenum, Polyp, Biopsy

Brunner gland proliferative lesion, negative for high-grade dysplasia or malignancy, see Comment.

Comment
Histologic sections show polypoid small bowel mucosa with a proliferation of Brunner glands separated into small lobules by smooth muscle. Brunner gland lesions are categorized as hyperplasia, hamartoma, or adenoma, but histologic distinction is frequently irresolvable, as in this case, and thus some experts use a simplified nomenclature of "Brunner gland proliferative lesion." Local excision is curative, as follow-up studies show no recurrence among lesions lacking overt high-grade dysplasia or malignancy.

References:
Levine JA, Burgart LJ, Batts KP, Wang KK. Brunner's gland hamartomas: clinical presentation and pathological features of 27 cases. *Am J Gastroenterol.* 1995;90(2):290-294.

Kim K, Jang SJ, Song HJ, Yu E. Clinicopathologic characteristics and mucin expression in Brunner's gland proliferating lesions. *Dig Dis Sci.* 2013;58(1):194-201.

KEY FEATURES: Brunner Gland Proliferative Lesions

- Brunner gland proliferative lesions encompass **hyperplasias, hamartomas, and adenomas**.
- These may be encountered as **nodules, polyps, or masses** in the duodenum.
- In large examples, patients present with GI bleed, obstruction, and jaundice, but up to **25% are found incidentally**.
- Histologically, Brunner glands are composed of cuboidal cells with clear foamy cytoplasm and small round or flattened nuclei basally located.
- In proliferative lesions, Brunner glands extend from the normal submucosal location to **involve the lamina propria** and may be **separated into lobules by smooth muscle and vascular septae**.
- Brunner gland **hyperplasia** can be **isolated** or, **when found with other features of peptic injury, should be reported as CPD**.
- Brunner gland **hamartomas** may include additional **hamartomatous elements, such as fat**.
- Brunner gland **adenomas** are cited to have **nuclear atypia**.
- **It can be impossible to differentiate these lesions** confidently, and an inclusive diagnosis of Brunner gland proliferative lesion is reasonable.
- In the absence of high-grade dysplasia or carcinoma, **local excision is curative**.

HAMARTOMATOUS POLYPS AND SYNDROMIC CONSIDERATIONS

Hamartomatous polyps result from disordered growth of tissues native to the site and can arise from any of the three embryonic layers. These lesions are frequently, but not universally, associated with a clinical syndrome. In the small bowel, such lesions have such highly characteristic and consistent features that even in the modern era of germline testing, histologic confirmation of hamartomatous polyps remains sufficient to meet clinical criteria for conditions such as Peutz-Jeghers syndrome or juvenile polyposis syndrome. As a result, familiarity with the morphologic features and diagnostic criteria is important for optimum management and outcomes for patients and their families. This section covers disease-defining hamartomatous polyps, also discussed in "Stomach" chapter, including Peutz-Jeghers syndrome, juvenile polyposis syndrome, Cronkhite-Canada syndrome, and Cowden (PTEN hamartoma tumor) syndrome.

Peutz-Jeghers Polyp

Peutz-Jeghers syndrome is characterized by hamartomatous polyps of the GI tract and melanocytic mucocutaneous hyperpigmentation.[24] Up to 25% of documented cases are sporadic, but this condition is best known as an autosomal dominant inherited syndrome, with 80% of affected families harboring a germline mutation in the *STK11/LKB1* gene.[25,26] Patients with Peutz-Jeghers syndrome have a 93% cumulative lifetime risk for cancer, including carcinomas of the GI tract, breast, ovary, and testis.[27-29] In this context, early recognition of the syndrome allows for appropriate screening and surveillance for patients and family members. World Health Organization (WHO) criteria for the clinical diagnosis of Peutz-Jeghers syndrome are:

1. Detection of three or more histologically confirmed Peutz-Jeghers polyps.
   or
2. The presence of *any number* of Peutz-Jeghers polyps in a patient with a family history of the syndrome.
   or
3. Detection of characteristic, prominent mucocutaneous pigmentation in the patient with a family history of the syndrome.
   or
4. Detection of *any number* of Peutz-Jeghers polyps in a patient with prominent mucocutaneous pigmentation.[30]

Three of the aforementioned four potential methods of diagnosis include histologic identification of Peutz-Jeghers polyps, making pathologic recognition a necessary skill. These hamartomatous polyps have an easy-to-recognize characteristic appearance, showing compactly spaced glands supported by an arborizing framework of well-developed smooth muscle that is contiguous with the muscularis mucosae (Figs. 3.42–3.51). The small bowel is the most common site for Peutz-Jeghers polyps (64%), followed by the colon (53%) and stomach (15% to 20%).[31] These lesions of the small bowel and colon are not only more common but also highly distinctive; their intact lamina propria with arborizing smooth muscle fibers helps differentiate them from juvenile polyps, unlike their gastric counterparts (discussed further in "Stomach" chapter), which are routinely indistinguishable from nonspecific gastric hyperplastic polyps or other syndromic gastric polyps.[32] This smooth muscle framework may result in a characteristic lobulated appearance of the otherwise normal-appearing background mucosa (Figs. 3.52–3.54).[33] Characteristic histology is less frequently seen in small (<1 cm) polyps, and these lesions can be indistinguishable from other hamartomatous lesions, such as juvenile polyps or inflammatory/retention polyps. Dysplasia is rarely found in these polyps (Figs. 3.55 and 3.56), but patients with the syndrome have significant risk for malignancy elsewhere, including gastric adenocarcinoma outside of the polyp.[34] These patients are important to recognize because of their high life-time risk of malignancy, including tubular GI carcinomas, pancreatic carcinoma, Sertoli cell tumors of the testes, minimal deviation adenocarcinoma (adenoma malignum) of the uterine cervix, sex cord tumor with annular tubules of the ovaries, and breast carcinomas. Screening and surveillance for these patients start at age 30 years with bidirectional endoscopy every 2 years and annual pelvic, testicular, and pancreatic ultrasound imaging with annual mammography.

FAQ: I have a patient with a single *classic* Peutz-Jeghers polyp, but this patient has no other polyps or family history of Peutz-Jeghers syndrome. What does this mean?

Rare instances of patients with isolated sporadic Peutz-Jeghers polyps have been documented. In nearly all instances, these patients had clinical histories suggesting Peutz-Jeghers syndrome (e.g., concurrent pancreatic cancer, family GI cancer history, metachronous tumors) but failed to meet the WHO criteria. Thus, isolated or sporadic Peutz-Jeghers polyps may occur, but clinicians should be advised that these patients seem to have a cumulative lifetime risk of malignancy similar to those with the syndrome.[35]

FAQ: Are Peutz-Jeghers polyps dysplastic?

Although patients with Peutz-Jeghers polyps have a near 90% life-time risk of malignancy, the malignancies do not arise within the hamartomatous polyps. These hamartomatous polyps are rarely dysplastic (Figs. 3.55 and 3.56).

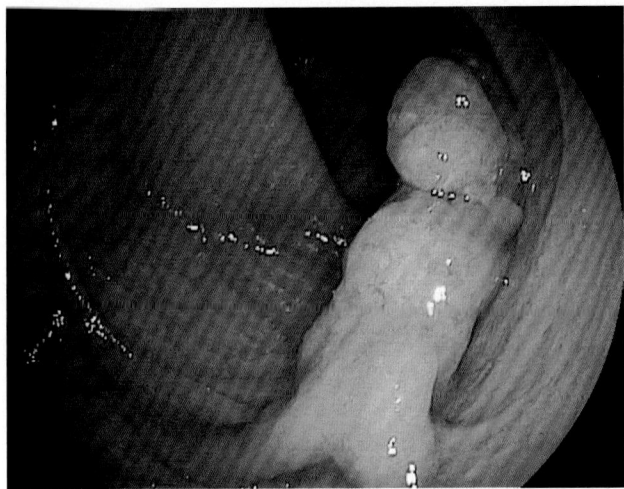

Figure 3-42. Peutz-Jeghers polyp, endoscopic photo. This small bowel polyp is multilobulated and appears to branch. Histologically, its central core will show an arborizing network of smooth muscle connected to the muscularis mucosae.

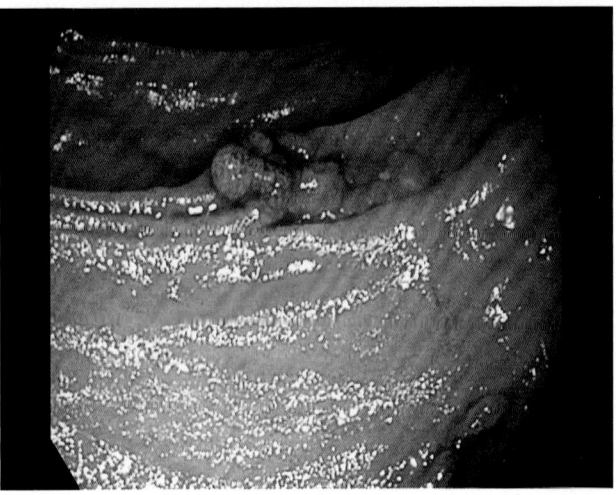

Figure 3-43. Peutz-Jeghers polyp, endoscopic photo. The archetypical lesion for this syndrome is found in the small bowel, where it shows a branching central core composed of smooth muscle. Endoscopically, these lesions may have a multilobulated appearance.

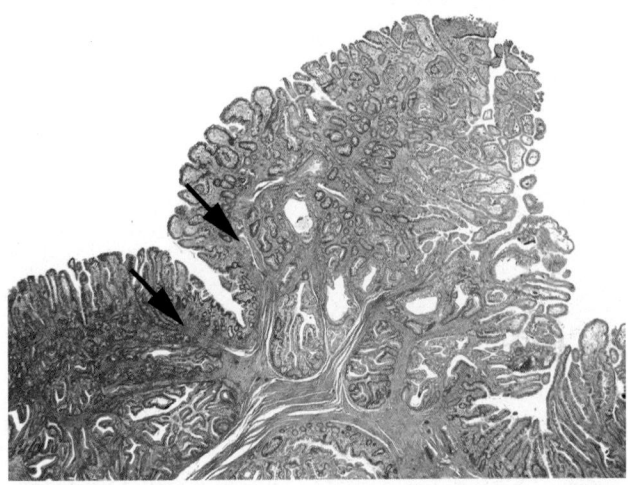

Figure 3-44. Peutz-Jeghers polyp. This example shows a lobulated architecture at low power, with bands of arborizing smooth muscle (arrows).

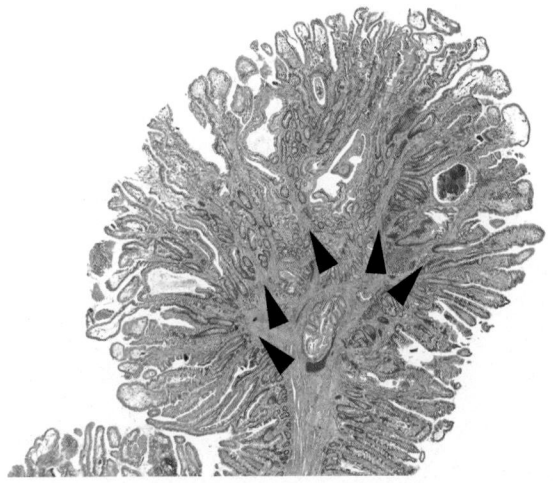

Figure 3-45. Peutz-Jeghers polyp. Lesions have a central core of smooth muscle that branches outward in many directions (arrowheads).

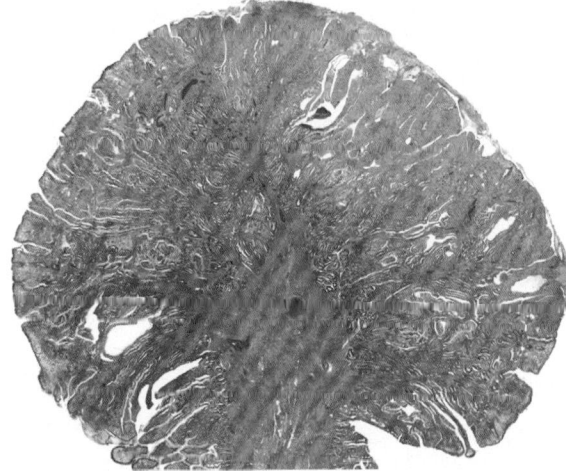

Figure 3-46. Peutz-Jeghers (PJ) polyp. This round PJ polyp has a thick central stalk with branches of smooth muscle extending outward, imparting a silhouette of an oak tree.

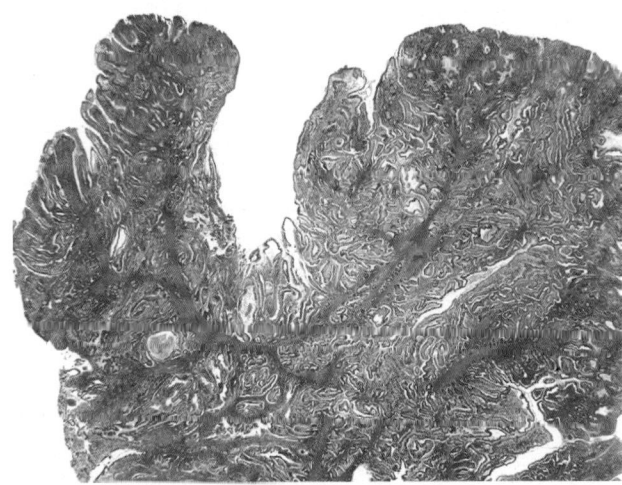

Figure 3-47. Peutz-Jeghers polyp. Branches of the smooth muscle may produce broad fingerlike projections. Despite variations in shape, the unifying feature is the branching smooth muscle core.

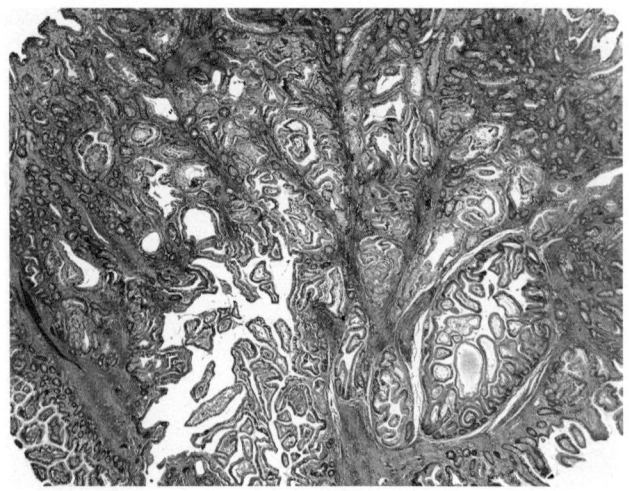

Figure 3-48. Peutz-Jeghers polyp. The smooth muscle is intimately associated with normal glandular structures. Although some may be dilated, there is a normal ratio of crypts to lamina propria.

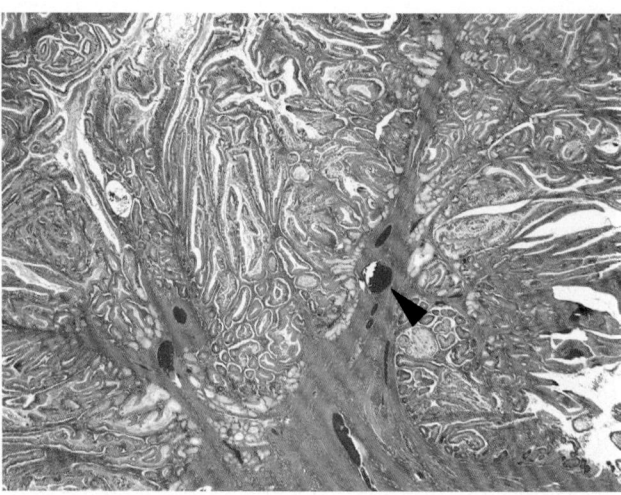

Figure 3-49. Peutz-Jeghers polyp. The smooth muscle core is connected to the muscularis mucosae and can contain larger vessels (*arrowhead*) than normally seen in the mucosa. Note that the ratio of glandular epithelium to lamina propria is within normal range, which is in contrast to other hamartomatous polyps that contain an excess of lamina propria (e.g., juvenile polyps and Cronkhite-Canada syndrome polyps).

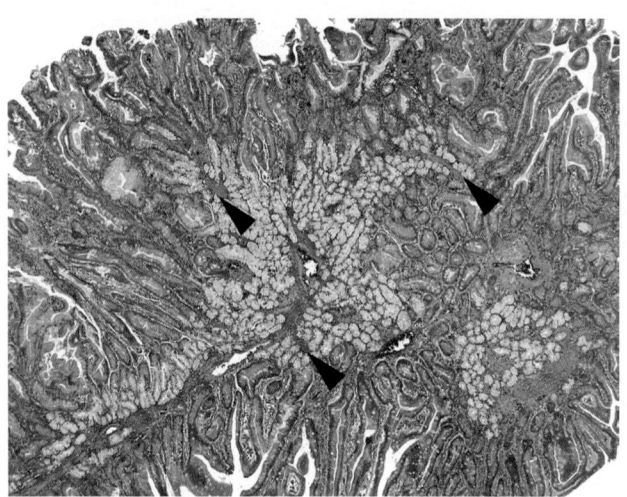

Figure 3-50. Peutz-Jeghers polyp. This polyp bears resemblance to the Brunner gland proliferative lesions discussed in the previous section, in particular Fig. 3.31, which contains a similar dense aggregate of intramucosal Brunner glands. This polyp, however, was resected from a patient with known Peutz-Jeghers syndrome and contains branching smooth muscle bands (*arrowheads*).

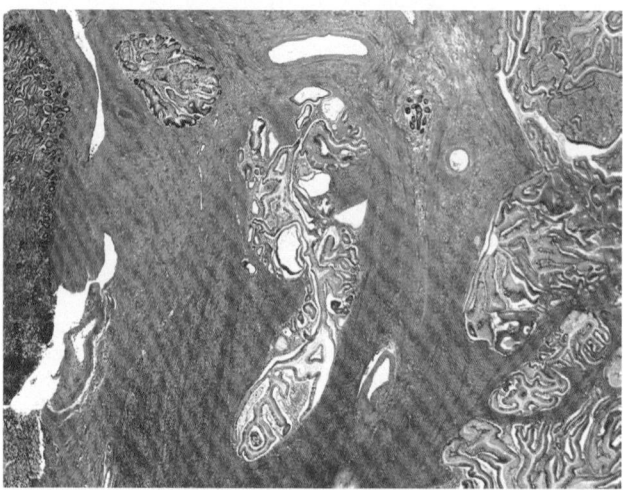

Figure 3-51. Peutz-Jeghers polyp. Entrapped crypts and lamina propria can be found at the polyp stalk. The bland and lobulated appearance is a clue to their benign nature.

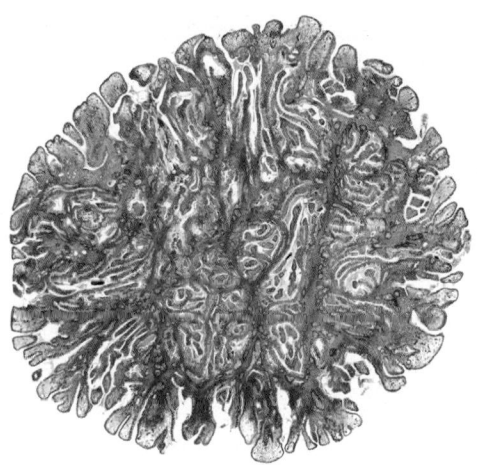

Figure 3-52. Peutz-Jeghers polyp. Transverse sections such as this one allow one to peer downward through the head of the polyp, which accentuates the characteristic lobulated appearance described in some studies.

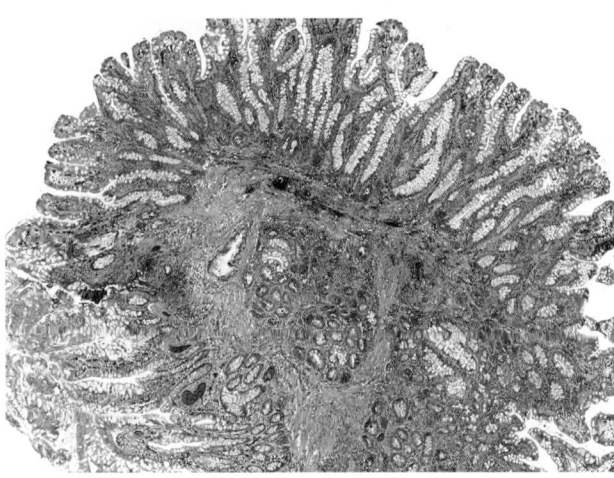

Figure 3-53. Peutz-Jeghers polyp. A tangential cut through a PJ polyp shows the arborizing smooth muscle wrapping around lobules of crypts and lamina propria.

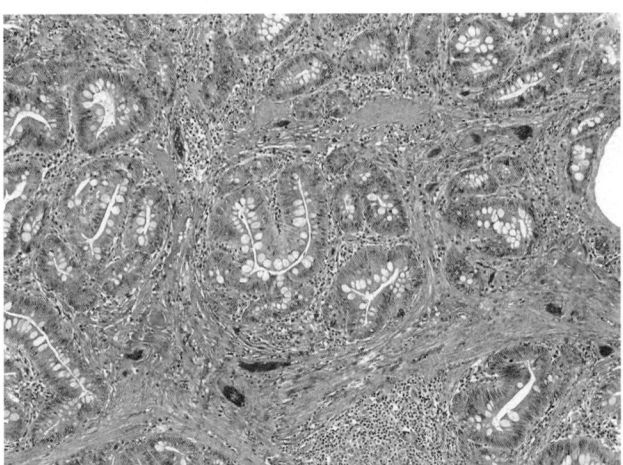

Figure 3-54. Peutz-Jeghers polyp. Small lobules of crypts are enveloped by bands of smooth muscle, a characteristic feature found in many PJ polyps.

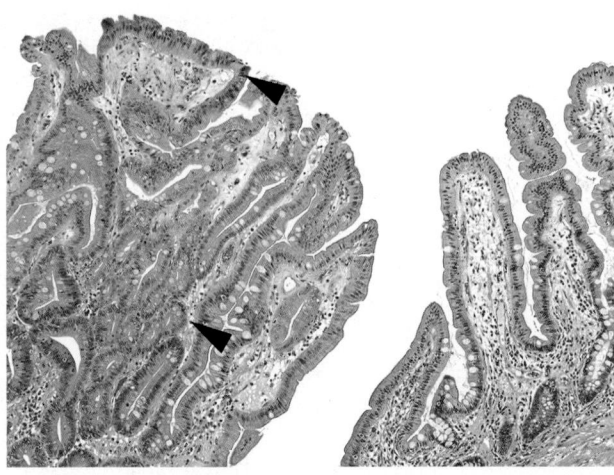

Figure 3-55. Low-grade dysplasia arising in a Peutz-Jeghers polyp. Dysplasia is rare in PJ polyps, but do not forget to look for it. The left side of this photo shows low-grade dysplasia arising within a PJ polyp, with nondysplastic small bowel mucosa for contrast to the right. The dysplastic area shows hyperchromasia, nuclear crowding, and nuclear stratification extending to the surface epithelium (*arrowheads*).

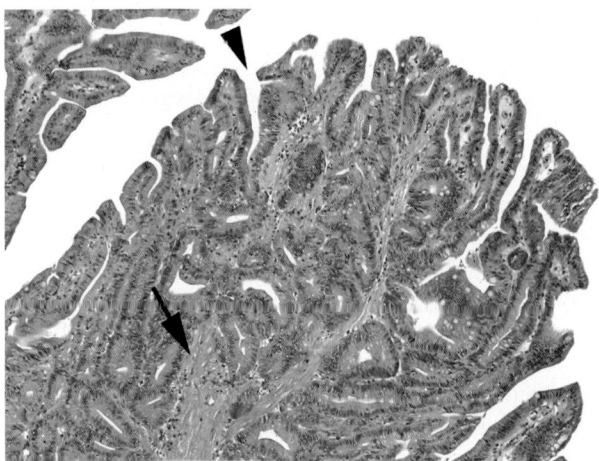

Figure 3-56. Low-grade dysplasia arising in a Peutz-Jeghers polyp. An abrupt transition (*arrowhead*) from nondysplastic to low-grade dysplasia is seen in this PJ polyp. Not the central core of arborizing smooth muscle (*arrow*).

SAMPLE NOTE: Isolated Peutz-Jeghers Polyp in a Patient Without Known Peutz-Jeghers Syndrome

Small Bowel, Polyp, Polypectomy

- Hamartomatous polyp, Peutz-Jeghers type, see Note.

Note: Histologic sections show classic morphology for Peutz-Jeghers polyp, including a central core of branching smooth muscle dividing lobular compartments of mucosa. Correlation with clinical findings, such as mucocutaneous pigmentation (perioral or intraoral) and any other GI polyps found on bidirectional endoscopy (including prior encounters) would be of interest to evaluate for Peutz-Jeghers syndrome. In one study, patients with isolated or sporadic Peutz-Jeghers polyps demonstrated a cumulative lifetime risk of malignancy similar to those with the syndrome.

Reference:
Burkart AL, Sheridan T, Lewin M, Fenton H, Ali NJ, Montgomery E. Do sporadic Peutz-Jeghers polyps exist? Experience of a large teaching hospital. *Am J Surg Pathol.* 2007;31(8):1209-1214.

PEARLS & PITFALLS

Oral mucocutaneous pigmentation characteristic of Peutz-Jeghers syndrome is often less prominent as individuals age. Careful examination of the intraoral mucosa may be required in older patients.

KEY FEATURES: Peutz-Jeghers Syndrome

- About **80%** of patients have defect in **STK11** (formerly *LKB1*) inherited **autosomal dominantly.**
- It most commonly affects the **small bowel**, but the polyps can occur anywhere along the GI tract.
- Hamartomatous syndromic polyps have a **central core of arborizing smooth muscle** dividing lobular compartments of otherwise normal-appearing mucosa.
- Classic morphology is uncommon in small polyps (<1 cm) or in gastric or colonic sites.
- There is **greater than 90% life-time risk of malignancy**, even among those who fail to meet criteria for the syndrome.
- **Hamartomatous polyps** *rarely* **contain dysplasia,** and malignancy associated with this syndrome are at other sites (tubular GI carcinomas, pancreatic carcinoma, Sertoli cell tumors of the testes, minimal deviation adenocarcinoma [adenoma malignum] of the uterine cervix, sex cord tumor with annular tubules of the ovaries, and breast carcinomas).

Juvenile Polyp

Juvenile polyposis syndrome, the most common of the hamartomatous polyposis syndromes, affects one in 100,000. The syndrome is largely sporadic but can be inherited as autosomal dominant familial syndrome (30%).[36] Both inherited and sporadic forms share similar genetics, with germline mutations in *SMAD4* (also known as *DPC4*) (15%) and the related gene *BMPR1A* (25%), whereas *ENG* is associated with early childhood presentation.[37,38] These genetic changes cause a disruption in the transforming growth factor beta signal transduction pathway and result in an increased risk of malignancy. The overall risk of GI malignancies in these patients is 55%, with colorectal cancer presenting at an average age of 37 years.[39,40] The characteristic hamartomatous polyps can be limited to the colorectum in some patients but can also be found anywhere along the GI tract, as reflected in the WHO criteria for diagnosis.

The following are the WHO criteria for the clinical diagnosis of juvenile polyposis syndrome:

1. More than three to five juvenile polyps of the colorectum.
or
2. Juvenile polyps throughout the GI tract.
or
3. Any number of juvenile polyps with a family history of juvenile polyposis.[41]

Like Peutz-Jeghers polyps, juvenile polyps are classified as hamartomatous lesions, but their histologic profiles differ. Juvenile polyps consist primarily of an excess of lamina propria and show abundant distorted and dilated glands (Figs. 3.57–3.60). The combination of lamina propria edema and abundance of distended, mucus-filled glands in combination with inflammatory cells is occasionally mistaken for "inflammatory" or "retention" polyp. This is understandable because solitary or sporadic juvenile polyps may be indistinguishable from inflammatory/retention polyps in either the upper or lower GI tract (Figs. 3.61–3.63). Fortunately, and in contrast to sporadic Peutz-Jeghers polyps, there is no documented increased lifetime risk for malignancy reported for sporadic juvenile polyps. Nevertheless, foci of dysplasia are regularly seen in juvenile polyps, underscoring their neoplastic potential and the value of recognition. In the absence of sufficient clinical history, and when the histology precludes definitive classification, patients benefit from a more inclusive diagnosis, such as "juvenile/inflammatory polyp" and a careful note. When multiple similar polyps are encountered, the possibility of a polyposis syndrome should be stated. Other syndromes involving hamartomatous GI polyps should be ruled out clinically or by pathologic examination.

PEARLS & PITFALLS: Juvenile Polyps Appear Similar to Cronkhite-Canada Syndrome

Juvenile polyps and polyps of Cronkhite-Canada syndrome are virtually impossible to differentiate histologically. Both contain an excess of lamina propria containing inflammatory cells and dilated glands. The key to differentiating these two conditions is found in the intervening nonpolypoid mucosa. This nonpolypoid mucosa is essentially normal in juvenile polyposis syndrome in contrast to that of Cronkhite-Canada syndrome, which appears edematous and similar to polypoid areas.

KEY FEATURES: Juvenile Polyposis Syndrome

- About **30%** of cases are inherited in an **autosomal dominant** pattern with defects in *SMAD4* **or** *BMPR1A*.
- Most cases are **sporadic.**
- Syndromic polyp is the **hamartomatous polyp/inflammatory-type polyp** with excessive lamina propria, inflammatory cells, and distorted glands.
- Polyps can be indistinguishable from the other syndromic and sporadic hamartomatous/inflammatory-type polyps.

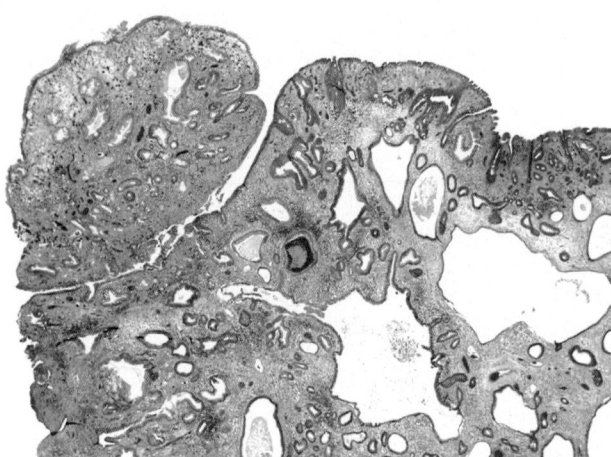

Figure 3-57. Juvenile polyp. At low magnification, these lesions may be multilobulated and have broad fingerlike projections. Crypts are dilated and distorted, with unusual shapes embedded within an excess of lamina propria.

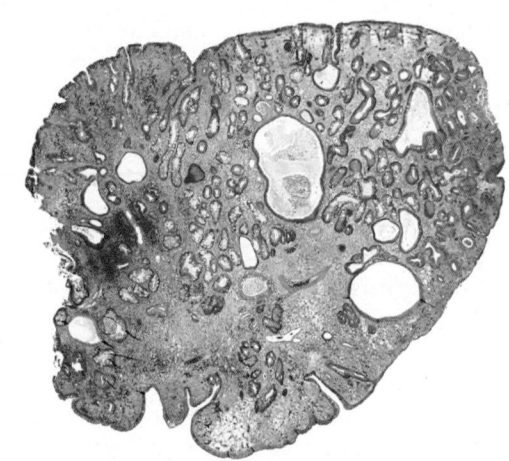

Figure 3-58. Juvenile polyp. Characteristic dilated distorted crypts are associated with excess pale lamina propria. The surface may be eroded with adjacent reactive/regenerative epithelial changes that appear hyperchromatic at low magnification.

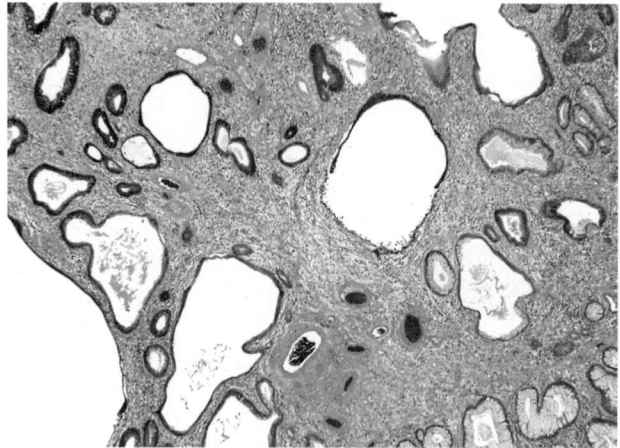

Figure 3-59. Juvenile polyp. The glandular epithelium is bland and surrounded by abundant lamina propria. The ratio of crypts to lamina propria is close to 1:1 in this example.

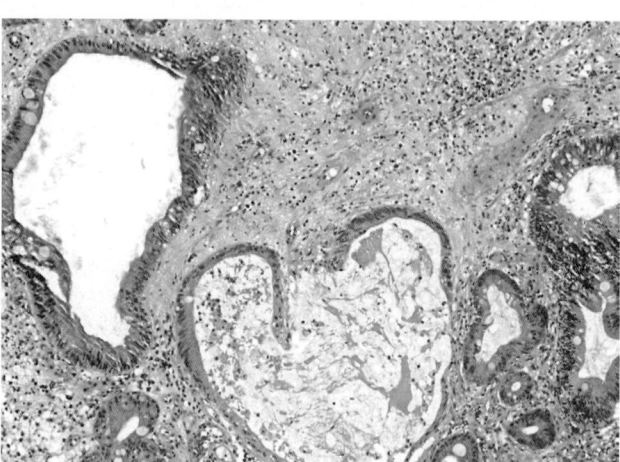

Figure 3-60. Juvenile polyp. The lamina propria appears edematous and contains a mixed inflammatory cell infiltrate of variable density.

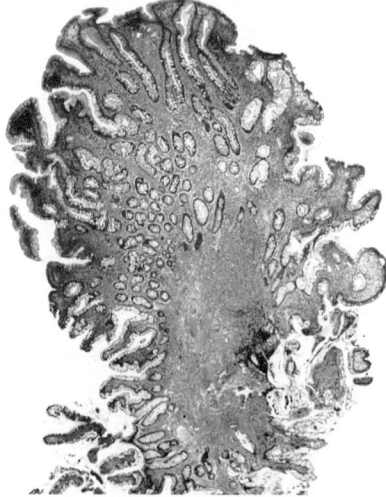

Figure 3-61. Juvenile polyp. Some juvenile polyps are indistinguishable from inflammatory polyps, as in this lesion, which was resected from a patient with documented juvenile polyposis syndrome. There is a slight excess of lamina propria and some mildly distorted crypts.

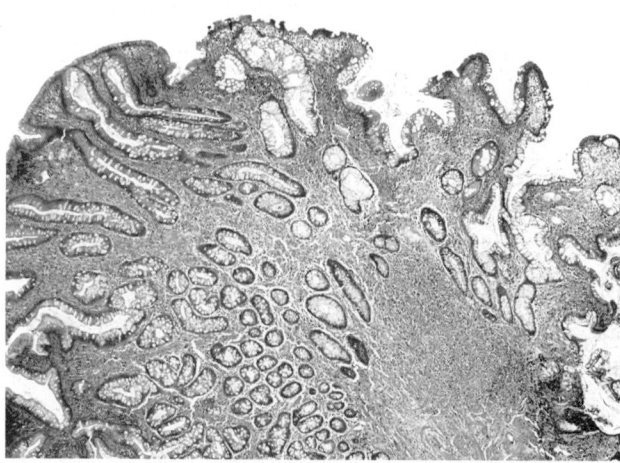

Figure 3-62. Juvenile polyp, higher magnification of the previous figure. The lamina propria contains a mixed inflammatory cell infiltrate, similar to the normal lamina propria constituents. Mild architectural distortion is present. In the absence of a documented syndrome, nonspecific polyps such as this may be diagnosed as "juvenile/inflammatory polyp."

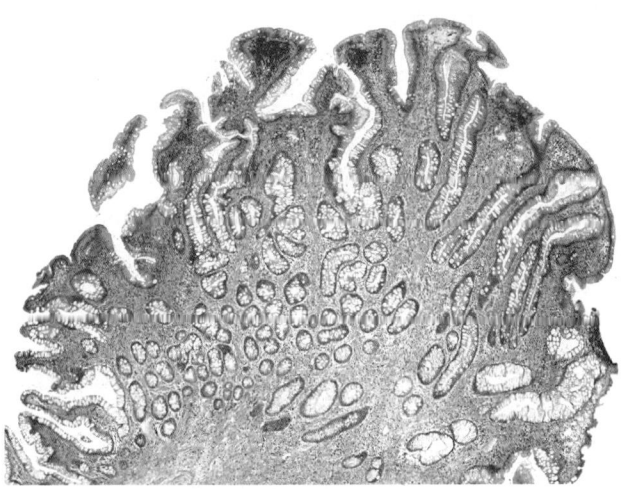

Figure 3-63. Juvenile/inflammatory polyp. Distinction between juvenile and inflammatory polyps may not be possible when lesions are small. Both may show mildly distorted crypts and a slightly expanded lamina propria containing mixed inflammatory cells.

Cronkhite-Canada Syndrome Polyps

Cronkhite-Canada syndrome is a rare, acquired clinical condition characterized by GI hamartomatous polyposis and the dermatologic triad of alopecia, onychodystrophy, and hyperpigmentation.[42,43] Patients present with diarrhea that rapidly progresses to intractable protein-losing enteropathy, and there have been no linked etiologic factors or genetic defects identified. Some studies report increased IgG4-positive plasma cells in this condition[44-46] and a response to immunosuppression, suggesting that the underlying cause may be immune dysregulation. Consider this syndrome when numerous biopsies show juvenile polyp–like features: cystically dilated and tortuous glands containing proteinaceous fluid or inspissated mucus with an excess of background lamina propria showing marked edema and chronic inflammation (Figs. 3.64–3.67).[47] Small bowel polyps have been associated with villous atrophy, crypt distortion, inflammation, and increased apoptotic bodies.[45] At first glance, the changes resemble inflammatory-type polyps and are nonspecific in the absence of clinical information, but the tip-off is the diffuse nature of the changes and the lack of intervening normal mucosa (Figs. 3.68–3.70).[48] If only the polyps are sampled, which is often the case, the histology is indistinguishable from sporadic or syndromic hamartomatous/inflammatory-type polyposis syndromes (Fig. 3.71),[49] such as juvenile polyposis syndrome, and further investigation into the clinical presentation (alopecia, onychodystrophy, and hyperpigmentation) is necessary to diagnose Cronkhite-Canada syndrome. In the diagnosis comment, one might suggest sampling the intervening flat mucosa should the patient receive follow-up endoscopy. Complications due to GI bleeding, sepsis, malnutrition, and heart failure result in a 55% 5-year mortality rate. First-line treatment is primarily supportive and trials of steroids, azathioprine, acid suppression, and antibiotics have not proven consistently effective. It is unnecessary to perform IgG4 immunohistochemical studies for diagnosis. First-line therapy is corticosteroids with cyclosporine suggested for steroid-resistant cases.[44,50]

PEARLS & PITFALLS: The Flat Mucosa Can Aid in a Diagnosis of Cronkhite-Canada Syndrome

As noted previously, juvenile polyps and polyps of Cronkhite-Canada syndrome are virtually impossible to differentiate histologically. Both share features with inflammatory polyps, including abundant lamina propria with inflammatory cells and dilated or atrophic glands. Clinical clues such as alopecia and onychodystrophy can aid in the diagnosis of Cronkhite-Canada syndrome, but this information is frequently unavailable to pathologists and sometimes not clinically evident, even when specifically addressed. A helpful clue is the intervening nonpolypoid mucosa, which in Cronkhite-Canada syndrome will show features identical to that seen in the polypoid mucosa.

KEY FEATURES: Cronkhite-Canada Syndrome

- This condition is a **noninherited polyposis** with **no known genetic defects.**
- There is **greater than 50% mortality rate.**
- Patients present with **diarrhea, protein-losing enteropathy, and ectodermal** changes, such as **alopecia, onychodystrophy, and hyperpigmentation.**
- Polyps are seen diffusely throughout the GI tract and consist of **hamartomatous/inflammatory-type polyps identical to juvenile polyps.**
- Key to diagnosis is the **intervening nonpolypoid mucosa, which is histologically identical to the polyps.**

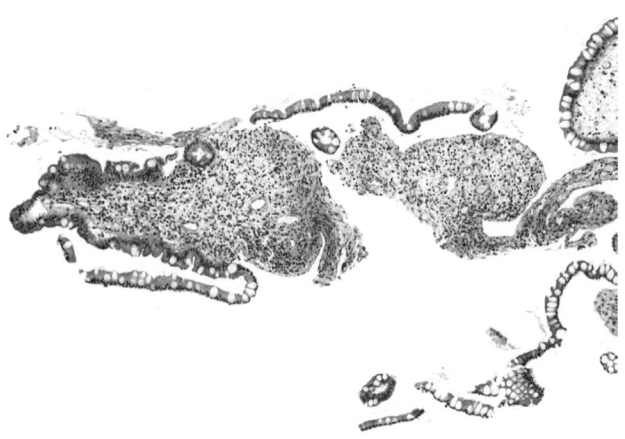

Figure 3-64. Cronkhite-Canada syndrome polyp. These biopsies show marked lamina propria edema and an absence of normal glandular architecture. At first glance, they resemble juvenile polyps. However, these changes are also found in random samples of nonpolypoid mucosa. One of the key diagnostic clues to Cronkhite-Canada syndrome is the involvement of nonpolypoid mucosa.

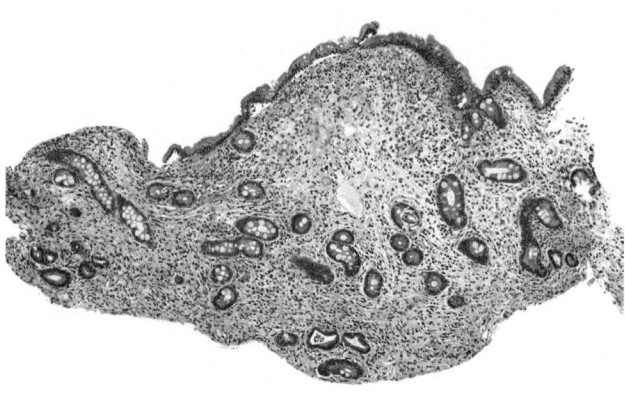

Figure 3-65. Cronkhite-Canada syndrome polyp. There is an excess of edematous lamina propria and dilated irregular crypts. In isolation, the findings suggest a juvenile polyp or inflammatory polyp. When these changes are found diffusely in both polypoid and nonpolypoid mucosa, consider Cronkhite-Canada syndrome and look for the clinical triad of alopecia, onychodystrophy (changes in nail color or quality), and hyperpigmentation.

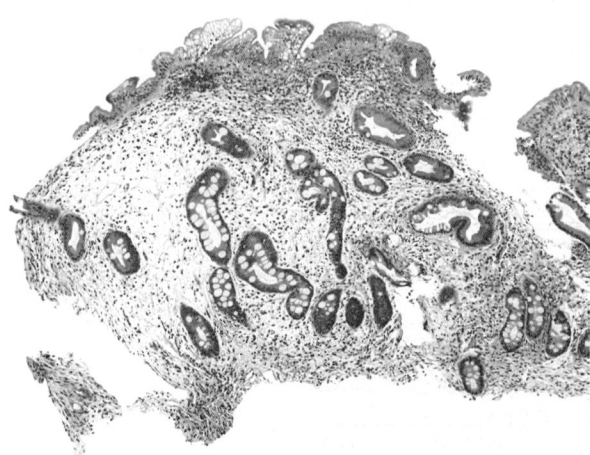
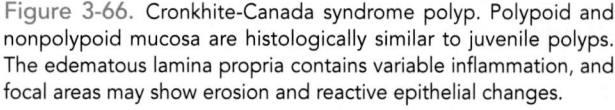

Figure 3-66. Cronkhite-Canada syndrome polyp. Polypoid and nonpolypoid mucosa are histologically similar to juvenile polyps. The edematous lamina propria contains variable inflammation, and focal areas may show erosion and reactive epithelial changes.

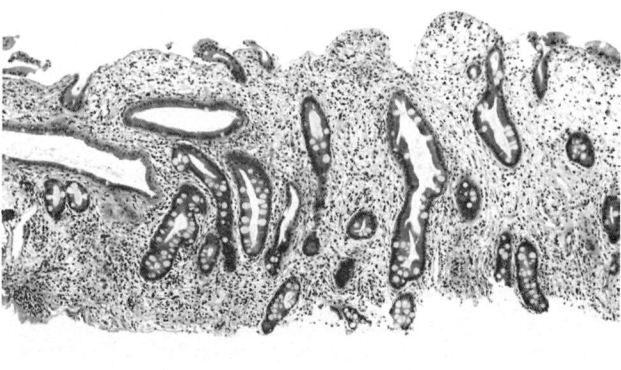

Figure 3-67. Cronkhite-Canada syndrome polyp. There is an excess of edematous lamina propria, and the crypts appear dilated and distorted. In isolation, this polyp biopsy could represent a juvenile polyp or an inflammatory polyp. Biopsies of the intervening flat mucosa are necessary to suggest Cronkhite-Canada syndrome and will show similar changes as those found in the polypoid mucosa.

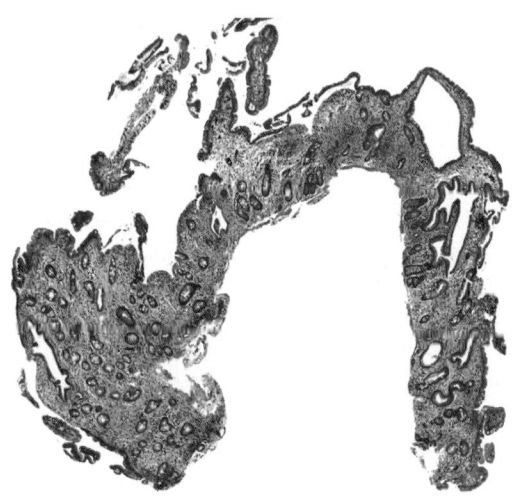

Figure 3-68. Cronkhite-Canada syndrome, flat mucosa. This intervening flat mucosa is abnormal, showing similar, although slightly subdued, features as those found in the polypoid mucosa. Note the dilated and distorted crypts and the expanded lamina propria.

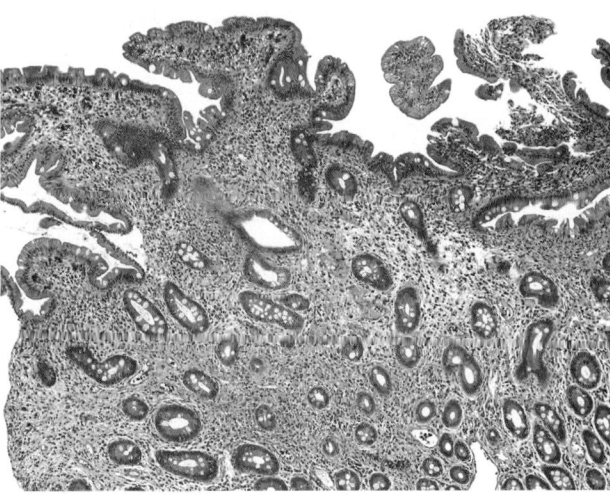

Figure 3-69. Cronkhite-Canada syndrome, flat mucosa. This small bowel mucosa shows distortion of the glandular architecture and edematous lamina propria with mixed inflammatory cells.

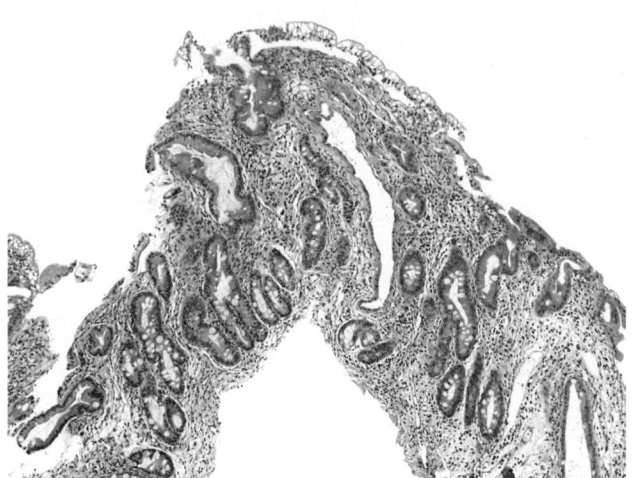

Figure 3-70. Cronkhite-Canada syndrome, flat mucosa. Another example of flat mucosa from a patient with Cronkhite-Canada syndrome features dilated and distorted crypts with villous atrophy and edematous lamina propria. The flat and polypoid mucosa shows similar features in this condition.

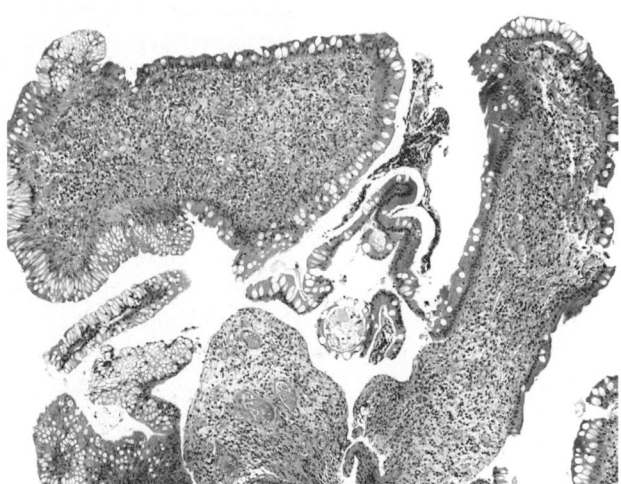

Figure 3-71. Cronkhite-Canada syndrome, polyp. The expanded lamina propria, distorted glandular architecture, and inflammation can be seen in several conditions, requiring more than just histology for diagnosis. For example, if this were an isolated incidental polyp, one might call it an inflammatory polyp. In a patient with SMAD4 germline mutation, it would be called a juvenile polyp. When found in a patient with diffuse mucosal changes, such as in this case, one would suggest the possibility of Cronkhite-Canada syndrome.

PTEN Hamartoma Tumor Syndrome and Cowden Syndrome Polyps

Cowden syndrome is inherited in an autosomal dominant fashion and is the best-described PTEN hamartoma tumor syndrome, the others of which include Bannayan-Riley-Ruvalcaba syndrome and adult Lhermitte-Duclose disease. These rare disorders are characterized by *PTEN* mutations, and patients have hamartomatous/inflammatory polyps throughout the GI tract, with 66% to 100% of affected individuals reported to have duodenal or gastric polyps.[51-53] Proteus and Proteuslike syndromes, although also belonging to the PTEN mutation family, do not feature GI hamartomas as a prominent finding. The range of clinical manifestations of Cowden syndrome is diverse and includes mucocutaneous and extracutaneous hamartomatous tumors in multiple organ systems and characteristic dermatologic manifestations, such as trichilemmomas, oral fibromas, and punctate palmoplantar keratoses. This syndrome is associated with high penetrance of carcinomas of the breast (cumulative risk as high as 85%), endometrium (13% to 28%), thyroid (3% to 35%), kidney (13% to 34%), and colorectum (66% to 93%).[52-54] The increased risk of malignancy underscores the importance of reporting any hamartomatous polyp within the GI tract, thus alerting clinicians to screen for a polyposis syndrome. A case report of primary small bowel adenocarcinoma has been associated with Cowden syndrome but this association has not been found in larger series.[55] Although adenomas may be encountered in patients with *PTEN* mutations, these are rare and most GI lesions comprise hamartomatous polyps, lipomas, ganglioneuromas, and inflammatory polyps (Figs. 3.72–3.74). In comparison with hamartomatous lesions of Peutz-Jeghers syndrome and juvenile polyposis syndrome, the polyps of Cowden syndrome usually lack erosions, contain fewer inflammatory cells in the lamina propria, and lack thick inspissated mucin; on the other hand, smooth muscle proliferation and lymphoid aggregates are common.[56] Syndromic patients may also present with diffuse glycogenic acanthosis of the esophagus,[53] another helpful clue and one of the minor criteria. Diagnosis of the syndrome should be left to clinical counterparts, as the rubric for diagnosis requires multidisciplinary knowledge of the patient's clinical findings (see Table 3.1 for a list of major and minor criteria), but any history of multiple cancers or ≥3 GI hamartomatous polyps, in particular ganglioneuromas, warrants mentioning this syndrome in a diagnosis comment to allow for further testing and genetic screening.

PEARLS & PITFALLS: When to Suggest Screening for PTEN Hamartoma Tumor Syndrome

The high risk of malignancy in patients with PTEN syndromes makes early identification critical for appropriate screening and surveillance. However, the clinical presentation can be diverse and the rubric for diagnosis is complex, utilizing a combination of major and minor criteria covering a spectrum of diverse organ systems. Thus, pathologists play a key role in suggesting screening for this (and other) syndrome(s), and one might consider including a note to this end when the following are encountered:

1. Multiple inflammatory or hamartomatous polyps anywhere in the GI tract, not otherwise associated with a known syndrome

2. Any intramucosal lipomas

3. Any ganglioneuromas[56]

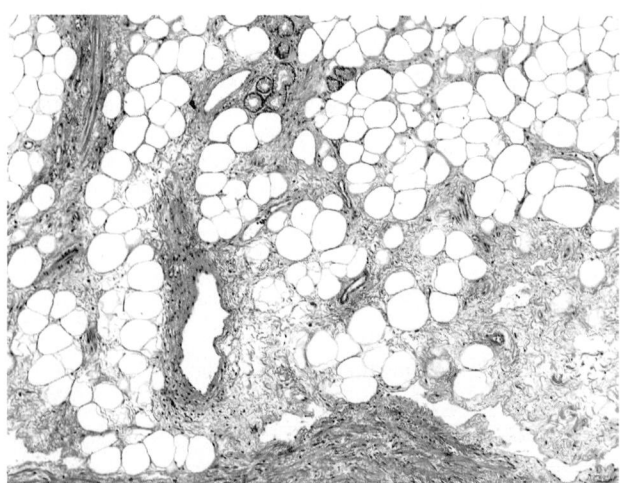

Figure 3-72. Hamartomatous polyp from Cowden syndrome. Polyps from patients with PTEN hamartoma tumor syndromes (e.g., Cowden syndrome) are variable and include hamartomatous polyps, lipomas, ganglioneuromas, and inflammatory polyps. This example shows intramucosal fat and smooth muscle and was classified as a hamartomatous lesion in a patient with known Cowden syndrome.

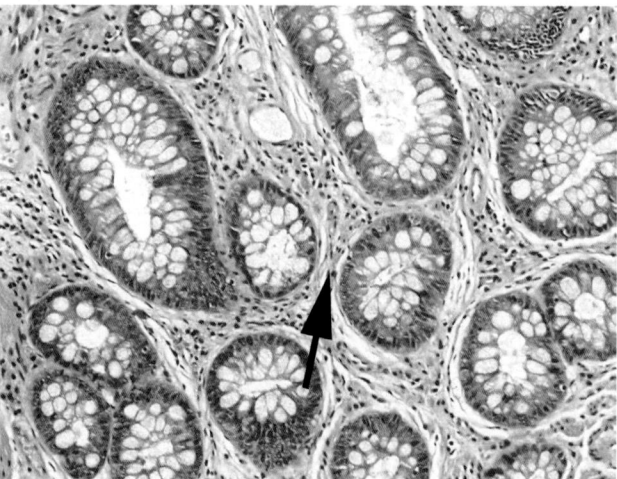

Figure 3-73. Hamartomatous polyp from Cowden syndrome. This polyp from a patient with Cowden syndrome was relatively unremarkable at low magnification, but higher magnification (shown here) reveals delicate smooth muscle strands (*arrow*) between crypts.

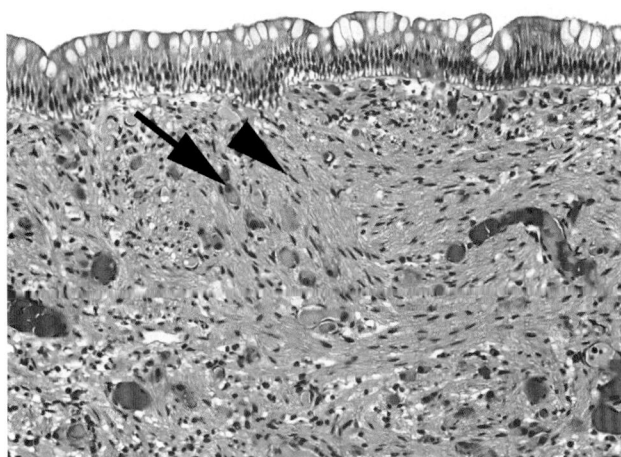

Figure 3-74. Mucosal ganglioneuroma. Gastrointestinal mucosal ganglioneuromas are composed of bland spindled Schwann cells (*arrowhead*) with a variable number of epithelioid ganglion cells (*arrow*) containing abundant amphophilic cytoplasm and round nuclei with prominent single nucleoli. Mucosal ganglioneuromas should raise suspicion for Cowden syndrome, particularly if multiple; isolated sporadic lesions are inconsequential.

SAMPLE NOTE: Multiple Hamartomatous Polyps in the GI Tract

Small Bowel, Polyps, Polypectomy

- Fragments of hamartomatous/inflammatory-type polyps, see Note.
- Negative for dysplasia

Note: Histologic sections show multiple fragments of hamartomatous/inflammatory-type polyps without definitive characteristic features. In the setting of multiple polyps, one might consider the possibility of a polyposis syndrome, such as Peutz-Jeghers syndrome, juvenile polyposis syndrome, Cronkhite-Canada syndrome, and *PTEN* hamartoma tumor syndrome. If Cronkhite-Canada syndrome is a clinical concern, biopsy of the intervening nonpolypoid mucosa is helpful should follow-up endoscopy be performed. Correlation with family history, physical examination, and genetic counselor evaluation/testing may be of interest.

KEY FEATURES: *PTEN* Hamartoma Tumor Syndrome and Cowden Syndrome

- PTEN hamartoma tumor syndrome is the result of a **defect in *PTEN***, which is transmitted **autosomal dominantly**
- The syndromes include **Cowden, Bannayan-Riley-Ruvalcaba** and adult **Lhermitte-Duclose** syndromes.
- **Proteus and Proteuslike syndromes** are also PTEN syndromes but **do not feature GI polyps.**
- Patients can have **diffuse glycogenic acanthosis** of the esophagus and **hamartomas polyps/inflammatory-type polyps** in the stomach, small bowel, and colorectum.
- Uncommon but specific features include **mucosal fat, ganglion cells, and nerve fibers.**
- Polyps can be indistinguishable from the other syndromic and sporadic hamartomatous/inflammatory-type polyps
- Diagnosis requires fulfilling major and minor criteria across multiple organ systems (see Table 3.1)
- Patients are at risk for **malignancy: breast > endometrium > kidney > colorectum.**

TABLE 3.1: Revised 2013 PTEN Hamartoma Tumor Syndrome Clinical Diagnostic Criteria

Diagnosis for an individual (either of the following):

1. Three or more major criteria, but one must include macrocephaly, Lhermitte-Duclos disease, or gastrointestinal hamartomas; or
2. Two major and three minor criteria.

Diagnosis for a family where one individual meets revised PTEN hamartoma tumor syndrome clinical diagnostic criteria or has a PTEN mutation:

1. Any two major criteria with or without minor criteria; or
2. One major and two minor criteria; or
3. Three minor criteria.

Major Criteria

Breast cancer
Endometrial cancer (epithelial)
Thyroid cancer (follicular)
Gastrointestinal hamartomas (including ganglioneuromas but excluding hyperplastic polyps; ≥3)
Lhermitte-Duclos disease (adult)
Macrocephaly (≥97 percentile: 58 cm for women, 60 cm for men)
Macular pigmentation of the glans penis
Multiple mucocutaneous lesions (any of the following):
  • Multiple trichilemmomas (≥3, at least one biopsy proven)
  • Acral keratoses (≥3 palmoplantar keratotic pits and/or acral hyperkeratotic papules)
  • Mucocutaneous neuromas (≥3)
  • Oral papillomas (particularly on tongue and gingiva), multiple (≥3); (biopsy proven OR dermatologist diagnosed)

Minor Criteria

Autism spectrum disorder
Colon cancer
Esophageal glycogenic acanthosis (≥3)
Lipomas (≥3)
Mental retardation (i.e., IQ ≤75)
Renal cell carcinoma
Testicular lipomatosis
Thyroid cancer (papillary or follicular variant of papillary)
Thyroid structural lesions (e.g., adenoma, multinodular goiter)
Vascular anomalies (including multiple intracranial developmental venous anomalies)

ADENOMATOUS POLYPS

Polypoid dysplasia in the small bowel is designated "adenoma" and can be divided into conventional (i.e., colonic-like) adenomas and pyloric gland adenomas. These lesions are far more common in the colon and stomach, respectively, and are covered in greater detail in "Stomach" and "Colon" chapters. This section discusses syndromic considerations, such as familial adenomatous polyposis (FAP) syndrome, and histologic features unique to this anatomic location. For these lesions, the degree of dysplasia is graded similar to other parts of the GI tract: low grade, high grade, or indefinite for dysplasia (Figs. 3.75–3.77).

Conventional Adenoma

Conventional small bowel adenomas are similar to their colonic counterparts and can be classified by architecture as tubular, villous, or tubulovillous adenomas (see "Colon" chapter for further illustration). Most small bowel adenomas are duodenal, with rare examples in the jejunum or ileum. Adenomatous lesions of the small bowel

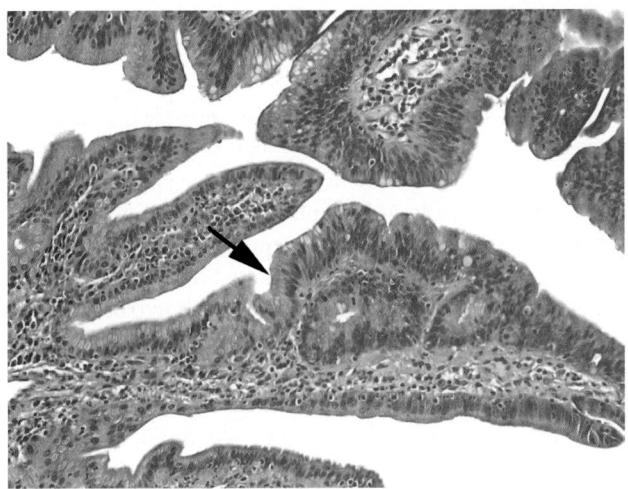

Figure 3-75. Small bowel adenoma, low-grade dysplasia. Similar to adenomatous lesions in other parts of the GI tract, small bowel adenomas show an abrupt transition between nondysplastic and low-grade dysplastic epithelium (*arrow*). Hyperchromasia is the result of nuclear crowding, stratification, and increased mitotic activity. The nuclei remain columnar in shape and retain polarity.

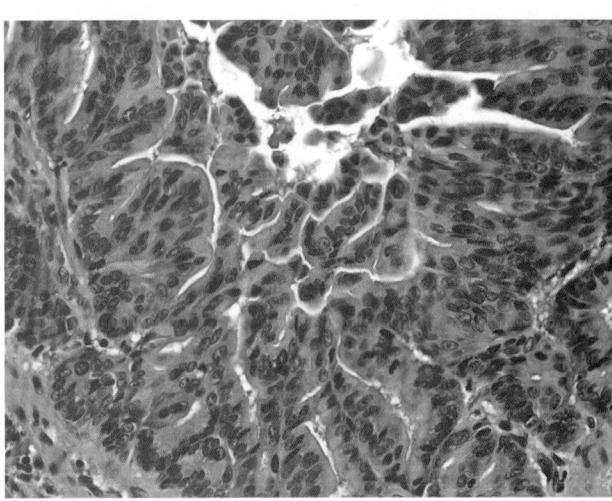

Figure 3-76. Small bowel adenoma, high-grade dysplasia. There is a higher degree of cellular crowding and overlap with cribriform architecture. Individual nuclei are rounder and many have lost a sense of polarity or direction.

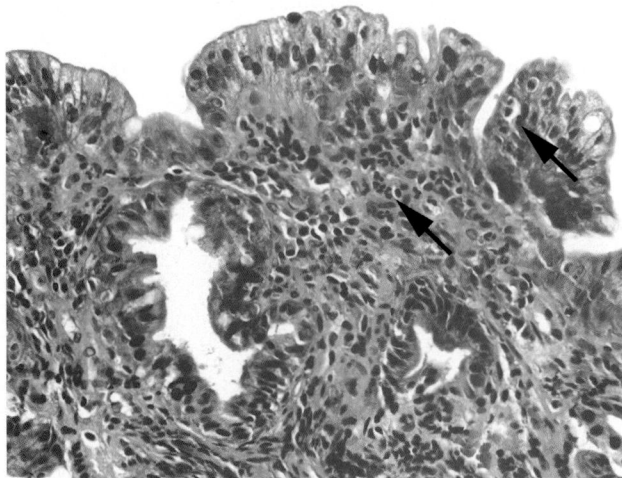

Figure 3-77. Small bowel mucosa, indefinite for dysplasia. When in doubt, a diagnosis of "indefinite for dysplasia" prevents overtreatment, and suggesting rebiopsy at a short interval provides additional material for review. This biopsy was signed out as "indefinite for dysplasia" because of its proximity to an ulcer and marked acute inflammation (*arrows*). The biopsy is atypical with crowding and overlapping of the nuclei along with some variation in nuclear size and hyperchromasia, but this sample remains challenging. Repeat biopsies following resolution of the ulcer showed unequivocal low-grade dysplasia.

are uncommon in the general population and usually solitary, with a prevalence of 0.2% to 0.4% among patients undergoing endoscopy.[57,58] Patients with duodenal adenomas are more likely to have colorectal adenomas (42%) as compared with the general population during screening colonoscopy.[57] When multiple duodenal adenomas are encountered, consider FAP or Lynch syndromes, as multiple lesions are seen almost exclusively in these settings. Duodenal adenomas are commonplace in FAP, are found in greater than 90% of these patients, and 4% progress to upper GI carcinoma, emphasizing the importance of surveillance endoscopy in this at-risk group.[59] Lesions are usually found incidentally or on surveillance endoscopy, but large adenomas may cause clinical symptoms such as abdominal pain, anemia, GI bleed, intussusception, and obstruction. Simple polypectomy or endoscopic mucosal resection is curative for endoscopically accessible lesions.

In most cases, diagnosis of dysplasia is straightforward, as lesions appear histologically similar to their colonic counterparts. However, the duodenal location presents several challenges in both overcalling and undercalling duodenal adenomas. Reactive epithelium is the most common pitfall for overdiagnosis of small bowel dysplasia, especially in areas near the duodenal bulb where acid from the stomach can cause peptic changes (e.g., gastric mucin cell metaplasia) and erosions, resulting in regenerative epithelium that can appear revved up enough to be concerning for dysplasia (Figs. 3.78–3.89). Clues to true dysplasia include an abrupt transition from nondysplastic areas (Figs. 3.90–3.93), diffuse hyperchromasia appreciable at low magnification (Figs. 3.94–3.96), and nuclear stratification (Figs. 3.97–3.101). One should maintain a high threshold for calling high-grade dysplasia, defined as architectural complexity (e.g., cribriform glands) with loss of nuclear polarity (Figs. 3.102–112), as this diagnosis results in aggressive surgical intervention that may include ampullectomy or pancreaticoduodenectomy (Whipple resection) if the ampullary area is involved. On the other hand, one must balance against underdiagnosis. Take care to avoid hastily attributing all changes to peptic injury when mucin cell metaplasia is found, as peptic duodenitis and dysplasia can certainly coexist (Fig. 3.92). Take a moment to look beyond the border of mucin metaplasia for additional epithelial atypia. When dysplasia and metaplasia are both present, they will each show abrupt transitions from normal, but at dyssynchronous locations. Therefore, finding two abrupt transitions, one for metaplasia and a separate one for dysplasia, can be a helpful tool to evaluate for small bowel adenomas.

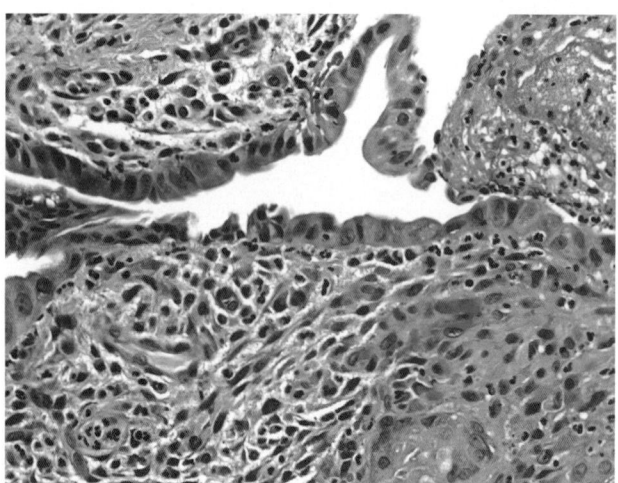

Figure 3-78. Small bowel mucosa, reactive changes. These epithelial cells show both anisonucleosis (variation in nuclear size) and pleomorphism (variation in shape) along with prominent nucleoli. The fibroinflammatory debris indicates proximity to an ulcer, and the cytologic changes are purely reactive.

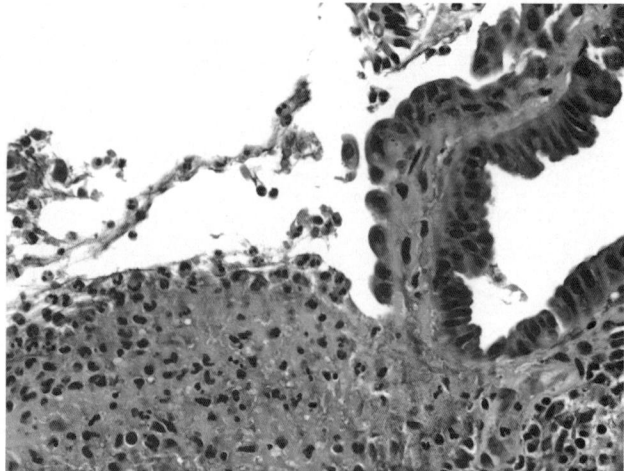

Figure 3-79. Small bowel mucosa, reactive changes. This example highlights the nondysplasia cytologic atypia that can be found adjacent to an erosion with marked acute inflammation. In the setting of acute inflammation, epithelial cells may show reactive and regenerative atypia, such as anisonucleosis, hyperchromasia, pleomorphism, and prominent nucleoli, all features that overlap with dysplasia. One should only call dysplasia if the findings are unequivocal.

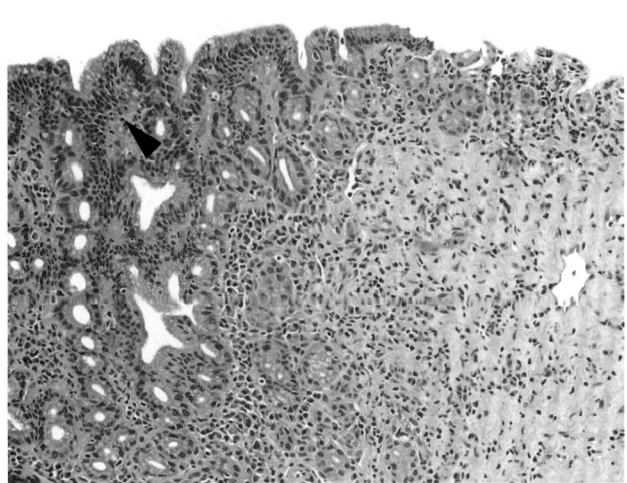

Figure 3-80. Small bowel mucosa, reactive and regenerative changes. Regenerative epithelial changes adjacent to an erosion (far right) can show cribriform architecture (far left) and may contain mitotic figures (*arrowhead*). This should not be mistaken for the cribriforming found in high-grade dysplasia, which is always accompanied by severe cytologic atypia (see Figs. 3.102–3.106 for comparison).

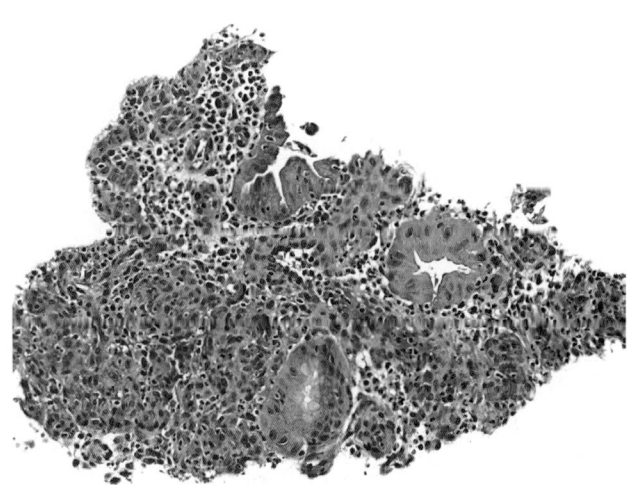

Figure 3-81. Small bowel mucosa, reactive changes. Minute samples with a backdrop of granulation tissue and marked acute inflammation should be treated with caution. Although the epithelial cells show cytologic atypia, with nuclear enlargement, prominent nucleoli, and eosinophilia of the cytoplasm, a sample of this size and with this degree of inflammation is not diagnostic. This example was handled as "Scant atypical glands in markedly inflamed granulation tissue, nondiagnostic for dysplasia or malignancy. Rebiopsy may be of interest, if clinically indicated."

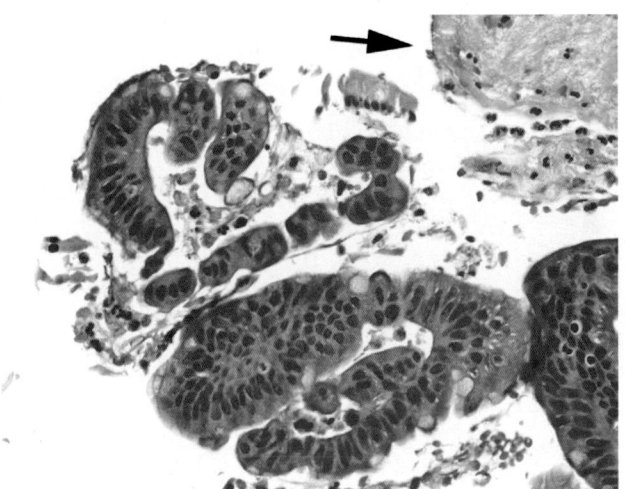

Figure 3-82. Small bowel mucosa, reactive changes. These detached epithelial strips show reactive changes, including hyperchromasia and nuclear variation in size and shape. When associated with fibroinflammatory debris indicating an adjacent ulcer (*arrow*), maintain a high threshold to diagnose dysplasia, especially if in the ampullary region. Requesting additional samples can prevent unnecessary surgery.

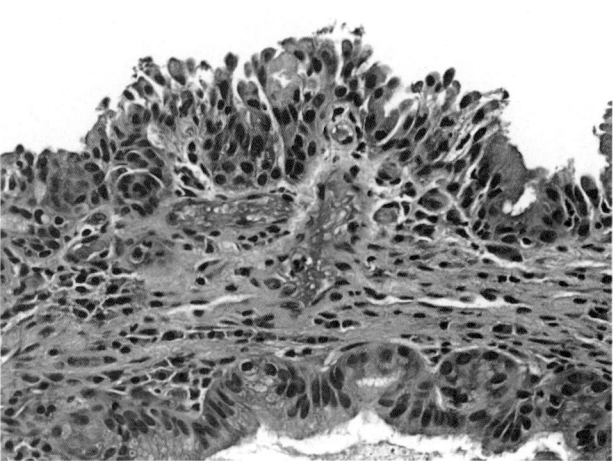

Figure 3-83. Small bowel mucosa, reactive changes. Reactive and regenerative changes can look alarming in isolation, so do not spend too much time at high magnification. This area shows stratification, increased nuclear to cytoplasmic ratio (compare with normal cells at the bottom), and jumbled up nuclei that one might argue represents loss of polarity and high-grade dysplasia. However, if one takes a step back to lower magnification (see next figure), this is a small area of epithelial regeneration adjacent to an ulcer.

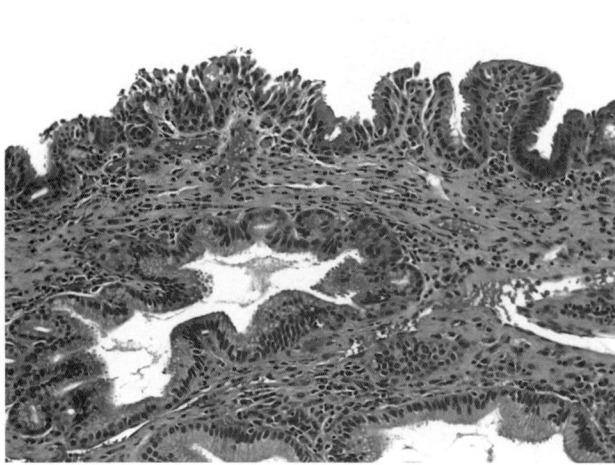

Figure 3-84. Small bowel mucosa, reactive changes, low power of the previous figure. At lower magnification, one can appreciate the gradual transition to an isolated area of atypia, rather than an abrupt transition to dysplasia. This sample showed additional metaplastic changes due to chronic ulceration (see the next two figures).

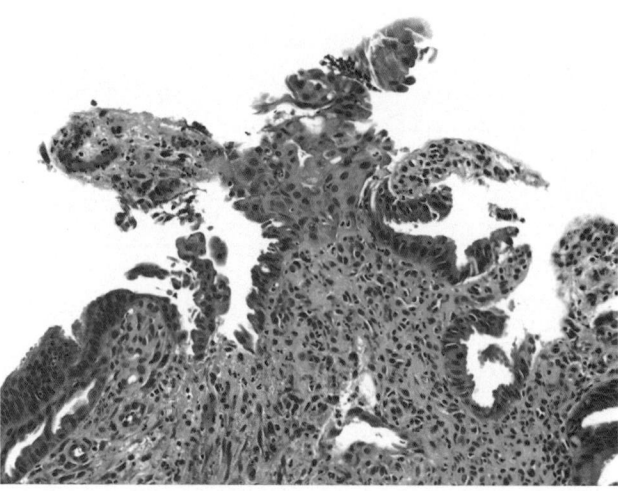

Figure 3-85. Small bowel mucosa, reactive changes. An area of ulceration shows squamoid metaplasia amid a backdrop of marked reactive and regenerative epithelial changes and acute inflammation.

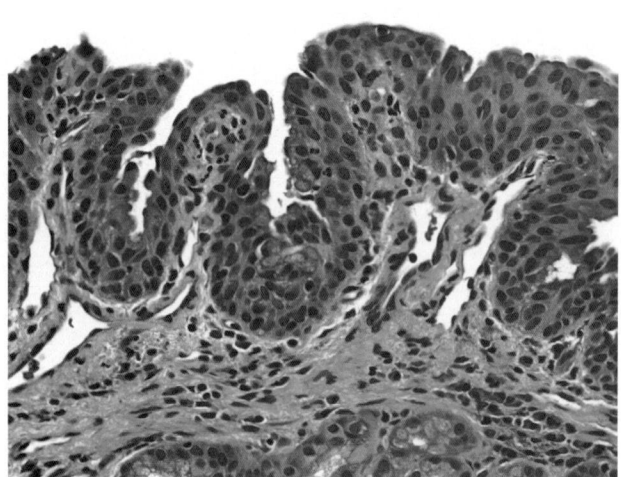

Figure 3-86. Small bowel mucosa, reactive changes. An isolated high-power field of metaplastic epithelium can be mistaken for high-grade dysplasia. Always confirm your high-power impression by checking for low-power hyperchromasia and an abrupt transition. Dysplasia is typically a low-power diagnosis.

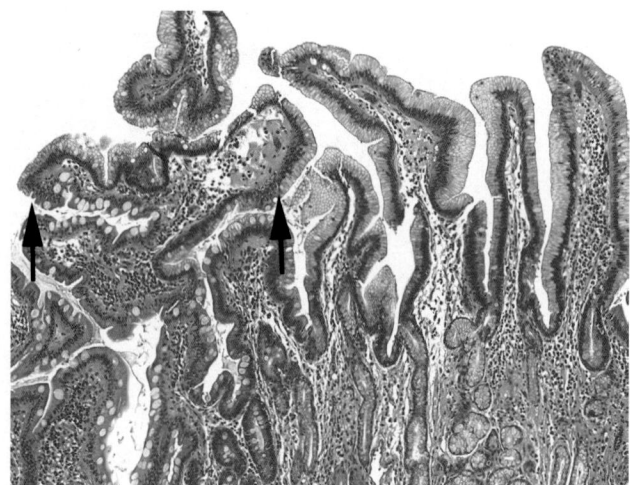

Figure 3-87. Small bowel mucosa, chronic peptic duodenitis. Abrupt transitions can be seen in benign nondysplastic conditions, such as seen here (*arrows*). The gastric foveolar metaplasia found in chronic peptic duodenitis should not be mistaken for dysplasia.

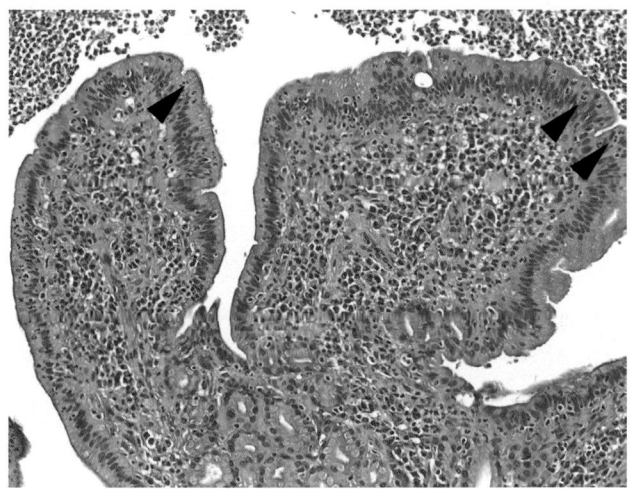

Figure 3-88. Small bowel mucosa, reactive changes. There is nuclear crowding and overlapping found in this example, but the backdrop of marked acute inflammation and the presence of intraepithelial neutrophils (*arrowheads*) indicate that these are reactive changes.

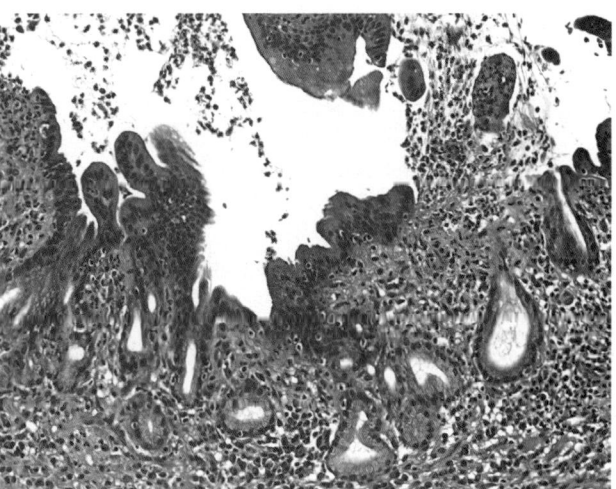

Figure 3-89. Small bowel mucosa, reactive changes. Note the marked nuclear crowding and overlapping found directly adjacent to this acute erosion. This example is clearly nondysplastic, but samples that are scant or composed of detached epithelial strips can be extremely challenging. Stay conservative when dealing with biopsies in the ampullary area where an overdiagnosis can result in radical surgery.

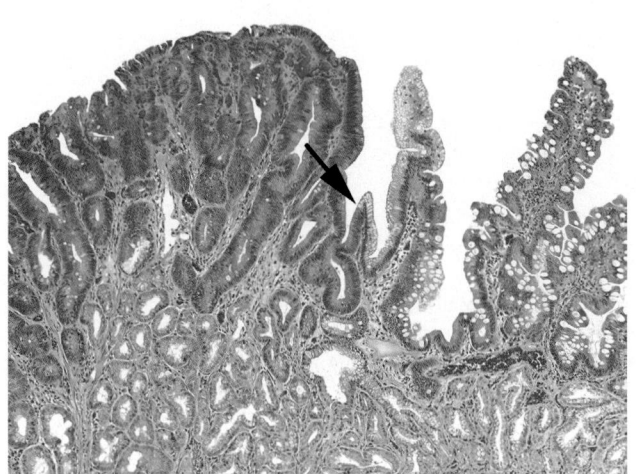

Figure 3-90. Duodenal adenoma. Like their colonic counterparts, conventional small bowel adenomas are visible at low magnification owing to their hyperchromasia and have a characteristic abrupt transition (*arrow*) from nondysplastic mucosa.

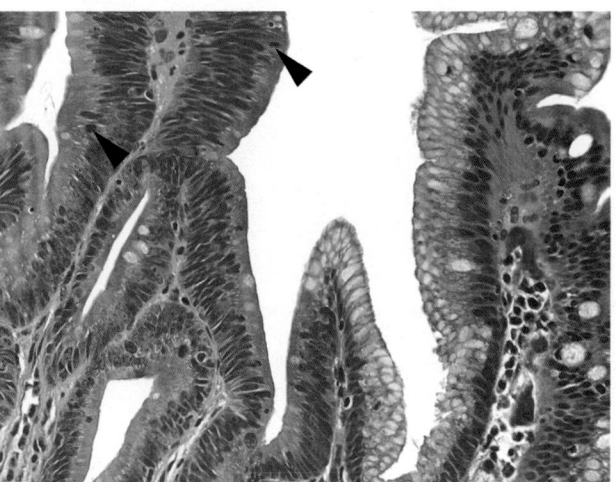

Figure 3-91. Duodenal adenoma, higher magnification of the previous figure. There is an abrupt transition to low-grade dysplasia. The dysplastic epithelium (left) shows nuclear crowding, stratification, and overlapping compared with the nondysplastic epithelium (right). Increased mitotic activity is common in dysplasia (*arrowheads*).

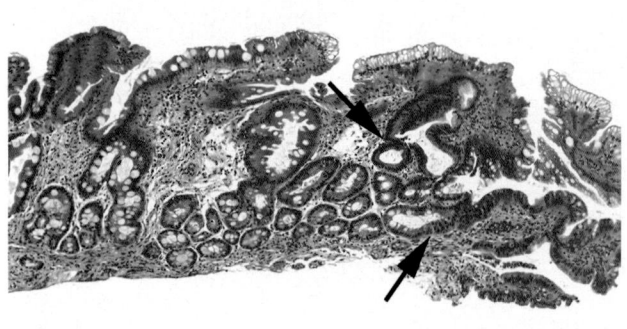

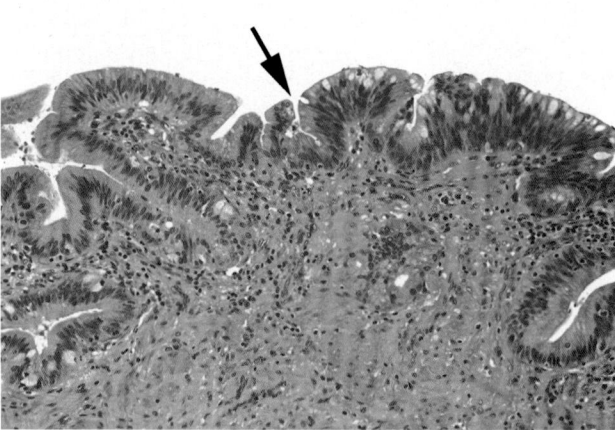

Figure 3-92. Duodenal adenoma. Dysplasia is a low-power diagnosis indicated by an abrupt transition to hyperchromasia and nuclear crowding (*arrows*). Note the clearing within the surface epithelial cells. This is a characteristic feature of small bowel adenomas caused by their inability to properly transport lipids (see also Figs. 3.113–3.115).

Figure 3-93. Duodenal adenoma. An abrupt transition (*arrow*) delineates the nondysplastic from dysplastic epithelium.

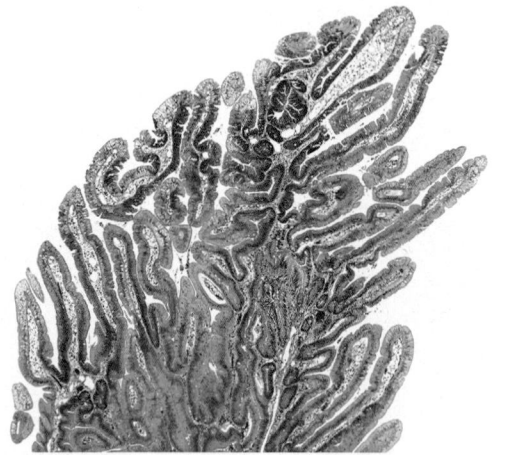

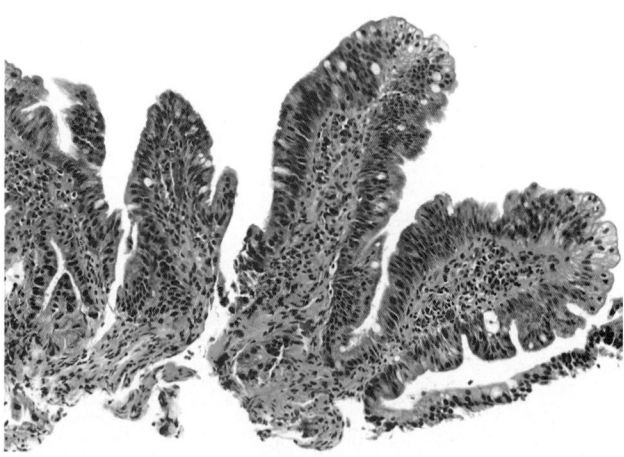

Figure 3-94. Duodenal villous adenoma. Small bowel adenomas can be classified by their low-power architecture, such as tubular adenoma, villous adenoma (pictured), and tubulovillous adenoma, the same as that of their colonic counterparts.

Figure 3-95. Small bowel adenoma. The nuclei of the surface enterocytes are crowded and many have moved away from the basement membrane toward the surface. This nuclear overlapping and stratification result in a low-power hyperchromasia distinctive to conventional low-grade dysplasia (see the next figure).

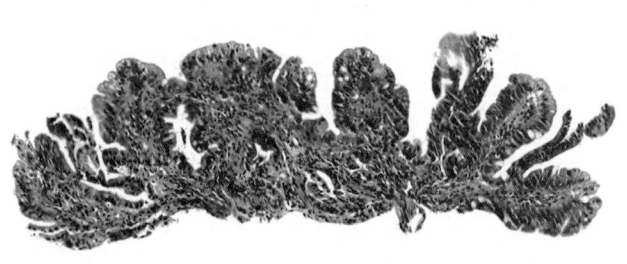

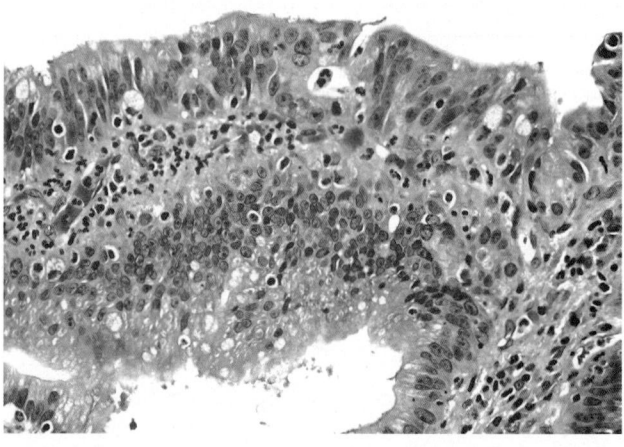

Figure 3-96. Small bowel adenoma, lower power of the previous figure. Like their colonic counterparts, conventional adenomas of the small bowel are readily identified at low magnification owing to their hyperchromasia.

Figure 3-97. Small bowel adenoma, low-grade dysplasia. Inflamed low-grade dysplasia can be difficult to differentiate from reactive changes (compare with Figs. 3.88 and 3.89). A single high-power field can be impossible to interpret. A diagnosis of dysplasia should be made with low-power support.

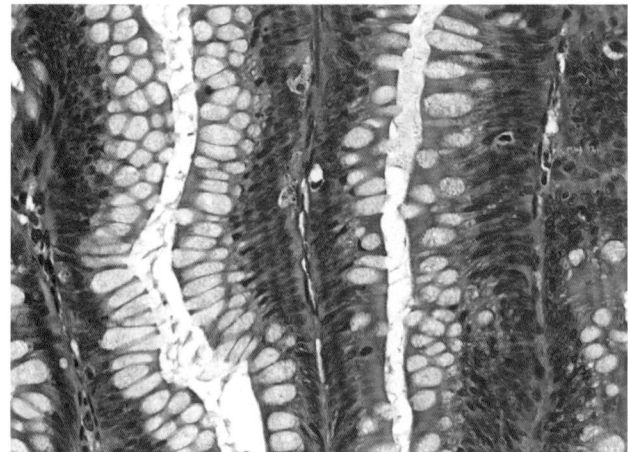

Figure 3-98. Small bowel adenoma, low-grade dysplasia. This example is rich in goblet cells. The nuclei are crowded, stratified, and overlapping.

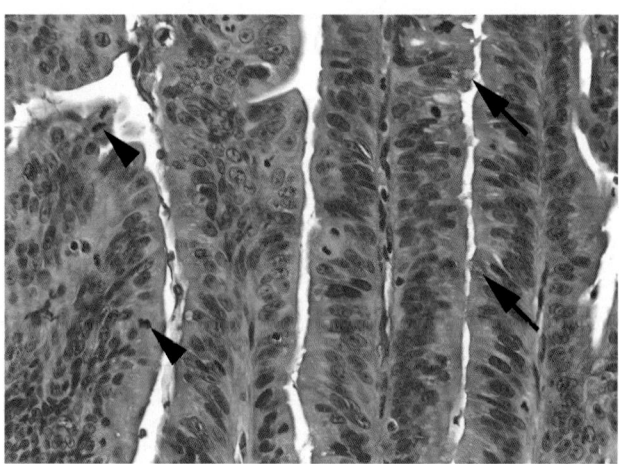

Figure 3-99. Small bowel adenoma, low-grade dysplasia. Compared with the previous figure, this example has sparse and inconspicuous goblet cells (*arrows*) but the nuclei show similar features of crowding, stratification, and overlapping. Mitotic figures are frequent (*arrowheads*).

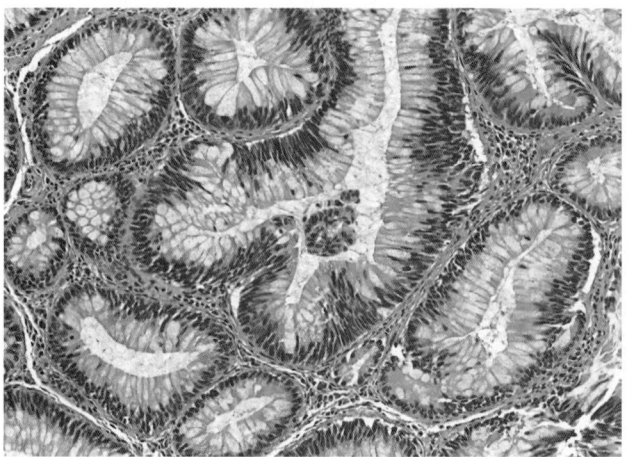

Figure 3-100. Small bowel adenoma, low-grade dysplasia. The nuclei remain basally located in this example rich with mucin but are crowded and overlapping.

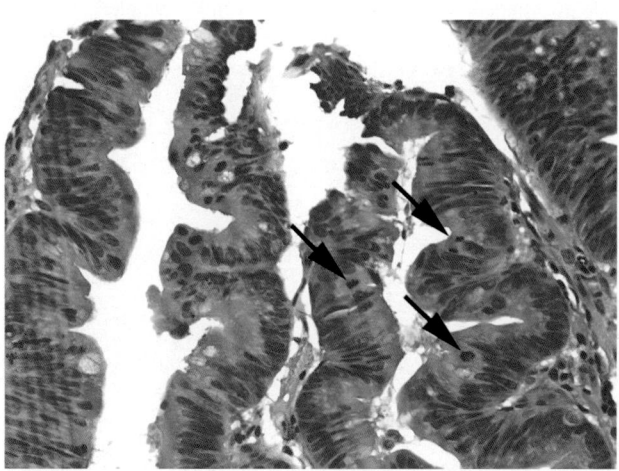

Figure 3-101. Small bowel adenoma, low-grade dysplasia. Crowded overlapping nuclei show stratification and mitotic activity (*arrows*).

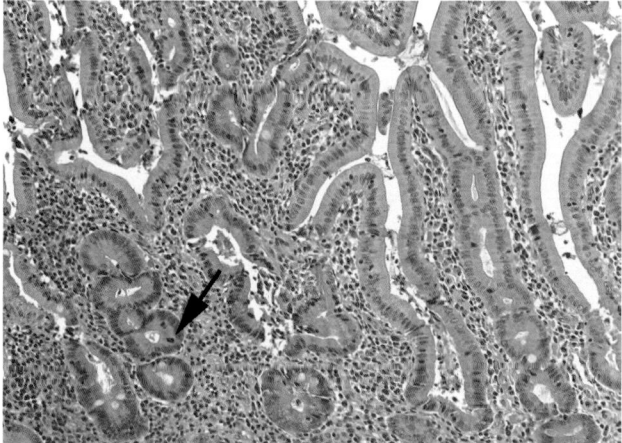

Figure 3-102. Small bowel reactive and regenerative changes. This area of small bowel is healing from previous injury and shows cribriform architecture and mitotic activity (*arrow*), but the nuclei remain evenly spaced and basally located. This example is benign regenerative change, but cribriform architecture combined with nuclear atypia can indicate high-grade dysplasia (see the next four figures).

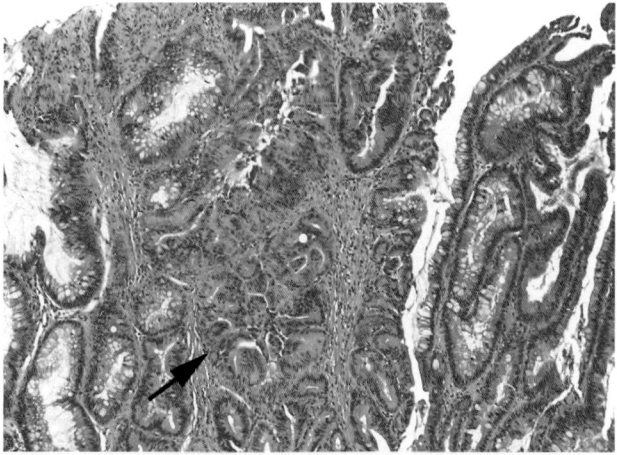

Figure 3-103. Small bowel adenoma, high-grade dysplasia. Architectural complexity, such as cribriforming (*arrow*), is a feature of high-grade dysplasia. The crowded nuclei should also show marked atypia and loss of nuclear polarity.

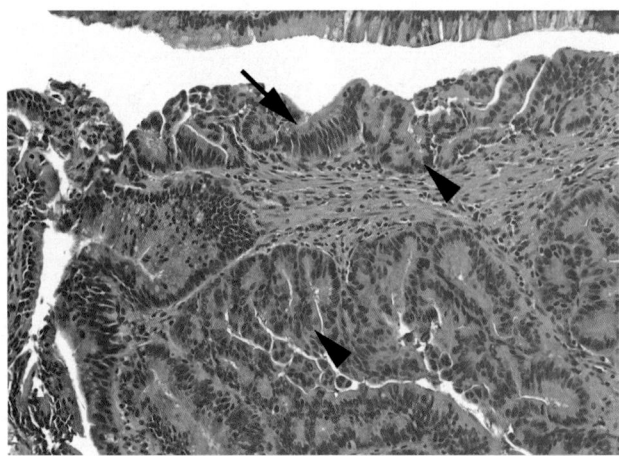

Figure 3-104. Small bowel adenoma, high-grade dysplasia. Compare the normal nondysplastic epithelium at the top to the surface low-grade dysplasia (LGD) (*arrow*) and high-grade dysplasia (HGD) (*arrowheads*). The nuclei of LGD are crowded and overlapping but retain their columnar appearance and basal location. By comparison, the nuclei of HGD appear rounder and show loss of polarity, whereas the overall architecture is more complex.

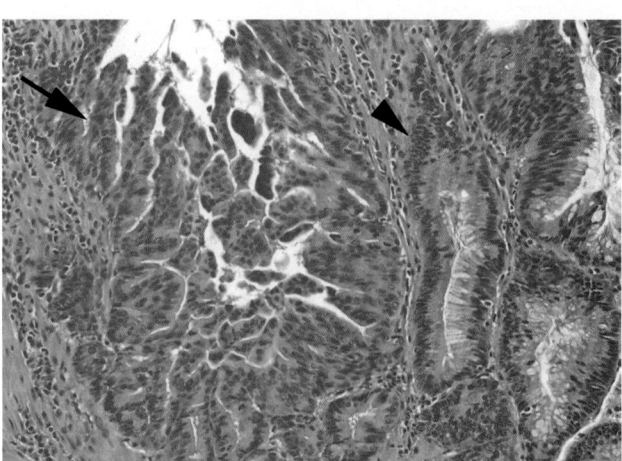

Figure 3-105. Small bowel adenoma, high-grade dysplasia. High-grade dysplasia (*arrow*) shows architectural complexity, and the nuclei are no longer aligned. Compared with this, the low-grade dysplasia (*arrowhead*) is much more organized and orderly despite its nuclear crowding.

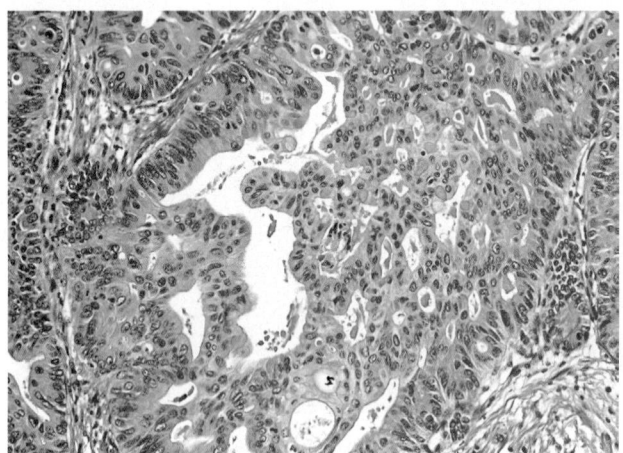

Figure 3-106. Small bowel adenoma, high-grade dysplasia. Cribriform architecture and marked cytologic atypia with loss of nuclear polarity make this a straightforward call of HGD.

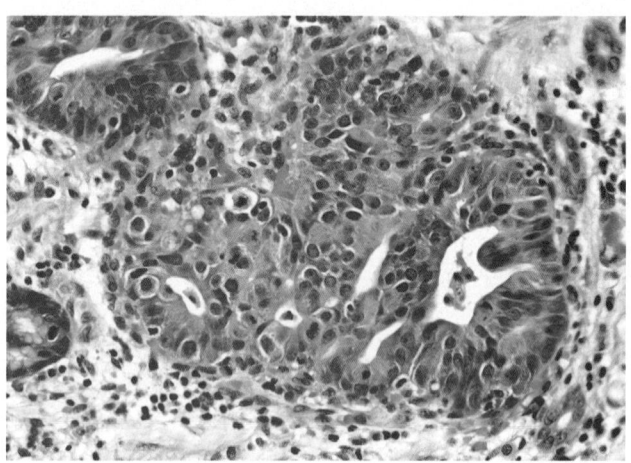

Figure 3-107. Small bowel adenoma, high-grade dysplasia. Criteria for high-grade dysplasia include complex architecture and cytologic atypia with loss of nuclear polarity, as seen here.

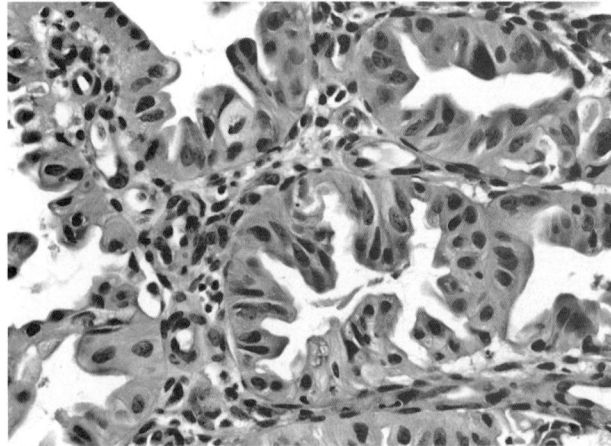

Figure 3-108. Small bowel adenoma, high-grade dysplasia. There is marked cytologic atypia among these cells with variation in nuclear size and shape, as well as loss of nuclear polarity.

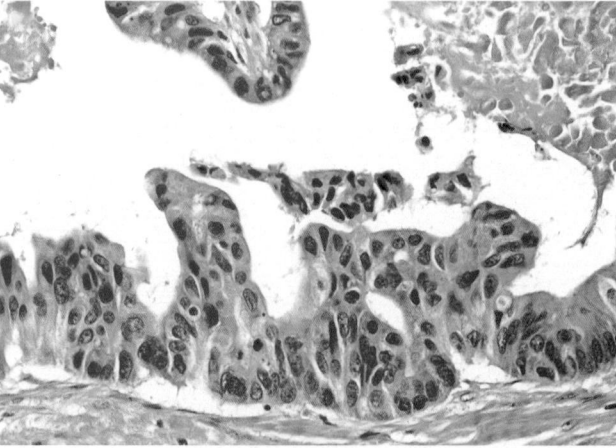

Figure 3-109. Small bowel adenoma, high-grade dysplasia. These nuclei show anisonucleosis (variation in size) and pleomorphism (variation in shape) along with crowding, overlapping, and loss of polarity. Necrosis is present (*top right*) with ghostlike outlines of dead cells, suggesting nearby adenocarcinoma.

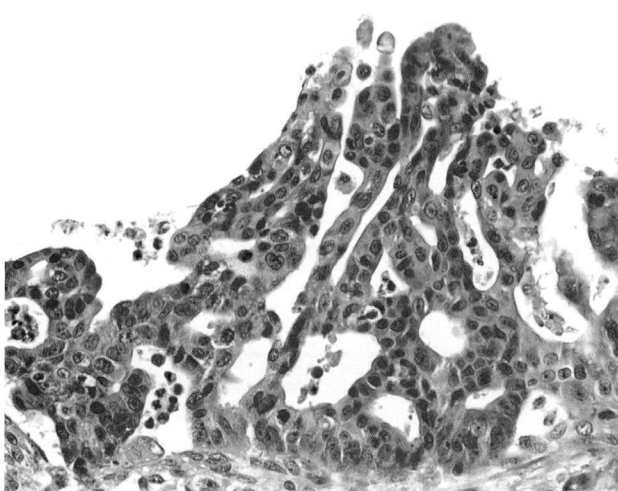

Figure 3-110. Small bowel adenoma, high-grade dysplasia. The architecture in this area is complex with cribriforming. The nuclei are highly atypical with crowding, variation in size and shape, and loss of polarity.

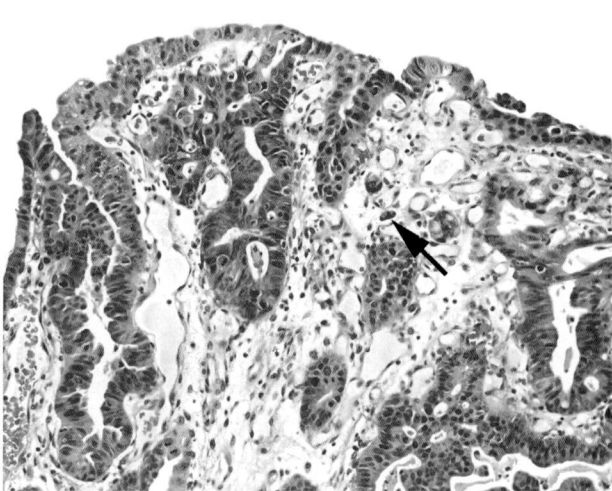

Figure 3-111. Small bowel early invasive adenocarcinoma. When encountering high-grade dysplasia, inspect for invasive foci (*arrows*). Recall, invasion into the lamina propria of the small bowel is a considered pT1 lesion with access to lymphatic and hematogenous metastasis.

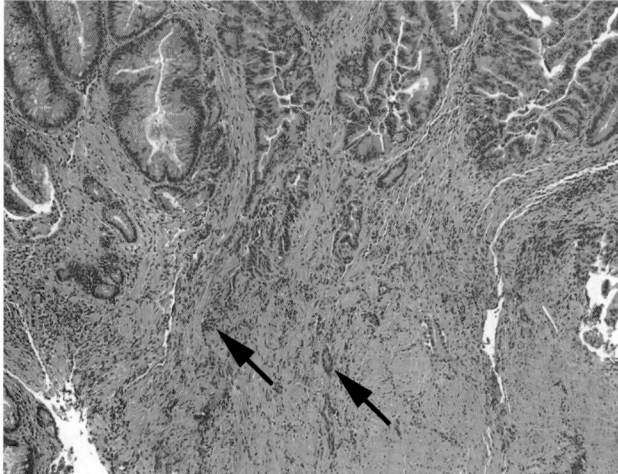

Figure 3-112. Small bowel invasive adenocarcinoma. Angulated glands and small clusters of cells infiltrate at the leading edge of this invasive adenocarcinoma (*arrows*) arising from the base of high-grade dysplasia.

Another histologic hazard in duodenal dysplasia is the inability of dysplastic enterocytes to properly transport lipid vacuoles, resulting in the accumulation of intracytoplasmic lipid and pale foamy cytoplasm along the surface of adenomas. This can be mistaken for mucin cell metaplasia (aka peptic duodenitis). To differentiate the two, observe the cellular location of foamy pallor: dysplastic cells with lipid vacuolization show diffuse cytoplasmic change (Figs. 3.113–3.115), whereas mucin cell metaplasia results in a single apical mucin vacuole (Fig. 3.116). Application of a PAS stain can also aid in differentiation, as PAS will highlight apical mucin but not intracytoplasmic lipid (Figs. 3.117 and 3.118). These surface challenges sometimes make duodenal dysplasia more readily identifiable *below* the surface, contrary to the traditional dogma of dysplasia always extending to involve the surface (Figs. 3.119–3.124). Again, examine the surrounding epithelium for clear-cut dysplastic changes away from these challenging areas.

The periampullary area can be a treacherous landscape because biopsies may capture small periampullary glands surrounded by splayed smooth muscle and can be mistaken for adenocarcinoma (Fig. 3.125). However, when benign, these glands maintain a lobular configuration (Fig. 3.126) despite the disorganized smooth muscle characteristic of this site.

One more word of caution about this location: do not forget that a neighboring pancreatic adenocarcinoma can extend through the small bowel wall and colonize the surface epithelium, mimicking a primary small bowel adenoma or adenocarcinoma. Small endoscopic biopsy samples may be extremely challenging if not downright duplicitous. These complicating factors in the proximal small bowel contribute to both intraobserver and interobserver variability in diagnosis, which is cited as fair to poor in one study.[60] Liberally sharing these cases with colleagues and obtaining consensus opinion is heartily recommended. Finally, some cases will simply be irresolvable, requiring a descriptive diagnosis, use of the indefinite for dysplasia category, and a note communicating a need for repeat biopsy.

PEARLS & PITFALLS: Metaplasia and Dysplasia Can Coexist

In most cases, pathologists are cautious to avoid over-calling dysplasia in the setting of peptic duodenitis, but recall that metaplasia and dysplasia are not mutually exclusive. When encountering a juicy nodular peptic duodenitis, take a moment to examine beyond the metaplastic border of mucin cell metaplasia for additional atypia or a second abrupt transition indicating dysplasia. Although these processes can coexist, their transformations are etiologically independent of one another and this is reflected histologically. So when dysplasia is present, its abrupt transition from normal will be dyssynchronous with the transition of metaplasia, a helpful clue.

PEARLS & PITFALLS: Adenomatous Epithelium Can Transport Lipid Into the Cell but Not Out Again

Enterocytes at the surface of adenomas often have pale foamy cytoplasm owing to the inability of cells to properly transport lipid. This can impart a bland appearance to the surface of adenomas or be mistaken for mucin cell metaplasia (aka CPD). Note that lipid vacuolization appears as a diffuse cytoplasmic pallor, whereas mucin cell metaplasia is seen as a single apical mucin vacuole (Figs. 3.113–3.116).

PEARLS & PITFALLS: Sometimes Duodenal Dysplasia Is More Easily Identified Below the Surface

The proximal small bowel bears the brunt of emptying gastric contents such as the acidic juices. Thus, it is not surprising that 39% of patients undergoing upper endoscopy show abnormalities in the duodenal bulb.[61] The small bowel, therefore, is one location where surface involvement by dysplasia can be hard to evaluate. Metaplasia, erosions, reactive/regenerative atypia, and lipid hang-up can all confound interpretation. Looking below the surface and away from these areas can clarify otherwise perplexing histology (Figs. 3.119–3.124).

PEARLS & PITFALLS: Metastatic Tumor Can Colonize the Surface and Mimic Adenomatous Epithelium

Always stay alert in the small bowel. Adenomatous epithelium can be mistaken when invasive tumor from adjacent sites, such as the pancreas (Fig. 3.127), or metastatic tumor from a distant site colonizes the surface. Endoscopic biopsies are small and often fraught with artifact. When in doubt, suggest correlation with endoscopic and imaging findings, and do not hesitate to request additional samples.

KEY FEATURES: Small Bowel Adenomas

- Conventional small bowel adenomas are **polypoid dysplasia** histologically **similar to colonic** adenomas.
- They are evaluated as **low-grade** dysplasia, **high-grade** dysplasia, and **indefinite for dysplasia**.
- Architectural patterns of **tubular adenoma, villous adenoma,** and **tubulovillous adenoma** are similar to those in the colon.
- **Sporadic adenomas are rare** (0.2% to 0.4%) and **solitary** but when encountered portend a likelihood for colonic adenomas (42%).
- **Multiple adenomas indicate a syndrome (FAP or Lynch).**
- Duodenal adenomas are found in **>90%** of **patients with FAP.**
- **Simple polypectomy or endoscopic mucosal resection** is curative when endoscopically amenable.
- Larger lesions may require surgical resection or **Whipple resection if involving the ampulla.**
- Pancreatic adenocarcinoma spreading to involve the small bowel can be a diagnostic pitfall.
- CPD and dysplasia can coexist.

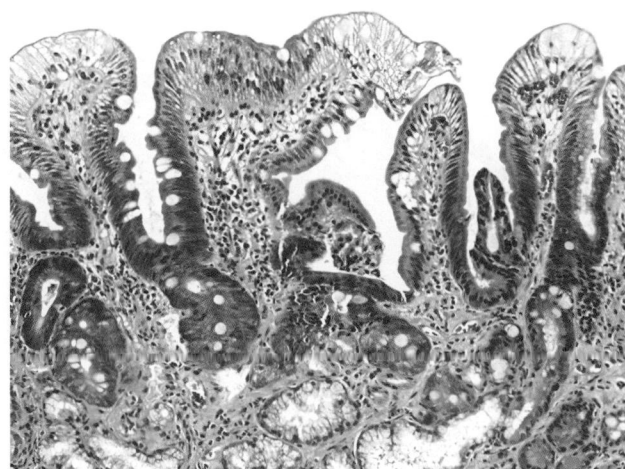

Figure 3-113. Duodenal adenoma, lipid hang-up. The surface of this adenoma appears pale rather than hyperchromatic because of the inability of dysplastic enterocytes to properly transport lipid vacuoles.

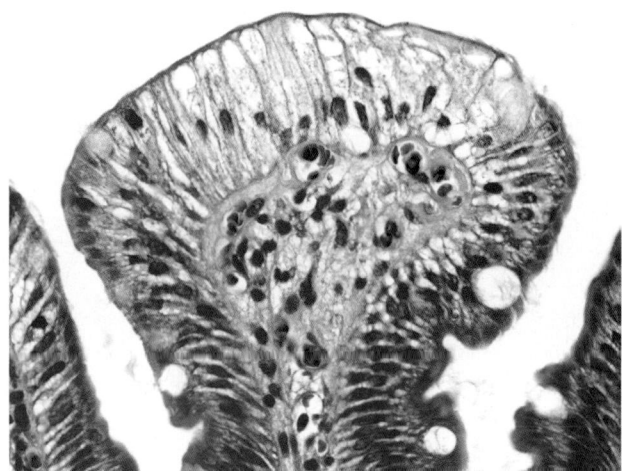

Figure 3-114. Duodenal adenoma, lipid hang-up, higher power of the previous figure. The dysplastic enterocytes are able to absorb lipid from the luminal contents but are unable to transport it out again. This results in lipid accumulation and pale foamy cytoplasm.

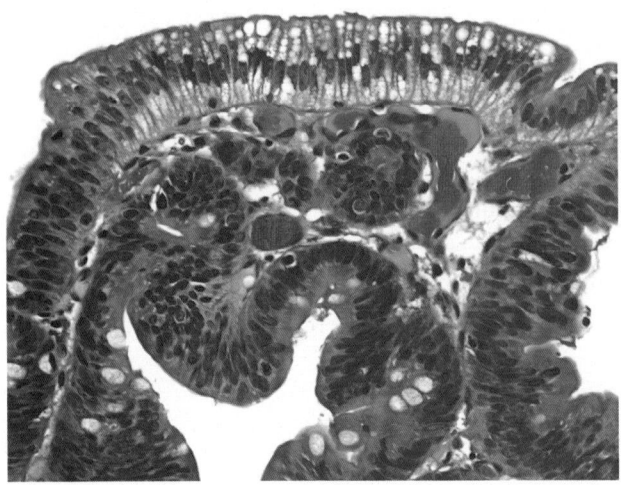

Figure 3-115. Duodenal adenoma, lipid hang-up. The cytoplasmic pallor of lipid hang-up is diffuse, and the cytoplasm can be composed of numerous small lipid droplets, as seen in this example. Do not mistake this for the nondysplastic chronic peptic duodenitis, which also shows surface pallor (see the next figure). An adenoma with lipid hang-up will still show hyperchromatic crowded nuclei, but one may need to look below the surface, as in this case.

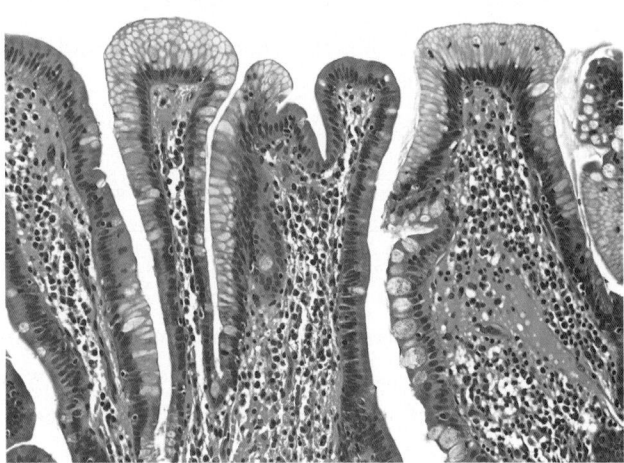

Figure 3-116. Chronic peptic duodenitis, gastric foveolar mucin cell metaplasia. A single apical mucin vacuole is present in gastric foveolar metaplasia. The superficial pallor and the abrupt transition are shared features with duodenal adenomas, but this lesion lacks the nuclear atypia and crowding, and is nondysplastic.

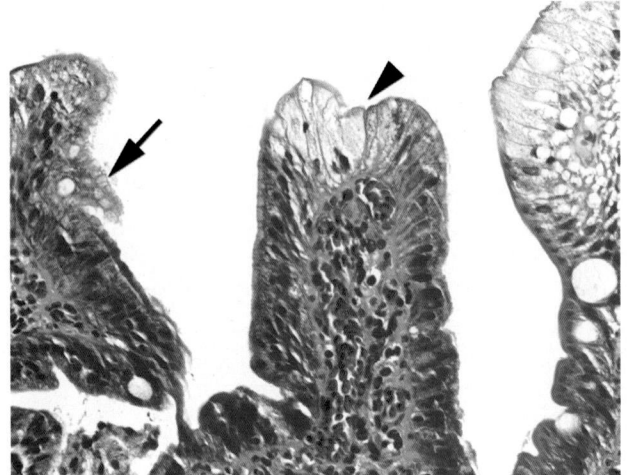

Figure 3-117. Duodenal adenoma, lipid hang-up. The surface epithelium appears pale and foamy owing to microvesicles of fat that cannot be properly transported in these dysfunctional and dysplastic cells (*arrowhead*). By comparison, foveolar metaplasia from peptic injury is composed of a single apical mucin vacuole (*arrow*). In challenging cases, a PAS stain may be helpful (see the next figure).

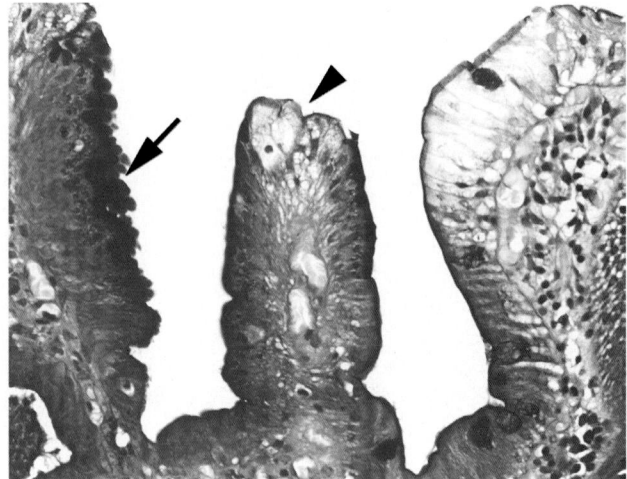

Figure 3-118. Duodenal adenoma, lipid hang-up, PAS stain of the previous figure. PAS highlights mucin within areas of foveolar metaplasia (*arrow*), whereas lipid is PAS negative and the cytoplasm of these dysplastic areas remains pale (*arrowhead*).

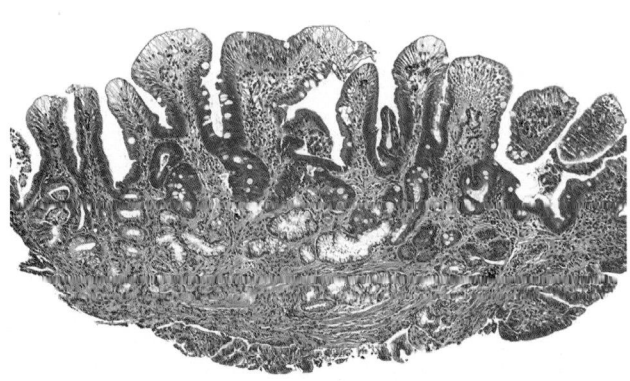

Figure 3-119. Duodenal adenoma, lipid hang-up. The lipid hang-up at the surface of duodenal adenomas imparts a superficial pallor. This can be a pitfall if one is accustomed to scanning the surface for dysplasia. In the small bowel, the hyperchromatic areas of dysplasia may be below the surface, but they are still evident at low magnification.

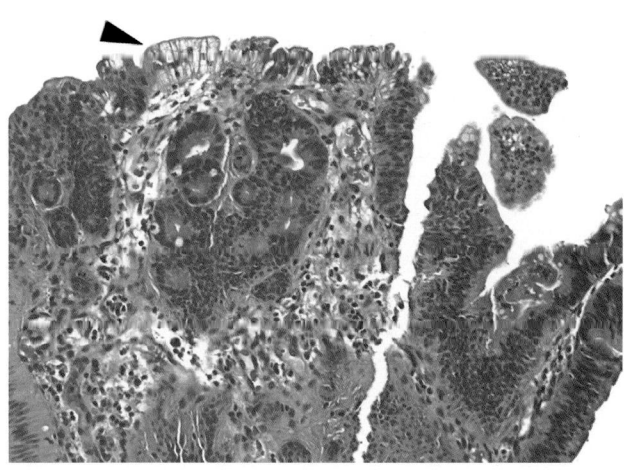

Figure 3-120. Duodenal adenoma, lipid hang-up. A focal area of surface pallor (*arrowhead*) is present in this adenoma due to dysfunctional lipid transport.

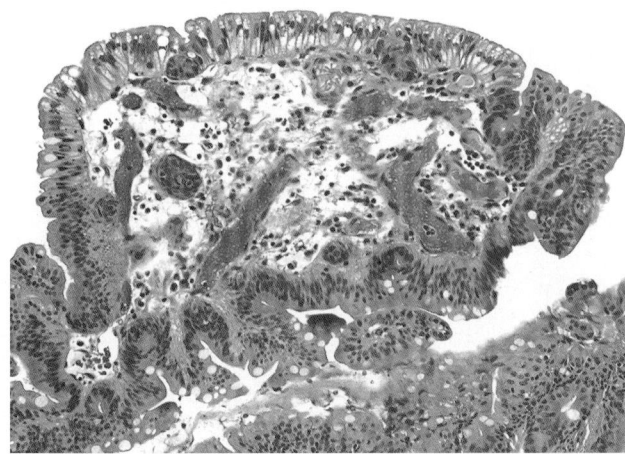

Figure 3-121. Duodenal adenoma, lipid hang-up. An adenoma with surface lipid hang-up can be easy to overlook if one is accustomed to scanning along the surface for hyperchromasia. Take a moment to look below the surface for the characteristic features of dysplasia, such as nuclear crowding, overlapping, and stratification.

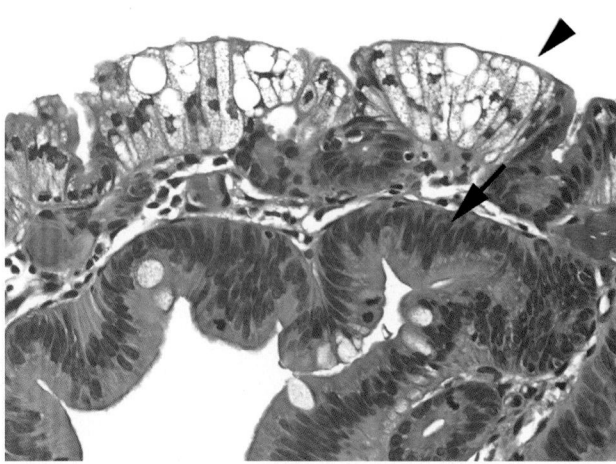

Figure 3-122. Duodenal adenoma, lipid hang-up. The surface epithelium lacks typical hyperchromasia because the pale foamy cytoplasm is filled with small fat droplets (*arrowhead*). Just below this surface, however, characteristic features of dysplasia (*arrow*) are seen, such as nuclear crowding, overlapping, and stratification along with mitotic activity.

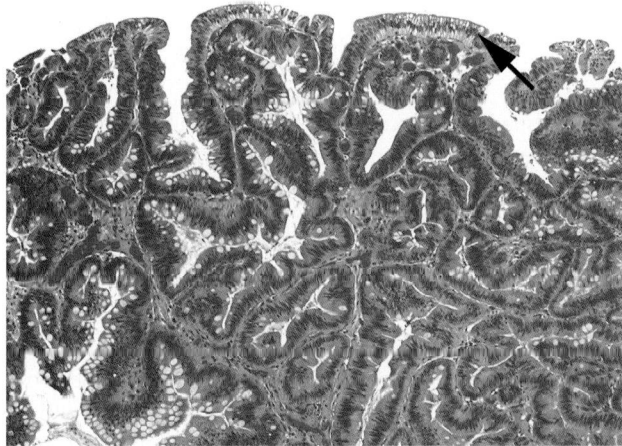

Figure 3-123. Duodenal adenoma. Adenomas are a low power diagnosis. Note the lipid hang-up along the surface of this lesion (*arrow*).

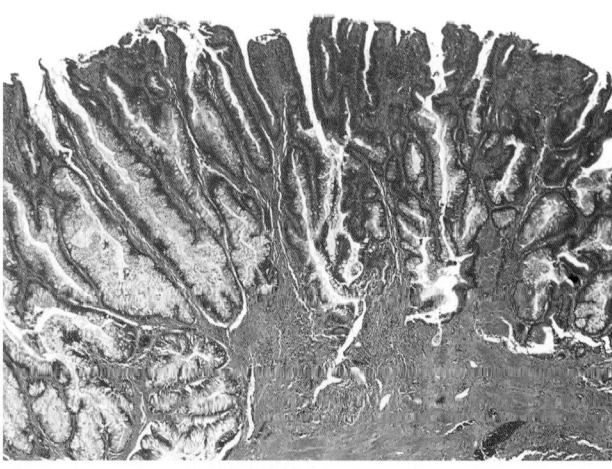

Figure 3-124. Duodenal adenoma. The surface is eroded in this example and can be difficult to interpret, but the deeper crypts show unequivocal low-grade dysplasia.

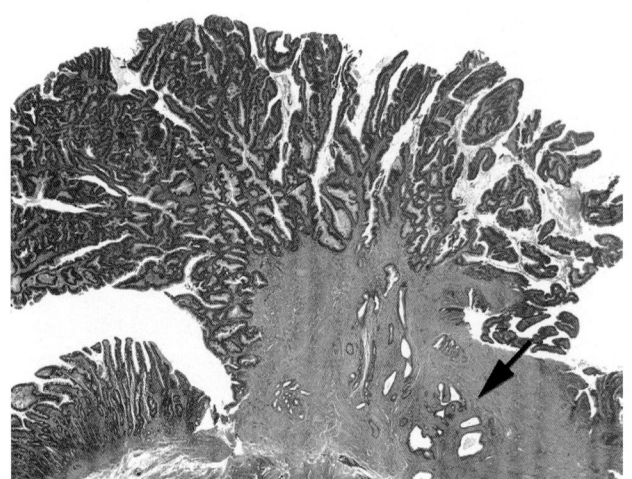

Figure 3-125. Duodenal adenoma with benign ampullary glands. In the periampullary area, smooth muscle bands and benign glands (*arrow*) are admixed and can appear disorganized histologically. Do not mistake these deep glands for adenocarcinoma. The lobulated and rounded configuration are clues to their benign nature.

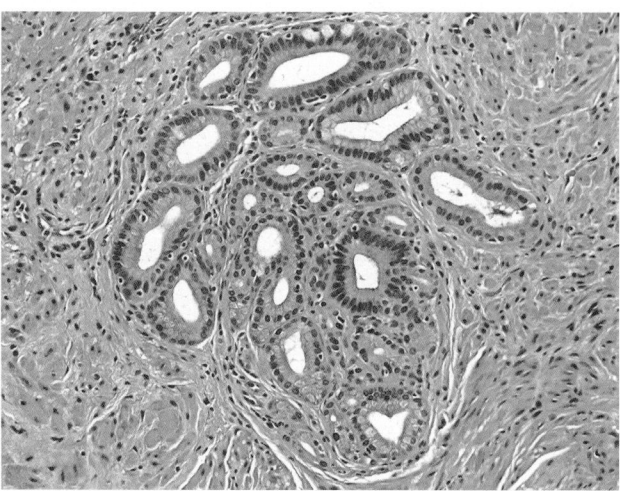

Figure 3-126. Benign ampullary glands, higher magnification of the previous figure. The lobular configuration and the bland epithelial cells confirm the benign nature of these glands. Note the basally located evenly spaced nuclei lack overlapping.

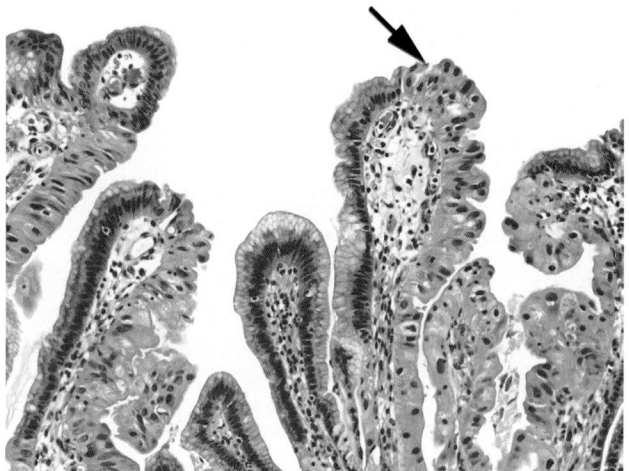

Figure 3-127. Small bowel mucosa colonized by adjacent malignancy. Although this may look like high-grade dysplasia involving the small bowel, a pancreatic adenocarcinoma has extended through the small bowel wall to colonize the surface epithelium (*arrow*). Beware of this pitfall when assessing for primary small bowel lesions.

Pyloric Gland Adenoma

Pyloric gland adenomas are best described in the stomach (see "Stomach" chapter) but can also occur in the small bowel. These are neoplastic lesions and are considered at least low-grade dysplastic, a view that has developed over time since earlier descriptions.[62] They can be found in a variety of GI sites, with the stomach being the most common, followed by duodenal bulb, bile duct, gallbladder, duodenum, and main pancreatic duct.[22,63] Histologically, they are composed of closely packed pyloric gland–like tubules with a bland monolayer of cuboidal or columnar epithelial cells containing round nuclei and pale ground glass eosinophilic cytoplasm (Figs. 3.128–3.134). These lesions can be histologically heterogenous, and this variability, in combination with the overall infrequency of these lesions, causes challenges in recognition. Application of immunohistochemical stains is helpful in problematic cases: PGAs coexpress MUC5AC (foveolar mucin marker) and MUC6 (pyloric mucin marker) and are nonreactive for MUC2 or CDX2 (both intestinal mucin markers) (Figs. 3.135–3.137).[64] Most centers, however, do not have these helpful MUC stains readily available, and so a good number of pathologists will rely upon routine hematoxylin-eosin (H&E) stains for this diagnosis. As noted earlier, all PGAs are considered at least low-grade dysplastic,[62] even in the absence of conventional low-grade dysplasia, which is seen in 63% of these lesions, or high-grade dysplasia, which is found in 51% (Figs. 3.138–3.142).[64] Adjacent adenocarcinoma is frequent (12% to 30%), underscoring the importance of adequate sampling[64]; complete excision is the treatment of choice. PGAs have been reported to occur in FAP syndrome (6% of patients), but these lesions show similar genetic background as sporadic PGAs (i.e., *KRAS* and *GNAS* mutations).[65-67]

KEY FEATURES: Pyloric Gland Adenoma

- **Low-grade dysplastic lesion, by definition**
- Most frequent locations: stomach > duodenal bulb > bile duct > gallbladder > duodenum > main pancreatic duct
- Closely packed tubules lined by monolayer of cuboidal **pyloric gland cells with ground glass cytoplasm**
- Frequently associated with **high-grade dysplasia** (51%) and **adenocarcinoma** (30%)
- Immunohistochemistry profile: **MUC5AC+, MUC6+,** MUC2−, CDX2−

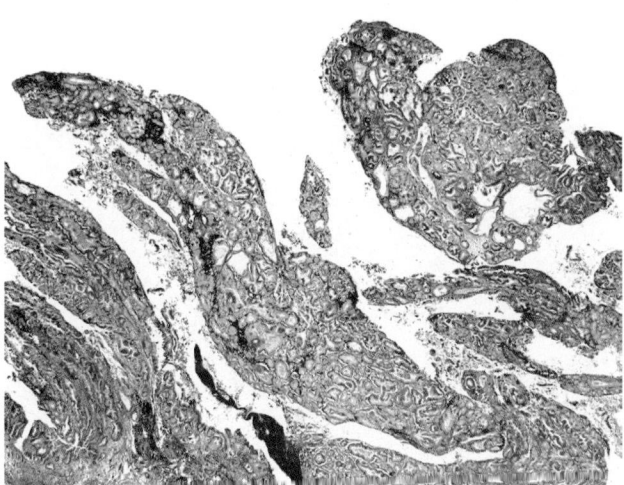

Figure 3-128. Pyloric gland adenoma. At low magnification, this PGA shows closely packed pyloric glandlike tubules, some of which are cystically dilated and distorted. The lesion lacks stroma-rich or edematous areas, and the presence of back-to-back glands indicates an epithelial proliferative process. PGAs, by definition, have at least low-grade dysplasia.

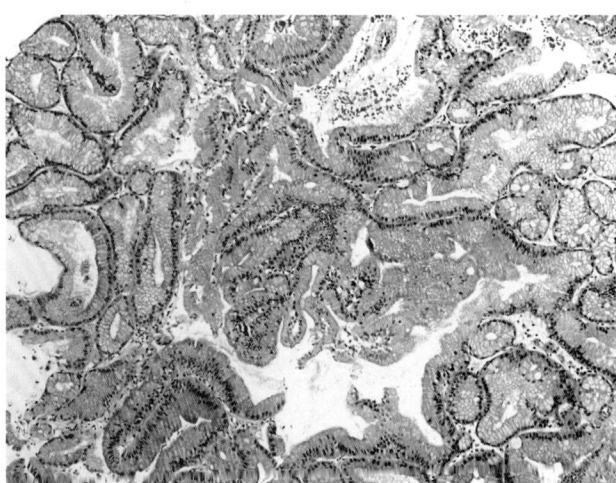

Figure 3-129. Pyloric gland adenoma. PGAs are composed of a monolayer of low columnar or cuboidal cells with abundant clear to foamy cytoplasm and basally located nuclei. These polyps are considered low-grade dysplasia despite the lack of conventional dysplasia (such as that seen in colon tubular adenomas).

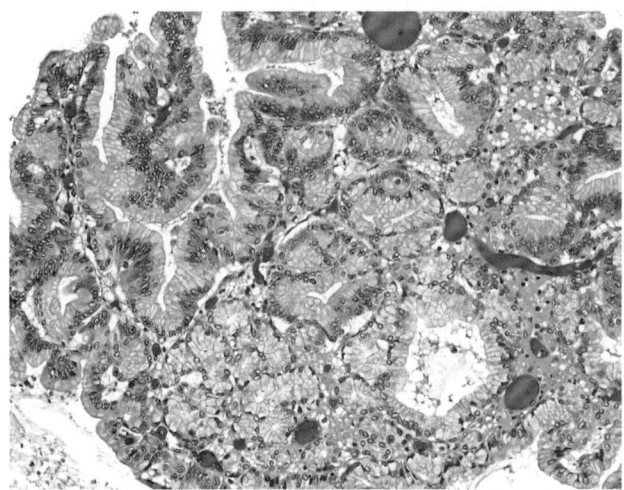

Figure 3-130. Pyloric gland adenoma. PGAs are heterogeneous, adding to diagnostic difficulty. Some areas have back-to-back well-formed tubules, whereas other areas have dilated and distorted glands. Epithelial cells range from low cuboidal with clear cytoplasm to columnar with eosinophilic cytoplasm. The field shown here contains variability in cells, but it all represents PGA.

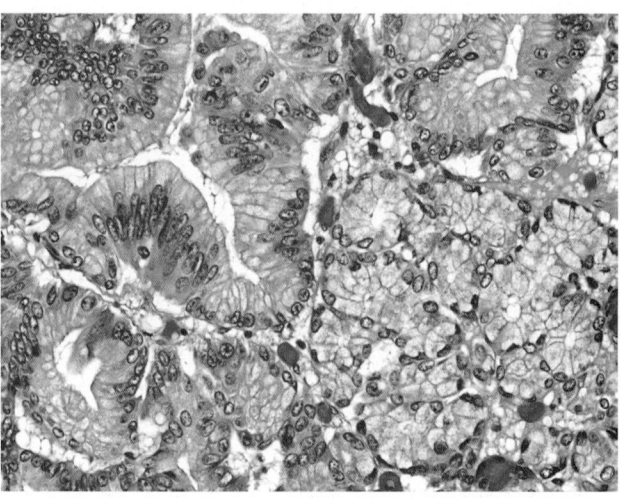

Figure 3-131. Pyloric gland adenoma. These back-to-back glands are composed of uniform low columnar to cuboidal cells with abundant ground glass or foamy cytoplasm. The nuclei are small and basally located. Original descriptions did not consider areas containing a monolayer of bland cells dysplastic, but this view has evolved over time, and all PGAs are now considered at least low-grade dysplasia regardless of whether conventional dysplasia is present.

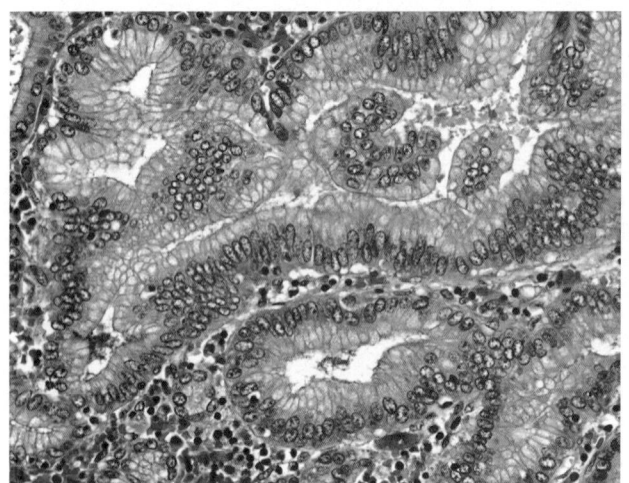

Figure 3-132. Pyloric gland adenoma. These cells are low columnar with round basally located nuclei. PGAs have eosinophilic to clear cytoplasm with ground glass or foamy appearance.

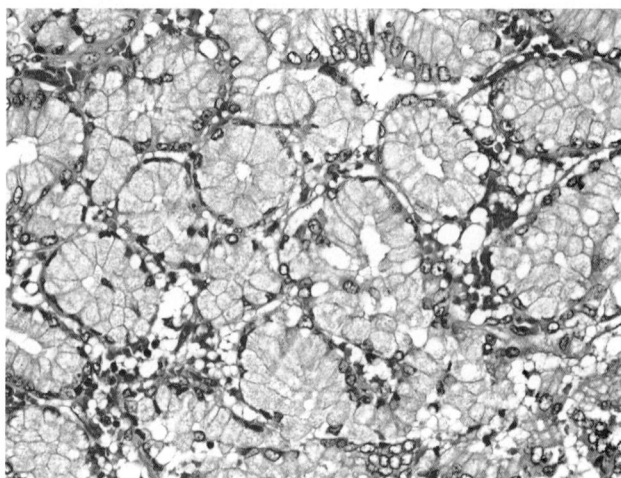

Figure 3-133. Pyloric gland adenoma. The proliferative tubules are pyloric gland-like, with uniform basally located small nuclei and abundant clear foamy cytoplasm. Despite their bland appearance, these cells are considered at least low-grade dysplastic.

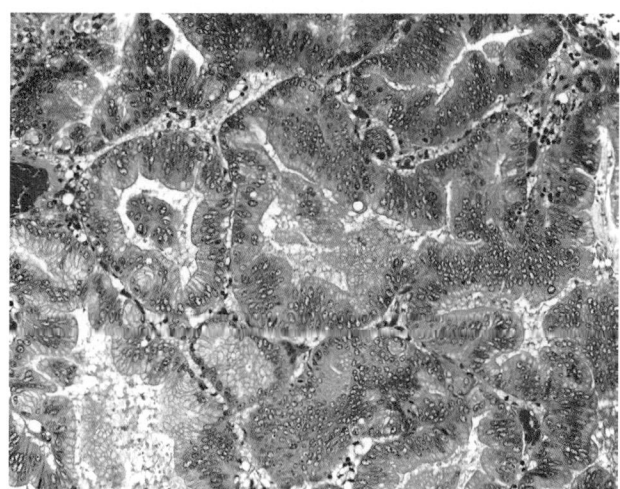

Figure 3-134. Pyloric gland adenoma. This example shows more cytologic atypia, and cells are overlapping with pseudostratification. There is some complexity in glandular architecture, but the nuclei maintain polarity and there is abundant cytoplasm. Although all PGAs are considered low-grade dysplasia, this example shows features similar to conventional dysplasia such as those seen in a typical colonic tubular adenoma.

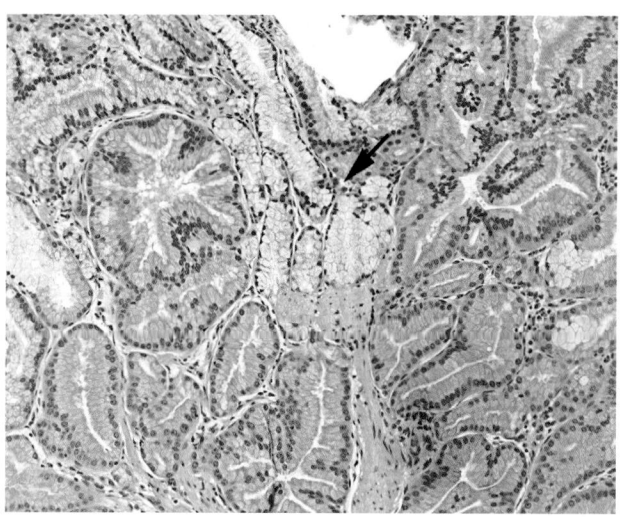

Figure 3-135. Pyloric gland adenoma. This pyloric gland adenoma has entrapped Brunner glands (arrow).

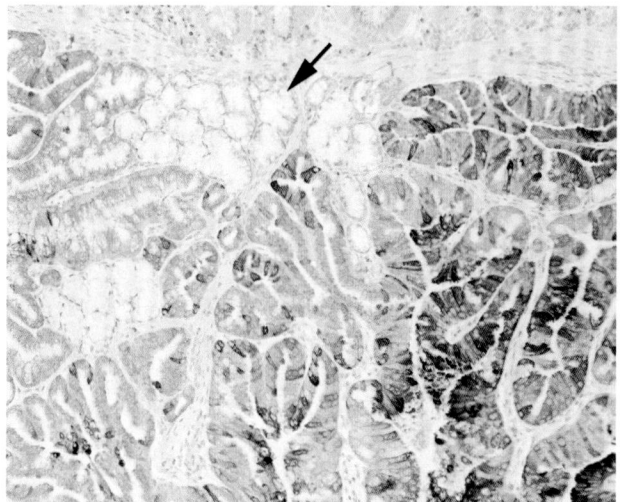

Figure 3-136. Pyloric gland adenoma, MUC5 immunostain of the previous figure. PGAs coexpress MUC5 (a foveolar mucin marker) and MUC6 (a pyloric mucin marker). The entrapped Brunner glands (arrow) in this example do not express MUC5. This immunoprofiling can be helpful in differentiated Brunner gland proliferative lesions from PGAs.

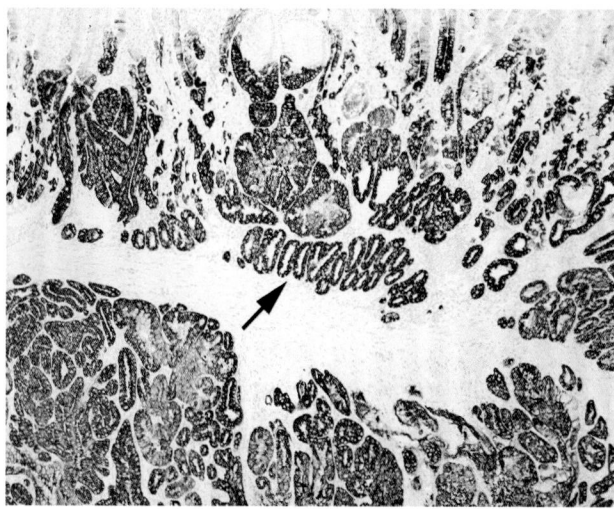

Figure 3-137. Pyloric gland adenoma, MUC6 immunostain. PGAs coexpress MUC5 (a foveolar mucin marker) and MUC6 (a pyloric mucin marker), whereas Brunner glands express MUC6 only. The entrapped Brunner glands (arrow) are seen in this example.

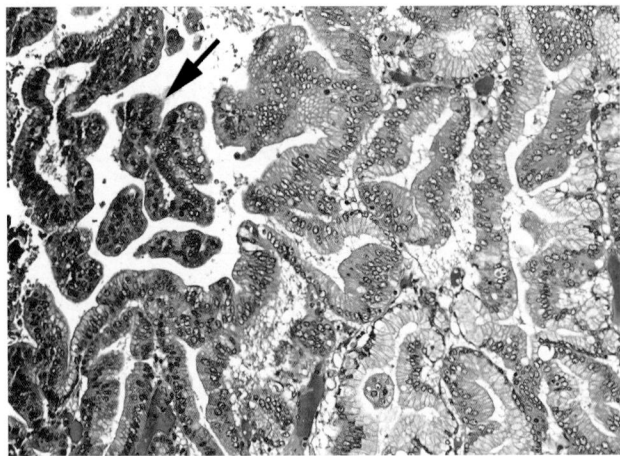

Figure 3-138. Pyloric gland adenoma, high-grade dysplasia. The focus of high-grade dysplasia (*arrow*) in this PGA is hyperchromatic and shows marked cytologic atypia. The nuclei in this example are highly atypical with variation in size and shape. They are no longer situated in an orderly fashion along the basement membrane but instead are haphazardly arranged. The columnar cells to the far right are low-grade dysplastic, as all PGAs are considered to have low-grade dysplasia.

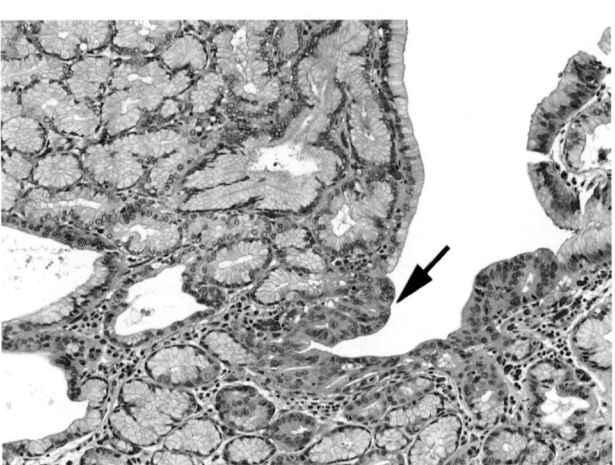

Figure 3-139. Pyloric gland adenoma, high-grade dysplasia. High-grade dysplasia (*arrow*) is found in half of PGAs and is highly associated with adjacent adenocarcinoma (up to 30% of cases). These cells have increased nuclear to cytoplasmic ratio and have lost nuclear polarity. Note the extremely bland monolayer of cells composing the remainder of this PGA; these areas are considered low-grade dysplasia by definition.

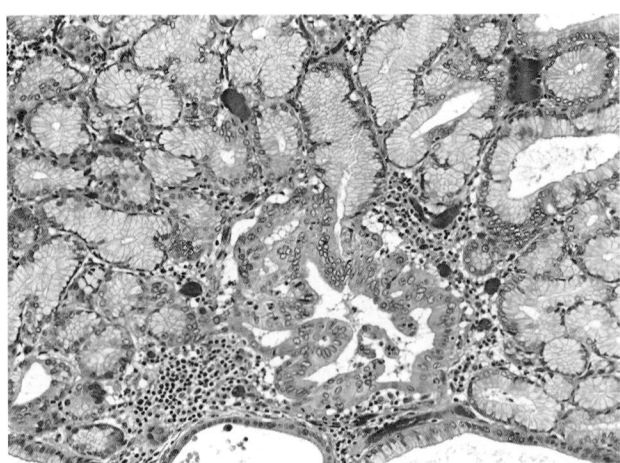

Figure 3-140. Pyloric gland adenoma, high-grade dysplasia. The glandular architecture is complex with crowding and cribriforming. The nuclei are not aligned along the basement membrane and are overlapping. This area of high-grade dysplasia is abruptly different from the background bland monolayer of cells.

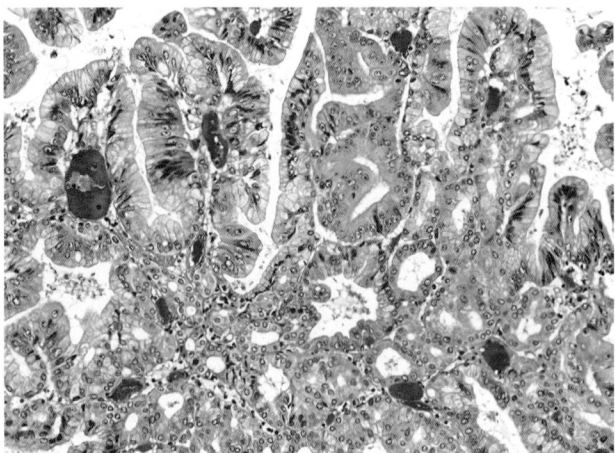

Figure 3-141. Pyloric gland adenoma, high-grade dysplasia. The glandular architecture is complex with crowding and cribriforming.

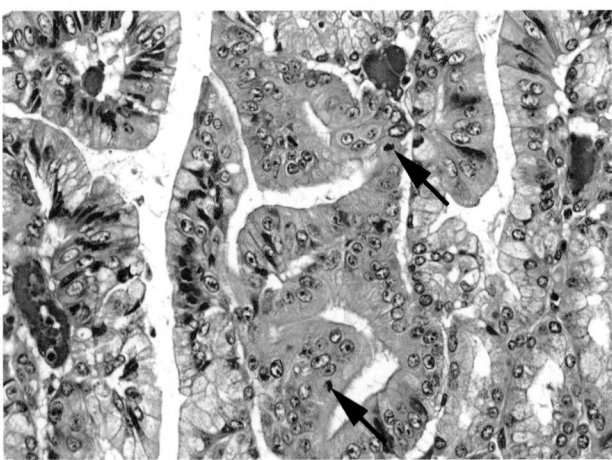

Figure 3-142. Pyloric gland adenoma, high-grade dysplasia. The nuclei show variation in size and shape, have irregular nuclear borders, and contain prominent nucleoli. Mitotic figures are frequent (*arrows*).

ADENOCARCINOMA

Despite the small bowel comprising more than 75% the length of the GI tract (Fig. 3.143), small intestinal adenocarcinoma is rare, accounting for less than 3% of all GI tract neoplasms.[68] In contrast to the colon where adenocarcinoma dominates, small bowel adenocarcinoma is the second most common lesion (25%) following neuroendocrine tumors.[69] To explain this comparative infrequency of small bowel adenocarcinoma, several hypotheses have been proposed based on differences in the small bowel environment compared with the colon. For example, the small bowel has more rapid transport resulting in decreased exposure to carcinogens, lower bacterial load resulting in lower conversion of bile acids to potential carcinogens, more dilute and liquid contents resulting in less mucosal irritation, higher concentrations of ingested carcinogens, and more lymphoid tissue with secretory IgA that provides a protective effect.[70,71] In 2018, the overall mortality rate was low (14%), resulting in less than 1% of all deaths due to GI cancers,[68] and this is partially attributable to improved detection methods and advanced endoscopic techniques.[72] The mean age at diagnosis is 65 years, with a slight male predominance (male to female ratio 1.5:1) and a higher reported incidence in blacks than whites.[73] Most small intestinal carcinomas arise in the duodenum (64%) in the periampullary area, followed by the jejunum (20%) and ileum (15%),[74] and about 10% are associated with a syndrome, such as FAP, Peutz-Jeghers, or Lynch syndromes. An exception to the predominantly proximal location is in the setting of Crohn disease. These patients have a predilection for adenocarcinoma to arise in the ileum (70% of cases) at the primary site of their chronic inflammatory disease. Clinical presentation is variable, with abdominal pain, nausea and vomiting, anemia, GI bleed, jaundice, intestinal obstruction, and less frequently perforation. Owing to the vague nature of these symptoms, 58% of patients are advanced stage at the time of diagnosis.[74] Stage remains the most important prognostic indicator, and proper staging requires identifying tumor location (e.g., small bowel vs ampullary) (Figs. 3.144–3.149). Histologically, the tumors are identical to those found in the colon (see "Colon" chapter). Special morphologic variants identified by WHO (e.g., mucinous, adenosquamous, medullary) (Table 3.2) have little impact on overall prognosis and therefore are not imperative in the diagnostic line, but documentation can aid in identifying the primary site when metastatic disease is encountered (Figs. 3.150–162). Histologic grading is identical to that of colonic adenocarcinoma:

Grade 1: Well differentiated, >95% tumor composed of glands
Grade 2: Moderately differentiated, 50% to 95% tumor composed of glands
Grade 3: Poorly differentiated, <50% tumor composed of glands
Grade 4: Undifferentiated, reserved for WHO undifferentiated and neuroendocrine carcinomas (NECs)

APPROACH TO THE BIOPSY

Tumor Location and Staging: Duodenal Versus Ampullary

Neoplasms in the proximal duodenum may originate from the pancreas, duodenum, distal common bile duct, or the structures of the ampullary complex. Although ampullary and pancreaticobiliary tumors are beyond the scope of this book, it is important to understand the anatomy of the periampullary area to separate duodenal carcinomas from ampullary carcinomas, which are staged differently (for example, an ampullary tumor invading into the pancreas is staged as pT3, whereas a duodenal primary is staged as pT4). Ampullary/periampullary tumors are neoplasms that arise in the vicinity of the ampulla of Vater, a mucosal papillary mound on the posteromedial wall of the proximal duodenum that forms the outlet for the distal common bile duct and main pancreatic duct which converge at this site (Fig. 3.144) and are surrounded by the sphincter of Oddi muscle. Ampullary carcinomas are defined as those that arise within this ampullary complex, distal to the confluence of the distal common bile duct and the pancreatic duct, and they may arise within the ampulla (intra-ampullary type) or on the duodenal surface of the papilla (periampullary type) or may involve both the intra-ampullary and periampullary regions (mixed type) (Figs. 3.145–118). Because of this, ampullary tumors may show biliary or intestinal features or a combination of the two. Consequently, it may

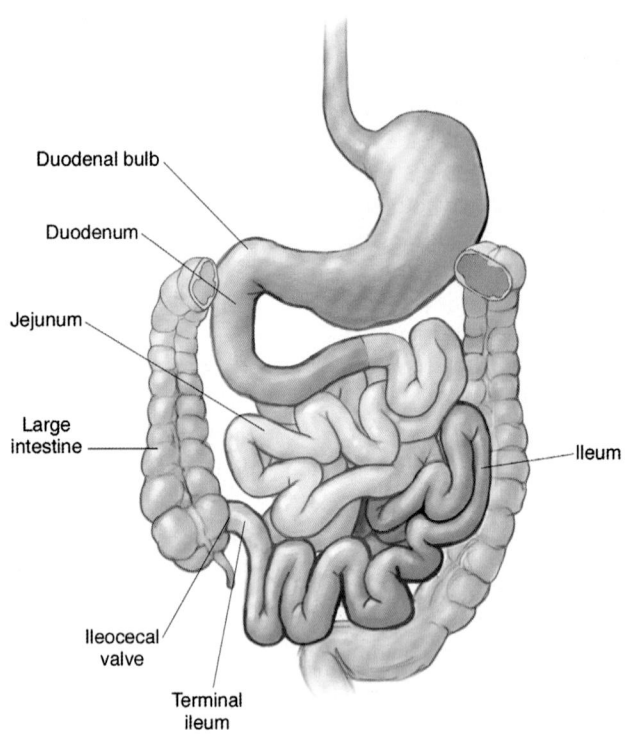

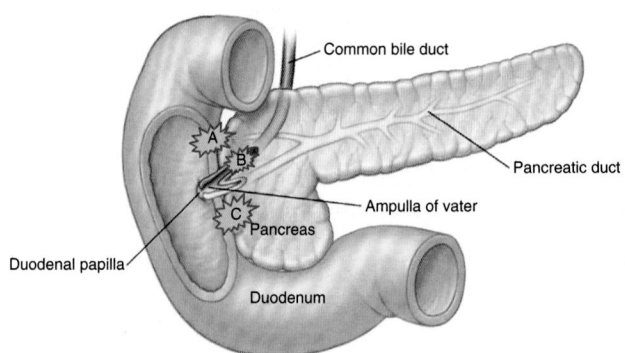

Figure 3-144. Criteria for tumor classification: Duodenum, bile duct, pancreas, and ampulla. Tumors in the proximal duodenum may originate from the pancreas, duodenum, common bile duct, or structures within the ampullary complex. These tumors are all staged differently, but the convergence of these organs at the ampulla can make distinction difficult. Classification is based on the epicenter of the tumor. For example, despite involving multiple organs, tumor A is staged as a duodenal primary, B is an extrahepatic bile duct primary, and C is a pancreatic primary.

Figure 3-143. The small bowel, starting at the duodenal bulb and extending to the ileocecal valve, comprises >75% the length of the entire GI tract, but small bowel adenocarcinoma accounts for <3% of all GI neoplasms. Nearly two-thirds of these lesions are found in the duodenum, with 20% in the jejunum and 15% in the ileum.

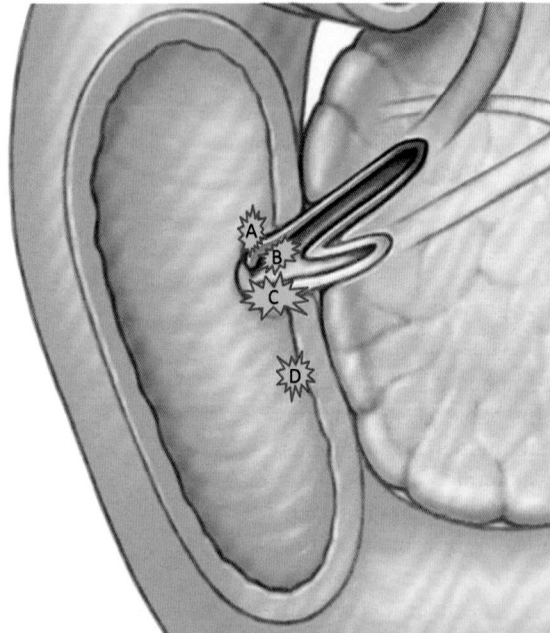

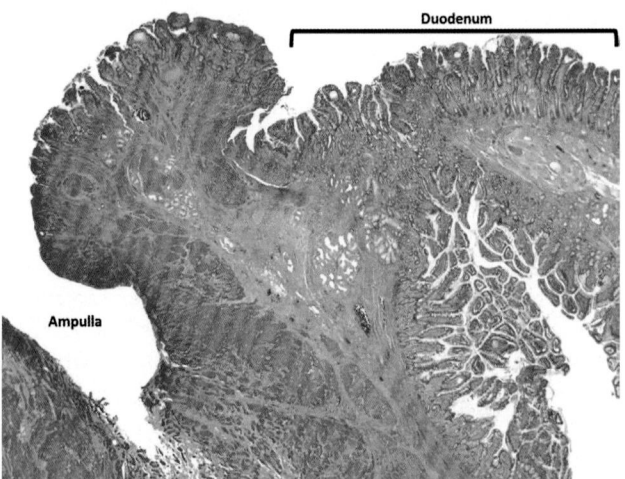

Figure 3-145. Criteria for tumor classification: duodenum versus ampulla. Ampullary carcinomas are defined as those that arise within the ampullary complex, distal to the confluence of the distal common bile duct and the pancreatic duct. They may arise on the duodenal surface of the papilla (periampullary type) (A), within the ampulla (intra-ampullary type) (B), or may involve both the intra-ampullary and periampullary regions (mixed type) (C). Tumors with epicenters in the duodenum are staged as duodenal tumors (D).

Figure 3-146. Intra-ampullary tumor. This tumor is arising from within the ampulla and should be classified and staged as an ampullary carcinoma.

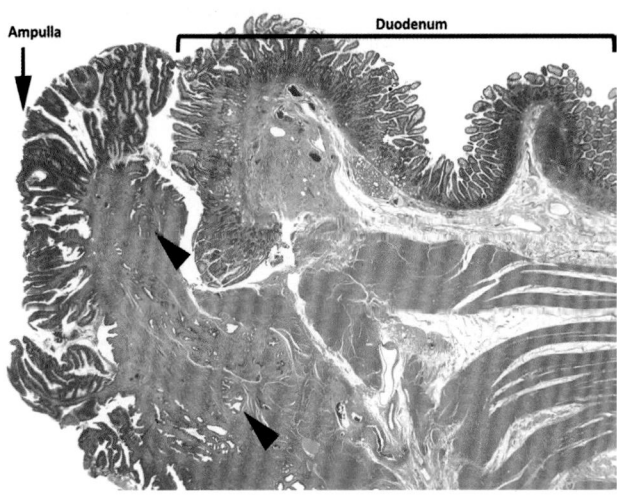

Figure 3-147. Intra-ampullary tumor. The lesion is arising from the intra-ampullary surface (*arrow*). On this resection specimen, the sphincter of Oddi is appreciable, but these disordered smooth muscle bundles and periampullary glands (*arrowheads*) complicate interpretation on small endoscopic biopsies.

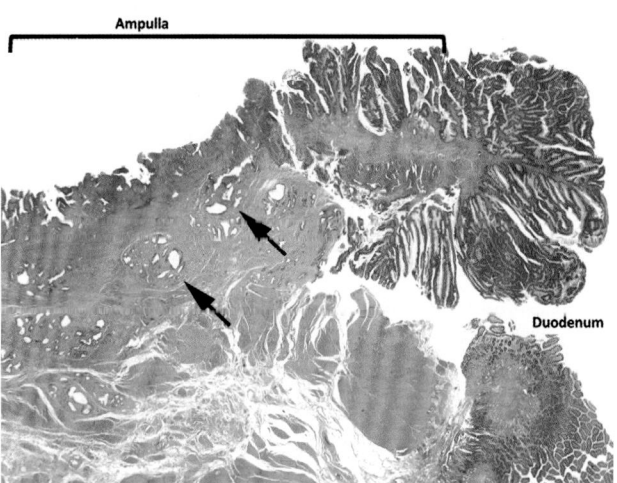

Figure 3-148. Mixed intra- and periampullary tumor. This ampullary tumor extends to involve both the intra-ampullary surface and the duodenal surface of the ampulla. Again note the thickened and disorganized smooth muscle bundles characteristic of this region and the lobules of periampullary glands (*arrows*).

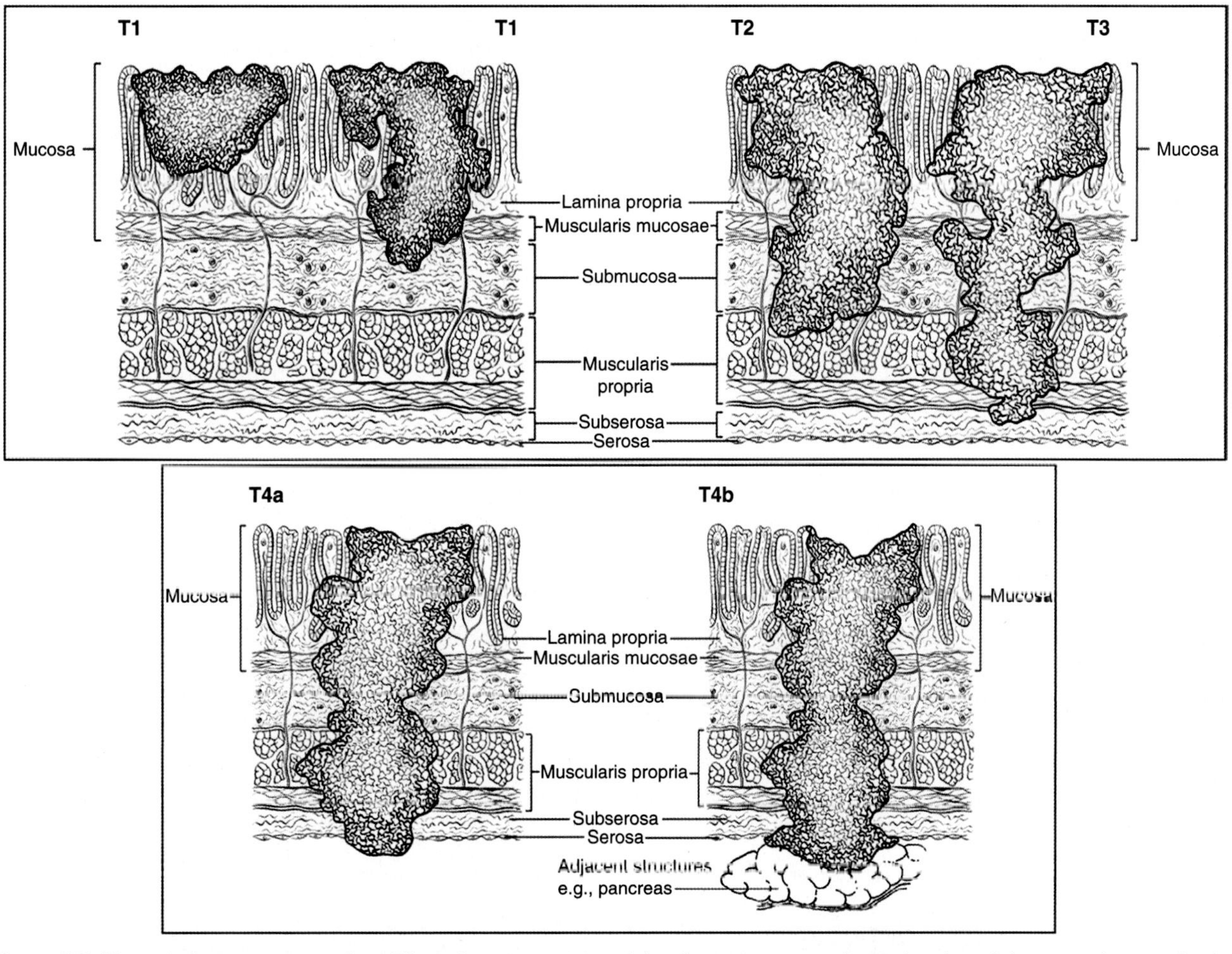

Figure 3-149. Pathologic T staging of small bowel cancer, AJCC eighth edition. Staging is identical to that of the stomach. T1 is divided into lamina propria invasion (pT1a) and invasion into submucosa (pT1b). Involvement of muscularis propria is pT2, whereas invasion beyond the muscularis propria into the subserosal tissue is pT3. Penetration of the serosa (visceral peritoneum) is pT4a, and when adjacent structures are involved the stage is designated pT4b. (Used with permission of the American Joint Committee on Cancer [AJCC], Chicago, IL. The original source for this material is the AJCC Cancer Staging Atlas [2006] edited by Greene FL, Compton C, Fritz AG, et al. and published by Springer Science and Business Media, LLC, www.springerlink.com.)

TABLE 3.2: WHO 2010 Classification of Small Bowel Carcinoma

Tumor Type	Histologic Features	
Adenocarcinoma, not otherwise specified		
Mucinous adenocarcinoma	>50% extracellular mucin pools May contain signet ring cells	
Signet-ring cell carcinoma	>50% signet ring cells containing a clear droplet of cytoplasmic mucin displacing the nucleus Infiltrating single cells or small aggregates	
Adenosquamous carcinoma	≥25% squamous component mixed with glandular	
Medullary carcinoma	Sheets of malignant cells with vesicular nuclei, prominent nucleoli, and abundant eosinophilic cytoplasm Prominent infiltration by intraepithelial lymphocytes	
Squamous cell carcinoma	Either keratinizing or nonkeratinizing	
Undifferentiated carcinoma	High-grade carcinoma not classifiable among other categories	
Neuroendocrine carcinoma (NEC)		
Large cell NEC	Poorly differentiated High grade Marked nuclear atypia Synaptophysin+ or chromogranin+	Cells are large and pleomorphic Moderate amount of cytoplasm Prominent nucleoli
Small cell NEC	May have: Focal necrosis Ki-67 >20% >20 mitoses per 10 HPF	Cells are small Finely granular chromatin (salt and pepper) Indistinct nucleoli
Mixed adenoneuroendocrine carcinoma (MANEC)		>30% each of gland-forming and neuroendocrine areas (Adenocarcinomas showing immunoreactivity for neuroendocrine markers is not sufficient for diagnosis)

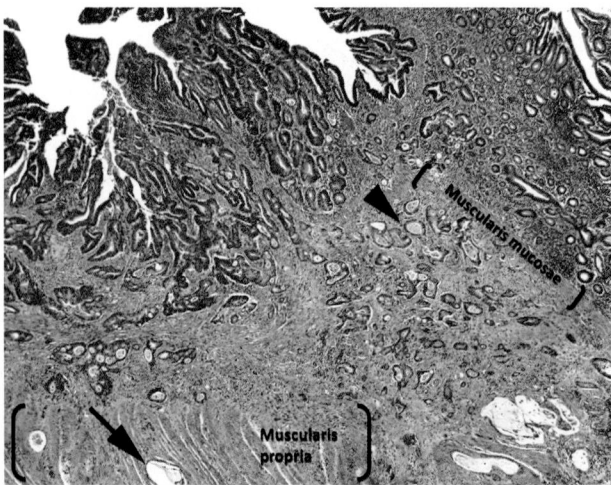

Figure 3-150. Small bowel adenocarcinoma, well differentiated. Arising from the overlying adenoma, the tumor cells of this invasive adenocarcinoma form glands (>95% glands = well differentiated) and extend through the submucosa (*arrowhead*) into at least the muscularis propria (*arrow*) and is at least stage pT2.

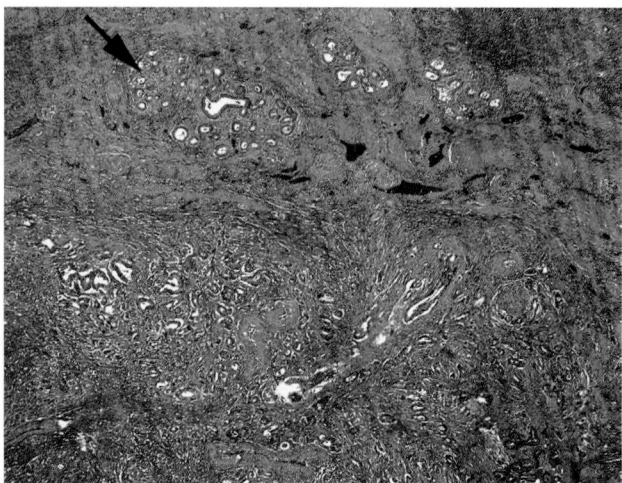

Figure 3-151. Moderately differentiated adenocarcinoma. The moderately differentiated adenocarcinoma seen at the bottom half of this photo is composed of sheets of tumor cells with gland formation (50%–95%). Compare this with the benign glands (*arrow*), which retain a lobular configuration at low magnification.

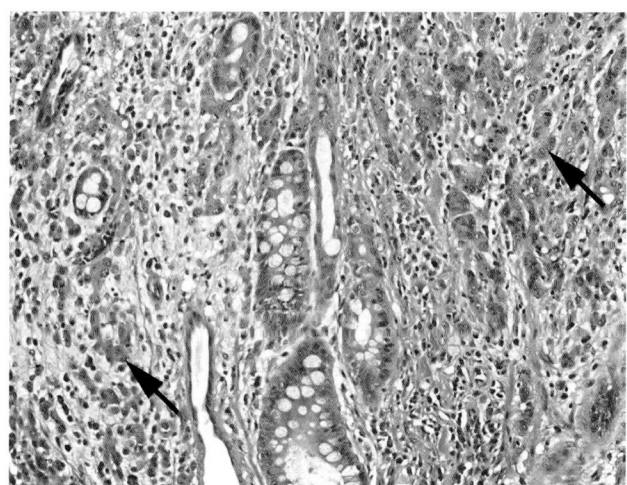

Figure 3-152. Poorly differentiated adenocarcinoma. The infiltrating cells of this adenocarcinoma (*arrows*) do not show any gland formation. Tumors with <50% gland formation are considered poorly differentiated.

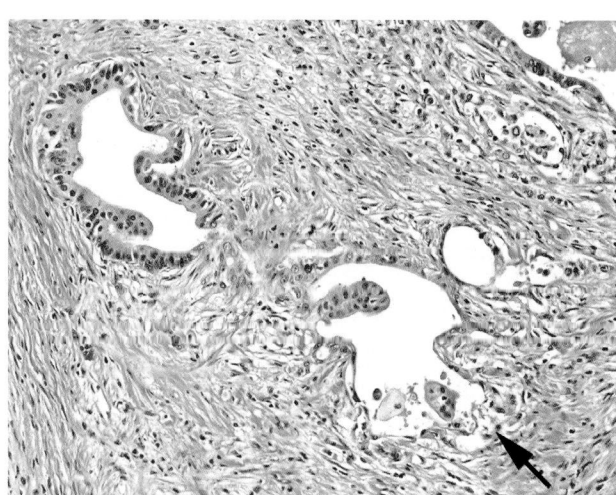

Figure 3-153. Small bowel adenocarcinoma. Malignant glands may show abortive or incomplete gland formation (*arrow*), whereas the stroma is slightly pale owing to desmoplastic response.

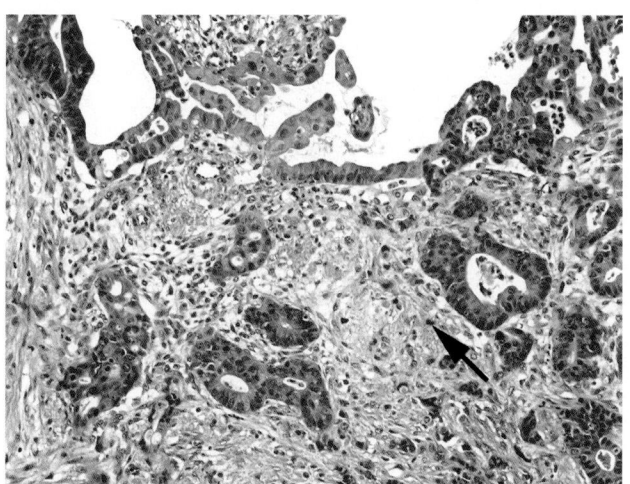

Figure 3-154. Small bowel adenocarcinoma. Single infiltrative cells (*arrow*) are a feature of poorly differentiated tumors.

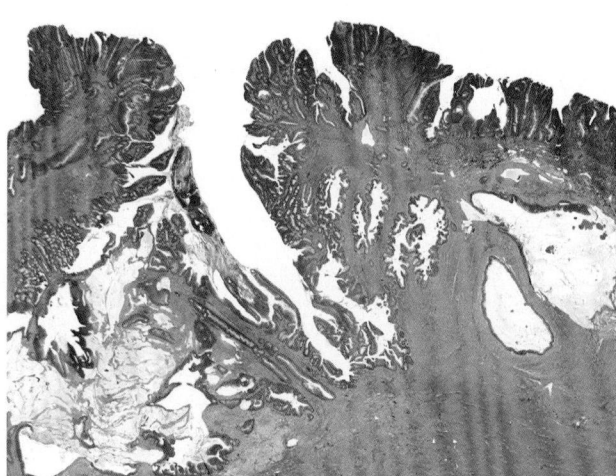

Figure 3-155. Small bowel adenocarcinoma with mucinous features. WHO subtypes, such as mucinous adenocarcinoma, do not affect prognosis but are worth mentioning in the event of metastatic disease.

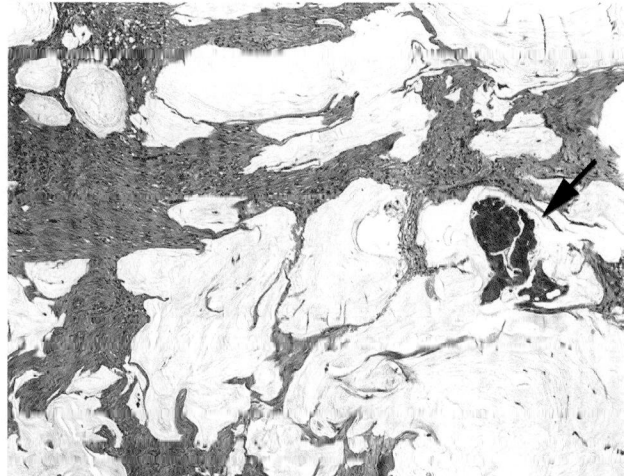

Figure 3-156. Mucinous adenocarcinoma. Single cells or strips of epithelium (*arrow*) may be seen floating in mucin pools, which compose >50% of mucinous adenocarcinoma.

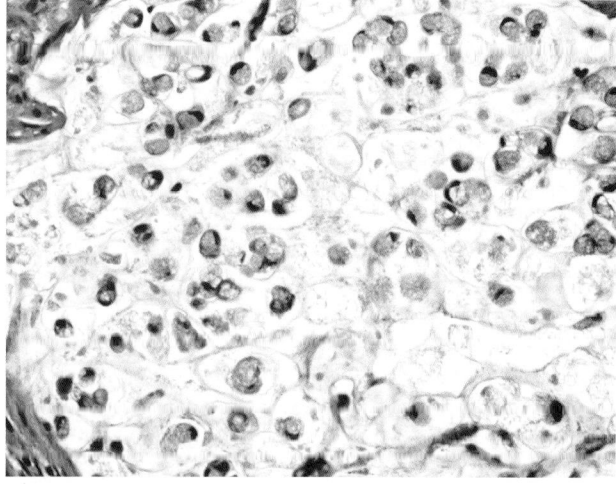

Figure 3-157. Mucinous adenocarcinoma with signet ring cells. Mucinous adenocarcinomas may also take on signet ring cell morphology.

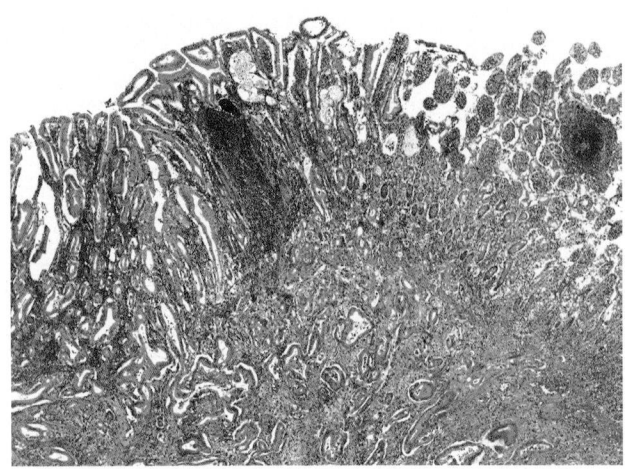

Figure 3-158. Adenocarcinoma extending from a pancreatic primary. On small endoscopic biopsy, this may appear to be a primary small bowel adenocarcinoma, but in the duodenum, always consider the possibility of extension from a nearby organ, such as ampulla, pancreas, and distal common bile duct. On biopsy material, it is best to sign out as simply: "Adenocarcinoma."

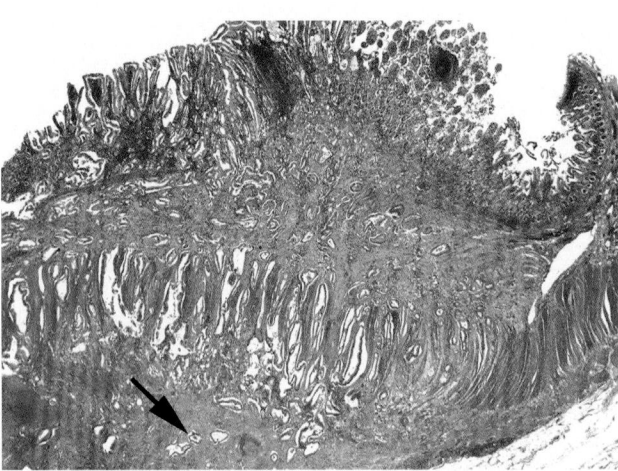

Figure 3-159. Adenocarcinoma extending from a pancreatic primary, lower power of the previous figure. At lower magnification, one can appreciate the transmural extension (*arrow*) of this pancreatic adenocarcinoma to involve the duodenal surface.

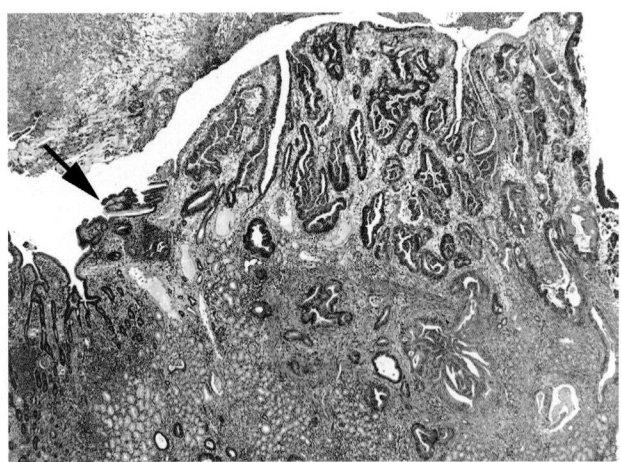

Figure 3-160. Adenocarcinoma at the ampulla. Endoscopic biopsies will not capture enough tissue for pathologists to make an informed diagnosis of the primary site. Ampullary adenocarcinomas, such as this, may extend to involve the small bowel (*arrow*).

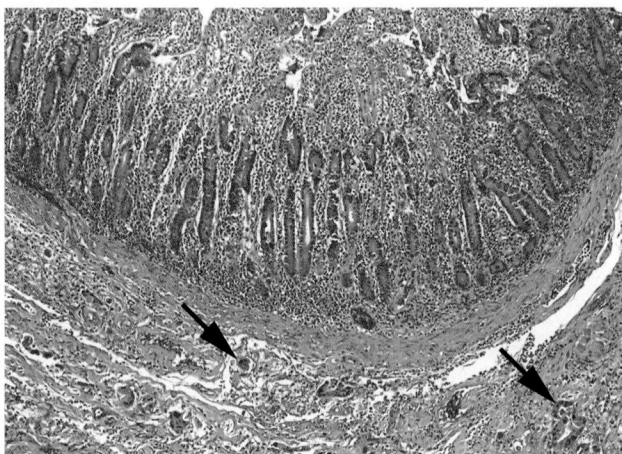

Figure 3-161. Adenocarcinoma undermining small bowel. The small bowel mucosa is eroded and reactive in this sample, but tumor cells extending from an adjacent site are found in the submucosa (*arrows*).

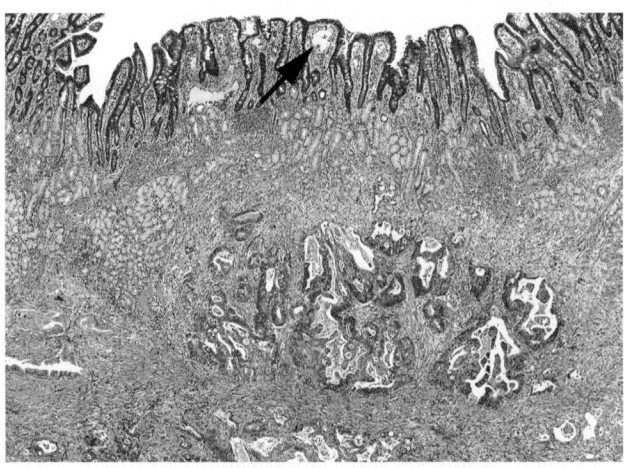

Figure 3-162. Dilated lacteals as a clue to underlying pathology. The dilated lymphatic spaces (*arrow*) in the mucosa are a clue to nearby pathology. In this case, there is an underlying adenocarcinoma.

be difficult, if not impossible, to differentiate these lesions from primary duodenal carcinomas on small endoscopic biopsies, especially when ampullary tumors are exophytic or colonize the duodenal mucosa. Correlation with imaging findings, such as endoscopic retrograde cholangiopancreatography, is necessary, and some cases may require surgical resection before suitable classification. On endoscopic biopsies, it is best to refrain from labeling a tumor as primary duodenal or ampullary, as treatment can range from a relatively conservative endoscopic mucosal resection or ampullectomy to a Whipple resection with greater morbidity.

FAQ: What anatomic landmark distinguishes duodenal from ampullary tumors?

No specific landmark differentiates duodenal tumors from ampullary tumors. Instead, the tumor epicenter defines the tumor type. For example, if the tumor epicenter is intra-ampullary and the lesion extends to involve the duodenal mucosa, this tumor should be considered ampullary and staged as such. Of course, it is impossible to discern the tumor epicenter from an endoscopic biopsy. For this reason, it is best to sign these cases as simply adenocarcinoma and leave the documentation of tumor type (duodenal vs ampullary) for the resection specimen.

For staging purposes, the duodenum and ampulla are differentiated by the American Joint Committee on Cancer (AJCC) Staging Manual (eighth edition).[75] Duodenal carcinomas are staged identical to gastric carcinomas based on depth of invasion and independent of tumor size. Any invasion into the lamina propria, muscularis mucosae, or submucosa is considered pT1. Recall, these intramucosal carcinomas have access to the rich lymphatics within the gastric lamina propria, allowing for lymphatic spread and lymph node metastases. The T1 category is further divided into pT1a (invasion into the lamina propria or muscularis mucosae) and pT1b (invasion into the submucosa). pT2 tumors invade the muscularis propria, pT3 penetrate the subserosal connective tissue or extend into the nonperitonealized perimuscular tissue (mesentery or retroperitoneum) without serosal penetration, and tumors that involve the visceral peritoneum are considered pT4. This last category is further subdivided as pT4a (involvement of the visceral peritoneum only) and pT4b (involvement of adjacent organs or structures, including the pancreas and other loops of bowel) (Fig. 3.149).

By comparison, ampullary tumors have a staging system that combines location of invasion with specific size criteria (Table 3.3). For example, pT1 is tumor that is limited to the ampulla or the sphincter of Oddi (pT1a) or extends to the duodenal submucosa (pT1b); pT2 is invasion into the muscularis propria of the duodenum; pT3 is invasion of the pancreas up to 0.5 cm (pT3a) or more (pT3b) or extension beyond the pancreas/duodenum without involvement of the celiac axis or superior mesenteric artery (pT3b); and pT4 is any involvement of the celiac axis, superior mesenteric artier, and/or common hepatic artery, irrespective of size. Again, one can see that a tumor invading into the pancreas is pT4 if considered a duodenal primary but pT3 if considered an ampullary primary, underscoring the importance of classifying these tumors correctly.

FAQ: Is invasion into the muscularis mucosae considered mucosal (pT1a) or submucosal (pT1b)?

The "e" at the end of "muscularis mucosae" indicates possession in this Latin derivative, and the phrase can be loosely translated as "muscle of the mucosa." Thus, the mucosa includes both the lamina propria and the muscularis mucosae layer, and invasion into either is staged as pT1a. By comparison, pT2 lesions must demonstrate invasion beyond this thin muscle layer into the submucosa (Fig. 3.149).

PEARLS & PITFALLS: Small Bowel Mucosa Can Be Colonized by Other Tumors

Colonization of the duodenal mucosa by neighboring disease (e.g., pancreatic or ampullary carcinoma) and metastatic carcinoma from distant sites can mimic primary duodenal carcinoma or adenoma (Figs. 3.163–3.165).[76] Always take a moment to consider mucosal colonization and exclude metastatic disease by immunohistochemistry if the patient has a known history of malignancy and the sample is sufficient. Suggesting correlation with imaging studies is always prudent (see the following Sample Note).

TABLE 3.3: Comparison of Small Bowel Versus Ampullary Carcinoma Staging by AJCC Eighth Edition

Stage	Ampulla	Small Bowel
pTx	Cannot be assessed	Cannot be assessed
pT0	No tumor	No tumor
pTis	HGD/CIS	HGD/CIS
pT1		
pT1a	Limited to ampulla of Vater or Sphincter of Oddi	Invades lamina propria
pT1b	Invades beyond sphincter of Oddi and/or Into duodenal submucosa	Invades submucosa
pT2	Invades muscularis propria of duodenum	Invades muscularis propria of duodenum
pT3		Invades through the muscularis propria into the subserosa or Extends into nonperitonealized perimuscular tissue (mesentery or retroperitoneum) without serosal penetration
pT3a	Directly invades pancreas ≤0.5 cm	
PT3b	Extends >0.5 cm into pancreas or Extends into peripancreatic tissue or periduodenal tissue or duodenal serosa without involvement of the celiac axis or superior mesenteric artery	
pT4	Involves celiac axis, superior mesenteric artery, and/or common hepatic artery, regardless of size	Tumor perforates the visceral peritoneum or Directly invades other organs or structures (e.g., other loops of bowel, mesentery by way of serosa, pancreas, or bile duct)

CIS, carcinoma in situ; HGD, high-grade dysplasia.

FAQ: Are there immunostains to identify primary small bowel carcinoma?

Short answer: No, but a panel can be helpful. CK7 and CK20 are the mainstays for triaging metastatic carcinoma from GI sites. Nearly all colorectal carcinomas express CK20+, and an immunoprofile of CK7–/CK20+ is highly consistent with colorectal primary. The opposite is true of small bowel adenocarcinoma, and a good rule of thumb to remember is that *95% of small bowel adenocarcinomas are CK7+* with CK20 variable (Figs. 3.166 and 3.167). Conegative CK7/CK20 is seen in 5% of small intestinal adenocarcinomas and almost never in colorectal carcinomas.[77] The challenge, however, is that other upper GI sites, such as the stomach and esophagus, can also show CK7+/CK20 variable reactivity, as can pancreaticobiliary tumors and metastatic tumors from distant sites, such as lung or kidney. The immunoprofile of small bowel mucosa includes strong and diffuse nuclear reactivity for CDX2, a transcription factor specific for intestinal differentiation (recall, all transcription factors localize to the nucleus). This stain is helpful but not specific to the small bowel, as CDX2 is expressed in any tumor with intestinal differentiation, including colonic, esophageal, extrahepatic biliary, and gastric carcinomas, and variably in lung, bladder, and other sites.[78] Villin, targeting a protein found in the brush border of microvilli, is another helpful but nonspecific marker. Thus, the key to differentiating small bowel adenocarcinoma from other tumors requires the use of an immunohistochemical panel comprising multiple stains. When considering primary versus metastatic disease, the following panels are cited as 75% predictive of primary sites[79]:

Colorectal:

   TTF-1–/CDX2+/CK7–/CK20+ or

   TTF-1–/CDX2+/CK7–/CK20–/(CEA+ or MUC2+)

Ovarian:

   CK7+/MUC5AC+/TTF-1–/CDX2–/CEA–/GCDFP-15–

Breast:

   GCDFP-15+/TTF-1–/CDX2–/CK7+/CK20– or

   ER+/TTF-1–/CDX2–/CK20–/CEA–/MUC5AC–

Lung:

   TTF-1+ or

   TTF-1–/CDX2–/CK7+/CK20–/GCDFP-15–/ER–/CEA–/MUC5AC–

Pancreaticobiliary:

   TTF-1–/CDX2–/CK7+/CEA+/MUC5AC+ or

   smad4–(DPC4)

Stomach:

   TTF-1–/CDX2+/CK7+/CK20–

SAMPLE NOTE: Adenocarcinoma Involving the Proximal Small Bowel

Small Bowel, Mass, Biopsy

• Adenocarcinoma, moderately differentiated, see Note.

Note: Histologic sections show small intestinal mucosa involved by an infiltrating adenocarcinoma. Tumors near the ampulla may represent primary duodenal, ampullary, biliary, or pancreatic origin due to mucosal colonization. Correlation with imaging studies (e.g., endoscopic retrograde cholangiopancreatography and computed tomography) is necessary to determine the origin of this tumor. Final classification and staging may be performed on the surgical specimen. Mismatch repair protein immunohistochemistry studies show intact/normal MLH1, PMS2, MSH2, and MSH6. Should additional ancillary testing be desired, sufficient tumor tissue is available in blocks A1 and A2.

KEY FEATURES: Adenocarcinoma of Small Bowel

- This is a rare (<3%) neoplasm of the GI tract with **low mortality** (14%) resulting in <1% of all GI cancer deaths.

- The mean age at diagnosis is **65 years**, with a slight male predominance.

- Most of the tumors arise in the **duodenum (64%)** in the periampullary area, followed by the jejunum (20%) and ileum (15%).

- About **10% are associated with a syndrome**, such as **FAP, Peutz-Jeghers, or Lynch syndrome.**

- Patients with **Crohn disease** have a predilection for **adenocarcinoma in the ileum.**

- About 58% of patients are **advanced stage at the time of diagnosis.**

- Histologically, the tumors are identical to those found in the colon and are graded similarly.

- Special morphologic variants (e.g., mucinous, adenosquamous, medullary) have little impact on prognosis.

- **Refrain from labeling a tumor as primary duodenal or ampullary**, as biopsies are not reliable and there are **no specific landmarks to differentiate** the two; instead, the **tumor epicenter** defines the tumor type.

- **Colonization** of the duodenal mucosa by neighboring disease (e.g., pancreatic or ampullary carcinoma) and metastatic carcinoma from distant sites **can mimic primary duodenal carcinoma** or adenoma.

- No specific immunostain identifies small bowel: **CK7+, CK20 variable, CDX2+, Villin+, TTF1-, GCDFP-, ER-, SMAD4 retained.**

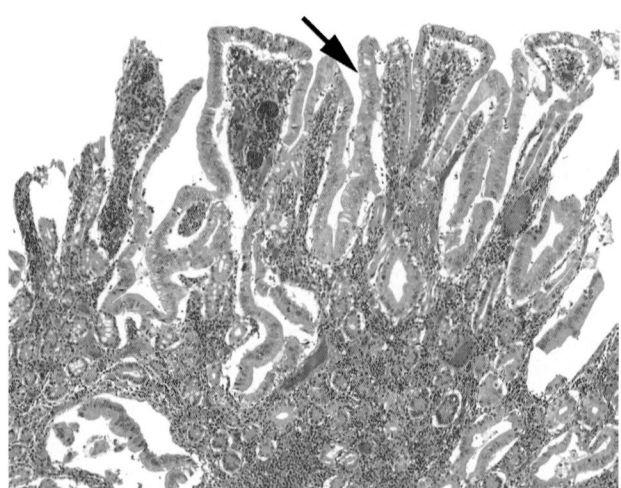

Figure 3-163. Small bowel mucosa colonization. Adjacent or metastatic tumor can colonize the surface epithelium, mimicking an in situ lesion (*arrow*). Always take a moment to consider mucosal colonization and exclude metastatic disease by immunohistochemistry if the patient has a known history of malignancy, such as the pancreatic ductal adenocarcinoma seen in this case.

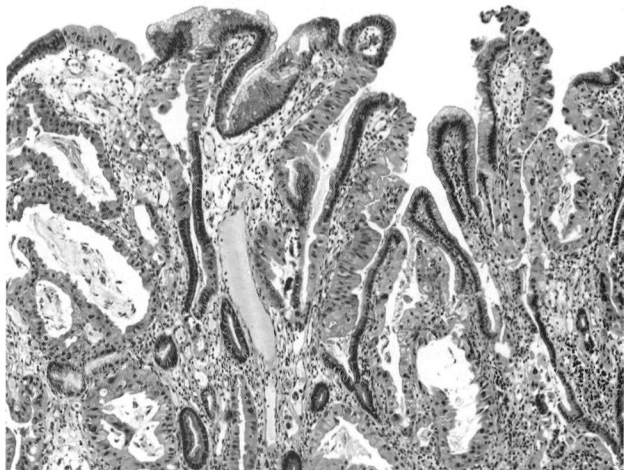

Figure 3-164. Small bowel mucosa colonization. The adjacent pancreatic cancer in this case invaded through the small bowel and colonizes the surface. On endoscopic biopsy material, it is best to simply state adenocarcinoma rather than elaborate on a primary site.

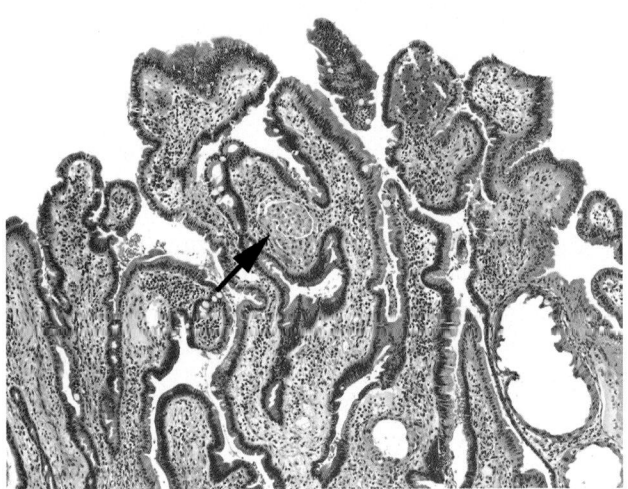

Figure 3-165. Intralymphatic tumor. Sneaky metastatic tumor (*arrow*) can be found in small bowel lacteals.

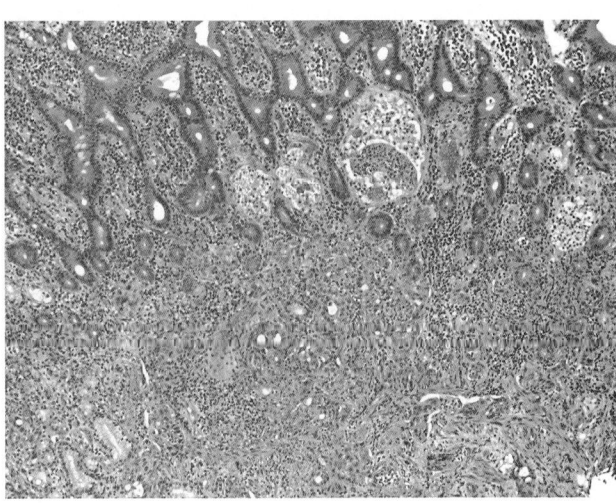

Figure 3-166. Small bowel adenocarcinoma. This small bowel mucosa looks primarily inflamed and reactive. The extent of this poorly differentiated adenocarcinoma is difficult to appreciate on H&E.

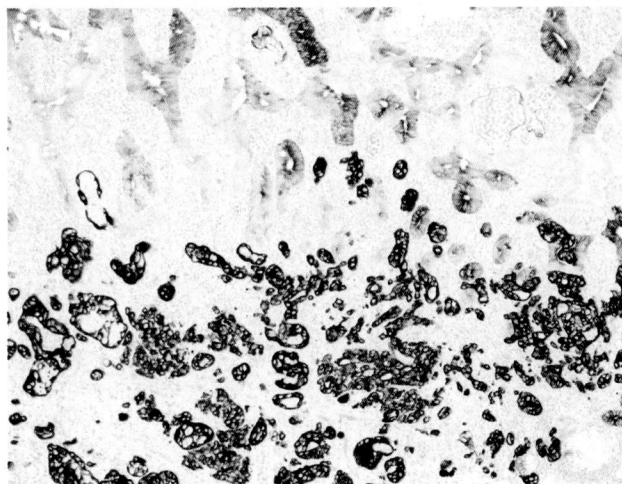

Figure 3-167. Small bowel adenocarcinoma, CK7 immunohistochemistry of the previous figure. A CK7 immunostain highlights extensive involvement. Greater than 95% of small bowel carcinomas are reactive for CK7, but these tumors are variable for CK20. No specific marker exists to differentiate small bowel from pancreaticobiliary or ampullary primaries. Although a panel of stains can be helpful, correlation with imaging studies is necessary.

NEUROENDOCRINE TUMORS AND NEUROENDOCRINE CARCINOMAS

WELL-DIFFERENTIATED NEUROENDOCRINE TUMORS (FORMERLY "CARCINOID")

Based on WHO 2017 classification, well-differentiated neuroendocrine tumors (WD-NETs) are distinguished from NECs by their morphologic features, independent of mitotic count or Ki-67 proliferative index. This is a departure from previous WHO 2010 classification for neuroendocrine neoplasms, in which tumors were stratified based solely on mitoses and Ki-67. The updated system not only more reliably indicates prognosis and response to therapy but is also more intuitive to pathologists. For example, tumors that are morphologically uniform are classified as WD-NETs, whereas NECs are classified by their poorly differentiated high-grade cytology and marked nuclear atypia. The morphologic distinction is important as NEC has a worse prognosis that more closely reflects adenocarcinoma and thus is staged as per adenocarcinoma guidelines.

Histologically WD-NET tumors are composed of nests (type A), trabeculae (type B), or acini (type C) of small, uniform, polygonal, or cuboidal cells with lightly eosinophilic and finely granular cytoplasm (Figs. 3.168–3.175). Some examples, particularly those that arise in the small bowel, are rich in Paneth cells (Fig. 3.176) and may display a palisading or picket-fence organization at the periphery or sheetlike growth, whereas others can mimic adenocarcinoma with prominent acini formation (Figs. 3.177 and 3.178). Although these tumors can have a broad spectrum of architectural features, the variations have no impact on prognosis. A shared feature of all WD-NETs is their bland uniform nuclei, which are round or oval with smooth nuclear borders containing stippled chromatin with indistinct nucleoli (Figs. 3.179–3.181). Prominent nucleoli are never a feature of WD-NETs and when encountered should prompt one to consider PD-NEC or other tumors, such as adenocarcinoma or melanoma. Immunohistochemistry with synaptophysin, chromogranin, or CD56 will highlight neuroendocrine differentiation.

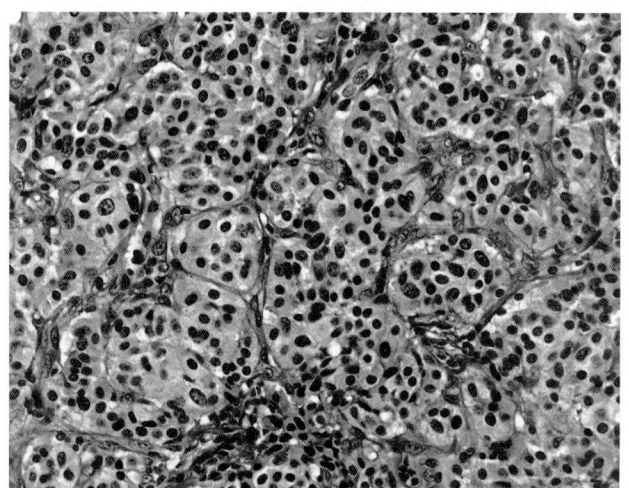

Figure 3-168. Well-differentiated neuroendocrine tumor, type A. The tumor cells in WD-NET have variable architectural patterns. In this example, they form small packets or nests.

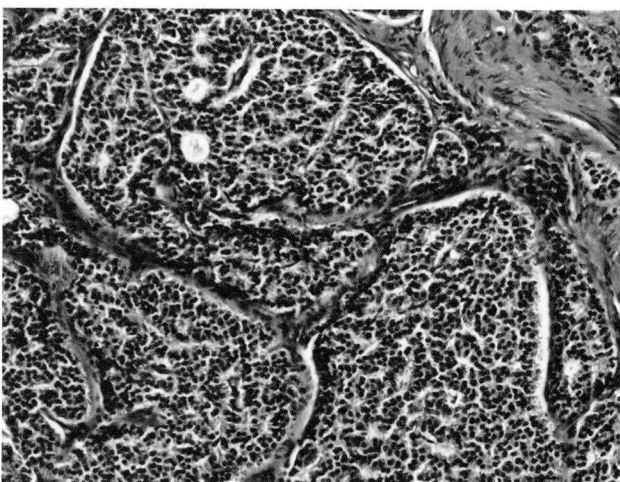

Figure 3-169. Well-differentiated neuroendocrine tumor, type B. Uniform tumor cells form sheets and trabeculae.

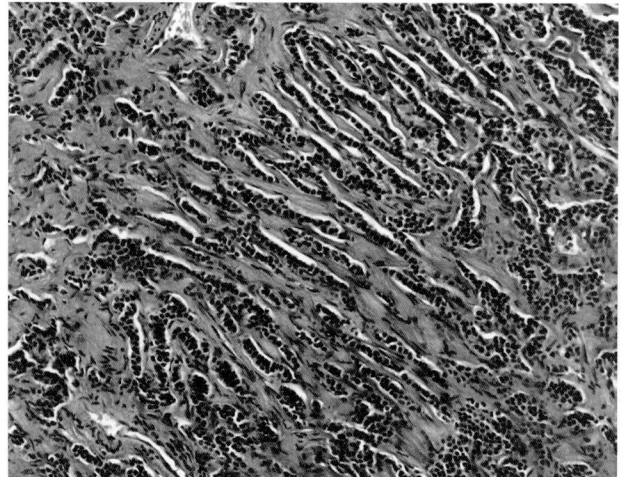

Figure 3-170. Well-differentiated neuroendocrine tumor, type B. The trabeculae are narrow, and some areas appear to have cells lined up in single file.

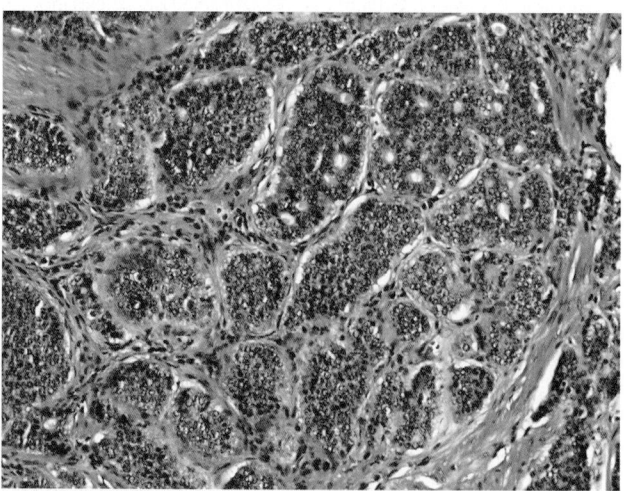

Figure 3-171. Well-differentiated neuroendocrine tumor, type C. Aside from sheets and nests, tumor cells can form acini. This example resembles mammary ductal carcinoma in situ.

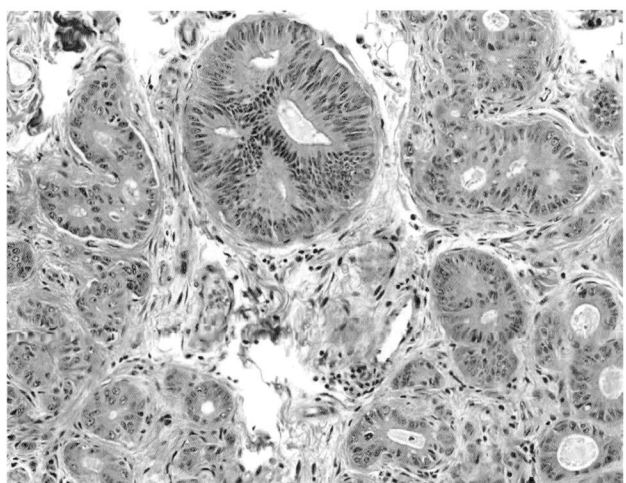

Figure 3-172. Well-differentiated neuroendocrine tumor, type C. When considering adenocarcinoma in the small bowel, always ask whether this could be an acinar variant of WD-NET, as the treatment and prognosis are different. The tumor pictured is in fact a WD-NET.

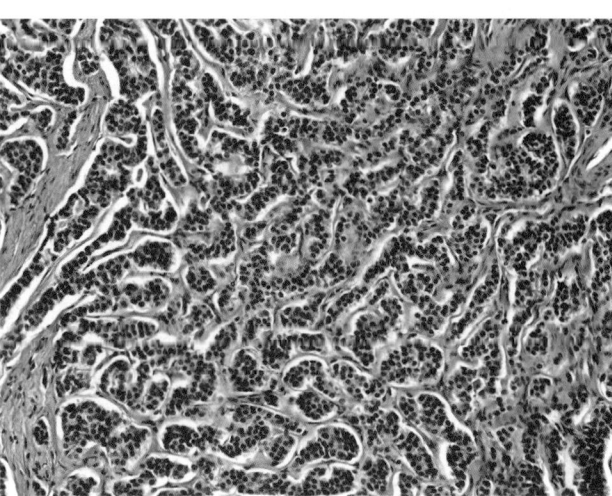

Figure 3-173. Well-differentiated neuroendocrine tumor. Architectural variations can occur within the same tumor; some areas show nested morphology and other areas are trabecular.

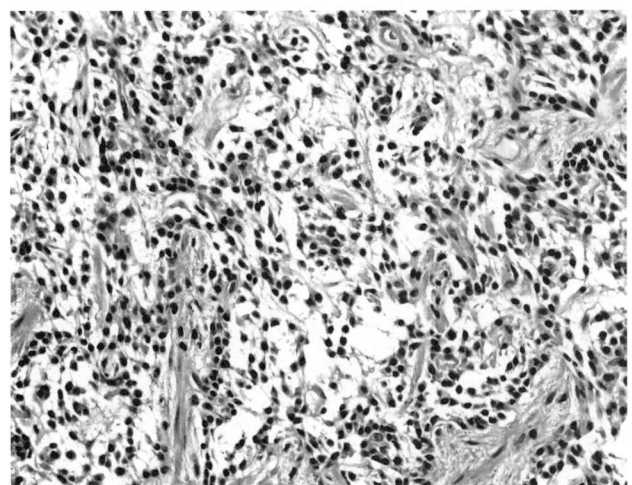

Figure 3-174. Well-differentiated neuroendocrine tumor. Other rare variants include a reticular pattern, as seen here.

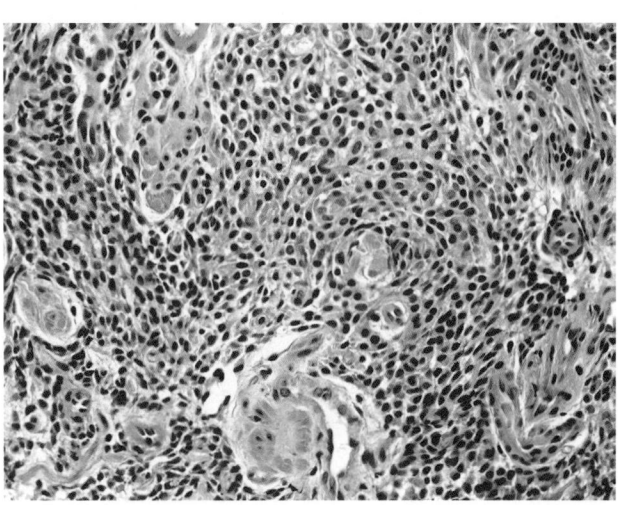

Figure 3-175. Well-differentiated neuroendocrine tumor. These tumor cells appear somewhat spindled, and their cell borders blend in a syncytial pattern.

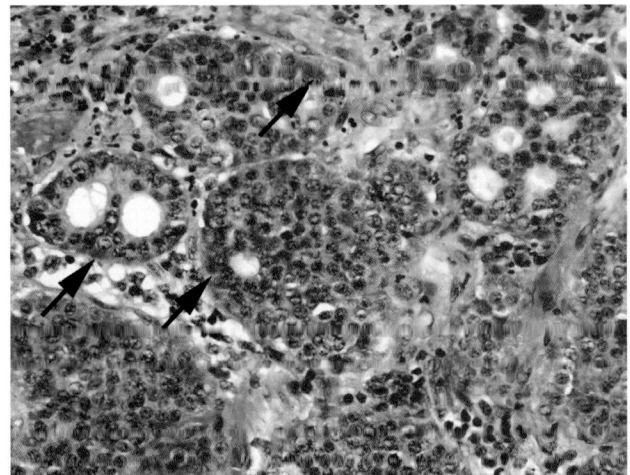

Figure 3-176. Well-differentiated neuroendocrine tumor. Small bowel NETs are often rich in Paneth cells (arrows), identified by the bright pink intracytoplasmic granules.

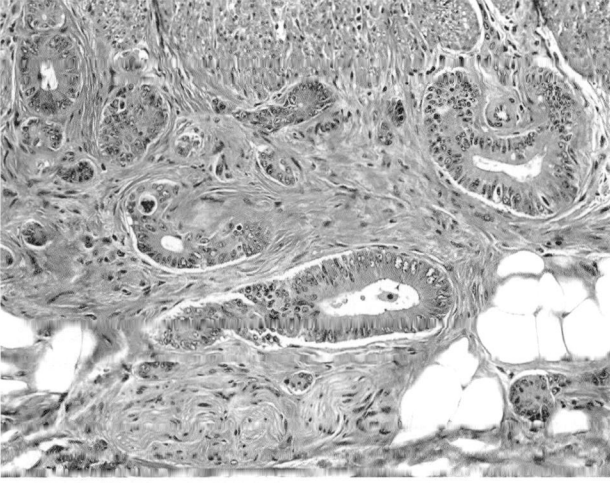

Figure 3-177. Well-differentiated neuroendocrine tumor, acinar variant. Although these look remarkably like glands from an adenocarcinoma, this tumor is diffusely reactive for synaptophysin (see the next figure).

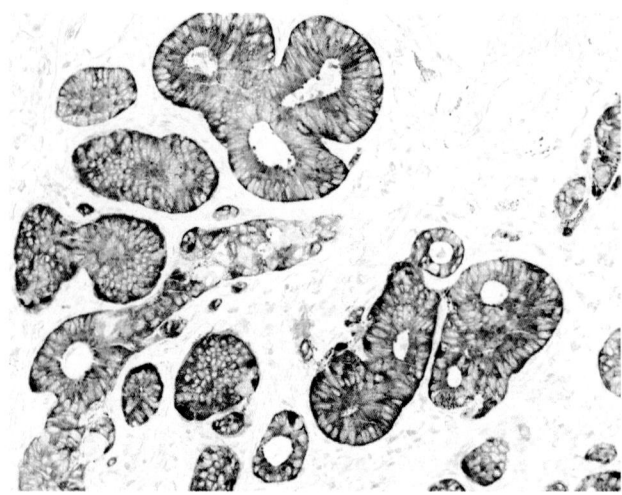

Figure 3-178. Well-differentiated neuroendocrine tumor, acinar variant, synaptophysin of the previous case.

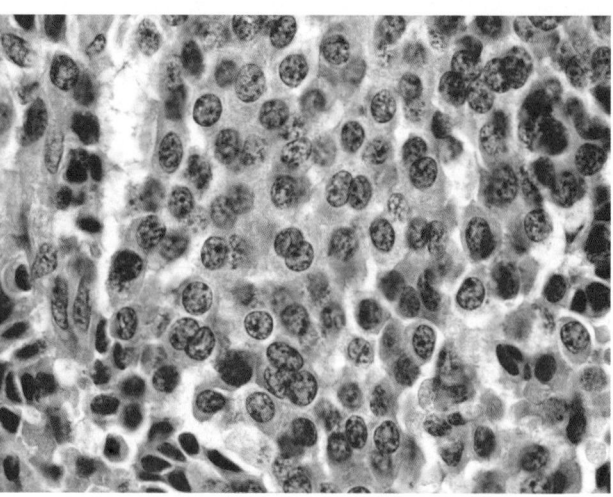

Figure 3-179. Well-differentiated neuroendocrine tumor. A shared feature of all WD-NETs is their bland uniform nuclei, which are round or oval with smooth nuclear borders containing stippled chromatin with indistinct nucleoli.

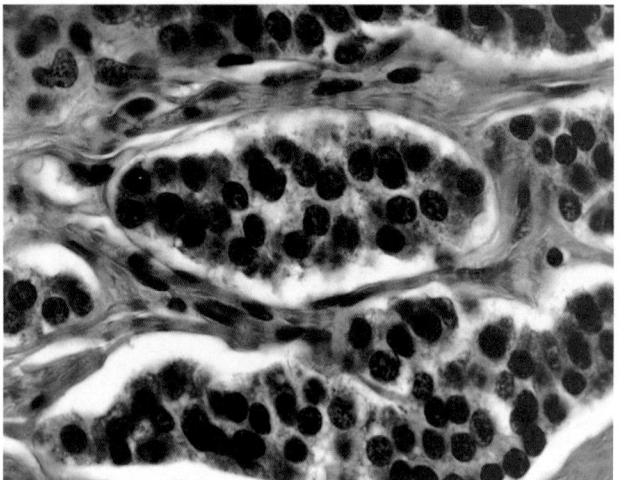

Figure 3-180. Well-differentiated neuroendocrine tumor. These nested tumor cells are uniform in size and shape and have smooth nuclear borders and a stippled chromatin.

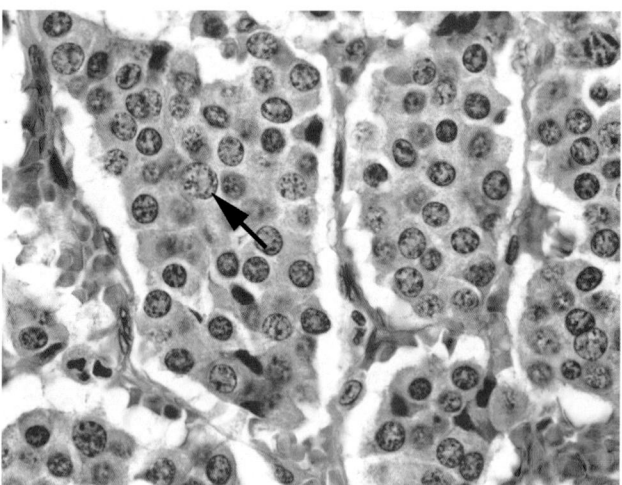

Figure 3-181. Well-differentiated neuroendocrine tumor. Differentiation of NETs is determined by the morphologic uniformity of the cells. Slight variation in nuclear size (*arrow*) and shape is acceptable for well-differentiated tumors, pictured here.

PEARLS & PITFALLS: NETs of the Small Bowel Exhibit Site-Related Differences (Proximal Versus Distal)

Proximal (duodenum) small bowel: Derived from the foregut, these NETs mainly produce **somatostatin** and **gastrin**, similar to ampullary and pancreatic neoplasms. These tumors may be functional or nonfunctional, and some have cited gastrinomas associated with Zollinger-Ellison syndrome as more aggressive than their nonfunctional counterparts.[80] In this location, NETs producing serotonin are rare, as are NECs and mixed neuroendocrine-nonneuroendocrine neoplasms (MiNEN). Only about 75% of proximal NETs show immunoreactivity for CDX2,[81] a tip worth remembering when dealing with metastatic NETs.

Distal (ileum and jejunum) small bowel: Derived from the midgut, these NETs are mainly composed of endocrine cells secreting **serotonin** and, less commonly, L-cells producing **glucagon**like peptide and **peptide-YY**. These tumors result in intermittent crampy abdominal pain and "carcinoid syndrome" in 5% to 7.7% of patients with EC-cell serotonin-producing NETs.[82] Nearly all distal NETs are reactive for CDX2.[83]

FAQ: What are the clinical syndromes associated with functional NETs?

Carcinoid syndrome: This syndrome is associated with 5% of NETs. Secretion of serotonin and bradykinin by NETs results in a catalytic cascade culminating in vasodilation and symptoms such as flushing, diarrhea, abdominal pain, bronchoconstriction, secondary restrictive cardiomyopathy due to serotonin-induced fibrosis, and nausea and vomiting.

Zollinger-Ellison syndrome: A gastrin-secreting tumor leads to elevated serum gastrin, which in turn causes uninhibited release of gastric acid ultimately resulting in refractory peptic ulcer disease. Tumors are most commonly in the duodenum but are also found in the pancreas (25%) and rarely in stomach, peripancreatic lymph nodes, liver, bile duct, ovary, and extra-abdominal (heart, small cell lung cancer) locations.[84,85] This condition is cured when the gastrinoma is resected. Should clinical symptoms persist, consider metastatic disease to a lymph node, a finding in nearly half of duodenal and pancreatic gastrinomas. By comparison, liver metastasis is rare in duodenal gastrinomas (5%).[86]

Somatostatinoma syndrome: This syndrome of diabetes mellitus, diarrhea, steatorrhea, hypochlorhydria or achlorhydria, anemia, and gallstones is the result of stomatostatin-producing NETs but is found almost exclusively in pancreatic somatostatinomas.[87] Tumors are proximal and often have psammomatous calcifications (Fig. 3.182).

FAQ: What is the significance of carcinoid syndrome in GI NETs?

Functional NETs secreting serotonin may be found in the lung or GI tract, but when affecting the latter, carcinoid syndrome does not occur until the disease is so advanced that it overwhelms the liver's ability to metabolize the released serotonin. NETs in the proximal small bowel, for example, only produce carcinoid syndrome following liver metastasis.[88]

FAQ: Is it necessary to perform gastrin or somatostatin immunohistochemistry for NETs?

No. When tumors are functional, clinical symptoms are apparent before resection and therefore immunohistochemistry is not required. Most NETs are nonfunctioning tumors, even if they label for gastrin or somatostatin by immunohistochemistry. For example, Zollinger-Ellison syndrome is found in only about 40% of gastrin-secreting NETs (gastrinoma) and is the only syndrome of neuroendocrine hyperfunction consistently observed in association with NETs of the duodenum and proximal jejunum.[86,89] Immunohistochemistry provides no additional prognostic information and is not necessary except to satisfy personal curiosity or if requested by the clinical team.

PEARLS & PITFALLS: Tubuloglandular and Trabecular Tumors Are More Likely to Be Somatostatinomas

Again, the morphologic variant is unimportant in the overall prognosis of NETs, and it is unnecessary to mention this in the reports. However, some histologic features are seen more commonly among NET subtypes, such as tubuloglandular architecture in somatostatinomas, and this clue can be helpful in identifying functional tumor types, especially if a clinical syndrome is questionable. Psammomatous calcifications, when present, are also characteristic of somatostatinomas (Fig. 3.182).

PEARLS & PITFALLS: Genetic Syndromes Are Highly Associated With NETs

Always consider genetic syndromes in the setting of NETs!

Multiple endocrine neoplasia type 1 (MEN1): Up to 30% of gastrinomas are found in association with MEN1.[90] This autosomal dominant syndrome is best known for the predisposition to tumors of the "3 Ps": parathyroid glands, pituitary gland, and pancreas. This mnemonic is catchy, but the clinical spectrum of this disorder is broad and includes duodenal gastrinomas, adrenal adenomas, and lipomas. Consider MEN1 in the setting of any duodenal gastrinoma.

Neurofibromatosis type I (NF1): There are three clinically and genetically distinct forms of neurofibromatosis, neurofibromatosis types 1 and 2 (NF1 and NF2) and schwannomatosis. NF1, also known as von Recklinghausen disease, is the most common type and is an autosomal dominant disorder caused by mutations in the *NF1* gene that encodes the protein neurofibromin. Patients with von Recklinghausen disease are at significant risk of developing ampullary and periampullary NETs.[91,92] When considering this syndrome, look for other hallmarks of NF1, such as multiple café-au-lait macules and cutaneous neurofibromas.

Von Hippel-Lindau (VHL) disease: VHL disease is an inherited, autosomal dominant syndrome manifested by a variety of benign and malignant tumors, including hemangioblastomas of the cerebellum and spine, retinal capillary hemangioblastomas, clear cell renal cell carcinomas, pheochromocytomas, endolymphatic sac tumors of the middle ear, serous cystadenomas and NETs of the pancreas, and papillary cystadenomas of the epididymis and broad ligament. Although pancreatic NETs are classic for this disease, NETs in these patients have been found outside of the pancreas, including the proximal duodenum.[93]

PEARLS & PITFALLS: Grading of WD-NET Requires Both Mitotic Count and Ki-67 Proliferative Index

WD-NETs are graded by both mitotic index and Ki-67 proliferation index (Figs. 3.183 and 3.184). Ki-67 index frequently results in a higher grade than mitotic count, and studies have shown these grade-discordant tumors more likely to have metastases to lymph nodes and distant sites, perineural invasion, small vessel invasion, and overall survival.[94] In cases for which grade results are discordant, *assign the higher grade.*

WHO 2017 Classification of Neuroendocrine Neoplasms:

WD-NET G1	<3% Ki-67	<2 mitoses/10 HPF
WD-NET G2	3%–20% Ki-67	2–20 mitoses/10 HPF
WD-NET G3	>20% Ki-67	>20 mitoses/10 HPF

FAQ: Can I eyeball the Ki-67?

No - a manual count is required. Numerous studies have demonstrated poor accuracy in eyeball estimates of the Ki-67 proliferation index.[95-97] Counting a minimum of 500 cells (suggested range 500 to 2000) is necessary to determine a reliable Ki-67 index, which is reported as the percent of positive tumor cells (e.g., 2.4%, or 12 of 500 cells). Manual counting is time consuming, and a number of studies have examined different techniques for Ki-67 index, including digitized automatic counting and eyeballing.[96] Digital image analysis software is not widely available and requires software modification to prevent inaccurate counting, for example, to exclude immunoreactive intratumoral or peritumoral lymphocytes (Figs. 3.185 and 3.186). Eyeballing in areas of the highest density "hot spots" is accurate in higher-grade lesions, but when tumors are close to grade cutoffs, *it is best to perform manual count.* One challenge, however, is how quickly one can lose track of which cells have been counted while attempting to tally up 500 to 2000 cells under the microscope. A simple and economical approach is to print out a photo or screenshot of a hotspot area and manually cross off each cell as it is counted (Fig. 3.187). Take care to exclude lymphocytes, which will skew the Ki-67 count higher.

PEARLS & PITFALLS: Cytotechnologists Can Aid in Ki-67 Manual Counts

Cytotechnologists are skilled morphologists accustomed to screening gynecologic and nongynecologic cytopathology specimens daily. In our practice, Ki-67 manual counts are performed by cytotechnologists, an approach that not only allows these professionals to perform at the top of their proficiency but also reclaims physician time. This method has been validated and shows near-perfect agreement between cytotechnologist and pathologist grading.[97] An example workflow is as follows:

1. Pathologist circles hot spot area for counting on Ki-67 slide.
2. Cytotechnologist captures two to three digital images at 20x from this area and prints out via color printer.
3. Cytotechnologist performs manual count by crossing off nonreactive cells and circling reactive cells with a target of 2000 cells minimum (Fig. 3.187).
4. Pathologist confirms results by reviewing original H&E, Ki-67 immunohistochemistry, and printed images before signout, assuring that cells marked appear appropriate.

PEARLS & PITFALLS: Grading by Mitotic Rate Requires Counting 50 HPF but Is Reported as per 10 HPF

The mitoses in 50 HPF should be counted to accurately grade the tumor. This number is divided by five to report mitoses per 10 HPF. These minimum requirements for grading (50 HPF for mitotic count and 500 to 2000 cells for Ki-67 index) presume there is enough tissue for accurate grading, but small biopsy material may be insufficient in many cases. See the following Sample Note.

SAMPLE NOTE: When Small Biopsies Contain Insufficient WD-NET for Mitotic Count or Ki-67 Index Grading

Small Bowel, Polyp, Biopsy

- Well-differentiated neuroendocrine tumor, see Comment.

Comment

There is insufficient tumor cell quantity to accurately grade this WD-NET (minimum requirement 50 HPF for mitotic count and 500 cells for Ki-67 proliferation index). Based on the available material, this tumor appears to be (G1, G2, G3). Final grading will be revised following review of a larger sample (e.g., excision specimen).

> **PEARLS & PITFALLS: Both Size and Depth of Invasion Are Considered in Staging of WD-NETs**
>
> Although depth of invasion defines most staging criteria, gastric WD-NETs are among the few that also take into account tumor size at the lower stages. For example, staging criteria by depth is fairly typical, with invasion into the lamina propria and submucosa staged as pT1, *but only if the tumor is ≤1 cm.* Any tumor >1 cm is automatically pT2 or higher, even if superficially invasive. Once tumors invade at least into the muscularis propria, the tumors are staged by depth regardless of size: pT2, involvement of muscularis propria; pT3, involvement of subserosa; pT4, invasion of serosa or adjacent tissue/organs (Fig. 3.188).

POORLY DIFFERENTIATED NEUROENDOCRINE CARCINOMA

NECs are classified as such by their poorly differentiated high-grade cytology and marked nuclear atypia, although this was not always the case. The now outdated WHO 2010 classification of neuroendocrine neoplasms defined three grades based purely on the mitotic rate and Ki-67 index, with the high-grade (G3) category defined as >20 mitoses per 10 HPF or Ki-67 proliferation index >20% without regard to histologic atypia.[80] This older WHO 2010 classification regarded G3 neoplasms as synonymous with poorly differentiated NECs (PD-NECs). However, when investigators divided the G3 group into morphologically well- and poorly differentiated tumors, the poorly differentiated tumors had different causes, genetic alterations, and response to treatment with worse survival outcomes.[98-102] For these reasons, the updated classification of endocrine tumors (WHO 2017) now relies first on morphologic features; a tumor should be identified as well-differentiated or poorly differentiated before further stratification by mitotic count and Ki-67 proliferative index. In the case of poorly differentiated morphology, characterized by nuclear pleomorphism, anisonucleosis, frequent mitotic activity, and necrosis, these tumors should always be classified as NECs and staged as carcinomas.[103] This group can be further divided into (1) small cell type, in which the cells are small with finely granular "salt and pepper" chromatin and inconspicuous nucleoli; (2) large cell type, in which the cells are large with a moderate amount of cytoplasm and prominent nucleoli (Figs. 3.189–3.192); and (3) MiNEN (previously "mixed adenoneuroendocrine carcinoma" or MANEC), in which the tumor is composed of at least 30% both neuroendocrine tumor and adenocarcinoma or other high-grade carcinoma (Figs. 3.193–3.195). Immunoreactivity for neuroendocrine markers within an adenocarcinoma does not indicate MiNEN.

> **FAQ: How does one differentiate NET from NEC?**
>
> Based on WHO 2017 classification, NECs are identified by their poorly differentiated high-grade morphology (Figs. 2.180 and 2.181) independent of mitotic count or Ki-67 proliferative index. This is a departure from previous WHO 2010 classification for neuroendocrine neoplasms, which stratified tumors based purely on mitoses and Ki-67. The updated system not only indicates prognosis and response to therapy more reliably but is also more intuitive to pathologists. Tumors that are morphologically well differentiated are classified as WD-NETs and can be further graded based on mitotic and Ki-67 cutoffs.

KEY FEATURES: Small bowel WD-NETs and PD-NECs

- WD-NETs and PD-NECs are **distinguished by their morphology, independent of the Ki-67 index and mitotic rate.**
- WE-NETs have uniform cells, whereas PD-NECs have marked pleomorphism and nuclear atypia.
- Histologic variants include **nested** (type A), **trabecular or insular** (type B), and **acinar** (type C) but have **no impact on prognosis.**

- **Proximal** small bowel NETs are almost exclusively **gastrinomas** or **somatostatinomas**.

- **Distal** small bowel NETs almost exclusively secrete **serotonin** or **glucagon**like peptide and **peptide-YY**.

- **Carcinoid syndrome** is caused by **serotonin-secreting tumors** and **indicates metastasis**.

- When encountering a small bowel NET, consider a genetic syndrome, such as **MEN1**, **NF1**, and **VHL**.

- **Grading requires both the mitotic count (50 HPFs) and Ki-67 index (500 to 2000 cells)**, with final grade being the higher of the two.

- Eyeball estimates of Ki-67 are unacceptable, but **cytotechnologists can aid with manual counts**.

- NETs can be subtle and deeper levels are advised when atypical cells are present (Figs. 3.196 and 3.197).

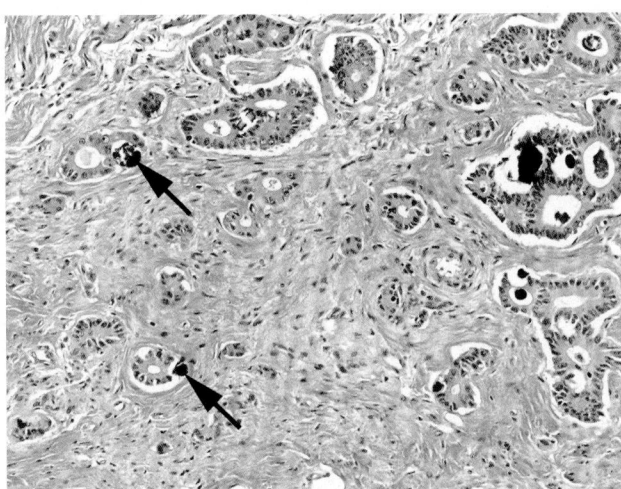

Figure 3-182. Somatostatinoma. Psammomatous calcifications (*arrows*) are characteristic of somatostatinomas.

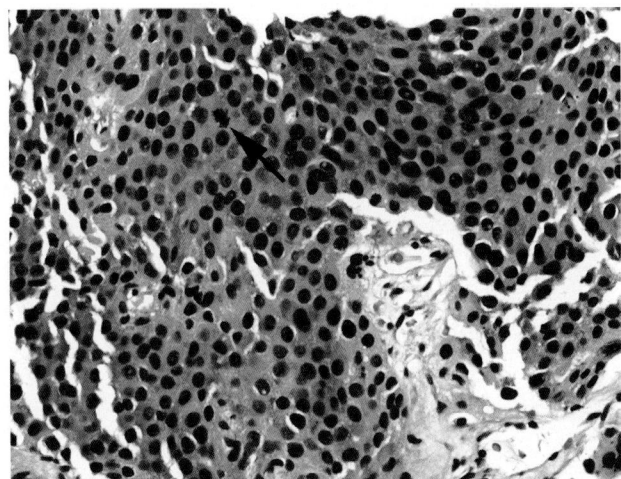

Figure 3-183. Well-differentiated neuroendocrine tumor, G3. Well-differentiated tumors can exhibit high grade. Differentiation is decided based on the uniformity of cells. Grade is decided based on the mitotic activity (*arrow*) and Ki-67 proliferation index.

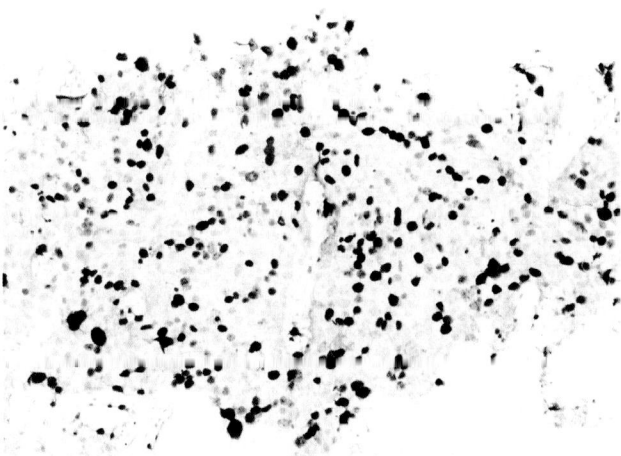

Figure 3-184. Well-differentiated neuroendocrine tumor, G3, Ki-67 immunohistochemistry of the previous figure. The Ki-67 proliferation index in this well-differentiated tumor is high, a finding not predictable based on the uniformity of the tumor cells on H&E.

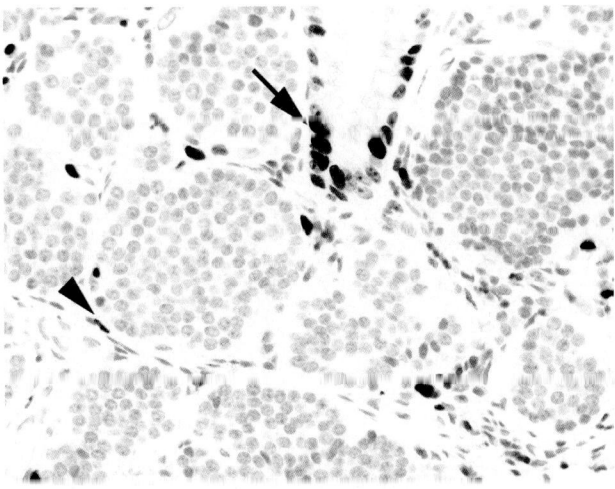

Figure 3-185. Well-differentiated neuroendocrine tumor, Ki-67 immunostain. When evaluating Ki-67 immunostains, take care not to count normal glandular epithelium (*arrow*) or stromal cells (*arrowhead*) that may light up. Always compare with the H&F for correlation.

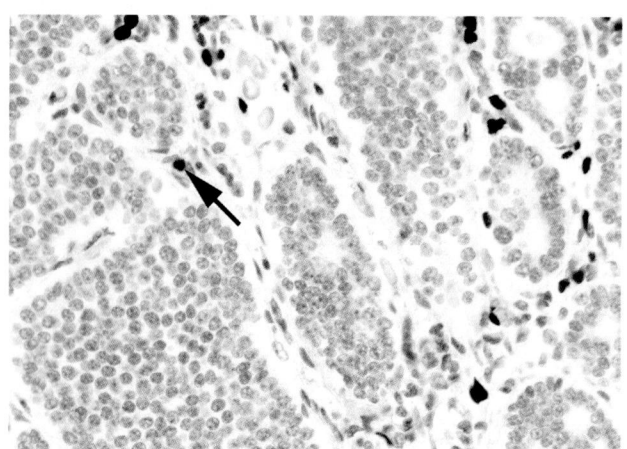

Figure 3-186. Well-differentiated neuroendocrine tumor, Ki-67 immunostain. Lymphocytes (*arrow*) will show reactivity and should not be counted in the Ki-67 proliferation index.

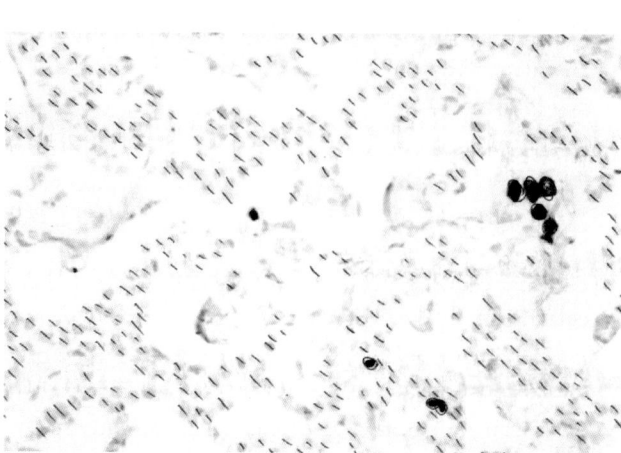

Figure 3-187. Well-differentiated neuroendocrine tumor, Ki-67 immunostain. The manual count for Ki-67 can be tedious, but printing out a snapshot can facilitate the process. Here, the negative cells are crossed off to prevent duplicate counting. This method can be taught to allied health professionals, such as cytotechnologists, to reduce the burden on physician time.

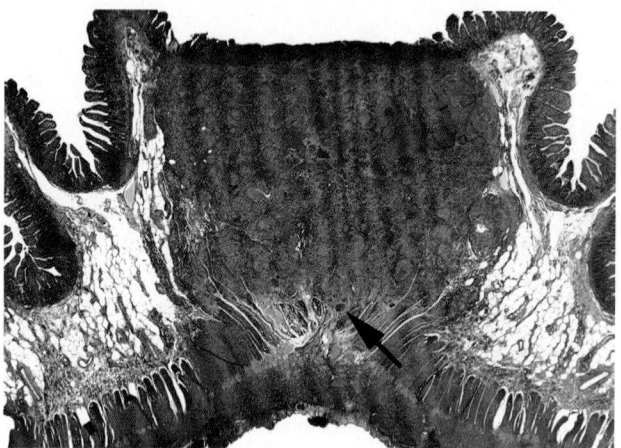

Figure 3-188. Well-differentiated neuroendocrine tumor, stage pT2. Involvement of the muscularis propria (*arrow*) is considered pT2 regardless of tumor size. However, even if only superficially invasive into the submucosa, any tumor >1 cm is automatically pT2.

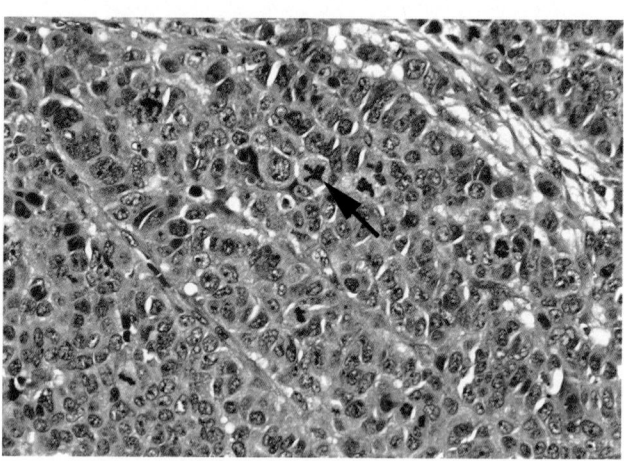

Figure 3-189. Poorly differentiated neuroendocrine carcinoma. The cells in this tumor are markedly pleomorphic and have prominent nucleoli and atypical mitosis (*arrow*).

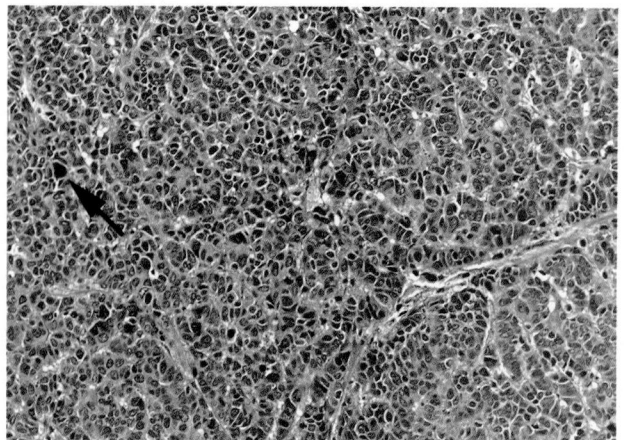

Figure 3-190. Poorly differentiated neuroendocrine carcinoma. The cells in this tumor show marked variation in size and shape. They appear angulated rather than round and uniform, and monster cells are visible (*arrow*). These findings warrant classification as a PD-NEC. These tumors have a prognosis similar to that of adenocarcinoma and are staged as such.

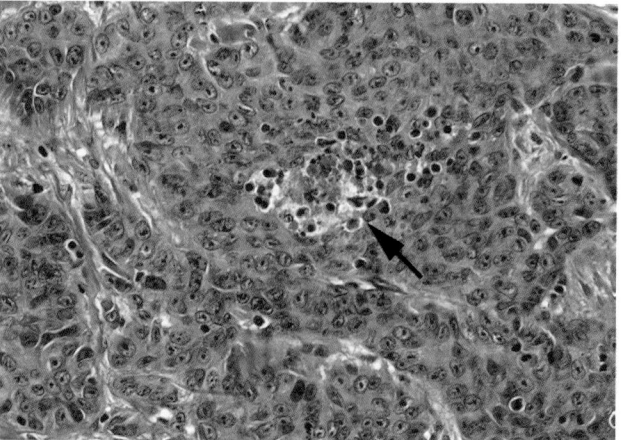

Figure 3-191. Poorly differentiated neuroendocrine carcinoma. These tumor cells are no longer uniform and display prominent nucleoli. An area of necrosis is present (*arrow*).

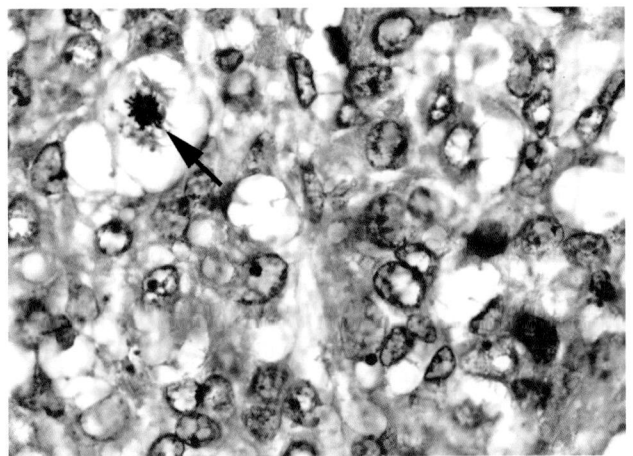

Figure 3-192. Poorly differentiated neuroendocrine carcinoma. At high magnification, the nuclei lack the typical stippled chromatin and show marked variation in size and shape. The mitotic figure (*arrow*) does not affect differentiation but is used instead for grade. PD-NECs are invariably G3.

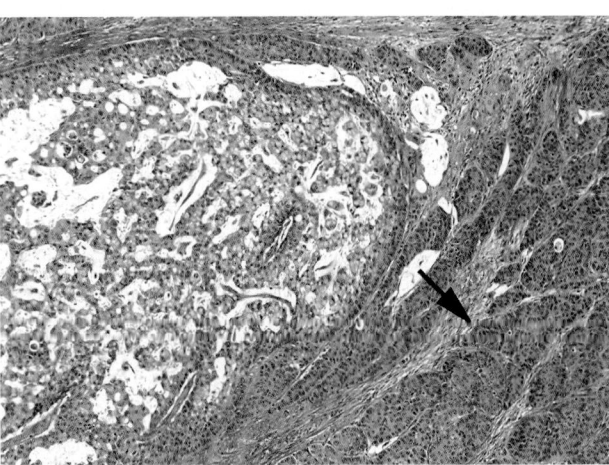

Figure 3-193. Mixed neuroendocrine-nonneuroendocrine neoplasm (MiNEN, previously known as MANEC). Immunoreactivity for neuroendocrine markers within an adenocarcinoma does not indicate MiNEN. Instead, this rare variant is composed of at least 30% neuroendocrine tumor (*arrow*) and adenocarcinoma (or other high-grade carcinoma), as seen here. Note the mucin produced by the adenocarcinoma.

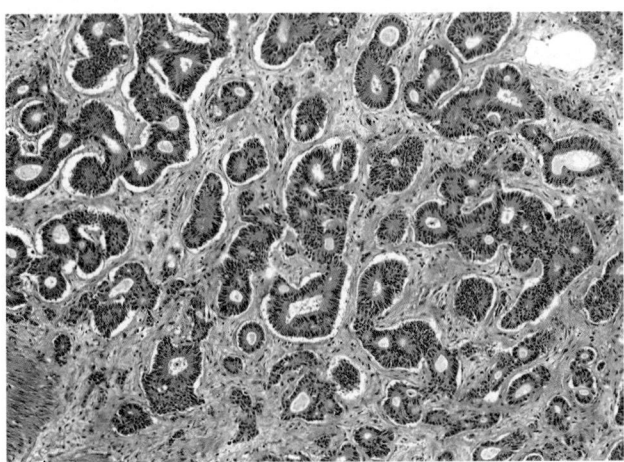

Figure 3-194. Neuroendocrine tumor, acinar type. Do not mistake acinar morphology in an NET for a mixed tumor, such as MiNEN. See the next figure.

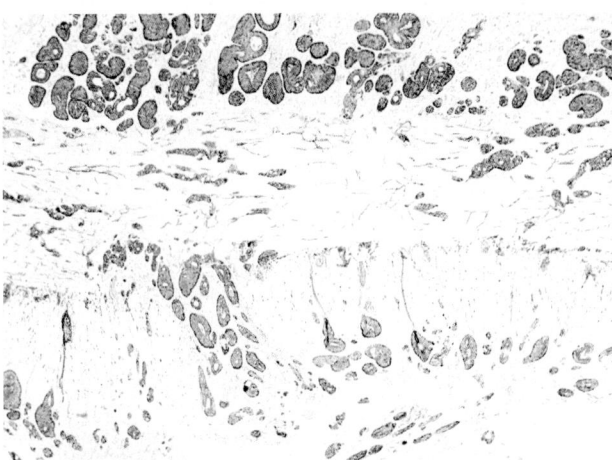

Figure 3-195. Neuroendocrine tumor, acinar type, synaptophysin of the previous tumor. This NET shows prominent acini formation, but the strong and diffuse synaptophysin reactivity confirms neuroendocrine differentiation.

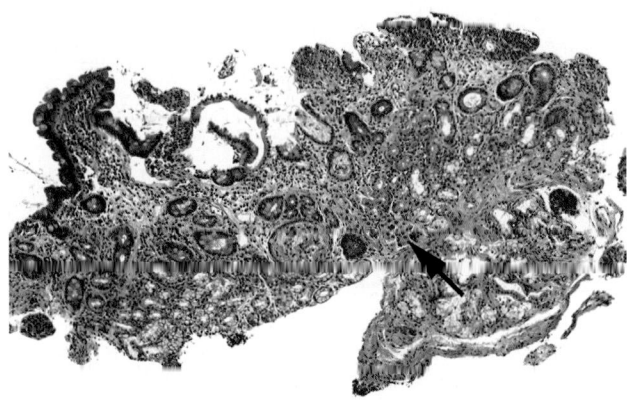

Figure 3-196. Sneaky neuroendocrine tumor. Neuroendocrine tumors are notoriously sneaky on small endoscopic biopsies, especially those that are busy appearing. This small focus (*arrow*) was atypical, and deeper levels were performed (see the next figure).

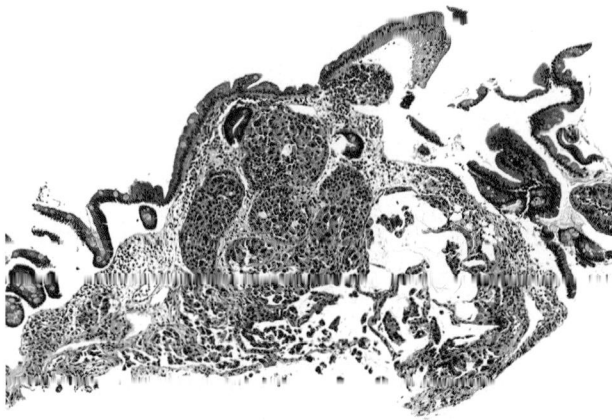

Figure 3-197. Sneaky neuroendocrine tumor, deeper level of the previous figure. Deeper levels reveal a poorly differentiated neuroendocrine carcinoma.

NEAR MISS

CRUSHED BRUNNER GLANDS

Crush artifact is common among endoscopic biopsies, and in the duodenum crushed Brunner glands can take on a unique appearance mimicking a neural tumor. Although one might initially consider a schwannoma or gangliocytic paraganglioma, always take into consideration the endoscopic findings and the low-power appearance of the biopsy. Ask yourself: Is there an expansile lesion? Is there crush artifact in the rest of the biopsy? Is there an endoscopic correlate, such as a mass lesion? Recall, GI schwannomas are accompanied by a peripheral lymphoid cuff, and the absence of this finding is another tip-off that one might be dealing with crushed Brunner glands rather than a true lesion (Figs. 3.198–3.202).

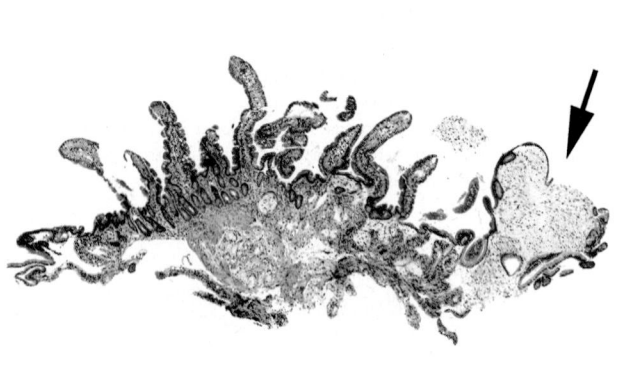

Figure 3-198. Crushed Brunner glands mimicking a tumor. At low magnification, the lamina propria appears to be involved by an expansile lesion (*arrow*).

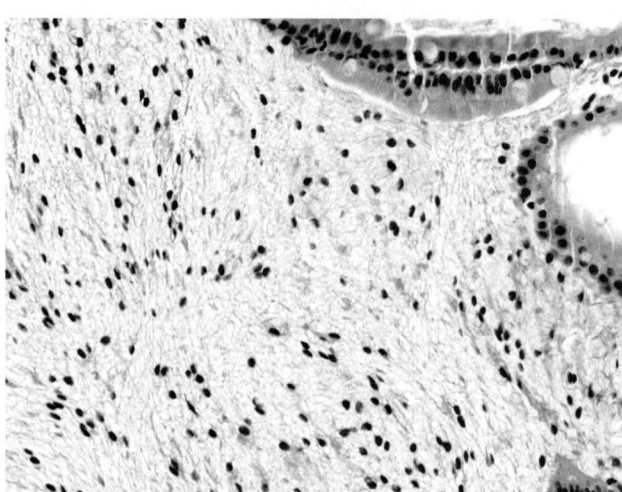

Figure 3-199. Crushed Brunner glands mimicking a tumor, higher magnification of the previous figure. Crushed Brunner glands fill the lamina propria. It is easy to see how one might mistake this for a neural proliferation. The crushed cells appear to be streaming and have slightly spindled nuclei with fake cytoplasmic processes.

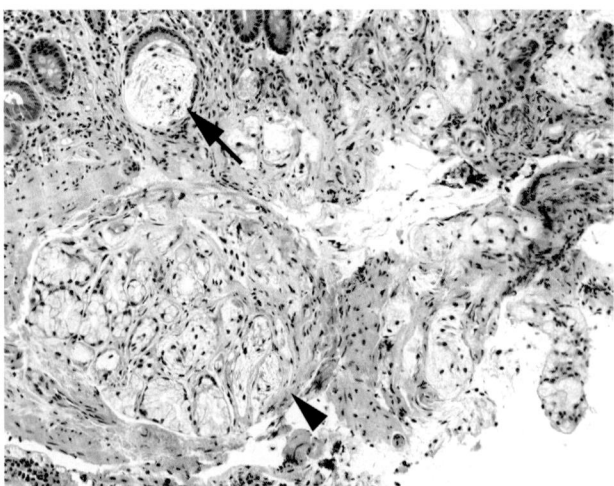

Figure 3-200. Crushed Brunner glands. This field shows areas of intact (*arrowhead*) and partially crushed Brunner glands (*arrow*). When confluent, these crushed areas can mimic a neural proliferation.

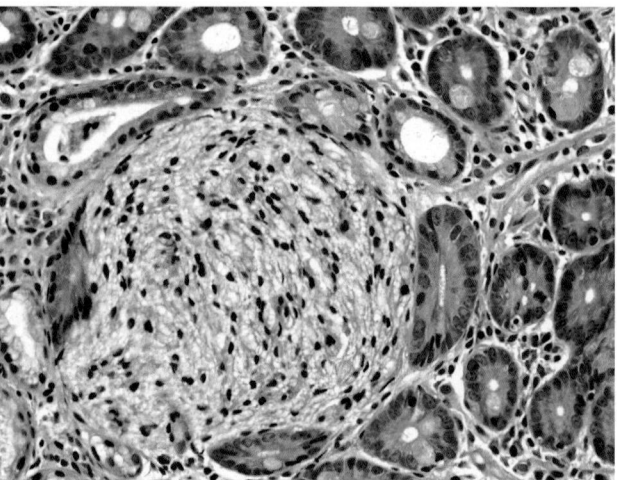

Figure 3-201. Crushed Brunner glands. In isolation, this small pocket of crushed Brunner glands resembles a neural or perineural proliferation. Take the entire biopsy into consideration and check for crush artifact elsewhere.

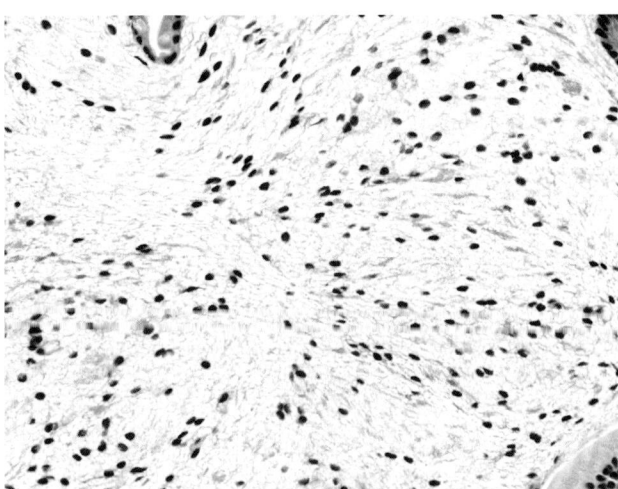

Figure 3-202. Crushed Brunner glands. The cytoplasmic contents of these ruptured cells are streaming, but do not mistake this for a neural proliferation. A PAS special stain will highlight the spilled mucin of crushed Brunner glands but not true neural proliferations.

ENDOMETRIOSIS

Endometriosis involving the GI tract is more commonly seen in the rectum and sigmoid colon (93%), and although a lesser percentage involves the small bowel (7%),[104,105] one should stay alert for this tricky diagnosis, especially in the ileocecal region. Clinical presentation can be vague, with abdominal pain, bloody diarrhea, and strictures that lead to obstruction, perforation, or mass, and often the working diagnosis is Crohn disease.[104,106] Diagnosis of endometriosis requires at least two of the three following histologic features: (1) endometrial glands, (2) endometrial stroma, or (3) evidence of chronic hemorrhage (i.e., hemosiderin deposition). The pitfall is overcalling these haphazard glands adenocarcinoma, especially when they show deep involvement in the bowel wall and the provided clinical history is "ileocecal mass" or Crohn disease. The overlying mucosa may show distorted glands or other submucosal changes mimicking true Crohn disease, such as neuronal hypertrophy and fibrosis, but take care not to mistake the associated spindled endometrial stroma for desmoplasia. The clue to diagnosis is the bland appearance of the glandular epithelium and absence of goblet cells. A low threshold to evaluate by immunohistochemistry will prevent overdiagnosis: CD10 immunohistochemistry is useful to highlight the endometrial stroma, and these lesions are reactive for both ER and PR. Excision or segmental resection may be necessary if patients are symptomatic, but these lesions are benign (Figs. 3.203–3.211).

LYMPHANGIOMA

Lacteals are blind-ended lymphatic channels and normal constituents of the small bowel lamina propria. Normally these delicate structures are difficult to discern at low power; on high power they appear as slightly expanded slits containing pale eosinophilic serum. When dilated, the engorged structures are more readily apparent and are a clue to underlying pathology such as lymphangioma, as seen in this case. Lymphangiomas are rare benign congenital malformations causing mass lesions in which the lymphatic channels fail to drain properly into the venous system and can occur at any age but are most commonly found in children and infants. Most (80% to 95%) occur in the head and neck, and the most frequent location for intra-abdominal lymphangiomas is the small bowel or small bowel mesentery (80%), which can present with intussusception and rarely with acute abdomen.[107] Diagnosis on endoscopic biopsies can be challenging, as superficial samples may reveal only the tip of this lesion. Consider this diagnosis whenever requisition forms include the buzz-words "milky fluid," and always check the base of biopsies for a subtle endothelial like lining whenever dilated lacteals are evident (Figs. 3.212–3.220). Other considerations include primary and secondary lymphangiectasia, obstruction, adjacent neoplasm, adhesions or strictures, and infection such as Whipple disease. For more discussion on nonneoplastic entities, see Volume 1 (*Atlas of Gastrointestinal Pathology: A Pattern Based Approach to Non-Neoplastic Biopsies*). The bland cytology of lymphangioma differentiates it from malignant vascular tumors, such as angiosarcoma and Kaposi sarcoma, which both show more cytologic atypia. Angiosarcoma is overtly malignant with plump hobnail endothelial cells. Kaposi sarcoma can be confirmed by HHV8 immunohistochemistry.

PEARLS & PITFALLS

Occult malignancies occasionally lurk in dilated lacteals. As a result, dilated lacteals can serve as precious clues to malignancy in an otherwise busy-appearing small bowel biopsy. Make sure to routinely check all lacteals, and check them twice in cases with a history of mass lesion or malignancy (Figs. 3.221–3.223).

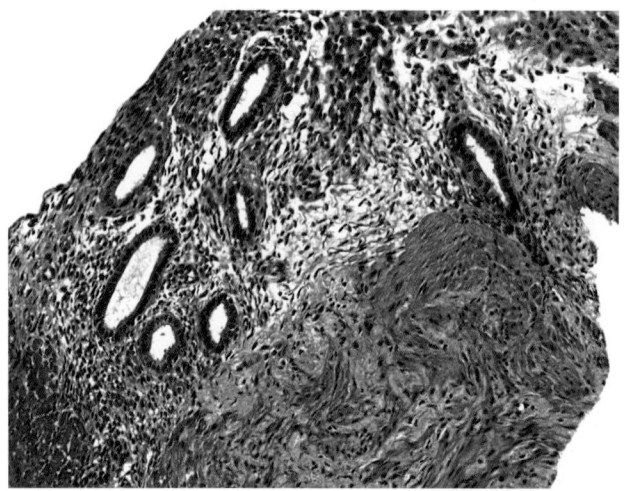

Figure 3-203. Endometriosis involving small bowel. These disordered glands in a spindled stroma raise concern for invasive adenocarcinoma. However, the epithelium is too uniform and the stroma is too cellular, both clues to a benign diagnosis, such as endometriosis.

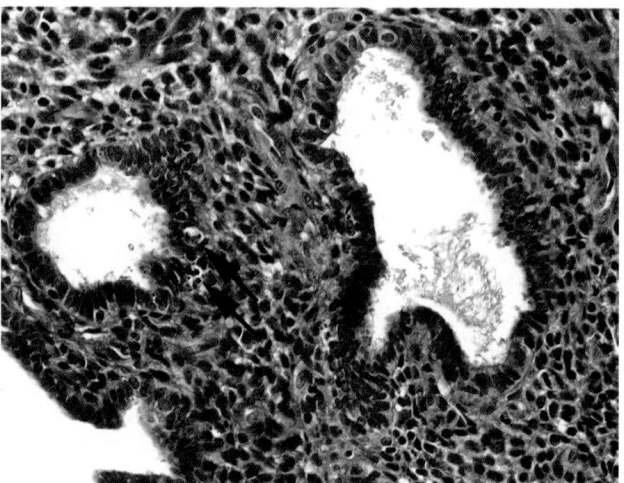

Figure 3-204. Endometriosis. The glandular epithelium shows crowded nuclei and overlapping cells with frequent apoptoses (*arrows*), all features considered atypical within the small bowel. However, pay attention to the cells surrounding this gland. Rather than the normal mixed inflammatory cells of lamina propria, the cells seen here comprise endometrial stroma.

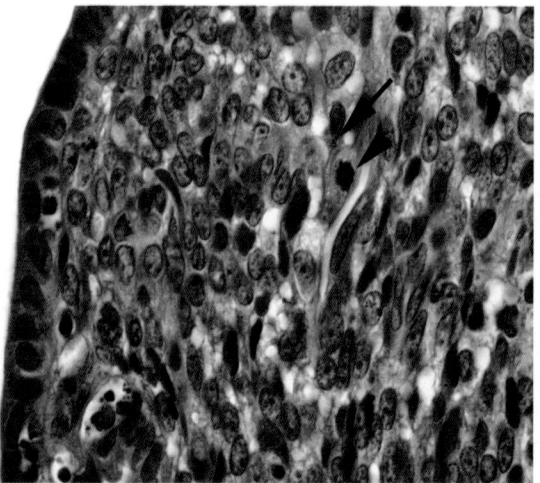

Figure 3-205. Endometriosis. Diagnosis of endometriosis requires three components: (1) endometrial glands; (2) endometrial stroma; (3) evidence of hemorrhage, such as hemosiderin deposition (*arrow*). Frequent mitoses (*arrowhead*) and apoptoses are characteristic for endometrium.

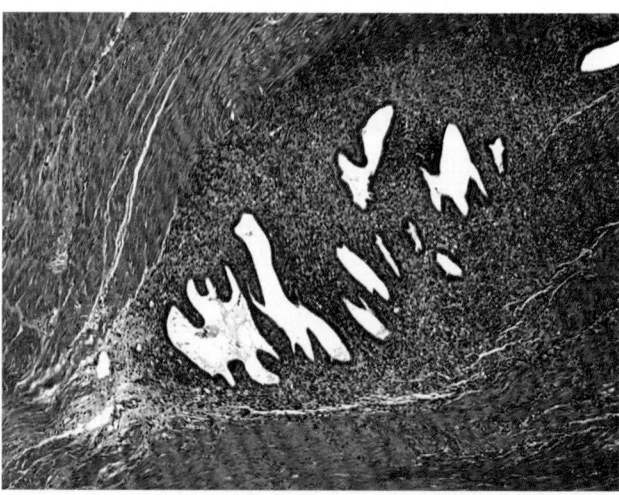

Figure 3-206. Endometriosis. This collection of endometrial glands and stroma is deep in the muscularis propria of the bowel wall. The glands are surrounded by a densely cellular endometrial stroma. This example is an easy diagnosis, but when the stroma is scant, cases can prove challenging (see the next four figures).

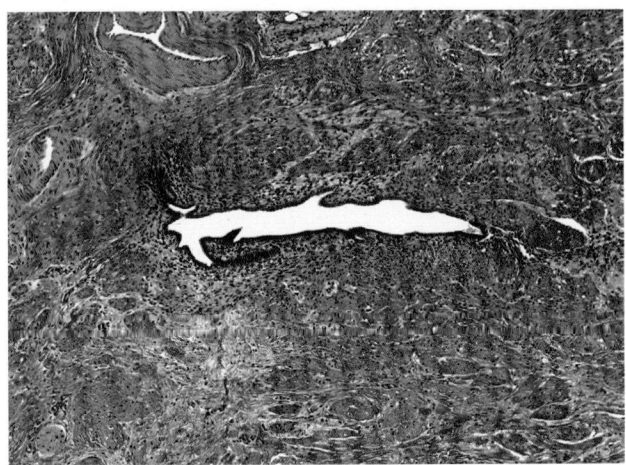

Figure 3-207. Endometriosis. Angulated glands in the deep bowel wall can raise concern for adenocarcinoma. The pallor imparted by the scant endometrial stroma can mimic desmoplasia. The key to diagnosis is remembering to think of this pitfall, but in challenging cases, application of immunohistochemistry can be helpful.

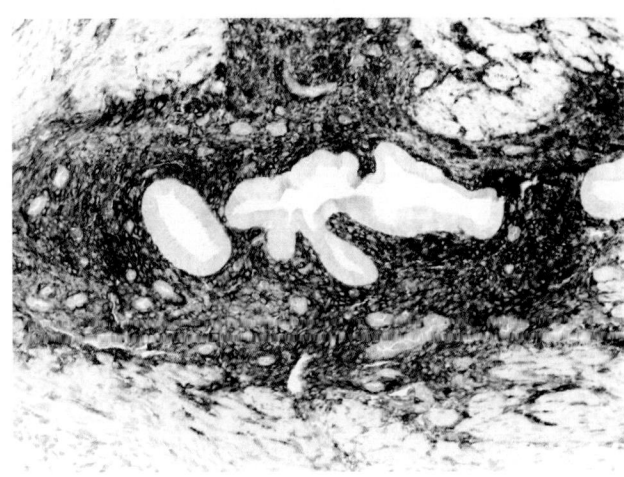

Figure 3-208. Endometriosis, CD10 immunohistochemistry. CD10 highlights the endometrial stroma, confirming the diagnosis of endometriosis.

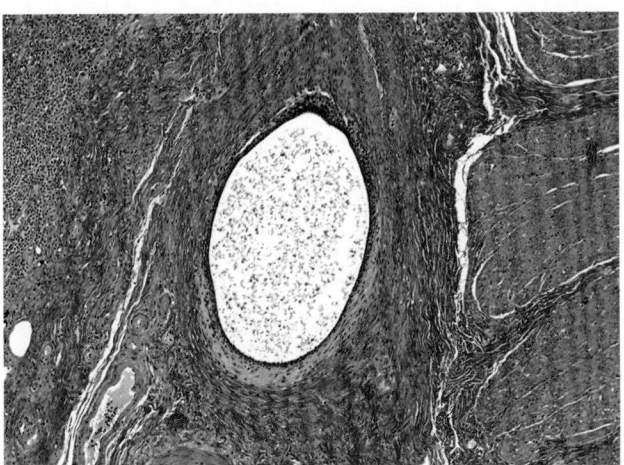

Figure 3-209. Endometriosis. Upon evaluation of a postneoadjuvant small bowel resection, this attenuated and atrophic gland was mistaken for residual treated tumor.

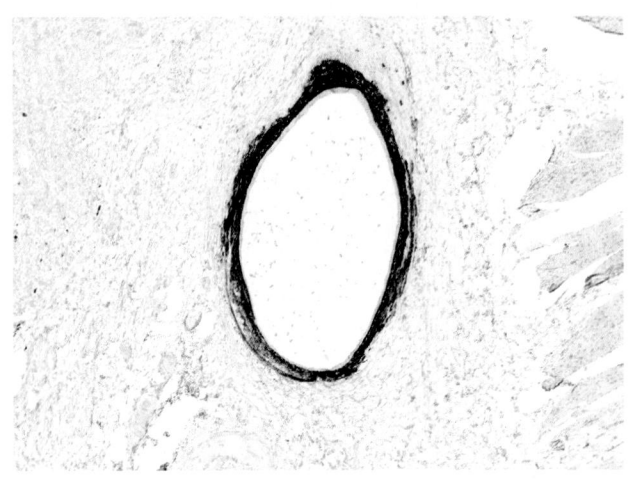

Figure 3-210. Endometriosis, CD10 immunohistochemistry of the previous figure. A CD10 immunostain highlights the scant endometrial stroma surrounding the gland, confirming that this is not residual adenocarcinoma.

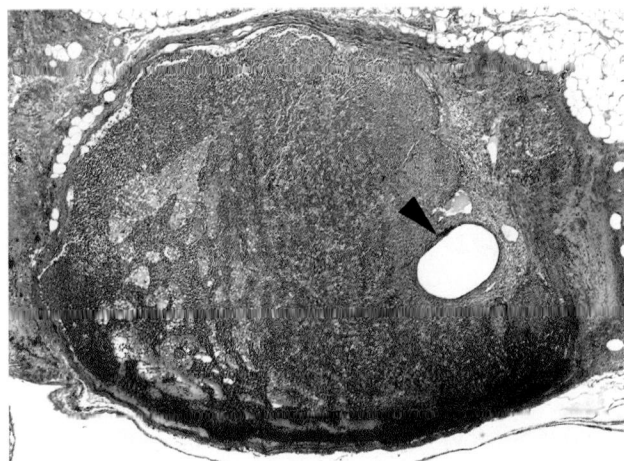

Figure 3-211. Endometriosis involving a lymph node. Endometriosis can affect distant organ systems and even lymph nodes. Take care not to call this metastatic adenocarcinoma (arrowhead).

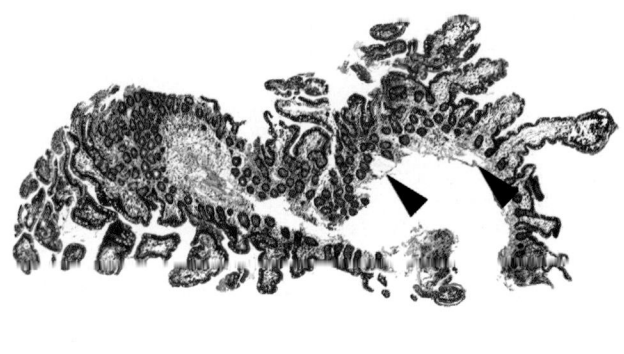

Figure 3-212. Lymphangioma/lymphangiectasia. Make a habit of systematically checking all the layers of a biopsy, and subtle findings are often found, such as these lymphatic spaces (arrowheads) at the base of otherwise unremarkable tissue.

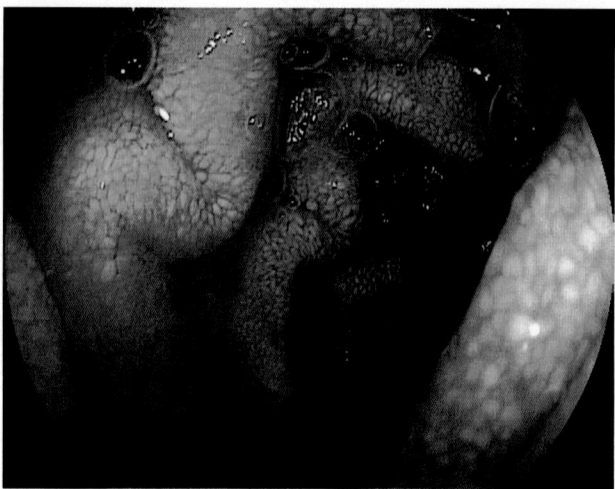

Figure 3-213. Dilated small bowel villi overlying a lymphangioma, endoscopic photo. A carpet of villi line the small bowel and, in this example, are markedly congested and dilated, a clue to underlying pathology.

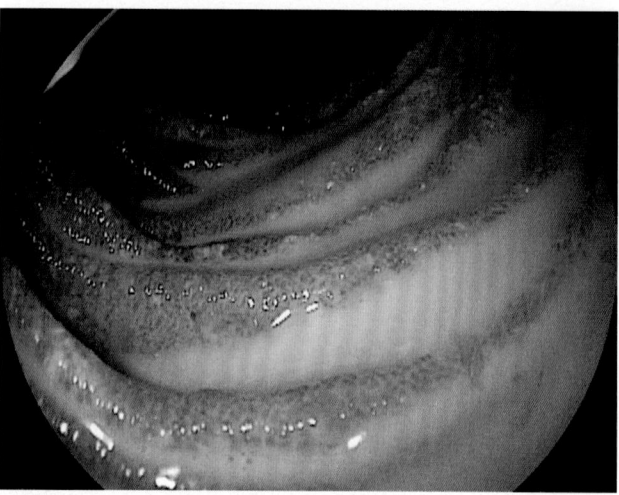

Figure 3-214. Lymphatic fluid, endoscopic photo. Characteristic "milky" fluid surround congested duodenal villi in this patient with an underlying lymphangioma.

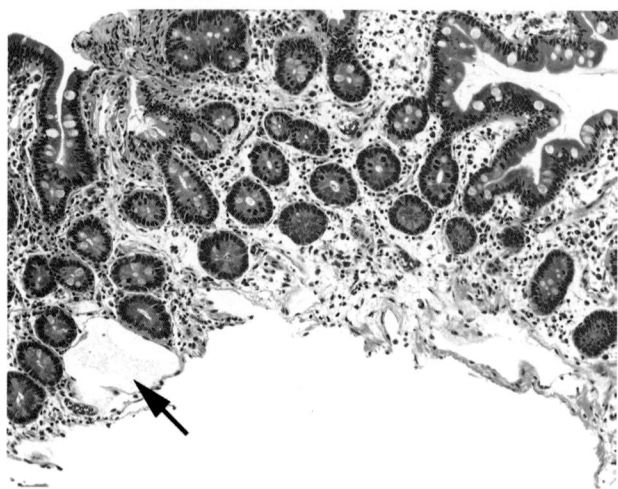

Figure 3-215. Lymphangioma/lymphangiectasia. The base of this biopsy shows endothelial lined spaces filled with acellular proteinaceous fluid (*arrow*).

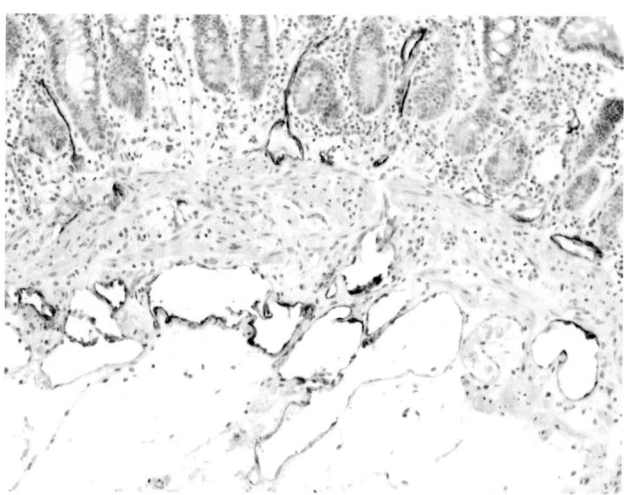

Figure 3-216. Lymphangioma/lymphangiectasia, D2-40 immunohistochemistry of the previous figure. The immunostain highlights lymphatic endothelial cells lining the lymphatic spaces.

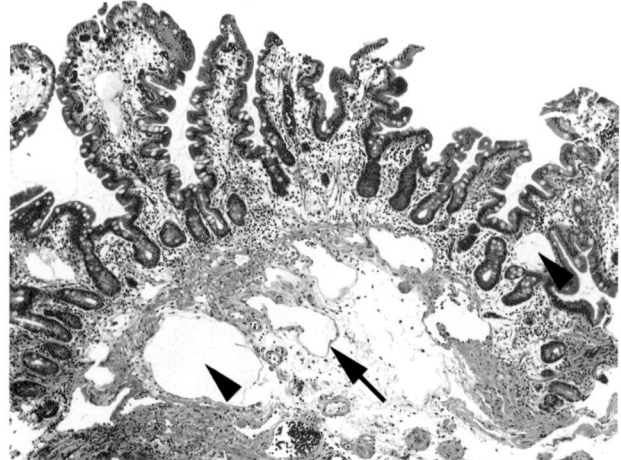

Figure 3-217. Lymphangioma/lymphangiectasia. The superficial mucosa is relatively unremarkable aside from dilated lacteals (*arrow*). The base of the specimen shows dilated lymphatic and vascular spaces within the submucosa. The proteinaceous lymph fluid (*arrowheads*) is acellular and lightly eosinophilic.

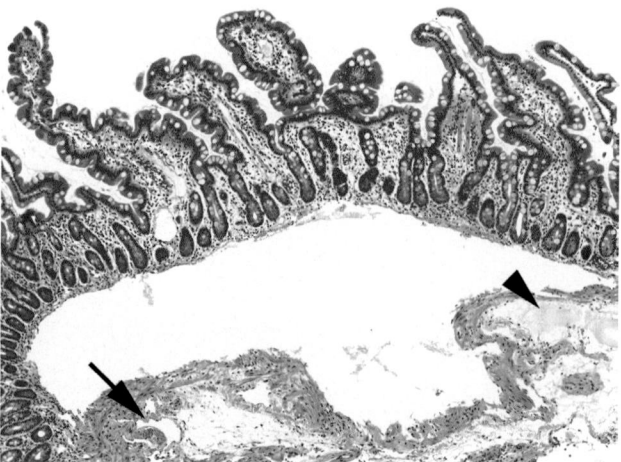

Figure 3-218. Lymphangioma/lymphangiectasia. These cases can be challenging, as the endothelial cell lining is fine and nondescript. This example could be written off as an artifactual split of the muscularis mucosae. The pale pink proteinaceous material (*arrowhead*) is a clue, along with other dilated lymphatic spaces (*arrow*) nearby.

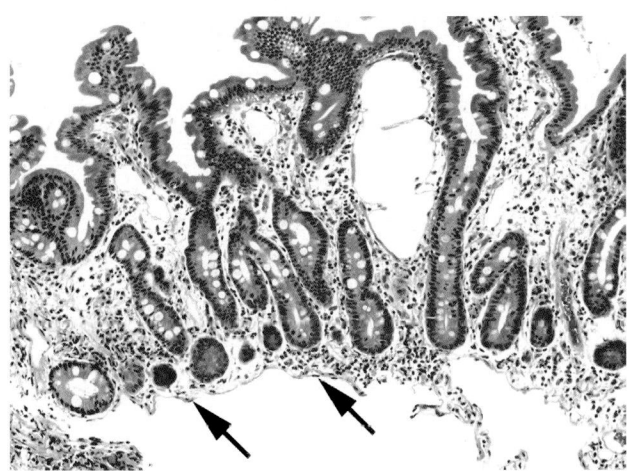

Figure 3-219. Lymphangioma/lymphangiectasia. On small superficial biopsies, one cannot distinguish a lymphangioma malformation from ectasia. The dilated lymphatic spaces are both lined by small flattened endothelial cells with inconspicuous spindled nuclei (*arrows*).

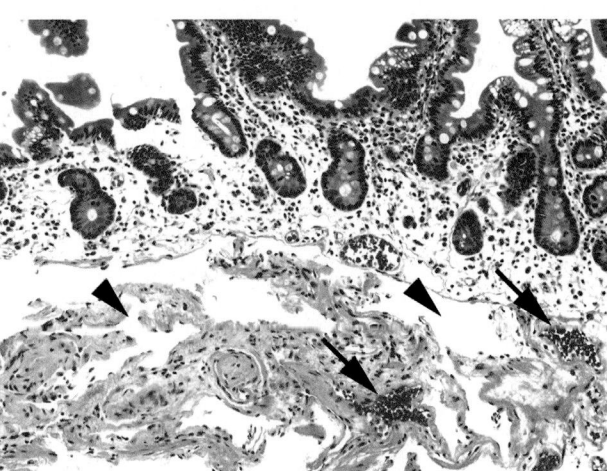

Figure 3-220. Lymphangioma. This lymphangioma shows anastomosing "empty" lymphatic channels (*arrowheads*) juxtaposed with blood vessels filled with red blood cells (*arrows*).

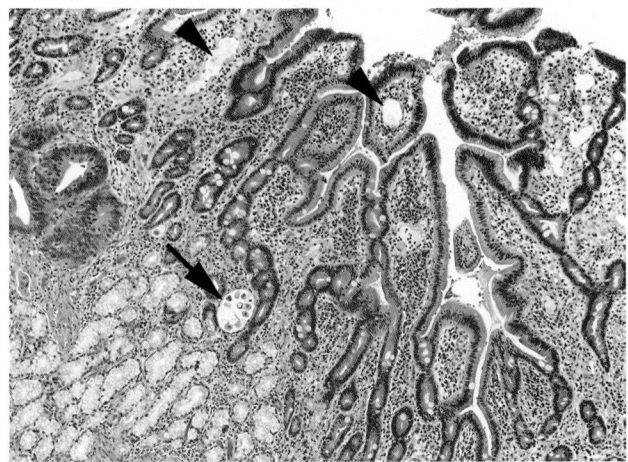

Figure 3-221. Intralymphatic tumor. Lymphatic channels provide a route for metastasis. Whenever dilated lymphatic channels are visible (*arrowheads*), take a moment to examine for intralymphatic tumor cells (*arrow*). This example is metastatic pancreatic ductal carcinoma.

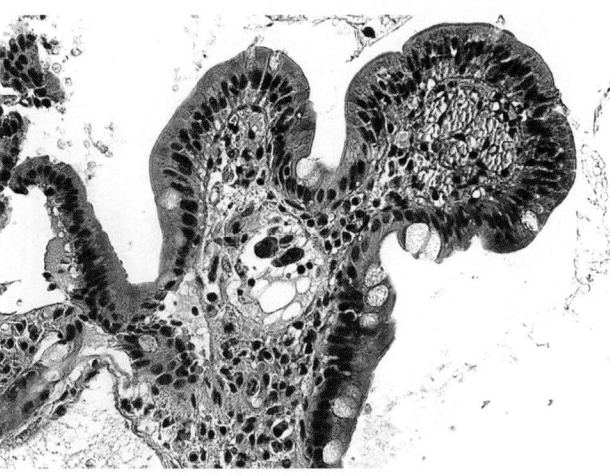

Figure 3-222. Intralymphatic tumor. Dilated lacteals in the small bowel can harbor tumor cells. This example is diffuse large B-cell lymphoma.

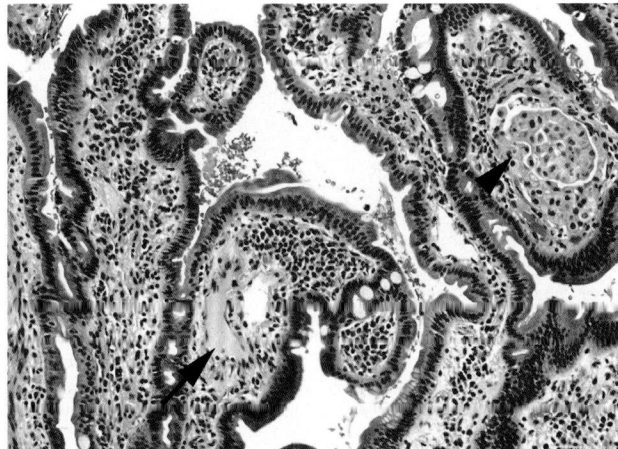

Figure 3-223. Intralymphatic tumor. Tumor cells plug up lymphatic spaces (*arrowhead*) and cause congestion of lymphatic flow resulting in adjacent or upstream dilated lacteals (*arrow*). These dilated spaces with acellular pale pink fluid are clues to adjacent pathology.

METASTATIC CLEAR CELL RENAL CELL CARCINOMA

Take an extra moment to scrutinize small and crushed endoscopic biopsies for sneaky metastatic disease, especially if they are accompanied by an endoscopic abnormality such as erosion or ulcer. At first glance, this mucosa shows acute ulceration and granulation tissue formation. The embedded clear cells masquerade as Brunner glands, and the atypical nuclei could easily be written off as reactive changes due to the overlying ulceration. When dealing with crushed biopsies, listen to your gut instincts and throw a keratin stain on the tissue if you have even a vague uneasiness. In this case, a PAX8 immunostain reveals extensive involvement by metastatic clear cell renal cell carcinoma (Figs. 3.224–3.228).

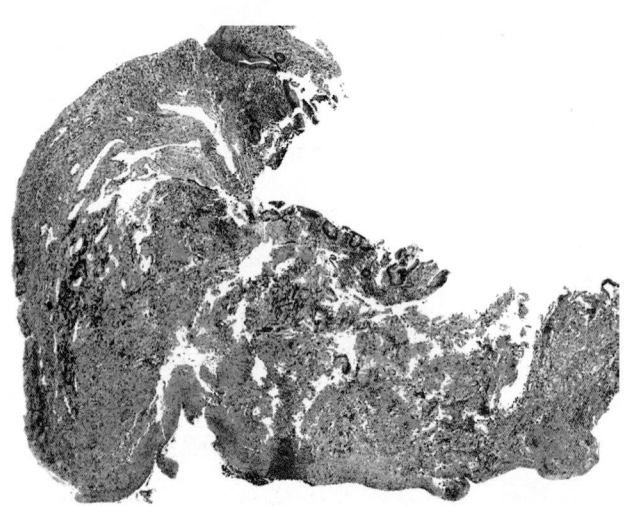

Figure 3-224. Metastatic clear cell renal cell carcinoma. Crushed, ulcerated, and inflamed biopsies can harbor unexpected lesions.

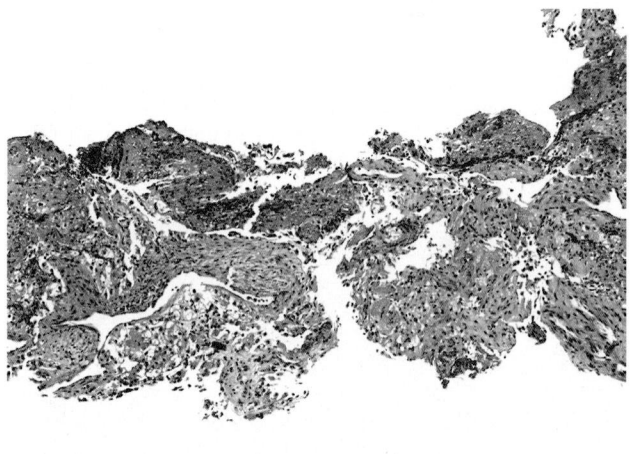

Figure 3-225. Metastatic clear cell renal cell carcinoma. This ulcer bed appears fairly unremarkable, but it is hiding metastatic tumor (see the next figure).

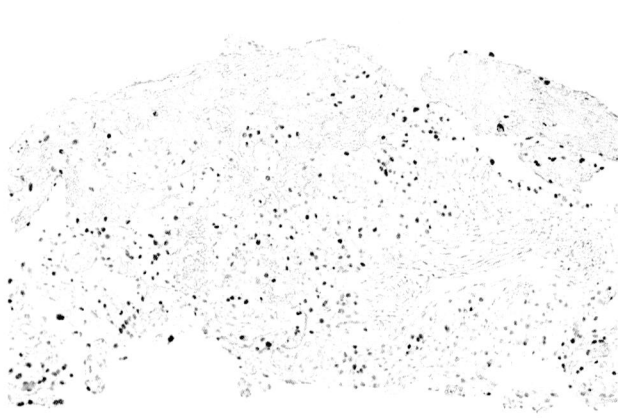

Figure 3-226. Metastatic clear cell renal cell carcinoma, PAX8 immunohistochemistry of the previous figure. Many of the cells from the previous figure show nuclear reactivity for PAX8, confirming the presence of metastatic clear cell RCC.

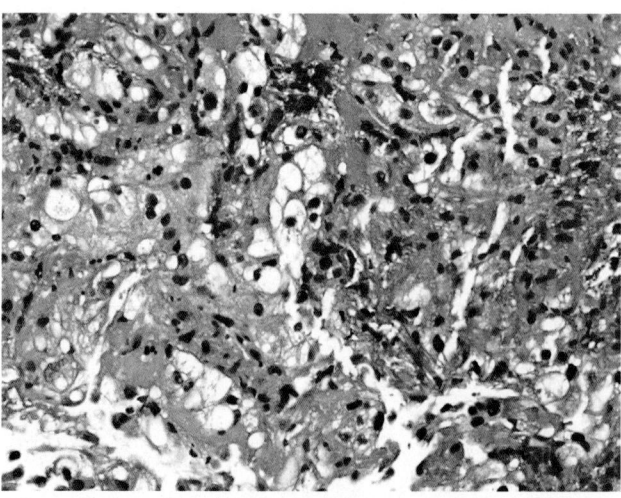

Figure 3-227. Metastatic clear cell renal cell carcinoma. At higher magnification, cells with clear cytoplasm are found within the ulcer base. They may appear similar to Brunner glands, but knowledge of a prior malignancy and a high level of suspicion can avoid a missed diagnosis.

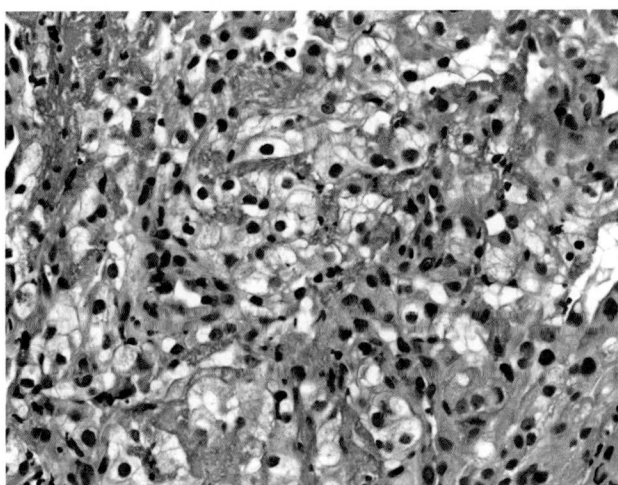

Figure 3-228. Metastatic clear cell renal cell carcinoma. In the base of an ulcer, one might mistake these cells as disorganized or disrupted Brunner glands with reactive atypia. However, keep a high level of suspicion for cells that look like they might not belong.

DUODENAL-TYPE FOLLICULAR LYMPHOMA

Lymphomas of the gut are beyond the scope of this text, as the authors are not hematopathologists. We encourage a low threshold for sharing lymphoid infiltrates with colleagues who have expertise. Most cases of gut lymphoma are mass forming or obviously malignant (e.g., diffuse large B-cell lymphoma, Burkitt lymphoma, enteropathy associated T-cell lymphoma). Primary intestinal follicular lymphoma (FL) is an exception and therefore worth mentioning because those of us who do not routinely evaluate hematopathology specimens worry most about missing a low-grade lymphoma. This rare variant of FL is confined to the intestine without nodal metastasis, typically presents as multiple small polyps, and is encountered in one of every 3000 to 7000 upper endoscopic procedures.[108-110] In contrast to FL of other sites that usually present with late-stage disease, duodenal-type FL is characteristically stage I-II and clinically indolent with 98% 5-year progression-free survival,[108,111] Duodenal-type follicular lymphoma (D-FL) (Fig. 3.229) is therefore regarded as a unique clinicopathologic entity in the 2016 WHO classification of lymphoid neoplasms.[108,112] Most cases are detected incidentally with unrelated indications for upper endoscopy, and mean age at presentation is 59 to 65 years without a predilection for men versus women.[108,111] Endoscopically, lesions appear as small polyps, nodules, or plaques and multifocal involvement is common (78% to 85%), including involvement of other segments of small bowel. Compared with other gut lymphomas that tend to involve the deep mucosa and submucosa, a peculiar histologic feature of D-FL is its involvement of small intestinal villi resulting in a lymphoid nodule that looks as if it is hanging out into the lumen (Fig. 3.230). The neoplastic cells are small and uniform, expressing CD20, CD79a, CD10, BCL-6, and aberrant expression of BCL-2 (Figs. 3.230–3.234). The cells are nonreactive for CD5, CD23, CD43, cyclin D1, and T-cell markers.[108,111] Ki-67 highlights a low proliferation index, and follicular dendritic cell markers (CD21 and CD23) show an abnormal meshwork of cells at the periphery occupying <10% of the neoplastic nodule (most other FL show two-thirds of the germinal center involved). Etiologically, D-FL shares some similarities with mucosa-associated lymphoid tissue (MALT) lymphoma as both are related to inflammation and antigen stimulation, but D-FL remains in the FL family as it expresses the hallmark translocation t(14;18)(q32;q21) affecting the genes immunoglobulin heavy chain (IgH) and B-cell leukemia/lymphoma (BCL2). Treatment is external beam radiotherapy, but this can lead to radiation-induced strictures and other complications. Some centers prefer instead to "watch and wait" because even when left untreated, D-FL usually does not develop tumorous growth, rarely disseminates, and does not transform into high-grade disease.[108]

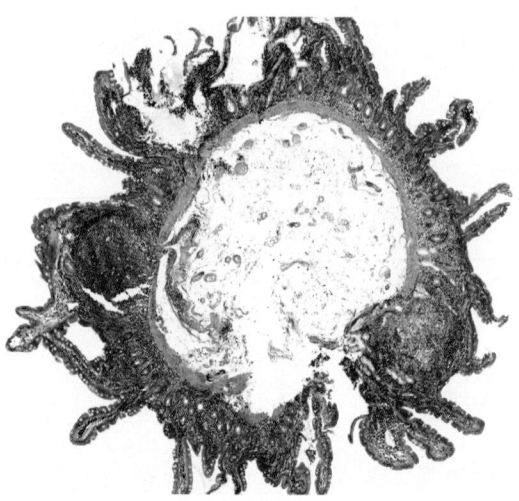

Figure 3-229. Duodenal-type follicular lymphoma. The GI tract is an immunologic organ, and it is common to see lymphoid aggregates within endoscopic mucosal biopsies. Knowledge of a few key points will help differentiate benign reactive aggregates from follicular lymphoma, such as seen here. Red flags in this example include the uniformity of the lymphoid follicles and the diffuse hyperchromasia of the lamina propria, which on higher magnification shows infiltration by a uniform monomorphic population of lymphocytes rather than the normal mixed inflammatory cells.

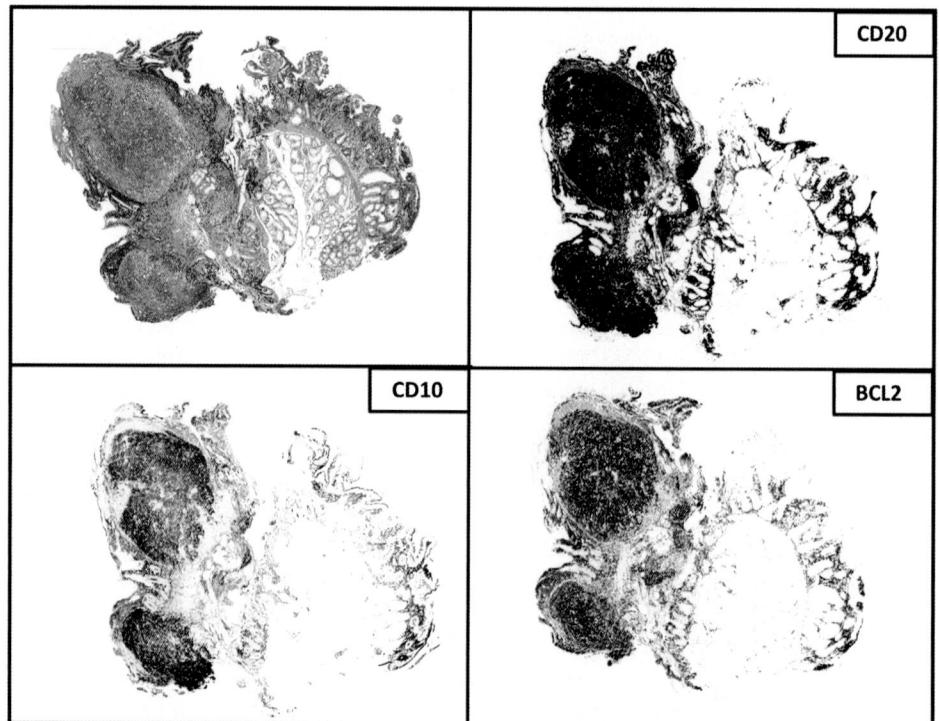

Figure 3-230. Duodenal-type follicular lymphoma. The size of this follicle is unusually large. Benign lymphoid aggregates typically involve the mucosa and submucosa, but the bulbous protrusion seen here is unusual. Follicular lymphomas involving the small bowel frequently involve the villi. The tumor is composed of CD20-positive B cells with expression of CD10 and BCL2.

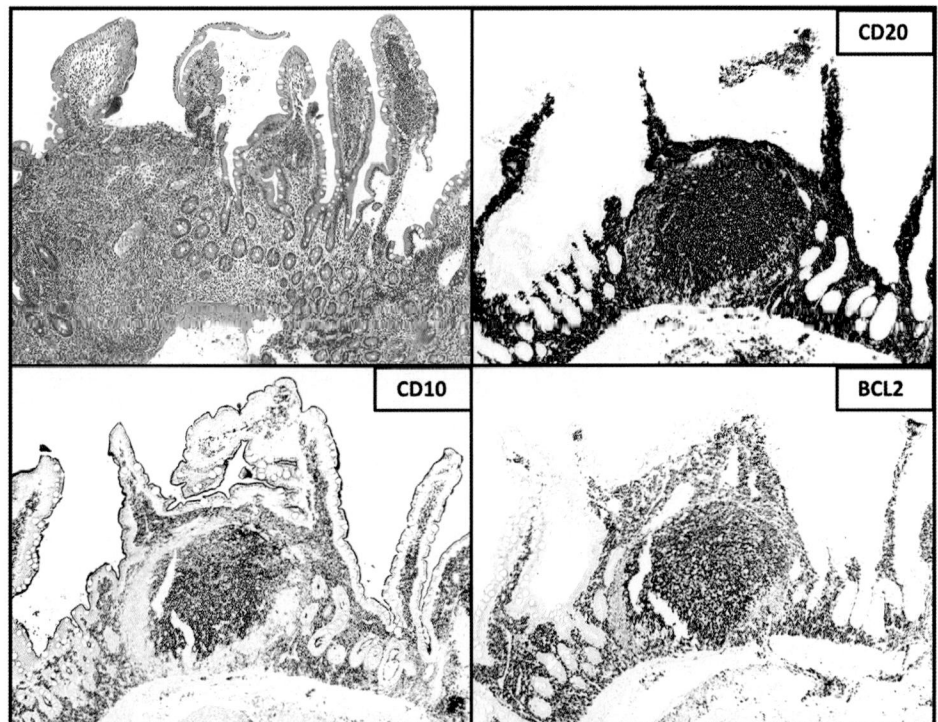

Figure 3-231. Duodenal-type follicular lymphoma. Architecturally, this small bowel is only slightly distorted. However, note the uniformity of cells within the lamina propria and filling the duodenal villi. The normal mixed inflammatory cells of the lamina propria are absent. Further immunohistochemical workup of this area shows a diffuse population of CD20-positive B cells with expression of CD10 and BCL2.

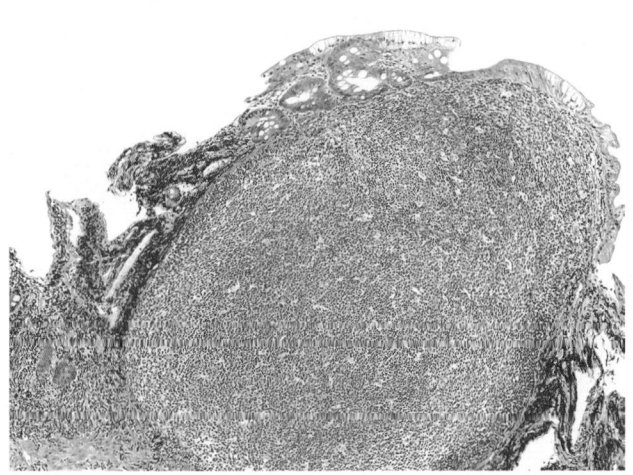

Figure 3-232. Duodenal-type follicular lymphoma. This lymphoid aggregate is abnormal because it is unusually large, protrudes into the lumen, lacks polarity (see Figs. 3.250 and 3.251 for comparison), contains a diffuse uniform population of cells, and lacks tingible body macrophages (see Figs. 3.235 and 3.236). These features warrant further workup.

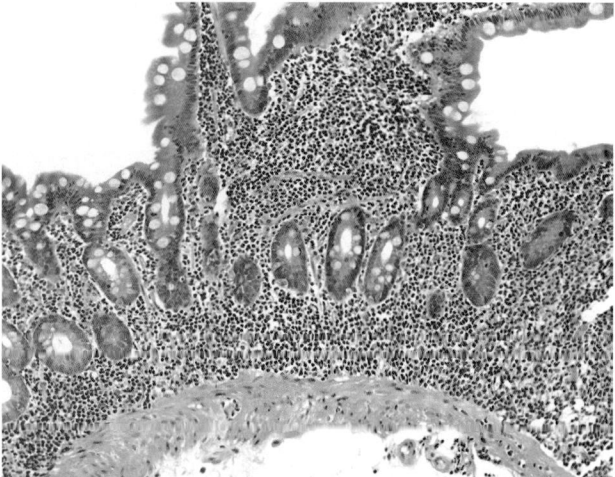

Figure 3-233. Duodenal-type follicular lymphoma. The normal lamina propria contains a mixed population of inflammatory cells (see Figs. 3.3 and 3.4). By comparison, this lamina propria is filled with a single population of monomorphic small lymphocytes.

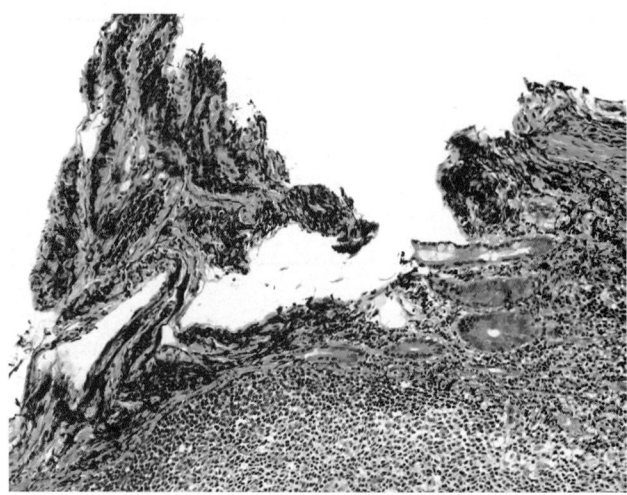

Figure 3-234. Duodenal-type follicular lymphoma. Crushed biopsies can be challenging, if not impossible, to interpret. A targeted panel of immunostains including cytokeratin and hematolymphoid markers can exclude a neoplastic process; the crushed cells remain immunoreactive despite their lack of nuclear detail. This area is from a case of follicular lymphoma.

PEARLS & PITFALLS: Key Features of Reactive Lymphoid Follicles

Reactive lymphoid follicles can impart a nodular endoscopic appearance and raise concern for a hematolymphoid malignancy, especially for those of us lacking in hematopathology experience. When encountering lymphoid nodules, look for these reassuring features of benign reactive follicles (Figs. 3.235 and 3.236):

- Germinal centers with variation in size and shape
- Eccentric low-power appearance, with polarized germinal center
- Tingible body macrophages
- Preserved follicular dendritic cell network (can be highlighted by CD21)

PEARLS & PITFALLS: Key Features of Malignant Hematolymphoid Lesions

When lymphoid aggregates exhibit the following features on H&E, it is worthwhile to seek additional workup or hematopathology expertise (Figs. 3.237–3.243):

- Mass formation or unusually large lymphoid aggregates
- Exquisitely uniform cell population, or
- Large atypical cells
- Destructive infiltration (involving muscularis mucosae or glandular epithelium)
- Unusual location (e.g., tip of villous or deep muscularis propria)

PEARLS & PITFALLS: A Dartboard Analogy for Hematopathology Markers

For those of us who do not routinely evaluate hematopathology specimens, it can be difficult to remember the significance of several of the similarly sounding hematopathology markers, particularly BCL-2, BCL-6, and CD 10. If you relate to these challenges, consider this dartboard analogy as a handy learning tool (Figs. 3.244–3.246). In the game of darts, a player is awarded more points for landing a dart at the prized center bull's eye owing to the challenging nature of this difficult shot, and fewer points for landing a dart in the periphery of the dart board. In this analogy, imagine the center bull's eye as a germinal center with the highest points awarded (BCL-6 and CD10). In contrast, the peripheral location outside of the germinal center is awarded fewer points (BCL-2). Importantly, this analogy works only for normal lymphoid aggregates! FL, for example, is characterized by BCL-2 reactive germinal centers owing to the t(14;18) rearrangement of *BCL-2* and the immunoglobin variable region heavy chain (IgH).

FAQ: My terminal ileum biopsy shows prominent lymphoid aggregates. How can I be sure I am not missing a sneaky hematolymphoid malignancy (Fig. 3.247)?

Answer: You are not alone. Prominent lymphoid aggregates can be especially alarming in the terminal ileum and, thus, are a common source of consultation. The small bowel serves as an essential component of the immune system through its perpetual surveillance of the passing luminal contents. Diligent immunosurveillance is facilitated through specialized epithelial cells (M-cells) that transport luminal antigens to the lymphoid aggregates (designated "Peyer patches" when seen in the terminal ileum). Hyperplastic lymphoid aggregates can be sufficiently large as to be visualized endoscopically (Fig. 3.248) and can also serve as intussusception lead points, especially in young children. The epicenter of lymphoid aggregates is in the mucosa, but especially prominent cases can feature extension into the submucosa, raising concerns for a hematolymphoid malignancy (Figs. 3.249 and 3.250). Alternatively, polypoid lymphoid hyperplasia can involve the villi mimicking FL of the small bowel (Figs. 3.251 and 3.252). Histologic features reassuring for a benign, reactive process include the presence of germinal centers, tingible body macrophages, and a polymorphous constituent lymphoid population (i.e., a variety of cell sizes represented). However, if the focus seems at all concerning, a quick immunohistochemical panel may be worthwhile (Table 3.4).

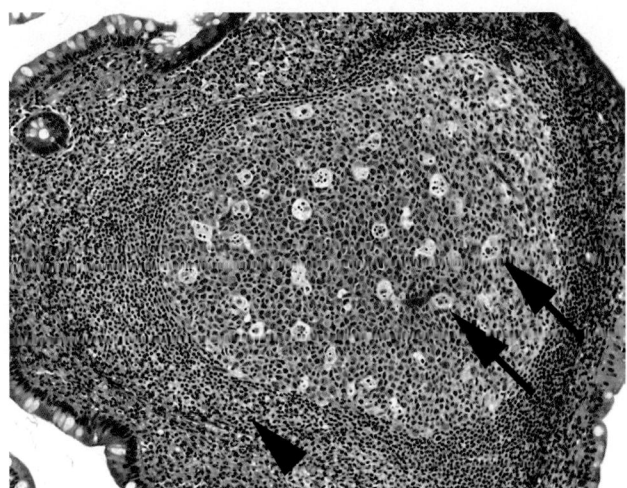

Figure 3-235. Benign reactive lymphoid follicle. Reactive follicles have variably sized germinal centers that are eccentric, giving the follicle a polarized appearance. The numerous tingible body macrophages (*arrows*) are visible at low magnification and are reassuring for a benign follicle. Not also the variation in cell sizes between the germinal center and mantle zone (*arrowhead*).

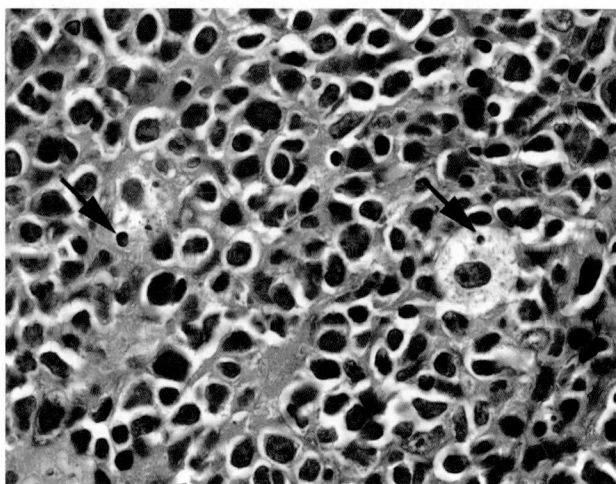

Figure 3-236. Tingible body macrophages. These macrophages are found in germinal centers of reactive follicles. They have phagocytized nuclear debris (*arrows*) from apoptotic cells. The word tingible means "stainable." Thus, these tingible body macrophages contain stainable bodies of condensed chromatin fragments.

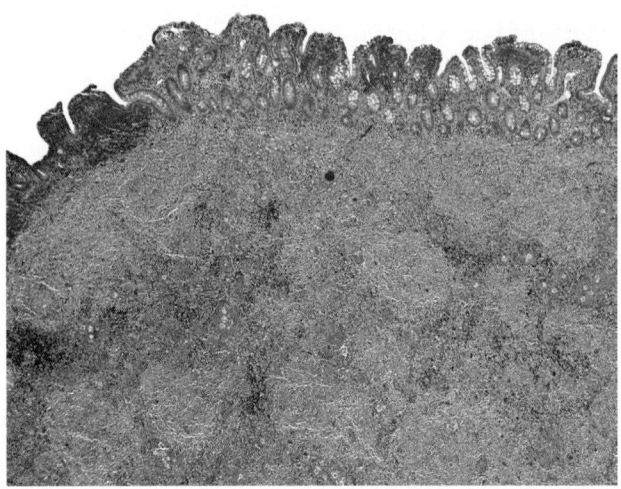

Figure 3-237. Mucosa-associated lymphoid tissue (MALT) extranodal marginal zone lymphoma. Mass formation or unusually large lymphoid aggregates are red flags to initiate a workup for lymphoma. In addition, the lymphoid aggregates in this mass lack germinal centers and tingible body macrophages and do not appear polarized. Instead, one can appreciate that the cells are uniform even in this low-power view.

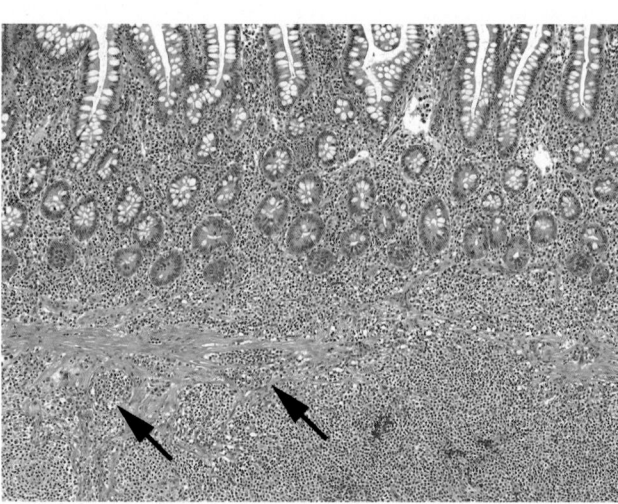

Figure 3-238. Mucosa-associated lymphoid tissue (MALT) extranodal marginal zone lymphoma. Benign lymphoid cells can cross the muscularis mucosae, but when a monomorphic lymphoid population is destructive and splays the muscle fibers apart (*arrows*), exclusion of a hematolymphoid malignancy is prudent.

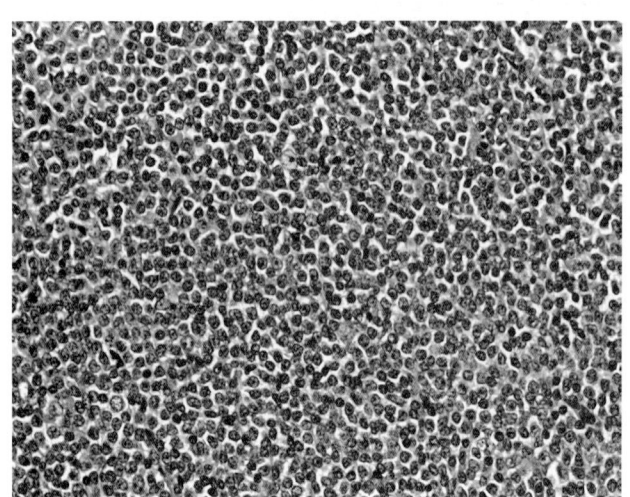

Figure 3-239. Mucosa-associated lymphoid tissue (MALT) extranodal marginal zone lymphoma. Normal reactive infiltrates show mixed cell populations. When an infiltrate is exquisitely uniform, lacking any variability in size and shape, beware of lymphoma.

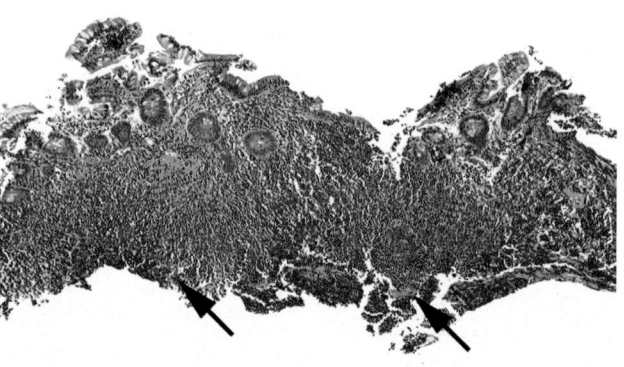

Figure 3-240. Mantle cell lymphoma. Several hallmark red flags are present in this biopsy, including the replacement of normal mixed inflammatory cells in the lamina propria by a dense population of small uniform cells, and there is active destruction of the muscularis mucosae with abnormal splaying of smooth muscle fibers (*arrows*).

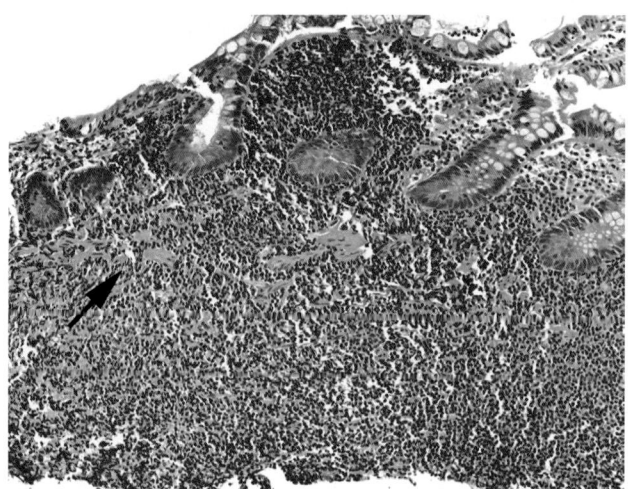

Figure 3-241. Mantle cell lymphoma. The normal lamina propria contains a mixed population that includes plasma cells and eosinophils in addition to lymphocytes. These cells are conspicuously lacking in this biopsy, which shows only a single monomorphic population of lymphocytes. The cells are also destroying the muscularis mucosae and splaying it apart (*arrow*).

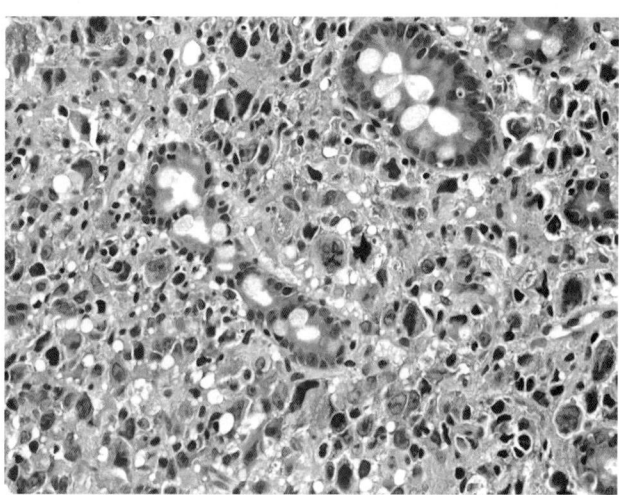

Figure 3-242. Diffuse large B-cell lymphoma. Large cell lymphomas are easy to spot, but their pleomorphic and atypical cells can mimic a carcinoma. A keratin immunostain will be negative, whereas CD20 will be strongly and diffusely reactive (see the next figure).

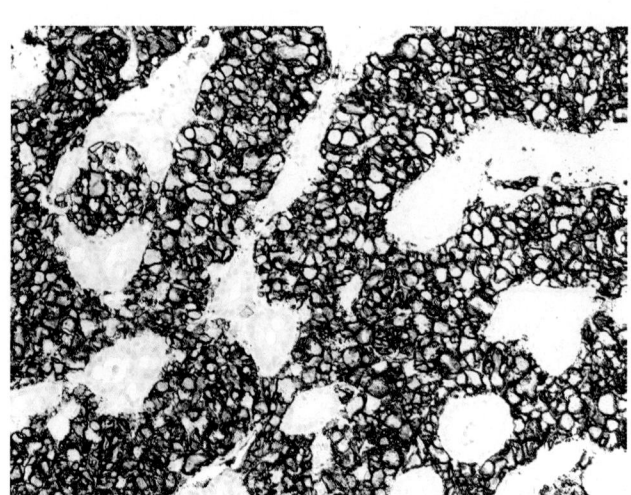

Figure 3-243. Diffuse large B-cell lymphoma, CD20 immunostain of the previous figure.

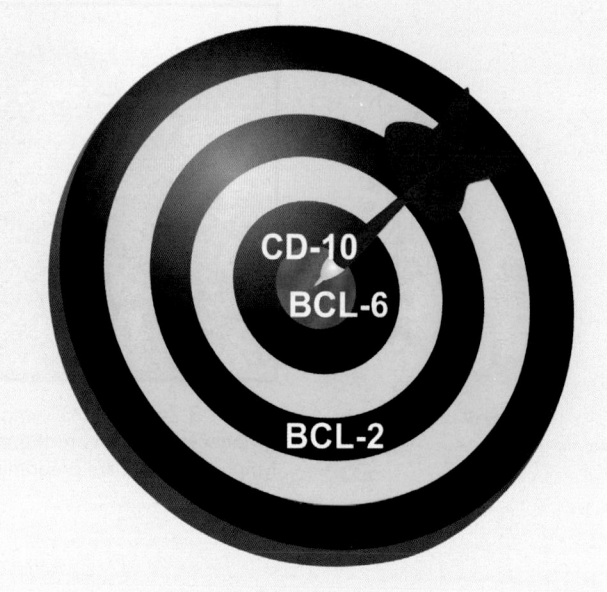

Figure 3-244. Dart game analogy. If it is difficult to remember the significance of BCL-2, BCL-6, and CD10 as they relate to normal lymphoid aggregate architecture, consider this dartboard analogy. In the game of darts, a player is awarded more points for landing a dart at the center bull's eye as compared with the periphery of the dartboard. In this analogy, imagine the bull's eye as a germinal center with the highest points awarded (BCL-6 and CD10). In contrast, the peripheral location is outside of the germinal center and fewer points are awarded for these less challenging shots (BCL-*2*).

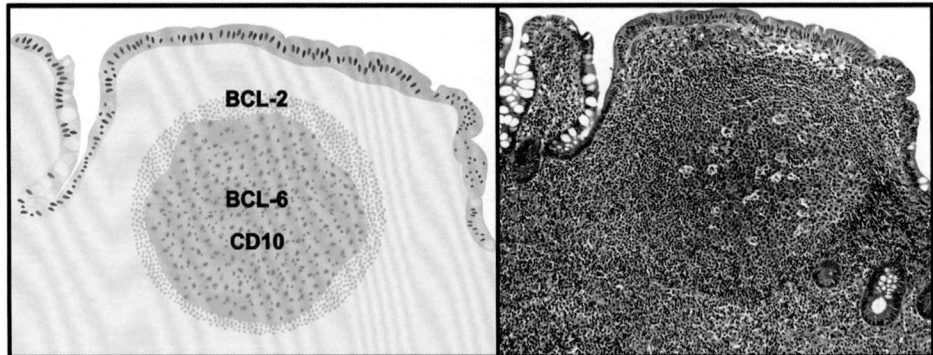

Figure 3-245. Normal lymphoid aggregate, illustration. In a normal lymphoid aggregate, the germinal center is highlighted by BCL-6 and CD10 (analogous to a dartboard's prized bull's eye) and is negative for BCL-2. Recall, normal B lymphocytes in the mantle zone surrounding the germinal center and normal T lymphocytes express BCL-2 (analogous to a dartboard's periphery). Therefore, interpretation of BCL-2 always requires concomitant interpretation of CD20 B-lymphocyte marker and CD3 T-lymphocyte marker for contrast.

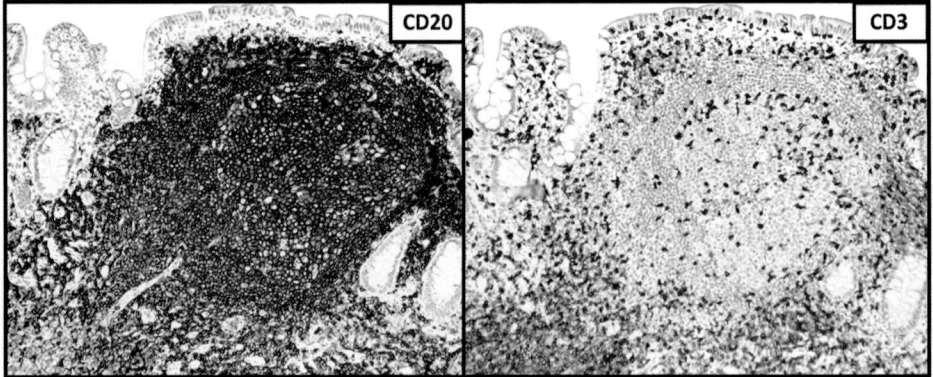

Figure 3-246. Normal lymphoid aggregate, CD20 and CD3 immunostains. A CD20 highlights B lymphocytes, which are the majority of the lymphoid constituents. A contrasting CD3 highlights T lymphocytes that are predominantly seen surrounding the germinal center.

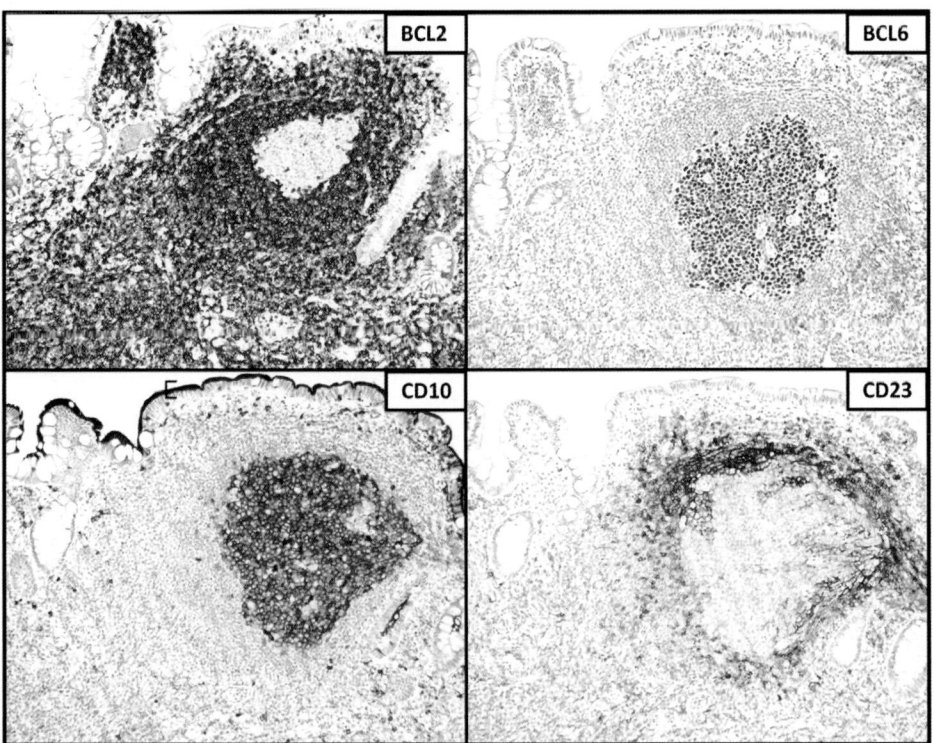

Figure 3-247. Normal lymphoid aggregate, BCL2, BCL6, CD10, CD23 immunostains. Normal germinal centers are BCL-2 negative. If the germinal center is BCL-2 reactive, consider follicular lymphomas, which are characterized by the t(14;18) rearrangement of BCL-2 and the immunoglobin heavy chain (IgH). Importantly, recall that normal B lymphocytes in the mantle zone surrounding the germinal center and normal T lymphocytes express BCL-2. Therefore, interpretation of BCL-2 always requires concomitant interpretation of CD20 B lymphocytes and CD3 T lymphocytes (see Fig. 3.246). BCL-6 and CD10 are equally helpful markers that highlight germinal centers. CD23 highlights the follicular dendritic cell meshwork surrounding the germinal centers, a feature of intact (normal) lymphoid aggregate architecture.

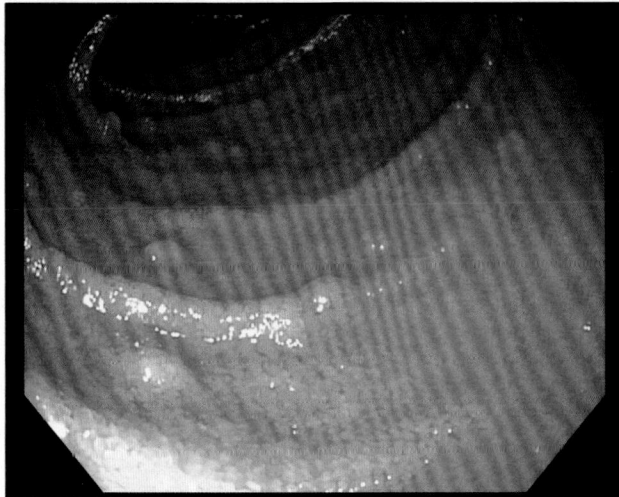

Figure 3-248. Lymphoid hyperplasia of small bowel, endoscopic photo. Nodular lymphoid hyperplasia and follicular lymphoma can have similar endoscopic appearances. Biopsy and immunohistochemical workup are necessary to differentiate these entities.

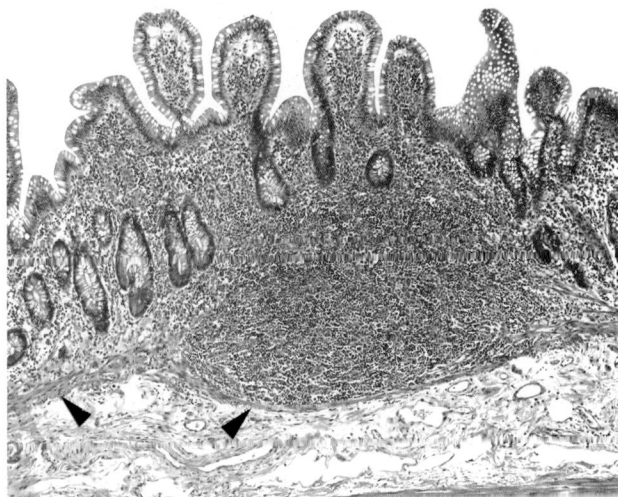

Figure 3-249. Normal terminal ileum. The overlying villi of the terminal ileum are characteristically shorter than those seen in the duodenum and jejunum. At low power, the prominent lymphoid aggregate is seen confined within the mucosa and respecting the narrow wisp of muscularis mucosae (*arrowheads*). The lymphoid aggregate gently pushes the crypts apart, which remain intact.

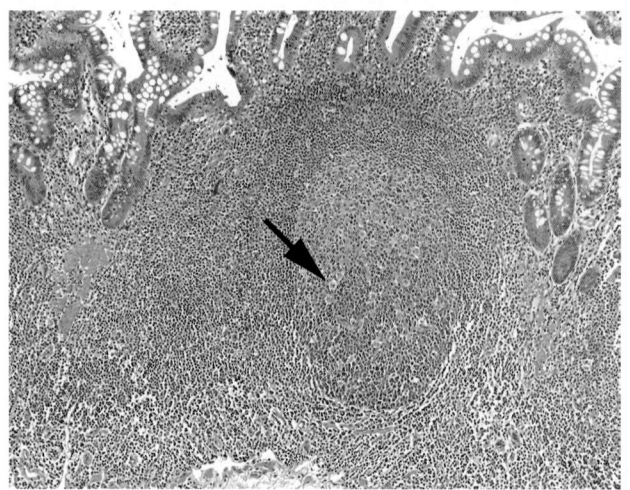

Figure 3-250. Normal terminal ileum. This large follicle is reassuring at low magnification because it is nondestructive and has an eccentric appearance, with a polarized germinal center and mantle zone. There is variability in cell size and shape, and tingible body macrophages are present (*arrow*).

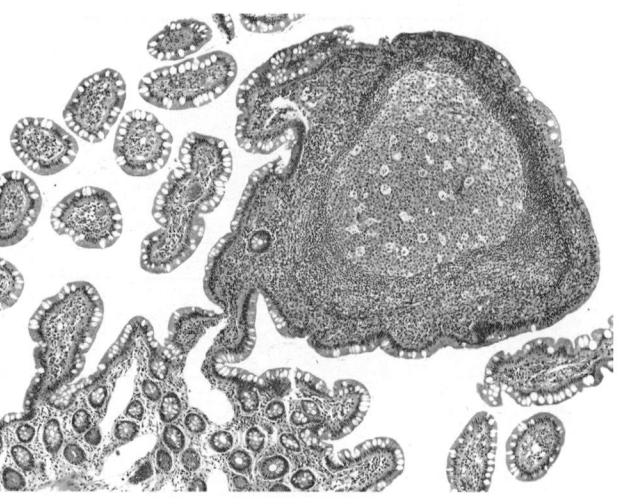

Figure 3-251. Polypoid lymphoid hyperplasia. Lymphoid nodules of the small bowel can involve the villi, causing a nodule to protrude or hang in the lumen. This peculiar feature is seen in, but not exclusive to, follicular lymphomas. This photo is an example of benign polypoid lymphoid hyperplasia found in the terminal ileum. The low-power features of benign follicles are seen here, such as eccentric germinal center, abundant tingible body macrophages, and polymorphous population.

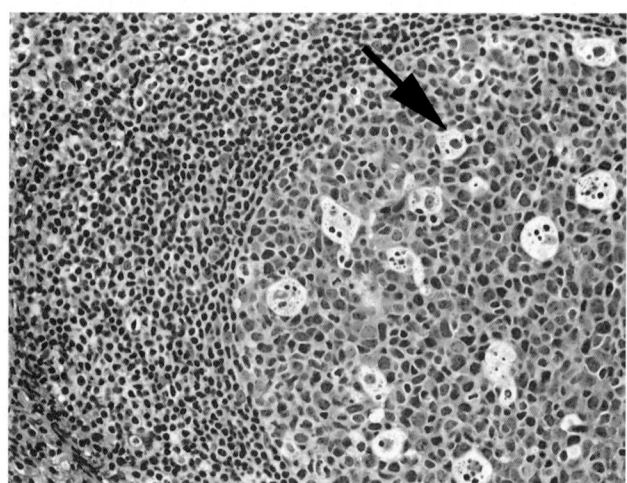

Figure 3-252. Benign reactive lymphoid follicle, higher power of the previous figure. The tingible body macrophages (*arrow*) contain engulfed fragments of nuclear debris from cells undergoing selective apoptosis. The peripheral mantle zone contains small lymphocytes, whereas the germinal center contains larger centroblasts, centrocytes, and follicular dendritic cells. This variability in size and shape of cells is reassuring for benign lymphoid follicles.

TABLE 3.4: Quick and Dirty Immunohistochemical Panel for Prominent Lymphoid Aggregates Versus Select Hematolymphoid Malignancies

Marker	Benign, Reactive Process	Hematolymphoid Malignancy
CD 3	T lymphocytes surround germinal centers (overall, T lymphocytes constitute the minority of lymphoid cells)	T lymphocytes may constitute the majority of lymphoid cells, are not confined to the perigerminal center location, and show nuclear pleomorphism
CD 20	B lymphocytes are present in the germinal center (overall, B lymphocytes constitute the majority of lymphocytes)	B lymphocytes may constitute almost all lymphoid cells present and can appear monotonous (small B lymphomas) or wildly atypical (diffuse large B-cell lymphoma)
CD 10	Highlights germinal center cells	Highlights germinal center cells
BCL-6	Highlights germinal center cells	Highlights germinal center cells
BCL-2	Germinal centers are BCL-2 negative; normal B lymphocytes in the mantle zone surrounding the germinal center and normal T lymphocytes express BCL-2	Germinal centers BCL-2 positive (small B lymphocytes = follicular lymphoma, CD5–/CD10+, t(14;18) involving *BCL2* and *IgH*; large B lymphocytes = diffuse large B-cell lymphoma, CD5/CD10 variable, *BCL6* most common translocation, *BCL2* translocation seen in 20%)
Cyclin D1/ BCL-1	Germinal centers negative	Germinal centers positive (small B lymphocytes = mantle lymphoma, CD5+/CD10–, t(11:14) involving *cyclin D1*
Extras		Extranodal marginal zone lymphoma of mucosa-associated lymphoid tissue (MALT lymphoma) is CD5–/CD10–, comprising monotonous B lymphocytes that typically aberrantly coexpress CD20 and CD43
		Burkitt lymphoma consists of medium-sized, monotonous B-lymphoid cells, prominent tingible body macrophages ("starry-sky"), CD10+, KI-67 near 100%, most have Ig heavy chain-*MYC* translocation
Pearls and **Pitfalls**		
		CD43 also highlights plasma cells
		Lymphomas treated with rituximab (anti-CD20) can be CD20 negative (use PAX5 to confirm B lymphocytes in these cases)

SYSTEMIC MASTOCYTOSIS

Mastocytosis is a clonal neoplastic proliferation of mast cells involving multiple organ systems and encompassing a heterogeneous group of disorders, including urticaria pigmentosa, telangiectasia macularis eruptiva perstans, diffuse cutaneous mastocytosis, solitary mastocytoma, and systemic mastocytosis (SM). GI dysfunction caused by release of mast cell mediators can occur in both cutaneous and systemic disease, with 80% of patients with SM reporting abdominal pain and diarrhea and 30% to 50% of patients experiencing duodenal ulceration.[113] The mucosa may be endoscopically normal (38%) or show erythema, granularity, and nodularity.[114] Patients with infiltration of the GI tract mucosa fulfill the WHO criteria for the diagnosis of SM, which requires the presence of either 1 major and 1 minor criterion or ≥3 minor criteria (Fig. 3.253):

Major criterion:
  • Multifocal dense aggregates of mast cells (≥15) detected in bone marrow or other extracutaneous organs (e.g., GI tract, lymph nodes, liver, or spleen) and confirmed by special stains

Minor criteria:
  • Greater than or equal to 25% of mast cells have atypical morphology or spindle shapes
  • Mast cells coexpress CD117 with CD2 and/or CD25
  • Detection of KIT point mutation at codon 816 in bone marrow, blood, or other extracutaneous organs
  • Serum total tryptase persistently >20 ng/mL

As one can see, a diagnosis of SM can be made on endoscopic biopsy alone when mast cell aggregates show aberrant expression of CD25 or have spindled/ovoid morphology (Figs. 3.254–3.259). Mucosal involvement can be remarkably subtle and easily overlooked, and the first clue to a neoplastic process may be a prominent eosinophilic infiltrate, found in nearly half of all cases (Figs. 3.256–3.262).[114] These nonneoplastic bystanders are drawn in by chemokines released from the neoplastic cells and warn pathologists to stay attentive. Histologically, look for ovoid to spindled cells with abundant pale granular cytoplasm aggregated in the lamina propria or forming a confluent band beneath the surface epithelium. Identification of SM in the GI tract should prompt further hematologic evaluation, such as bone marrow biopsy. The prognosis and treatment of SM varies widely from indolent with symptomatic treatment by medical pharmacotherapy (e.g., antihistamines, antileukotrienes) to advanced disease requiring cytoreductive therapy or hematopoietic stem cell transplantation.

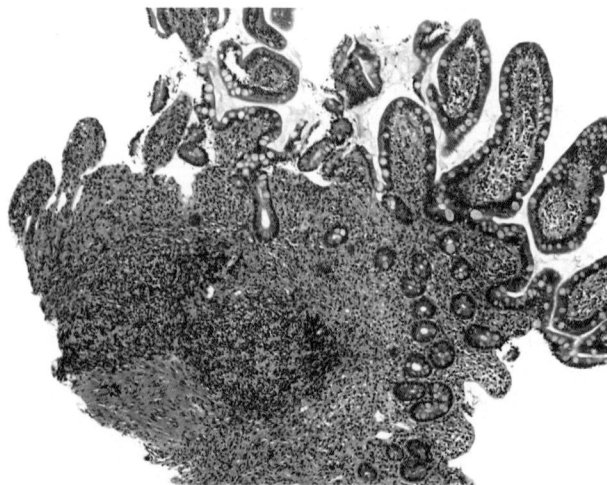

Figure 3-253. Systemic mastocytosis. GI tract involvement by systemic mastocytosis can be remarkably subtle. The clonal proliferation of mast cells is pale at low magnification and blends in with the normal lamina propria.

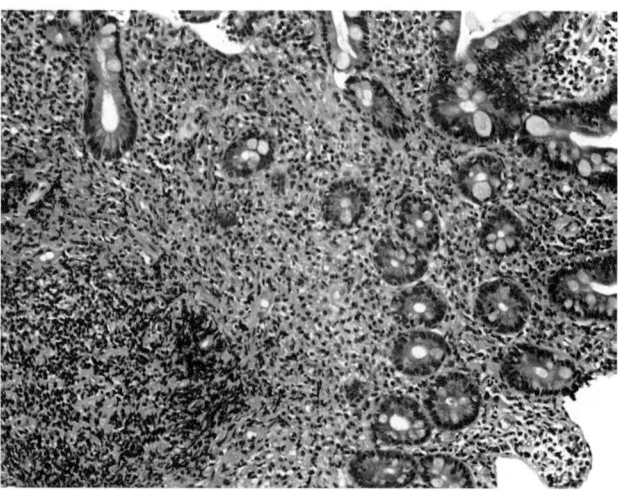

Figure 3-254. Systemic mastocytosis, higher magnification of the previous figure. Even at higher magnification, the mast cell proliferation is inconspicuous. The tumor cells are arranged back to back and have replaced the normal mixed inflammatory cell constituents of the lamina propria. Scattered eosinophils are present but not extensive. A helpful clue is the area of slight pallor as compared with normal lamina propria.

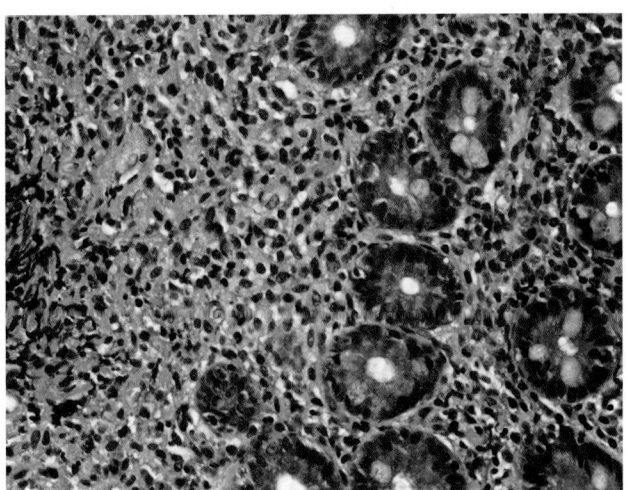

Figure 3-255. Systemic mastocytosis, higher magnification of the previous figure. At high magnification, the neoplastic cells are nondescript, and one might overlook them. The round to oblong nuclei are normochromatic, and the cells have abundant pale cytoplasm. The admixed eosinophils are drawn in by chemokines released from the mast cells and can be the first clue to the diagnosis.

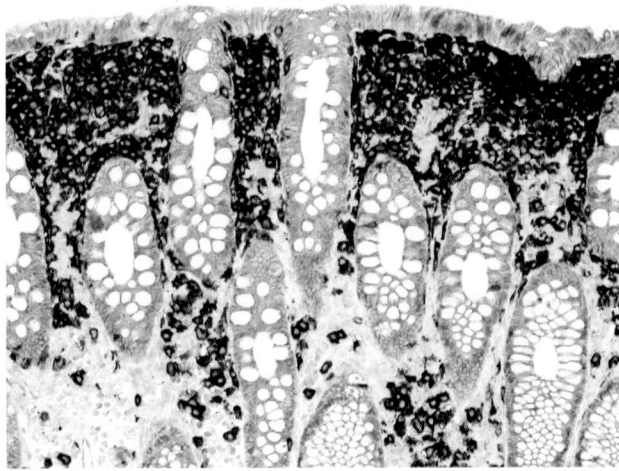

Figure 3-256. Systemic mastocytosis, CD117 immunostain. Mast cells show strong and diffuse reactivity for CD117, the best immunohistochemical marker. Although tryptase also highlights mast cells, at least one study has shown that a subset of tumor cells may be negative for tryptase.

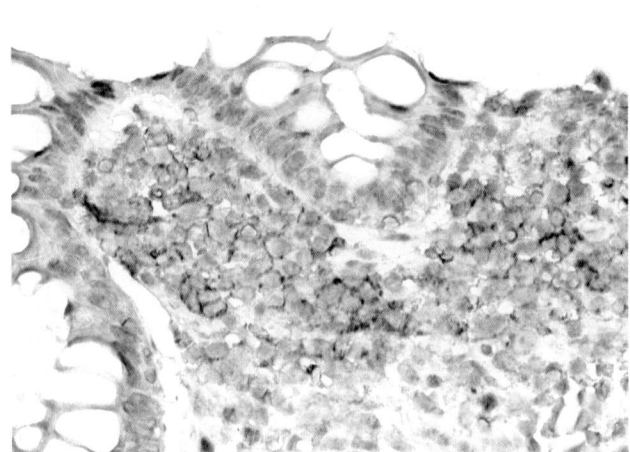

Figure 3-257. Systemic mastocytosis, CD25 immunostain. Aberrant expression of CD25 (membranous) by mast cells is a WHO minor criterion. This, combined with the WHO major criterion of a dense aggregate of ≥15 mast cells in an extracutaneous site (such as GI tract), is sufficient for a diagnosis of systemic mastocytosis.

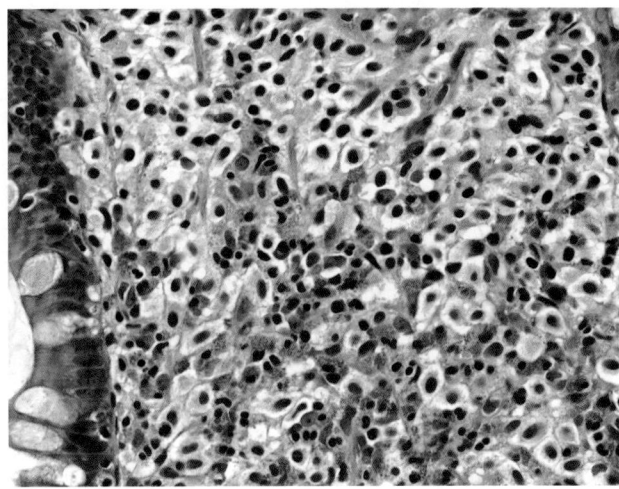

Figure 3-258. Systemic mastocytosis. The mast cells have a fried egg appearance with abundant finely granular cytoplasm that ranges from amphophilic to eosinophilic. Note the intimately admixed clusters of eosinophils, which are nonneoplastic bystanders.

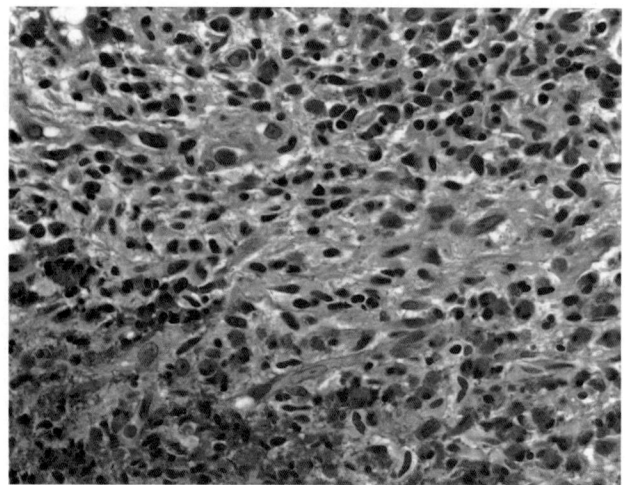

Figure 3-259. Systemic mastocytosis. The mast cells in this example show atypical morphology with spindled profiles. This spindled appearance contributes to diagnostic difficulty if one is looking for the typical fried egg appearance of normal mast cells. The dense infiltrate of eosinophils is characteristic and sometimes is the first clue to an associated pathologic process.

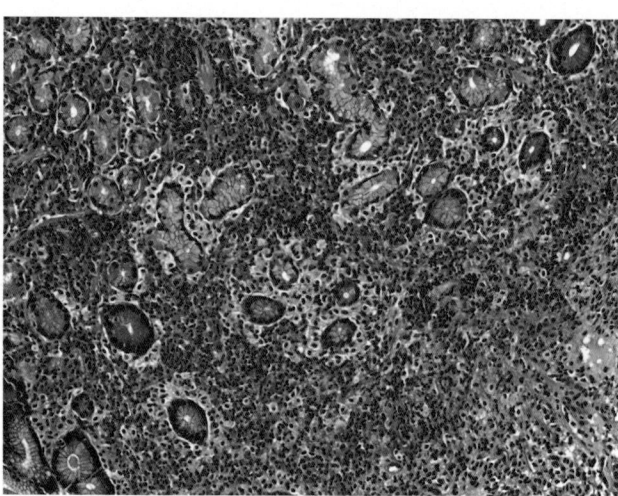

Figure 3-260. Systemic mastocytosis. The dense eosinophilic infiltrate is striking and should prompt one to examine for other pathology. Pale aggregates of mast cells surround these glands.

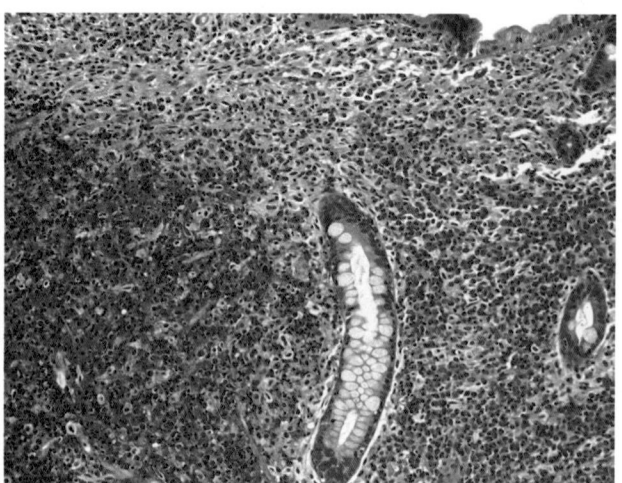

Figure 3-261. Systemic mastocytosis. Sheets of eosinophils create a dramatic impression. Note the admixed pale cells, many of which are also forming sheets in the backdrop. Some of these pale mast cells display spindled morphology, a feature characteristic of systemic mastocytosis and a WHO minor criterion for diagnosis.

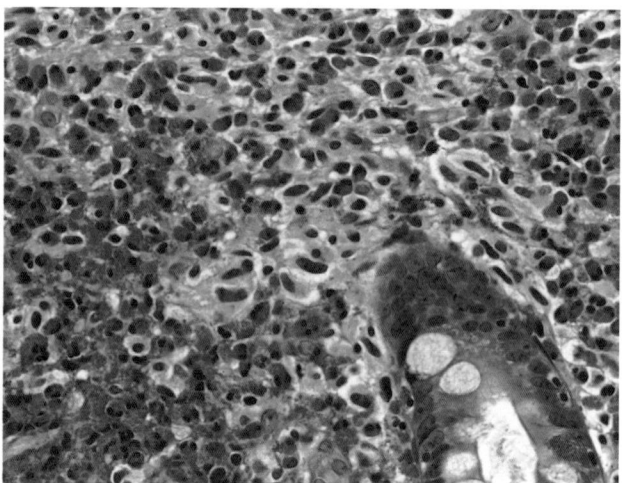

Figure 3-262. Systemic mastocytosis, higher magnification of the previous figure. The spindled neoplastic cells may be difficult to recognize as mast cells, as they are normally epithelioid with round nuclei and finely granular abundant cytoplasm. Any time one spots dense eosinophils such as this, examine for neoplasia such as systemic mastocystosis.

FAQ: Which stain is best for mast cells: CD117 or tryptase, or both?

CD117 is the best stain to highlight mast cells in the GI tract and will show diffuse membranous reactivity. Although tryptase also targets mast cells, one study found mast cell tryptase to have variable expression in SM, where 79% of cases showed positive staining in only a subset of the neoplastic mast cells.[114] Staining for both CD117 and tryptase is unnecessary (Figs. 3.256 and 3.263). However, if mast cells are confluent and SM is a consideration, then CD25 should be performed to evaluate for aberrant coexpression.

PEARLS & PITFALLS: Eosinophils Can Be a Clue to Surrounding Neoplasia

These nonneoplastic inflammatory bystanders are drawn in by chemokines released from the neoplastic cells or infectious parasitic processes and warn pathologists to stay attentive (Figs. 3.258–3.262). Tumors highly associated with eosinophilic infiltrates include SM, Langerhans cell histiocytosis, and inflammatory fibroid polyps, all of which can have remarkably subtle histologic appearances or a limited sample by endoscopic approach. When encountering dense mucosal eosinophils without an obvious cause, follow these sensible rules:

1. Rule out neoplasia with immunostains:

    a. CD117 and CD25 for SM

    b. S100 for Langerhans cell histiocytosis

    c. CD34 for inflammatory fibroid polyp

2. Rule out parasites with deeper levels and exhaust the tissue if necessary

3. Review the clinical history for other clues of disorders associated with eosinophilia (e.g., food allergies, vasculitides, drug reaction, inflammatory bowel disease, idiopathic eosinophilic enteritis). For more discussion on nonneoplastic entities, see Volume 1 (*Atlas of Gastrointestinal Pathology: A Pattern Based Approach to Non-Neoplastic Biopsies*).

FAQ: Do I need to count mast cells?

No. Staining for mast cells in the GI tract is performed for two conditions: (1) SM and (2) mast cell activation syndrome (MCAS), neither of which is diagnosed based on a mast cell count.

SM involving the GI tract requires the presence of extramedullary *confluent* sheets of CD117+ mast cells (WHO major criterion) showing aberrant expression of CD25 *or* atypical spindled morphology (WHO minor criteria).[114,115] Thus, single and scattered mast cells provide no support for SM (Fig. 3.264). Rarely, aberrant expression of CD25 is found among single scattered mast cells, which represents minimal involvement by SM, but these cases are always accompanied by concurrent biopsies showing obvious histologic involvement.[114] Again, aggregates of mast cells are required for a diagnosis, and mast cell counts do not figure in as a diagnostic criterion for SM.

MCAS diagnosis is clinical and has *no histologic correlate* and therefore does not require counting of mast cells.[116] Diagnostic criteria include all of the following:

1. Patients have at least four signs and symptoms of mast cell degranulation (abdominal pain, diarrhea, flushing, dermatographism, memory and concentration difficulties, headache)

2. Laboratory tests show increased mast cell mediators (serum tryptase, serum mature tryptase, urine histamine, serum/plasma prostaglandin 2)

3. Response to medications targeting mast cell mediators

4. Patients do not meet WHO criteria of SM or other clonal disorder

Mast cell staining in the evaluation of MCAS is *not* for the purposes of counting mast cells but rather to exclude the possibility of SM.

SAMPLE NOTE: Systemic Mastocytosis Confirmed

Small Bowel, Biopsy

- Small intestinal mucosa involved by systemic mastocytosis, see Note.

Note: Biopsies show confluent sheets of CD117+ mast cells with atypical spindled morphology and aberrant coexpression of CD25. The presence of abnormal mast cell clusters in an extracutaneous site fulfills diagnostic criteria for systemic mastocytosis (WHO, one major and one minor criterion).

SAMPLE NOTE: CD117 Shows Single Scattered Mast Cells

Small Bowel, Biopsy

- Small intestinal mucosa with nondiagnostic findings, see Note.

Note: CD117 immunostain (clinical request) highlights single, scattered mast cells without confluence or aberrant coexpression of CD25. These findings provide no evidence for systemic mastocytosis.

SAMPLE NOTE: Biopsies for Evaluation of Mast Cell Activation Syndrome

Small Bowel, Biopsy

- Small intestinal mucosa with nondiagnostic findings.
- CD117 immunostain (clinical request) highlights single, scattered mast cells with no evidence for systemic mastocystosis.
- See Note.

Note: Noted is the clinical concern for MCAS. The histologic sections show single scattered mast cells (confirmed by <tryptase/CD117> immunohistochemical stains) without confluence. The diagnosis of MCAS is clinical and requires that (1) patients have clinical signs and symptoms of mast cell degranulation, (2) laboratory tests show increased mast cell mediators, (3) patients demonstrate a clinical response to medication targeting mast cell mediators, and (4) patients do not have evidence of a mast cell malignancy or clonal disorder (e.g., systemic mastocytosis).

Based on our current understanding of the literature, mast cell density in mucosal biopsies is not useful in the diagnosis of MCAS but the biopsies are helpful to exclude systemic mastocytosis. The current biopsies confirm exclusion of systemic mastocytosis and aid in fulfilling the fourth requirement toward a clinical diagnosis of MCAS. Correlation with clinical presentation, serologic study, and response to medication is required.

Reference:
Hamilton MJ, Hornick JL, Akin C, Castells MC, Greenberger NJ. Mast cell activation syndrome: a newly recognized disorder with systemic clinical manifestations. *J Allergy Clin Immunol.* 2011;128(1):147.

SAMPLE NOTE: Clinician Asks for Mast Cell Counts

Small Bowel, Biopsy

- Small intestinal mucosa with nondiagnostic findings.
- CD117 immunostain (clinical request) highlights single, scattered mast cells with no evidence for systemic mastocystosis.
- See Note.

Note: Mast cell density in mucosal biopsies has been addressed by several studies that conclude that mast cell counts are not useful in the diagnosis or evaluation of patients with chronic diarrhea of unknown cause, chronic intractable diarrhea, diarrhea-predominant irritable bowel syndrome, or MCAS. However, some authors suggest that patients with these conditions may show symptomatic improvement with mast cell stabilizers. The current biopsies confirm exclusion of systemic mastocytosis and aid in fulfilling the fourth requirement toward a clinical diagnosis of MCAS should this be a clinical concern. Correlation with clinical presentation, serologic study, and response to medication is required.

References:

Doyle LA, Sepehr GJ, Hamilton MJ, Akin C, Castells MC, Hornick JL. A clinicopathologic study of 24 cases of systemic mastocytosis involving the gastrointestinal tract and assessment of mucosal mast cell density in irritable bowel syndrome and asymptomatic patients. *Am J Surg Pathol.* 2014;38(6):832-843.

Hamilton MJ, Hornick JL, Akin C, Castells MC, Greenberger NJ. Mast cell activation syndrome: a newly recognized disorder with systemic clinical manifestations. *J Allergy Clin Immunol.* 2011;128(1):147.

Sethi A, Jain D, Roland BC, Kinzel J, Gibson J, Schrader R, Hanson JA. Performing colonic mast cell counts in patients with chronic diarrhea of unknown etiology has limited diagnostic use. *Arch Pathol Lab Med.* 2015;139(2):225-232.

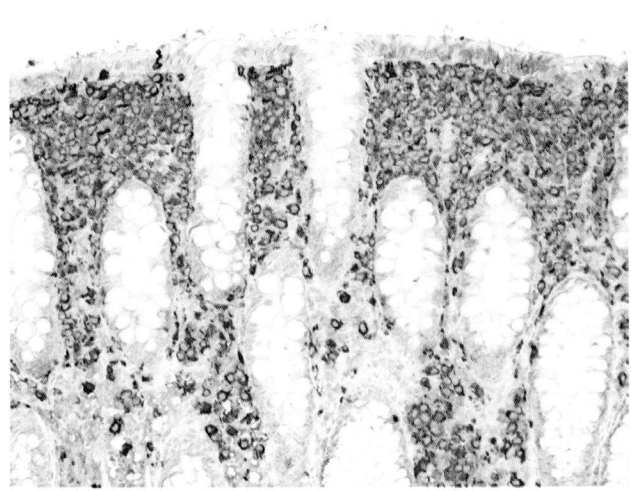

Figure 3-263. Systemic mastocytosis, tryptase immunostain. Tryptase is a sensitive marker for mast cells. However, CD117 is the preferred immunostain for systemic mastocytosis, as tryptase may be negative in a subset of tumor cells.

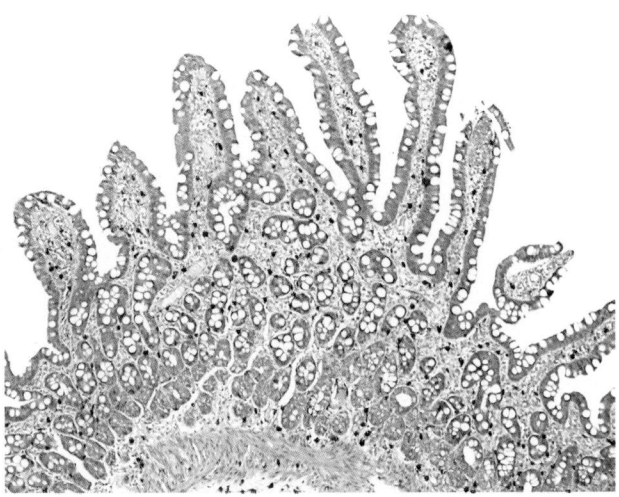

Figure 3-264. Normal small bowel, CD117 immunostain. Mast cells are normally distributed evenly and singly throughout the small bowel lamina propria. Some cases may have increased density, particularly in patients with unexplained diarrhea or irritable bowel syndrome, but there is no cutoff threshold for normal range, as it overlaps extensively with disease processes. All cases of systemic mastocytosis will show dense aggregates or sheets rather than single, scattered mast cells, as seen here.

References

1. Holmes R, Hourihane DO, Booth CC. The mucosa of the small intestine. *Postgrad Med J.* 1961;37:717-724.

2. Dobbins WO III. The intestinal mucosal lymphatic in man. A light and electron microscopic study. *Gastroenterology.* 1966;51(6):994-1003.

3. Rubin W. The epithelial "membrane" of the small intestine. *Am J Clin Nutr.* 1971;24(1):45-64.

4. Robertson HE. The pathology of Brunner's glands. *Arch Pathol Lab Med.* 1941(31):112-130.

5. Zhang Y, Sun X, Gold JS, et al. Heterotopic pancreas: a clinicopathological study of 184 cases from a single high-volume medical center in China. *Hum Pathol.* 2016;55:135-142.

6. Genta RM, Kinsey RS, Singhal A, Suterwala S. Gastric foveolar metaplasia and gastric heterotopia in the duodenum: no evidence of an etiologic role for Helicobacter pylori. *Hum Pathol.* 2010;41(11):1593-1600.

7. Wolff M. Heterotopic gastric epithelium in the rectum: a report of three new cases with a review of 87 cases of gastric heterotopia in the alimentary canal. *Am J Clin Pathol.* 1971;55(5):604-616.

8. Hoedemaeker PJ. Heterotopic gastric mucosa in the duodenum. *Digestion.* 1970;3(3):165-173.

9. Lessells AM, Martin DF. Heterotopic gastric mucosa in the duodenum. *J Clin Pathol.* 1982;35(6):591-595.

10. Conlon N, Logan E, Veerappan S, McKiernan S, O'Briain S. Duodenal gastric heterotopia: further evidence of an association with fundic gland polyps. *Hum Pathol.* 2013;44(4):636-642.

11. Nasir A, Amateau SK, Khan S, Simpson RW, Snover DC, Amin K. The many faces of intestinal tract gastric heterotopia; a series of four cases highlighting clinical and pathological heterogeneity. *Hum Pathol.* 2018;74:183-187.

12. So CS, Jang HJ, Choi YS, et al. Giant Brunner's gland adenoma of the proximal jejunum presenting as iron deficiency anemia and mimicking intussusceptions. *Clin Endosc.* 2013;46(1):102-105.

13. Levine JA, Burgart LJ, Batts KP, Wang KK. Brunner's gland hamartomas: clinical presentation and pathological features of 27 cases. *Am J Gastroenterol.* 1995;90(2):290-294.

14. Jansen JM, Stuifbergen WN, van Milligen de Wit AW. Endoscopic resection of a large Brunner's gland adenoma. *Neth J Med.* 2002;60(6):253-255.

15. Lu L, Li R, Zhang G, Zhao Z, Fu W, Li W. Brunner's gland adenoma of duodenum: report of two cases. *Int J Clin Exp Pathol.* 2015;8(6):7565-7569.

16. Marinacci LX, Manian FA. Brunner gland adenoma. *Mayo Clin Proc.* 2017;92(11):1737-1738.

17. Akino K, Kondo Y, Ueno A, et al. Carcinoma of duodenum arising from Brunner's gland. *J Gastroenterol.* 2002;37(4):293-296.

18. Kamei K, Yasuda T, Nakai T, Takeyama Y. A case of adenocarcinoma of the duodenum arising from Brunner's gland. *Case Rep Gastroenterol.* 2013;7(3):433-437.

19. Kitagori K, Miyamoto S, Sakurai T. Image of the month. Adenocarcinoma derived from Brunner's gland. *Clin Gastroenterol Hepatol.* 2010;8(4):A26.

20. Koizumi M, Sata N, Yoshizawa K, Kurihara K, Yasuda Y. Carcinoma arising from Brunner's gland in the duodenum after 17 Years of observation - a case report and literature review. *Case Rep Gastroenterol.* 2007;1(1):103-109.

21. Ohta Y, Saitoh K, Akai T, Uesato M, Ochiai T, Matsubara H. Early primary duodenal carcinoma arising from Brunner's glands synchronously occurring with sigmoid colon carcinoma: report of a case. *Surg Today.* 2008;38(8):756-760.

22. Vieth M, Kushima R, Borchard F, Stolte M. Pyloric gland adenoma: a clinico-pathological analysis of 90 cases. *Virchows Arch.* 2003;442(4):317-321.

23. Vieth M, Montgomery EA. Some observations on pyloric gland adenoma: an uncommon and long ignored entity! *J Clin Pathol.* 2014;67(10):883-890.

24. Beggs AD, Latchford AR, Vasen HF, et al. Peutz-Jeghers syndrome: a systematic review and recommendations for management. *Gut.* 2010;59(7):975-986.

25. Hemminki A, Markie D, Tomlinson I, et al. A serine/threonine kinase gene defective in Peutz-Jeghers syndrome. *Nature.* 1998;391(6663):184-187.

26. Volikos E, Robinson J, Aittomaki K, et al. LKB1 exonic and whole gene deletions are a common cause of Peutz-Jeghers syndrome. *J Med Genet.* 2006;43(5):e18.

27. Giardiello FM, Welsh SB, Hamilton SR, et al. Increased risk of cancer in the Peutz-Jeghers syndrome. *N Engl J Med.* 1987;316(24):1511-1514.

28. Hearle N, Schumacher V, Menko FH, et al. Frequency and spectrum of cancers in the Peutz-Jeghers syndrome. *Clin Cancer Res.* 2006;12(10):3209-3215.

29. Jeghers H, Mc KV, Katz KH. Generalized intestinal polyposis and melanin spots of the oral mucosa, lips and digits; a syndrome of diagnostic significance. *N Engl J Med.* 1949;241(26):1031-1036.

30. Offerhaus GJA BM, Gruber SB. Peutz-Jeghers syndrome. In: Bosman FT, Carneiro F, Hruban RH, et al, eds. *Tumors of the Digestive System.* Lyon, France: IACR; 2010:160-170.

31. Latchford AR, Phillips RK. Gastrointestinal polyps and cancer in Peutz-Jeghers syndrome: clinical aspects. *Fam Cancer.* 2011;10(3):455-461.

32. Lam-Himlin D, Park JY, Cornish TC, Shi C, Montgomery E. Morphologic characterization of syndromic gastric polyps. *Am J Surg Pathol.* 2010;34(11):1656-1662.

33. Tse JY, Wu S, Shinagare SA, et al. Peutz-Jeghers syndrome: a critical look at colonic Peutz-Jeghers polyps. *Mod Pathol.* 2013;26(9):1235-1240.

34. Giardiello FM, Brensinger JD, Tersmette AC, et al. Very high risk of cancer in familial Peutz-Jeghers syndrome. *Gastroenterology.* 2000;119(6):1447-1453.

35. Burkart AL, Sheridan T, Lewin M, Fenton H, Ali NJ, Montgomery E. Do sporadic Peutz-Jeghers polyps exist? Experience of a large teaching hospital. *Am J Surg Pathol.* 2007;31(8):1209-1214.

36. Burt RW, Bishop DT, Lynch HT, Rozen P, Winawer SJ. Risk and surveillance of individuals with heritable factors for colorectal cancer. WHO Collaborating Centre for the Prevention of Colorectal Cancer. *Bull World Health Organ*. 1990;68(5):655-665.

37. Howe JR, Roth S, Ringold JC, et al. Mutations in the SMAD4/DPC4 gene in juvenile polyposis. *Science*. 1998;280(5366):1086-1088.

38. Sweet K, Willis J, Zhou XP, et al. Molecular classification of patients with unexplained hamartomatous and hyperplastic polyposis. *JAMA*. 2005;294(19):2465-2473.

39. Howe JR, Mitros FA, Summers RW. The risk of gastrointestinal carcinoma in familial juvenile polyposis. *Ann Surg Oncol*. 1998;5(8):751-756.

40. Giardiello FM, Hamilton SR, Kern SE, et al. Colorectal neoplasia in juvenile polyposis or juvenile polyps. *Arch Dis Child*. 1991;66(8):971-975.

41. Offerhaus GJA HJ. Juvenile polyposis. In: Bosman FT, Carneiro F, Hruban RH, et al, eds. *WHO Classification of Tumors of the Digestive System*. Lyon, France: IARC; 2010:166-167.

42. Cronkhite LW Jr, Canada WJ. Generalized gastrointestinal polyposis; an unusual syndrome of polyposis, pigmentation, alopecia and onychotrophia. *N Engl J Med*. 1955;252(24):1011-1015.

43. Nakamura M, Kobashikawa K, Tamura J, et al. Cronkhite-Canada syndrome. *Intern Med*. 2009;48(17):1561-1562.

44. Sweetser S, Ahlquist DA, Osborn NK, et al. Clinicopathologic features and treatment outcomes in Cronkhite-Canada syndrome: support for autoimmunity. *Dig Dis Sci*. 2012;57(2):496-502.

45. Bettington M, Brown IS, Kumarasinghe MP, de Boer B, Bettington A, Rosty C. The challenging diagnosis of Cronkhite-Canada syndrome in the upper gastrointestinal tract: a series of 7 cases with clinical follow-up. *Am J Surg Pathol*. 2014;38(2):215-223.

46. Fan RY, Wang XW, Xue LJ, An R, Sheng JQ. Cronkhite-Canada syndrome polyps infiltrated with IgG4-positive plasma cells. *World J Clin Cases*. 2016;4(8):248-252.

47. Daniel ES, Ludwig SL, Lewin KJ, Ruprecht RM, Rajacich GM, Schwabe AD. The Cronkhite-Canada Syndrome. An analysis of clinical and pathologic features and therapy in 55 patients. *Medicine (Baltimore)*. 1982;61(5):293-309.

48. De Petris G, Chen L, Pasha SF, Ruff KC. Cronkhite-Canada syndrome diagnosis in the absence of gastrointestinal polyps: a case report. *Int J Surg Pathol*. 2013;21(6):627-631.

49. Burke AP, Sobin LH. The pathology of Cronkhite-Canada polyps. A comparison to juvenile polyposis. *Am J Surg Pathol*. 1989;13(11):940-946.

50. Yamakawa K, Yoshino T, Watanabe K, et al. Effectiveness of cyclosporine as a treatment for steroid-resistant Cronkhite-Canada syndrome; two case reports. *BMC Gastroenterol*. 2016;16(1):123.

51. Heald B, Mester J, Rybicki L, Orloff MS, Burke CA, Eng C. Frequent gastrointestinal polyps and colorectal adenocarcinomas in a prospective series of PTEN mutation carriers. *Gastroenterology*. 2010;139(6):1927-1933.

52. Kato M, Mizuki A, Hayashi T, et al. Cowden's disease diagnosed through mucocutaneous lesions and gastrointestinal polyposis with recurrent hematochezia, unrevealed by initial diagnosis. *Intern Med*. 2000;39(7):559-563.

53. Levi Z, Baris HN, Kedar I, et al. Upper and lower gastrointestinal findings in PTEN mutation-positive Cowden syndrome patients participating in an active surveillance program. *Clin Transl Gastroenterol*. 2011;2:e5.

54. Tan MH, Mester JL, Ngeow J, Rybicki LA, Orloff MS, Eng C. Lifetime cancer risks in individuals with germline PTEN mutations. *Clin Canc Res*. 2012;18(2):400-407.

55. de Leon MP, Di Gregorio C, Giunti L, et al. Duodenal carcinoma in a 37-year-old man with Cowden/Bannayan syndrome. *Dig Liver Dis*. 2013;45(1):75-78.

56. Shaco-Levy R, Jasperson KW, Martin K, et al. Morphologic characterization of hamartomatous gastrointestinal polyps in Cowden syndrome, Peutz-Jeghers syndrome, and juvenile polyposis syndrome. *Hum Pathol*. 2016;49:39-48.

57. Genta RM, Hurrell JM, Sonnenberg A. Duodenal adenomas coincide with colorectal neoplasia. *Dig Dis Sci*. 2014;59(9):2249-2254.

58. Genta RM, Feagins LA. Advanced precancerous lesions in the small bowel mucosa. *Best Pract Res Clin Gastroenterol*. 2013;27(2):225-233.

59. Wallace MH, Phillips RK. Upper gastrointestinal disease in patients with familial adenomatous polyposis. *Br J Surg*. 1998;85(6):742-750.

60. Allard FD, Goldsmith JD, Ayata G, et al. Intraobserver and interobserver variability in the assessment of dysplasia in ampullary mucosal biopsies. *Am J Surg Pathol.* 2018;42(8):1095-1100.

61. Stoven SA, Choung RS, Rubio-Tapia A, et al. Analysis of biopsies from duodenal bulbs of all endoscopy patients increases detection of abnormalities but has a minimal effect on diagnosis of celiac disease. *Clin Gastroenterol Hepatol.* 2016;14(11):1582-1588.

62. Choi WT, Brown I, Ushiku T, et al. Gastric pyloric gland adenoma: a multicentre clinicopathological study of 67 cases. *Histopathology.* 2018;72(6):1007-1014.

63. Bakotic BW, Robinson MJ, Sturm PD, Hruban RH, Offerhaus GJ, Albores-Saavedra J. Pyloric gland adenoma of the main pancreatic duct. *Am J Surg Pathol.* 1999;23(2):227-231.

64. Chen ZM, Scudiere JR, Abraham SC, Montgomery E. Pyloric gland adenoma: an entity distinct from gastric foveolar type adenoma. *Am J Surg Pathol.* 2009;33(2):186-193.

65. Hackeng WM, Montgomery EA, Giardiello FM, et al. Morphology and genetics of pyloric gland adenomas in familial adenomatous polyposis. *Histopathology.* 2017;70(4):549-557.

66. Hashimoto T, Ogawa R, Matsubara A, et al. Familial adenomatous polyposis-associated and sporadic pyloric gland adenomas of the upper gastrointestinal tract share common genetic features. *Histopathology.* 2015;67(5):689-698.

67. Wood LD, Salaria SN, Cruise MW, Giardiello FM, Montgomery EA. Upper GI tract lesions in familial adenomatous polyposis (FAP): enrichment of pyloric gland adenomas and other gastric and duodenal neoplasms. *Am J Surg Pathol.* 2014;38(3):389-393.

68. Siegel RL, Miller KD, Jemal A. Cancer statistics, 2018. *CA Cancer J Clin.* 2018;68(1):7-30.

69. Hatzaras I, Palesty JA, Abir F, et al. Small-bowel tumors: epidemiologic and clinical characteristics of 1260 cases from the Connecticut Tumor Registry. *Arch Surg.* 2007;142(3):229-235.

70. Chow WH, Linet MS, McLaughlin JK, Hsing AW, Chien HT, Blot WJ. Risk factors for small intestine cancer. *Cancer Causes Control.* 1993;4(2):163-169.

71. Weiss NS, Yang CP. Incidence of histologic types of cancer of the small intestine. *J Natl Cancer Inst.* 1987;78(4):653-656.

72. Aparicio T, Zaanan A, Svrcek M, et al. Small bowel adenocarcinoma: epidemiology, risk factors, diagnosis and treatment. *Dig Liver Dis.* 2014;46(2):97-104.

73. Haselkorn T, Whittemore AS, Lilienfeld DE. Incidence of small bowel cancer in the United States and worldwide: geographic, temporal, and racial differences. *Cancer Causes Control.* 2005;16(7):781-787.

74. Howe JR, Karnell LH, Menck HR, Scott-Conner C. The American College of Surgeons Commission on cancer and the American cancer Society. Adenocarcinoma of the small bowel: review of the National Cancer Data Base, 1985-1995. *Cancer.* 1999;86(12):2693-2706.

75. Amin MB, Greene FL, Edge SB, et al. The Eighth Edition AJCC Cancer Staging Manual: continuing to build a bridge from a population-based to a more "personalized" approach to cancer staging. *CA Cancer J Clin.* 2017;67(2):93-99.

76. Estrella JS, Wu TT, Rashid A, Abraham SC. Mucosal colonization by metastatic carcinoma in the gastrointestinal tract: a potential mimic of primary neoplasia. *Am J Surg Pathol.* 2011;35(4):563-572.

77. Chen ZM, Wang HL. Alteration of cytokeratin 7 and cytokeratin 20 expression profile is uniquely associated with tumorigenesis of primary adenocarcinoma of the small intestine. *Am J Surg Pathol.* 2004;28(10):1352-1359.

78. Werling RW, Yaziji H, Bacchi CE, Gown AM. CDX2, a highly sensitive and specific marker of adenocarcinomas of intestinal origin: an immunohistochemical survey of 476 primary and metastatic carcinomas. *Am J Surg Pathol.* 2003;27(3):303-310.

79. Park SY, Kim BH, Kim JH, Lee S, Kang GH. Panels of immunohistochemical markers help determine primary sites of metastatic adenocarcinoma. *Arch Pathol Lab Med.* 2007;131(10):1561-1567.

80. Bosman FT, Carneiro F, Hruban RH, et al, eds. *WHO Classification of Tumours of the Digestive System.* 4th ed. Lyon: WHO Press; 2010.

81. La Rosa S, Rigoli E, Uccella S, Chiaravalli AM, Capella C. CDX2 as a marker of intestinal EC-cells and related well-differentiated endocrine tumors. *Virchows Arch.* 2004;445(3):248-254.

82. Godwin JD II. Carcinoid tumors. An analysis of 2,837 cases. *Cancer.* 1975;36(2):560-569.

83. Srivastava A, Hornick JL. Immunohistochemical staining for CDX-2, PDX-1, NESP-55, and TTF-1 can help distinguish gastrointestinal carcinoid tumors from pancreatic endocrine and pulmonary carcinoid tumors. *Am J Surg Pathol.* 2009;33(4):626-632.

84. Norton JA, Alexander HR, Fraker DL, Venzon DJ, Gibril F, Jensen RT. Possible primary lymph node gastrinoma: occurrence, natural history, and predictive factors: a prospective study. *Ann Surg.* 2003;237(5):650-657; discussion 657-659.

85. Jensen RT, Cadiot G, Brandi ML, et al. ENETS Consensus Guidelines for the management of patients with digestive neuroendocrine neoplasms: functional pancreatic endocrine tumor syndromes. *Neuroendocrinology.* 2012;95(2):98-119.

86. Donow C, Pipeleers-Marichal M, Schroder S, Stamm B, Heitz PU, Kloppel G. Surgical pathology of gastrinoma. Site, size, multicentricity, association with multiple endocrine neoplasia type 1, and malignancy. *Cancer.* 1991;68(6):1329-1334.

87. Garbrecht N, Anlauf M, Schmitt A, et al. Somatostatin-producing neuroendocrine tumors of the duodenum and pancreas: incidence, types, biological behavior, association with inherited syndromes, and functional activity. *Endocr Relat Cancer.* 2008;15(1):229-241.

88. Stamm B, Hedinger CE, Saremaslani P. Duodenal and ampullary carcinoid tumors. A report of 12 cases with pathological characteristics, polypeptide content and relation to the MEN I syndrome and von Recklinghausen's disease (neurofibromatosis). *Virchows Arch a Pathol Anat Histopathol.* 1986;408(5):475-489.

89. Burke AP, Sobin LH, Federspiel BH, Shekitka KM, Helwig EB. Carcinoid tumors of the duodenum. A clinicopathologic study of 99 cases. *Arch Pathol Lab Med.* 1990;114(7):700-704.

90. Norton JA. Neuroendocrine tumors of the pancreas and duodenum. *Curr Probl Surg.* 1994;31(2):77-156.

91. Burke AP, Sobin LH, Shekitka KM, Federspiel BH, Helwig EB. Somatostatin-producing duodenal carcinoids in patients with von Recklinghausen's neurofibromatosis. A predilection for black patients. *Cancer.* 1990;65(7):1591-1595.

92. Klein A, Clemens J, Cameron J. Periampullary neoplasms in von Recklinghausen's disease. *Surgery.* 1989;106(5):815-819.

93. Karasawa Y, Sakaguchi M, Minami S, et al. Duodenal somatostatinoma and erythrocytosis in a patient with von Hippel-Lindau disease type 2A. *Intern Med.* 2001;40(1):38-43.

94. McCall CM, Shi C, Cornish TC, et al. Grading of well-differentiated pancreatic neuroendocrine tumors is improved by the inclusion of both Ki67 proliferative index and mitotic rate. *Am J Surg Pathol.* 2013;37(11):1671-1677.

95. Young HT, Carr NJ, Green B, Tilley C, Bhargava V, Pearce N. Accuracy of visual assessments of proliferation indices in gastroenteropancreatic neuroendocrine tumours. *J Clin Pathol.* 2013;66(8):700-704.

96. Tang LH, Gonen M, Hedvat C, Modlin IM, Klimstra DS. Objective quantification of the Ki67 proliferative index in neuroendocrine tumors of the gastroenteropancreatic system: a comparison of digital image analysis with manual methods. *Am J Surg Pathol.* 2012;36(12):1761-1770.

97. Cottenden J, Filter ER, Cottreau J, et al. Validation of a cytotechnologist manual counting service for the Ki67 index in neuroendocrine tumors of the pancreas and gastrointestinal tract. *Arch Pathol Lab Med.* 2018;142(3):402-407.

98. Tang LH, Untch BR, Reidy DL, et al. Well-differentiated neuroendocrine tumors with a morphologically apparent high-grade component: a pathway distinct from poorly differentiated neuroendocrine carcinomas. *Clin Cancer Res.* 2016;22(1):1011-1017.

99. Yachida S, Vakiani E, White CM, et al. Small cell and large cell neuroendocrine carcinomas of the pancreas are genetically similar and distinct from well-differentiated pancreatic neuroendocrine tumors. *Am J Surg Pathol.* 2012;36(2):173-184.

100. Basturk O, Yang Z, Tang LH, et al. The high-grade (WHO G3) pancreatic neuroendocrine tumor category is morphologically and biologically heterogenous and includes both well differentiated and poorly differentiated neoplasms. *Am J Surg Pathol.* 2015;39(5):683-690.

101. Raj N, Valentino E, Capanu M, et al. Treatment response and outcomes of grade 3 pancreatic neuroendocrine neoplasms based on morphology: well differentiated versus poorly differentiated. *Pancreas.* 2017;46(3):296-301.

102. Sorbye H, Welin S, Langer SW, et al. Predictive and prognostic factors for treatment and survival in 305 patients with advanced gastrointestinal neuroendocrine carcinoma (WHO G3): the NORDIC NEC study. *Ann Oncol.* 2013;24(1):152-160.

103. Lloyd RV, Osamura RY, Kloppel G, Rosai J. WHO Classification of Tumours of Endocrine Organs Vol 10. 4th ed. Lyon: IARC; 2017.

104. Yantiss RK, Clement PB, Young RH. Endometriosis of the intestinal tract: a study of 44 cases of a disease that may cause diverse challenges in clinical and pathologic evaluation. *Am J Surg Pathol*. 2001;25(4):445-454.

105. Jiang W, Roma AA, Lai K, Carver P, Xiao SY, Liu X. Endometriosis involving the mucosa of the intestinal tract: a clinicopathologic study of 15 cases. *Mod Pathol*. 2013;26(9):1270-1278.

106. Tong YL, Chen Y, Zhu SY. Ileocecal endometriosis and a diagnosis dilemma: a case report and literature review. *World J Gastroenterol*. 2013;19(23):3707-3710.

107. Kumar B, Bhatnagar A, Upadhyaya VD, Gangopadhyay AN. Small intestinal lymphangioma presenting as an acute abdomen with relevant review of literature. *J Clin Diagn Res*. 2017;11(6):PD01-PD02.

108. Schmatz AI, Streubel B, Kretschmer-Chott E, et al. Primary follicular lymphoma of the duodenum is a distinct mucosal/submucosal variant of follicular lymphoma: a retrospective study of 63 cases. *J Clin Oncol*. 2011;29(11):1445-1451.

109. Yoshino T, Miyake K, Ichimura K, et al. Increased incidence of follicular lymphoma in the duodenum. *Am J Surg Pathol*. 2000;24(5):688-693.

110. Shia J, Teruya-Feldstein J, Pan D, et al. Primary follicular lymphoma of the gastrointestinal tract: a clinical and pathologic study of 26 cases. *Am J Surg Pathol*. 2002;26(2):216-224.

111. Takata K, Okada H, Ohmiya N, et al. Primary gastrointestinal follicular lymphoma involving the duodenal second portion is a distinct entity: a multicenter, retrospective analysis in Japan. *Cancer Sci*. 2011;102(8):1532-1536.

112. Swerdlow SH, Campo E, Pileri SA, et al. The 2016 revision of the World Health Organization classification of lymphoid neoplasms. *Blood*. 2016;127(20):2375-2390.

113. Cherner JA, Jensen RT, Dubois A, O'Dorisio TM, Gardner JD, Metcalfe DD. Gastrointestinal dysfunction in systemic mastocytosis. A prospective study. *Gastroenterology*. 1988;95(3):657-667.

114. Doyle LA, Sepehr GJ, Hamilton MJ, Akin C, Castells MC, Hornick JL. A clinicopathologic study of 24 cases of systemic mastocytosis involving the gastrointestinal tract and assessment of mucosal mast cell density in irritable bowel syndrome and asymptomatic patients. *Am J Surg Pathol*. 2014;38(6):832-843.

115. Hahn HP, Hornick JL. Immunoreactivity for CD25 in gastrointestinal mucosal mast cells is specific for systemic mastocytosis. *Am J Surg Pathol*. 2007;31(11):1669-1676.

116. Hamilton MJ, Hornick JL, Akin C, Castells MC, Greenberger NJ. Mast cell activation syndrome: a newly recognized disorder with systemic clinical manifestations. *J Allergy Clin Immunol*. 2011;128(1):147.e142-152.e142.

CHAPTER OUTLINE

THE UNREMARKABLE COLON

The large intestine consists of the right colon (cecum, ascending, transverse), left colon (descending, sigmoid), and rectum. Specimens can be submitted with these regional site specifications or as a centimeter distance from the anus. Familiarity with both designations is important for correct polyp classification, approaching chronic colitis, and staging (Fig. 4.1). For example, serrated polyps are most often sessile serrated adenomas/polyps (SSA/Ps) in the cecum through and including the transverse colon (or between 85 and 40 cm). In contrast, serrated polyps are most often hyperplastic polyps from the distal to the transverse colon (or between 40 and 0 cm). See also "Serrated Polyps" section.

The colonic wall includes the mucosa, submucosa, muscularis propria, and serosa (Fig. 4.2). The mucosa is composed of a single cell layer of columnar cells lining colonic crypts, the investing lamina propria, and a delicate slip of smooth muscle—the muscularis mucosae. The surface epithelium consists of varying proportions of absorptive columnar cells and mucus-secreting goblet cells, depending on the colonic location (Figs. 4.3–4.5). The right colon has more absorptive cells to facilitate water absorption (Fig. 4.3), and the left colon has more goblet cells to facilitate lubrication of the luminal contents (Fig. 4.4). Other regional differences include increased inflammatory cells in the lamina propria of the right colon, compared with the left. Endocrine and Paneth cells can be easy to confuse at first but are important to distinguish because endocrine cells are normal crypt constituents throughout the colon, and Paneth cells are only normal in the crypt bases through and including the transverse colon (Fig. 4.6). The normal colonic architecture is analogous to test tubes in a test tube rack whether viewed in profile (Figs. 4.7 and 4.8) or en face (Figs. 4.9 and 4.10). This orderly arrangement is due to the similar size and distribution of the crypts, which abut neatly on the muscularis mucosae.

The submucosa sits between the mucosa and the muscularis propria. Unlike those within the mucosa, the larger submucosal lymphovascular channels can facilitate lymphovascular spread of tumor cells.[1] Other submucosal cells include adipocytes,

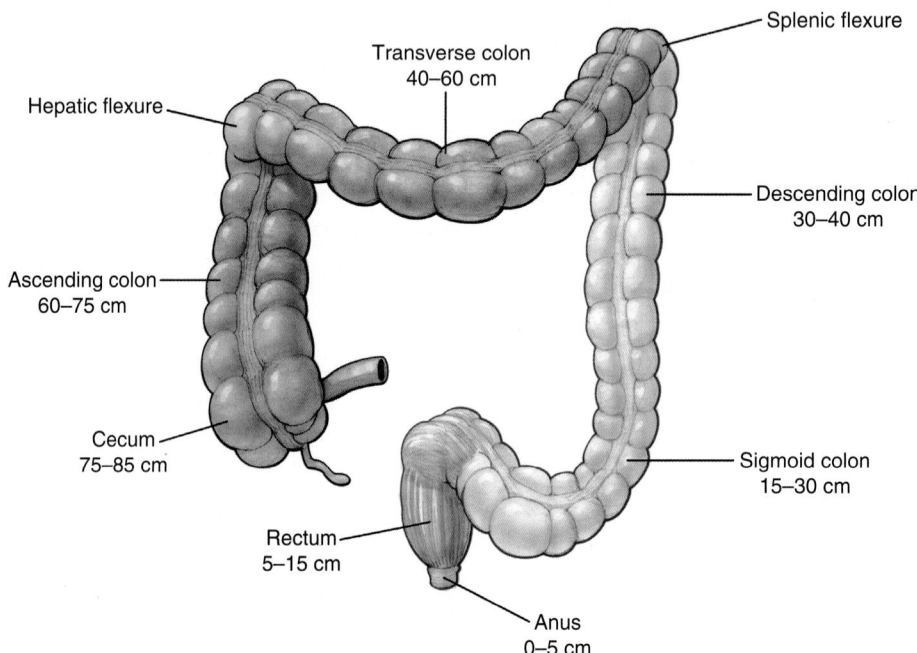

Figure 4-1. Major colonic landmarks. Colonic landmarks are designated as distance from the anus (0 cm). For most patients, the anus is approximately at 0–5 cm, the rectum is at 5–15 cm, the sigmoid is at 15–30 cm, the descending colon is at 30–40 cm, the transverse colon is at 40–60 cm, the ascending colon is at 60–75 cm, and the cecum is at 75–85 cm.

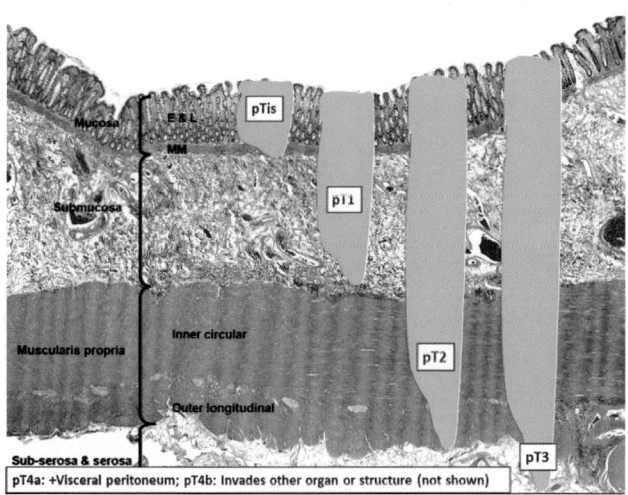

pT4a: +Visceral peritoneum; pT4b: Invades other organ or structure (not shown)

Figure 4-2. Normal colon. This resection specimen illustrates the four main layers of the colon: mucosa, submucosa, muscularis propria, and serosa. The mucosa consists of the epithelium (E), lamina propria (L), and muscularis mucosae (MM). The submucosa sits between the muscularis mucosae and the muscularis propria and consists of loose fibroconnective tissue and lymphovascular channels. The muscularis propria consists of inner circular and outer longitudinally oriented muscle fibers. This is covered by subserosal fibroadipose tissue and the outermost serosa. Invasion limited to the mucosa but not beyond the muscularis mucosae is pTis; invasion into but not beyond the submucosa is pT1; invasion into but not beyond the muscularis propria is pT2; invasion beyond the muscularis propria is pT3; involvement of the visceral peritoneum is pT4a; invasion into another organ or structure is pT4b (not shown).

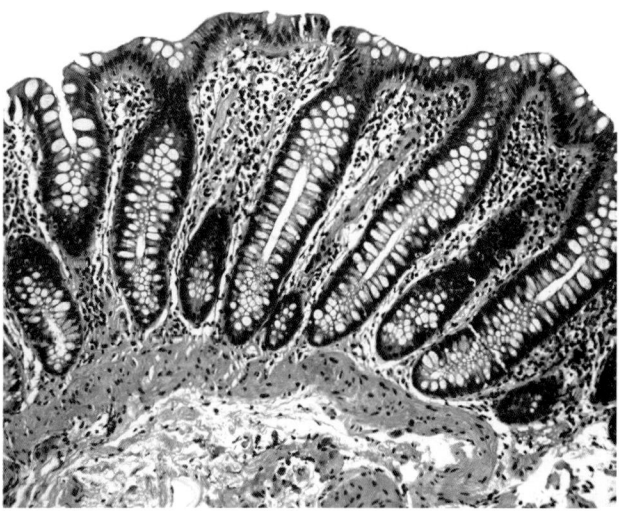

Figure 4-3. Normal right colon. Compared with the left colon (Fig. 4.4), the normal right colon has more mixed chronic inflammatory cells in the lamina propria, more absorptive cells, and fewer goblet cells and Paneth cells (not shown) are normal only in the proximal colon (right, cecum, ascending, and through and including the transverse colon). The crypts are superimposable because of their similar size and spacing and sit directly on the muscularis mucosae, as seen here.

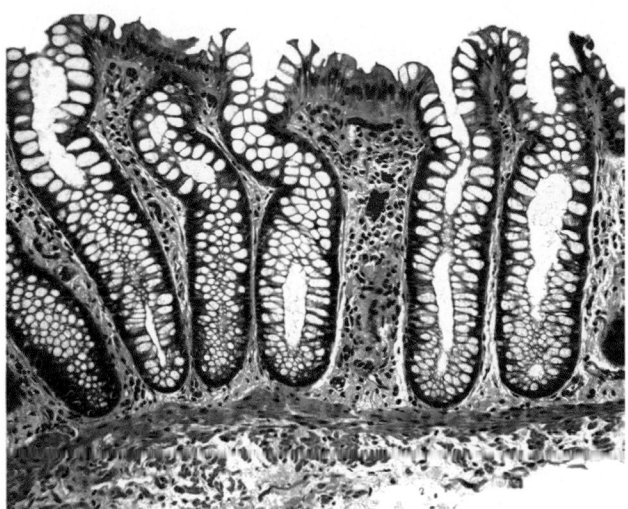

Figure 4-4. Normal left colon. Compared with the right colon (Fig. 4.3), the normal left colon contains fewer lamina propria inflammatory cells, fewer absorptive cells, and more goblet cells and Paneth cells are absent in the distal colon (left, descending, rectosigmoid). The crypts are superimposable because of their similar size and spacing and sit directly on the muscularis mucosae, as seen here.

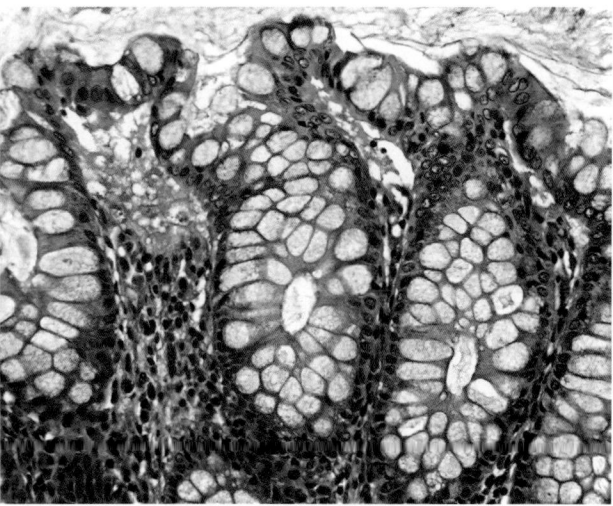

Figure 4-5. Normal colon, surface epithelium. A high-power view of normal colon shows normochromatic chromatin and small basally oriented nuclei. The bland nuclei comprise approximately less than 10% of the overall cell volume. Apoptotic bodies and mitotic figures are not seen.

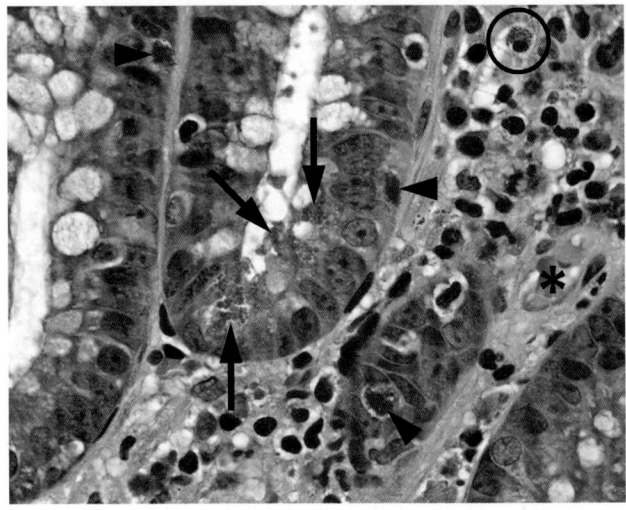

Figure 4-6. Normal colon, Paneth cell versus endocrine cell. The Paneth cell (*arrows*) contains larger, coarse, *pink* granules. These contents relate to innate immunity and are released toward the crypt lumen to combat luminal organisms. In contrast, the endocrine cell (*arrowheads*) contains small, fine, reddish granules containing hormones, which are released toward the crypt basement membrane, nearest the surrounding capillaries (*asterisk*). The granules of the eosinophil (*circle*) are *bright orange* and intermediate in size between those of the Paneth and endocrine cell. Paneth cells in the distal colon (left, descending, and rectosigmoid) are abnormal and a feature of chronic injury.

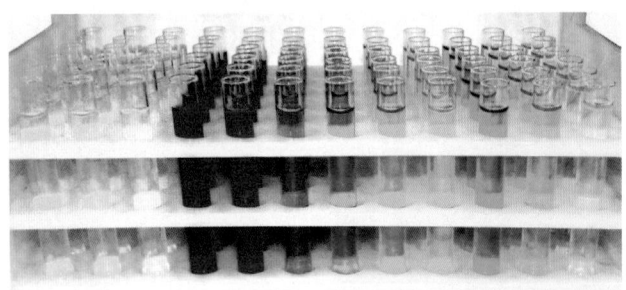

Figure 4-7. Test tubes in a rack, profile view. Normal colonic architecture is analogous to a profile view of test tubes in a test tube rack. Each test tube is U-shaped and superimposable upon its neighbor based on uniform size and distribution.

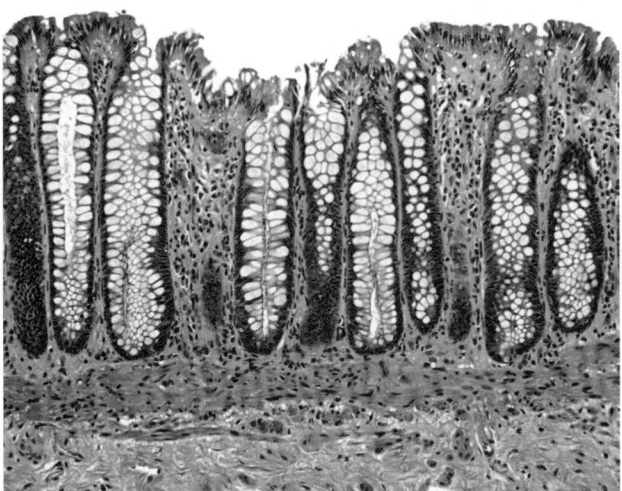

Figure 4-8. Normal colon, profile view. Analogous to a profile view of test tubes in a rack (Fig. 4.7), a well-oriented colon section in profile illustrates the same orderly architecture. The crypts are U-shaped, evenly spaced, and arranged in parallel. The crypt bases extend down to sit neatly on the muscularis mucosae.

ganglion cells, and nerve axons of the superficial Meissner plexus and the deeper Henle plexus. The muscularis propria is the large smooth muscle layer investing the outer aspects of the colon. The myenteric plexus of Auerbach is sandwiched between its inner circular and outer longitudinal muscular layers. Externally, the subserosal connective tissue and the mesothelial-derived serosa encase the bowel. This connective tissue is termed "adventitia" at sites not entirely covered by serosa: the posterior surface of the

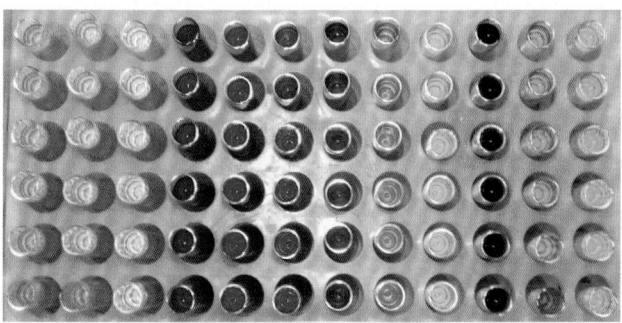

Figure 4-9. Test tubes in a rack, en face view. When viewed from above, the round test tubes are superimposable upon their neighbors based on uniform size and distribution.

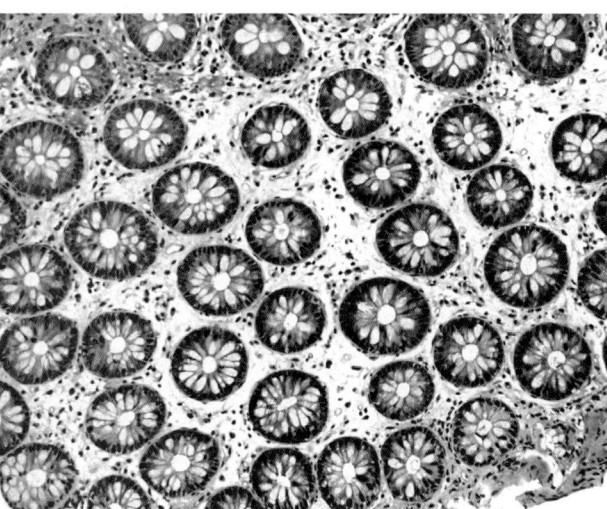

Figure 4-10. Normal colon, en face view. Analogous to an en face view of test tubes in a rack (Fig. 4.9), a well-oriented colon section en face illustrates the same orderly architecture. The crypts are round, evenly spaced, and arranged in orderly rows.

ascending and descending colon and portions of the rectum (posterior aspect of the upper third, posterior and lateral aspects of the middle third, and the lower third), features important for assessing radial margins in resection specimens of colonic neoplasms. Grossly visible through the serosa are the external longitudinal layers of the muscularis propria, which appear as three distinct bands, or taenia coli, on the right colon and become confluent on the left.

An understanding of the layers of the colonic wall is important to understand colorectal cancer staging (Fig. 4.2).

- pTis = invasion limited to the mucosa (invasion within the mucosa but not beyond the muscularis mucosae)
- pT1 = invasion into but not beyond the submucosa
- pT2 = invasion into but not beyond the muscularis propria
- pT3 = invasion beyond the muscularis propria
- pT4a = involvement of the visceral peritoneum
- pT4b = invasion into another organ or structure (not shown)

For a more detailed discussion of the unremarkable colon, see also "Colon" chapter in *Atlas of Gastrointestinal Pathology: A Pattern Based Approach to Non-Neoplastic Biopsies.*

POLYPS

This book starts with this particular topic because polyps are fun and the mainstay of work for pathologists who deal with gastrointestinal (GI) pathology with any regularity. Accurate diagnosis is important to help guide the next steps in clinical management and to prevent malignant progression, in the case of neoplastic polyps. Polyps are satisfyingly simple when the tissue is well oriented and the morphology is classic. However, not all cases are easy, and the evolving clinical management nuances offer their own challenges. To help approach these very common diagnoses, this section features a quick and dirty approach to all the usual suspects along with practical clinical guidelines, handy diagnostic algorithms, and sample notes. Bon appetit!.

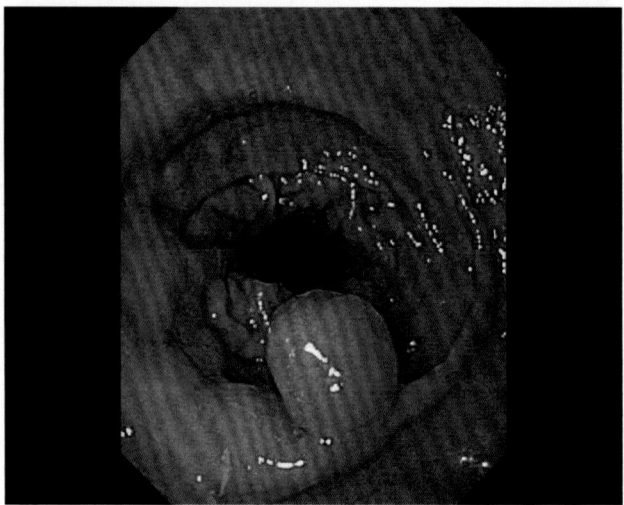

Figure 4-11. Endoscopic view of a colon polyp. The routinely encountered colon polyp requires histologic evaluation for diagnosis.

CONVENTIONAL ADENOMATOUS POLYPS

Classification

Conventional adenomatous polyps comprise up to 65% of all colorectal polyps.[2] They consist of tubular adenomas (TAs), tubulovillous adenomas (TVAs), and villous adenomas (VAs). Unfortunately, there are no universally accepted criteria for classification of the adenomas, and the assessment of high-grade dysplasia (HGD), intramucosal carcinoma (IMC), and invasive adenocarcinoma is controversial. The following is our practical approach, but be aware that your institutional practices may differ, and it is worthwhile to discuss thresholds with colleagues for consistent reporting.

The subjective amount of villous component determines the subclassification of the conventional adenoma, such as TA, TVA, or VA. A villus can be defined as a structure at least twice as long as it is wide. TAs are up to 25% villous (and up to 75% tubules); TVAs are between 25% and 75% villous (and between 75% and 25% tubules), and VAs are greater than 75% villous (and up to 25% tubules; [Fig. 4.12]).[3] Designation as a TVA or a VA has important clinical implications because these polyps are considered high-risk adenomas and have an abbreviated surveillance interval of 3 years (Table 4.1).[4] Histologically, conventional adenomas are synonymous with low-grade dysplasia (LGD); the columnar cells have pseudostratified nuclei, basophilia due to increased nuclear to cytoplasmic ratios, hyperchromasia, and increased mitotic and apoptotic bodies (compare normal colon [Fig. 4.5] with conventional adenomas [Figs. 4.13–4.17]). These changes are typically accompanied by an abrupt transition between the normal and dysplastic epithelium (Fig. 4.13), a feature not seen with reactive changes (Figs. 4.18–4.24). See also Pearls and Pitfalls: Distinguishing Reactive Changes from Dysplasia. Importantly, the atypia must involve the surface to qualify for a diagnosis of a conventional adenoma (synonymous with dysplasia). Atypia restricted to the crypt bases could be a reactive change, the normal proliferative compartment of a hyperplastic polyp, or a tangential section of a conventional adenoma in which the surface cannot be visualized. In the latter case, deeper sections are helpful to demonstrate that the atypical changes extend to the surface.

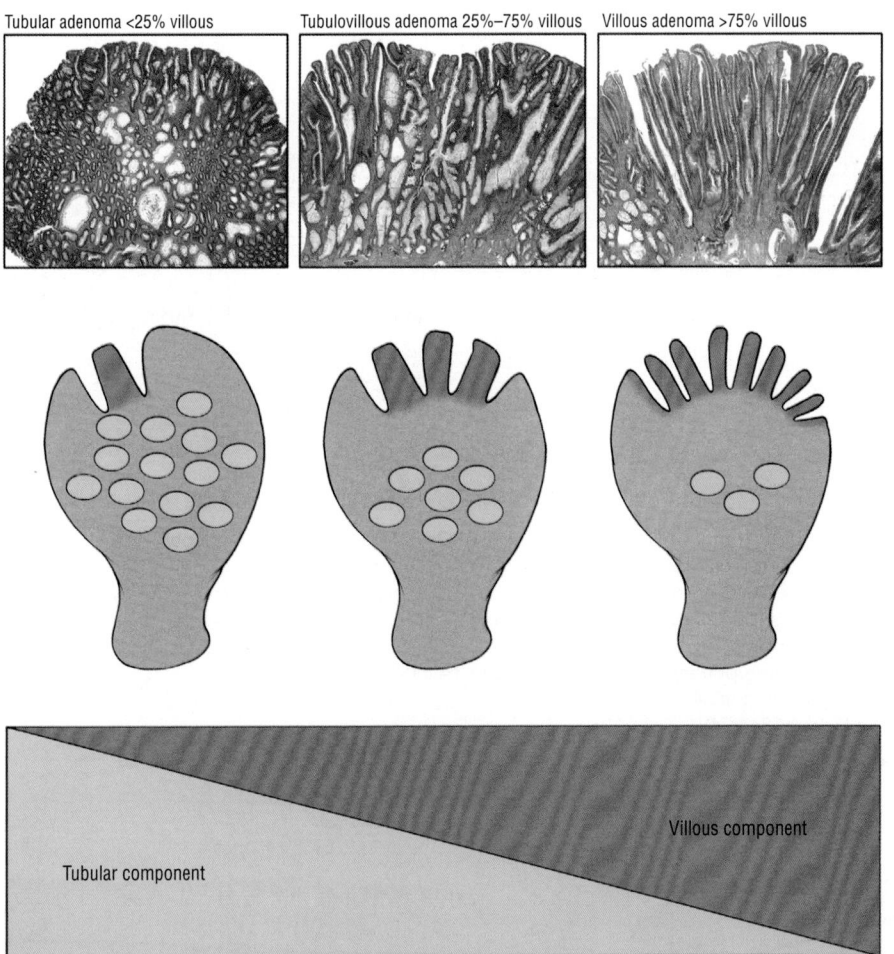

Figure 4-12. Conventional adenomas, composite illustration. Conventional adenomatous polyps are synonymous with LGD and subclassified as TA, TVA, or VA based on the subjective amount of villous component present: TA are less than 25% villous, TVA are between 25%–75% villous, and VA are greater than 75% villous, where a villus is defined as a structure with a height at least twice its width. In the cartoon version of the photomicrographs, the villous component is illustrated with triangles and the tubular component is illustrated with circles.

TABLE 4.1: 2012 Recommendations for Surveillance and Screening Intervals in Individuals With Baseline Average Risk[4]

		Baseline Colonoscopy	Surveillance Interval (Years)
		No polyps	10
		Small (<10 mm) hyper-plastic polyps in rectum or sigmoid	10
Low-risk adenoma		1–2 small (<10 mm) TA	5–10
High-risk adenoma		3–10 TA	3
High-risk adenoma		>10 Adenomas	<3
High-risk adenoma	Advanced neoplasia	At least one TA ≥10 mm	3
High risk adenoma	Advanced neoplasia	At least one TVA or VA	3
High risk adenoma	Advanced neoplasia	Adenoma with high grade dysplasia	3

TA, tubular adenoma; TVA, tubulovillous adenoma; VA, villous adenoma.

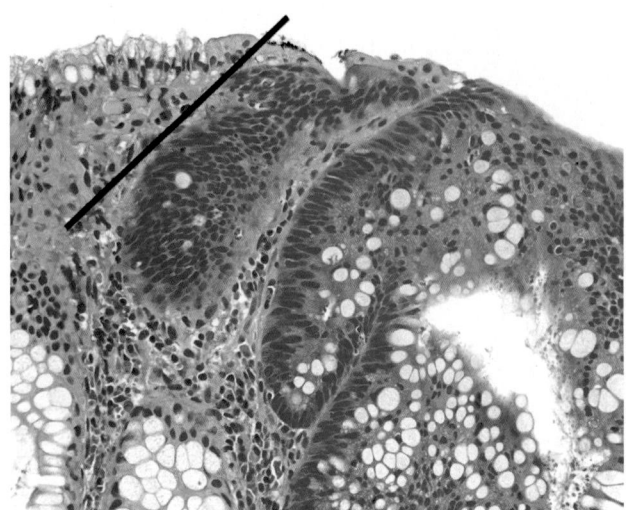

Figure 4-13. Conventional tubular adenoma (TA) (synonymous with LGD). Compared with a high-power view of normal colonic epithelium (Fig. 4.5), high power of conventional adenomas shows columnar cells with pseudostratified nuclei, basophilia due to increased nuclear to cytoplasmic ratios, and hyperchromasia. A helpful feature in diagnosing dysplasia is noting an abrupt transition between the normal and the adenomatous epithelium (*line*), a feature not seen with reactive epithelium (see Figs. 4.18–4.24).

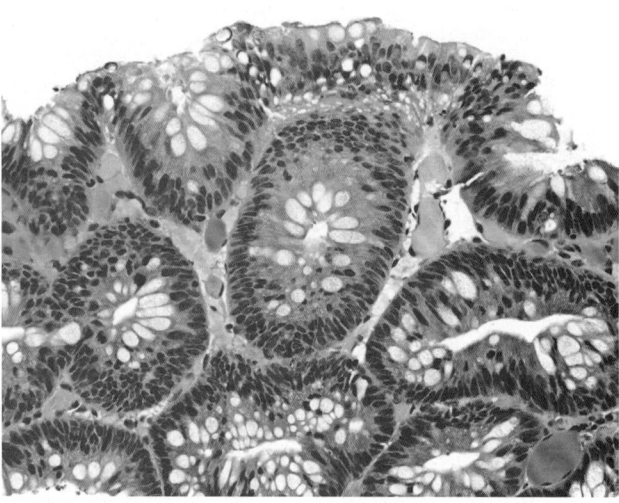

Figure 4-14. Conventional TA (synonymous with LGD). Typical features of a conventional adenoma include a "dark look" due to increased nuclear to cytoplasmic ratios and hyperchromasia. These changes must be present at the surface to satisfy the criteria for conventional adenoma, as seen here. Retained nuclear polarity supports a diagnosis of TA (LGD).

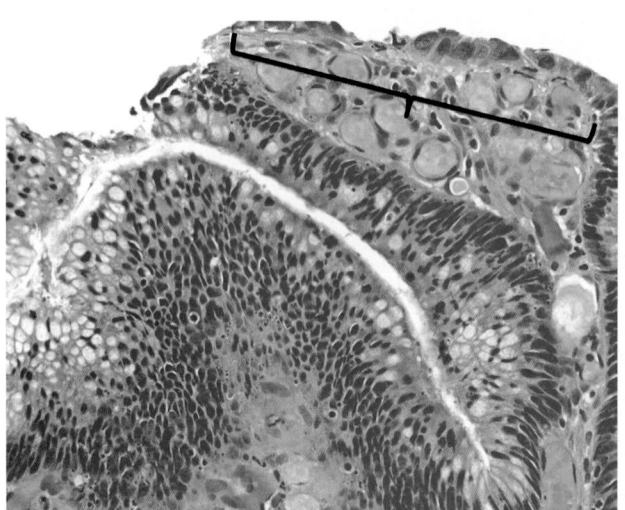

Figure 4-15. Conventional TA (synonymous with LGD). This photomicrograph illustrates an important caveat of dysplasia grading in the conventional adenomas: HGD requires both cytologic (loss of nuclear polarity) and architectural complexity (cribriforming). The *bracketed* focus shows marked atypia but is within the spectrum of LGD for a conventional adenoma because it lacks architectural complexity (*bracket*). These atypical changes are commonly encountered on the surface of large polyps, theoretically because these large polyps are mechanically abused as they flop among the luminal contents.

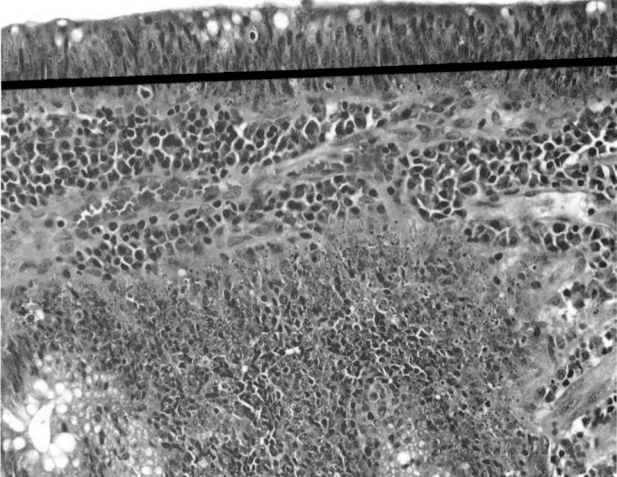

Figure 4-16. Conventional TA (synonymous with LGD). As seen in this case, atypia must be present at the surface for a diagnosis of conventional adenoma. These columnar cells are quite dark because of the increased nuclear to cytoplasmic ratios and hyperchromasia. The elongated nuclei are pseudostratified with preserved nuclear polarity: a *line* drawn through the basal aspect of the dysplastic cells shows that essentially 100% of the nuclei are on the *black line*.

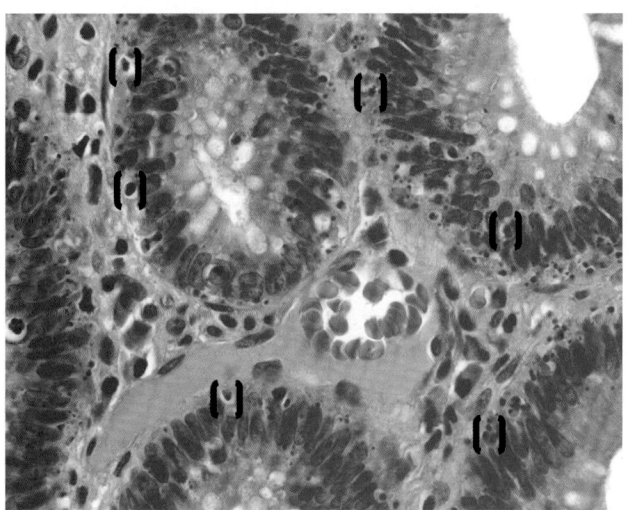

Figure 4-17. Conventional TA (synonymous with LGD). A common feature of conventional adenomas is increased apoptotic bodies (occasional apoptotic bodies are highlighted with *brackets*). Apoptotic bodies are variably sized bits of nuclear debris. This handy trick can be helpful in challenging cases, such as small or cauterized TAs.

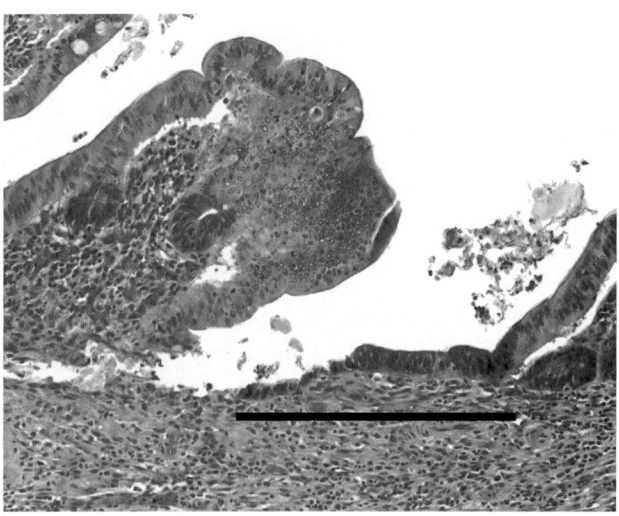

Figure 4-18. Reactive colonic epithelium, negative for dysplasia. The wildest reactive changes are often seen overlying a healing erosion or ulcer that is in the process of re-epithelization, as in this case (*line*). Although these changes are eye-catching, they are reactive because of the underlying healing erosion/ulcer, in addition to the blurred transition between the normal and the reactive epithelium (compare with Fig. 4.13).

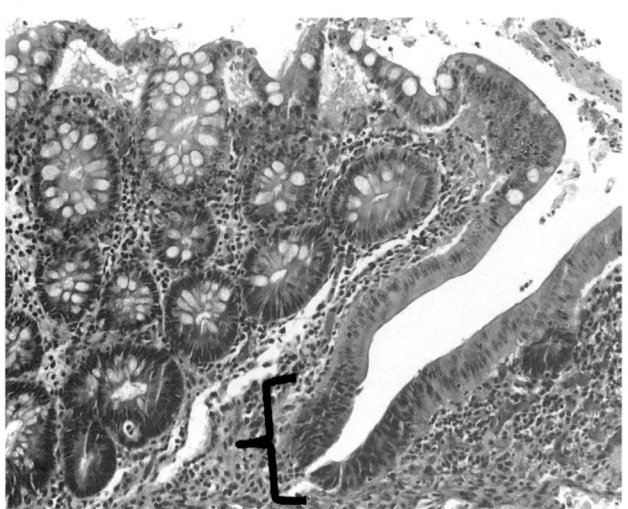

Figure 4-19. Reactive colonic epithelium, negative for dysplasia. The *bracket* highlights epithelium with pseudostratification and hyperchromasia. These changes are restricted to the crypt base, and mature epithelium is seen at the surface, supporting the diagnosis of reactive changes. Further support of reactive changes includes the blurred or gradual transition between the normal and the reactive epithelium and absence of prominent apoptotic bodies (compare with Figs. 4.13 and 4.17).

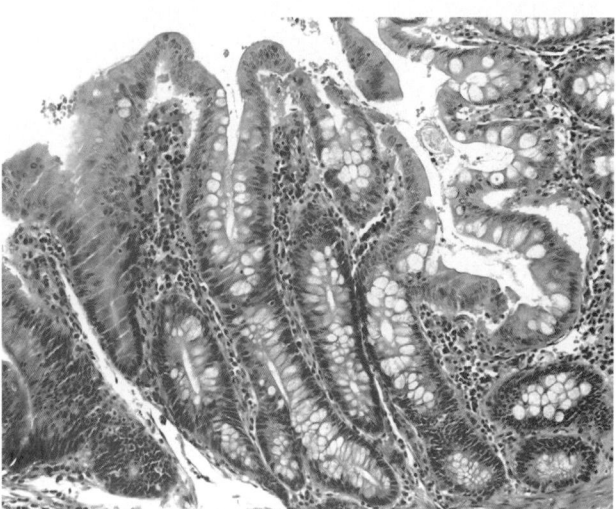

Figure 4-20. Reactive colonic epithelium, negative for dysplasia. In contrast to the dark look of a conventional adenoma (Figs. 4.12–4.17), reactive changes have a *pinkish* low-power appearance because the nuclei are normochromatic and there is abundant cytoplasm.

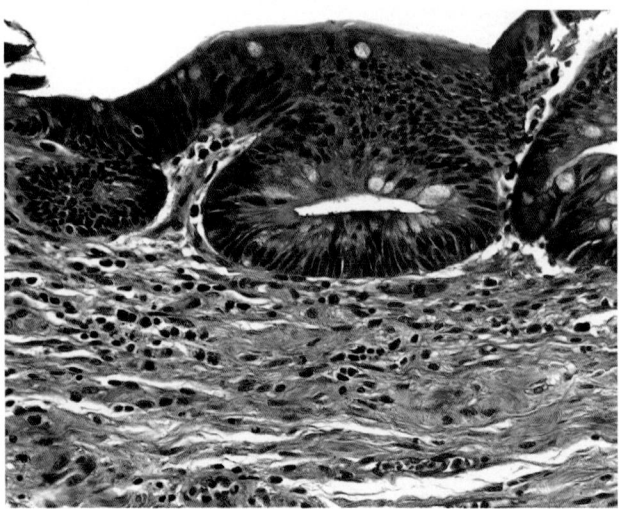

Figure 4-21. Reactive colonic epithelium, negative for dysplasia. On high power, these atypical changes look very similar to those in a conventional adenoma (synonymous with LGD) because the nuclei are dark, pseudostratified, and the changes extend to the surface. However, no apoptotic bodies are seen.

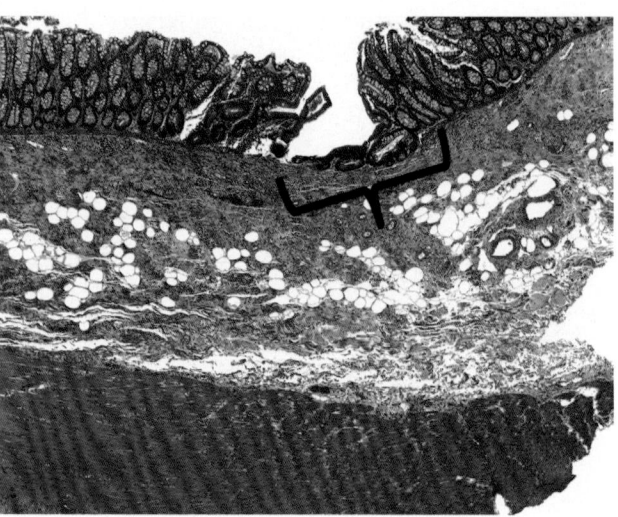

Figure 4-22. Reactive colonic epithelium, negative for dysplasia. Lower power of the previous figure shows that the atypical changes are in an area of healing erosion or ulceration (*bracket*). Other features of reactive epithelium include a blurred transition between the normal and the reactive epithelium.

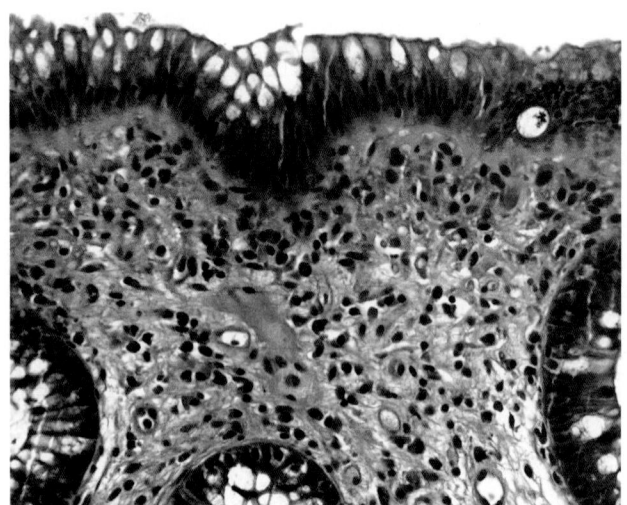

Figure 4-23. Reactive colonic epithelium, negative for dysplasia. This is an example of a thick section. The thick sectioning imparts a dark and atypical nuclear appearance. Features favoring reactive include the blurred transition zone between the normal and reactive epithelium and the absence of prominent apoptotic bodies. Deeper (thinner) sections were reassuring for reactive.

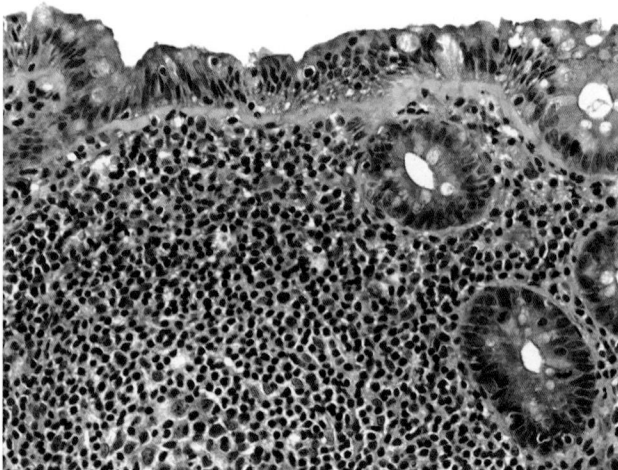

Figure 4-24. Reactive colonic epithelium overlying a lymphoid aggregate, negative for dysplasia. The epithelium overlying lymphoid aggregates often appears mildly atypical and can raise concerns for a conventional adenoma. Deeper sections often resolve the issue, and, in our experience, the majority are classified as reactive. This case features the usual reassuring features of reactive change: a blurred transition between the normal and the reactive epithelium and absence of prominent apoptotic bodies.

PEARLS & PITFALLS: Distinguishing Reactive Changes From Dysplasia

Distinguishing reactive changes from dysplasia is a common reason for consultation cases because these cases are difficult, and the differing diagnoses lead to differing management: dysplasia often requires further management, and reactive diagnoses often do not. Common settings that can account for reactive changes include healing erosions or ulcerations, acute inflammation, ischemia, recent procedure, stent placement, medication-associated injury, and viral infections. Thick sections and the epithelium overlying lymphoid aggregates can also appear atypical. In these cases, deeper (thinner) sections are helpful in resolving the issues. Keep in mind that improved endoscopic techniques allow clinicians to identify and remove ever smaller polyps that might not yet have their diagnostic features in full bloom. To address these issues, know the following dirty little secrets of recognizing dysplasia in the GI tract. These tips can be applied to the three illustrated tiny, early TAs that had been initially overlooked and reported as negative for dysplasia in Figs. 4.25–4.30.

1. Dysplasia should grab you at low power (4×)! At low power, cells with distinct hyperchromasia are seen that stand out from their neighbors (Figs. 4.25, 4.27, and 4.29). Avoid looking for dysplasia at 40× because everything looks atypical on high power.

2. Prominent apoptotic bodies are clues to dysplasia (Figs. 4.26, 4.28, and 4.30). If on the fence between reactive and dysplasia, the presence of prominent apoptotic bodies is a helpful feature that favors dysplasia.

3. Dysplasia is characterized by abrupt transitions between the normal and dysplastic zones. These zones are so crisply distinct that a line can be drawn between them (Figs. 4.26 and 4.28). In contrast, reactive changes are characterized by an indistinct blur of transition from normal to reactive that does not permit a line to be drawn between these zones (Figs. 4.18–4.24).

4. Dysplasia requires the typical changes to extend to the surface, with the exception of the esophagus where basal atypia justifies a diagnosis of so-called basal crypt dysplasia, a term that is used even though the structures are best regarded as pits! See also "Esophagus" chapter 1.

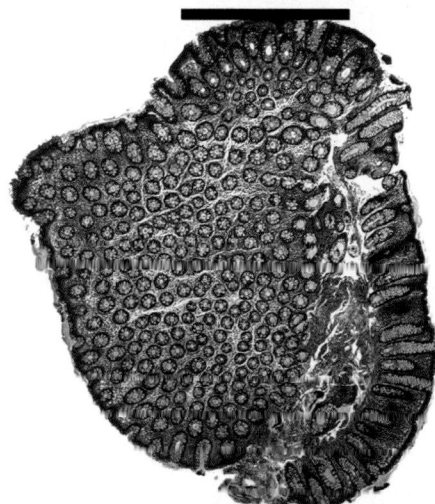

Figure 4-25. Early TA at 4×. Distinguishing reactive changes from dysplasia is one of the most difficult areas in GI pathology. Handy tip #1: Dysplasia should grab you at low power (1×) (line).

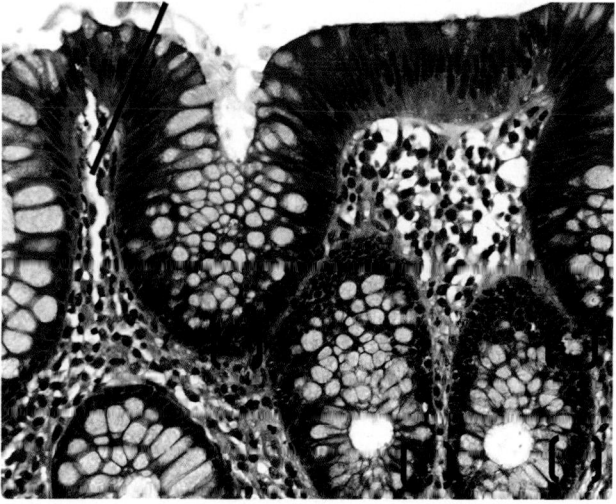

Figure 4-26. Early TA at 40×. Higher power of the previous figure. Handy tip #2 & 3: dysplasia has prominent apoptotic bodies (brackets) and abrupt transitions between the normal and dysplastic zones (line). Remember diagnosing dysplasia in the colon requires that the atypical changes extend to the surface.

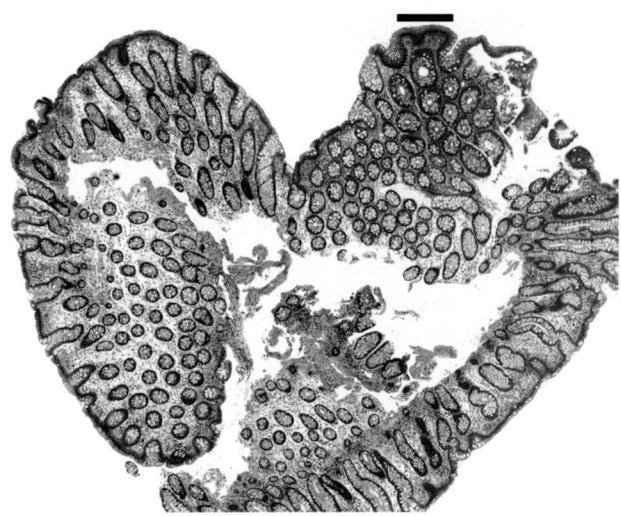

Figure 4-27. Early TA at 4×. Even focal bits of dysplasia should grab you at low power (*line*).

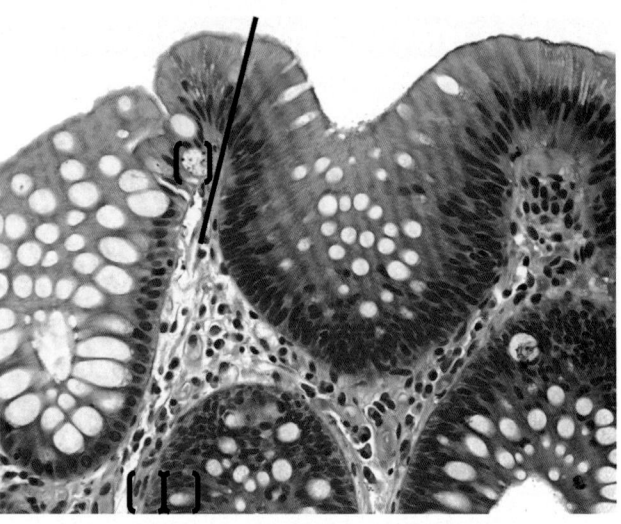

Figure 4-28. Early TA at 40×. Higher power of the previous figure. A reliable clue to dysplasia is abrupt transitions between the normal and dysplastic zones (*line*) and prominent apoptotic bodies (*brackets*).

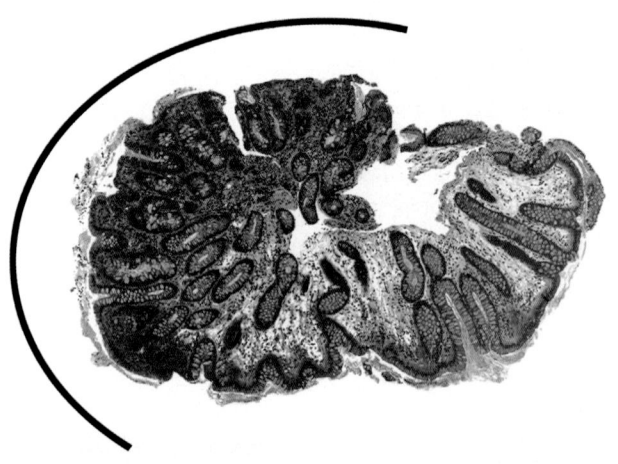

Figure 4-29. Early TA at 4×. Dysplasia (*arc*) is a low-power diagnosis.

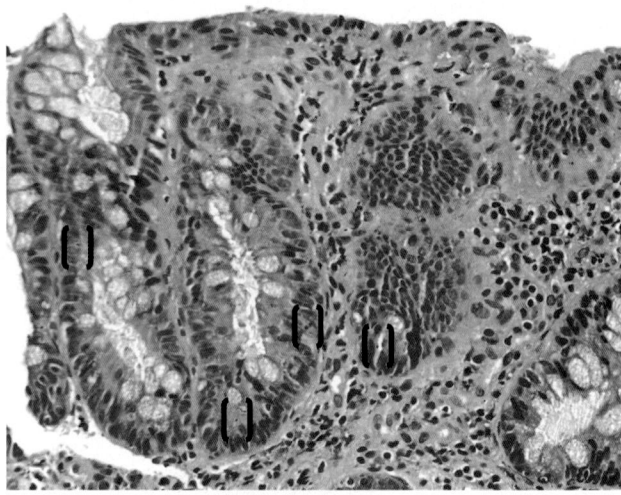

Figure 4-30. Early TA at 40×. In tough cases, a quick tip to 40× can be reassuring to identify prominent apoptotic bodies (*brackets*).

FAQ: The pathology report says TA but there is no mention of dysplasia. Is this polyp dysplastic?

Answer: This is a common question from junior clinicians and trainees. Because conventional adenomas are synonymous with LGD, the concise diagnosis is simply tubular adenoma (LGD is implied). Although not exactly incorrect, a diagnosis of tubular adenoma with low-grade dysplasia is redundant; it is similar to saying low-grade dysplasia with low-grade dysplasia and better simplified to tubular adenoma. However, if a higher-grade lesion is seen, the highest grade should be specified first. For example, high-grade dysplasia arising in a TA or invasive adenocarcinoma arising in a TA is the preferred nomenclature.

Dysplasia Grading

Once convinced of definitive dysplasia, the next step is to properly classify the dysplasia as LGD (synonymous with the diagnosis of "conventional adenoma"), HGD, IMC, or invasive adenocarcinoma. There are many schools of thought on how to classify, but let us keep it simple. LGD shows retained nuclear polarity. Retained nuclear polarity can be illustrated by drawing a line through the basal aspect of the cells and finding that essentially 100% of the nuclei are on the line (Fig. 4.16). HGD in conventional adenomas requires both cytologic atypia and architectural complexity (Figs. 4.31–4.36).[3] Cytologic atypia is best exemplified by a loss of nuclear polarity (Figs. 4.32, 4.34, and 4.36). Loss of nuclear polarity can be illustrated by drawing a line through the basal aspect of the cells and finding that many of the cells are not on the line (Fig. 4.32). Architectural complexity is best exemplified by cribriform architecture (Figs. 4.31, 4.33, and 4.35). Because the term conventional adenoma is synonymous with LGD, when more advanced dysplasia is seen, the higher grade

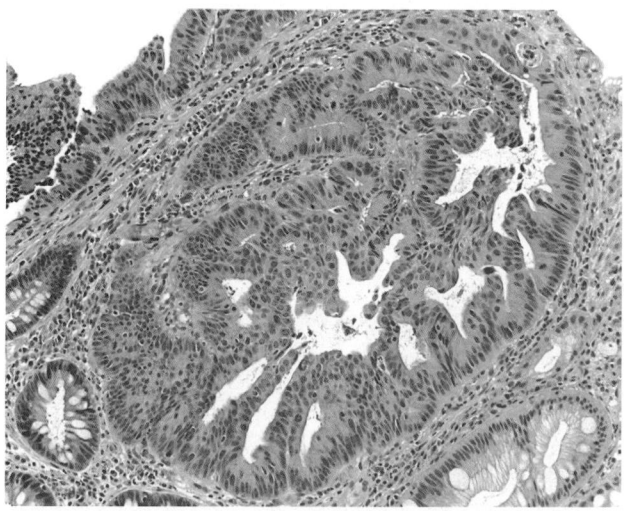

Figure 4-31. High-grade dysplasia (HGD) in a conventional tubular adenoma (TA), negative for invasion. Diagnosing HGD in conventional adenomas requires both cytologic (loss of nuclear polarity) and architectural complexity (cribriform architecture). Architectural complexity is best seen at intermediate power, as depicted here.

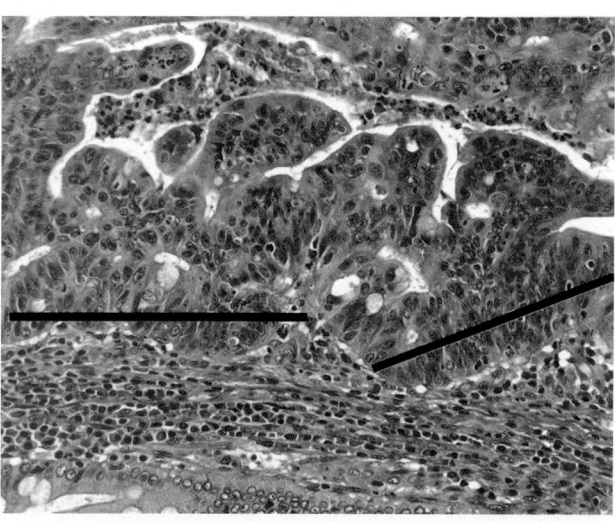

Figure 4-32. HGD in a TA, negative for invasion. Higher power of the previous figure. Loss of nuclear polarity can be illustrated by drawing *lines* through the basal aspect of the dysplastic cells, parallel to the basement membrane, and finding that many nuclei are no longer present on the *lines*, as seen here.

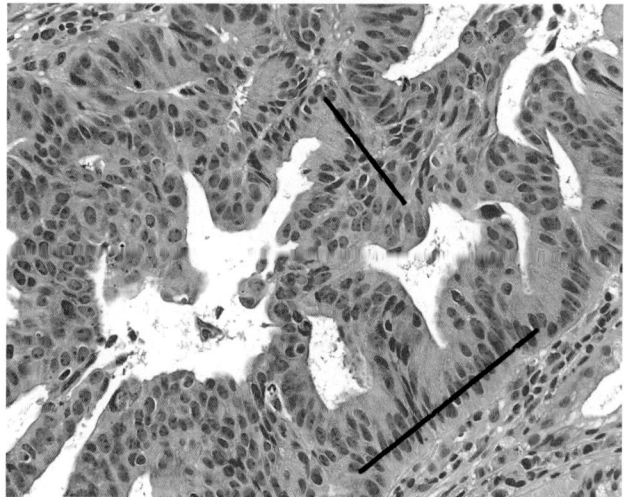

Figure 4-33. HGD in a TA, negative for invasion. A cribriform pattern is a feature of architectural complexity and often seen with glandular crowding and depletion of the intervening lamina propria, as in this case. The lack of desmoplasia is evidence of a noninvasive lesion, and this pertinent negative should be included in the report as "negative for invasion" (compare with desmoplasia seen in invasive adenocarcinoma [Figs. 4.43–4.45]). *Lines*, as described in Fig. 4.32.

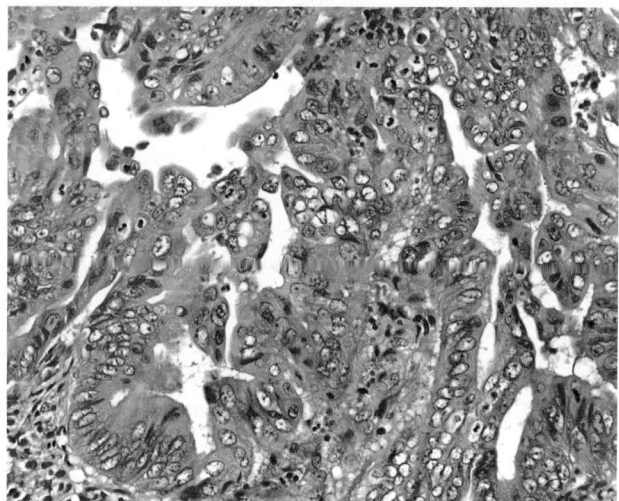

Figure 4-34. HGD in a TA, negative for invasion. Higher power of the previous figure shows loss of nuclear polarity. Note that the preferred diagnosis is HGD in a TA (and not TA with HGD) so that the most important diagnosis is listed first.

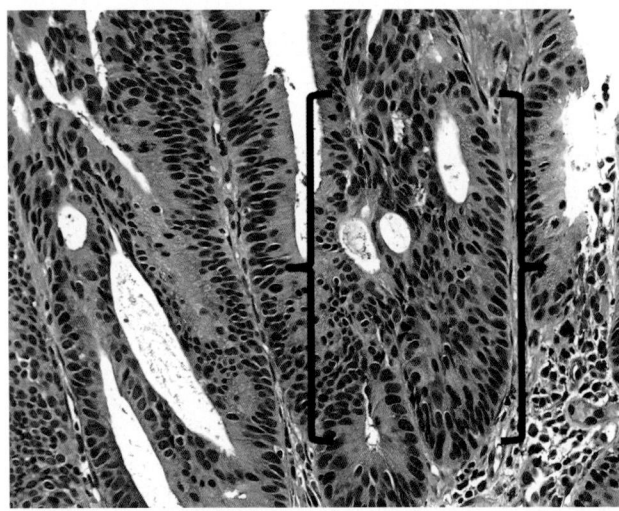

Figure 4-35. HGD in a TA, negative for invasion. Cribriform architecture is easily seen at this power (*brackets*). Make sure to carefully examine such cases for single cell invasion and/or desmoplasia, which indicates at least submucosal invasion, neither of which are seen here.

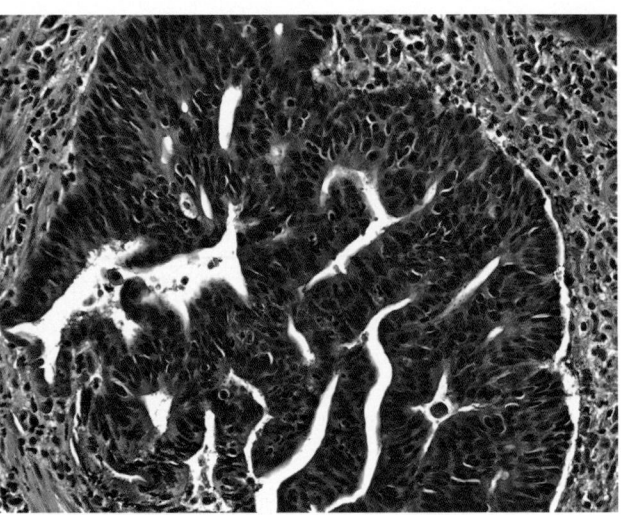

Figure 4-36. HGD in a TA, negative for invasion. Higher power of the previous figure. Loss of nuclear polarity is a required feature of HGD in conventional adenomas, in addition to architectural complexity.

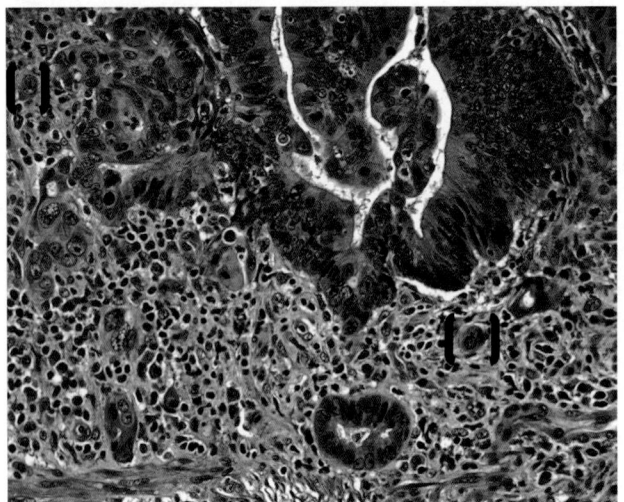

Figure 4-37. Intramucosal carcinoma (IMC) in a conventional tubulovillous adenoma (TVA). Diagnosing IMC requires identification of individual cell infiltration (*brackets*) through the basement membrane into the lamina propria or into the muscularis mucosae but not beyond the muscularis mucosae.

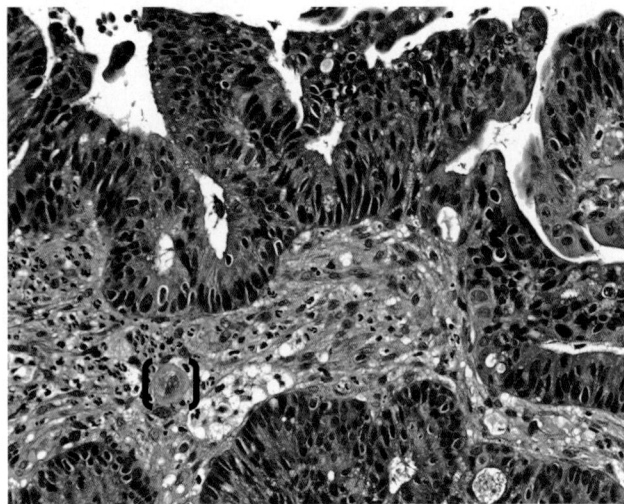

Figure 4-38. At least IMC in a TVA. The minimum criterion for IMC is a single neoplastic cell extending beyond the basement membrane but not into the submucosa, as seen here. Thorough evaluation of these specimens for that single wayward cell (*bracket*) can take some time. The background lamina propria appears a bit desmoplastic, justifying the qualification of at least IMC in the case.

is listed first on the diagnostic line. For example, HGD in a TA is the preferred phrase-ology to avoid the clinician's missing the most important aspect of the diagnosis. Cases with HGD that are negative for invasion should include the pertinent negative line diagnosis of negative for invasion. IMC involves individual cells infiltrating through the basement membrane into the lamina propria or into, but not beyond, the muscularis mucosae (Figs. 4.37–4.42).[8] In the colon, IMC is staged as pTis because of a lack of sufficiently large lymphovascular spaces to support metastasis.[5-7] The term invasive adenocarcinoma is reserved for colorectal carcinoma (CRC) cases with invasion beyond the muscularis mucosae into at least the submucosa and is staged as at least pT1 (Fig. 4.2). Note that this staging approach differs from the rest of the tubular GI tract where a diagnosis of IMC is associated with metastatic potential and is, accordingly, staged as pT1.[8] Very rarely, a specimen is received

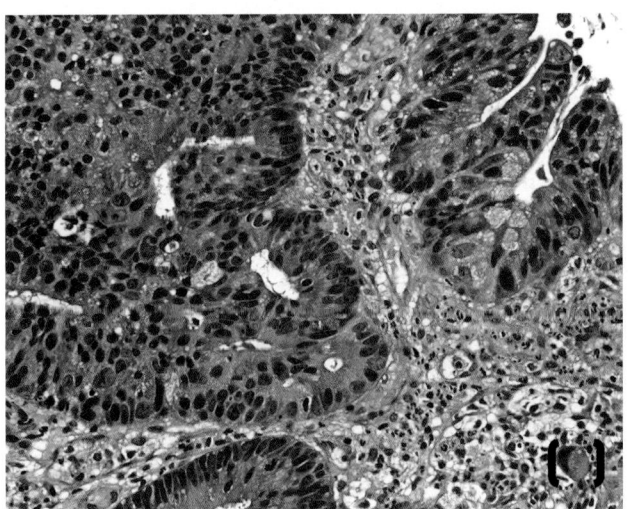

Figure 4-39. IMC in a TVA. Clues to slow down to look for IMC (*bracket*) include a backdrop of a large TVA, HGD (seen here), or clinical designation of the specimen as a mass.

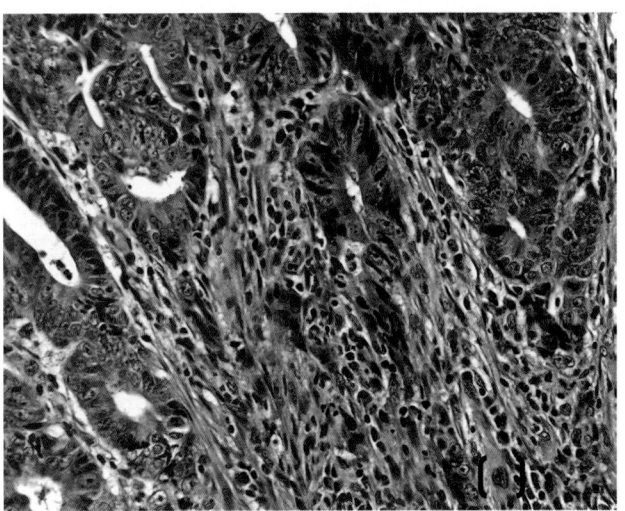

Figure 4-40. IMC in a TVA (*bracket*). Unique to the colon, IMC is staged as pTis because of a lack of sufficiently large lymphovascular spaces to support metastasis.[5-7] IMC in the rest of the GI tract is staged as pT1.

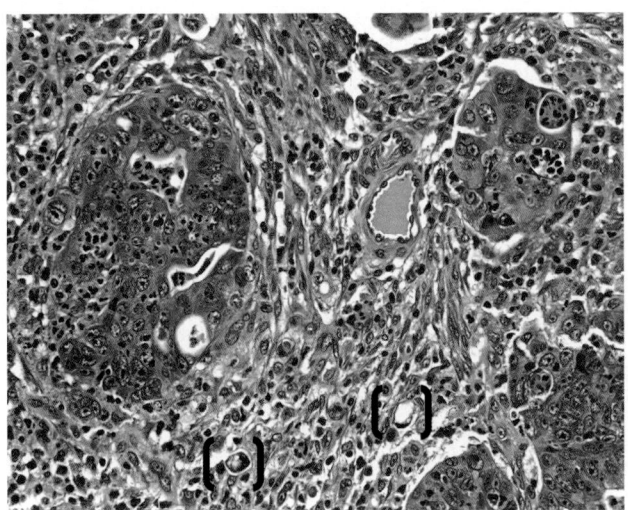

Figure 4-41. IMC in a TVA (*brackets*).

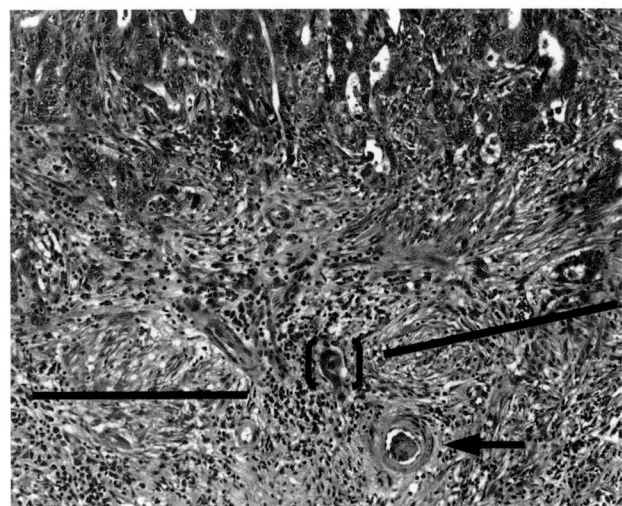

Figure 4-42. At least IMC in a TVA. This was a difficult case to assess for the depth of invasion, despite deeper sections. A single neoplastic gland (*bracket*) is seen at the level of the muscularis mucosae (*lines*). Technically, this focus is no more than IMC because it does not extend beyond the muscularis mucosae. However, it was signed out as at least IMC with a note that the neoplastic cells were in an area focally devoid of muscularis mucosae, in close proximity to a muscularized vessel (*arrow*), and in a backdrop of angulated glands and with a suggestion of desmoplasia; early submucosal invasion could not be excluded.

perfectly oriented, permitting easy assessment of submucosal invasion (Fig. 4.43). More often than not, the specimen is poorly oriented and evaluating it requires a bit of imagination to piece together the bounds of the mucosa (Fig. 4.44). In these cases, one can approach the case by first identifying the definitive muscularis mucosae and then drawing an imaginary line to visualize the suspected boundaries of the mucosa. Invasion in the mucosa up to that line is IMC, and invasion beyond the line is invasive adenocarcinoma. Other submucosal landmarks include muscularized, large vessels and a lack of investing lamina propria around the invading glands. Most commonly, the biopsy is impossibly oriented. In these cases, identifying desmoplasia is helpful because desmoplasia signifies

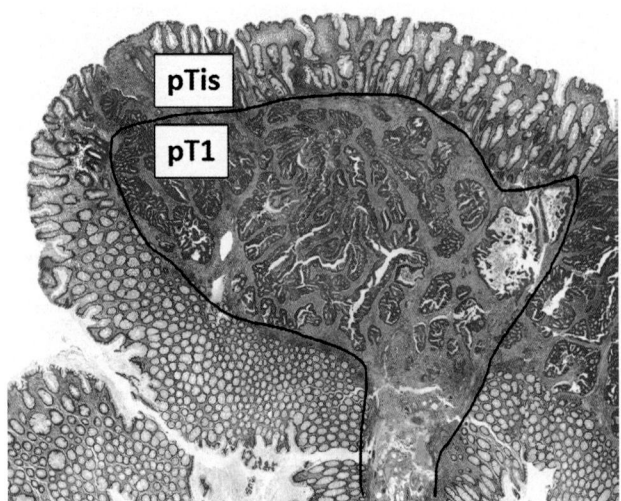

Figure 4-43. Invasive adenocarcinoma. Invasive adenocarcinoma refers to (at least) submucosal invasion. The *line* denotes the muscularis mucosae. Unique to the colon, mucosal invasion (above the *line*) is designated as pTis and submucosal invasion (below the *line*) is designated as pT1. Although the margins were uninvolved and the specimen was negative for lymphovascular invasion, a subsequent resection showed two lymph nodes with metastatic adenocarcinoma.

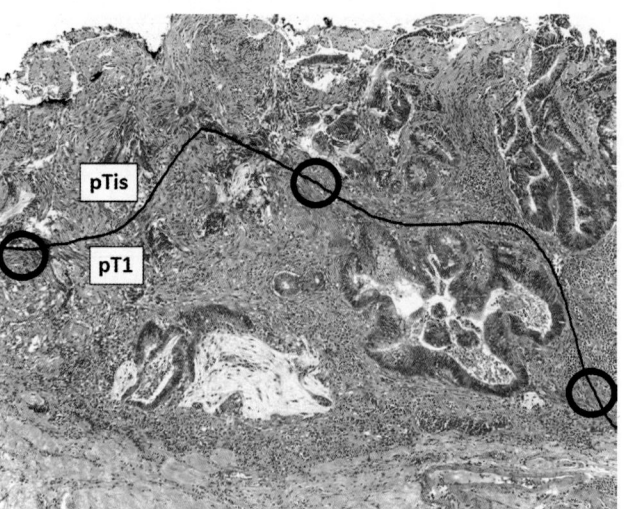

Figure 4-44. Invasive adenocarcinoma. The preceding case is a beautiful, but rare, example of a real-life case. In routine practice, a bit of imagination is required to properly evaluate the depth of invasion for most specimens. As in this case, first identify the definitive bits of muscularis mucosae *(circles)*, and then draw a *line* between the circles to visualize the boundaries of the mucosa. Invasion in the mucosa up until that *line* is intramucosal carcinoma (pTis), and invasion beyond the *line* is invasive adenocarcinoma into at least the submucosa (at least pT1). Other clues to invasion include desmoplasia, angulated neoplastic glands that lack investing lamina propria, and the identification of neoplastic glands near large, muscularized vessels (not featured). Large-caliber, muscularized vessels are generally only seen in the submucosa and beyond.

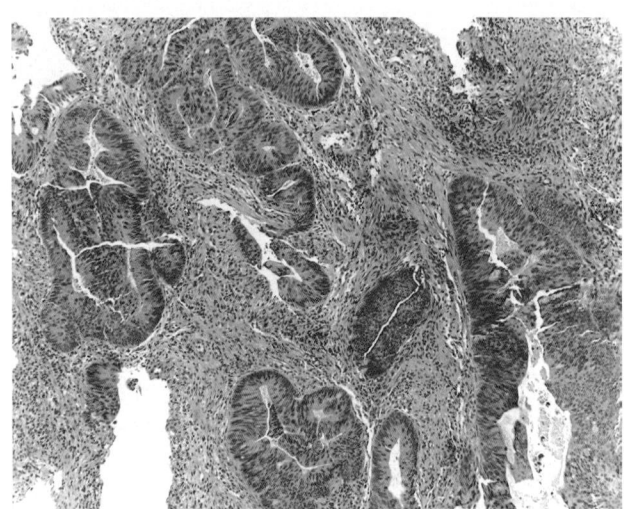

Figure 4-45. Invasive adenocarcinoma. Most real-life cases are impossibly oriented. Thankfully, the diagnostic process can be simplified by knowing that desmoplasia signifies at least submucosal invasion. Desmoplasia imparts a *light blue* pallor to the background lamina propria and submucosa, as seen here. Desmoplasia is best seen on low power.

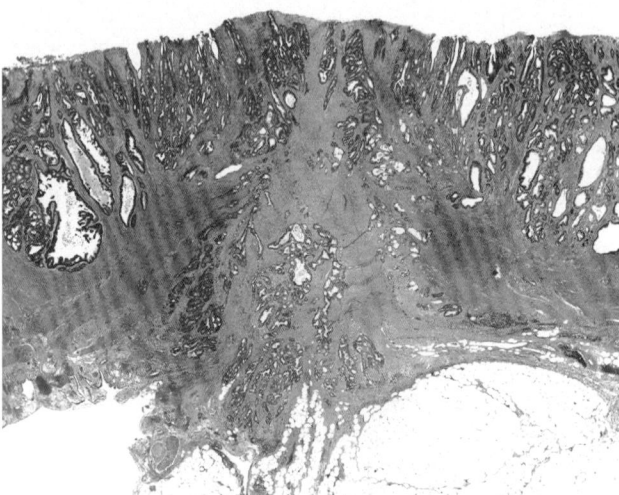

Figure 4-46. Invasive adenocarcinoma, resection. This is the resection from the patient whose biopsy appears in the previous figure. The adenocarcinoma is seen infiltrating through the muscularis propria (pT3).

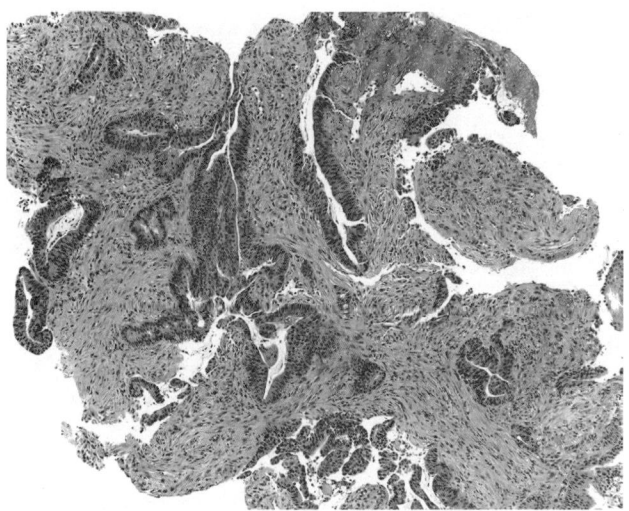

Figure 4-47. Invasive adenocarcinoma. This tiny biopsy is diagnostic of invasive adenocarcinoma based on the presence of desmoplasia.

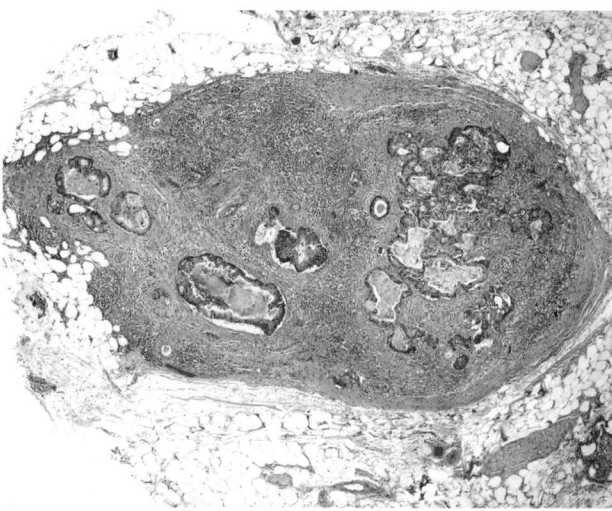

Figure 4-48. Positive lymph node with metastatic adenocarcinoma. This positive lymph node is from the resection of the prior case.

(at least) submucosal invasion (Figs. 4.43–4.48).[9] Desmoplasia imparts a light blue tint to the background mucosa and submucosa and represents a tissue reaction to the (at least) submucosal invasion. Cases with invasive adenocarcinoma should include a comment on the presence or absence of lymphovascular space invasion, whether the invasive carcinoma is poorly differentiated, and entirely excised. See Pearls and Pitfalls: Controversies in Classifying Conventional Adenomas and Dysplasia Grading and Checklist: Approach to the Malignant Polyp.

See Fig. 4.49 for a side-by-side composite of the dysplasia grades in conventional adenomas.

The Microanatomy of a Malignant Polyp (Fig. 4.50)

Staging of cancer in a polyp is similar to staging of cancer in a colorectal resection specimen: IMC is staged as pTis, and invasion into the submucosa is staged as pT1. IMC is presumed to have negligible metastatic potential and, thus, is sufficiently treated by polypectomy alone if it is completely excised with at least 1 mm surgical margin clearance, and is negative for lymphovascular invasion and a poorly differentiated or an undifferentiated component.[8,10] The following checklist is useful for a complete report of carcinoma in a polyp.

CHECKLIST: Approach to the Malignant Polyp

☐ Histologic type of cancer
☐ Presence or absence of a poorly differentiated or undifferentiated component
☐ Depth of invasion
☐ Evaluation of margins for dysplasia and carcinoma
☐ Distance of carcinoma from the deep margin
☐ Presence or absence of lymphovascular invasion
☐ Presence or absence of perineural invasion
☐ Background polyp or colitis, if applicable

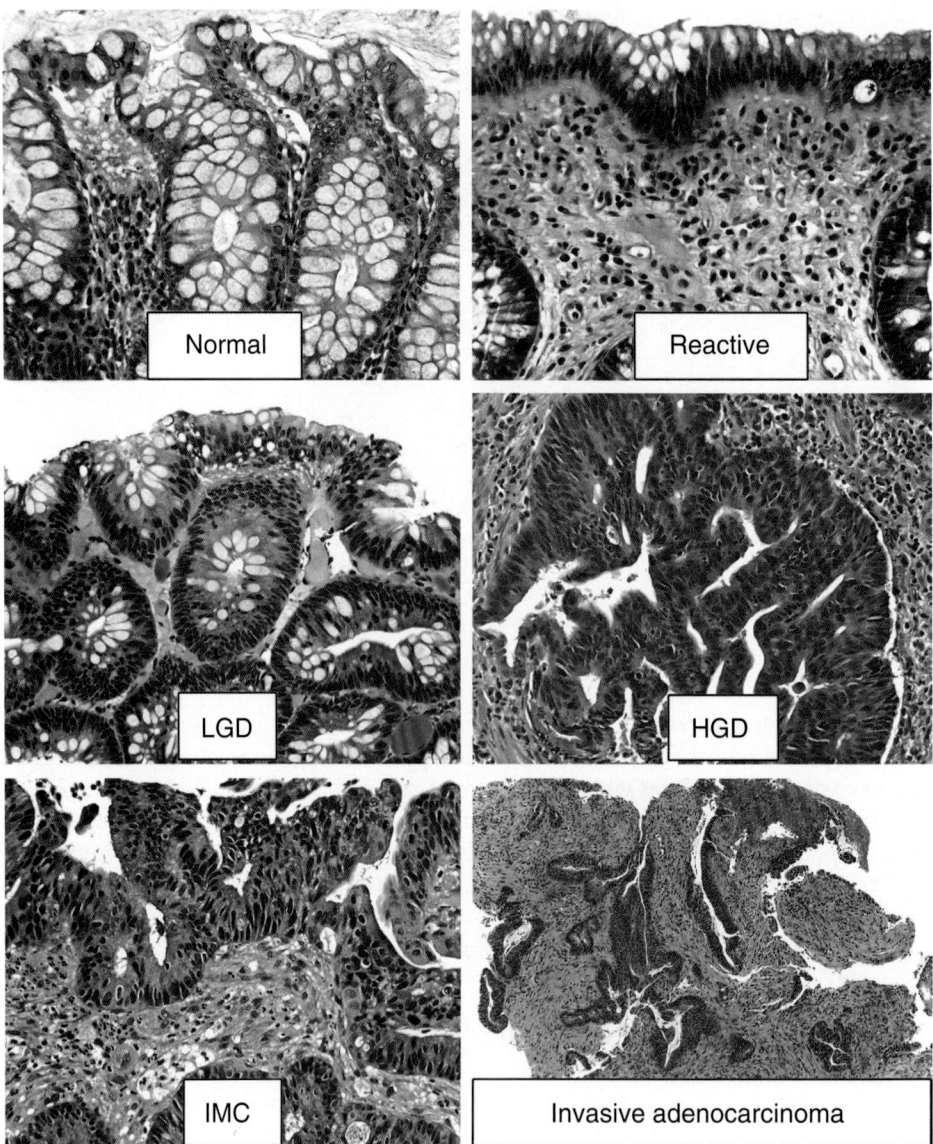

Figure 4-49. A composite image of dysplasia categories in conventional adenomas. Normal (without adenoma): tiny, basally oriented nuclei with normochromatic chromatin, abundant cytoplasm, and negative for pleomorphism and prominent apoptotic bodies and mitotic figures. Reactive: an indistinct blur of transition from normal to atypia and negative for prominent apoptotic bodies and mitotic figures. Dysplasia is eye-catching at low power with abrupt transitions between the normal and dysplastic epithelium and prominent apoptotic bodies, and the atypical changes involve the surface. LGD: retained nuclear polarity. HGD: cytologic atypia (loss of nuclear polarity) and architectural complexity (cribriforming). IMC: individual cells infiltrating the mucosa but not through the muscularis mucosae. Invasive adenocarcinoma: at least submucosal invasion, which is evidenced by desmoplasia.

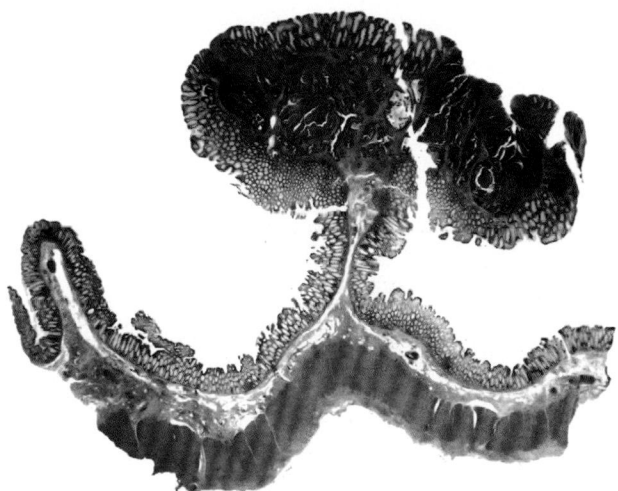

Figure 4-50. The microanatomy of a malignant polyp. Staging of cancer in a polyp is similar to staging of cancer in a colorectal resection specimen. A surgically resected polyp is shown here as an example of invasive adenocarcinoma into the submucosa arising in a TA. A checklist approach to the malignant polyp is useful to include all the usual pertinent data points, such as the histologic type of cancer, depth of invasion, the presence or absence of a poorly differentiated or undifferentiated component, margin status, distance of malignancy from the margin (s), presence or absence of lymphovascular invasion and perineural invasion, and background polyp classification or colon pathology, if applicable.

PEARLS & PITFALLS: Controversies in Classifying Conventional Adenomas and Dysplasia Grading

Based on a lack of well-accepted criteria, some pathologists do not subclassify conventional adenomas as TA, TVA, or VA, and some do not report HGD or IMC. For these pathologists, this conservative approach in the colon is to avoid potential overaggressive resections and chemotherapy for lesions that lack significant risk of metastasis, assuming the lesion was entirely removed. Others lump HGD and IMC together, as both are staged pTis in the colon; the colonic mucosa is devoid of sufficiently large lymphovascular spaces to support metastasis.[1] This peculiarity of the colon may be unfamiliar to some clinical colleagues, and in an attempt to avoid potential overtreatment, some pathologists abstain entirely from using IMC in the colon and instead call it HGD. Others avoid this clinical hazard by including a note that clearly states the staging status for IMC. See the following Sample Note.

SAMPLE NOTE: Intramucosal Carcinoma Arising in a Tubular Adenoma

Colon, Polyp, Polypectomy

- IMC arising in a TVA (pTis at this site), see Note
- IMC 0.5 cm to the inked resection margin
- Inked resection margin negative for dysplasia

Note: IMC arising in colonic adenomas is biologically equivalent to HGD (pTis) and lacks metastatic potential. Complete polypectomy is considered adequate management. Endoscopic assurance of complete excision is recommended.

SAMPLE NOTE: Intramucosal Carcinoma Arising in a Tubular Adenoma, Alternative Reporting

Colon, Polyp, Polypectomy
- HGD arising in a TA
- Inked resection margin negative for dysplasia

Epithelial Misplacement as a Mimic of Invasion

A diagnosis of invasive adenocarcinoma will sometimes result in aggressive management and needs to be distinguished from its benign mimic, epithelial misplacement (also known as pseudoinvasion). Epithelial misplacement occurs as a polyp enlarges and adenomatous glands are displaced into the submucosa or between prolapsed muscle bundles, simulating invasion. In a study of 256 polyps with epithelial misplacement, 78.9% originated from the rectosigmoid colon.[11] Although the sigmoid is the most common site for epithelial misplacement because of its narrow lumen and propensity for diverticular disease, epithelial misplacement can occur in any region of the bowel with sufficiently large polyps. Typical histologic features of epithelial misplacement include a lobular glandular architecture surrounded by lamina propria, hemosiderin-laden macrophages, a lack of desmoplasia, and cytologic atypia similar to that of the overlying (nonmisplaced) adenomatous epithelium[12-14] (Figs. 4.51–4.58). Another reassuring feature of epithelial misplacement, when present, is a lack of HGD or IMC in the remaining polyp because true invasion is less likely to occur in its absence. Mechanical stress of these squished misplaced glands can result in gland rupture and extruded mucin and can raise concerns for a mucinous adenocarcinoma (Fig. 4.59). Keep in mind that a recent biopsy can also result in epithelial misplacement.[14] In these cases, awareness of the recent procedure is helpful, along with identifying the usual features of epithelial misplacement. Some advocate Ki67 and p53 to demonstrate strong, diffuse nuclear immunolabeling in true invasion and weak/negative immunoreactivity in epithelial misplacement.[14] Routine use of these adjunct stains is not required; deeper sections and sharing with a colleague resolves most diagnostic dilemmas.

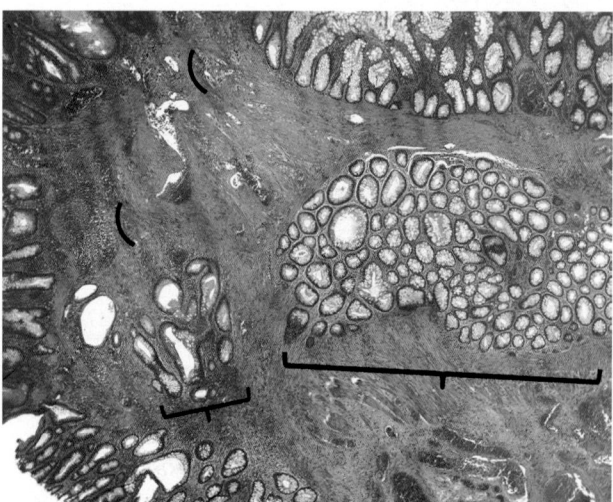

Figure 4-51. Epithelial misplacement. Epithelial misplacement occurs as a polyp enlarges and adenomatous glands are pushed into the submucosa (*brackets*), mimicking submucosal invasion, as seen here. Clues to epithelial misplacement include a lobular glandular architecture of the displaced glands and presence of surrounding lamina propria; cancer does not organize itself into lobules and does not travel with its lamina propria. Other helpful clues to misplacement include finding hemosiderin-laden macrophages (*arcs*), a lack of desmoplasia, and cytologic atypia similar to that in the overlying mucosal component of the adenoma.

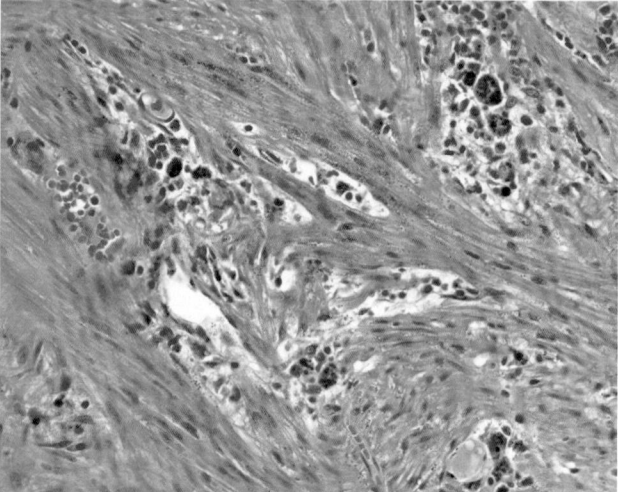

Figure 4-52. Epithelial misplacement. Although not seen in every case of epithelial misplacement, hemosiderin-laden macrophages can be a helpful clue to benign epithelial misplacement, as seen here.

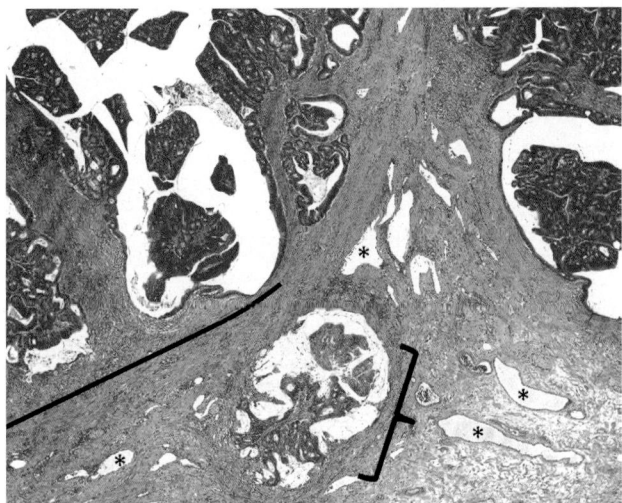

Figure 4-53. Epithelial misplacement. Epithelial misplacement is a common finding in large polyps. The *bracket* highlights adenomatous epithelium that has herniated beyond the muscularis mucosae (*line*) into the submucosa. The large vessels (*asterisks*) are clues to the submucosal location. This focus represents benign epithelial misplacement because the glands are lobular, surrounded by lamina propria, and unaccompanied by desmoplasia.

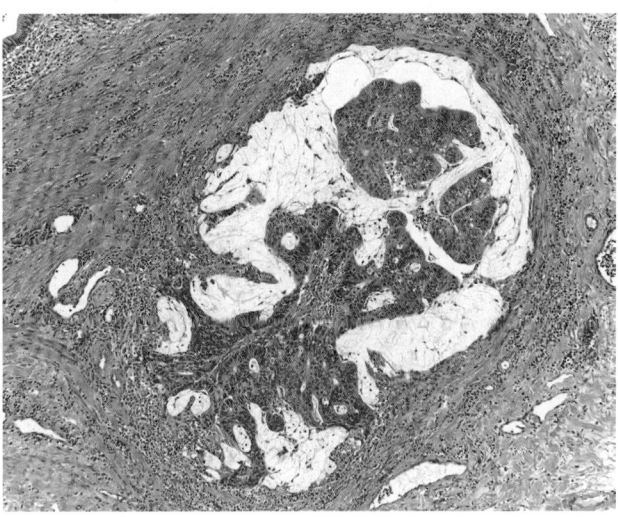

Figure 4-54. Epithelial misplacement. Higher power of the previous figure. Note the lobular architecture and investing lamina propria, clues to the diagnosis of epithelial misplacement.

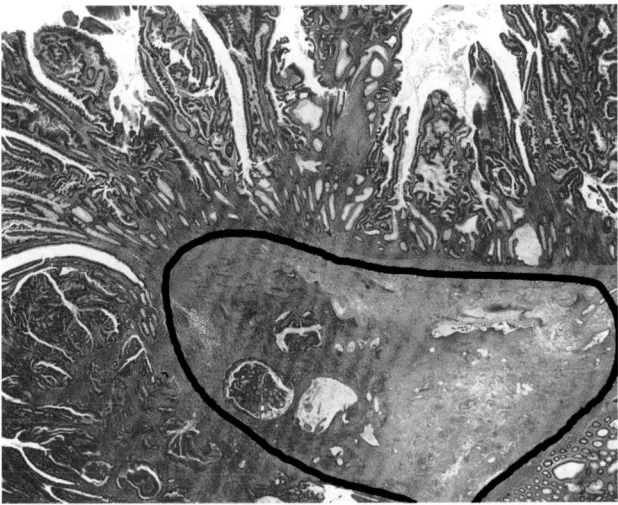

Figure 4-55. Epithelial misplacement. The *line* denotes the boundaries of the mucosa. The glands within the submucosa represent epithelial misplacement because of their lobular architecture, surrounding lamina propria, and lack of desmoplasia. Tangential sections, such as this one, have mucosa on all edges of the polyp and commonly show epithelial misplacement.

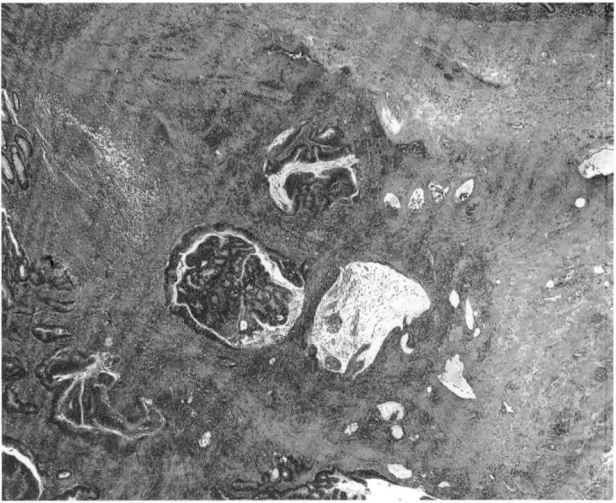

Figure 4-56. Epithelial misplacement. Higher power of the previous figure. Note the lobular architecture, surrounding lamina propria, and lack of desmoplasia.

Squamous Morules as a Mimic of Invasion

Squamous morules (also known as squamous metaplasia or microcarcinoids) are another mimic of HGD and invasive adenocarcinoma. In contrast to neuroendocrine tumors (NETs) (formerly carcinoids) that grossly present as polyps, nodules, or masses, these are microscopic collections of cells with variable neuroendocrine and squamous differentiation. They have been described in the stomach and small bowel[15] but are most commonly encountered intermingled within large, colonic TVAs with HGD, epithelial misplacement, and serrated features.[16] Given the associated high-risk adenoma features, it is understandable that squamous morules can raise concerns for invasive poorly differentiated carcinoma, particularly

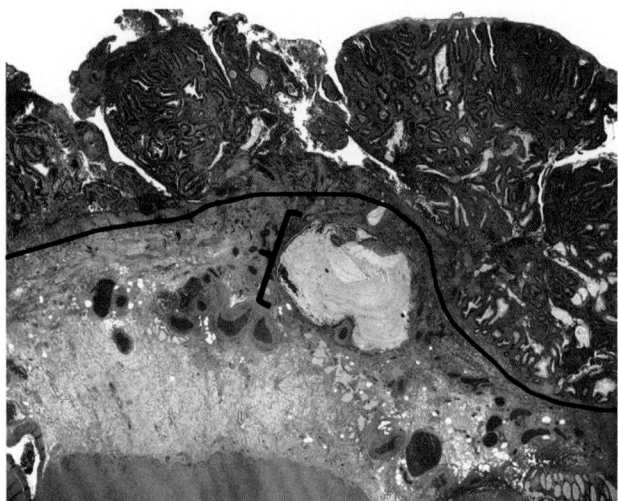

Figure 4-57. Epithelial misplacement. This low-power image shows a focus of adenomatous epithelium (*bracket*) that has been displaced beyond the mucosa (*line*) into the submucosa. The lobular architecture and lack of desmoplasia are low-power clues to benign epithelial misplacement.

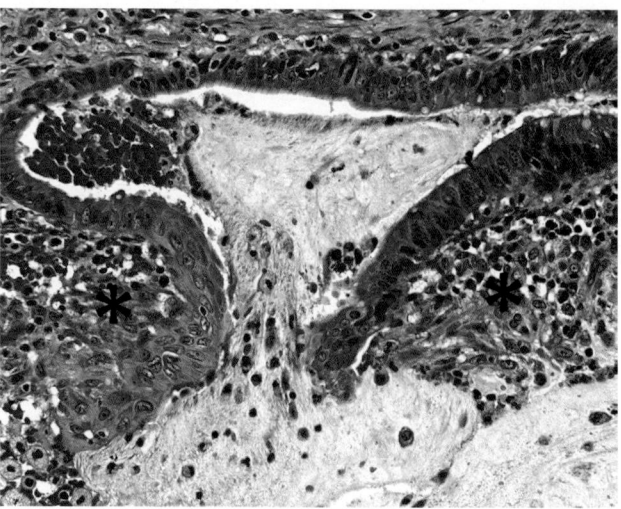

Figure 4-58. Epithelial misplacement. On higher power, the epithelium shows only LGD with preserved nuclear polarity and surrounding lamina propria (*asterisks*), features that support benign epithelial misplacement. This case features prominent extruded mucin, a common finding when the misplaced glands are mechanically squeezed, leading to gland rupture and spillage of the mucin into the surrounding tissue.

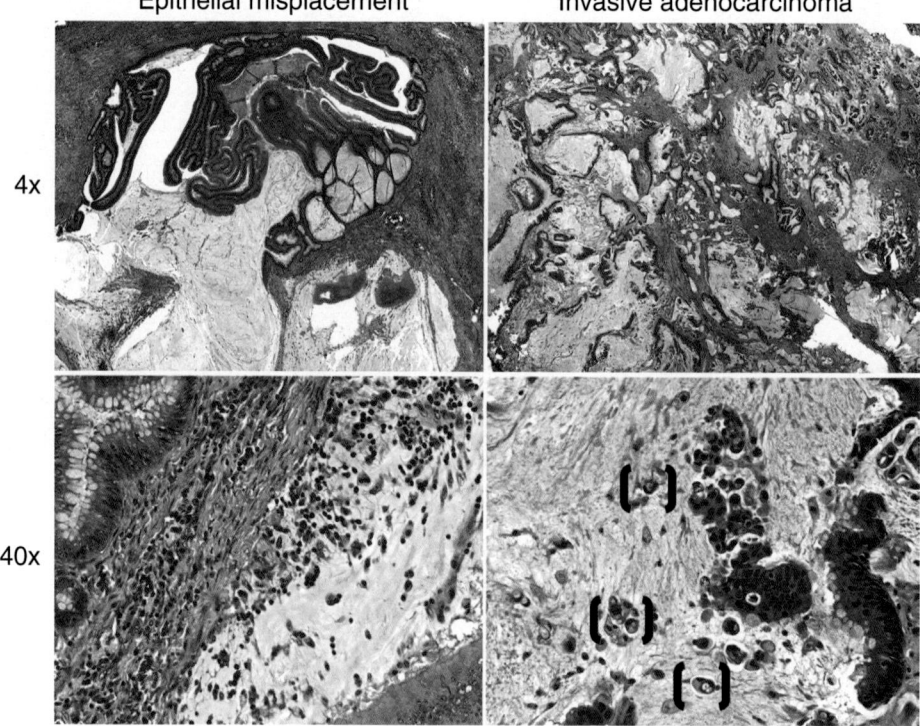

Figure 4-59. Extruded mucin in epithelial misplacement versus dissecting mucin of an invasive adenocarcinoma. The extruded mucin seen in epithelial misplacement can raise concerns for an invasive adenocarcinoma. Clues to epithelial misplacement include a low-power view (upper left) of retained lobular architecture with wisps of surrounding lamina propria and a high-power view (lower left) showing only inflammation seen suspended within the mucin pools. In contrast, a low-power view (upper right) of infiltrating adenocarcinoma shows disorganized mucin that dissects the tissue and a high-power view (lower right) shows neoplastic cells with high-grade nuclear features and signet ring cells floating within the mucin pool (*brackets*).

when individual cells are seen in the lamina propria and the background stromal changes mimic desmoplasia. Typical features of squamous morules include their distinctly bland morphology compared with that of the associated adenoma (compare Figs. 4.60–4.65 with 4.16). These small, cuboidal cells lack pleomorphism, mitotic figures, and apoptotic bodies, and they appear pink because of abundant eosinophilic cytoplasm. They aggregate in lobular collections and occasionally connect to the adjoining adenoma. They consistently immunolabel with nuclear β-catenin and have variable staining for neuroendocrine (synaptophysin and chromogranin) and squamous markers (p63 and CK 5/6) with negligible p53 and Ki67 immunolabeling.[16] Squamous morules sparsely intermingled within an adenoma can be classified as composite intestinal adenoma-microcarcinoid, and those that comprise a more substantial component of the adenoma can be classified as combined intestinal adenoma-microcarcinoid. To avoid unnecessary patient and clinician anxiety, the term squamous morules is preferred over microcarcinoids; they are unnecessary to report, especially if they

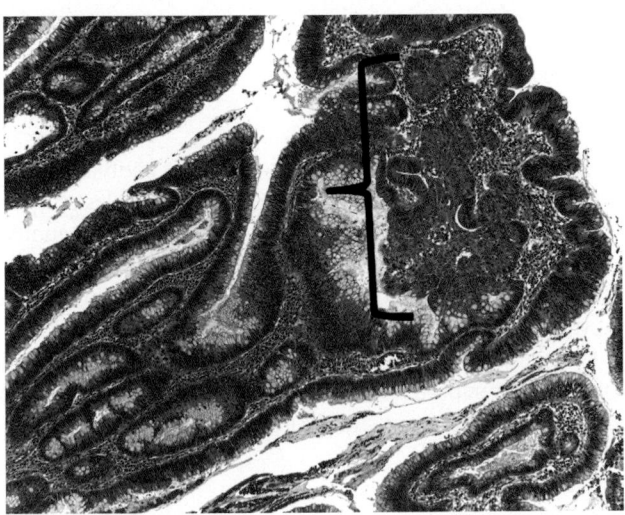

Figure 4-60. Squamous morules. Squamous morules are another mimic of invasive adenocarcinoma. They are most commonly seen in large, colonic tubulovillous adenomas with HGD, epithelial misplacement, and serrated features. On low power, they (*bracket*) look different from the surrounding adenoma and sometimes can raise concerns for focal HGD or a focus of invasive adenocarcinoma.

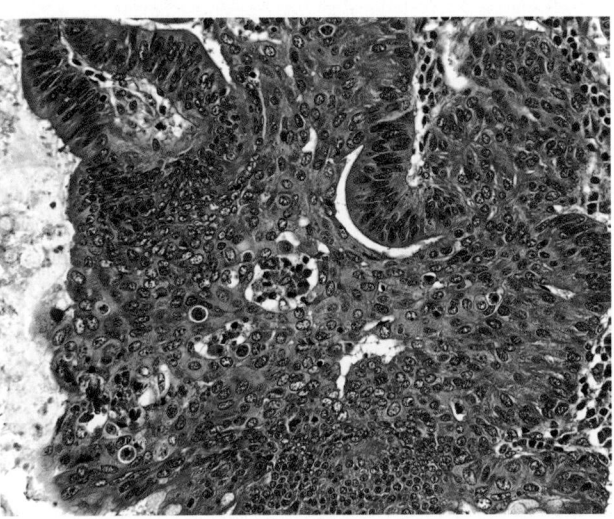

Figure 4-61. Squamous morules. Higher power of the previous figure shows that the cells forming squamous morules are more cuboidal in shape with small round, normochromatic nuclei, in comparison with the adjoining adenoma.

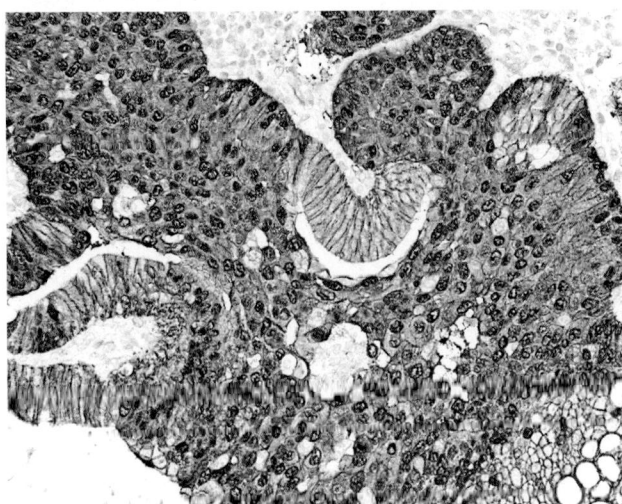

Figure 4-62. Squamous morules (β-catenin). Although squamous morules are easily identified on H&E alone, β-catenin can be helpful in challenging cases. As seen here, squamous morules demonstrate strong, nuclear β-catenin immunolabeling.

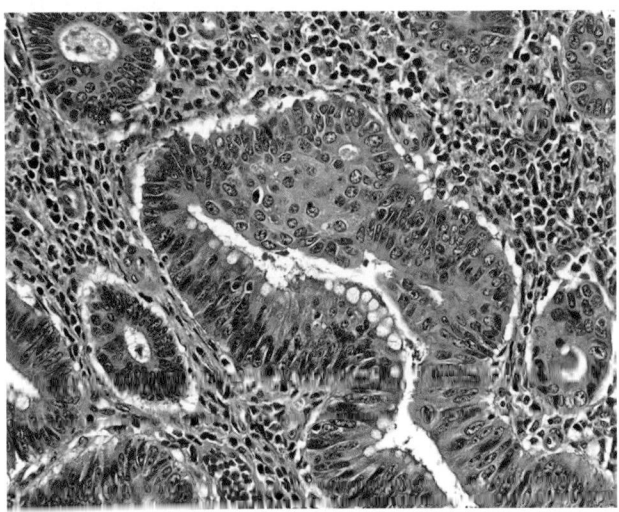

Figure 4-63. Squamous morules. As seen here, squamous morules can have solid growth and occasionally connect to the adenoma. They are uniformly small, cuboidal, and lack pleomorphism, mitotic figures, and apoptotic bodies.

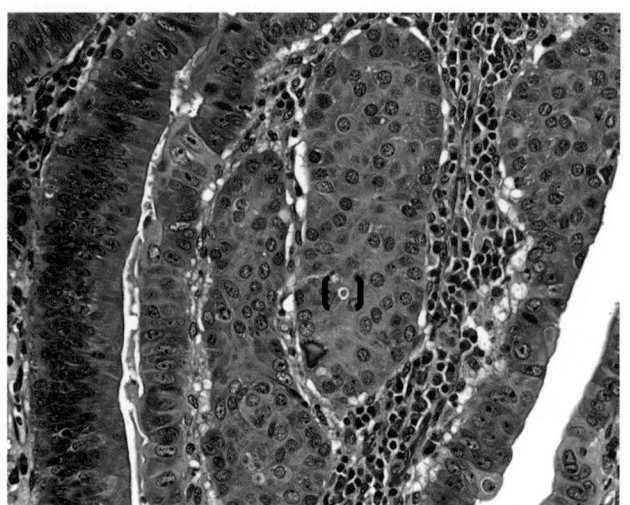

Figure 4-64. Squamous morules. Rarely, what appears as intracytoplasmic mucin can be seen (*brackets*).

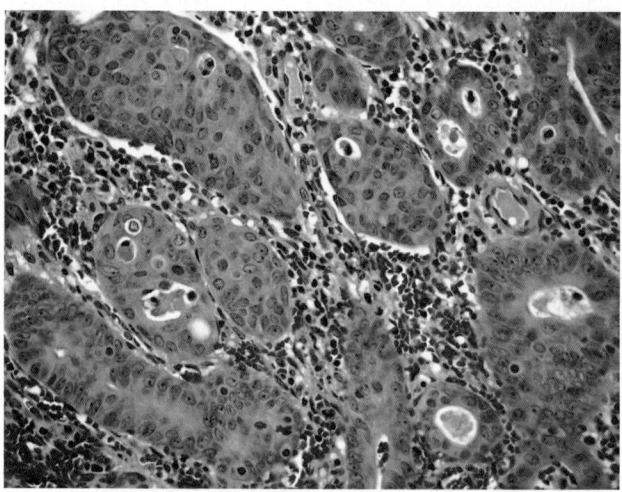

Figure 4-65. Squamous morules. We do not routinely mention squamous morules in reports to avoid unnecessary clinician and patient anxiety.

are very focal and completely excised. The importance of being aware of this entity is to simply avoid misdiagnosis as an invasive carcinoma. There is a single report of this lesion with infiltrative growth into the submucosa and metastatic high-grade neuroendocrine carcinoma to a lymph node.[15] It is unclear whether the metastasis derived from the squamous morule or the associated adenoma.[17,18] Regardless, reporting squamous morules may be of use when they are especially prominent, if they display unusual features such as infiltration, if they appear incompletely excised, or if a colleague submits them for consultation with a concern for carcinoma. Cases of adenomas that show submucosal invasion of their squamous morules would likely benefit from a carefully crafted note suggesting at least close surveillance.[15]

FAQ: What are low- and high-risk conventional adenomas?

Answer: These terms are designated by clinicians (Table 4.1). Low-risk refers to patients with up to 2 small (<10 mm) TAs, and the surveillance interval is 5 to 10 years, assuming all polyps were completely removed. High risk refers to patients with at least three TAs, *or* at least one adenoma ≥10 mm, *or* at least one adenoma designated as either a TVA or a VA, *or* an adenoma with HGD. These patients have a shortened surveillance interval of 3 years, assuming all polyps were completely removed at the initial endoscopy. Advanced neoplasia refers to a conventional adenoma of ≥10 mm, *or* designated as either a TVA or a VA, *or* with HGD.[4] As we have noted, there is subjectivity in classifying HGD and how much of a lesion is villous, but fortunately this is not as concerning as one might think, because it is large adenomas that tend to have HGD or be villous and the endoscopy colleague is well aware of the size of the polyp that has been resected.

FAQ: Because the surveillance interval is based on the number and size of adenomas, should I report the size and number of polyps?

Answer: For the most part, leave these particulars to the clinician. Although practice patterns may differ, high-volume services often cannot sustain the time-intensive process of piecing together the endoscopy report, the gross evaluation, and the pathology diagnoses. Attempting to do so puts the pathologist at risk for inaccurate reporting owing to factors such as incomplete endoscopic reports, piecemeal resections, and tissue fragmentation within the laboratory. Overcounting or undercounting conventional adenomas can change surveillance intervals (e.g., the difference between two and three TAs can result in 5- or 3-year surveillance intervals, respectively). Thus, it is best left to the clinician to tally the polyp type, number, and size to accurately determine the surveillance interval. An exception can be made for the (rare) straightforward case in which the number of polyps is designated and matches the number of tissue fragments received. In these cases, the polyps are listed by priority of surveillance: for example, a TA is listed before a hyperplastic polyp because a TA has a shortened surveillance interval (Table 4.1). When in doubt, simply describe what is seen, see the following Sample Notes.

SAMPLE NOTE: One Polyp Designated on the Requisition, One Fragment Received

Colon Polyp × 1, Biopsy
- Tubular adenoma

SAMPLE NOTE: Three Polyps Designated on the Requisition, Three Fragments Received; Polyps Are Listed in Priority of Surveillance

Colon Polyps × 3, Biopsy
- Tubular adenoma ×2
- Separate hyperplastic polyp ×1

SAMPLE NOTE: Unclear How Many Polyps Submitted, Multiple Fragments Received; Polyps Are Listed in Priority of Surveillance

Colon, Polyps, Biopsy
- Fragments of TA
- Separate fragments of hyperplastic polyp

FAQ: What is the trigger to pursue deeper sections if the initial sections of the submitted polyp appear histologically normal?

Answer: In a study of 733 polyps over 6 months, 22% were histologically unremarkable or had only a lymphoid aggregate. Deeper sections of these polyps uncovered additional diagnoses in 22%, prompting the investigators to recommend deeper sections for histologically unremarkable polyps or polyps with only lymphoid aggregates on initial sections.[19] Similar findings were reported by others.[20,21] In the interest of optimal turnaround times and reducing laboratory expenses, one rational approach is to only pursue deeper sections if the results will affect the subsequent surveillance interval. For example, if a patient has two polyps and one is a TA and the other consists of unremarkable colonic mucosa, one would not pursue deeper sections because this patient will be on an adenoma protocol regardless of the results of the deeper sections (Table 4.1). On the other hand, if the patient has two clinical polyps that are histologically unremarkable, one might pursue deeper sections of both polyps based on a potential change to the subsequent surveillance interval: the surveillance interval for a nondiagnostic polyp is 10 years, whereas a TA has a 5-year interval. In essence, deeper sections should be pursued if the initial sections are ambiguous and deeper sections could lead to change to the surveillance interval. Common scenarios include mild atypia overlying a lymphoid aggregate or thick sections, in which case deeper sections usually resolve the issues.

FAQ: When is margin status on a polyp specified in the report?

Answer: Most biopsies are received fragmented with no discernable margin, and, consequently, most reports are issued without a comment on margin, as outlined earlier in the Sample Notes. In these cases, the clinicians generally remove all visible polyp in piecemeal fashion and submit the fragments for a tissue diagnosis only. When the clinicians resect a larger polyp and submit it intact, they are generally expecting a comment on margins. Beware, cautery (and ink) can be misleading and extend to the tops and sides of the polyps, making it important to rely on discernable polyp stalks, careful grossing and embedding, and effective communication with the clinician when the margin remains histologically unclear. In the case of a single polyp submitted with no clearly identified margin because of grossing or embedding mishaps, for example, we have to settle for just doing our best by reporting "where assessable (embedding artifact), the margin is negative (or positive)" or "margin not assessable due to embedding artifact."

KEY FEATURES: Conventional Adenomas

- Designation as TA, TVA, or VA is based on the amount of villous component: TAs are up to 25% villous, TVAs are between 25% and 75% villous, and VAs are greater than 75% villous.
- TVA and VA result in shorter surveillance interval than TA.
- Conventional adenomas are synonymous with LGD.
- LGD has retention of the nuclear polarity.
- HGD requires both cytologic (loss of nuclear polarity) and architectural (cribriforming) complexity.
- IMC involves individual cells infiltrating into the lamina propria or into, but not through, the muscularis mucosae and is staged as pTis.
- IMC and HGD result in the same surveillance; as such, some practices avoid using the term IMC to prevent potential confusion. Invasive adenocarcinoma is reserved for invasion into at least the submucosa and is staged as at least pT1.
- Common mimics of invasion include epithelial misplacement and squamous morules.

SERRATED POLYPS

Diagnosis of serrated polyps is one of the most perplexing areas in GI pathology. Difficulties arise from their similar sounding names, evolving histologic criteria and nomenclature in some areas, wholly absent criteria in other areas, and overlapping morphologic features. Despite these challenges, proper classification is essential because it directs divergent surveillance intervals. For example, a patient with only a small, rectal hyperplastic polyp has a surveillance interval of 10 years, but the same sized SSA/P at the same site has a 5-year interval, and a slightly larger SSA/P of 10 mm has a 1-year interval. In our attempts to simplify the diagnostic process, this subsection starts with classic examples of the usual suspects and then segues to real-life cases, which are usually far from pretty. The (few) existing guidelines are emphasized and supplemented by our diagnostic algorithms created in partnership with our clinicians with a bit of common sense and a splash of consideration of the existing surveillance recommendations for the remaining gray zones.

Classification: Unwinding the Serrated Polyp Nomenclature

Serrated polyps comprise approximately 35% of colorectal polyps.[2] The term serrated polyp is an umbrella term that encompasses a family of heterogeneous polyps with variable morphology, molecular alterations, and neoplastic potential. This family includes the hyperplastic polyp (30% of all colorectal polyps), SSA/P (4% of all colorectal polyps), traditional serrated adenoma (TSA, 0.7% of all colorectal polyps), and serrated polyp, unclassifiable (Tables 4.2 and 4.3).

TABLE 4.2: Serrated Polyp Classification

Hyperplastic Polyp	
Microvesicular Goblet cell rich Mucin poor	
Sessile Serrated Adenoma/Polyp (SSA/P)	Without cytological dysplasia With LGD cytological dysplasia With HGD cytological dysplasia
Traditional Serrated Adenoma (TSA) Flat Filiform Mucinous	Without cytological dysplasia With LGD cytological dysplasia With HGD cytological dysplasia
Serrated Polyp, Unclassifiable	

Adapted from Snover DC, Ahnen DJ, Burt RW, et al. *Serrated Polyps of the Colon and Rectum and Serrated Polyposis.* Lyon, France: IARC Press; 2010; Limketkai BN, Lam-Himlin D, Arnold MA, Arnold CA. The cutting edge of serrated polyps: a practical guide to approaching and managing serrated colon polyps. *Gastrointest Endosc.* 2013;77(3):360-375.

Hyperplastic Polyps

Up to 85% of serrated polyps are hyperplastic polyps.[2] These are left colon predominant and less than 5 mm in the greatest dimension.[24] For academic purposes, they can be subclassified as microvesicular, goblet cell rich, or mucin poor,[22,24] although reporting of the precise subclassification is unnecessary because it lacks clinical significance. Hyperplastic polyps are pale pink owing to their abundant cytoplasm, many have a prominent subepithelial collagen table and increased neuroendocrine cells,[24] their superficial crypts often feature star-shaped lumens, and their small crypt bases are narrow and lack serrations (Table 4.3). The microvesicular subtype comprises the vast majority of hyperplastic polyps (Figs. 4.66–4.77). It has a delicate, frothy, jagged surface, similar to the jagged surface of a serrated knife (Fig. 4.67). The goblet cell–rich subtype is almost exclusively seen in the rectosigmoid colon (Figs. 4.78–4.83), and typical features are subtle, even on a good day. To avoid missing this polyp, consider this entity when a biopsied rectosigmoid polyp has

TABLE 4.3: Serrated Polyp Overview

Features	Hyperplastic Polyp	Sessile Serrated Adenoma (SSA)/Sessile Serrated Polyp (SSP)	Traditional Serrated Adenoma (TSA)
Classic Morphology			
Previous nomenclature (no longer used)	N/A	Giant hyperplastic polyp, variant hyperplastic polyp, or serrated polyp with abnormal proliferation. Dysplastic SSA/Ps have been referred to as mixed hyperplastic adenomatous polyp, mixed polyp, hybrid polyp, hyperplastic polyp with adenoma, or advanced SSA/P	Serrated adenoma
Most frequent colon site	Left	Right	Left
Shape	Sessile	Sessile	Pedunculated
Average size	<5 mm	>5 mm	>5 mm
Prominent subepithelial collagen table and neuroendocrine cells	+	–	–
Ectopic crypt foci	–	–	+++
Cytoplasm eosinophilia	+	+	+++
Dilated crypt bases	–	+++	–
BRAF mutation	+/–	+	+/–
KRAS mutation	+/–	–	+/–
Other	Variants include microvesicular (MVHP), goblet cell rich (GCHP), and mucin poor (MPHP)	The uncomplicated SSA lacks dysplasia; when dysplasia is present, the preferred terminology is low- or high-grade cytologic dysplasia in an SSA/P	Variants include flat, filiform, and mucinous; the uncomplicated TSA lacks dysplasia; when dysplasia is present, the preferred terminology is low- or high-grade conventional dysplasia arising in a TSA
Malignant potential	Absent	+	+

N/A, not applicable; SSA, sessile serrated adenoma; SSP, sessile serrated polyp; TSA, traditional serrated adenoma.

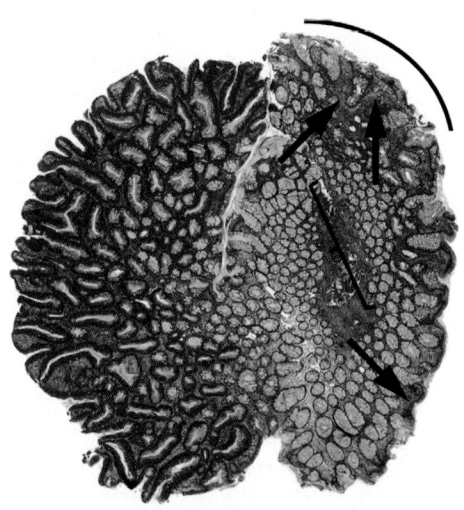

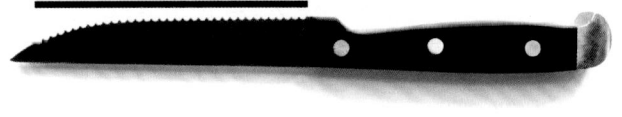

Figure 4-66. TA and hyperplastic polyp. This unusual specimen was submitted as two rectal polyps and consists of a TA (left) compressed against a hyperplastic polyp (right). Note the sharp contrast in color of the two polyps at low power; this is an important clue to the diagnoses. The TA is dark owing to increased nuclear to cytoplasmic ratios and hyperchromatic chromatin, and the hyperplastic polyp is *pink* owing to abundant eosinophilic cytoplasm and normochromatic chromatin. As expected for hyperplastic polyps, the hyperplastic polyp on the right has a serrated surface (*arc*), the crypt bases are narrow and lack serrations (*bracket*), and a subepithelial collagen table is apparent (*arrows*).

Figure 4-67. A serrated knife. Serrated polyps (including hyperplastic polyps, sessile serrated adenomas/polyps, and traditional serrated adenomas) have a variably ruffled surface that is similar to the serrated edge (*line*) of a knife, as seen here.

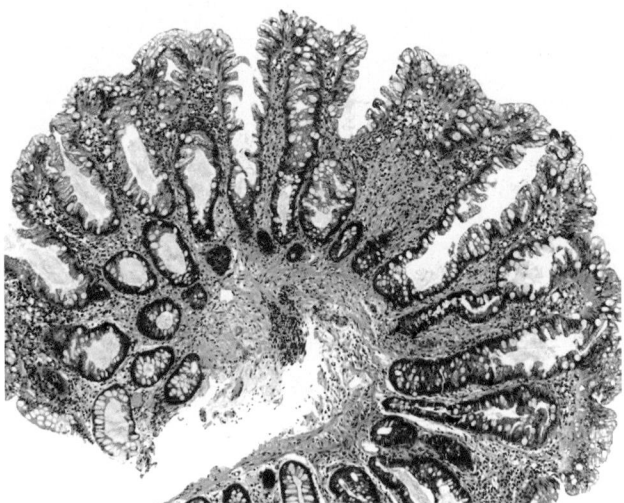

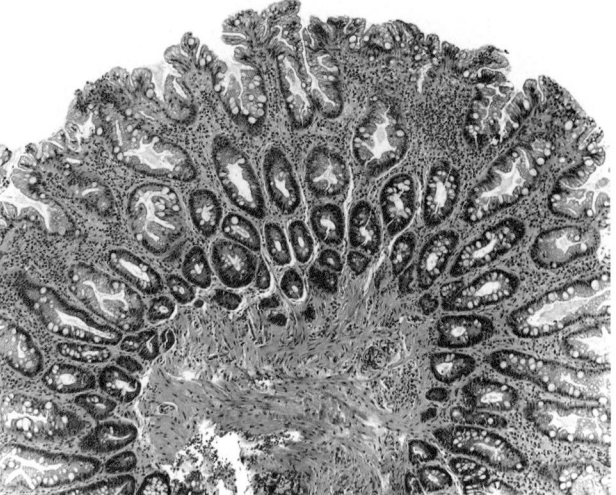

Figure 4-68. Hyperplastic polyp, microvesicular subtype. Most hyperplastic polyps are of the microvesicular subtype. On low power, note the defining features of a hyperplastic polyp with surface serrations and narrowed crypt bases that lack serrations. Compared with the other hyperplastic polyp subtypes, the microvesicular subtype has especially prominent surface serrations with abundant delicate, frothy cytoplasm.

Figure 4-69. Hyperplastic polyp, microvesicular subtype. Because all serrated polyps generally have a serrated surface, it is important to evaluate the crypt bases to correctly classify the serrated polyps. Hyperplastic polyps have narrowed crypt bases that lack serrations (as in this case), and SSA/Ps have dilated crypt bases with serrations (Figs. 4 108–4,116).

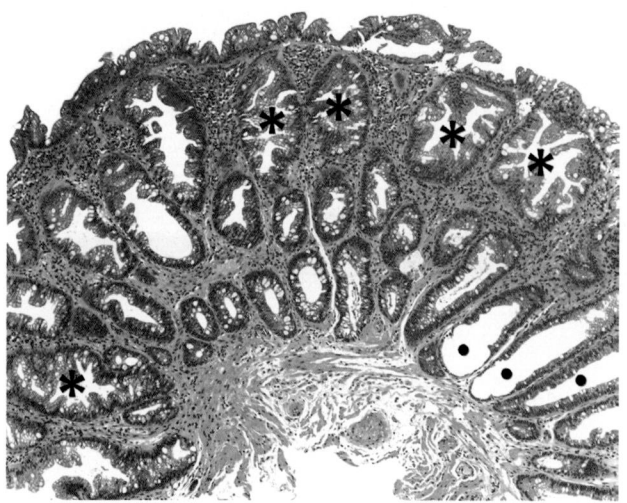

Figure 4-70. Hyperplastic polyp, microvesicular subtype. Hyperplastic polyps can have dilated crypts with serrations in the superficial aspects of the polyp (*asterisks*), but the crypt bases must be narrowed and lack serrations. Note that some of the crypt bases are dilated (*dots*), but these dilated crypts lack serrations and, consequently, the lesion is best classified as a hyperplastic polyp based on the history of a 0.2-cm rectal polyp (see also Fig. 4.135).

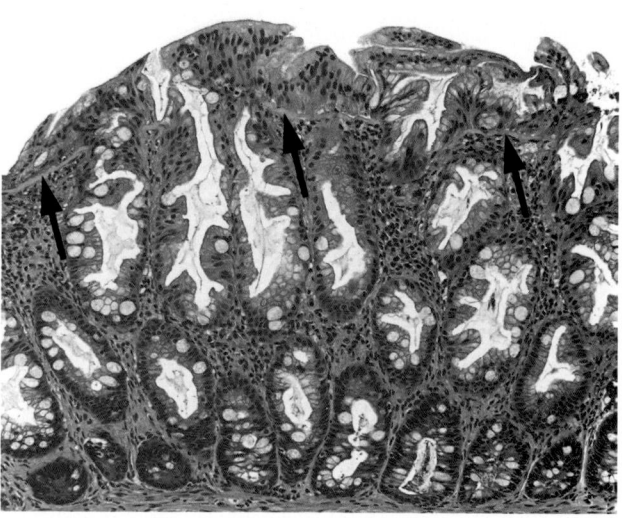

Figure 4-71. Hyperplastic polyp, microvesicular subtype. Another helpful clue to a diagnosis of hyperplastic polyp is the presence of a prominent subepithelial collagen table (*arrows*) in addition to the surface serrations and narrowed crypt bases that lack serrations, as seen here.

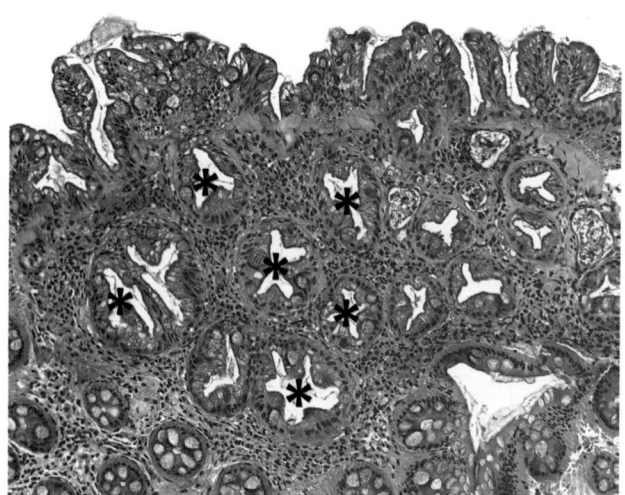

Figure 4-72. Hyperplastic polyp, microvesicular subtype. This microvesicular hyperplastic polyp has all the usual features: surface serrations, prominent subepithelial collagen table, and superficial crypts with star-shaped lumina (*asterisks*).

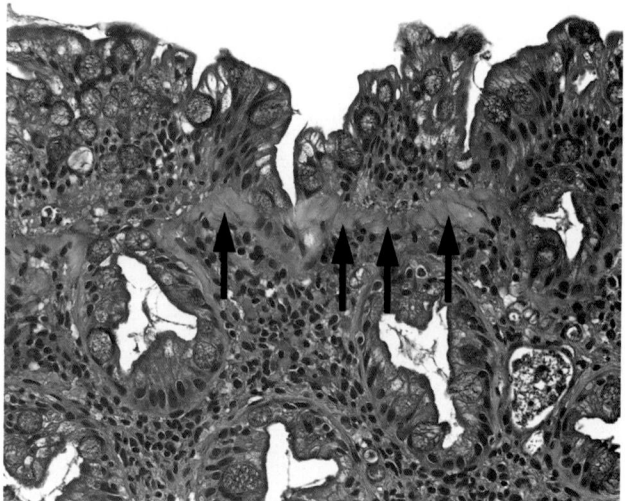

Figure 4-73. Hyperplastic polyp, microvesicular subtype. Higher power of the previous figure shows the prominent subepithelial collagen table (*arrows*) and star-shaped lumina characteristic of hyperplastic polyps.

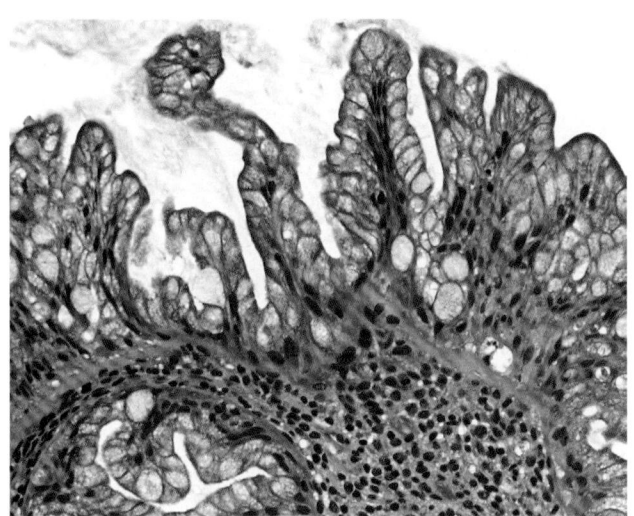

Figure 4-74. Hyperplastic polyp, microvesicular subtype. The high-power views show the surface of microvesicular hyperplastic polyps with abundant delicate surface serrations. These images appear *pink* because of the abundant frothy, eosinophilic cytoplasm, which allows distinction of the microvesicular subtype from the goblet cell–rich and mucin-poor subtypes. Beware, the identical surface can be seen with a sessile serrated adenoma/polyp. As a result, evaluation of the crypt bases is critical for the correct diagnosis: hyperplastic polyps have narrowed crypt bases that lack serrations (as in this case) and SSA/P have dilated crypt bases with serrations.

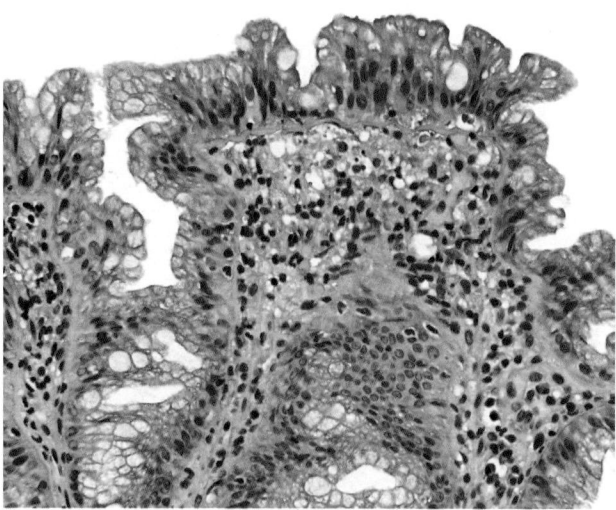

Figure 4-75. Hyperplastic polyp, microvesicular subtype. High power of the surface of a microvesicular hyperplastic polyp shows abundant delicate surface serrations and a prominent subepithelial collagen table. It is unnecessary to subclassify the hyperplastic polyp variants in diagnostic reports, although it is useful to be aware of their morphology for accurate diagnosis.

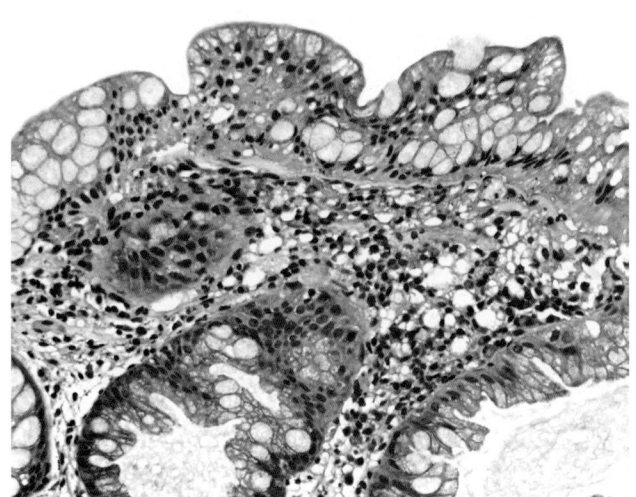

Figure 4-76. Hyperplastic polyp, microvesicular subtype. High power of the surface of a microvesicular hyperplastic polyp shows abundant delicate surface serrations. A prominent subepithelial collagen table, as seen here, is common to all hyperplastic polyp subtypes.

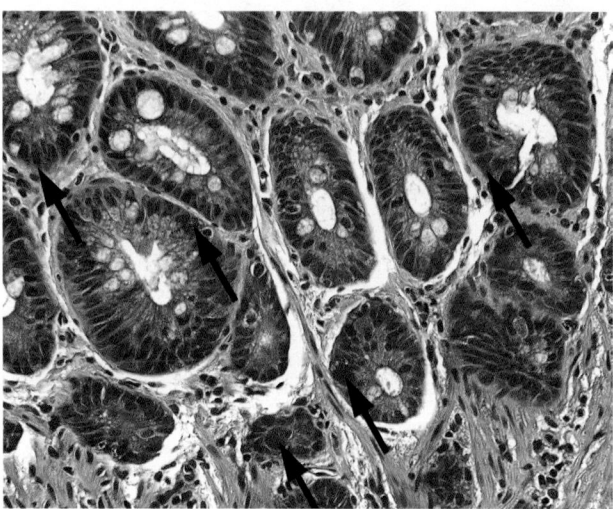

Figure 4-77. Hyperplastic polyp, microvesicular subtype. High power of the base of a microvesicular hyperplastic polyps shows narrowed crypt bases that lack serrations and prominent neuroendocrine cells (*arrows*), features common to all hyperplastic polyp subtypes.

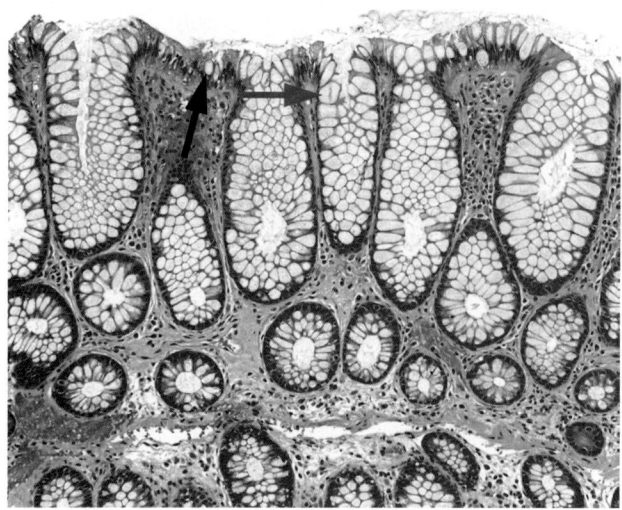

Figure 4-78. Hyperplastic polyp, goblet cell–rich subtype. Typical features include usually minimal surface serrations and prominent large back-to-back goblet cells. The large size of the lesional goblet cell (*red arrow*) is best appreciated after spotting a normal-sized goblet cell (*black arrow*) as a reference point. As is typical for hyperplastic polyps, narrowed crypt bases lacking serrations are seen.

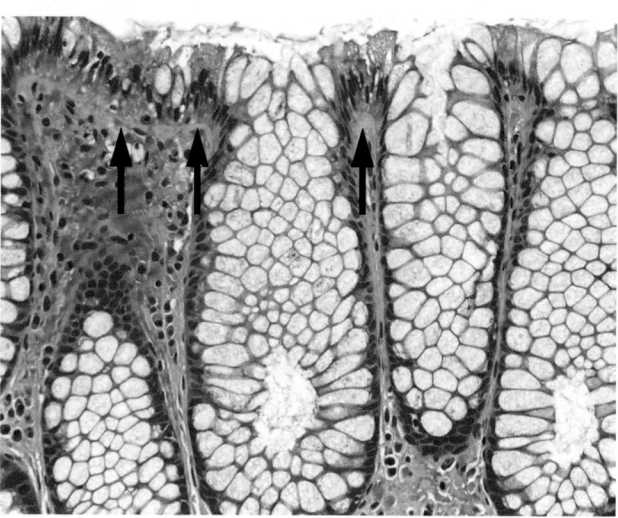

Figure 4-79. Hyperplastic polyp, goblet cell–rich subtype. Higher power of the previous figure. The prominent subepithelial collagen table is a reassuring clue to the diagnosis of hyperplastic polyp (*arrows*); the prominent goblet cells are clues to the diagnosis of goblet cell–rich subtype.

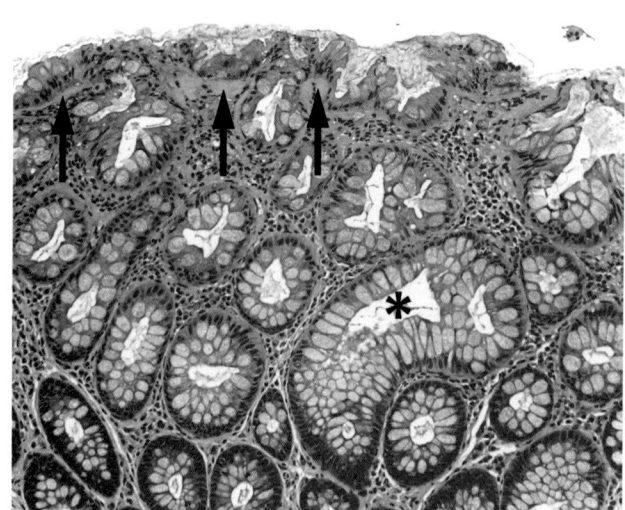

Figure 4-80. Hyperplastic polyp, goblet cell–rich subtype. Another low-power example showing the typical features of a goblet cell–rich subtype with its almost flat surface and prominent, large goblet cells. The single dilated crypt base (*asterisk*) is within the spectrum of a hyperplastic polyp in light of the lack of serrations, the presence of a prominent subepithelial collagen table (*arrows*), and based on the size and location of this 0.2-cm rectal polyp (Fig. 4.135).

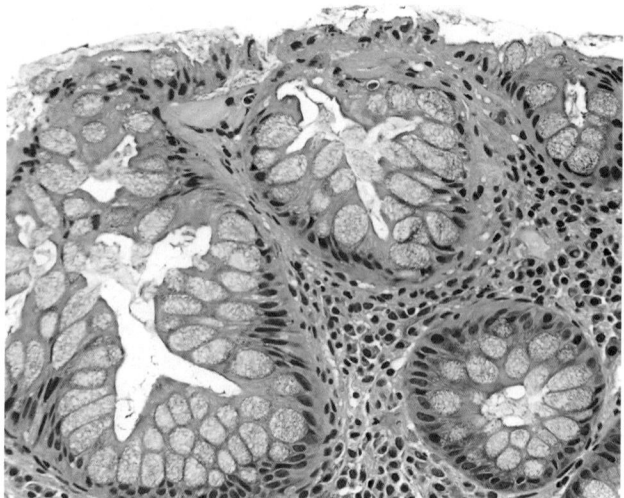

Figure 4-81. Hyperplastic polyp, goblet cell–rich subtype. Higher power of the previous figure shows the prominent subepithelial collagen table, large lesional goblet cells, and star-shaped crypt lumina.

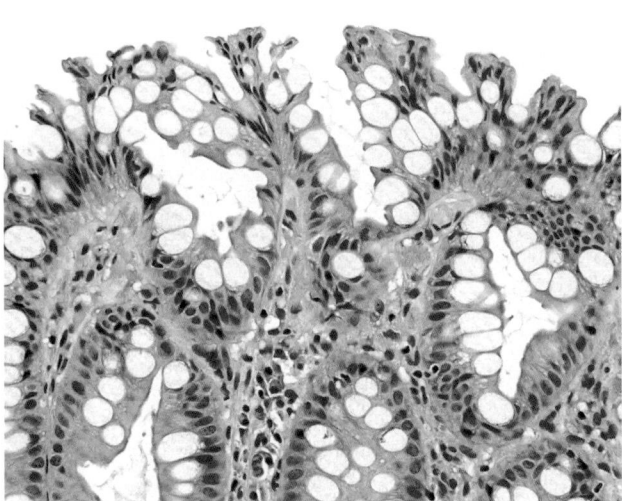

Figure 4-82. Hyperplastic polyp, goblet cell–rich subtype.

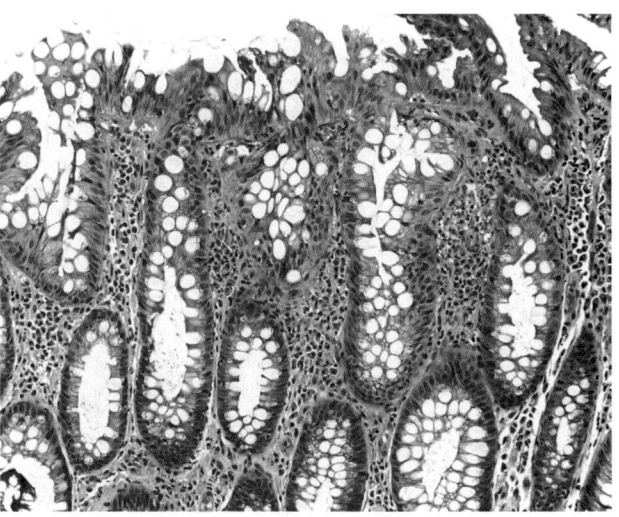

Figure 4-83. Hyperplastic polyp, goblet cell–rich subtype. Another typical example of the easy-to-miss goblet cell–rich subtype. If the biopsy is labeled as a rectosigmoid polyp and no obvious polyp is present, consider the goblet cell–rich hyperplastic polyp. This 0.3-cm rectal polyp shows minimal surface serrations with large goblet cells, narrowed crypt bases (not shown), and prominent neuroendo-crine cells (not shown).

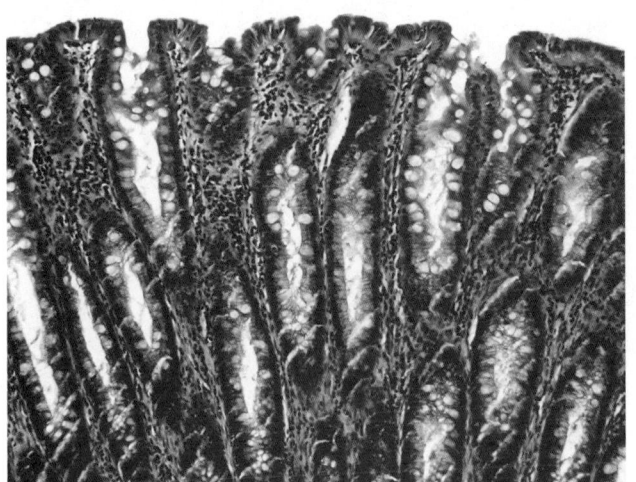

Figure 4-84. Hyperplastic polyp, mucin-poor subtype. This is a rarely encountered polyp. This particular example is a very thick section of a 0.2-cm rectal polyp. Although it is dark, the lesional cells are small and the basophilia is imparted by thick tissue and mucin loss.

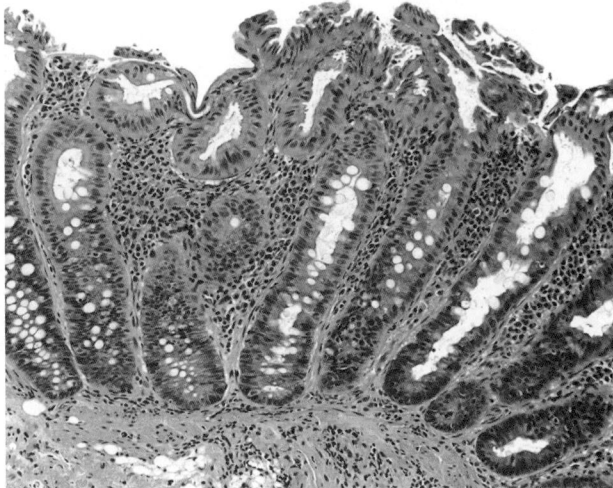

Figure 4-85. Hyperplastic polyp, mucin-poor subtype. Another example of a small sigmoid polyp. Surface serrations (top right) and narrowed crypt bases satisfy the criteria for a hyperplastic polyp, and the mucin-depleted lesional cells satisfy the criteria for the mucin-poor subtype. Although we do not subclassify for reporting purposes, it is useful to be aware of the spectrum of morphology.

no apparent diagnostic counterpart when you review the slide. The surface serrations are minimal, if at all present, and the lesional cells consist of back-to-back large goblet cells. The large size of the lesional goblet cell is best appreciated after spotting a normal-sized goblet cell in the adjoining nonpolypoid tissue as a reference point and the area in question is thicker than fragments that you are sure show normal mucosa. The mucin-poor subtype is the rarest subtype (Figs. 4.84–4.88). It often looks dark and can raise concerns for a TA. However, these polyps are not dysplastic. They merely appear dark because of mucin loss and the reactive and regenerative appearance of their nuclei. In contrast to dysplastic nuclei,

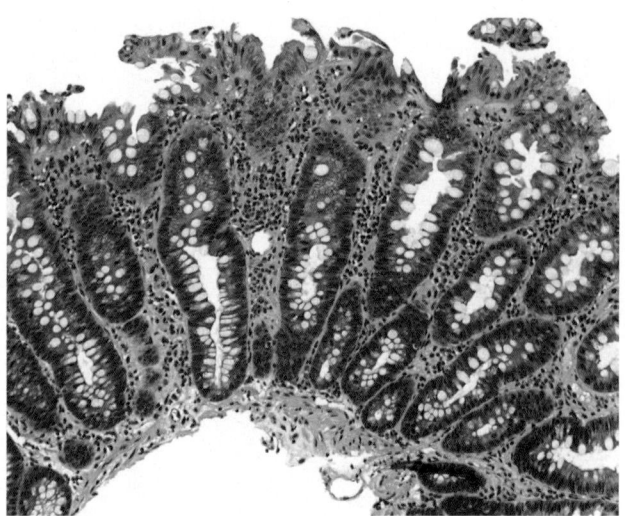

Figure 4-86. Hyperplastic polyp, mucin-poor subtype.

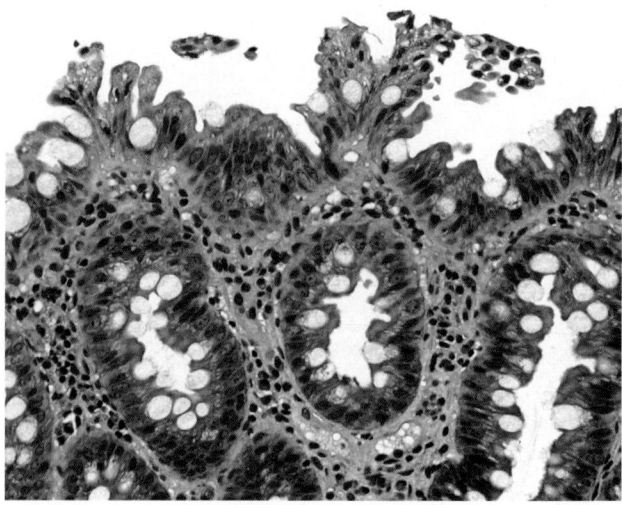

Figure 4-87. Hyperplastic polyp, mucin-poor subtype. Higher power of the previous figure. Although these lesions are characteristically dark, note that they are not dysplastic. These nuclei are tiny with light chromatin and lack pseudostratification, pleomorphism, and apoptotic bodies (compare with the usual features of the TA Figs.4.13–4.17).

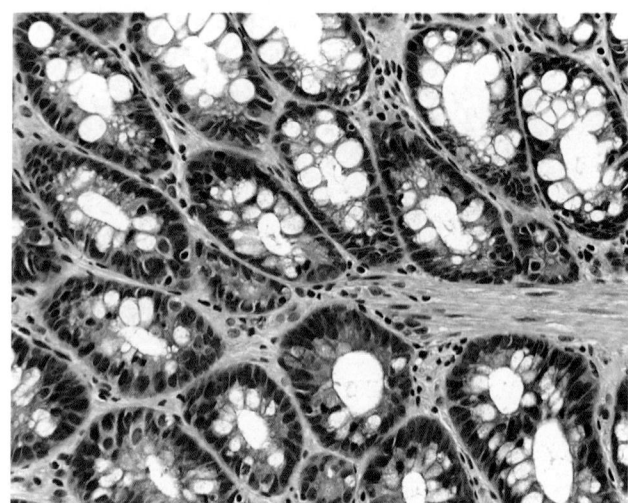

Figure 4-88. Hyperplastic polyp, mucin-poor subtype. Other reassuring features include a prominent subepithelial collagen table (not shown), narrowed crypt bases, and prominent neuroendocrine cells, as seen here.

these nuclei are tiny and lack pseudostratification and pleomorphism (compare with the usual features of the TA [Figs. 4.13–4.17]). Some theorize that the mucin-poor subtype is a damaged version of the microvesicular hyperplastic polyp.[24] Beware new game-changing guidelines: According to the 2012 Expert Recommendations, hyperplastic polyps >10 mm proximal to the sigmoid are clinically managed as SSA/P; all proximal serrated polyps should be fully excised; rectosigmoid serrated polyps >5 mm should be fully excised.[25]

See also Fig. 4.89 for a side-by-side comparison of normal versus the hyperplastic polyp subtypes and the following Pearls and Pitfalls to learn how these guidelines simplify the diagnostic approach.

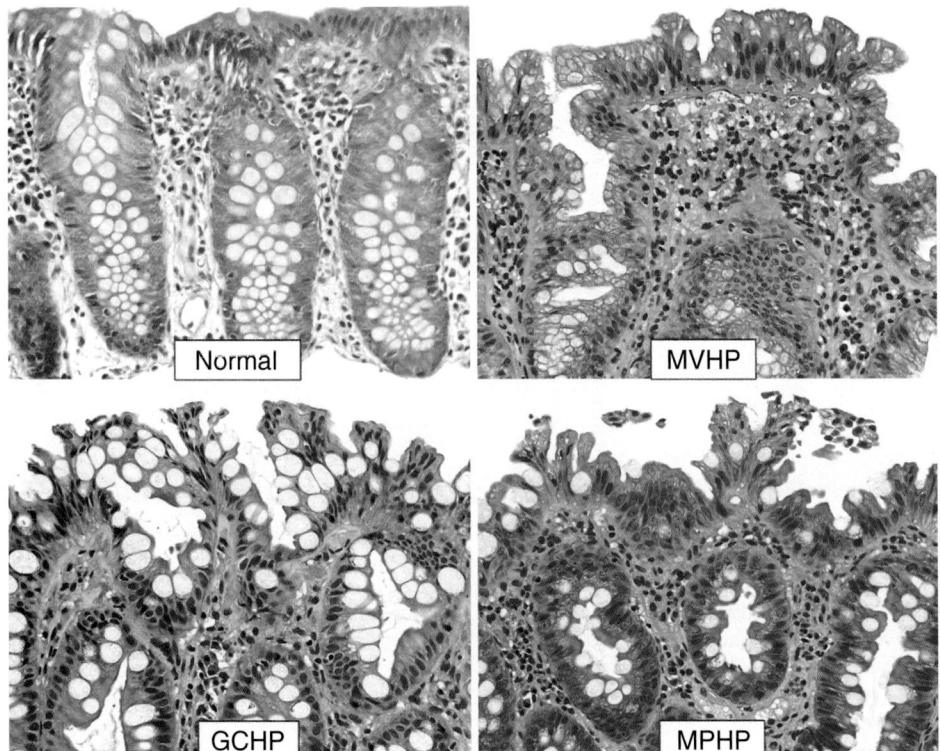

Figure 4-89. Composite of the hyperplastic polyp variants. Normal without hyperplastic polyp: colonic mucosa with a flat surface and nuclei with minimal cytoplasm. Defining features of hyperplastic polyps include a serrated surface and narrow crypt bases that lack serrations. Many have prominent subepithelial collagen table, increased neuroendocrine cells, and star-shaped crypt lumens. Microvesicular hyperplastic polyp (MVHP): distinctive delicate, frothy cytoplasm. Goblet cell–rich hyperplastic polyp (GCHP): prominent, large goblet cells. Mucin-poor hyperplastic polyp (MPHP): dark, regenerative appearance due to its loss of mucin.

PEARLS & PITFALLS: Avoid Overcalling the Proliferative Compartment of a Hyperplastic Polyp as a TA

Beware that the normal proliferative compartment of the hyperplastic polyp is an important mimic of a conventional adenoma. This compartment is normally dark with mitoses, slight hyperchromasia, and sometimes pseudostratification, but these changes do not involve the surface, and, therefore, are not dysplasia (compare the hyperplastic polyp proliferative compartment [Figs. 4.90–4.93] with the usual features of the TA [Figs. 4.13–4.17]).

PEARLS & PITFALLS: Avoid Undercalling Superficial Sections of a TA as the Proliferative Compartment of a Hyperplastic Polyp

Similarly, avoid overlooking a TA by assuming the dark center is always the proliferative compartment of a hyperplastic polyp. This undercall will lead to inappropriate management: a small hyperplastic polyp has a subsequent surveillance interval of 10 years, and a TA has a subsequent surveillance interval of 5 years.[4] Triggers to consider superficial sections of a TA include prominent apoptotic bodies, hyperchromasia greater than that typically seen in the proliferative compartment of a hyperplastic polyp, and the absence of a prominent subepithelial collagen table and neuroendocrine cells (Figs. 4.94–4.100). Deeper sections are enormously helpful in resolving these cases, as they may demonstrate that the atypical changes extend to the surface and thus satisfy the criteria for dysplasia.

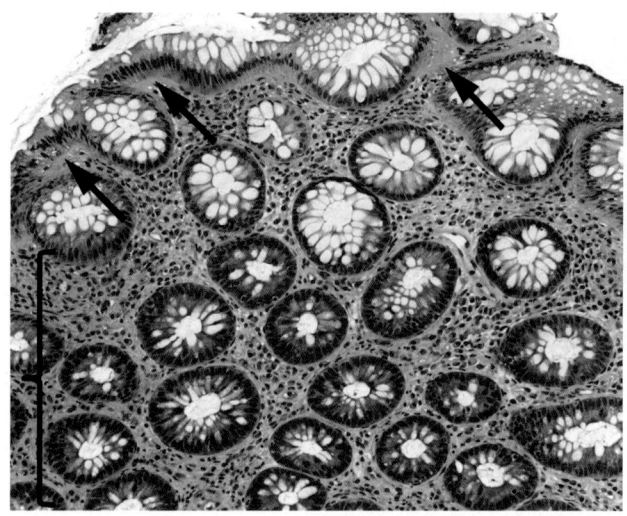

Figure 4-90. The normal proliferative compartment of a hyperplastic polyp, goblet cell–rich subtype. Occasionally, the normal proliferative compartment of the hyperplastic polyp is misdiagnosed as a TA. This compartment is responsible for normal cellular proliferation and is expected to be a bit dark with mitoses, slight hyperchromasia, and sometimes pseudostratification (*bracket*). Because these changes do not involve the surface, they are not dysplastic (compare with the usual features of the TA [Figs. 4.13–4.17]). The prominent subepithelial collagen table is another clue to the diagnosis of hyperplastic polyp (*arrows*).

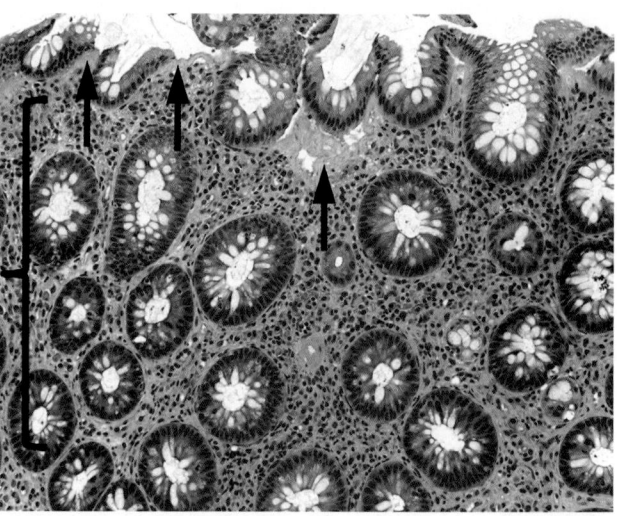

Figure 4-91. The normal proliferative compartment of a hyperplastic polyp, goblet cell–rich subtype. A separate case showing the slightly dark proliferative compartment (*bracket*) of a hyperplastic polyp. The prominent subepithelial collagen table is another clue to the diagnosis of hyperplastic polyp (*arrows*).

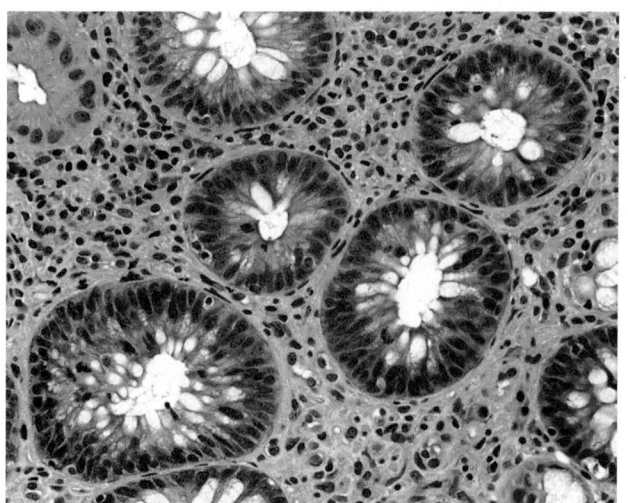

Figure 4-92. The normal proliferative compartment of a hyperplastic polyp, goblet cell–rich subtype. Higher power of the previous figure. Note the absence of prominent apoptotic bodies. In contrast, conventional adenomas have prominent apoptotic bodies (Fig. 4.17).

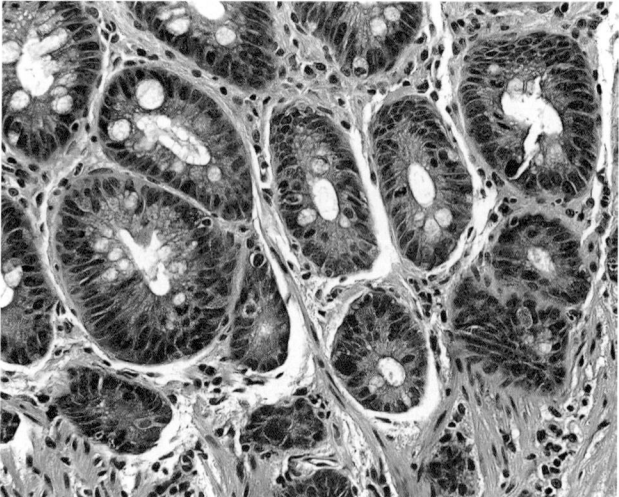

Figure 4-93. The normal proliferative compartment of a hyperplastic polyp, goblet cell–rich subtype. Higher power of another hyperplastic polyp's proliferative compartment. The prominent neuroendocrine cells and absent apoptotic bodies are reassuring features of a hyperplastic polyp (in addition to the surface serrations, not shown). If the atypical findings are concerning, deeper sections can often be helpful to demonstrate that the atypical changes do not extend to the surface.

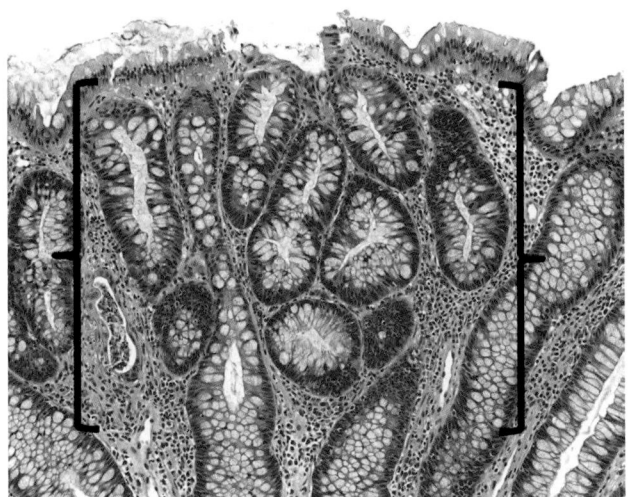

Figure 4-94. Superficial sections of a TA. Initial sections show atypia that does not definitively involve the surface (*brackets*). This focus represents either the proliferative compartment of a hyperplastic polyp or superficial sections of a TA. Features that favor that it is a TA include the qualitatively increased nuclear hyperchromasia and atypia over that expected for the normal proliferative compartment and the absence of a subepithelial collagen table.

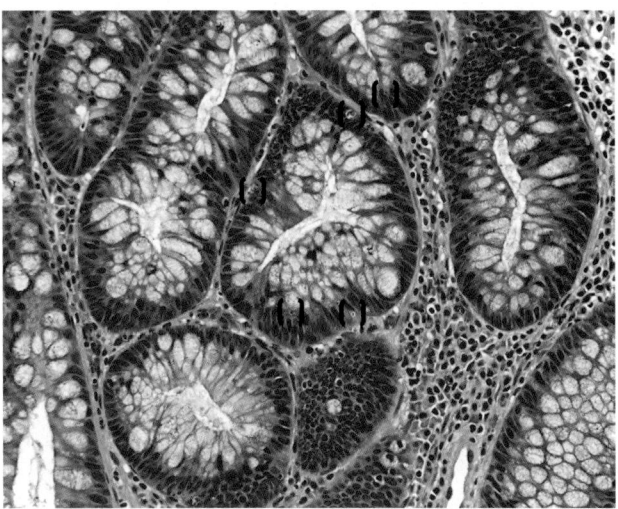

Figure 4-95. Superficial sections of a TA. Higher power of the previous figure shows prominent apoptotic bodies (*brackets*), further raising concerns for a TA.

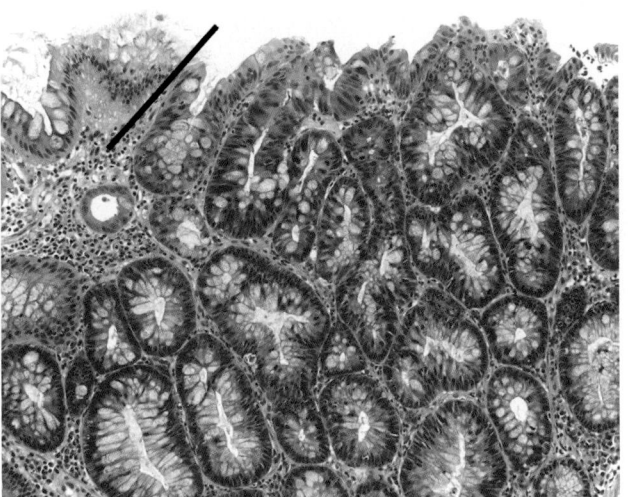

Figure 4-96. Superficial sections of a TA. Deeper sections of the previous figure demonstrate definitive surface involvement by the prominent hyperchromasia, pseudostratified nuclei, and an abrupt transition between normal and atypia (*line*). As a result, this case was signed out as a TA.

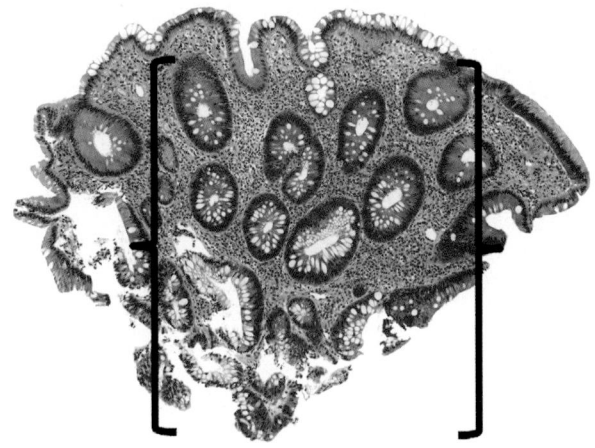

Figure 4-97. Superficial sections of a TA. This case had been previously signed out as a hyperplastic polyp, presumably because the atypia seems to be mostly beneath the serrated epithelium (*brackets*).

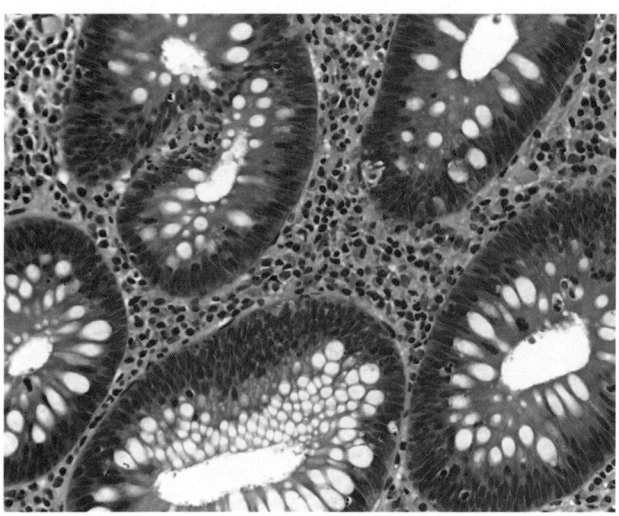

Figure 4-98. Superficial sections of a TA. Higher power of the previous figure shows prominent apoptotic bodies, clues to a diagnosis of a TA.

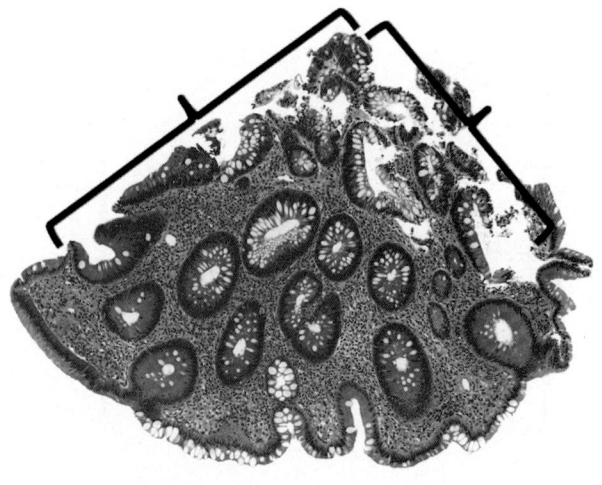

Figure 4-99. Superficial sections of a TA. Upon rotating the polyp, it is easier to see that the atypia does extend to the surface (*brackets*), supporting the revised diagnosis of a TA.

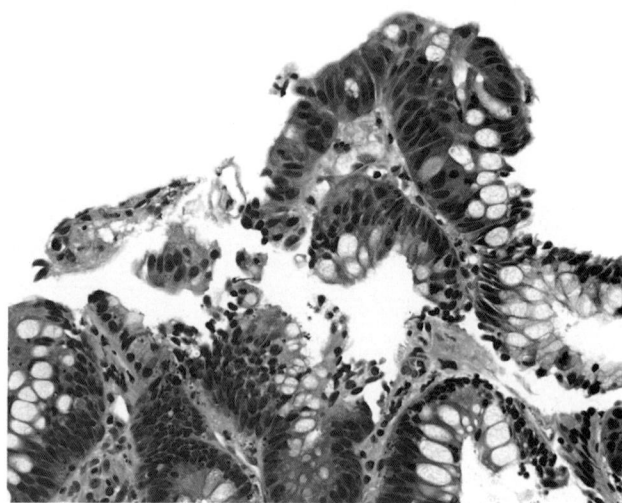

Figure 4-100. Superficial sections of a TA. Higher power of the previous figure.

Sessile Serrated Adenomas/Polyps

Here is where this topic gets a lot more interesting. Most serrated polyps were just hyperplastic polyps until 1996, when investigators noted an association with adenocarcinoma in patients with these historically benign, previously diagnosed "hyperplastic polyps."[26] Investigators pursued thorough studies of these peculiar serrated polyps and eventually reclassified a subset as sessile serrated adenomas/polyps[24,26] to acknowledge their malignant potential and help ensure appropriate clinical management. Today, SSA/P comprise approximately 11% of all serrated polyps, making the difficult issue of distinguishing hyperplastic polyps from SSA/P a daily occurrence.[2] Both hyperplastic polyps and SSA/P appear pale pink because of the abundant pale cytoplasm, and both have surface serrations (Table 4.3). As of 2012, the minimum diagnostic criterion for the SSA/P changed to requiring "at least one unequivocal architecturally distorted, dilated, and/or horizontally branched crypt, particularly if it is associated with inverted maturation."[25] An unequivocally diagnostic crypt base is dilated with serrations that are out of proportion to those associated with confounding factors such as mucosal prolapse, absent muscularis mucosae, or tangential or superficial sections. Although SSA/Ps are typically large and proximal colon predominant, one unequivocal distorted crypt base is sufficient for a diagnosis of SSA/P in a polyp of any size and at any site. For example, Figs. 4.101–4.116 qualify for a diagnosis of SSA/P based on an unequivocal crypt base(s), even if the polyp were a 0.2-cm rectal polyp.

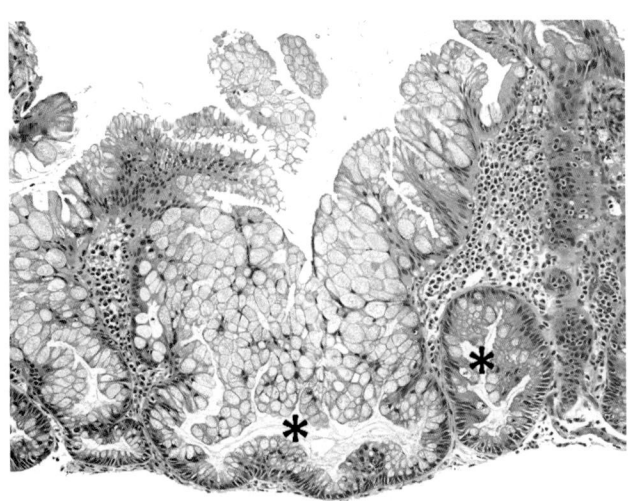

Figure 4-101. Sessile serrated adenoma/polyp (SSA/P). SSA/Ps have a serrated surface, lack a prominent subepithelial collagen table and neuroendocrine cells, and have at least one unequivocal architecturally distorted, dilated, and/or horizontally branched crypt (*asterisks*). This polyp would be classified as an SSA/P regardless of location or size based on this typical histology.

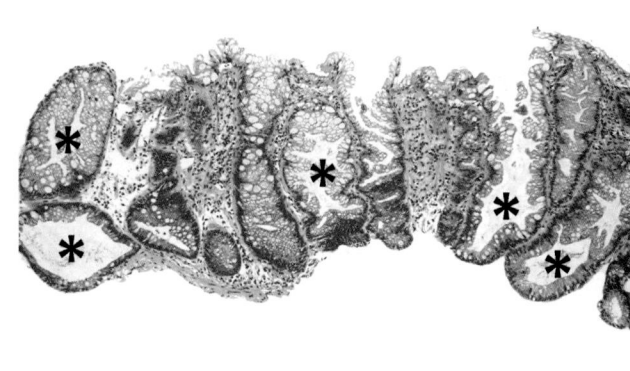

Figure 4-102. Sessile serrated adenoma/polyp. "Unequivocal crypt bases" are both dilated and contain serrations (*asterisks*), as seen in this example.

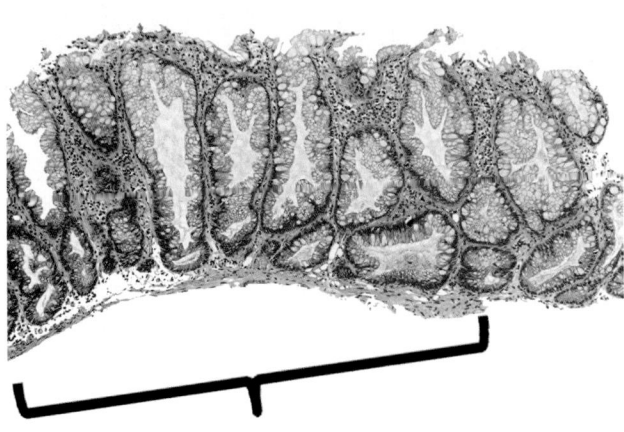
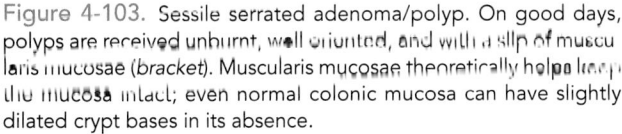

Figure 4-103. Sessile serrated adenoma/polyp. On good days, polyps are received unburnt, well oriented, and with a slip of muscularis mucosae (*bracket*). Muscularis mucosae theoretically helps keep the mucosa intact; even normal colonic mucosa can have slightly dilated crypt bases in its absence.

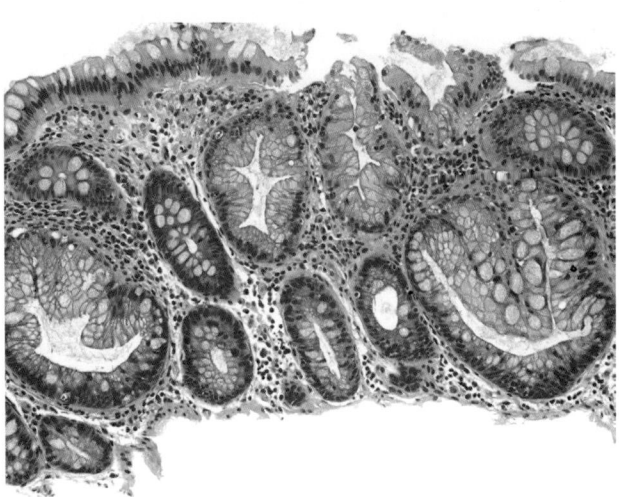

Figure 4-104. Sessile serrated adenoma/polyp. Compared with hyperplastic polyps, SSA/Ps are larger and more common in the proximal colon.

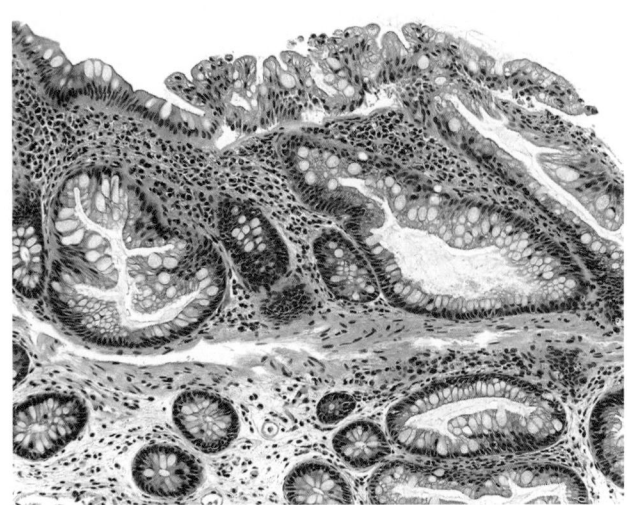

Figure 4-105. Sessile serrated adenoma/polyp. A minimum of only one unequivocal aberrant crypt base is needed to satisfy the minimum diagnostic criteria for the SSA/P.

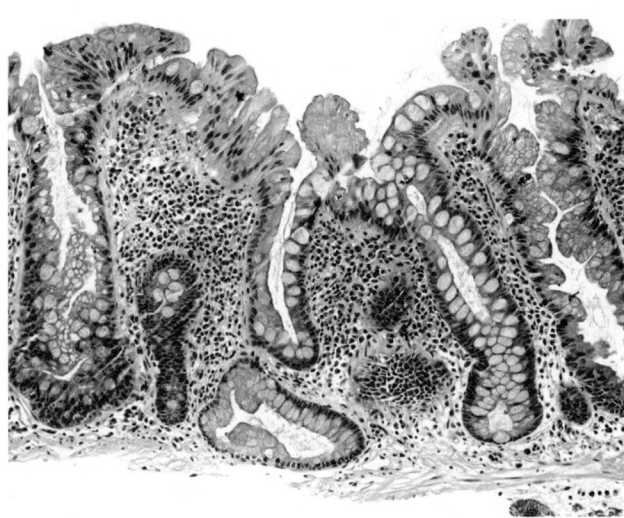

Figure 4-106. Sessile serrated adenoma/polyp.

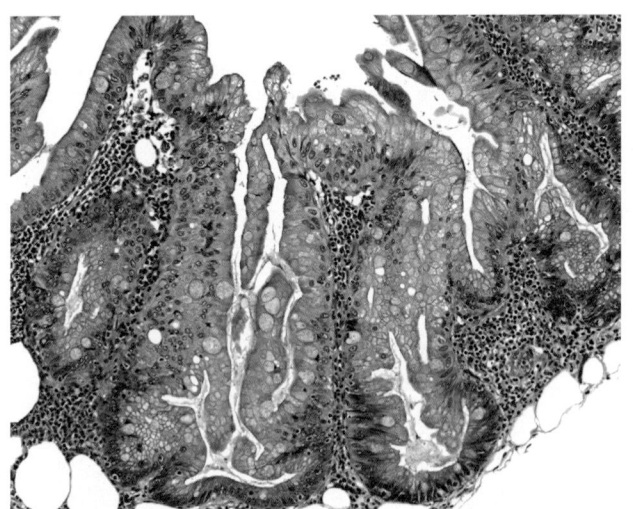

Figure 4-107. Sessile serrated adenoma/polyp.

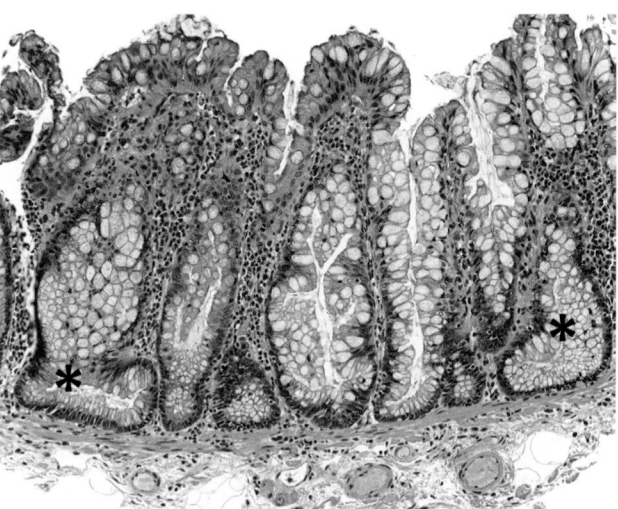

Figure 4-108. Sessile serrated adenoma/polyp. Other helpful features of unequivocal crypt bases include these examples of crypts that appear boot shaped or J-, L-, or inverted T-shaped because the crypt base extends horizontally along the muscularis mucosae (*asterisks*).

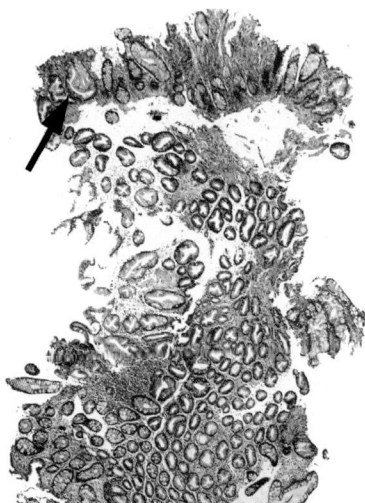

Figure 4-109. An unequivocal distorted crypt base diagnostic of an SSA/P. This 0.4-cm cecal polyp was submitted with a prior diagnosis of hyperplastic polyp. Although this is a small polyp, it is an SSA/P based on the single unequivocally distorted crypt base (*arrow*).

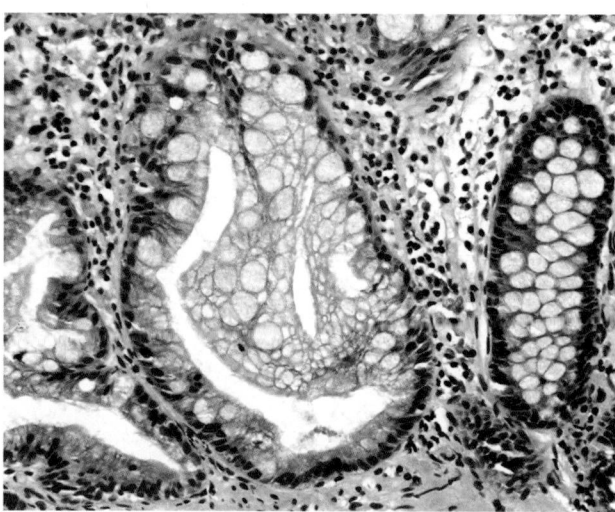

Figure 4-110. An unequivocal distorted crypt base diagnostic of an SSA/P. Higher power of the previous figure shows the requisite single unequivocally distorted crypt base necessary for the revised diagnosis of SSA/P.

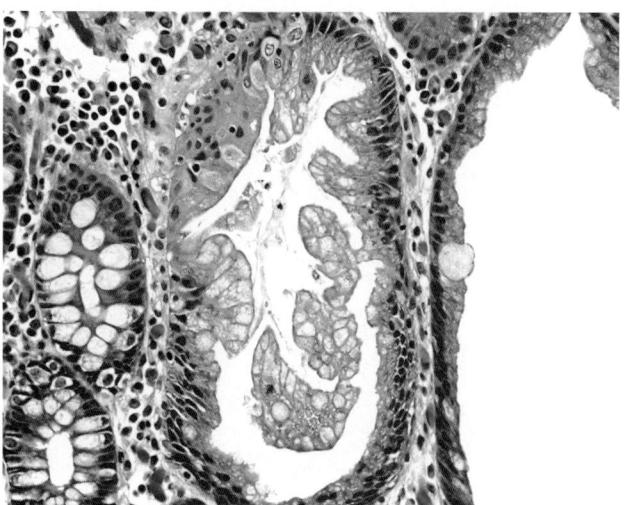

Figure 4-111. An unequivocal distorted crypt base diagnostic of an SSA/P. An unequivocally distorted crypt base is dilated and contains serrations, as seen here.

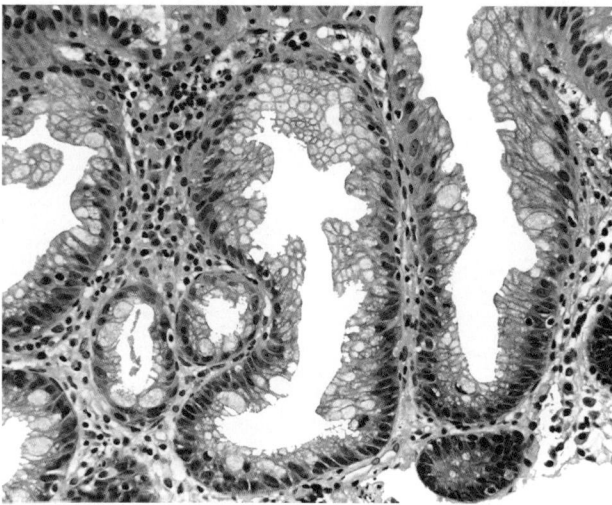

Figure 4-112. An unequivocal distorted crypt base diagnostic of an SSA/P. As seen here, an unequivocally distorted crypt base often is boot-shaped or J-, L-, or inverted T-shaped because the crypt base extends horizontally along the muscularis mucosae.

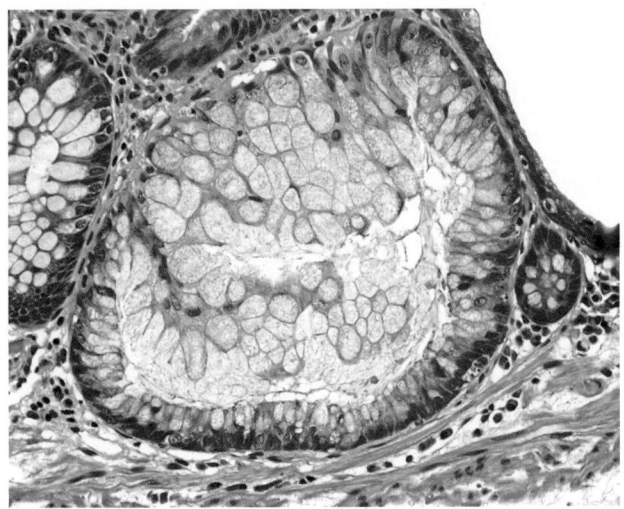

Figure 4-113. An unequivocal distorted crypt base diagnostic of an SSA/P.

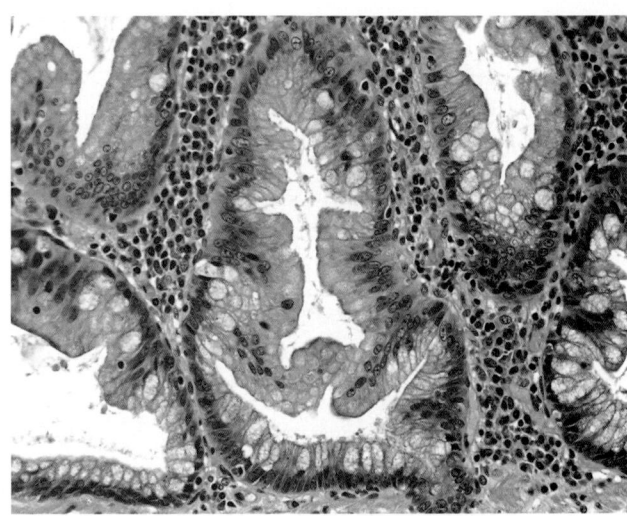

Figure 4-114. An unequivocal distorted crypt base diagnostic of an SSA/P.

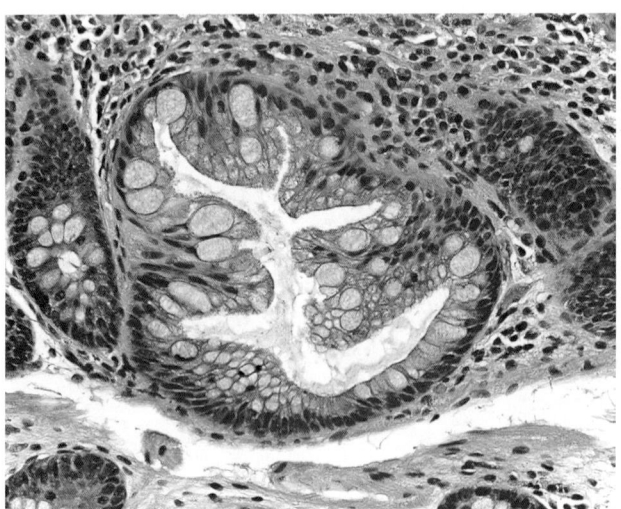

Figure 4-115. An unequivocal distorted crypt base diagnostic of an SSA/P.

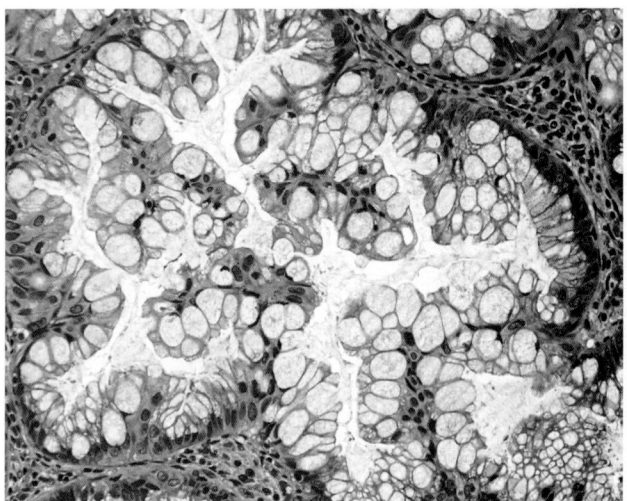

Figure 4-116. An unequivocal distorted crypt base diagnostic of an SSA/P. An unequivocally distorted crypt base justifies the diagnosis of SSA/P regardless of the polyp's site or size. Although SSA/Ps are usually large and in the proximal colon, this crypt base would justify a diagnosis of SSA/P in a polyp of any site or size.

The term unequivocal sounds straightforward, but it is not. This sentiment is confirmed in the subsequent sentence that follows the minimum SSA/P criteria in the 2012 consensus recommendations: "In clinical practice, there is substantial interobserver variation among pathologists in the differentiation of SSA/P from HP, and agreement between pathologists is moderate at best, including between experts."[25] Examples of *equivocal* distorted crypts include slightly dilated crypts that lack serrations and slightly dilated crypts that are in proportion to the background mucosal prolapse or absent muscularis mucosae (Figs. 4.117–4.122). Other examples of equivocal serrated polyps include those associated with prominent mucosal prolapse, large

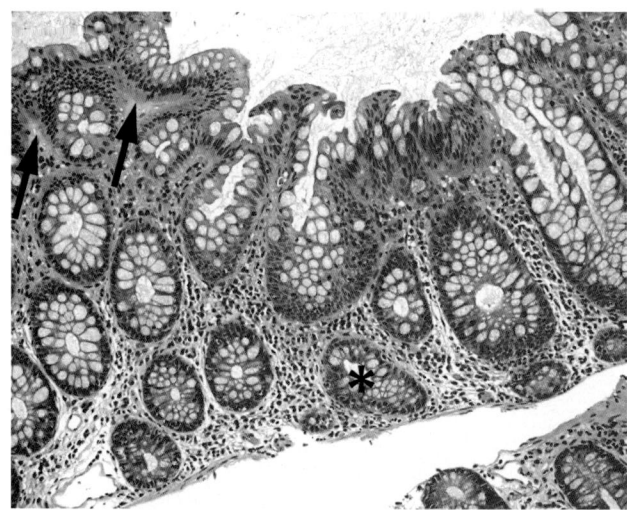

Figure 4-117. An equivocal distorted crypt in a hyperplastic polyp, goblet cell–rich subtype. This example of a 0.3-cm rectal polyp shows a small dilated crypt base (*asterisk*). The crypt is equivocal because, although it is slightly dilated, it lacks serrations. Based on the small size, distal location, and focally prominent subepithelial collagen table (*arrows*), this polyp is best classified as a hyperplastic polyp.

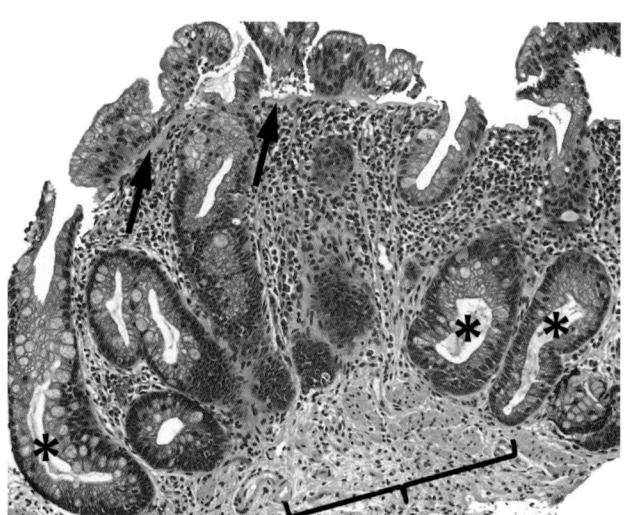

Figure 4-118. Equivocal distorted crypts in a hyperplastic polyp, microvesicular subtype. This 0.2-cm rectal polyp was previously diagnosed as an SSA/P. The crypts are equivocally dilated (*asterisks*) because there are no serrations, and the dilatation is in proportion to the prolapse (*bracket*). This tiny rectal polyp is best classified as a hyperplastic polyp based on its size, location, prominent subepithelial collagen table (*arrows*) and equivocally distorted crypt bases in proportion to the background prolapse. This exact polyp in the proximal colon would be diagnosed as a serrated polyp with features of both SSA/P and hyperplastic polyp based on the lower SSA/P threshold in the proximal colon. If site was not submitted, the polyp would have been classified as serrated polyp. Note: The classification depends on the polyp location. If the polyp arose in the left, descending, sigmoid, or rectum, it is a hyperplastic polyp. If the polyp arose in the right, cecum, ascending, or transverse colon, it is a serrated polyp with features of an SSA/P and hyperplastic polyp.

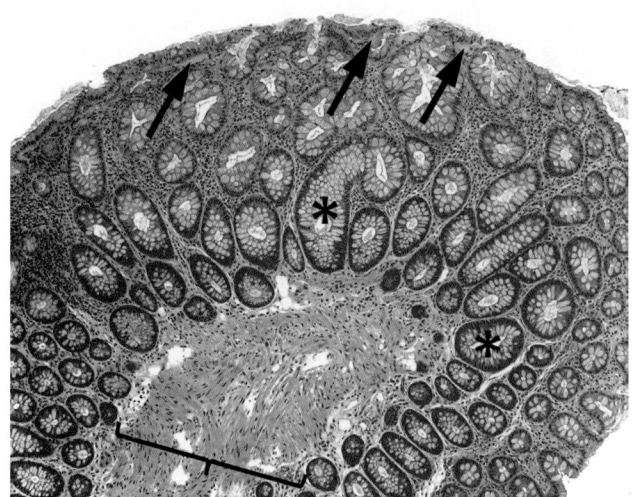

Figure 4-119. Equivocal distorted crypts in a hyperplastic polyp, goblet cell–rich subtype. This 0.3-cm rectal polyp was also initially misdiagnosed as an SSA/P. Similar to those in the prior case, the crypts are equivocally distorted because there are no serrations (*asterisks*) and there is mucosal prolapse (*bracket*). This tiny rectal polyp is best classified as a hyperplastic polyp based on its size, location, prominent subepithelial collagen table (*arrows*) and equivocally dilated crypt bases in proportion to the background prolapse.

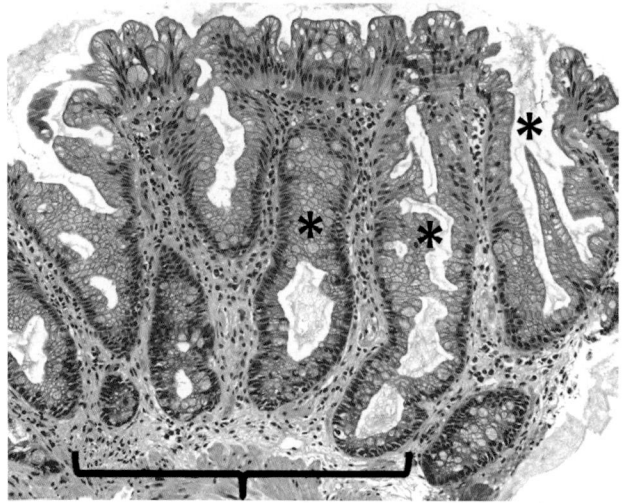

Figure 4-120. Equivocal distorted crypts in a hyperplastic polyp, microvesicular subtype. This 0.2-cm rectal polyp case is another example of an overcalled SSA/P. Only equivocal crypt dilatation is seen, which is in proportion to the associated prolapse in the distal colon. The tops of the crypts have serrations (*asterisks*), but they do not count for an SSA/P because they do not extend to the crypt base (*bracket*). Based on the polyp size, location, prominent subepithelial collagen table, and background prolapse, this polyp is best classified as a hyperplastic polyp in the rectum. This exact polyp in the proximal colon would be diagnosed as a serrated polyp with features of both SSA/P and hyperplastic polyp based on the lower SSA/P threshold in the proximal colon.

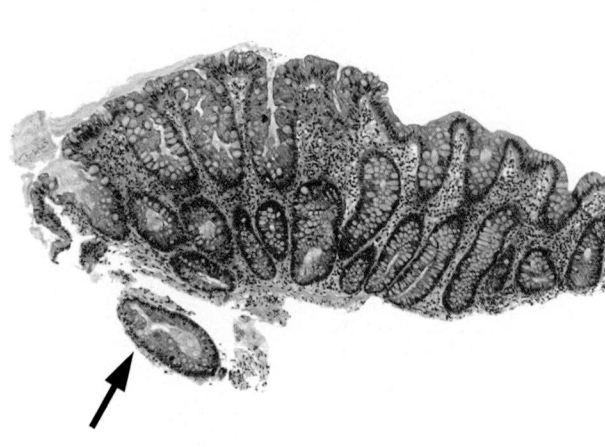

Figure 4-121. An equivocal distorted crypt in a hyperplastic polyp, microvesicular subtype. This small rectal polyp illustrates that colonic mucosa not tethered to a muscularis mucosae can appear artifactually dilated. Such examples are only equivocal and insufficient for a diagnosis of SSA/P in small rectal polyps (*arrow*). This exact polyp in the proximal colon would be diagnosed as a serrated polyp with features of both SSA/P and hyperplastic polyp based on the lower SSA/P threshold in the proximal colon.

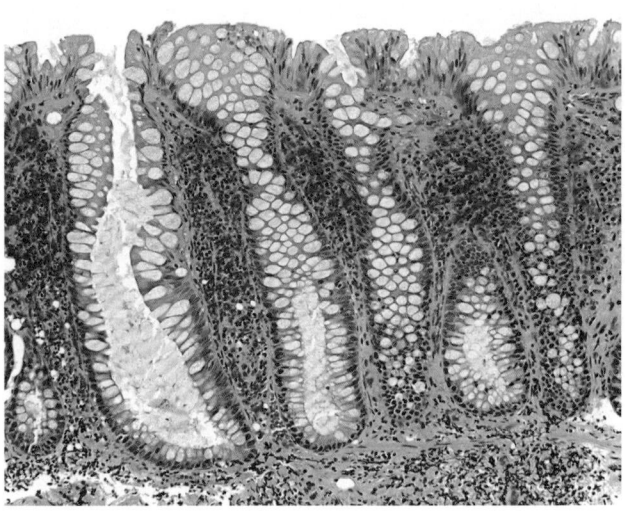

Figure 4-122. Equivocal distorted crypts in a hyperplastic polyp, microvesicular subtype. This small rectal polyp has only equivocal crypt dilatations (no serrations present in the crypt base) and is best classified as a hyperplastic polyp.

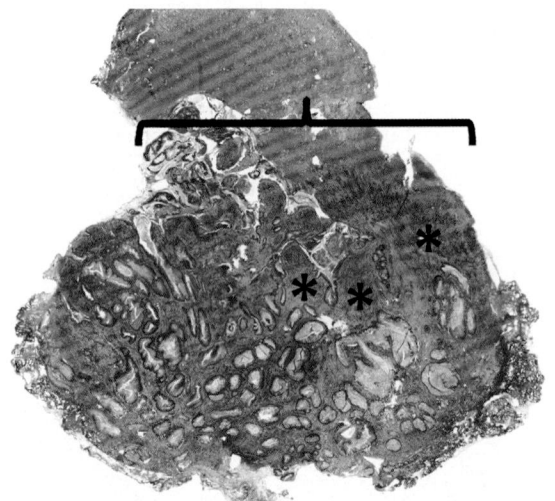

Figure 4-123. Equivocally distorted crypts in a hyperplastic polyp with prominent prolapse. This is a 0.5-cm rectal polyp with heavy cautery artifact. It was initially misdiagnosed as an SSA/P based on the dilated crypts seen throughout. Note the erosion (*bracket*) and prominent *pink* lamina propria (*asterisks*).

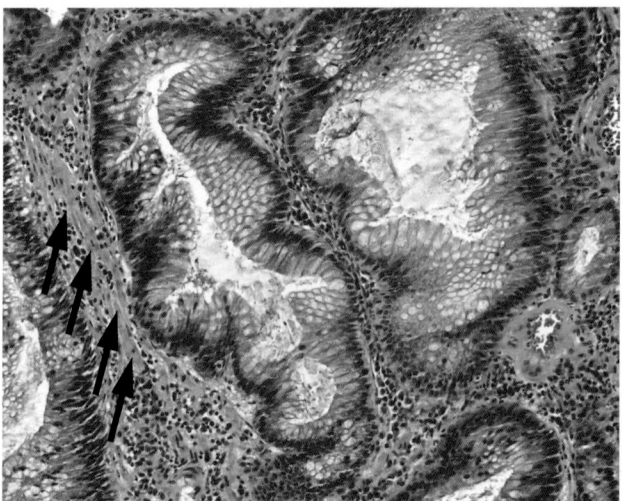

Figure 4-124. Equivocally distorted crypts in a hyperplastic polyp with prominent prolapse. Higher power of the previous figure shows the prominent smooth muscle ingrowth (*arrows*) characteristic of mucosal prolapse. Normal colonic mucosa is devoid of smooth muscle ingrowth into the lamina propria (Fig. 4.8). In this case, the crypt dilatation is in proportion to the prolapse and insufficient for the diagnosis of an SSA/P. Based on the size, location, and equivocal crypt dilatation, this lesion was ultimately classified as a hyperplastic polyp with prominent prolapse. Note that this exact polyp in the proximal colon would be diagnosed as a serrated polyp with features of SSA/P, hyperplastic polyp, and prolapse based on the lower SSA/P threshold in the proximal colon.

serrated polyps over 1.0 cm, and those that are tangentially embedded (Figs. 4.123–4.134). In these imperfect, real-life scenarios, polyp site and size are used to render a useful diagnosis (Fig. 4.135). In general, for serrated polyps, it is good practice to give preference to SSA/P in the proximal colon, hyperplastic polyp in the distal colon, and simply "serrated polyp, not further classified" in the remaining minority of cases. A diagnosis of serrated polyp, not further classified

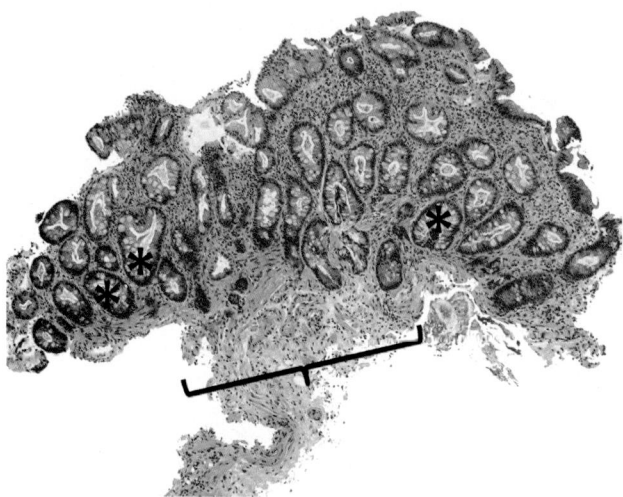

Figure 4-125. Equivocally distorted crypts in a hyperplastic polyp with prominent prolapse. Another case initially misdiagnosed as a rectal SSA/P based on an overcall of the equivocally dilated crypt bases (*asterisks*). The crypt base dilatation is equivocal because it is in proportion to the background prolapse (*bracket*).

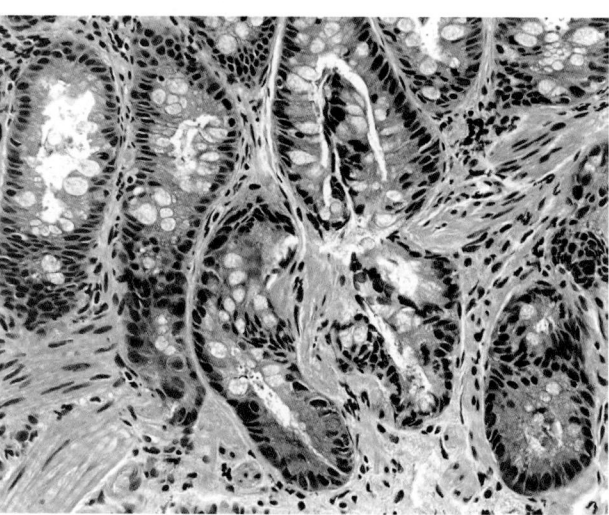

Figure 4-126. Equivocally distorted crypts in a hyperplastic polyp with prominent prolapse. Higher power of the previous figure shows squished crypts herniating through the prolapsed muscle. The prominent neuroendocrine cells are a reassuring feature of a hyperplastic polyp and not seen in SSA/P.

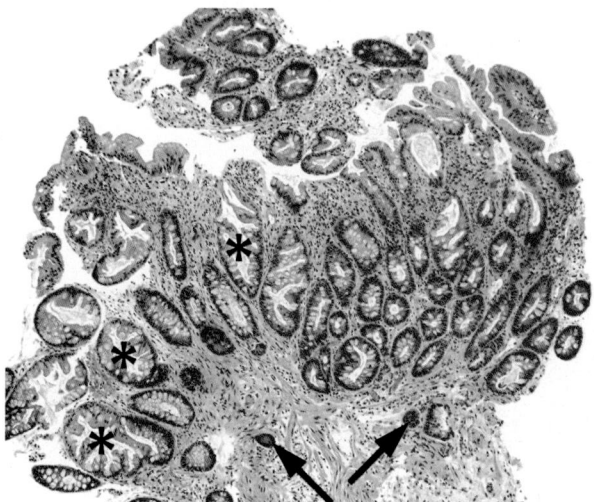

Figure 4-127. Equivocally distorted crypts in a hyperplastic polyp with prominent prolapse. The dilatation is equivocal because the serrated dilated crypts are superficial (*asterisks*), there is prominent smooth muscle ingrowth, and crypts are seen herniating into the smooth muscle ingrowth (*arrows*). Based on the size, site, equivocal crypt dilatation, and prolapse, this case was diagnosed as a hyperplastic polyp with prolapse. This exact polyp in the proximal colon would be diagnosed as a serrated polyp with features of SSA/P, hyperplastic polyp, and prolapse based on the lower SSA/P threshold in the proximal colon

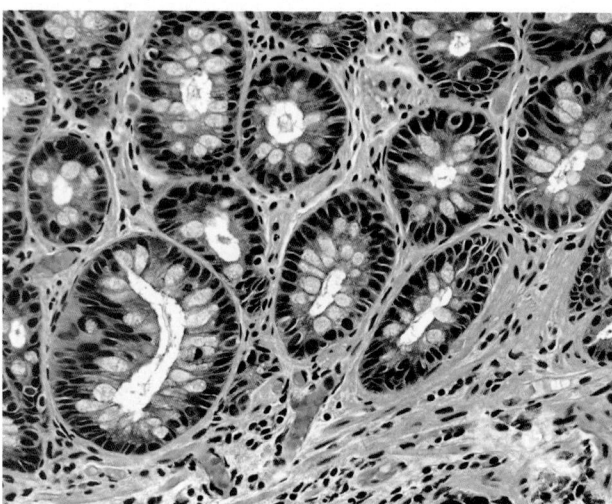

Figure 4-128. Equivocally distorted crypts in a hyperplastic polyp with prominent prolapse. Higher power of the previous figure shows squished crypts, prominent smooth muscle, and increased neuroendocrine cells, supporting the diagnosis of hyperplastic polyp with prolapse.

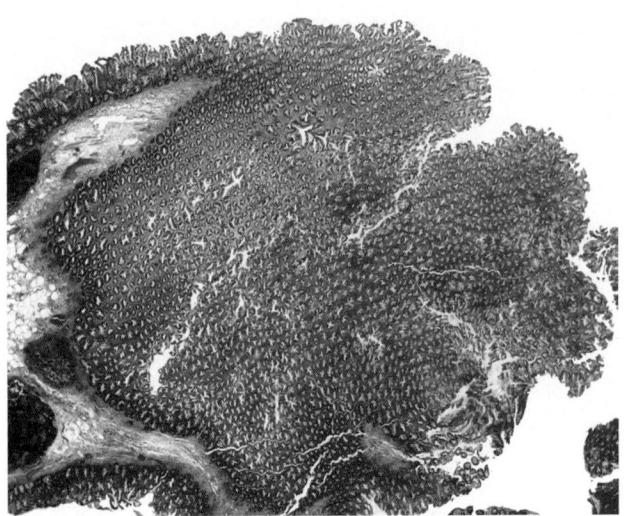

Figure 4-129. Equivocally distorted crypts in a 1.5-cm proximal serrated polyp. Based on size and site this should be an SSA/P, but there is no unequivocal crypt dilatation. Imperfect cases such as these are best diagnosed with proper management in mind. Based on the discussed 2012 recommendations, hyperplastic polyps more than 10 mm in the proximal colon are clinically managed as per SSA/P. As such, this case was diagnosed as a serrated polyp with features of SSA/P (size and site) and hyperplastic polyp (morphology). The same diagnosis would have been rendered in the distal colon based on the size. This diagnosis will prompt follow-up as per SSA/P in most centers.

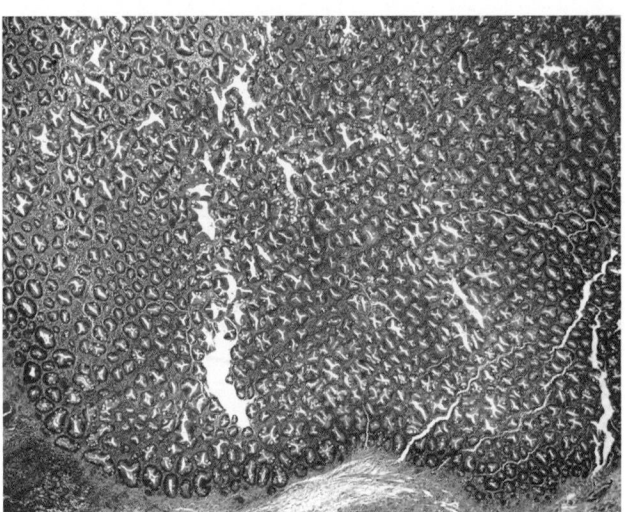

Figure 4-130. Equivocally distorted crypts in a 1.5-cm proximal serrated polyp. Higher power of the previous figure. The crypt bases are equivocally dilated because they contain no serrations. However, a hyperplastic polyp should be less than 0.5 cm and must have perfect morphology in the proximal colon.

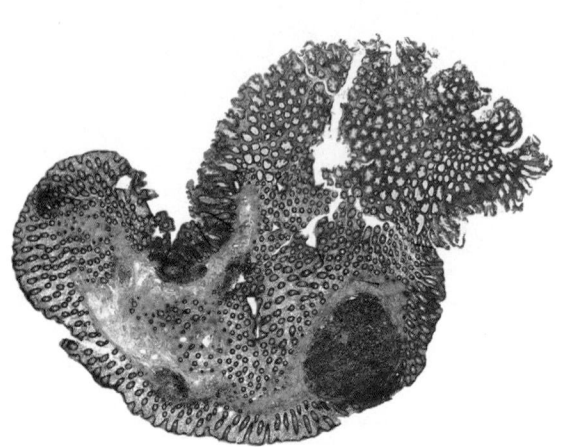

Figure 4-131. Equivocally distorted crypts in a 1.0-cm proximal serrated polyp. This case resembles the Twitter bird logo. It was also signed out as a serrated polyp with features of SSA/P (size and site) and hyperplastic polyp (morphology). The same diagnosis would have been rendered in the distal colon based on the size.

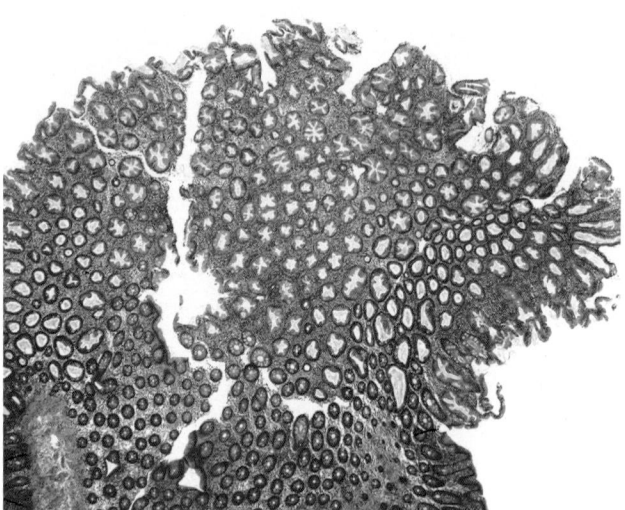

Figure 4-132. Equivocally distorted crypts in a 1.0-cm proximal serrated polyp. Higher power of the previous figure. In one of the author's first years of practice (CAA), she routinely delayed the case a day to cut deeper into the block until she inevitably found the unequivocal crypt dilatation in large, proximal serrated polyps to satisfy the diagnosis of SSA/P. Now, she releases such cases without deeper sections and report them descriptively as "serrated polyp with features of SSA/P." Because a diagnosis of serrated polyp with features of SSA/P is managed as an SSA/P in most centers, deeper sections do not change management. Skipping on the deeper sections saves time and resources for the laboratory, clinician, and patient.

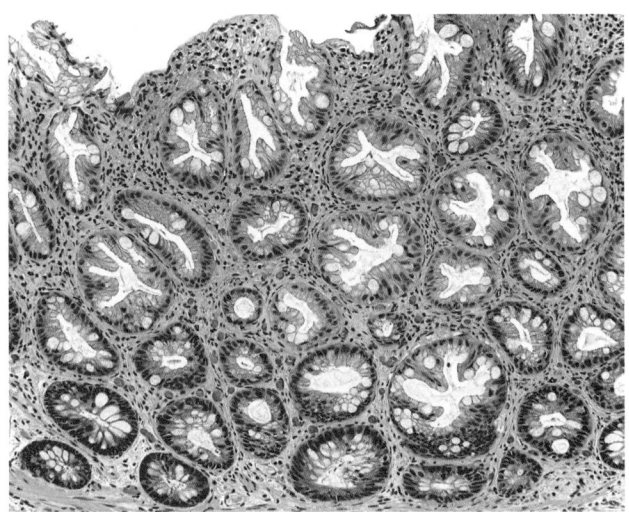

Figure 4-133. Equivocally distorted crypts in a 0.5-cm cecal serrated polyp. Based on its size, location, and morphology, it was signed out as a serrated polyp with features of SSA/P and hyperplastic polyp.

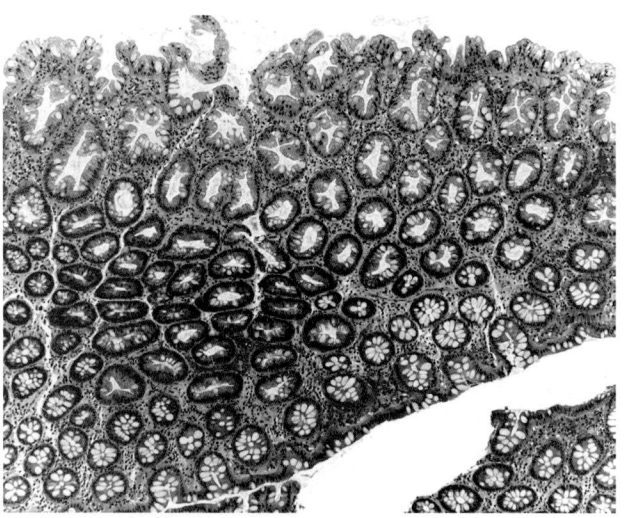

Figure 4-134. Equivocally distorted crypts in a 0.6-cm rectal serrated polyp. Tangential sections are another common reason for the descriptive diagnosis of serrated polyp with features of both SSA/P and hyperplastic polyp, as in this case. This case features surface on three aspects of the small rectal polyp (not shown), such that the crypt bases are not visible, precluding a more definitive diagnosis.

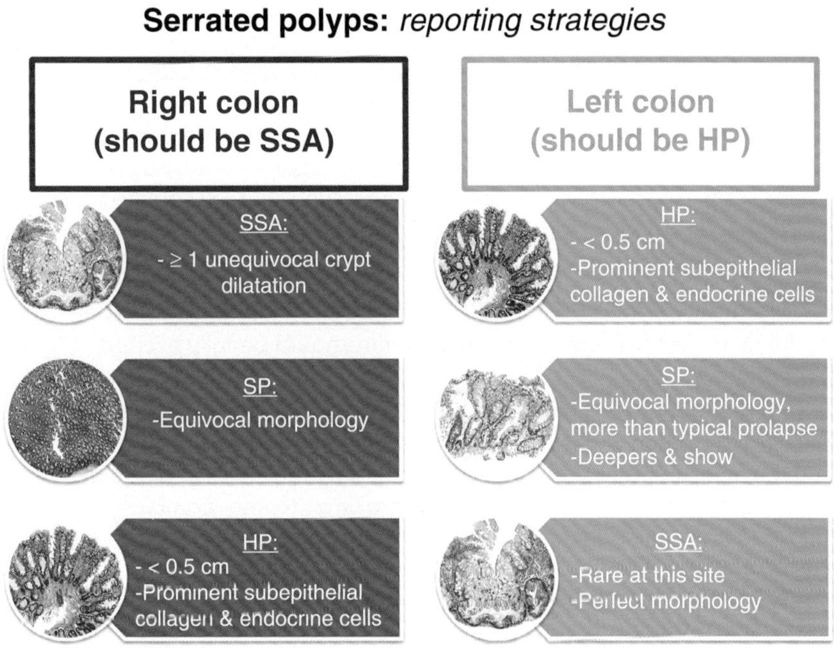

Serrated polyps: *reporting strategies*

Right colon (should be SSA)

SSA:
- ≥ 1 unequivocal crypt dilatation

SP:
-Equivocal morphology

HP:
- < 0.5 cm
-Prominent subepithelial collagen & endocrine cells

Left colon (should be HP)

HP:
- < 0.5 cm
-Prominent subepithelial collagen & endocrine cells

SP:
-Equivocal morphology, more than typical prolapse
-Deepers & show

SSA:
-Rare at this site
-Perfect morphology

Figure 4-135. A practical diagnostic algorithm for approaching serrated polyps. In brief, SSA/Ps are more common than hyperplastic polyps in the proximal colon (right, cecum, ascending, and transverse colon), larger in size, and lack a subepithelial collagen table and prominent neuroendocrine cells. Well-oriented serrated polyps with perfect SSA/P morphology are diagnosed as SSA/P, regardless of site. Similarly, serrated polyps with perfect hyperplastic polyp morphology are diagnosed as a hyperplastic polyp, regardless of site in well-oriented tissue cut sufficiently deep. Unfortunately, most serrated polyps have imperfect morphology, and many are not submitted with site designation. A low threshold for an SSA/P is recommended in the proximal colon based on its typical distribution, and a high threshold for SSA/P is recommended in the left colon based on the probability of confounding prolapse. For these imperfect cases, the term serrated polyp is used. Deeper sections and sharing with a colleague can be helpful because this diagnosis results in management as per SSA/P in most centers.

will be followed as per an SSA/P in most centers. Distal SSA/P and proximal HP exist, but their morphology at these atypical sites must be perfect in well-oriented tissue that is cut sufficiently deeply. Admittedly, some of the unpleasantness of serrated polyps is because the diagnosis does not rest solely on morphology. This imperfect approach to these imperfect polyps hopefully simplifies the diagnostic approach and helps with the ultimate goal of preventing CRC. See the following Pearls and Pitfalls and FAQ for more on this approach.

FAQ: Which term is correct—Sessile serrated adenoma (SSA) or sessile serrated polyp (SSP)?

Answer: Practice patterns differ at different centers, but according to the 2010 WHO both terms are correct and can be used interchangeably.[22] Some pathologists are passionate about one term over the other, depending on where they trained and their personal experience. Those who prefer SSA prefer to include the designation of adenoma to ensure proper clinical management because clinicians universally understand that adenoma has malignant potential. Those who prefer SSP are nomenclature purists who point to the convention that the term adenoma implies LGD and should not be applied to polyps lacking dysplasia, such as the SSA/P. Some of these pathologists describe patients overaggressively managed by a diagnosis of SSA by clinicians unfamiliar with the term. Our advice is to know your clinicians and institutional preferences and incorporate the term that is most likely to ensure appropriate clinical management and reporting consistency.

PEARLS & PITFALLS: 2012 Recommendations on Serrated Colorectum Lesions From an Expert Panel

The most common issue in serrated polyps is distinguishing the hyperplastic polyp (generally, 10-year surveillance interval) from the SSA/P (as little as 1-year surveillance interval). In attempts to optimize clinical management and outcomes, clinical and pathology experts convened in 2012 and issued these recommendations[25]:

1. Hyperplastic polyps >10 mm proximal to the sigmoid colon can be clinically managed as SSA/P.

2. All serrated polyps proximal to the sigmoid should be fully excised.

3. All rectosigmoid serrated polyps >5 mm should be fully excised.

These recommendations reflect the importance of recognizing the SSA/P despite the inherent difficulties of endoscopically identifying and pathologically diagnosing the polyp. A few caveats of this recommendation are that (1) it is not clear if the measurement should be determined by the clinician or the pathologist and (2) these recommendations refer to proximal to the *sigmoid* colon (which therefore includes the right, cecum, ascending, transverse, *and* descending colon). These recommendations can simplify sign-out if pathologists incorporate morphology, site, and size to ensure appropriate follow-up: large proximal serrated polyps >10 mm should be SSA/P, and small distal serrated polyps should be hyperplastic polyps (Fig. 4.135). As an important departure from the 2012 recommendations, in our practice, we define proximal serrated polyps as polyps that arise only in the proximal colon (right, cecum, ascending, transverse colon) and exclude the left/descending colon. This evolving approach was at the request of our clinicians who saw an increase in distal SSA/P diagnoses immediately after the 2012 recommendations, triggering increased repeat endoscopies and patient anxiety for clinically presumed small hyperplastic polyps with confounding prolapse (Figs. 4.123–4.128).

FAQ: Because the diagnosis of the serrated polyps is influenced by site and size, do distal SSA/P and proximal hyperplastic polyps exist? What if the morphology is equivocal or my clinician did not disclose the polyp location?

Answer: Distal SSA/P and proximal HP exist, but their diagnosis relies on strong morphology in these atypical sites in well-oriented tissue that is cut sufficiently deep. As a result, it is important to know polyp location and size at the time of sign-out.

A low threshold for diagnosing SSA/P in the proximal colon is suggested, and this is supported by the 2012 recommendations specified earlier.[25] Hyperplastic polyps in the proximal colon do exist, but they are rare and their morphology should be perfect. They should be small (<5 mm), completely excised, have prominent subepithelial collagen and neuroendocrine cell proliferation, and narrow crypt bases in well-oriented tissue that is cut sufficiently deeply to avoid an undercall that would result in undermanagement of the patient. Deeper sections of a presumed proximal hyperplastic polyp can be helpful in some cases to ensure that the original sections are not superficial sections of an SSA/P. If the size or morphology remains equivocal or the polyp site is unavailable, a diagnosis of serrated polyp, not further classified is appropriate and will lead to management as an SSA/P (Fig. 4.135).

Similarly, a low threshold for diagnosing a hyperplastic polyp in the distal colon is suggested because hyperplastic polyps and mucosal prolapse feature more prominently at this site. SSA/Ps in the distal colon do exist but are rare and their morphology should be perfect to avoid an overcall that would result in overmanagement of the patient. As at any site, distal SSA/P should have at least 1 unequivocal crypt base (Figs. 4.101–4.116). In the distal colon, it is critical to beware of the potential for confounding mucosal prolapse, which is a result of fecal firmness, intraluminal pressures, and constipation-related straining. Mucosal prolapse is characterized by the ingrowth of thick muscle bundles that can mechanically "squeeze" the ensnarled crypt bases and result in bizarre crypt shapes. In the rectum, prolapse changes with ulceration are often clinically termed solitary rectal ulcer syndrome. This name is misleading, however, because these lesions can be multiple and the identical morphology can be seen anywhere along the tubular GI tract with large enough polyps. For example, the identical process is termed inflammatory cloacogenic polyp in the anus (see also "Anus" chapter). Regardless of terminology, if these distorted crypt shapes are in proportion to the investing muscle, these changes are regarded as equivocal crypt dilatations and, consequently, insufficient for a diagnosis of SSA/P (Figs. 4.117–4.128). In difficult distal cases, it is good practice to cut deeper into the block and show a colleague, which resolves most such cases as hyperplastic polyp with prolapse. In the rare case that remains unclear, a diagnosis of serrated polyp, not further classified is appropriate, but beware this will translate into management as an SSA/P and should be used sparingly in the left colon (Fig. 4.135).

SAMPLE NOTE: Serrated Polyp With Equivocal Features and No Location Provided; It Would Be Classified as an SSA/P in the Proximal Colon and Hyperplastic Polyp With Prolapse in the Distal Colon

Colon Polyp × 1, Site not Specified, Biopsy
- Serrated polyp, not further classified
- See Note

Note: According to the 2012 expert recommendations written by both clinical and pathology experts, the diagnosis of serrated polyps depends on polyp site, size, and morphology. The submitted polyp is a serrated polyp, not further classifiable. If this polyp arose in the proximal colon (right, cecum, ascending, transverse colon), it represents an SSA/P. If this polyp arose in the distal colon (left, descending, sigmoid, rectum), it represents a hyperplastic polyp with prolapse.

Reference:
Rex DK, Ahnen DJ, Baron JA, et al. Serrated lesions of the colorectum: review and recommendations from an expert panel. *Am J Gastroenterol.* 2012.

FAQ: Does anyone actually use the term serrated polyp, unclassifiable?

Answer: Yes!! The terms serrated polyp, unclassifiable or simply serrated polyp are unavoidable diagnostic terms that are equally vague and, consequently, equally disliked by both pathologists and clinicians. Although it is important to try to sort these polyps into discrete diagnostic categories, sometimes the polyps have ambiguous morphology, the histologic embedding or staining artifacts preclude a more specific diagnosis, or the polyp location is lacking. In support of this position, the term serrated polyp, unclassifiable was specifically listed in the 2012 consensus statement on serrated polyps written by both clinical and pathology experts as an acknowledgment to the unavoidable usefulness of this term.[25]

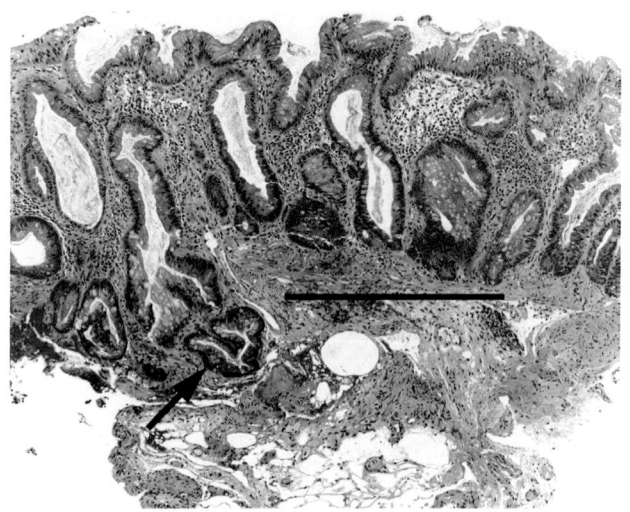

Figure 4-136. SSA/P epithelial misplacement. Sometimes SSA/P crypts (*arrow*) herniate beneath the muscularis mucosae (*line*) into the submucosa, as in this case. This focus is not invasive carcinoma because there is no desmoplasia. Other reassuring features of epithelial misplacement include a lack of overlying dysplasia and the presence of investing lamina propria.

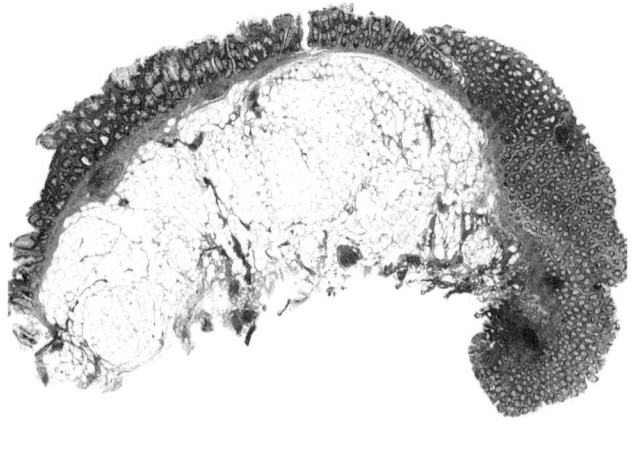

Figure 4-137. SSA/P overlying fat. SSA/P not uncommonly overlie prominent fat, as in this case.

SSA/P Odds and Ends

Sometimes the SSA/P crypts are displaced into the submucosa where they can raise concerns for invasive carcinoma (Fig. 4.136). Reassuring features of a noninvasive process include a lack of desmoplasia and the presence of investing lamina propria. A lack of overlying dysplasia, when present, and deeper sections to show a connection to the overlying surface can also be reassuring. Mesenchymal tissue can sometimes tag along with the SSA/P. It is not uncommon for SSA/P to overlie prominent fat (Figs. 4.137–4.139). It is unclear if this represents benign fat in the often fatty right colon or if there is a more sophisticated epithelial-mesenchymal interaction. A subset of hyperplastic polyps and SSA/P harbor a

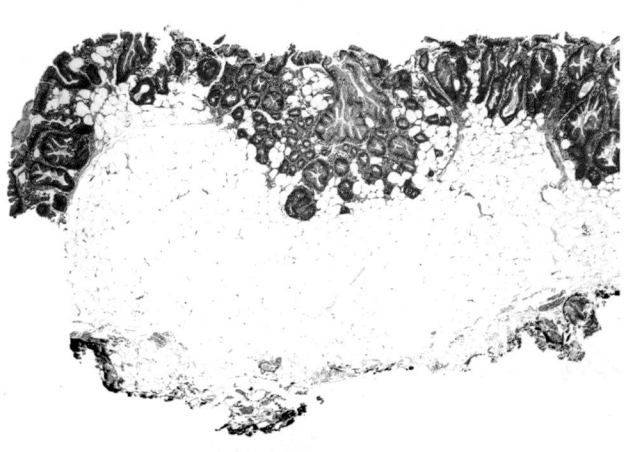

Figure 4-138. SSA/P overlying fat. It is unclear if the underlying fat is due to increased fat in the proximal colon or if there is a more complicated epithelial-mesenchymal interaction.

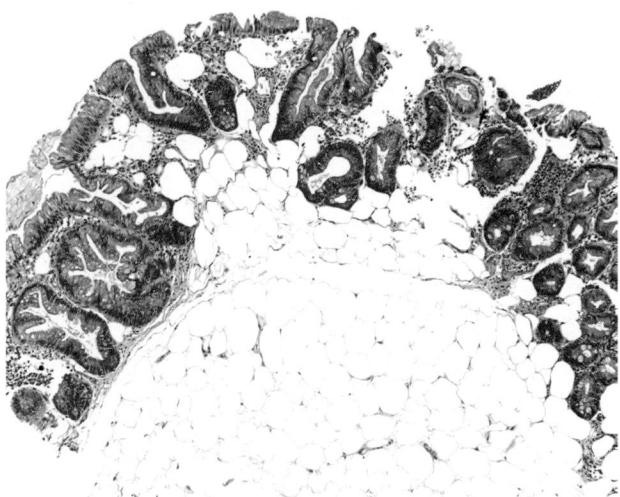

Figure 4-139. SSA/P overlying fat. Although this case would qualify for a diagnosis of an SSA/P at any location based on the perfect morphology, prominent underlying fat can be a helpful clue to an SSA/P in proximal serrated polyps with equivocal features.

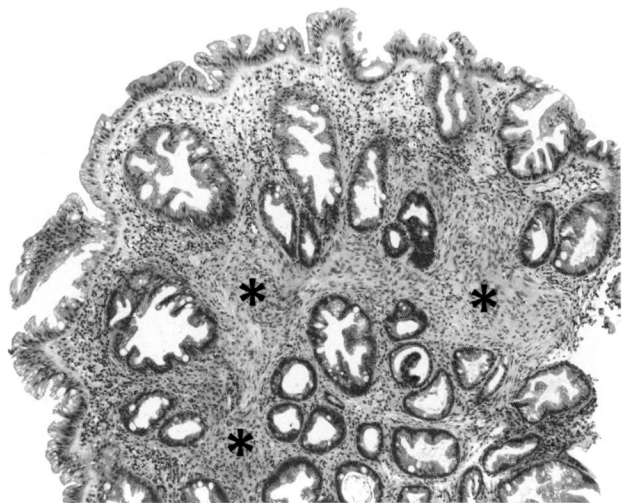

Figure 4-140. Proximal SSA/P with perineurioma. Colonic perineuriomas (*asterisks*) are frequently found intermingled with a hyperplastic polyp or SSA/P. At first, the perineurioma may appear similar to the smooth muscle of prolapse on low power, as seen here.

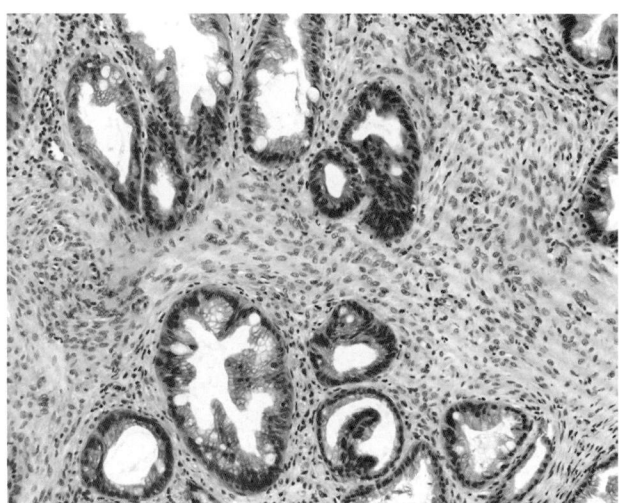

Figure 4-141. Proximal SSA/P with perineurioma. Intermediate power of the previous figure shows that the perineural cells are paler with smaller nuclei than smooth muscle (compare with Figs. 4.123–4.128).

perineurioma (also known as benign fibroblastic polyp) The perineurial cells are bland, spindled, and often arranged in a whorled configuration with small-ovoid nuclei and occasional intranuclear inclusions (Figs 4.140–4.149).[27-30] The perineurioma is easy to miss because it is usually only local, or it may be quickly dismissed as native smooth muscle. The good news is that there is no consequence to overlooking it! The cells can be highlighted with EMA (very, very weakly), Claudin-1, Glut-1, or collagen IV. These cells are S100 protein nonreactive, distinguishing them from Schwann cell hamartoma, a benign lesion unassociated with serrated polyps (Figs. 4.150–4.155).

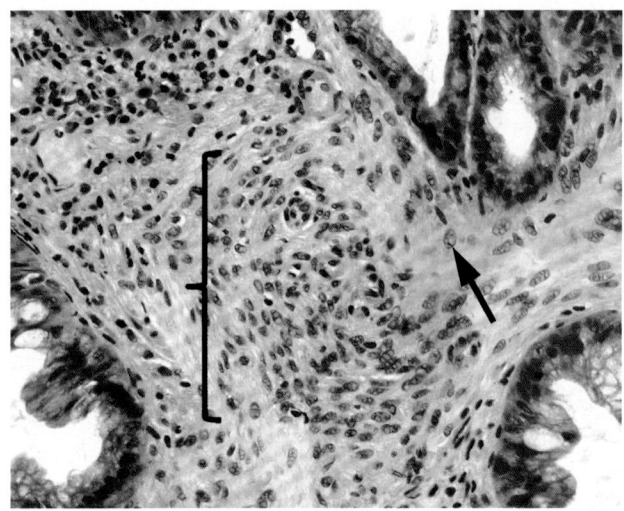

Figure 4-142. Proximal SSA/P with perineurioma. High power of the previous figure shows the typical morphology of a perineurioma. The small, spindled cells have abundant pale cytoplasm and are often arranged in a whorled configuration (*bracket*). The nuclei are small and ovoid, and intranuclear inclusions are seen (*arrow*).

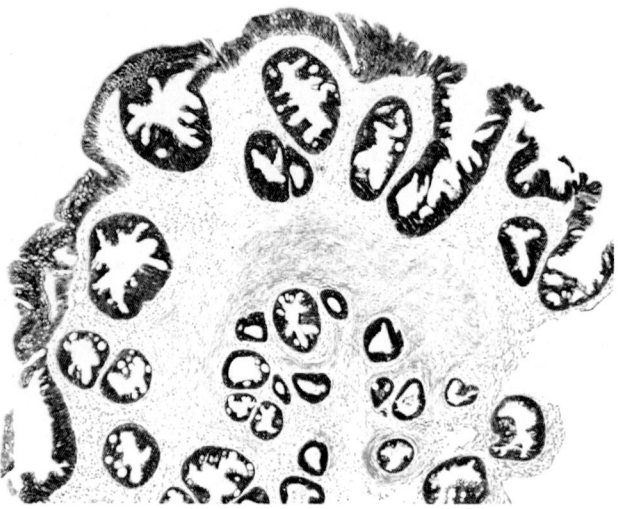

Figure 4-143. Proximal SSA/P with perineurioma (EMA). Perineuriomas are (very weakly) EMA reactive and S100 protein nonreactive. Because the EMA can be so difficult to interpret, it is our habit to order both EMA and S100 protein immunohistochemical stains at the same time to differentiate the perineurioma (EMA+, S100 protein–) from the Schwann cell hamartoma (EMA–, S100 protein +).

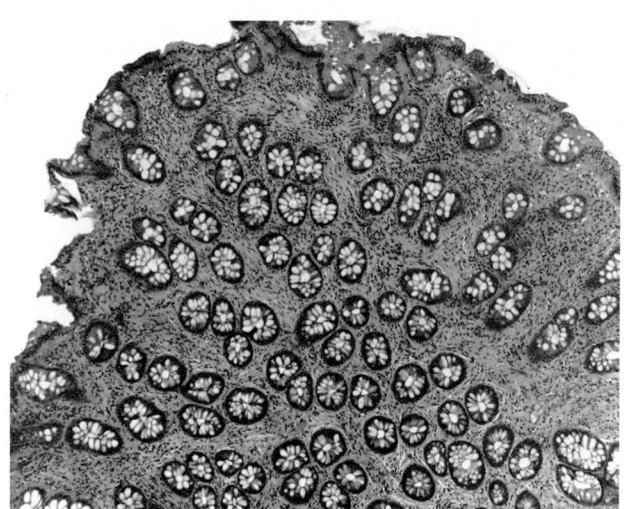

Figure 4-144. Perineurioma.

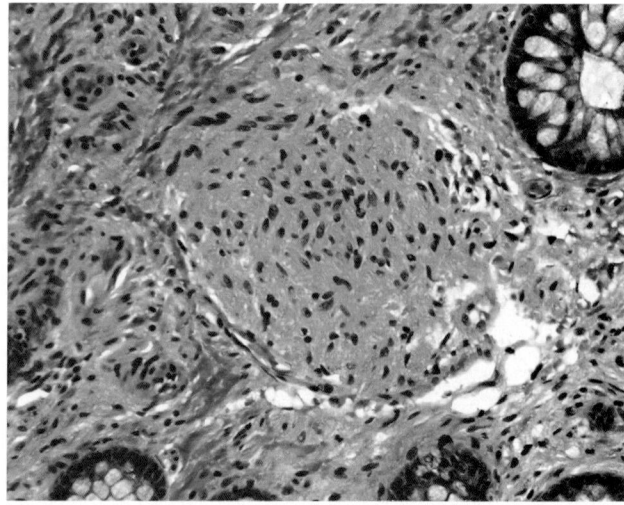

Figure 4-145. Perineurioma. Higher power of the previous figure showing the whorled appearance of the perineurioma. This focus was EMA reactive and S100 protein nonreactive.

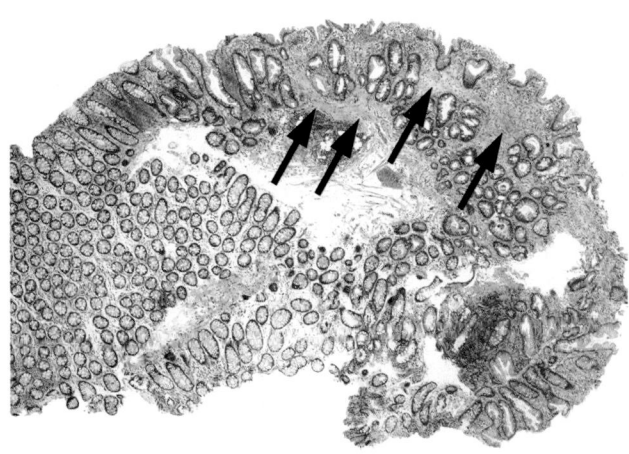

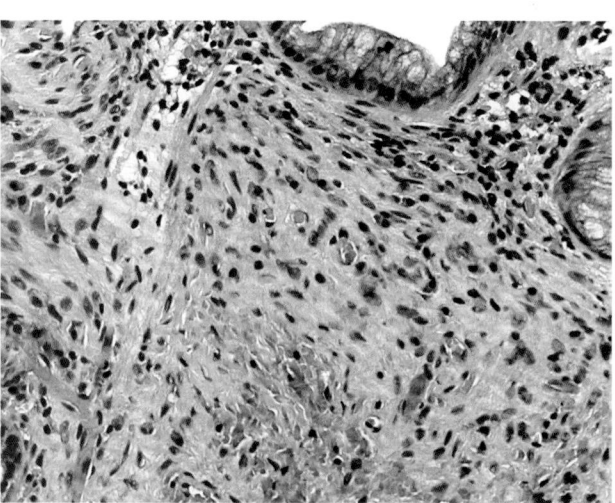

Figure 4-146. SSA/P with perineurioma. The perineural cells are often only focally distributed (*arrows*). This 1.0-cm cecal polyp was classified as an SSA/P based on its size and location despite the equivocal crypt dilatation.

Figure 4-147. SSA/P with perineurioma. Higher power of the previous figure.

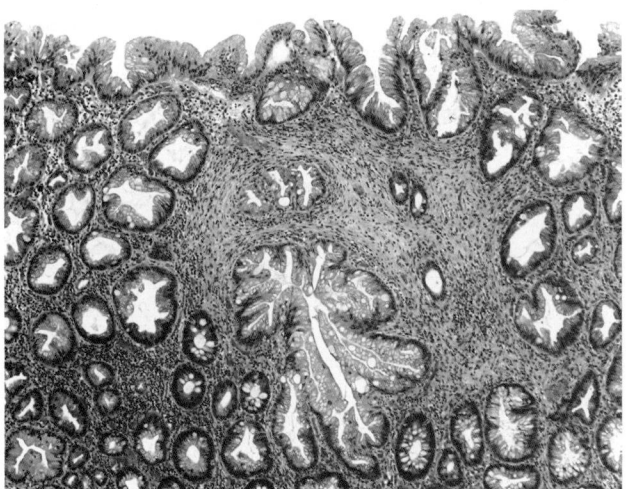

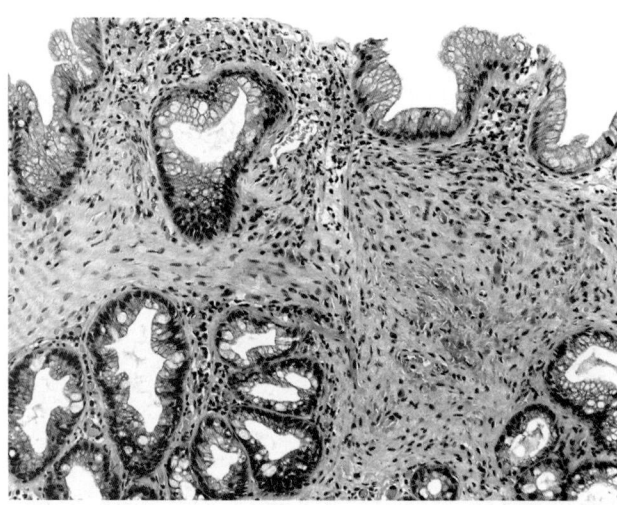

Figure 4-148. SSA/P with perineurioma.

Figure 4-149. SSA/P with perineurioma. Higher power of the previous figure.

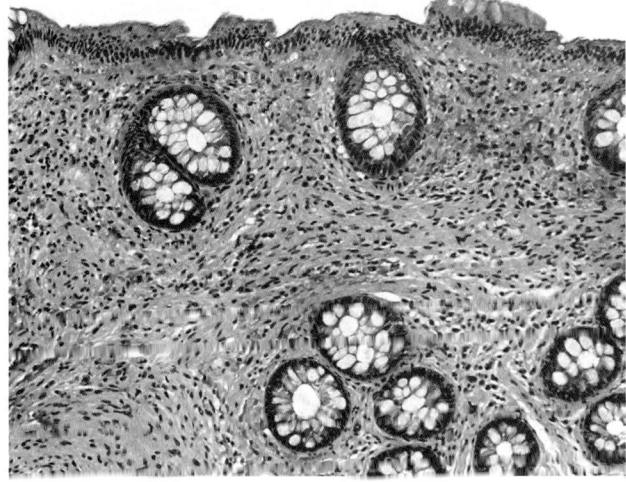

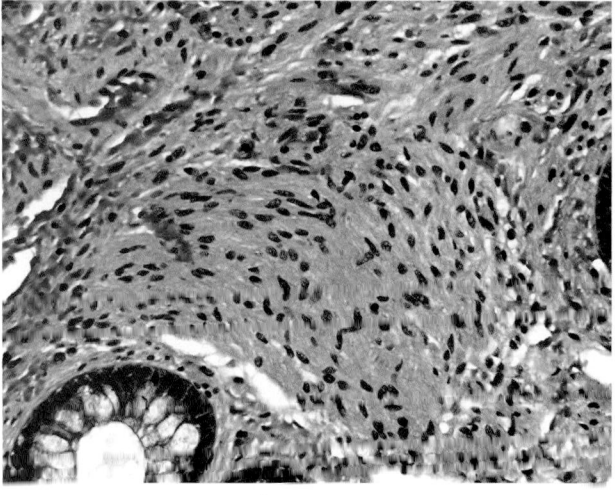

Figure 4-150. Schwann cell hamartoma This benign polyp is unassociated with serrated polyps, a feature that contrasts with the colonic perineuriomas.

Figure 4-151. Schwann cell hamartoma. Higher power of the previous figure.

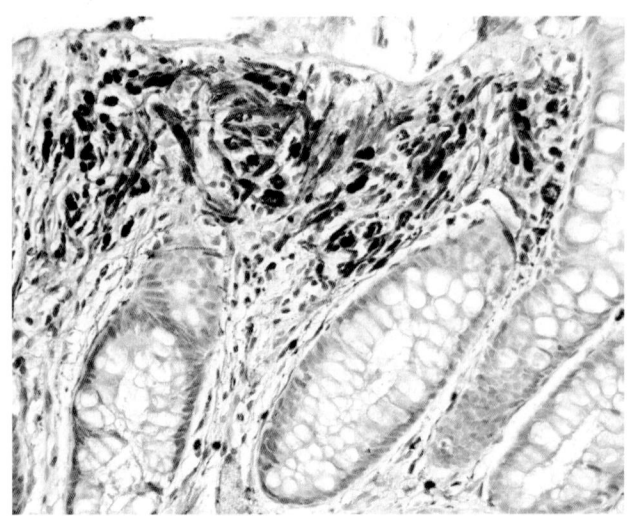

Figure 4-152. Schwann cell hamartoma (S100 protein). Schwann cell hamartomas are S100 protein reactive, as seen here, and EMA nonreactive (not shown).

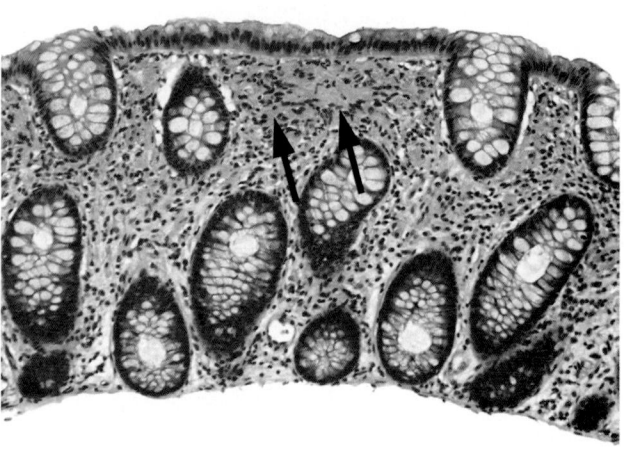

Figure 4-153. Schwann cell hamartoma. On H&E, it can be challenging to distinguish a Schwann cell hamartoma (*arrows*) from a perineurioma, although the cytoplasm in Schwann cell hamartomas is more fibrillary and brightly eosinophilic than the cytoplasm of perineurioma and there is often a suggestion of nuclear palisading in Schwann cell hamartomas. Perineurioma can be favored on H&E if there is an associated serrated polyp. EMA and S100 protein immunohistochemistry can be ordered for definitive diagnosis, but both spindle cell proliferations are benign.

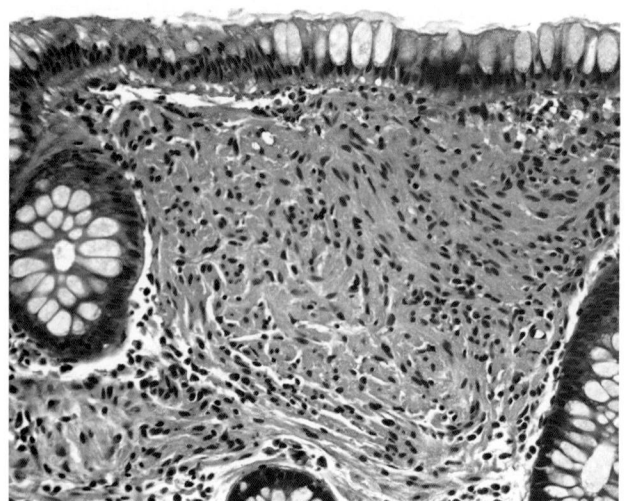

Figure 4-154. Schwann cell hamartoma.

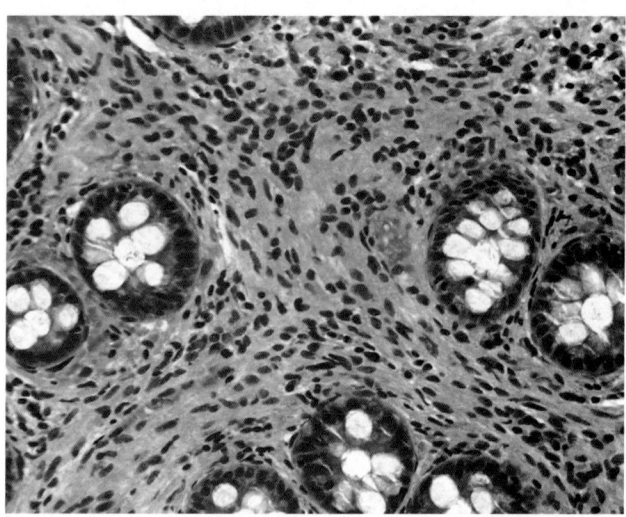

Figure 4-155. Schwann cell hamartoma.

Traditional Serrated Adenoma

The TSA was first described in 1990.[31] It is the least common of the serrated polyps, accounting for only 2% of all serrated polyps and 0.7% of all colon polyps.[2] Most (about 70%) arise in the left colon,[32] and they are usually >5 mm and protuberant or pedunculated (Table 4.3). Their lobular architecture is imparted by floppy villi with edematous lamina propria. The characteristic bright cytoplasmic eosinophilia is so striking that the diagnosis is often suggested from looking at the glass slide without a microscope (Figs. 4.156–4.159). Other signature features of the TSA include its luminal serrations, pencillate nuclei, and

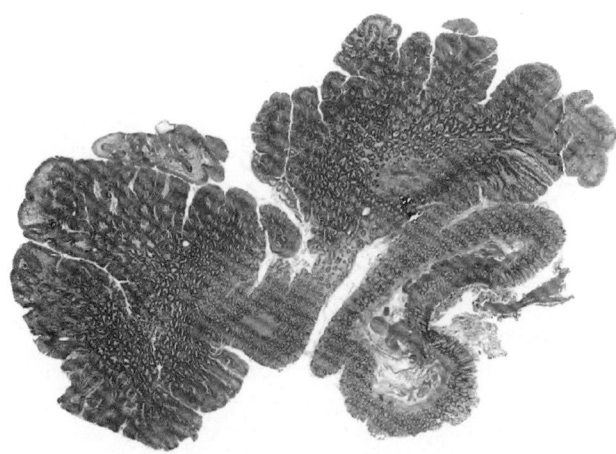

Figure 4-156. Traditional serrated adenoma (TSA). TSAs have bright eosinophilia that is best seen at 1× (without a microscope). The villi are usually broad with edematous lamina propria, as seen here.

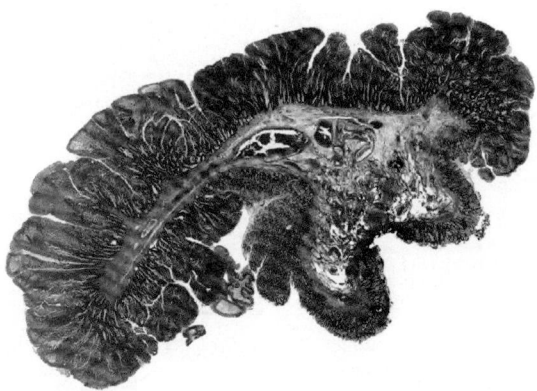

Figure 4-157. Traditional serrated adenoma. Another low-power view of a TSA with its characteristic bright eosinophilia and broad villi.

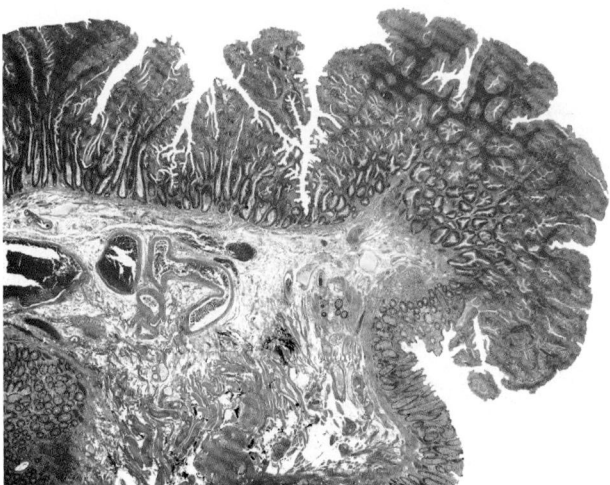

Figure 4-158. Traditional serrated adenoma. TSA are usually >5 mm and protuberant.

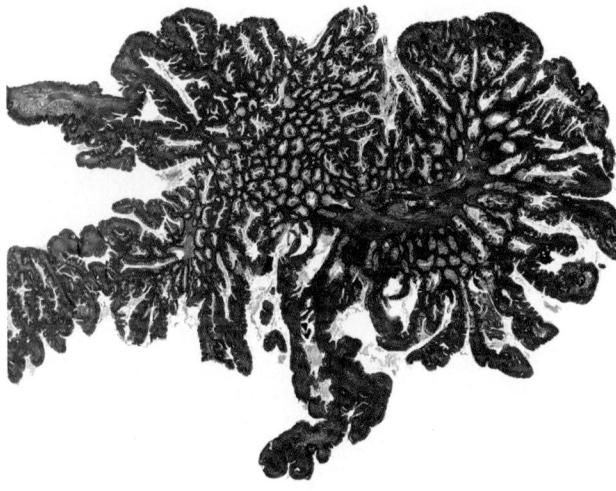

Figure 4-159. Traditional serrated adenoma. TSA are distal colon predominant.

ectopic crypt foci (ECF). ECF are small invaginations of the surface epithelium that lack a connection to the muscularis mucosae. They have been described as cryptlike, whorled eddies, buds, or clefts (Figs. 4.160–4.164).[31,33-35] The TSA is sometimes confused for a TVA, but the nuclei of the TSA are distinctly blander and smaller, more evenly spaced, less hyperchromatic and pleomorphic, and usually lack mitoses and apoptotic bodies. Three TSA variants have been described: filiform, flat, and mucin-rich. The filiform TSA is usually larger, with more prominent villiform projections[36] than that those associated with the

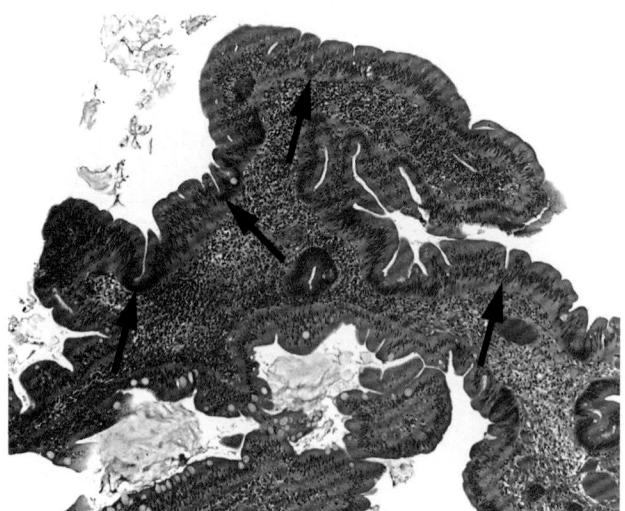

Figure 4-160. Traditional serrated adenoma. On intermediate power, TSAs appear similar to small bowel epithelium with bright eosinophilia and luminal serrations. Also seen at this power are ectopic crypt foci (ECF). ECF are small invaginations of the surface epithelium that appear similar to whorled eddies, buds, or clefts (*arrows*).

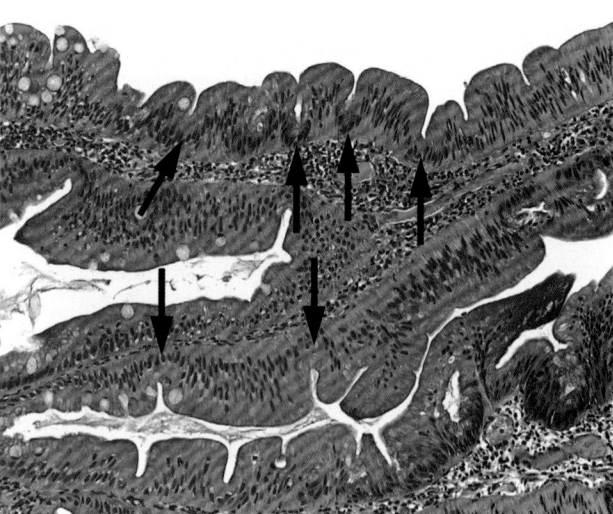

Figure 4-161. Traditional serrated adenoma. On higher power, the ECF are more easily seen (*arrows*), along with the pencillate nuclei characteristic of the TSA.

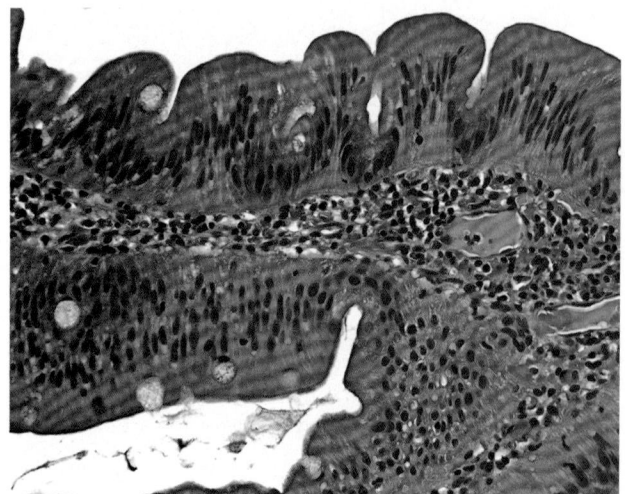

Figure 4-162. Traditional serrated adenoma. Highest power of the previous figure. These pencillate nuclei are longer than the epithelium of normal colonic mucosa (Fig. 4.5), the hyperplastic polyp (Fig. 4.74), and the SSA/P (Fig. 4.167). They are also distinctly blander than those in a conventional adenoma (Fig. 4.14). Compared with a conventional adenoma, these TSA pencillate nuclei are smaller, more evenly spaced, and less hyperchromatic, and no mitoses and apoptotic bodies are seen.

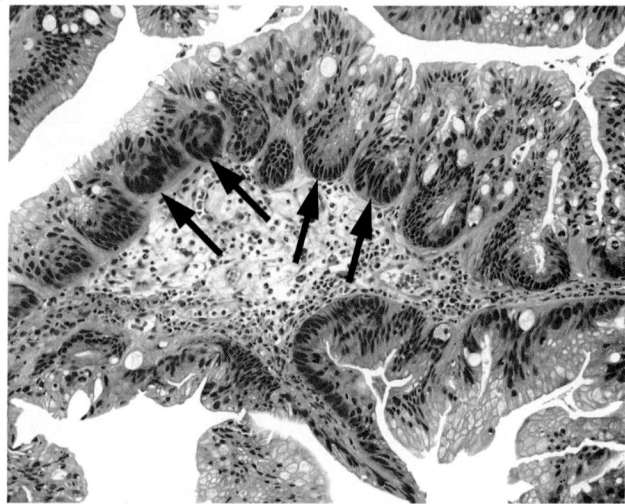

Figure 4-163. Traditional serrated adenoma. TSA characteristically have ECF (*arrows*) and pencillate nuclei, as seen here.

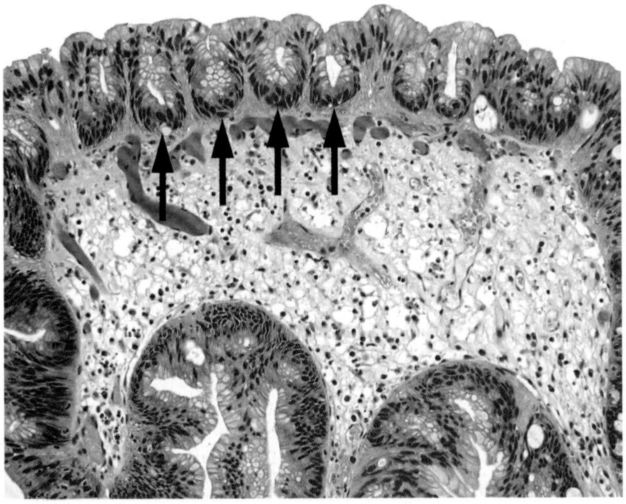

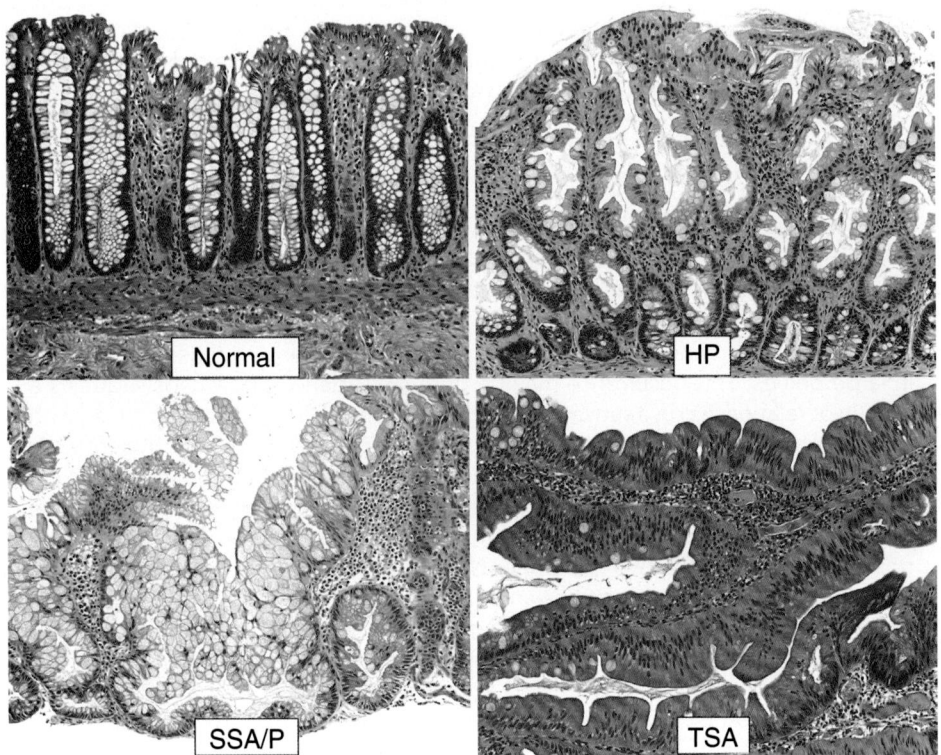

Figure 4-164. Traditional serrated adenoma. *Arrows* highlight the ECF.

Figure 4-165. A composite of the serrated polyp family. Normal colon mucosa with no lesion: flat surface and narrowed crypt bases. Hyperplastic polyp (HP): luminal serrations, superficial star-shaped crypt lumina, prominent epithelial collagen table and neuroendocrine cells (not shown), and narrowed crypt bases. SSA/P: surface serrations and at least one unequivocally distorted crypt base. TSA: bright eosinophilia, ECF, and pencillate nuclei.

other types. The flat TSA comprises 38% of TSAs. Its height is less than twice the height of the adjacent normal mucosa, and it lacks villiform projections.[32] The mucin-rich subtype is composed of at least 50% mucinous or goblet cells. Because these variants lack clinical significance and this difficult area is already plagued with nomenclature issues and poor interobserver agreement, it is adequate to report all TSA as simply TSA without routinely subclassifying the variants.

See also Fig. 4-165 for a side-by-side comparison of normal colonic mucosa, hyperplastic polyp, SSA/P, and TSA.

FAQ: What is the minimum diagnostic criterion for the TSA?

Answer: Unlike for the SSA/P, there is no minimum single diagnostic criterion for the TSA. Some have suggested the minimum criteria be its characteristic small bowel–like appearance with eosinophilic color, slitlike surface serrations, and pencillate nuclei.[35] Although ECF were once considered pathognomonic for TSA, they are not required for the diagnosis, and some report that they are entirely absent in up to 38% of TSAs.[37] Such TSAs tend to be small, flat, and right colon predominant.[32] Our experience is that ECF can be a bit promiscuous, as demonstrated by their identification in up to 6.5% of conventional TAs, 53.8% of TVAs, and 100% of VAs.[38,39] Although practice patterns vary, we diagnose TSA based on a constellation of features that includes cytoplasmic eosinophilia, ECF, slitlike surface serrations, and pencillate nuclei.

FAQ: Why has the term mixed polyp been abandoned?

Answer: The term mixed polyp was retired because it originally referred to polyps containing features of both conventional adenomas and hyperplastic polyps. Based on their unique morphology and molecular profiles, these polyps are today best classified by the modern terms TSA or dysplastic SSA/P.

FAQ: Because the term mixed polyp is out of date, what is the reporting approach for polyps with multiple components?

Answer: Encountering polyps with multiple features is fairly common, particularly in large polyps. This occurrence may be pure coincidence or perhaps suggests a precursor relationship in a subset. For example, up to 52% of TSA are admixed with other polyps, and some have suggested that its precursors are the hyperplastic polyp and SSA/P based on the intimate intermingling and often similar molecular profiles.[32,37,38,40] TSAs have also been described in association with conventional adenomas, although some report that this relationship is defined by more abrupt transitions between the two components.[40] We descriptively report hybrid polyps in order of the priority for surveillance and then by the more substantial component of the polyp. For example, "Serrated polyp with features of SSA/P, TSA, and hyperplastic polyp." In this example, SSA/P and TSA are listed first because their neoplastic potential requires an abbreviated surveillance interval over that for the hyperplastic polyp (Table 4.4). Another common example includes "TVA with focal TSA features" for the fairly common polyp that is mainly a conventional TVA with only focal TSA features. Some prefer the term "serrated tubulovillous adenoma" for this morphology.[41] In a study of 412 conventional TVAs, serrated TVA comprised 11% and were described as predominantly conventional TVA with at least 50% serrated architecture and less than 10% TSA-type cytology and slitlike serrations.[41] In the interest of clarity and to avoid compounding nomenclature issues, we prefer "TVA with focal TSA features" for such polyps.

TABLE 4.4: Serrated Polyp Surveillance[4,25]

Histology	Size (mm)	Number	Location	Interval (Years)
HP	<10	Any	Rectosigmoid	10
HP	≤5	3	Proximal to sigmoid	10
HP	Any	≥4	Proximal to sigmoid	5
HP	>5	≥1	Proximal to sigmoid	5
SSA/P or TSA	<10	<3	Any	5
SSA/P or TSA	≥10	1	Any	3
SSA/P or TSA	<10	≥3	Any	3
SSA/P	≥10	≥2	Any	1–3
Dysplastic SSA	Any	Any	Any	1–3
Serrated polyposis				1

FAQ: Are there any useful ancillary studies to help establish a diagnosis as hyperplastic polyp, SSA, or TSA?

Answer: The short answer is that there is no perfect marker. Our position is that these decisions are too important to rely on imperfect studies that have not been vetted through multiple, independent, multicenter data. Instead, we rely on the H&E, size, location, and morphology (Fig. 4.135). In challenging cases, deeper sections and sharing with a colleague can be helpful, but we do not use ancillary studies such as immunolabeling or molecular methods. It is handy to be aware of the expanding list of potential markers so that when the clinician inevitably requests them, a reasonable response is that, although you are aware of the ancillary tools, the H&E is best. An abbreviated list of proposed ancillary studies includes the following: RNF43, PTPRK-RSPO3, Annexin A10, Ki67, MUC2, MUC5AC, MUC6, Maspin, Hes1, MLH1, Cathepsin E, Trefoil factor 1, BRAF V600F mutation specific antibody VE1, *KRAS*, CpG island methylator phenotype (CIMP) status, and *MUC5AC* mucin gene hypomethylation.

Dysplastic Serrated Polyps

Unfortunately, almost everything on the topic of dysplastic serrated polyps is contentious. One practical approach is summarized in Fig. 4.166, but understand that there are widely divergent views on this topic. In this approach, the terms SSA/P and TSA imply that the polyp is negative for conventional dysplasia of the type seen in conventional adenomas; the redundant phrase negative for dysplasia is unnecessary. When dysplasia is seen, the correct nomenclature is low- (or high-) grade cytologic dysplasia arising in an SSA/P or TSA. The 2010 WHO recommends the distinct term cytologic dysplasia because this dysplasia can be morphologically, molecularly, and biologically distinct from the dysplasia seen in conventional adenomas.[11] Dysplasia in SSA/P and TSA can be further subclassified as conventional-type or serrated-type dysplasia. Conventional type dysplasia is more similar to that seen with conventional adenomas with columnar cells, pseudostratified nuclei, basophilia due

Classification of dysplastic serrated polyps

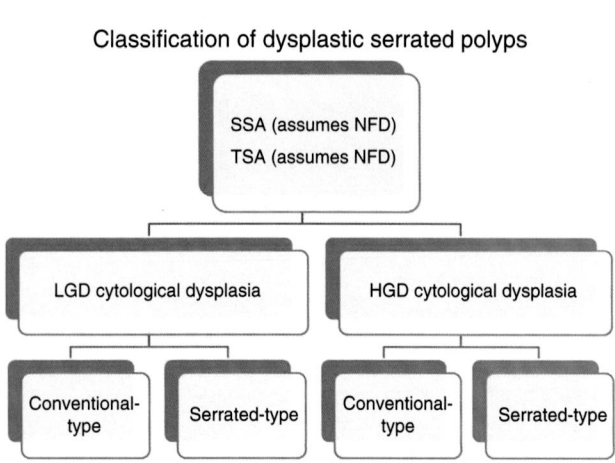

Figure 4-166. A practical approach to dysplasia classification in serrated polyps. Although dysplasia classification is a contentious subject, in our approach the terms SSA/P and TSA imply that the polyp is negative for dysplasia. When dysplasia is seen, the correct nomenclature is low- (or high-) grade cytologic dysplasia arising in an SSA/P or TSA. Dysplasia in SSA/P and TSA can be further subclassified as conventional-type or serrated-type dysplasia.

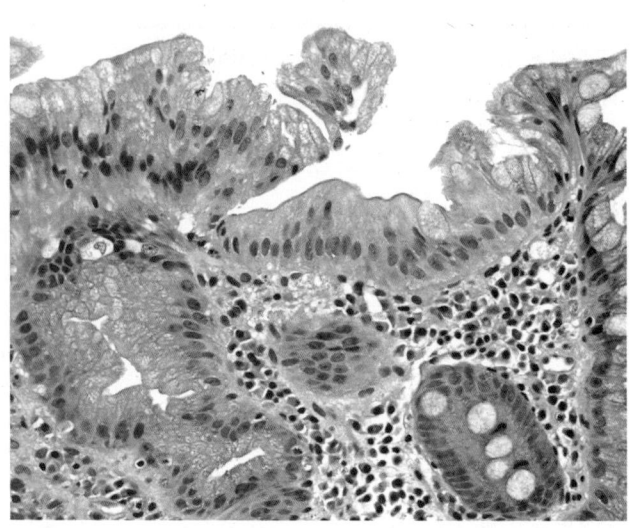

Figure 4-167. Normal colonic mucosa for comparison. A high-power view of normal colon shows normochromatic chromatin and small basally oriented nuclei. The bland nuclei comprise approximately less than 10% of the overall cell volume. Apoptotic bodies and mitotic figures are not seen.

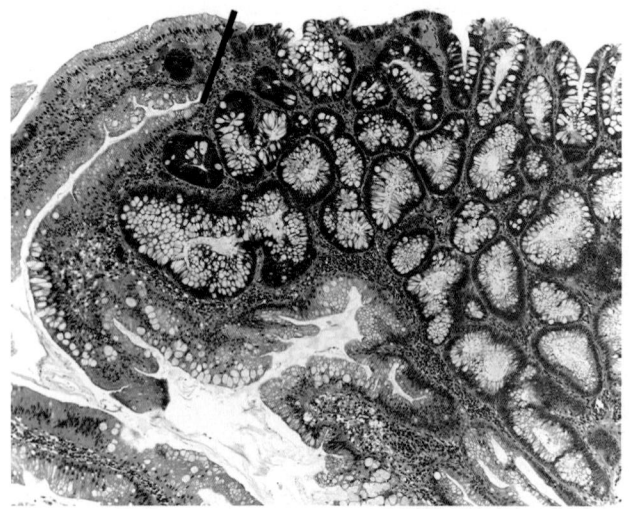

Figure 4-168. Low-grade cytologic dysplasia (conventional type) arising in an SSA/P. Dysplasia is a low-power diagnosis (right side of polyp) with an abrupt transition between normal and atypia (line), and the atypia involves the surface, as in this case. In general, avoid assessing dysplasia at 40× because everything looks atypical at 40×.

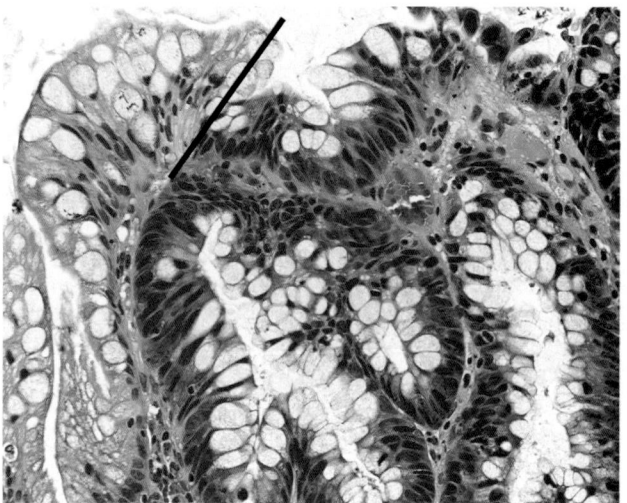

Figure 4-169. LGD cytologic dysplasia (conventional type) arising in an SSA/P. Higher power of the previous figure. The line illustrates the abrupt transition between normal and dysplasia, a characteristic feature of dysplasia. This type of dysplasia can be subclassified as conventional type because it appears similar to that seen in conventional adenomas (Figs. 4.13–4.17).

to increased nuclear to cytoplasmic ratios, and hyperchromasia[42] (compare the nuclei of a nondysplastic serrated polyp [Fig. 4.167] with the nuclei of conventional adenomas [Figs. 4.13–4.24] and the nuclei of dysplastic serrated polyps with conventional-type dysplasia [Figs. 4.168–4.174]). Serrated-type dysplasia is subtle and very easy to miss, and so a close look at 10× at all SSA/P and TSA is worthwhile. It is characterized by small cuboidal cells whose eosinophilia is imparted by pink cytoplasm, and their rounded nuclei contain open chromatin and prominent nucleoli and lack pseudostratification (compare the nuclei of a nondysplastic serrated polyp [Fig. 4.167] with the nuclei of a serrated polyps with conventional-type dysplasia [Figs. 4.168–4.174] and the nuclei of a dysplastic serrated polyp with serrated-type dysplasia [Figs. 4.175–4.181]). At this point, there is no clinical significance of distinguishing conventional-type from serrated-type dysplasia, but it may be worthwhile to specify to alert the subsequent pathologists to the pattern present and for ongoing academic projects. As an example, "low-grade cytologic dysplasia (conventional-type) arising in an SSA/P."

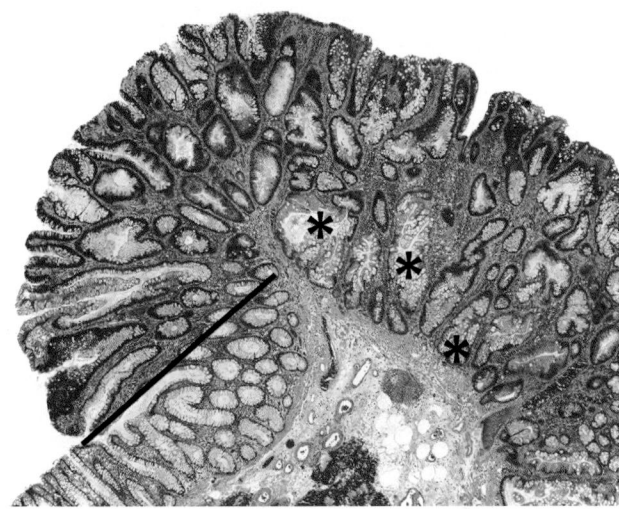

Figure 4-170. Low-grade cytologic dysplasia (conventional type) arising in an SSA/P. Unequivocal distorted crypts of the background SSA/P (*asterisks*) are seen along with low-grade cytologic dysplasia. The *line* highlights the abrupt transition between normal and dysplasia, as expected for dysplasia.

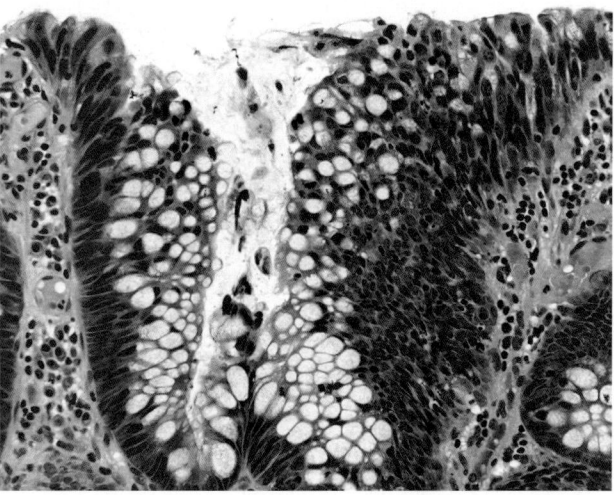

Figure 4-171. Low-grade cytologic dysplasia (conventional type) arising in an SSA/P. Higher power of the previous figure. Low-grade dysplasia is defined by retention of the nuclear polarity (most of the nuclei are positioned toward the basement membrane).

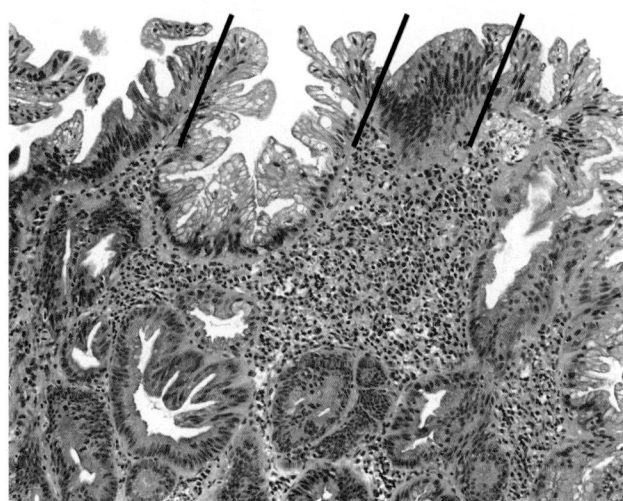

Figure 4-172. Low-grade cytologic dysplasia (conventional type) arising in an SSA/P. Because dysplasia can be focal (*lines*), it is important to carefully examine these polyps.

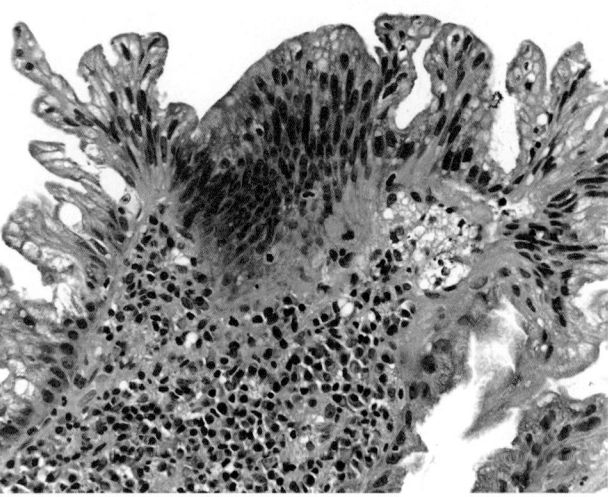

Figure 4-173. Low-grade cytologic dysplasia (conventional type) arising in an SSA/P. Higher power of the previous figure.

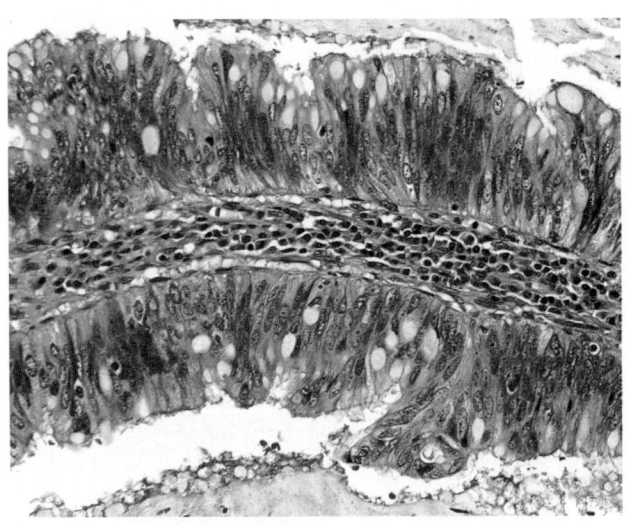

Figure 4-174. Low-grade cytologic dysplasia (conventional type) arising in a TSA. The diagnostic features of this TSA are not apparent at this power, but this photomicrograph shows low-grade conventional-type dysplasia identical to that seen in conventional adenomas.

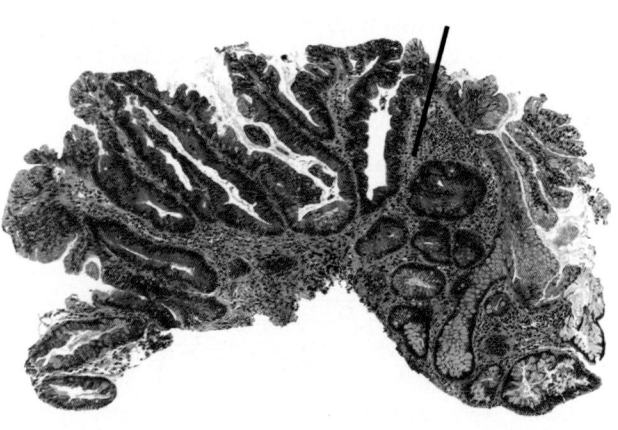

Figure 4-175. Low-grade cytologic dysplasia (serrated type) arising in an SSA/P. Serrated-type dysplasia is easy to miss because the cytoplasm is *pink* and the nuclei are cuboidal, in contrast to the basophilia and pseudostratified nuclei seen in conventional-type dysplasia (compare with Figs. 4.168–4.174). A *line* denotes the abrupt transition between normal and low-grade cytologic dysplasia.

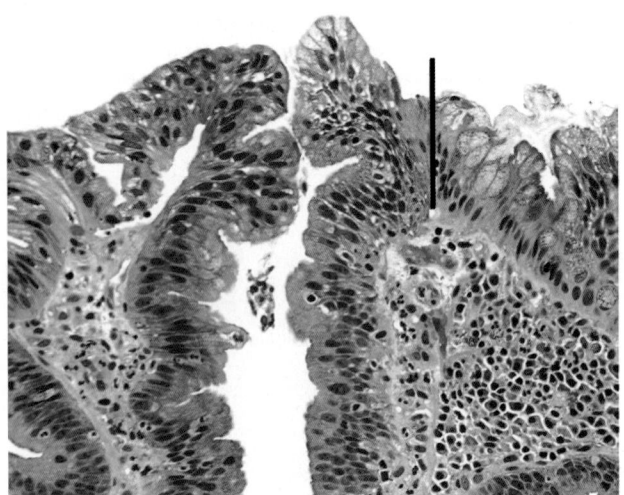

Figure 4-176. Low-grade cytologic dysplasia (serrated type) arising in an SSA/P. Higher power of the previous figure with the *line* denoting the abrupt transition between normal and dysplastic epithelium. Although serrated-type dysplasia is subtle, it must be recognized because dysplastic serrated polyps need to be entirely removed and because of their sometimes rapid progression to colorectal carcinoma.

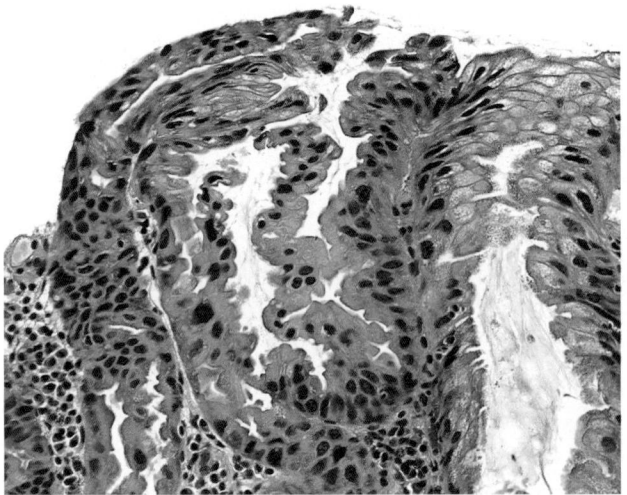

Figure 4-177. Low-grade cytologic dysplasia (serrated type) arising in an SSA/P. A careful 10× inspection and familiarity with the characteristic morphology are helpful tips for recognizing sneaky serrated-type dysplasia.

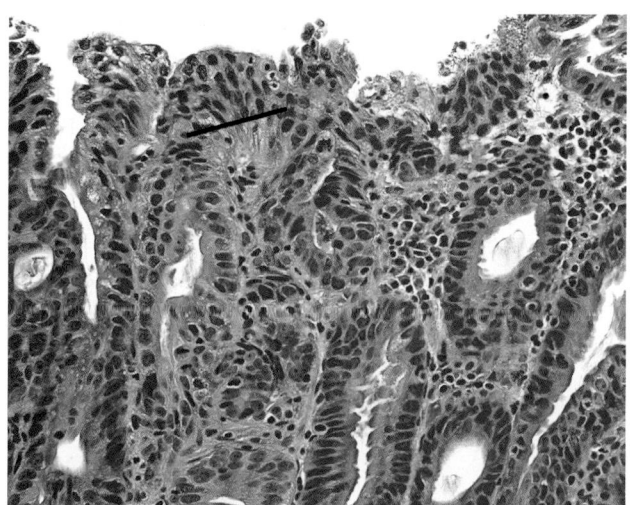

Figure 4-178. High-grade cytologic dysplasia (conventional type) arising in an SSA/P. In contrast to conventional adenomas, for which a diagnosis of high-grade dysplasia requires both high-grade cytology (loss of polarity) and architectural complexity (cribriforming), only high-grade cytology is needed for a diagnosis of high-grade dysplasia in serrated polyps. Loss of nuclear polarity is demonstrated by drawing a *line* through the basal aspect of the dysplastic cells showing that many of the nuclei are no longer on the *line*, as seen here. The underlying glands are crowded with minimal intervening lamina propria.

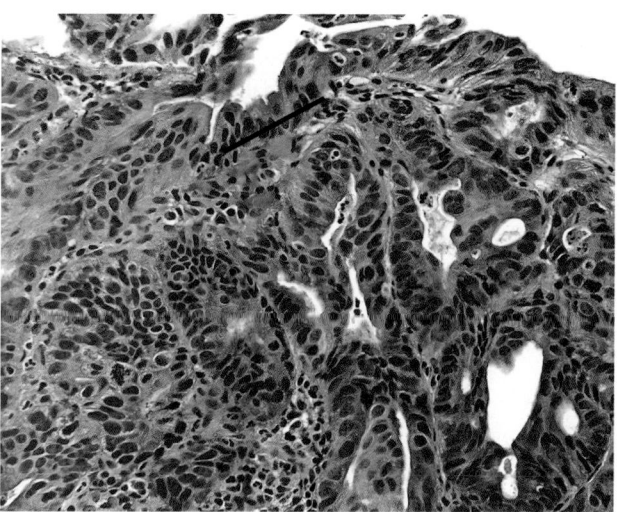

Figure 4-179. High-grade cytologic dysplasia (conventional type) arising in an SSA/P. The *line* demonstrates loss of nuclear polarity. Architectural complexity is not needed for a diagnosis of high-grade dysplasia in serrated polyps.

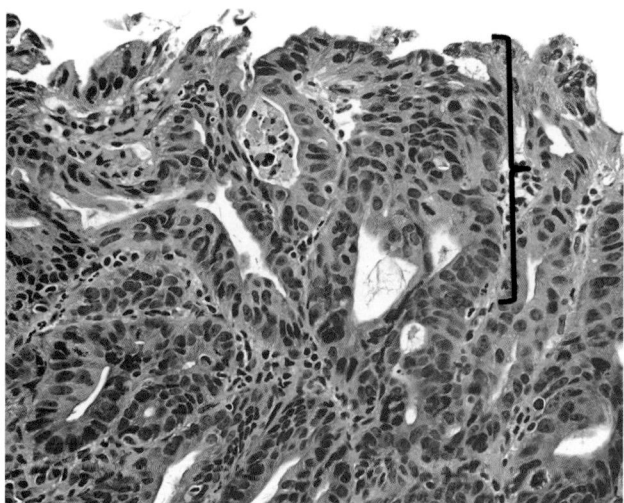

Figure 4-180. High-grade cytologic dysplasia (conventional type) arising in a TSA (*bracket*).

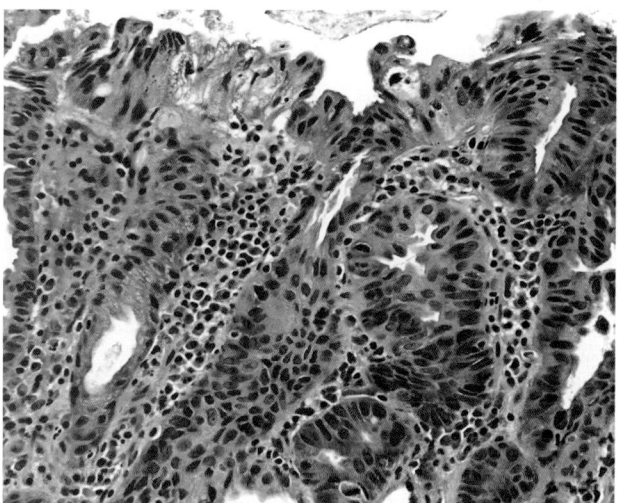

Figure 4-181. High-grade cytologic dysplasia (conventional type) arising in a TSA.

Once dysplasia is recognized, it is graded similarly to grading in the rest of the GI tract: LGD maintains nuclear polarity (Figs. 4.168–4.177), HGD shows cytologic atypia with loss of nuclear polarity (Figs. 4.178–4.184) (note that architectural changes are not required to diagnose HGD in serrated polyps), IMC has individual cells infiltrating through the basement membrane into the lamina propria but not beyond the muscularis mucosae (akin to IMC arising in a conventional adenoma [Figs. 4.37–4.42]), and invasive adenocarcinoma is reserved for cases with invasion beyond the muscularis mucosae into at least the submucosa and shows well-formed desmoplasia (Figs. 4.185–4.189).[9] Similar to conventional adenomas, IMC arising in serrated polyps is staged as pTis because of presumed negligible malignant potential,[5-7] and invasive adenocarcinoma into the submucosa is staged as pT1.

See Fig. 4.190 for a side-by-side comparison of normal, low-grade cytologic dysplasia, high-grade cytologic dysplasia, and invasive adenocarcinoma.

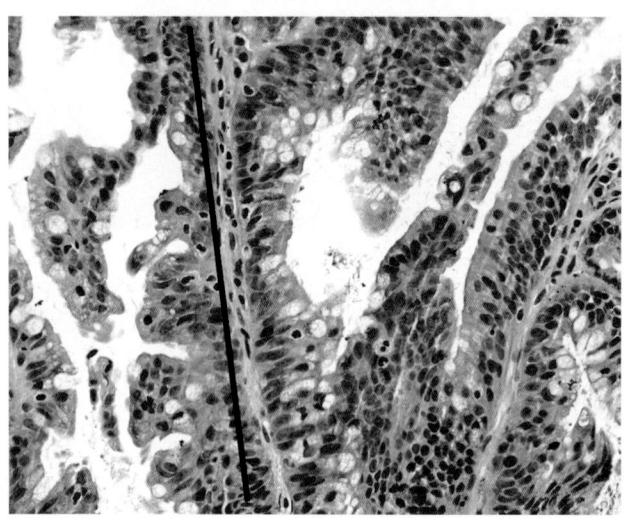

Figure 4-182. High-grade cytologic dysplasia (serrated type) arising in an SSA/P. Loss of nuclear polarity is demonstrated by drawing a *line* through the basal aspect of the cells and finding that many of the cells are not on the *line*. Serrated-type dysplasia is *pink* with smaller, more cuboidal nuclei than those in conventional-type dysplasia.

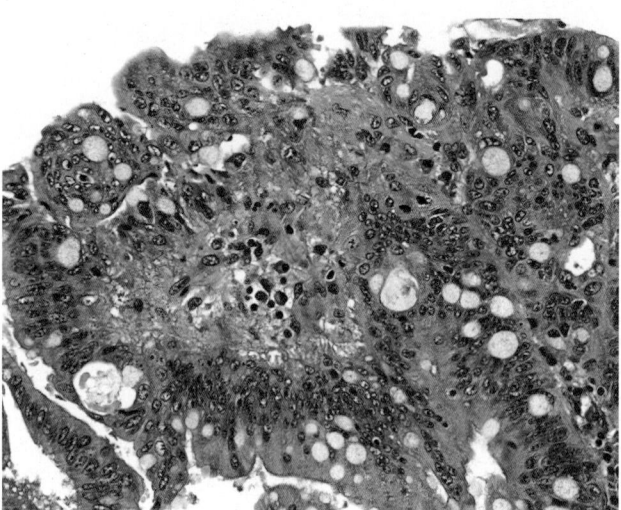

Figure 4-183. High-grade cytologic dysplasia (serrated type) arising in a TSA. The surface epithelium is jumbled with patchy loss of polarity. Serrated dysplasia is *pink* with cuboidal cells.

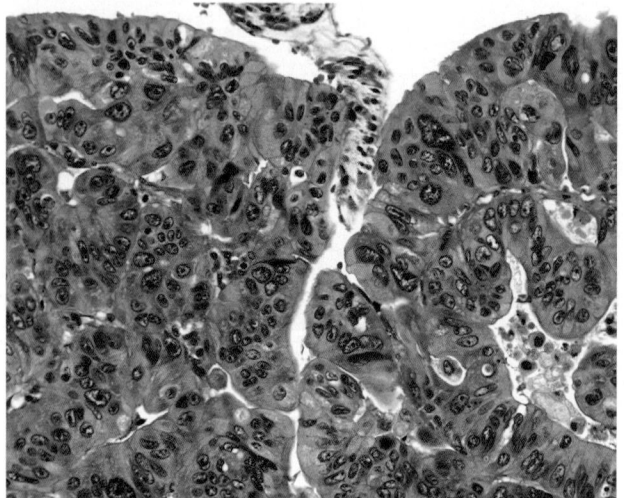

Figure 4-184. High-grade cytologic dysplasia (serrated type) arising in a TSA.

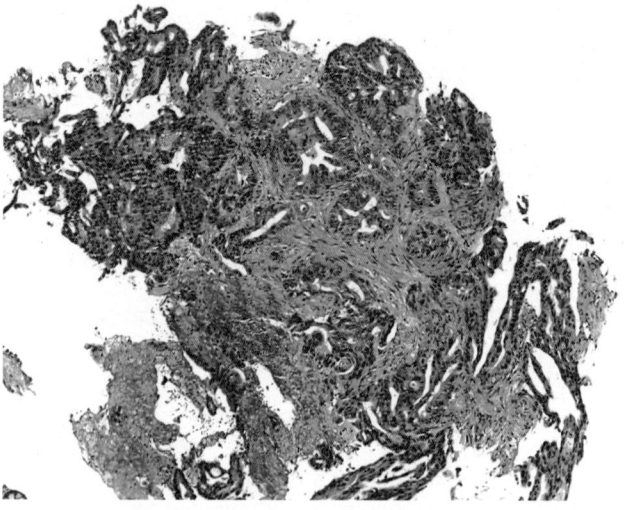

Figure 4-185. Invasive adenocarcinoma. Desmoplasia imparts a *light blue* pallor to the background lamina propria and signifies at least submucosal invasion.

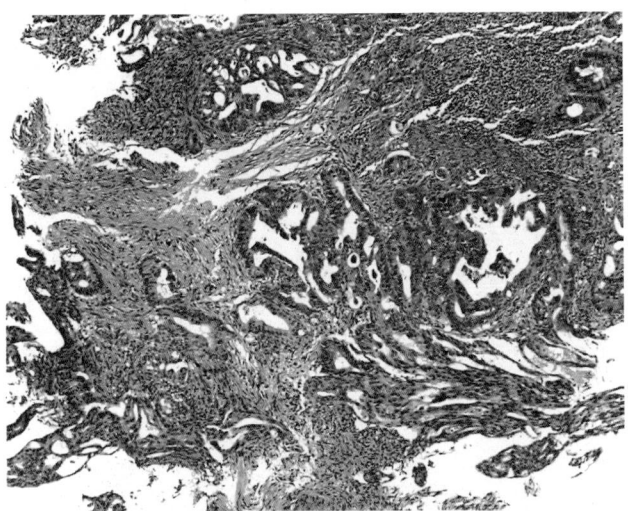

Figure 4-186. Invasive adenocarcinoma. Desmoplasia is best seen on low power; it is almost impossible to appreciate on 40×.

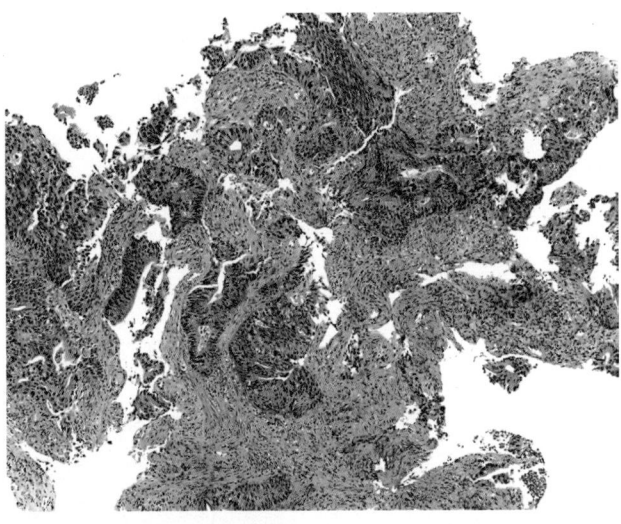

Figure 4-187. Invasive adenocarcinoma. The term invasive adenocarcinoma is reserved for cases with invasion beyond the muscularis mucosae into at least the submucosa. Similar to invasive adenocarcinomas arising from conventional adenomas, invasive adenocarcinoma in serrated polyps is also staged as (at least) pT1.

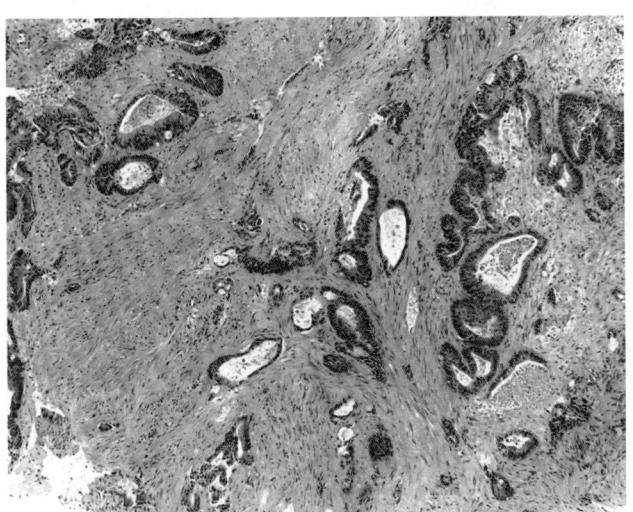

Figure 4-188. Invasive adenocarcinoma.

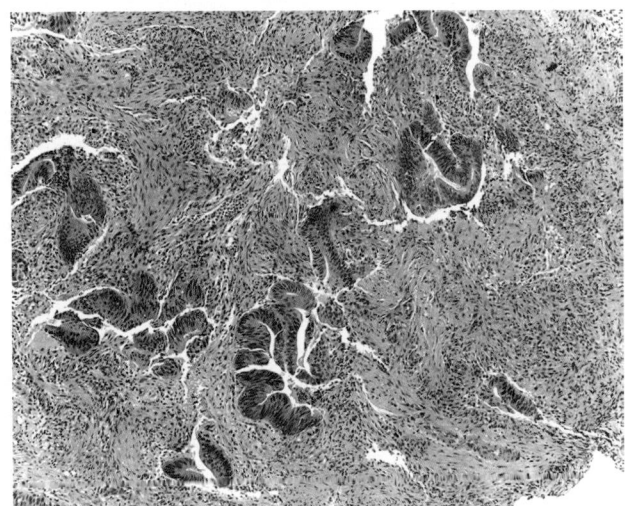

Figure 4-189. Invasive adenocarcinoma.

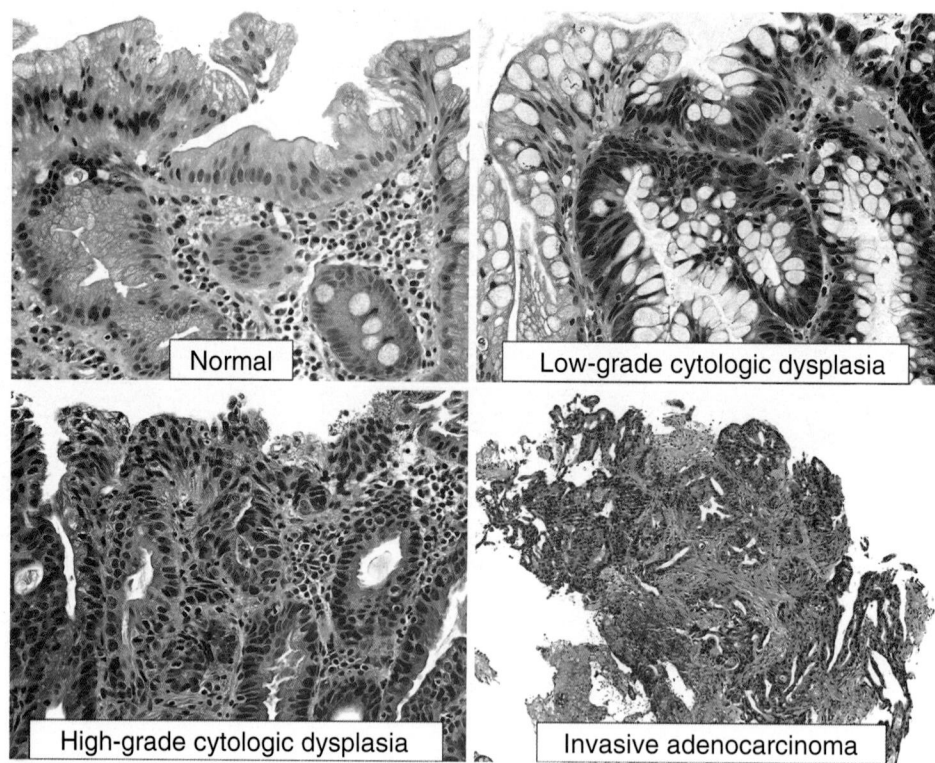

Figure 4-190. A composite image of cytologic dysplasia categories in serrated polyps. Normal colon: tiny, basally oriented nuclei, normochromatic chromatin, abundant cytoplasm, and negative for pleomorphism and prominent apoptotic bodies and mitotic figures. Dysplasia is eye-catching at low power with abrupt transitions between the normal and dysplastic epithelium, and the atypia involves the surface. Low-grade cytologic dysplasia (conventional type): retained nuclear polarity. High-grade cytologic dysplasia: loss of nuclear polarity. Architectural complexity (cribriforming) is not required for a diagnosis of high-grade dysplasia in serrated polyps. Intramucosal carcinoma (not shown) involves individual cells infiltrating the mucosa but not through the muscularis mucosae (as per IMC arising in a conventional adenoma [Figs. 4.37–4.42]). Invasive adenocarcinoma: at least submucosal invasion and signified by desmoplasia.

FAQ: How are dysplastic serrated polyps clinically managed?

Answer: The surveillance interval can be fairly clinician specific. As seen in Table 4.4, dysplastic SSA/Ps are seen in 1 to 3 years (Table 4.4).[25] Beware: this assumes the polyp was completely excised at the time of initial endoscopy. Many of our clinicians repeat the endoscopy within 3 to 6 months after removal of a dysplastic serrated polyp to confirm that the polyp was entirely removed and to exclude recurrence. Large dysplastic serrated polyps that are not amenable to endoscopic resection should be completely excised by whatever means necessary. This means that a right hemicolectomy is appropriate treatment of a large right-sided lesion with dysplasia. Less invasive endoscopic mucosal resection has high success rates when performed by skilled endoscopists at tertiary care centers, but the incidence of perforation is higher with these broad flat lesions in a difficult to maneuver right-sided location. Notice that the guidelines do not specify low-versus high-grade dysplasia in the SSA/P. These experts recommend all dysplastic SSA/P be managed analogously as a conventional adenoma with HGD, Table 4.1.[25] Also notice that the dysplastic TSA is absent from the guidelines. Some argue that the TSA is not truly dysplastic based on its negligible mitotic counts and Ki67 proliferation index, and, instead, argue the atypical changes are metaplastic or senescence related.[22,32,35] Until this controversial topic is well vetted, one can continue to grade the dysplasia in the TSA and SSA/P similarly, although this grading in the TSA has no official impact on surveillance guidelines at this time.

KEY FEATURES: Serrated Polyps

- The term serrated polyp includes the hyperplastic polyp, SSA/P, TSA, and serrated polyp, unclassifiable
- Hyperplastic polyps
  - Left colon predominant and less than 5 mm
  - Can be subclassified as microvesicular, goblet cell rich, or mucin poor, but this is not for clinical purposes and only a construct to recognize all such polyps!
  - Pale pink with a serrated surface, prominent subepithelial collagen table and increased neuroendocrine cells, superficial star-shaped crypts, and their small, narrow crypt bases lack serrations
- SSA/P
  - Right colon predominant and usually more than 5 mm
  - Pale pink with a serrated surface, at least one unequivocal architecturally distorted, dilated, and/or horizontally branched crypt base
  - Commonly seen with submucosal fat or perineurioma (EMA+, S100–)
- TSA
  - Left colon predominant and more than 5 mm
  - Bright eosinophilia, floppy villi, edematous lamina propria, luminal serrations, pencillate nuclei, and ECF
- Dysplastic SSA/P and TSA
  - The terms SSA/P and TSA imply negative for dysplasia
  - Dysplasia diagnostic categories include low- or high-grade cytologic dysplasia
  - Dysplasia can be further subcategorized as conventional-type (similar to that in conventional adenomas) or serrated-type (small cuboidal cells with eosinophilia)
  - Dysplasia of any grade indicates an advanced lesion that should be removed by whatever means necessary

UGLY CAUTERIZED POLYPS

Ugly cauterized polyp (UCP) is an unofficial diagnostic category (Fig. 4.191). Although this term should never be used in reports, it is a handy term for polyps with extensive cautery artifact. Thermal cautery is clinically used to remove some polyps. An unintentional consequence of this tissue searing is that everything, even normal mucosa (Figs. 4.192–4.196), appears dark and pseudostratified, raising concerns for dysplasia. Knowledge of a few dirty little secrets, deeper sections, and showing a colleague will resolve most cases. TAs have increased apoptotic bodies, and hyperplastic polyps typically have a prominent subepithelial collagen table and increased neuroendocrine cells. These features persist despite cautery and can be used reliably to resolve the vast majority of UCP into specific diagnostic categories (Figs. 4.197–4.210). If the diagnosis remains unclear despite these efforts, these cases are descriptively signed out as "cauterized polyp, favor X" or "cauterized polyp, not further classifiable" (Fig. 4.211).

See Fig. 4.212 for a side-by-side comparison of cauterized normal mucosa, a cauterized conventional adenoma, a cauterized hyperplastic polyp, and a cauterized polyp not further classifiable.

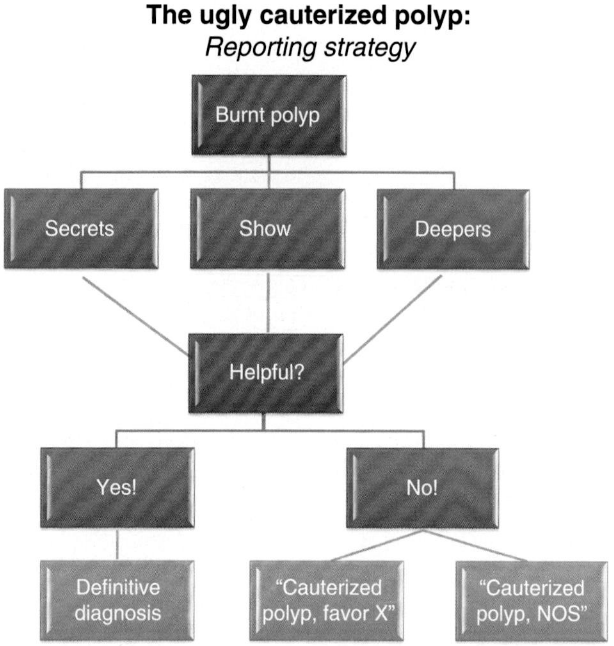

The ugly cauterized polyp:
Reporting strategy

Burnt polyp

Secrets — Show — Deepers

Helpful?

Yes! — No!

Definitive diagnosis — "Cauterized polyp, favor X" — "Cauterized polyp, NOS"

Figure 4-191. A practical approach to ugly cauterized polyps (UCPs). This approach resolves almost all UCPs into definitive diagnostic categories. First, know the dirty little secrets of UCP: conventional adenomas have increased apoptotic bodies, and hyperplastic polyps typically have a prominent subepithelial collagen table and increased neuroendocrine cells. Second, if ambiguity persists, cutting deeper into the block often helps move past the cautery. Showing a colleague is also helpful. In the rare case for which these steps are unhelpful, the case is best descriptively signed out as "cauterized polyp, favor X" or "cauterized polyp, not further classifiable."

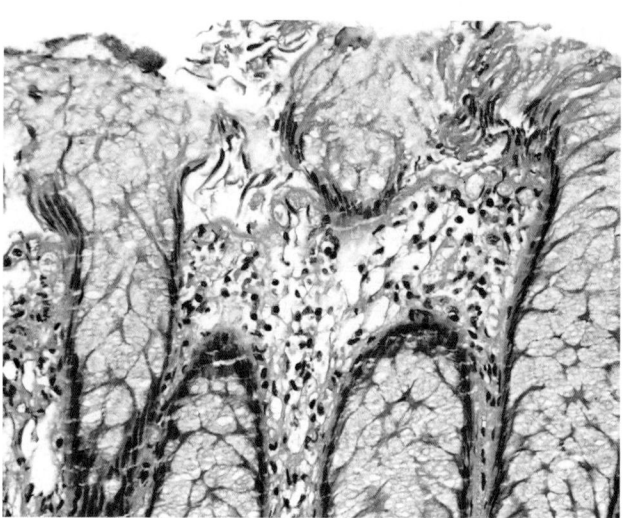

Figure 4-192. Cauterized normal colonic mucosa. UCP is not an official diagnostic category but is encountered on a daily basis and can make polyps sometimes impossible to classify because it makes everything darker and more pseudostratified. As a result, it is important to have a familiarity with the expected range of atypia due to cautery alone for accurate diagnosis and optimum clinical management.

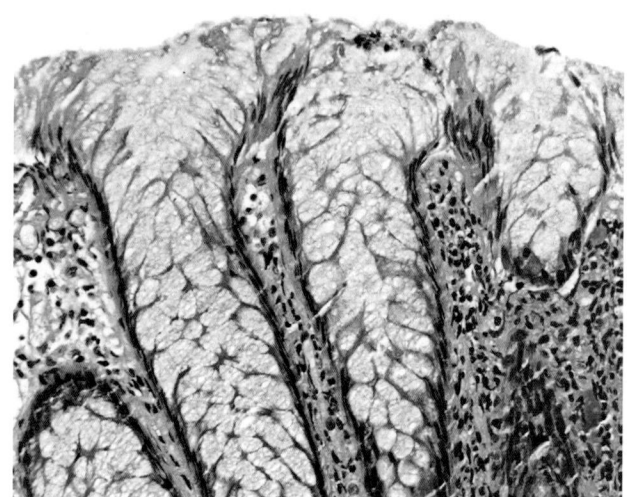

Figure 4-193. Cauterized normal colonic mucosa. These examples of cauterized, normal colonic mucosa originate from colonic resections performed for diverticular disease. The depicted nondysplastic nuclei are smeared and stretched and can raise concerns for a conventional adenoma. Helpful features of normal mucosa include normal chromasia; note that the appearance of the chromatin of the epithelium is similar (or slightly lighter) to that of the chromatin of the lymphocytes in the lamina propria.

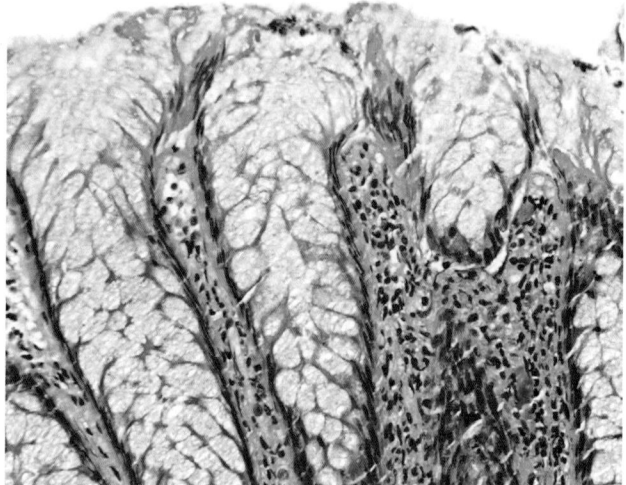

Figure 4-194. Cauterized normal colonic mucosa. Other reassuring features of nondysplastic epithelium include the lack of pleomorphism and apoptotic bodies and that the cauterized nuclei are tiny and account for only a small fraction of the overall cell volume.

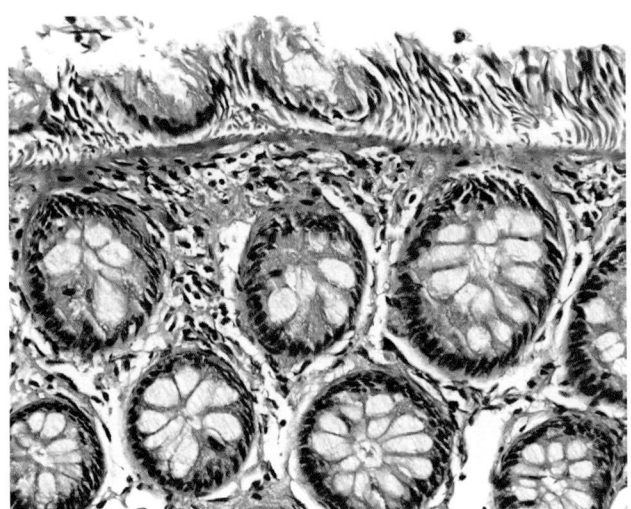

Figure 4-195. Cauterized normal colonic mucosa. It is important to be aware of the expected morphology of cauterized normal colonic mucosa so that a UCP is not overcalled as a TA, because this could lead to unnecessary overmanagement of the patient.

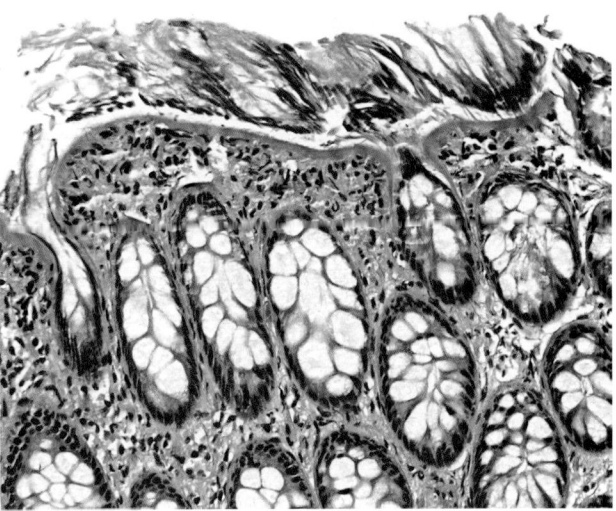

Figure 4-196. Cauterized normal colonic mucosa.

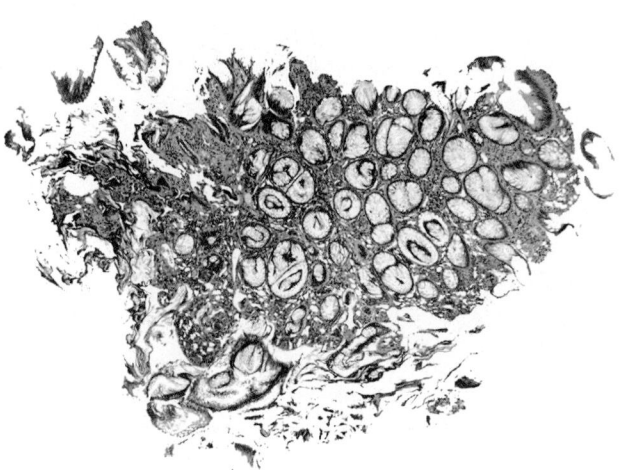

Figure 4-197. Ugly cauterized polyp (UCP), conventional tubular adenoma (TA). On low power, this seems like a polyp impossible to classify based on the extensive cautery artifact and tangential embedding.

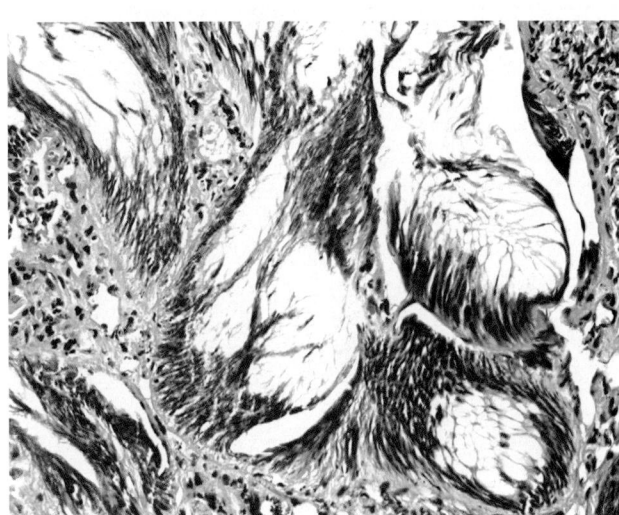

Figure 4-198. UCP, conventional TA. On high power, these nuclei are darker and more pseudostratified than can be explained by cautery alone (compare with cauterized normal colonic mucosa [Figs. 4.192–4.196]). These atypical changes involved the polyp surface and are in keeping with a diagnosis of cauterized TA.

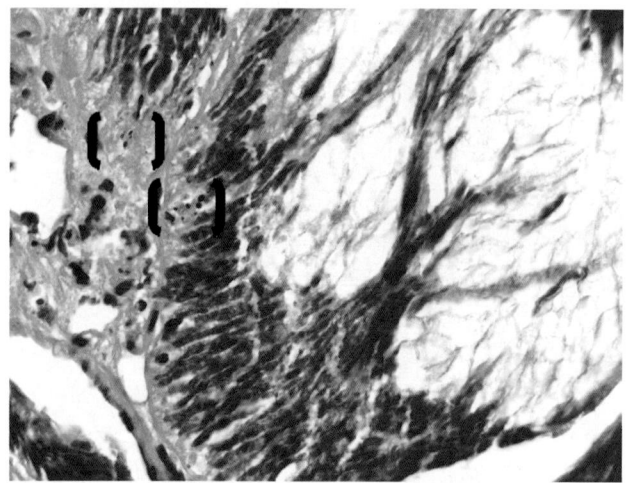

Figure 4-199. UCP, conventional TA. Another high-power field of the same case. Note the prominent apoptotic bodies (*brackets*) and the hyperchromasia and pseudostratification that is more than can be explained by cautery alone (compare with cauterized normal colonic mucosa [Figs. 4.192–4.196]).

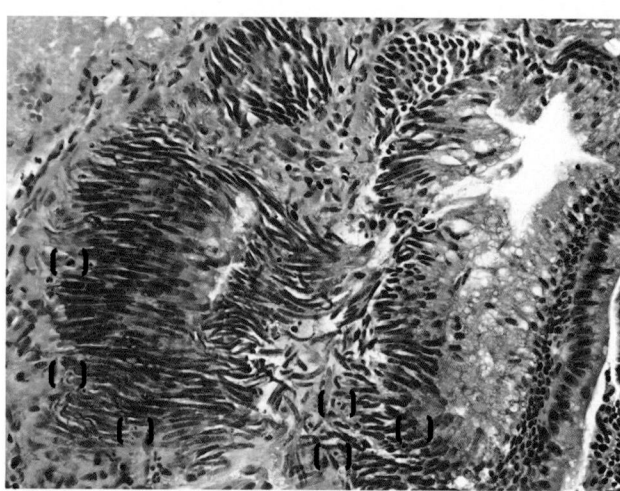

Figure 4-200. UCP, conventional TA. This degree of hyperchromasia and pseudostratification is far more than can be explained by cautery alone. The prominent apoptotic bodies (*brackets*) support the diagnosis of cauterized TA.

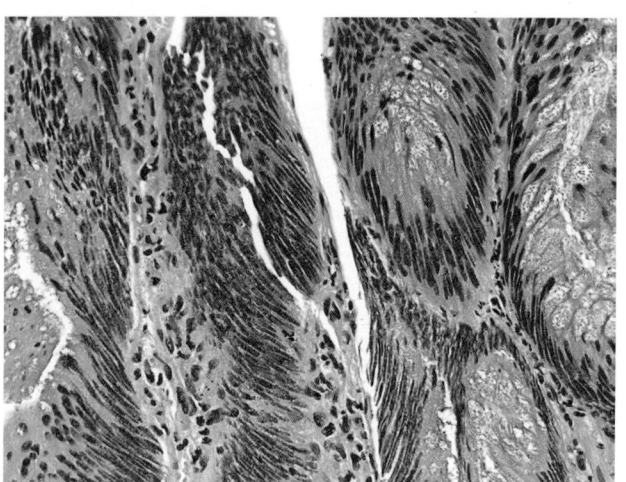

Figure 4-201. UCP, conventional TA.

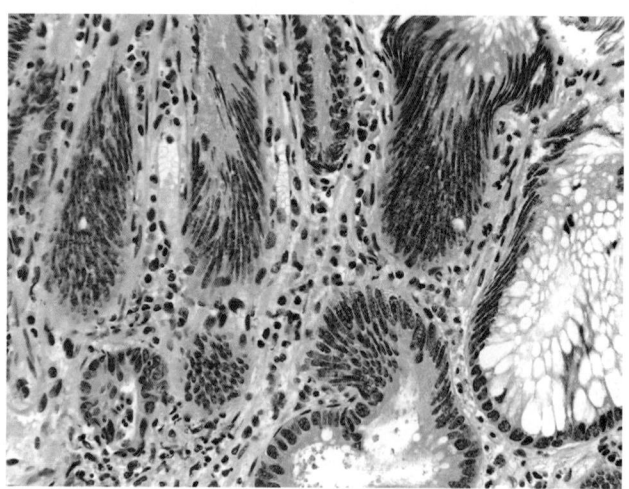

Figure 4-202. UCP, conventional TA.

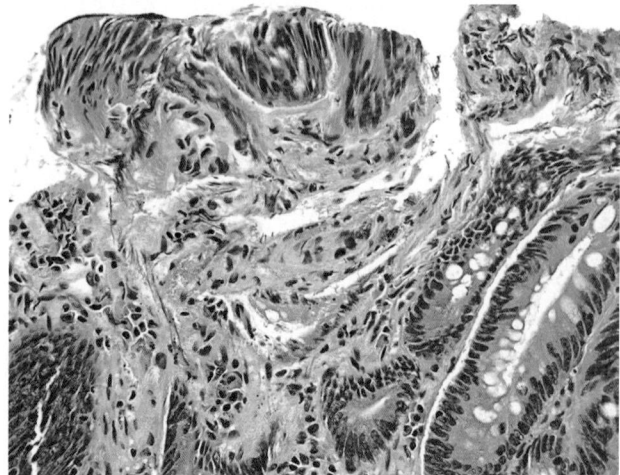

Figure 4-203. UCP, conventional TA. It is important to see the atypical changes at the polyp surface, as in this case, because dysplasia must have surface involvement. If the atypia is restricted to the crypt bases, it could be reactive, the normal proliferative compartment, or superficial sections of a conventional adenoma.

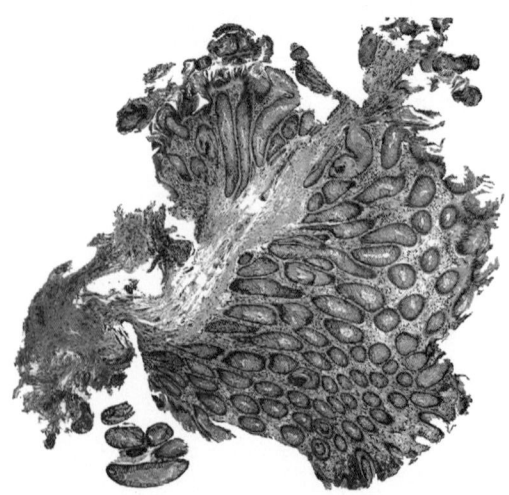

Figure 4-204. UCP, hyperplastic polyp. This 0.3-cm rectal polyp seems impossible to classify at this power based on the extensive cautery artifact and tangential embedding.

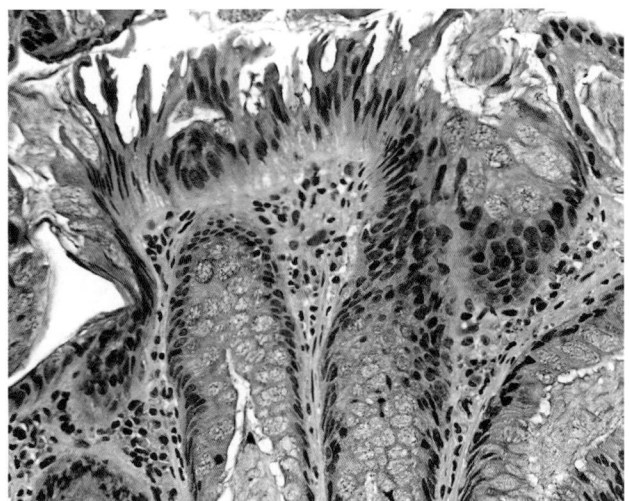

Figure 4-205. UCP, hyperplastic polyp. Higher power of the previous figure shows a prominent subepithelial collagen table and subtle serrations.

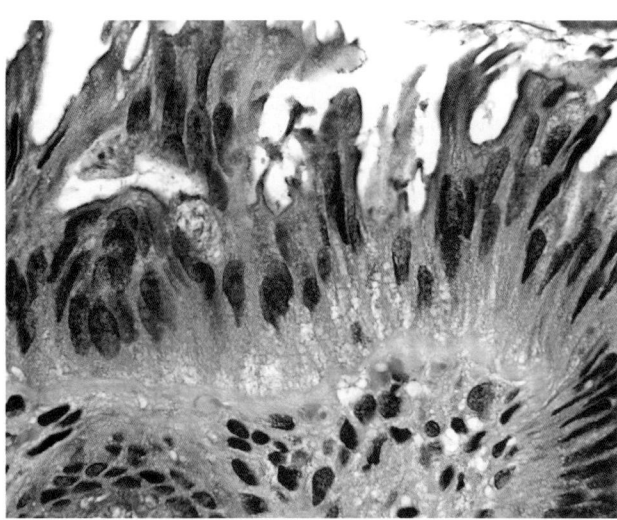

Figure 4-206. UCP, hyperplastic polyp. At this magnification, the subepithelial collagen table and subtle surface serrations are more easily seen. These cauterized nuclei are normochromatic (they appear less dark than the lamina propria lymphocytes) and bland.

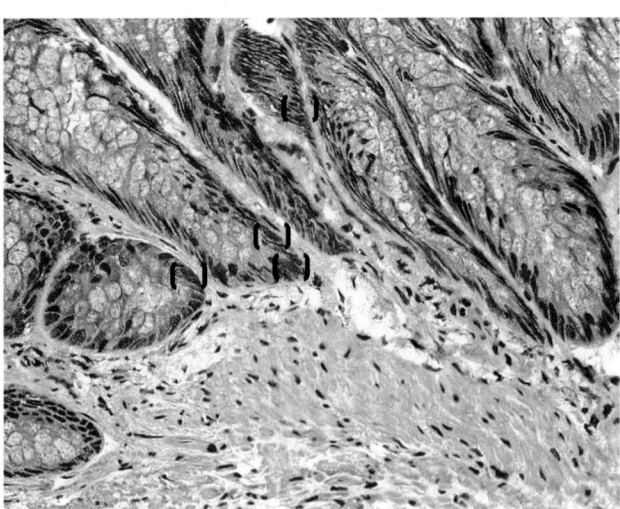

Figure 4-207. UCP, hyperplastic polyp. Another high-power field of the previous figure shows prominent neuroendocrine cells (*brackets*), narrow crypt bases, and prominent smooth muscle, supporting the diagnosis of a cauterized hyperplastic polyp.

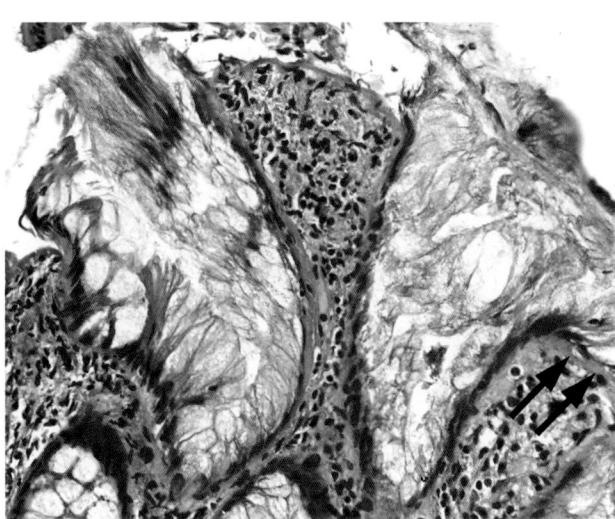

Figure 4-208. UCP, hyperplastic polyp. This cauterized 0.1-cm rectal polyp shows surface serrations, the nuclei are small and bland, and a prominent subepithelial collagen table is seen (*arrows*), in keeping with a cauterized hyperplastic polyp. The crypt bases were narrow (not shown).

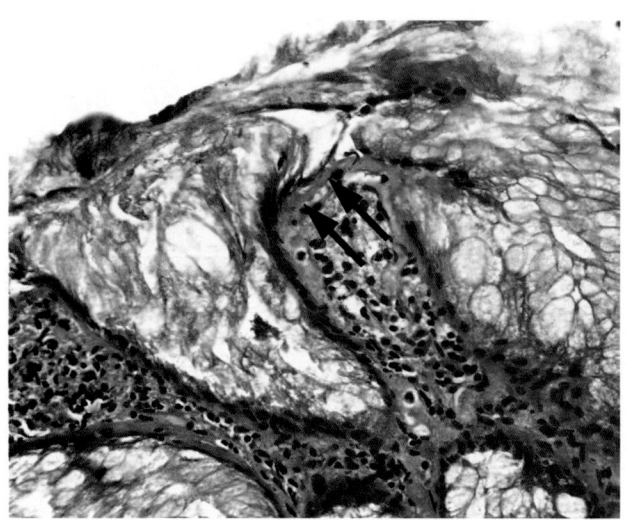

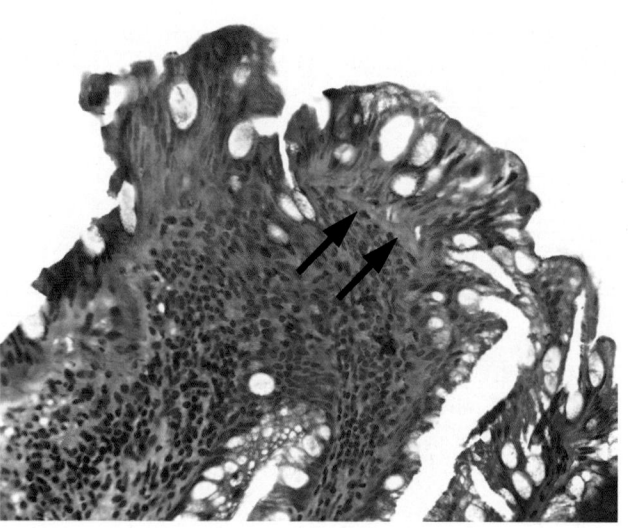

Figure 4-209. UCP, hyperplastic polyp. This cauterized 0.1-cm rectal polyp shows surface serrations, the nuclei are small and bland, and a prominent subepithelial collagen table is seen (*arrows*), as expected for a cauterized hyperplastic polyp. The crypt bases were narrow (not shown).

Figure 4-210. UCP, hyperplastic polyp. *Arrows* highlight the prominent (and burned) subepithelial collagen table, supporting the diagnosis of a cauterized hyperplastic polyp in this 0.2-cm rectal polyp (crypt bases were narrow, not shown).

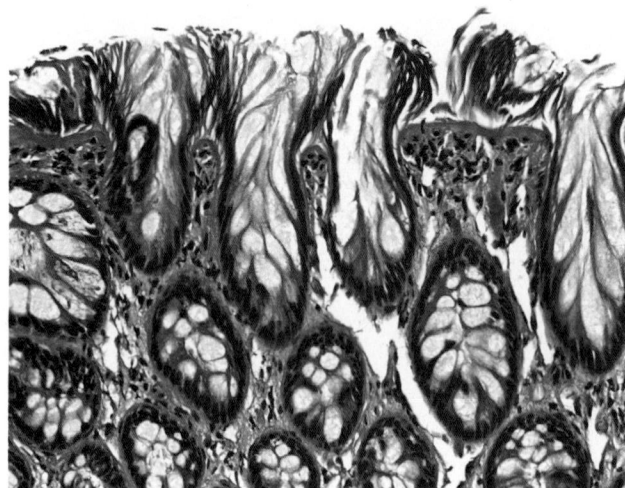

Figure 4-211. UCP, not otherwise classifiable. This type of unsatisfying case is encountered very rarely (approximately once a year). The surface is a bit darker than normal, but everything is dark and there are no apoptotic bodies to definitively diagnose a conventional adenoma. Deeper sections were pursued but were noncontributory. In the interest of not letting this patient fall out of surveillance for 10 years from a diagnosis of normal, it was signed out as cauterized polyp, not otherwise classifiable (marked cautery artifact). One hopes this feedback is received constructively to improve endoscopic technique; time will tell.

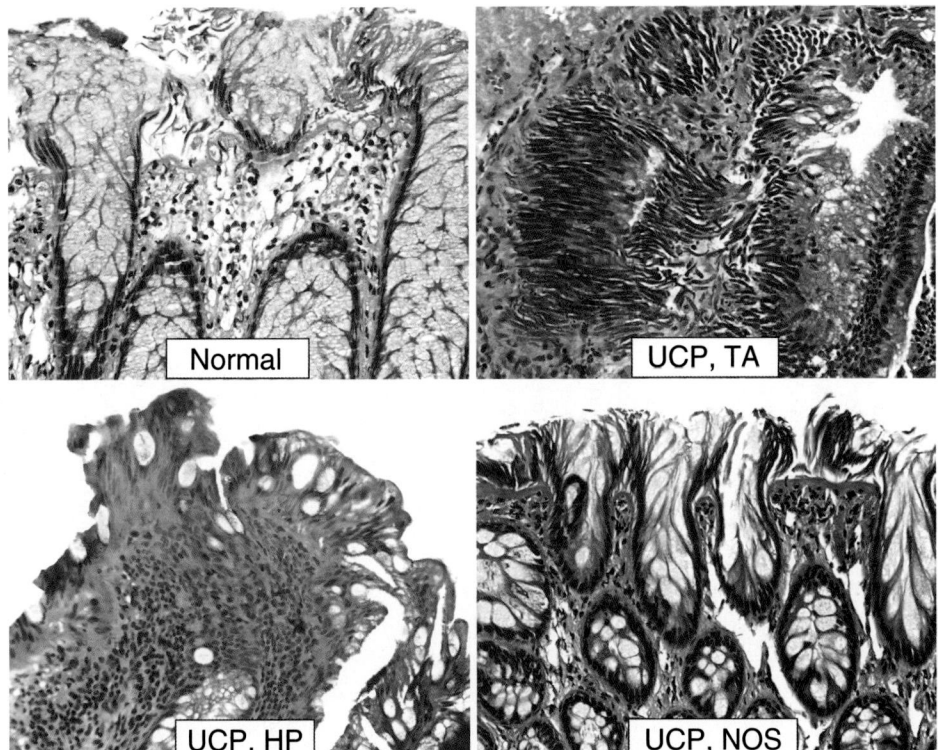

Figure 4-212. A composite of UCP diagnostic categories. Cauterized normal colon: normochromasia, lack of pleomorphism and apoptotic bodies, and the nuclei are tiny and comprise only a small fraction of the overall cell volume. Cauterized TA: hyperchromatic, pseudostratified nuclei with prominent apoptotic bodies and these changes extend to the polyp surface. Cauterized hyperplastic polyp: a serrated surface, a *pink* overall appearance, small/bland nuclei, and a prominent subepithelial collagen table; the crypt bases were narrow in this 0.2-cm rectal polyp (not shown). Cauterized polyp not otherwise classifiable: mixed features, dark (maybe a TA?) but no apoptotic bodies (maybe just cautery and a thick H&E section?). These types of diagnoses are not well received by clinicians or patients and are best avoided, if at all possible. We only release such an unhelpful diagnosis after deeper sections have been reviewed by a colleague with no better diagnosis possible.

SYNDROMIC CONSIDERATIONS

Although most polyps are sporadic, it is worthwhile to keep in mind that a subset represents a syndromic process, a diagnosis of which may trigger a genetic counselor evaluation, genetic testing, and initiation into a surveillance protocol. Alternatively, failing to recognize these syndromes may put the patient and their families at risk for preventable neoplasia by the lack of appropriate clinical management. These syndromes are easy to recognize in the dramatic presentation of a young patient with numerous polyps or carcinoma, but some cases are subtler. See the following text for a brief approach to the most common syndromic considerations (Table 4.5).

Lynch Syndrome

One of every 35 patients with CRC has Lynch syndrome (LS), making it the most common heritable form of CRC (Table 4.5).[54] Syndromic patients are at highest risk for colorectal and endometrial carcinoma but are also at risk for sebaceous tumors and malignancies of the renal pelvis/ureter, stomach, small bowel, ovary, brain, and hepatobiliary system. LS is an autosomal dominantly inherited defect in the genes encoding for mismatch repair (MMR) proteins: MLH1, PMS2, MSH2, MSH6, EPCAM, and MLH3. The diagnosis is established by demonstrating the presence of deleterious defects in MMR genes through (1) germline defects in the DNA MMR genes, *or* (2) germline methylation of the MLH1 promoter, *or* (3) inactivation of MSH2 due to deletion of the 3′ exons of the EPCAM (TACSTD1) gene. As a result of these MMR defects, the associated colorectal and endometrial carcinomas have microsatellite instability (MSI-high). The precursor polyp is the conventional adenoma. Most Lynch-associated CRC are in the proximal colon, and the characteristic morphology

TABLE 4.5: Overview of Select Syndromes

Syndrome	Age at clinical onset	Gene (Chromosome)	Gene Function	Polyp Distribution — Stomach	Polyp Distribution — Small bowel	Polyp Distribution — Colon	Polyp Histology	Clinical manifestations	Diagnostic criteria	Prognosis
Lynch syndrome (formerly hereditary nonpolyposis colorectal cancer, HNPCC)	45–50 years	MutL homologue 1 (MLH1:3p21-p23), mutS homologue 2 (MSH2:2p21), mutL homolog 6 (MSH6:2p21), postmeiotic segregation increased 2 (PMS2:7p22), Epithelial cell adhesion molecule (EpCAM:2p21), MutS Homolog 3: MLH3 (14q24)	Tumor suppressor (mismatch Repair)	Autosomal dominant	Usually low polyp burden	Usually low polyp burden	Usually low polyp burden	The precursor polyp is the conventional tubular adenoma in the small bowel and or colon; can also see gastric pyloric gland adenomas	60% of colorectal carcinomas occur in the proximal colon 18% have synchronous or metachronous colorectal carcinomas. Typical colorectal carcinomas are MSI-H with prominent tumor infiltrating lymphocytes, Crohn-like peritumoral reaction, and a mucinous, medullary, or poorly-differentiated component. Muir-Torre syndrome: Lynch Syndrome with sebaceous gland tumors or keratoacanthoma and other Lynch syndrome-type malignancies Turcot syndrome: Lynch Syndrome with brain tumors (glioblastomas) and multiple colorectal conventional tubular adenomas	1. Germline defects in the DNA MMR genes, OR 2. Germline methylation of the MLH1 promoter, OR 3. Inactivation of MSH2 due to deletion of the 3′ exons of the EPCAM (TACSTD1) gene	10-53% colorectal carcinoma risk 15-44% endometrial carcinoma risk Others: renal pelvis/ureter, stomach, small bowel, ovary, brain, hepatobiliary, and sebaceous tumors

| Familial adenomatous polyposis (FAP) | 15-20 years | Adenomatous polyposis coli (APC:5q21) | Tumor Suppressor (Negative regulator of cell adhesion, signal transduction, and activation; mutations lead to nuclear accumulatoin of B-catenin and growth promotion) | Autosomal dominant | 80% | 10% | 100% | The precursor polyp is the conventional tubular adenomas in the small bowel and colon. Gastric fundic gland polyps with or without dysplasia, gastric foveolar adenomas, and pyloric gland adenomas are also seen | Classic form: ≥100 polyps. Attenuated form: <100 polyps. Turcot syndrome: FAP with brain tumors (medulloblastoma) and hypertrophy of retinal pigment epithelium. Gardner syndrome: FAP with epidermoid cysts, mandibular osteomas, desmoids, and thyroid tumors | FAP 1. At least 100 or more colorectal adenomas, OR 2. A germline pathogenic-causing mutation of the APC gene, OR 3. Family history of FAP and any number of adenomas at a young age. Attenuated FAP 1. Fewer than 100 colorectal polyps 2. A germline disease-causing mutation of the APC gene | Colon, duodenal, and/or thyroid carcinomas 80-100% gastrointestinal cancer risk |

(Continued)

TABLE 4.5: Overview of Select Syndromes (Continued)

Syndrome	Age at clinical onset	Gene (Chromosome)	Gene Function	Inheritance	Polyp Distribution	Polyp Histology	Clinical manifestations	Diagnostic criteria	Prognosis
MUTYH-associated polyposis (MAP; previously MYH-associated polyposis)	45 years	MutY homologue (MUTYH; 1p34)	Tumor suppressor (base excision repair)	Autosomal recessive	Can have low polyp burden	Most are colon and small bowel conventional tubular adenomas, but also seen are hyperplastic polyps, SSA/Ps, and gastric fundic gland polyps and adenomas	Heterogeneous presentation: can have only a few polyps or 1000, the majority have less than 100 polyps Associated with sebaceous tumors Polyps and colorectal carcinomas are predominantly right colon and can show MSI-H, prominent tumor infiltrating lymphocytes, Crohn-like peritumoral reaction, and a mucinous, medullary, or poorly-differentiated component	1. > 10 synchronous colorectal adenomas 2. Lack of APC gene germline mutation, AND 3. A pedigree suggestive of an autosomal recessive inheritance	High-risk of small bowel cancer 2.5-fold increased risk of colorectal cancer 40% risk of extra-intestinal neoplasia with no predominant tumor type

Serrated polyposis syndrome (previously hyperplastic polyposis syndrome)	44-62 years	Unknown	Unknown	Unclear	0%	0%	100%	The precursor serrated polyps are limited to the colorectum and include hyperplastic polyp, SSA/P with and without dysplasia, TSA with and without dysplasia, and serrated polyp unclassifiable. Conventional tubular adenomas are seen as well.	Large polyps are usually proximal to the sigmoid colon. 64% of colorectal carcinomas are proximal to the sigmoid colon	1. At least 5 serrated lesions proximal to the sigmoid colon with 2 or more of these being greater than 10 mm, OR 2. Any number of serrated lesions proximal to the sigmoid colon in an individual who has a first-degree relative with serrated polyposis, OR 3. Greater than 20 serrated lesions of any size, but distributed throughout the colon	Up to 50% risk of colorectal carcinoma. Up to 26% of patients have a synchronous/metachronous colorectal carcinoma. First degree relatives have a 5.4% increased risk of colorectal carcinoma

(Continued)

TABLE 4.5: Overview of Select Syndromes (Continued)

Syndrome	Age at clinical onset	Gene (Chromosome)	Gene Function	Inheritance	Polyp Distribution		Polyp Histology	Clinical manifestations	Diagnostic criteria	Prognosis
Juvenile polyposis	18.5 years	Signaling effectors mothers against decapentaplegic protein 4 (SMAD4; 18q21) or bone morphogenetic protein receptor 1A (BMPR1A; 10q23)	Tumor suppressor (encodes for a protein involved in the transforming growth factor-beta family of signal transduction)	Autosomal dominant	14%	<10%	100%	The typical polyp is hamartomatous /inflammatory-type with surface erosions and edematous and inflamed lamina propria surrounding ectatic and inflamed crypts Dysplasia can be seen within the syndromic polyps	Rectal bleeding and intussception common Most present with colorectal syndromic polyps, ranging from 3-200 polyps Gastric and small bowel syndromic polyps can also be seen	1. More than 3 juvenile polyps of the colorectum, OR 2. Juvenile polyps throughout the GI tract, OR 3. Any number of juvenile polyps with a family history of juvenile polyposis	39% lifetime risk of colorectal carcinoma 10-15% risk of gastric, small bowel, and pancreas carcinoma

| Peutz-Jeghers syndrome | 10-30 years | Liver kinase B1 or serine/threonine kinase 11 (LKB1/STK1; 19p13) | Tumor Suppressor (Regulates cell polarity and energy metabolism) | Autosomal dominant | 15-30% | 64-96% | 25-53% | The typical polyp is hamartomatous and consists of a central core of arborizing smooth muscle dividing compartments of normal appearing mucosa Dysplasia in the hamartomatous polyp is uncommon Classic histology best seen in the small bowel, but polyps can also be seen in the stomach and colorectum | Freckle-like hyperpigmentation of the oral mucosa and lips, can also see gastric and colorectal polyps Polyps are most common in the small bowel, where they can cause intussusception | 1. Detection of three or more histologically confirmed Peutz-Jeghers polyps, OR 2. The presence of any number of Peutz-Jeghers polyps in a patient with a family history of the syndrome, OR 3. Detection of characteristic, prominent mucocutaneous pigmentation in the patient with a family history of the syndrome, OR 4. Detection of any number of Peutz-Jheghers polyps in a patient with prominent mucocutaneous pigmentation | 90% lifetime risk of malignancy 39-57% risk of colorectal carcinoma 29% lifetime risk of gastric adenocarcinoma 36% Pancreatic carcinoma Sertoli cell tumors in testes Minimal deviation adenocarcinoma (adenoma malignum) of the uterine cervix Sex cord tumor with annular tubules (SCTATs) of the ovaries Breast carcinomas pigmentation |

Adapted from Giardello FM, Burt RW, Jarvinen J, et al. *Familial Adenomatous Polyposis.* 4th ed. Lyon, France: IARC Press; 2010; Morreau H, Riddell R, Aretz S. *MUTYH-Associated Polyposis.* 4th ed. Lyon, France: IARC Press; 2010; Rosty C, Buchanan DD, Walsh MD, et al. Phenotype and polyp landscape in serrated polyposis syndrome: a series of 100 patients from genetics clinics. *Am J Surg Pathol.* 2012;36(6):876-882; Rosty C, Walsh MD Walters RJ, et al. Multiplicity and molecular heterogeneity of colorectal carcinomas in individuals with serrated polyposis. *Am J Surg Pathol.* 2013;37(3):434-442; Crowder CD, Sweet K, Lehman A, Frankel WL. Serrated polyposis is an underdiagnosed and unclear syndrome: the surgical pathologist has a role in improving detection. *Am J Surg Pathol.* 2012;36(8):1178-1185; Offerhaus G, Howe J. *Juvenile Polyposis.* 4th ed. Lyon, France: IARC; 2010; Campos FG, Figueiredo MN, Martinez CA. Colorectal cancer risk in hamartomatous polyposis syndromes. *World J Gastrointest Surg.* 2015;7(3):25-32; Offerhaus G, Billaud M, Gruber SB. *Peutz-Jeghers Syndrome.* 4th ed. Lyon, France: IARC 2010; Pai RK. A practical approach to the evaluation of gastrointestinal tract carcinomas for Lynch syndrome. *Am J Surg Pathol.* 2016;40(4):e17-e34; Lam-Himlin D, Arnold CA, DePetris G. Gastric polyps and polyposis syndromes. *Diagn Histopathol.* 2014;20:1-11; Seshadri D, Karagiorgos N, Hyser MJ. A case of Cronkhite-Canada syndrome and a review of gastrointestinal polyposis syndromes. *Gastroenterol Hepatol (N Y).* 2012;8(3):197-201.

includes prominent tumor infiltrating lymphocytes, Crohn-like peritumoral reaction, and a mucinous, medullary, or poorly differentiated component (see also "Adenocarcinoma" section, "Microsatellite Instability Pathway" subsection).[55] High-yield board examination fodder includes that Muir-Torre syndrome refers to patients with LS with sebaceous gland tumors or keratoacanthoma and other LS-type malignancies, and Turcot syndrome refers to patients with LS with brain tumors (glioblastomas) and multiple colorectal conventional adenomas. See also Turcot syndrome in the "Familial Adenomatous Polyposis" section.

In 1991, the Amsterdam criteria outlined the diagnostic requirements for LS based solely on clinical criteria. The 2004 revised Bethesda Guidelines offered an improved strategy for Lynch screening by directing select CRC for further microsatellite instability (MSI) testing (Table 4.6).[56] According to these guidelines, CRC that satisfied any of the specified criteria should be subject to MSI testing or MMR protein immunohistochemistry (MMR IHC) followed by germline confirmatory testing.[56] In 2008, universal LS screening was proposed because the Bethesda criteria failed to identify one in four (28%) of patients with LS.[54] These investigators concluded that MMR IHC is almost equally sensitive as MSI and that MMR IHC is easier to incorporate into most laboratories. Beware that the LS screening protocol varies by institution. Our center's (CAA) approach is discussed in depth in the "Adenocarcinoma" section, "Microsatellite Instability Pathway" subsection, this chapter.

TABLE 4.6: The Revised Bethesda Guidelines for Selection of Colorectal Tumors for Microsatellite Instability (MSI) Testing[56]

1. Colorectal carcinoma diagnosed in a patient <50 years of age
2. Presence of synchronous or metachronous colorectal or other Lynch syndrome–associated tumors,[a] regardless of age
3. Colorectal carcinoma with MSI-high[b] histology[c] in a patient who is <60 years of age
4. Colorectal carcinoma or Lynch syndrome–associated tumor diagnosed <50 years of age in at least one first-degree relative
5. Colorectal carcinoma or Lynch syndrome–associated tumor diagnosed at any age in two first- or second-degree relatives

---

[a]Lynch syndrome–associated tumors include colorectal, endometrial, stomach, ovarian, pancreas, ureter or renal pelvis, biliary tract, brain (usually glioblastoma), sebaceous gland adenomas and keratoacanthomas in Muir-Torre syndrome, and small bowel carcinomas.
[b]MSI-H in tumors refers to changes in two or more of the five US National Cancer Institute–recommended panels of microsatellite markers.
[c]MSI-H histology refers to the presence of tumor-infiltrating lymphocytes, Crohn disease–like lymphocytic reaction, mucinous or signet ring differentiation, or medullary growth pattern.

Biannual colonoscopy is recommended for those with an established diagnosis of LS.[57] Total colectomy is recommended for established CRC, with prophylactic colectomies recommended in some settings.[57-59] Similarly, prophylactic hysterectomy with bilateral salpingo-oophorectomy can be offered to women when fertility is no longer desired or by age 40 years, whichever comes first.[57,59,60] Annual endometrial biopsy, urine cytology, and ultrasound screening for upper urologic cancers starts at age 30 years.[57,61] Upper GI endoscopic screening can start at age 30 years and be repeated at 3- to 5-year intervals in patients with a family history of upper GI malignancy.[57]

FAQ: Is the term hereditary nonpolyposis colorectal cancer still used?

Answer: In 1984, the term hereditary nonpolyposis colorectal cancer (HNPCC) was introduced to distinguish patients with LS from those with familial adenomatous polyposis (FAP). The term HNPCC has fallen out of favor because patients with LS can have extracolonic neoplasms and an increased incidence of colorectal polyps compared with nonsyndromic patients, even though they manifest fewer adenoma than patients with FAP.[62]

PEARLS & PITFALLS

A popular misconception is that the precursor lesion in LS is the SSA/P because SSA/P-related CRCs are also MSI-high. However, the precursor polyp in LS is the conventional adenoma. See also "Adenocarcinoma" section, "Microsatellite Instability Pathway" subsection.

KEY FEATURES: LS

- There is an autosomal dominantly inherited defect in the genes encoding for MMR proteins.
- LS-associated CRCs are MSI-high.
- The precursor polyp is the conventional adenoma.
- Muir-Torre syndrome = patients with LS with sebaceous gland tumors or keratoacanthoma and other LS-type malignancies.
- Turcot syndrome = patients with LS with brain tumors (glioblastomas) and multiple colorectal conventional adenomas.
- Universal LS screening on CRC via MSI or MMR IHC is suggested.
- The term HNPCC should be avoided because patients with LS can have extracolonic neoplasms and an increased incidence of colorectal polyps compared with nonsyndromic patients.

Familial Adenomatous Polyposis

FAP is an autosomal dominantly inherited defect in the *APC* gene (Table 4.5). It clinically manifests as at least 100 colorectal polyps and imparts a 100% risk of CRC, if prophylactic colectomy is not performed. Patients are also at risk for small bowel and thyroid malignancies. Most of the colon and small intestine polyps are conventional TAs, and gastric polyps include fundic gland polyps with or without dysplasia, gastric foveolar adenomas, and pyloric gland adenomas.[63] FAP diagnostic criteria include (1) at least 100 or more colorectal adenomas, *or* (2) a germline pathogenic-causing mutation of the *APC* gene, *or* (3) family history of FAP and any number of adenomas at a young age. FAP screening involves genetic testing with a definitive FAP diagnosis requiring confirmation of a germline *APC* gene mutation, and the absence of the mutation excludes the diagnosis of FAP.[43] Variants include Turcot syndrome, which describes patients with FAP with brain tumors (medulloblastoma) and hypertrophy of retinal pigment epithelium (although many such patients probably would now be classified with biallelic MMR deficiency, also known as constitutional MMR deficiency usually a product of consanguity[64]), and Gardner syndrome, which describes patients with FAP with epidermoid cysts, mandibular osteomas, desmoids, and thyroid tumors. Attenuated FAP is characterized by fewer than 100 colorectal polyps and a germline *APC* gene mutation. Annual colonoscopic screening starts at puberty and continues until completion colectomy.[57] Indications for colectomy include the following: (1) suspected carcinoma, (2) significant symptoms, (3) multiple adenomas >6 mm, (4) a significant increase in polyp number, (5) presence of HGD, or (6) inability to adequately survey the colon because of numerous polyps.[57] Endoscopic screening for gastric and small bowel neoplasms starts at age 25 years and is repeated at 6-month to 4-year intervals depending on the findings. LGD in fundic gland polyps is common and does not require surgical intervention; resection is indicated for HGD or carcinoma.[57] Annual thyroid screening by ultrasound is recommended.[57]

KEY FEATURES: FAP

- There is an autosomal dominantly inherited defect in the *APC* gene.
- It clinically manifests as at least 100 colorectal polyps and has a 100% risk of CRC.
- Precursor polyp is the conventional adenoma.
- Turcot syndrome = patients with FAP with brain tumors (medulloblastoma) and hypertrophy of retinal pigment epithelium—some of these would be classified today as constitutional MMR deficiency, usually a product of consanguity.

- Gardner syndrome = patients with FAP with epidermoid cysts, mandibular osteomas, desmoids, and thyroid tumors.
- Attenuated FAP = fewer than 100 colorectal polyps and a germline *APC* gene mutation.

MUTYH-Associated Polyposis

MUTYH-associated polyposis is an autosomal recessively inherited defect in the *MUTYH* gene (Table 4.5).[65] The *MUTYH* gene product functions in base excision repair and protects against oxidative stress. The clinical presentation varies widely and can overlap with that of LS, attenuated FAP, serrated polyposis syndrome, and sporadic cases. Some patients with *MUTYH*-associated polyposis present with only a few colorectal polyps and others have >1000, but generally they present with fewer than 100 polyps. Most polyps are colon and small bowel conventional adenomas, but hyperplastic polyps and SSA/P are also seen. Colon polyps and CRCs are typically right sided and can show MSI-high, prominent tumor infiltrating lymphocytes, Crohn-like peritumoral reaction, and a mucinous, medullary, or poorly differentiated component, demonstrating further overlap with LS. Duodenal polyposis, gastric fundic gland polyps, and gastric adenomas can be seen, and there are also reports of associated urothelial carcinoma and sebaceous tumors. The diagnostic criteria include (1) >10 synchronous colorectal adenomas, (2) lack of *APC* gene germline mutation, *and* (3) a pedigree suggestive of an autosomal recessive inheritance.[44] Patients have an increased risk of small bowel and colon cancer, as well as a 40% risk of extraintestinal neoplasia.[44,66] Biannual colonoscopy starts at age 18 years, and gastroduodenoscopy starts at age 25 years with predictive genetic testing suggested. Indications for colectomy and upper GI and thyroid screening recommendations are identical to those described for patients with FAP.[57]

KEY FEATURES: MUTYH-Associated Polyposis

- There is autosomal recessively inherited defect in the *MUTYH* gene and lack of *APC* gene mutation.
- The clinical presentation overlaps with that of LS, attenuated FAP, serrated polyposis syndrome, and sporadic cases.
- Most have fewer than 100 polyps, and most are conventional adenomas, but one can also see hyperplastic polyps and SSA/Ps.

Serrated Polyposis Syndrome

Serrated polyposis syndrome is characterized by increased colorectal hyperplastic polyps, SSA/P, TSA, and serrated polyps, not further classifiable (Table 4.5). Polyps identical to conventional TA are also seen,[45] but it is unclear if they are typical conventional TAs or if they were once serrated polyps that have been entirely overrun by dysplasia. Syndromic patients have up to a 50% risk of CRC, and those under surveillance have a 7% cumulative risk of CRC at 5 years.[67] Although *BRAF*, *KRAS*, MMR, *TP53*, and *CTNNB1*/β-catenin have been studied,[45,46] the underlying genetic defect and the mode of inheritance remain unknown. The 2010 WHO diagnostic criteria for serrated polyposis syndrome include the following: (1) at least 5 serrated lesions proximal to the sigmoid colon with 2 or more of these being greater than 10 mm, *or* (2) any number of serrated lesions proximal to the sigmoid colon in an individual who has a first-degree relative with serrated polyposis, *or* (3) greater than 20 serrated lesions of any size but distributed throughout the colon.[22] Polyps are limited to the colorectum, making colonoscopy an important surveillance tool. Annual colonoscopic screening is recommended for syndromic patients with the goal to remove all serrated polyps proximal to the sigmoid colon or all serrated lesion ≥5 mm if there are numerous diminutive polyps. First-degree relatives have a 5.4-fold increased risk of colorectal cancer[68] and benefit from surveillance colonoscopy starting at age 40 years or beginning at 10 years younger than the youngest affected relative and repeated at 5-year intervals, or more frequently if polyps are identified.[25] Two types of serrated polyposis have been described, but it is not necessary to discriminate these types in pathology reports. Type 1 has at least five proximal, large SSA/P, *BRAF* mutations, CpG island promoter hypermethylation, and a relatively higher risk of CRC than type 2. Type 2 has at least 20 smaller polyps distributed uniformly throughout the colon, *KRAS* mutations, and a relatively lower incidence of colorectal cancer than type 1. Total colectomy is advocated by some over local resection based on an increased risk of metachronous neoplasia.[57] Colectomy indications include carcinoma or a polyp burden that cannot be managed endoscopically.[57]

PEARLS & PITFALLS

Unfortunately, this syndrome is easy to overlook because most syndromic patients satisfy the criteria only after multiple colonoscopies.[69] As a result, pathologists and clinicians should stay vigilant. Clinicians should be aware of the family history and maintain an accurate life-time tally of the polyp type, number, and location. Pathologists should peek at the prior pathology to assess the polyp burden over time and have a low threshold to direct the clinician to consider this syndrome. In a recent study, of the 17 patients who met the WHO criteria for serrated polyposis syndrome, only 1 was clinically suspected of the syndrome,[47] emphasizing the difficulty in prospective recognition. In another study, all syndromic patients who presented with CRC developed cancer before or at the same time that they satisfied the WHO criteria for serrated polyposis syndrome.[69] To help better recognize and manage these syndromic patients, some have suggested that clinicians use a cutoff of at least two serrated polyps to serve as a trigger point for syndromic consideration.[69]

SAMPLE NOTE: Typical Case of Patient With Unrecognized Serrated Polyposis Syndrome

Colon Polyps, Biopsy
- Fragments of SSA/P
- Separate fragments of hyperplastic polyp
- See Note

Note: From review of the prior pathology reports, the patient's history of several large, proximal serrated polyps at each colonoscopy is noted. In this case, it may be worthwhile considering serrated polyposis syndrome whose diagnostic criteria include a cumulative life-time finding of the following: (1) at least 5 serrated lesions proximal to the sigmoid colon with 2 or more of these being greater than 10 mm, *or* (2) any number of serrated lesions proximal to the sigmoid colon in an individual who has a first-degree relative with serrated polyposis, *or* (3) greater than 20 serrated lesions of any size but distributed throughout the colon. *MUTYH*-associated polyposis is another consideration, and the diagnostic criteria include the following: (1) >10 synchronous colorectal adenomas, (2) lack of *APC* gene germline mutation, and (3) a pedigree suggestive of an autosomal recessive inheritance.

References:

Snover DC, Ahnen DJ, Burt RW, et al. *Serrated Polyps of the Colon and Rectum and Serrated Polyposis.* Lyon, France: IARC Press; 2010.

Morreau H, Riddell R, Aretz S. *MUTYH-Associated Polyposis.* Lyon, France: IARC Press; 2010.

PEARLS & PITFALLS

Keep in mind that polyposis syndromes can show heterogeneity, and many have overlapping presentations. LS, attenuated FAP, *MUTYH*-associated polyposis, serrated polyposis syndrome, and sporadic cases can have similar presentations. In these cases, a careful family history, physical examination, and genetic testing are essential.

SAMPLE NOTE: Endoscopy Shows a Mass and 40 Colon Polyps

Colon, Polyps (Biopsy)
- Invasive adenocarcinoma arising in association with fragments of TAs, SSA/Ps, and hyperplastic polyps
- See Note

Note: The history of 40 polyps is noted. Although this could represent sporadic CRC, it may be worthwhile considering the possibility of a predisposing syndrome, such as LS, attenuated FAP, *MUTYH*-associated polyposis, or serrated polyposis syndrome, among others. Correlation with a careful family history, physical examination, and genetic counselor evaluation/testing is a consideration.

KEY FEATURES: Serrated Polyposis Syndrome

- Genetics are unclear.
- Syndromic polyps are colorectal hyperplastic polyps, SSA/P, TSA, and serrated polyps, not further classifiable.
- Syndromic patients have up to a 50% risk of CRC.

Hamartomatous/Inflammatory-type Polyp Syndromes

Hamartomas are collections of disorganized normal tissue constituents native to that particular site. The Peutz-Jeghers polyp is a common example, and it consists of a central core of smooth muscle dividing lobular compartments of mucosa native to the site from which it arises. Inflammatory-type polyps also have mucosa native to the site from which they arise, but the important distinction is their prominent inflammation. In most textbooks there is a clear delineation between hamartomas and inflammatory-type polyps, but in real life, these polyps exist on a morphologic spectrum and can show considerable overlap. Despite these challenges, histology alone is sufficient to satisfy diagnostic criteria for some syndromes. As a result, a familiarity with the morphologic spectrum, a broad differential diagnosis, and a carefully crafted note are important for optimum management and outcome. Below is a discussion of the major syndromes lumped together by their similar appearing hamartomatous/inflammatory-type polyps: juvenile polyposis, Peutz-Jeghers, Cronkite-Canada, and *PTEN* hamartoma tumor syndromes (PHTS) (Table 4.5).

Juvenile Polyposis

Juvenile polyposis is an autosomal dominantly inherited cancer predisposition syndrome most commonly associated with *SMAD4* or *BMPR1A* genetic defects (Table 4.5). The hamartomatous polyps are most commonly found in the colon but can also arise in the stomach and small bowel. As true for all hamartomas, these syndromic polyps are lined by mucosa native to their site. Typical features include surface erosions overlying granulation tissue and inflamed and edematous lamina propria surrounding ectatic and inflamed crypts (Figs. 4.213–4.219).[70] Dysplasia may be seen in these polyps; these hamartomatous polyps harbor malignant potential for gastric, small bowel, and colorectal carcinomas. The polyps can be indistinguishable from those found in the other hamartomatous/inflammatory-type polyp syndromes (Peutz-Jeghers syndrome, PHTS, and Cronkhite-Canada syndrome [CCS]) and sporadic inflammatory-type polyps, especially those that are small or those that arise in the stomach[71] and small bowel. The 2010 WHO criteria include the following: (1) more than three juvenile polyps of the colorectum, *or* (2) juvenile polyps throughout the GI tract, *or* (3) any number of juvenile polyps in a patient with a family history of juvenile polyposis, assuming other causes of hamartomatous polyposis have been excluded.[48] Upper and lower endoscopy starts at age 15 years or at the time of first symptoms and is repeated every 2 to 3 years.[49] Prophylactic resection is considered for patients with significant polyp-related symptoms, for those whose polyp burden cannot be managed endoscopically, or in those with a strong family history of cancer.

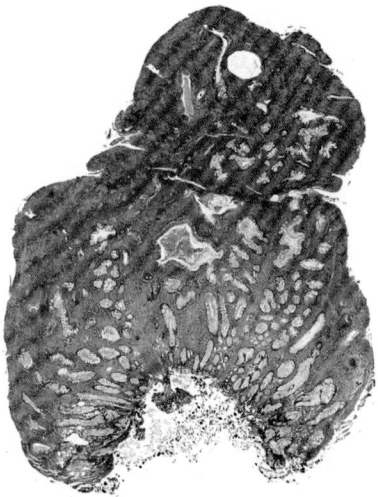

Figure 4-213. Colonic hamartoma/inflammatory-type polyp, juvenile polyposis syndrome. This polyp originated from a patient later confirmed to have juvenile polyposis and a *SMAD4* genetic defect. These syndromic polyps consist of mucosa native to their site with surface erosions, inflamed and edematous lamina propria, and ectatic and inflamed crypts, as seen here.

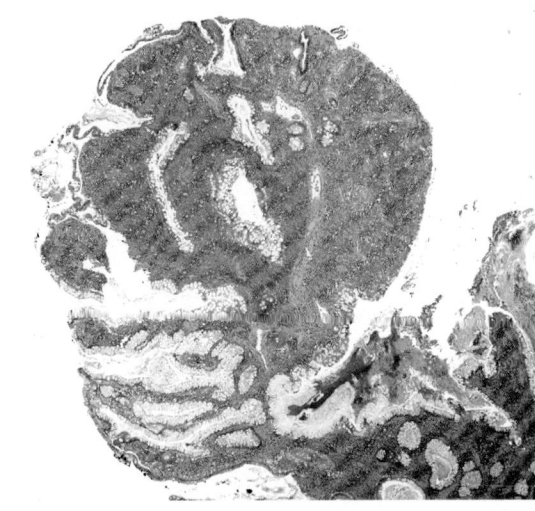

Figure 4-214. Colonic hamartoma/inflammatory-type polyp, juvenile polyposis syndrome. Juvenile polyps can be indistinguishable from the other syndromic or sporadic hamartomatous/inflammatory-type polyps.

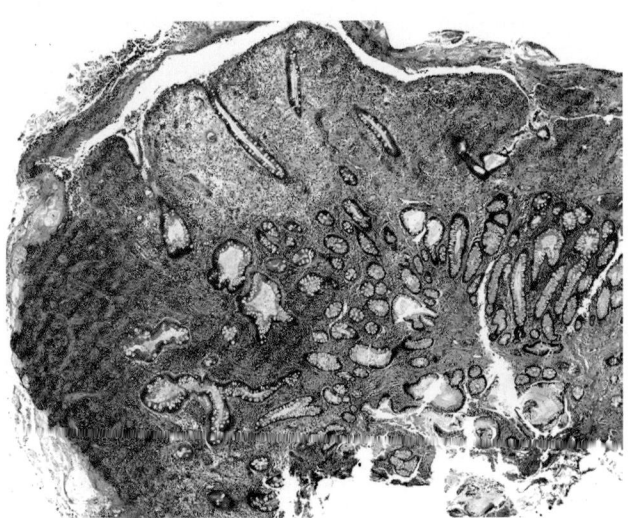

Figure 4-215. Colonic hamartoma/inflammatory-type polyp, juvenile polyposis syndrome. Typical features include surface erosions, inflamed and edematous lamina propria, and ectatic and inflamed crypts, as seen here.

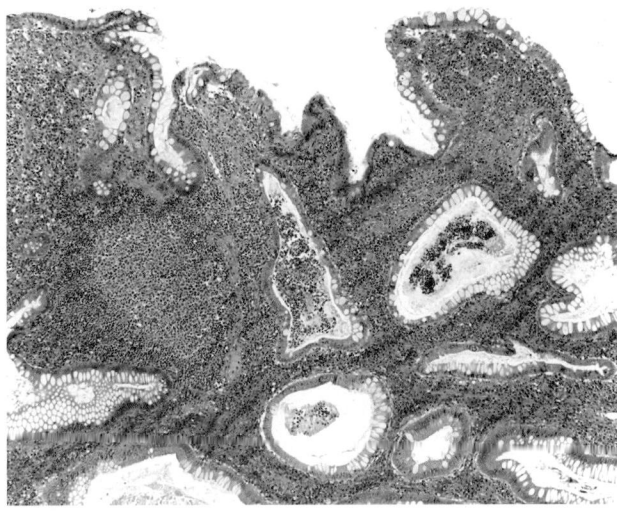

Figure 4-216. Colonic hamartoma/inflammatory-type polyp, juvenile polyposis syndrome. Higher power shows the inflamed lamina propria and ectatic and inflamed crypts. As seen here, the surface epithelium can look a bit undulating or serrated.

KEY FEATURES: Juvenile Polyposis

- There is an autosomal dominantly inherited defect in *SMAD4* or *BMPR1A*.
- Syndromic polyp is the hamartomatous polyp/inflammatory-type polyp.
- Polyps can be indistinguishable from the other syndromic and sporadic hamartomatous/inflammatory-type polyps.

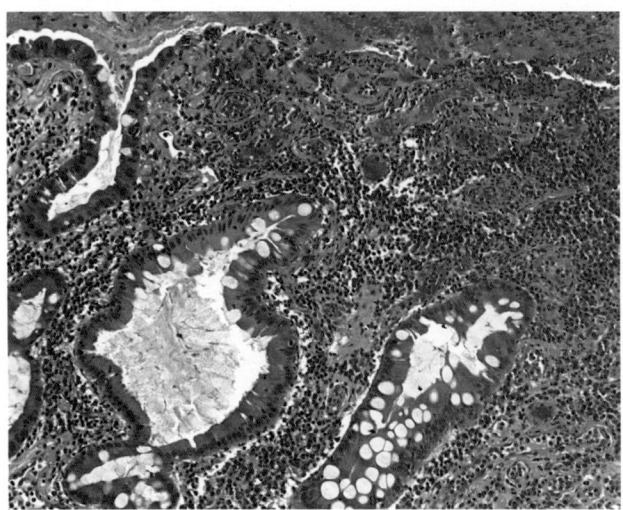

Figure 4-217. Colonic hamartoma/inflammatory-type polyp, juvenile polyposis syndrome. Surface erosions are common in juvenile polyps. Juvenile polyposis syndrome is autosomal dominantly inherited.

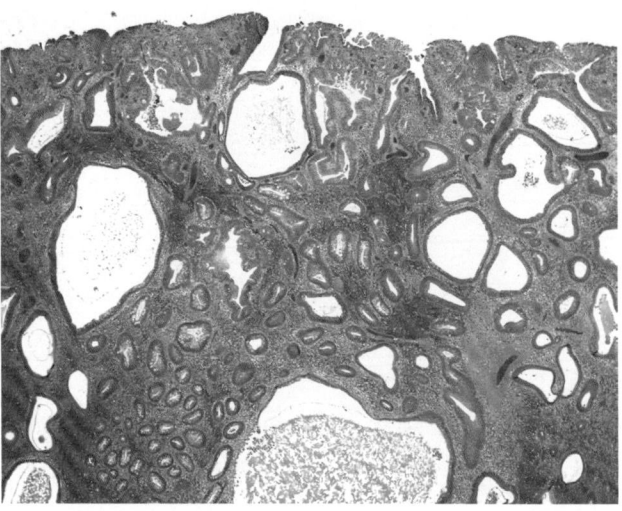

Figure 4-218. Low-grade dysplasia in a juvenile polyp. These polyps can appear visually busy because of the prominent inflammation. Make sure to take time to look carefully for dysplasia, seen best in the next image.

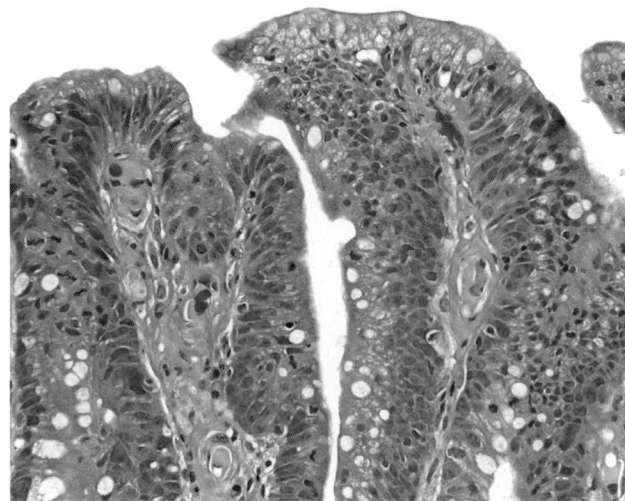

Figure 4-219. Low-grade dysplasia in a juvenile polyp. Higher power of the previous figure shows low-grade dysplasia with pseudostratified nuclei, hyperchromasia, and retained nuclear polarity.

Peutz-Jeghers Syndrome

Peutz-Jeghers syndrome most commonly manifests as small bowel polyps, but the polyps can occur anywhere along the GI tract (Table 4.5). It results from an autosomal dominantly inherited defect in *STK11* (formerly *LKB1*), a tumor suppressor gene encoding for a protein regulator of cell polarity and energy metabolism. Characteristically the patients present with frecklelike hyperpigmentation of the oral mucosa, but this pigmentation can fade over time. The typical syndromic polyp is a hamartoma with a central core of arborizing smooth muscle dividing lobular compartments of normal-appearing mucosa (Figs. 4.220–4.225).[72] Importantly, although this characteristic morphology is typical in the small bowel, it is uncommon in small polyps less than 1.0 cm or in gastric or colonic Peutz-Jeghers polyps (Figs. 4.224 and 4.225).[71,73] In the colon, a lobular crypt architecture is a more reliable clue than smooth muscle arborization for a diagnosis of Peutz-Jeghers polyp, and although investigators have shown that this can be highlighted with a desmin immunohistochemical stain, it is not necessary for diagnosis.[73] This lobular accentuation is not seen in the Peutz-Jeghers mimics, including polypoid mucosal prolapse, hyperplastic polyps, conventional adenomas, and juvenile polyps. For unknown reasons, this pattern is also not seen in small bowel Peutz-Jeghers but is rarely a diagnostic challenge based on the more obvious morphology in the small bowel. These patients are important to recognize because of their high life-time risk of malignancy, including tubular GI carcinomas, pancreatic carcinoma, Sertoli cell tumors of the testes, minimal deviation adenocarcinoma (adenoma malignum) of the uterine cervix, sex cord tumor with annular tubules of the ovaries, and breast carcinomas. The 2010 WHO diagnostic criteria include the following: (1) detection of three or more histologically confirmed Peutz-Jeghers polyps, *or* (2) the presence of any number of Peutz-Jeghers polyps in a patient with a family history of the syndrome, *or* (3) detection of characteristic, prominent mucocutaneous pigmentation in the patient with a family history of the syndrome, *or* (4) detection of any number of Peutz-Jeghers polyps in a patient with prominent mucocutaneous pigmentation.[50] Starting at age 30 years, syndromic patients enter an every 2-year upper and lower endoscopic surveillance program and an annual pelvic, testicular, and pancreatic ultrasound imaging with annual mammography.[49] See also "Small Bowel" chapter.

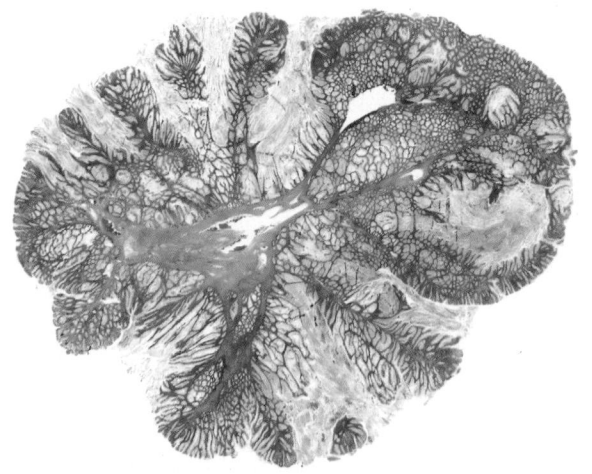

Figure 4-220. Colonic hamartoma, Peutz-Jeghers syndrome. Peutz-Jeghers polyps can often be spotted at scanning magnification. The typical syndromic polyp is a hamartoma with a central core of arborizing smooth muscle dividing lobular compartments of normal appearing mucosa, as seen here.

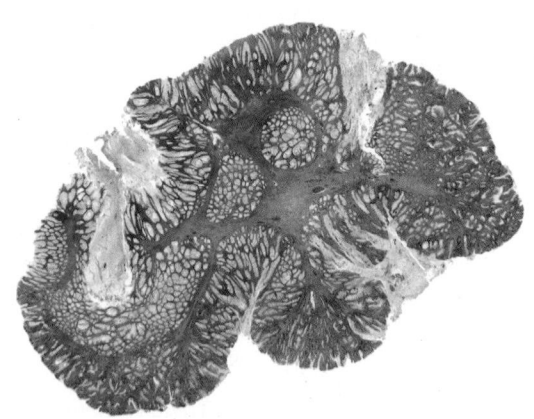

Figure 4-221. Colonic hamartoma, Peutz-Jeghers syndrome. Another scanning magnification showing a hamartoma with a central core of arborizing smooth muscle dividing lobular compartments of normal appearing mucosa. Peutz-Jeghers most commonly affects the small bowel, but the polyps can occur anywhere along the tubular GI tract.

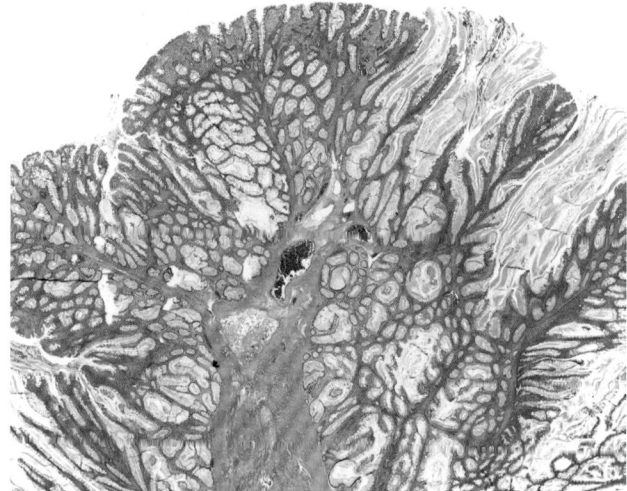

Figure 4-222. Colonic hamartoma, Peutz-Jeghers syndrome. The characteristic polyps are described as treelike with the central core of smooth muscle similar to a tree trunk, the peripheral smooth muscle tendrils similar to tree branches, and the normal hamartomatous mucosa similar to tree leaves.

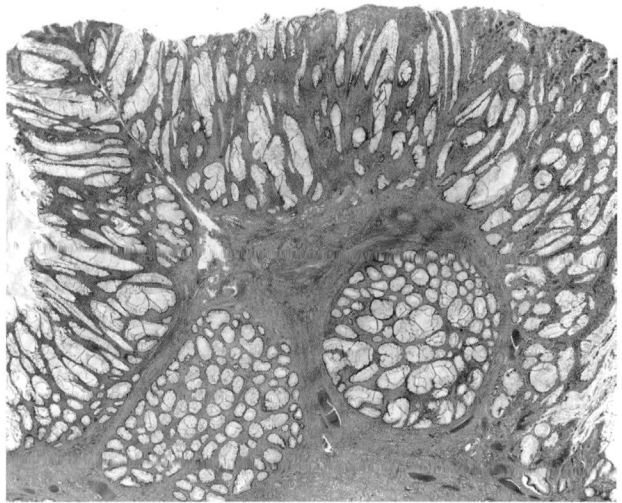

Figure 4-223. Colonic hamartoma, Peutz-Jeghers syndrome. Peutz-Jeghers can be sneaky to recognize, especially in small polyps and those that arise in the colon or stomach. In the colon, a lobular crypt architecture is a more reliable clue than smooth muscle arborization for a diagnosis of Peutz-Jeghers polyp, as highlighted in this case.

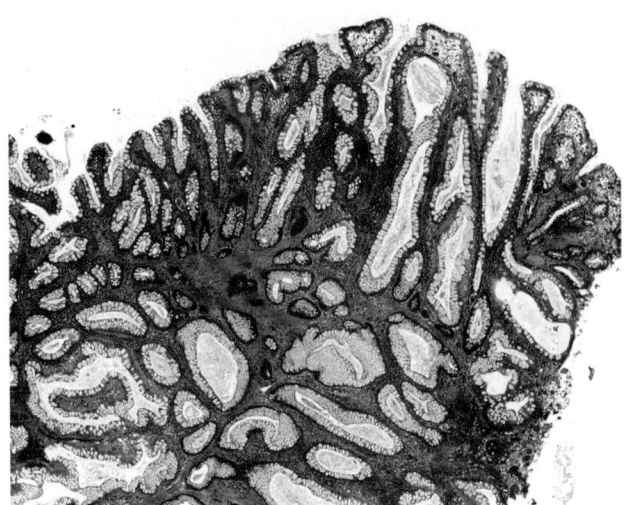

Figure 4-224. Colonic hamartoma, Peutz-Jeghers syndrome. Another not so obvious Peutz-Jeghers polyp. These polyps are critical to recognize because the patients have >90% lifetime risk of neoplasia, regardless of whether they arise in the sporadic or syndromic setting.

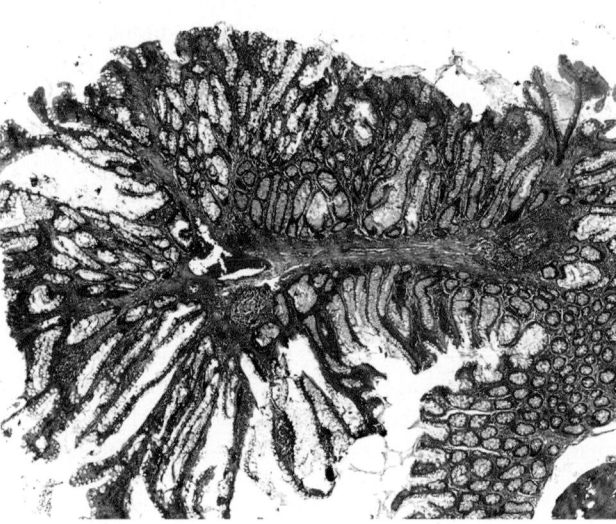

Figure 4-225. Colonic hamartoma, Peutz-Jeghers syndrome. Another not so obvious Peutz-Jeghers polyp. Peutz-Jeghers is an autosomal dominantly inherited defect in *STK11*, and the patients present with frecklelike hyperpigmentation of the oral mucosa.

> **PEARLS & PITFALLS**
>
> Although patients with Peutz-Jeghers syndrome have a near-90% life-time risk of malignancy, the malignancies do not arise within the hamartomatous polyps. These hamartomatous polyps are rarely dysplastic.

KEY FEATURES: Peutz-Jeghers Syndrome

- There is an autosomal dominantly inherited defect in *STK11* (formerly *LKB1*).
- It most commonly affects the small bowel, but the polyps can occur anywhere along the GI tract.
- Syndromic polyp is a hamartoma with a central core of arborizing smooth muscle dividing lobular compartments of normal-appearing mucosa.
- Polyps can be indistinguishable from the other syndromic and sporadic hamartomatous/inflammatory-type polyps.
- The classic morphology is uncommon in small polyps or in gastric or colon sites.
- There is a near-90% life-time risk of malignancy, regardless of sporadic or syndromic.
- Malignancies do not arise within the hamartomatous polyps.

PTEN *Hamartoma Tumor Syndrome*

PHTS refers to a group of syndromes molecularly defined by an autosomal dominantly inherited defect in *PTEN*: Cowden, Bannayan-Riley-Ruvalcaba, and Lhermitte-Duclose syndromes. The varied clinical presentations involve multiple organs from all three germ-cell layers and have led to equally complex diagnostic criteria, first outlined by the International Cowden Consortium in 1996 (Table 4.5).[74] The 2013 revisions include that Lhermitte-Duclose is now a pathognomic criterion, endometrial carcinoma is now a major criterion, and renal cell carcinoma is now a minor criterion.[75] Patients can have hamartomas polyps/inflammatory-type polyps in the stomach, small bowel, and colorectum (Figs. 4.226–4.233). In a study of 375 polyps, Cowden polyps usually lacked erosions with only mildly inflamed lamina propria; smooth muscle proliferation and lymphoid aggregates were common.[70] Uncommon but specific features included mucosal fat, ganglion cells, and nerve fibers. In contrast to the hamartomatous/inflammatory-type polyps seen in juvenile polyposis, Peutz-Jeghers syndrome, and sporadic inflammatory-type polyps, the polyps in Cowden syndrome do not tend to display prominent, thick inspissated mucin.[70]

Syndromic patients also can present with diffuse glycogenic acanthosis of the esophagus (Figs. 4.234–4.236). Because the clinical and pathologic presentations of these syndromic patients can be diverse, the following serve as indications to consider PHTS: (1) multiple GI hamartomas, especially ≥2 hamartomas, (2) any intramucosal lipomas (Fig. 4.237), or (3) any ganglioneuromas (Figs. 4.238 and 4.239).[76] Breast and thyroid carcinomas are the most frequent, with neoplasms also seen in the endometrium, colorectum, genitourinary system, and skin. As a result, screening for breast, thyroid, uterine, kidney, stomach, small bowel, colon, and skin neoplasms has been recommended, although no specific surveillance interval has been specified.[57]

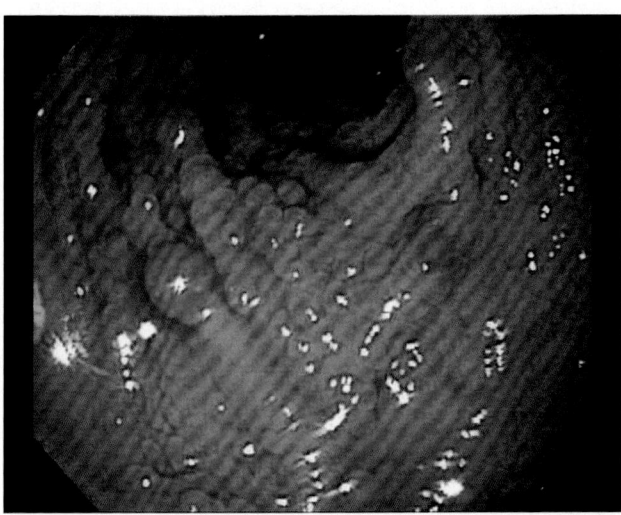

Figure 4-226. Colonic hamartoma/inflammatory-type polyp, *PTEN* hamartoma tumor syndrome (PHTS). An endoscopic view of the colon shows diffuse polyposis in this patient with confirmed Cowden syndrome and a *PTEN* mutation.

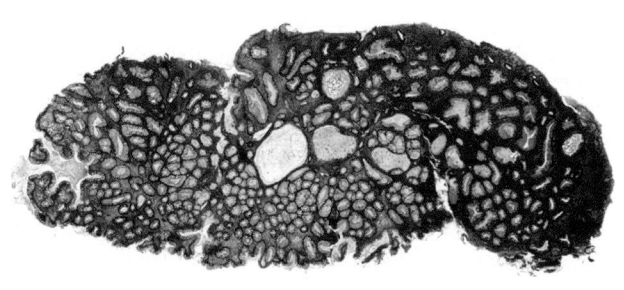

Figure 4-227. Colonic hamartoma/inflammatory-type polyp, PHTS. The low-power image shows the typical nondescript nature of these syndromic polyps: this colonic hamartomatous polyp has colonic mucosa with mildly inflamed lamina propria, as seen here.

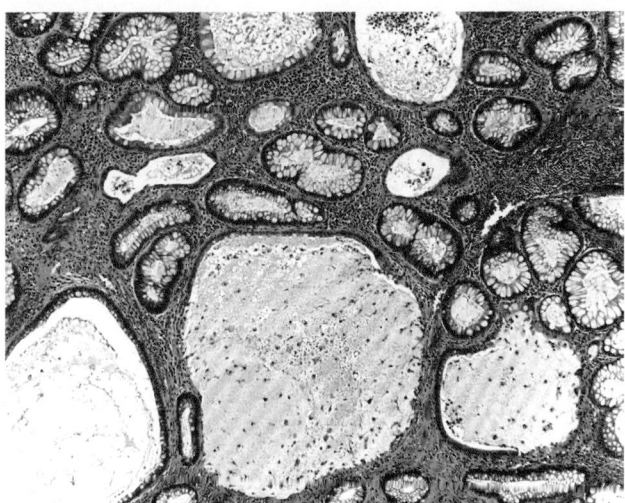

Figure 4-228. Colonic hamartoma/inflammatory-type polyp, PHTS. Higher power of the previous figure shows the ectatic, inflamed crypts with mildly inflamed lamina propria. On its own, this image is indistinguishable from a sporadic hamartoma/inflammatory-type polyp, or a juvenile polyp, among others. A good history is key to the specific diagnosis of Cowden polyp, as in this case.

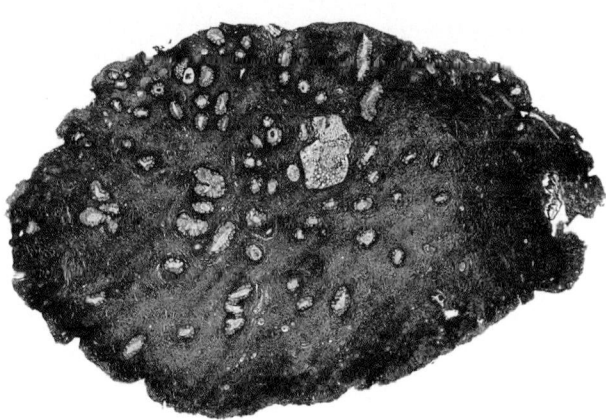

Figure 4-229. Colonic hamartoma/inflammatory-type polyp, PHTS. A polyp from another patient with confirmed Cowden syndrome.

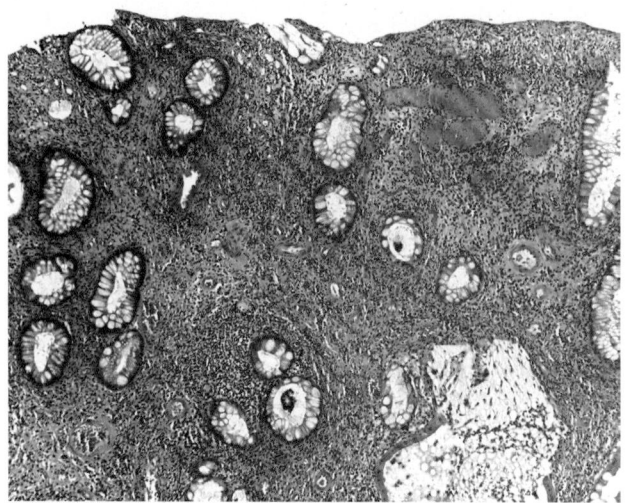

Figure 4-230. Colonic hamartoma/inflammatory-type polyp, PHTS. Higher power of the previous figure shows the ectatic, inflamed crypts with mildly inflamed lamina propria. Some have suggested that Cowden polyps are more likely to have lymphoid aggregates than other hamartomatous/inflammatory-type polyps.[70]

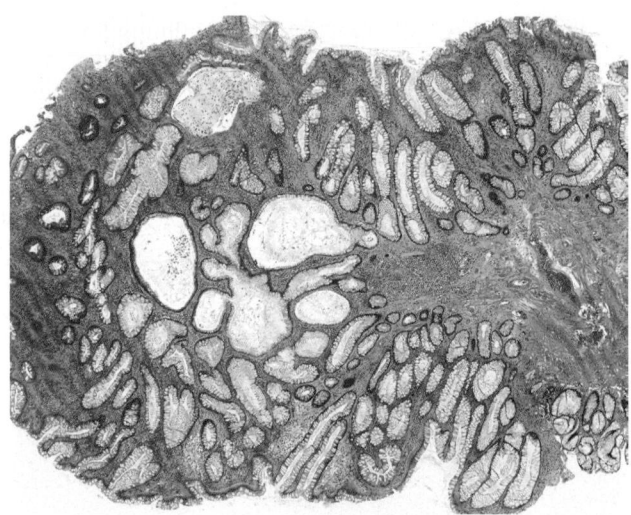

Figure 4-231. Colonic hamartoma/inflammatory-type polyp, PHTS. A polyp from another patient with confirmed Cowden syndrome. Some have suggested that these syndromic polyps are less likely to have erosions and inspissated mucin and more likely to have smooth muscle proliferation, mucosal fat, ganglion cells, and nerve fibers (not shown).[70]

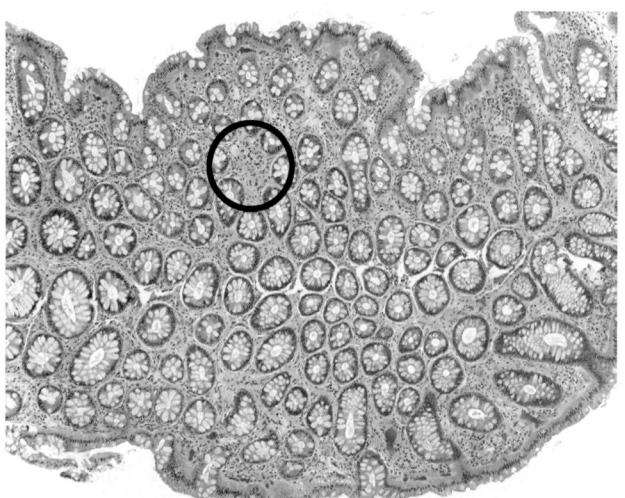

Figure 4-232. Colonic hamartoma/inflammatory-type polyp, PHTS. This polyp would be easy to overlook as normal in the absence of any history. This patient had a number of polyps throughout the colon, and all looked similar to this polyp. The entrapped neural elements (*circle*) in a patient with a polyposis syndrome should invoke consideration of PHTS. This patient was later confirmed to have Cowden syndrome.

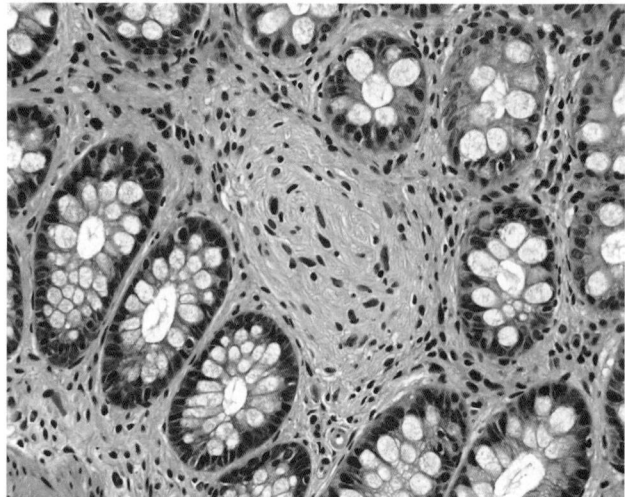

Figure 4-233. Colonic hamartoma/inflammatory-type polyp, PHTS. Higher power of the previous figure shows the focal neural elements.

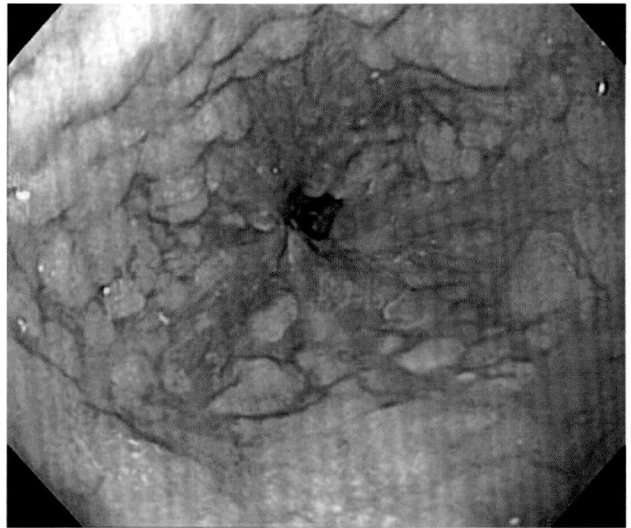

Figure 4-234. Diffuse esophageal glycogenic acanthosis, PHTS. This patient with confirmed Cowden syndrome had dramatic esophageal endoscopic findings with diffuse white patches, as seen here.

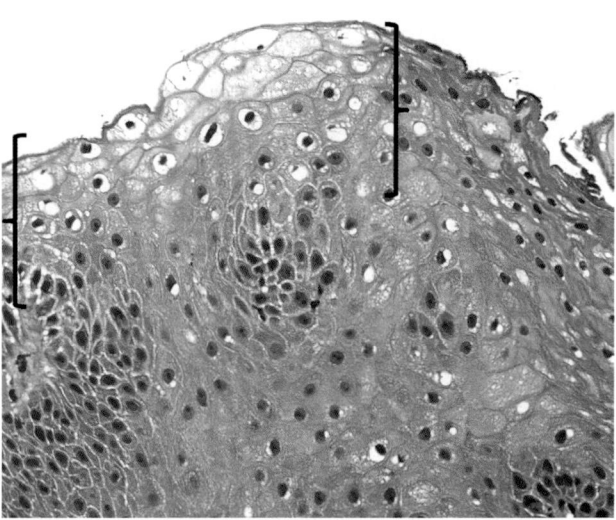

Figure 4-235. Diffuse esophageal glycogenic acanthosis, PHTS. Corresponding biopsies of the previous case show squamous mucosa with abundant cytoplasmic clearing (*brackets*). These changes do not involve the basal layer and are suggestive of glycogenic acanthosis on H&E.

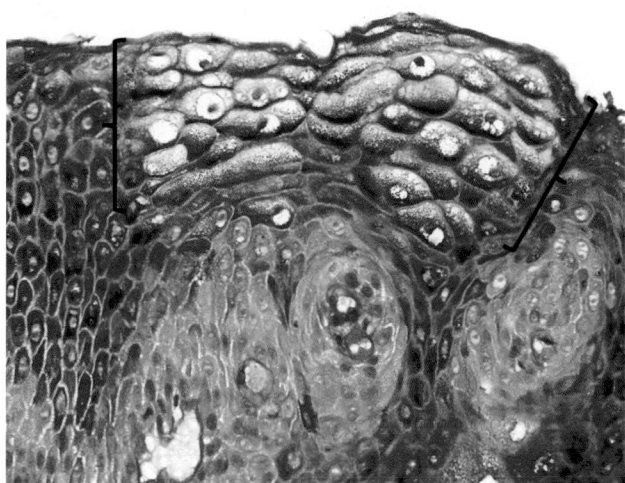

Figure 4-236. Diffuse esophageal glycogenic acanthosis, PHTS (PAS). A PAS shows a two-toned coloration (*brackets*) that confirms the diagnosis of glycogenic acanthosis.

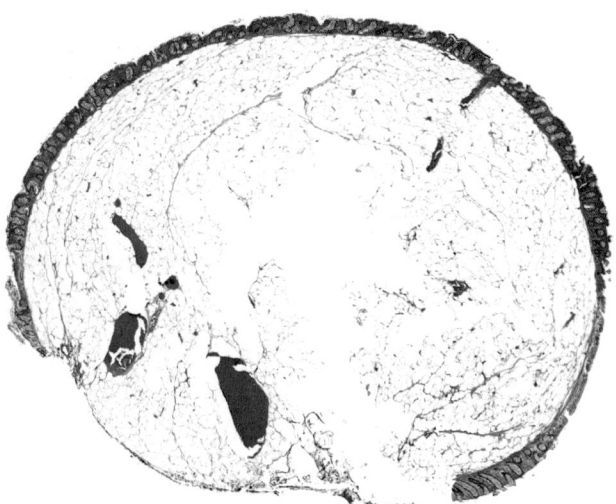

Figure 4-237. Colonic lipoma, PHTS. Colonic lipomas are technically hamartomas. An isolated lipoma is most often sporadic but can be a clue to PHTS.

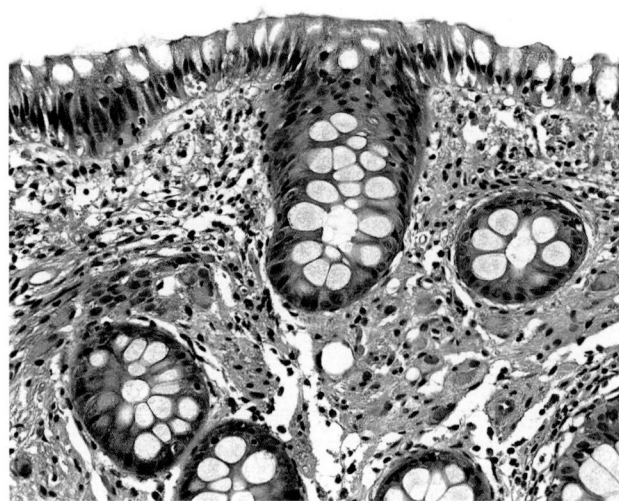

Figure 4-238. Colonic ganglioneuroma, PHTS. Isolated ganglioneuromas are most often sporadic in nature but can be a clue to PHTS.

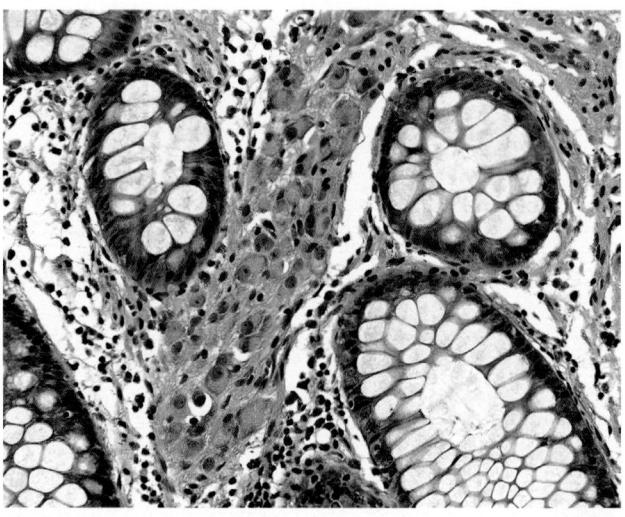

Figure 4-239. Colonic ganglioneuroma, PHTS. Higher power of the previous figure. Syndromic considerations for ganglioneuroma polyposis include the PHTS, neurofibromatosis type 1, and multiple endocrine neoplasia type IIB.

PEARLS & PITFALLS: Ganglioneuromas and Syndromic Considerations

Isolated ganglioneuromas are most often sporadic in nature, but the following syndromes should be considered in the setting of ganglioneuroma polyposis: PHTSs, neurofibromatosis type 1, and multiple endocrine neoplasia type IIB. The diagnostic distinctions are best left to the clinician to correlate with the family history, clinical examination, and molecular testing.

KEY FEATURES: PHTS

- There is an autosomal dominant defect in *PTEN*.
- It includes Cowden, Bannayan-Riley-Ruvalcaba, and Lhermitte-Duclose syndromes.
- Patients can have diffuse glycogenic acanthosis of the esophagus and hamartomas polyps/inflammatory-type polyps in the stomach, small bowel, and colorectum.
- Uncommon but specific features included mucosal fat, ganglion cells, and nerve fibers.
- Polyps can be indistinguishable from the other syndromic and sporadic hamartomatous/inflammatory-type polyps.

Cronkhite-Canada Syndrome

Unlike the aforementioned polyposis syndromes, CCS is a sporadic polyposis with no known genetic defects (Table 4.5). This syndrome is generally unassociated with neoplasia, but CCS is important to recognize because of a potentially high mortality of up to 50%.[77] Syndromic patients present with malabsorption, protein-losing gastroenterocolopathy, diarrhea, diffuse GI hamartomatous/inflammatory-type polyps, and ectodermal changes such as alopecia, onychodystrophy, and hyperpigmentation. GI polyps can be seen throughout the GI tract except the esophagus and consist of hamartomatous/inflammatory-type polyps with edematous lamina propria, an eosinophilic-rich mixed inflammatory infiltrate, and architectural changes with gland dilatation and withering (Figs. 4.240–4.245).[78] Small bowel polyps have been associated with villous atrophy, crypt distortion, inflammation, and increased apoptotic bodies.[78] The intervening nonpolypoid mucosa shows identical findings to the polyps and serves as essential diagnostic clue.[81] Unfortunately, if only the polyps are submitted, these polyps alone cannot be distinguished from sporadic or syndromic hamartomatous/inflammatory-type polyposis syndromes,[82] but CCS can still be suggested in combination with a compatible clinical presentation. Patients with CCS are severely ill, and the phone will be ringing off the hook for a diagnosis because they are so ill—patients with similar-appearing juvenile polyps, for example, are not ill with protein-losing diarrhea! Based on reported increased IgG4 staining[78-80] and a response to immunosuppressive therapy, the underlying cause is presumed immune dysregulation related. It is unnecessary to perform IgG4 immunohistochemical studies for diagnosis. First-line therapy is corticosteroids with cyclosporine suggested for steroid-resistant cases.[79,83]

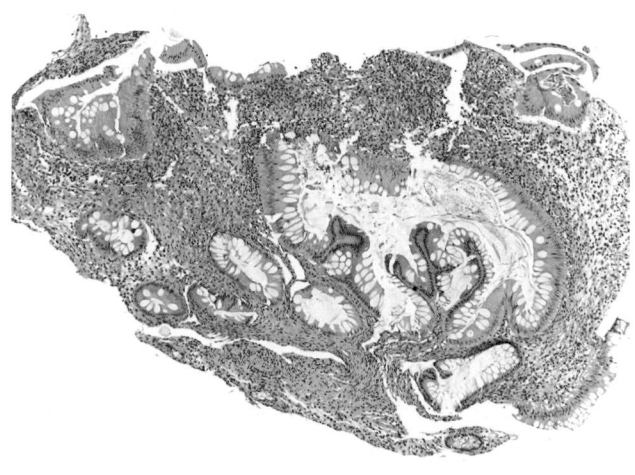

Figure 4-240. Colonic hamartoma/inflammatory-type polyp, Cronkhite-Canada syndrome (CCS). CCS is a sporadic polyposis with no known genetic defects. Inflamed lamina propria is seen surrounding ectatic crypts with scattered lymphoid aggregates. In isolation, the polyps are indistinguishable from sporadic or syndromic hamartomatous/inflammatory-type polyps, as seen here.

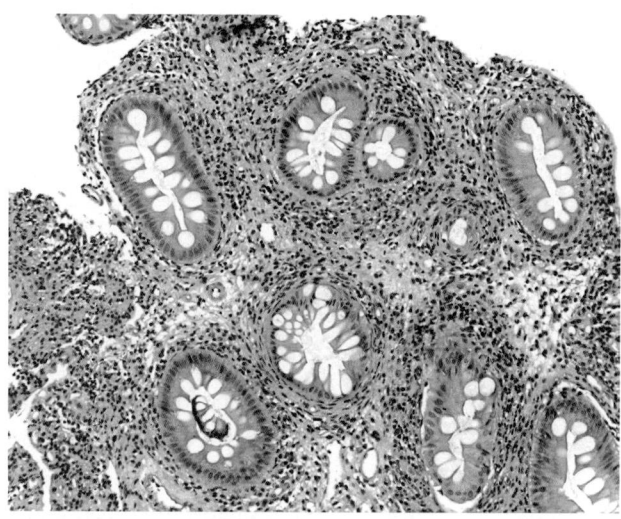

Figure 4-241. Biopsy of the flat mucosa in between the colonic polyps, CCS. Essential keys to a diagnosis of CCS include a pertinent history (malabsorption, protein-losing enteropathy, diarrhea, diffuse GI hamartomatous/inflammatory type polyps, and ectodermal changes) and similar histologic changes in the *intervening* nonpolypoid mucosa, as seen here.

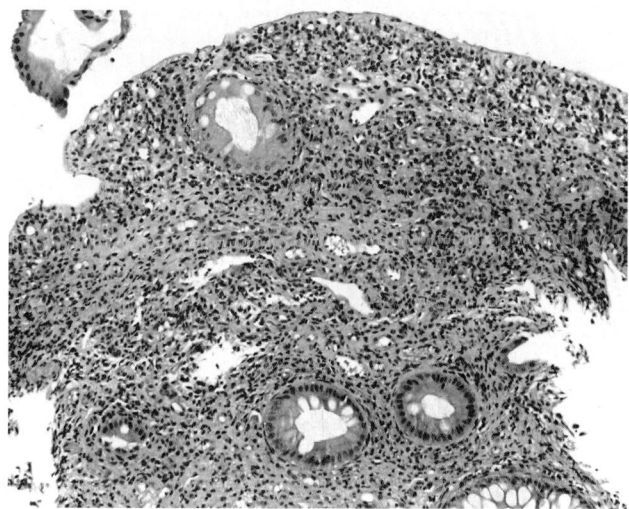

Figure 4-242. Colonic hamartoma/inflammatory-type polyp, CCS. This syndrome is unassociated with neoplasia but is important to recognize because of a potentially high mortality.

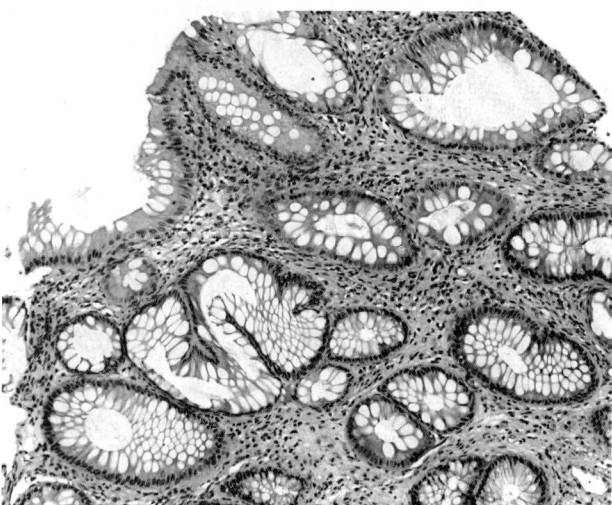

Figure 4-243. Biopsy of the flat mucosa in between the colonic polyps, CCS. A diagnosis of CCS requires that the same histologic changes seen in the polyps are also seen in the intervening nonpolypoid mucosa, as seen here.

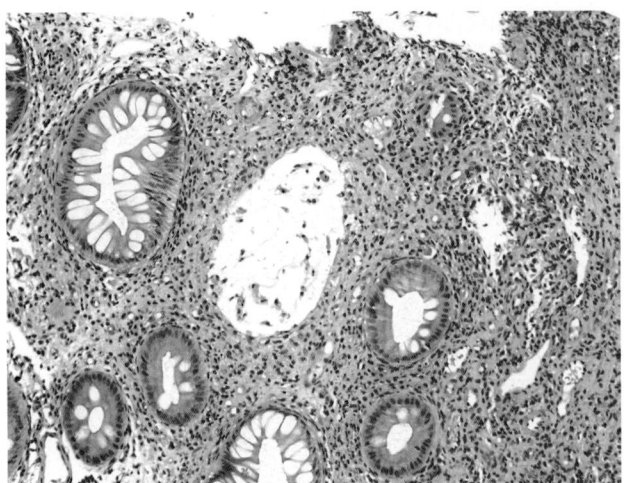

Figure 4-244. Colonic hamartoma/inflammatory-type polyp, CCS. Some investigators have found that these polyps have increased IgG4 staining[78-80] and that such patients response to corticosteroid therapy, suggesting the underlying cause is presumed immune dysregulation related.

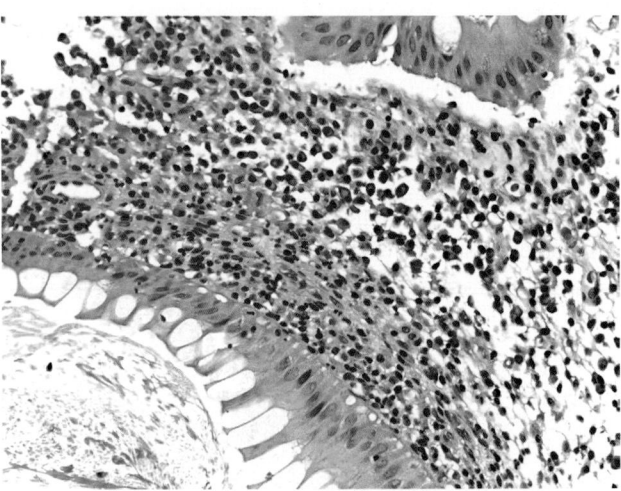

Figure 4-245. Colonic hamartoma/inflammatory-type polyp, CCS. High power shows the typical mixed lamina propria inflammatory infiltrate seen in CCS in both the polyps and intervening nonpolypoid mucosa. Eosinophils are often conspicuous, as in this case.

KEY FEATURES: CCS

- There is a sporadic polyposis with no known genetic defects.
- This condition has a mortality of up to 50%.
- Syndromic patients present with malabsorption, protein-losing gastroenterocolopathy, diarrhea, and ectodermal changes such as alopecia, onychodystrophy, and hyperpigmentation.
- GI polyps can be seen throughout the GI tract except the esophagus and consist of hamartomatous/inflammatory-type polyps.
- The intervening nonpolypoid mucosa shows identical findings to the polyps.
- Polyps can be indistinguishable from the other syndromic and sporadic hamartomatous/inflammatory-type polyps, but the clinical history is very different.

PEARLS & PITFALLS: Hamartomatous and Inflammatory-Type Polyps Are Often Indistinguishable

Beware that syndromic hamartomatous and inflammatory-type polyps are often indistinguishable from their sporadic counterparts. When in doubt, craft a careful note or reach out to the clinician to share your concerns. See the following Sample Notes.

SAMPLE NOTE: A 60-Year-Old Woman Is Found to Have 25 Small Polyps Throughout the Colon

Colon, Polyps (Biopsy)
- Fragments of hamartomatous/inflammatory-type polyps
- Negative for dysplasia
- See Note

Note: The history of 25 small colorectal polyps is noted. The polyps histologically consist of hamartomatous/inflammatory-type polyps. Consideration of cancer predisposition syndromes is worthwhile, such as juvenile polyposis, Peutz-Jeghers syndrome, PHTS, and CCS, among others. If CCS is a clinical concern, biopsy of the intervening nonpolypoid mucosa may be helpful if repeat endoscopy is planned. Correlation with a careful family history, physical examination, and genetic counselor evaluation/testing is a consideration.

SAMPLE NOTE: A 30-Year-Old Woman With Known Cowden Syndrome Is Found to Have 25 Small Polyps Throughout the Colon

Colon, Polyps (Biopsy)
- Fragments of hamartomatous/inflammatory-type polyps
- Negative for dysplasia
- See Note

Note: The submitted polyps are compatible with the established history of Cowden syndrome.

DYSPLASIA IN INFLAMMATORY BOWEL DISEASE
CLINICAL CONSIDERATIONS

Inflammatory bowel disease (IBD) is a high-risk condition that predisposes one to CRC. Historically, ulcerative colitis was thought to have a relatively higher risk of neoplasia than Crohn disease. More recently, an essentially similar relative risk of twice the background population has been described in patients with ulcerative colitis and Crohn disease, when adjusted for duration of disease and extent of involvement.[84-89] A meta-analysis of 116 ulcerative colitis studies reported the cumulative probabilities of CRC as 2% at 10 years, 8% at 20 years, and 18% at 30 years of disease.[90] This risk is directly associated with the extent and duration of the inflammatory injury with the highest risk seen in pancolitis, intermediate risk seen with left-sided restricted disease, and nominal risk seen in those with isolated proctitis.[91,92] Patients with ulcerative colitis with concomitant primary sclerosing cholangitis carry a marked increased risk for CRC of up to 50% at 25 years after ulcerative colitis diagnosis,[93,94] as well as an increased risk of cholangiocarcinoma. Other factors that increase the risk for CRC include a positive family history of sporadic CRC, inflammation, and (for ulcerative colitis) colonic strictures, a shortened colon, and/or multiple inflammatory-type polyps.[95] Endoscopic surveillance is a hallmark of IBD management. Its effectiveness is because IBD-related neoplasia generally parallels the distribution of inflammatory injury.[89,91] The details of endoscopic management vary by expert society, but an oft-cited study indicates that 33 biopsy specimens are needed to detect dysplasia with 90% probability, and at least 64 biopsies are needed to reach a probability of 95%.[96] In the United States, most centers follow the 2010 American College of Gastroenterology recommendations[85,95]:

1. Screening colonoscopy begins a maximum of 8 years after the onset of symptoms to assess for the extent of microscopic disease. Most colleagues submit at least 33 random biopsies generated from four quadrant biopsies from every 10 cm of the colon in patients with pancolitis. Fewer biopsies can be submitted with a targeted biopsy approach from clinicians with expertise in chromoendoscopy owing to its higher sensitivity for dysplasia detection. Regardless, random biopsies still play an important role in assessing for endoscopically invisible neoplasia.[97]
2. Surveillance colonoscopy is ideally performed during clinical disease remission.
3. Patients with isolated ulcerative proctitis or ulcerative proctosigmoiditis have a nominal risk for CRC and are subsequently managed similarly to average-risk patients.
4. Patients with pancolitis or left-sided colitis begin surveillance within 1 to 2 years after the initial screening colonoscopy.
5. After two colonoscopies negative for dysplasia and carcinoma, subsequent surveillance examinations occur every 1 to 3 years.
6. These recommendations also apply to patients with Crohn disease involving at least one-third of the length of the colon.

7. Patients with Crohn disease and ulcerative colitis with primary sclerosing cholangitis begin surveillance colonoscopy at the time of diagnosis and subsequently undergo yearly colonoscopy.

8. More frequent surveillance colonoscopy may be beneficial for patients with a first-degree relative with CRC, active endoscopic or histologic inflammation, shortened colon, stricture, or multiple inflammatory-type polyps.

PEARLS & PITFALLS: "Dysplasia-Associated Lesion or Mass" and "Flat Dysplasia" Are Terms That Should Be Abandoned by Pathologists

The above-mentioned recommendations are largely based on the older literature derived from random biopsy techniques with white light endoscopy. In 2015, the SCENIC consensus statement on IBD surveillance was issued to reflect improved endoscopic techniques, such as chromoendoscopy with high-definition colonoscopy.[97] The most notable recommendations state that the term dysplasia-associated lesion or mass (DALM) should be abandoned by pathologists and clinicians, and the term flat dysplasia should be abandoned by pathologists. DALM and flat dysplasia were terms historically considered an indication for resection. However, today's improved endoscopic techniques allow for some flat dysplasia to be endoscopically visible and, therefore, amenable to endoscopic surveillance or even endoscopic resection. Hence, the critical issue today is to determine if the lesion is endoscopically visible, regardless of whether the architecture of the lesion is polypoid, ulcerated, sessile, pedunculated, superficially elevated, flat, depressed, or ulcerated. If the lesion is endoscopically visible, it can be conservatively managed by endoscopy in the following settings:

1. The lesion must have distinct margins.

2. One must have endoscopic confirmation that the lesion was completely removed.

3. One must have histologic confirmation that the lesion was completely removed.

4. Biopsies immediately adjacent to the resection site must be free of dysplasia by histologic confirmation.

According to the 2015 SCENIC guidelines, endoscopically invisible lesions should be referred to a GI specialized pathologist for histologic confirmation. Those with confirmed dysplasia are referred to an IBD-specialized endoscopist with expertise in chromoendoscopy with high-definition colonoscopy to inform the next management steps. The following recommendations are adapted from the 2015 SCENIC guidelines and 2010 AGA recommendations as a starting point for discussion (Table 4.7).[85,95,97] In practice, the discussion of surveillance versus colectomy is a highly personal decision that is ultimately made by the patient and informed by the collective recommendations of that center's endoscopist, surgeon, and oncologist. With improved endoscopic surveillance and optimized medical and surgical management, CRC rates are decreasing in Crohn disease and ulcerative colitis.[86,88,98] Unfortunately, these decreases have been accompanied by increased risks of infection, lymphoma, and melanoma owing to the IBD-related anti-inflammatory medical therapies.[98-101]

TABLE 4.7: Adapted Recommendations for IBD Dysplasia Management[85,95,97]

Diagnosis	Management
Negative for dysplasia	Repeat colonoscopy in 1–2 years
Indefinite for dysplasia, favor negative	Repeat colonoscopy within 6–12 months
Indefinite for dysplasia, favor positive	Repeat colonoscopy within 3–6 months
Visible low- or high-grade dysplasia (colitis-associated or sporadic)	Complete endoscopic removal sufficient, consider colectomy if not endoscopically resectable
Invisible low-grade dysplasia	Colectomy or repeat colonoscopy within 6 months and colectomy recommended if persistent or multifocal, invisible low-grade dysplasia
Invisible high-grade dysplasia	Colectomy

DYSPLASIA GRADING

Although various IBD dysplasia grading schemes exist, most in the United States use Riddell's three-category classification system: negative for dysplasia, indefinite for dysplasia, and positive for dysplasia (low or high grade).[102] Introduced in 1983, this 37-page manuscript features more than 40 composite images on the spectrum of changes seen in IBD, suggested management guidelines, and suggested tissue preparation techniques. The author line is analogous to the Hollywood Walk of Fame, featuring Riddell, Goldman, Appelman, Fenoglio, Haggitt, Hamilton, and Yardley, to name but a few. Dysplasia was defined as an unequivocal neoplastic alteration of the colonic epithelium, and its atypia was beyond that acceptable for inflammation alone. Sorting out these diagnostic categories is a difficult task, especially in the setting of florid inflammation, re-epithelialization of an eroded or ulcerated focus, a denuded surface, or concomitant cytomegalovirus (CMV), for example. For these authors, atypia restricted to the crypt bases with a normal surface is regarded as reactive (compare normal colonic mucosa in IBD [Fig. 4.246] with reactive epithelial change [Figs. 4.247–254]). Reactive epithelium can have surface atypia, but it is usually mild, in proportion to the background inflammation or adjoining erosion or ulceration, and is characterized by a gradual transition from normal to atypia (Figs. 4.247–254). Cases with equivocal morphology are best classified as indefinite for dysplasia (Figs. 4.255–260). Riddell lectured at USCAP 2017 that if the answer to both of the following questions is "No," then the case is best classified as indefinite for dysplasia: (1) Is the atypia unequivocally dysplastic? (2) Is the atypia unequivocally negative for dysplasia? This indefinite category can be further specified, for example, as indefinite for dysplasia, favor LGD or indefinite for dysplasia, favor reactive, depending on the degree of atypia and accompanied inflammation.

Dysplasia most typically resembles a conventional adenoma with columnar cells, pseudostratified nuclei, basophilia due to increased nuclear to cytoplasmic ratios, hyperchromasia, and increased mitotic and apoptotic bodies. Recall that dysplasia is a low-power diagnosis with abrupt transitions and must involve the surface. LGD has preserved nuclear polarity (Figs. 4.261–4.267), and HGD has loss of nuclear polarity (Figs. 4.268–4.273). Architectural complexity, such as cribriform architecture, can be seen in HGD but is not required for a diagnosis of HGD in IBD. This contrasts with the criteria for HGD in conventional adenomas, which requires both cytologic and architectural complexity. See also "Conventional Adenomatous Polyps" section, "Dysplasia Grading" subsection. The presence of single cell infiltration signifies at least IMC (pTis) (similar to Figs. 4.37–4.42), and well-developed desmoplasia suggests at least submucosal invasion (pT1) (Figs. 4.274–4.279).

See Fig. 4.280 for a side-by-side comparison of the dysplasia categories in IBD.

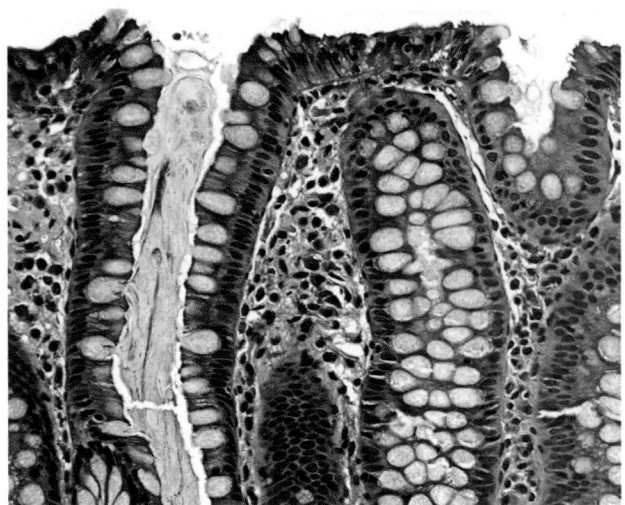

Figure 4-246. Normal colonic mucosa, inflammatory bowel disease (IBD). A high-power view of normal colon shows normochromatic chromatin and small basally oriented nuclei. The bland nuclei comprise approximately less than 10% of the overall cell volume. Apoptotic bodies and mitotic figures are not seen.

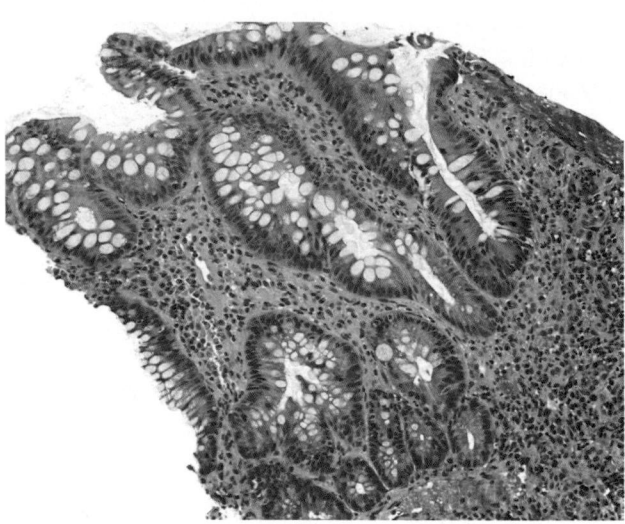

Figure 4-247. Reactive epithelial change, negative for dysplasia, IBD. This epithelium shows findings within the expected range of reactive epithelial changes. A nearby erosion is not featured.

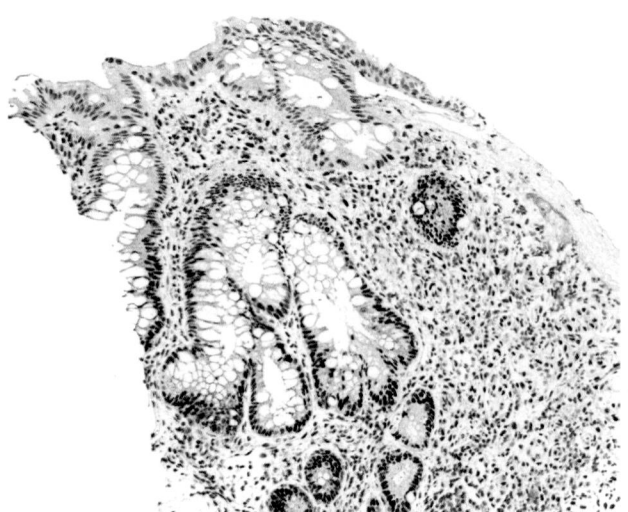

Figure 4-248. Reactive epithelial change, negative for dysplasia, IBD (p53). This pattern of p53 supports the diagnosis of negative for dysplasia. Normal and reactive epithelium show diffuse weak p53 reactivity in the proliferative compartment, as seen here. The surface lacks distinct, strong nuclear p53 reactivity (compare with p53 immunoreactivity in dysplasia Figs. 4.266–4.271).

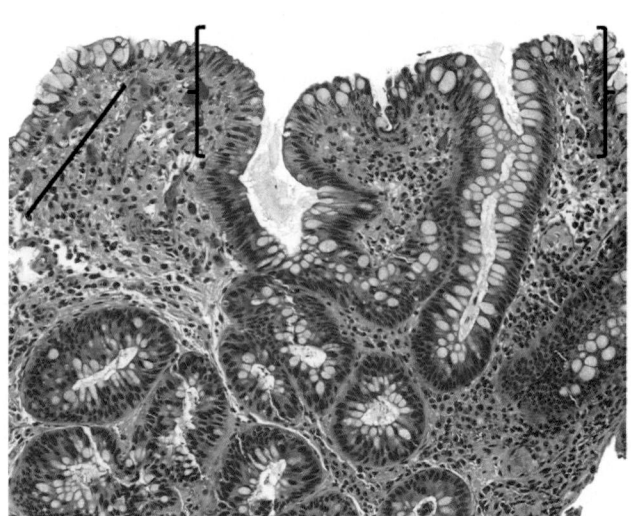

Figure 4-249. Reactive epithelial change, negative for dysplasia, IBD. The atypia of this case is predominantly in the crypts, supporting the diagnosis of reactive changes. A portion of the surface has slightly larger and darker nuclei (*brackets*) than the normal colonic mucosa (*line*). These changes are reactive because the atypia is very mild, and there is a gradual transition from normal to reactive. In contrast, dysplasia is characterized by abrupt transitions between normal and atypia (Figs. 4.256–4.258).

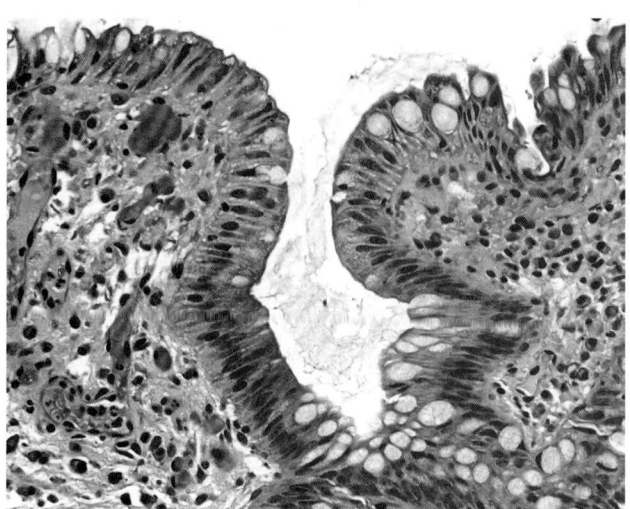

Figure 4-250. Reactive epithelial change, negative for dysplasia, IBD. Higher power of the previous figure.

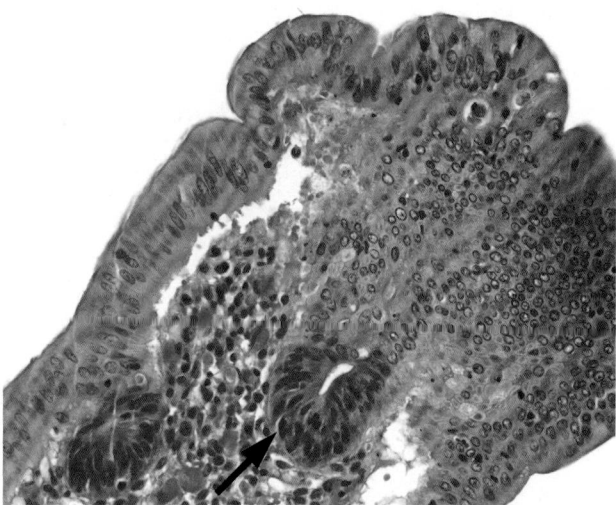

Figure 4-251. Reactive epithelial change, negative for dysplasia, IBD. Even though these crypts are dark, pseudostratified, and a mitotic figure is present (*arrow*), the changes are reactive because they do not extend to the surface.

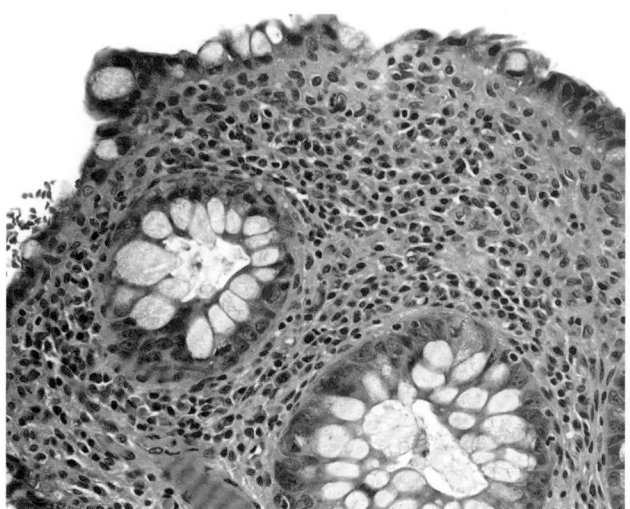

Figure 4-252. Reactive epithelial change, negative for dysplasia, IBD. The epithelium is dark, the nuclear to cytoplasmic ratio is high, and some of the nuclear contours are irregular. These atypical changes were adjacent to a healing ulcer (not shown) and interpreted as reactive because the atypia is in proportion to the adjacent ulcer. Although the cells are dark, they are dark because of mucin depletion; the chromatin is approximately the expected normochromasia, and there are no abrupt zones of transition between the atypia and normal, supporting the diagnosis of reactive changes.

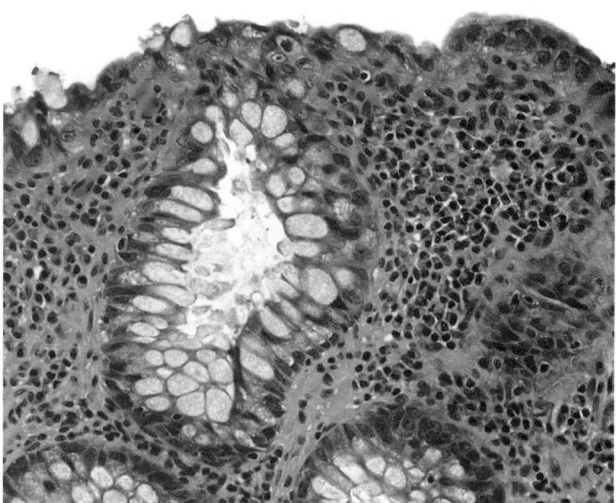

Figure 4-253. Reactive epithelial change, negative for dysplasia, IBD. A separate atypical focus adjoining a nearby erosion (not shown). A useful trick for assessing hyperchromasia is to establish the lymphocyte or endothelial cell chromatin as a baseline. If the atypical nuclei in question are lighter than the lymphocyte nuclei, then they are normochromatic and in keeping with reactive, as seen here.

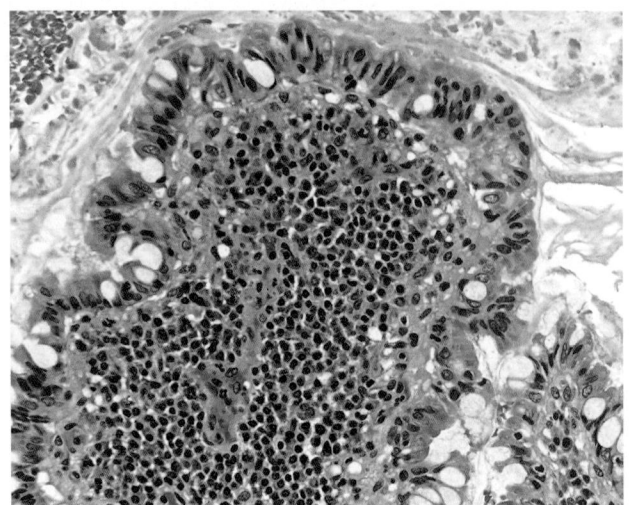

Figure 4-254. Reactive epithelial change, negative for dysplasia, IBD. Atypia is difficult to assess in IBD because of common confounding issues, such as florid inflammation, re-epithelialization of an eroded or ulcerated focus, or concomitant CMV. A familiarity with the spectrum of morphology comes with time and gray hair and is most helpful in sorting out the dysplasia categories.

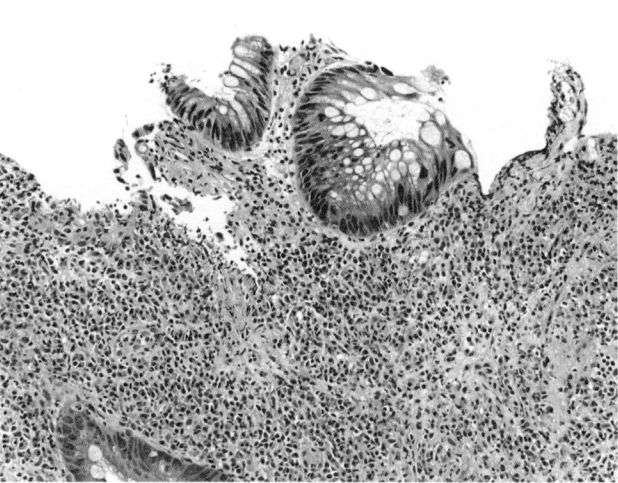

Figure 4-255. Indefinite for dysplasia, IBD. The presence of intact surface is important to determine if the atypical changes are restricted to the base (and reactive) or extend to the surface. The absence of intact mucosa in an area of atypia makes it impossible to assess the surface and, therefore, is one indication for classifying as indefinite for dysplasia, as in this case.

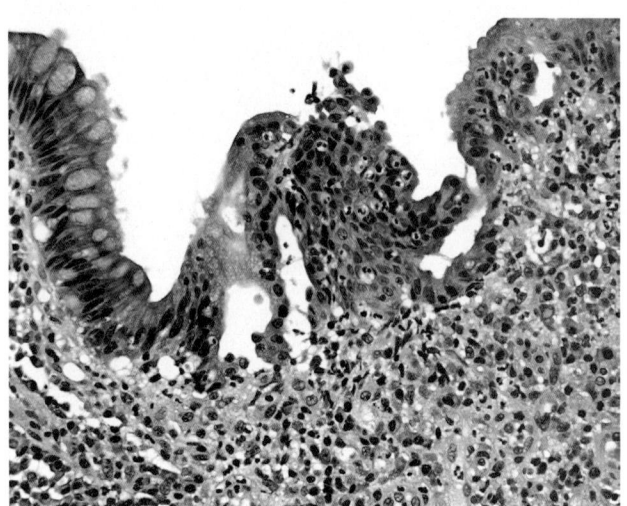

Figure 4-256. Indefinite for dysplasia, IBD. Another common indication for classifying as indefinite for dysplasia is the presence of florid inflammation, as in this case.

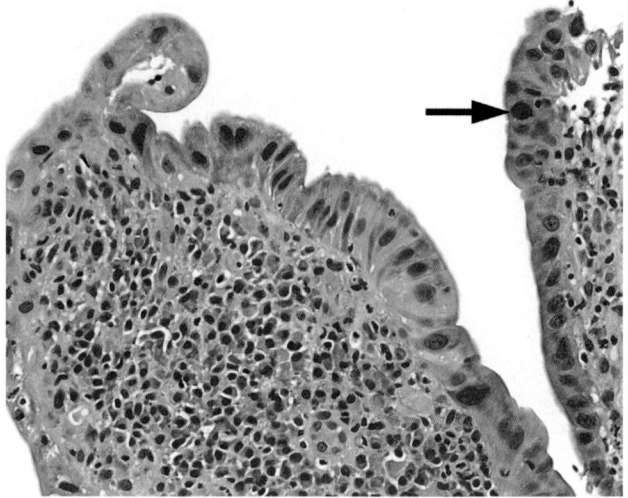

Figure 4-257. Indefinite for dysplasia, IBD. This case shows epithelial atypia in the form of mucin depletion, enlarged nuclei, and one hyperchromatic cell versus superficial mitotic figure (arrow). This case lacked florid inflammation or a nearby erosion or an ulcer to explain the atypia. Accordingly, this atypia was classified as indefinite for dysplasia.

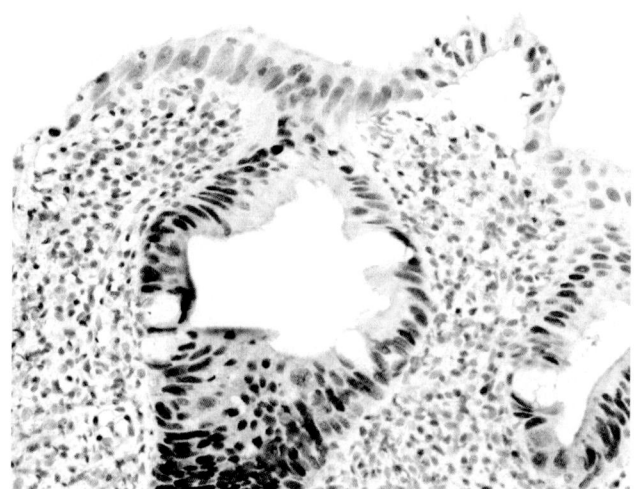

Figure 4-258. Indefinite for dysplasia, IBD (p53). The accompanied p53 shows predominantly crypt-restricted reactivity. The atypia was classified as indefinite for dysplasia (IFD) based on the H&E findings.

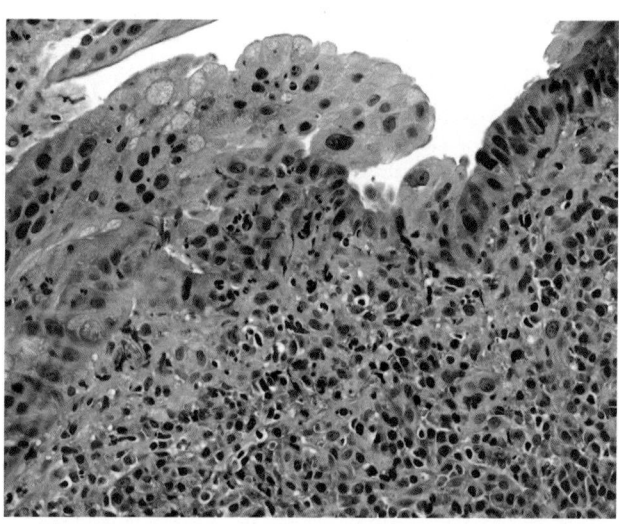

Figure 4-259. Indefinite for dysplasia, IBD. This case shows epithelial atypia in the form of mucin depletion, enlarged nuclei, a luminal mitotic figure, prominent nucleoli, and a loss of polarity. However, these changes were seen in all 10 biopsy sites of the same biopsy series and only in areas involved by inflammation. Dysplasia is unlikely to diffusely involve the colon and would be expected to have hyperchromasia and strong p53 reactivity (not shown). Accordingly, this atypia fell short of dysplasia and was classified as indefinite for dysplasia based on the atypia that seemed more than that expected from inflammation alone.

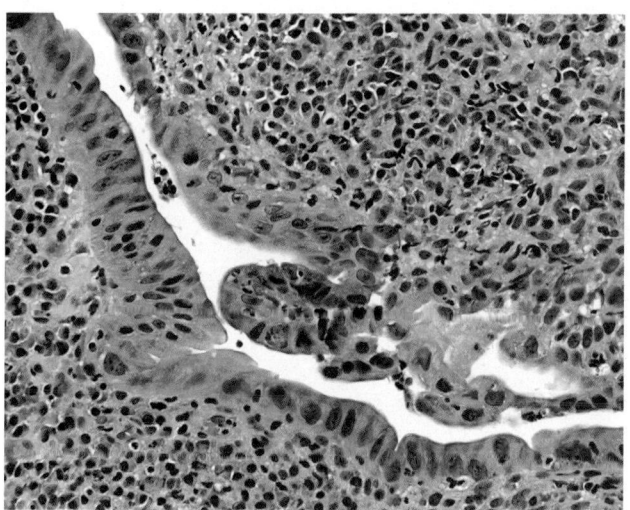

Figure 4-260. Indefinite for dysplasia, IBD. Another biopsy site from the same patient.

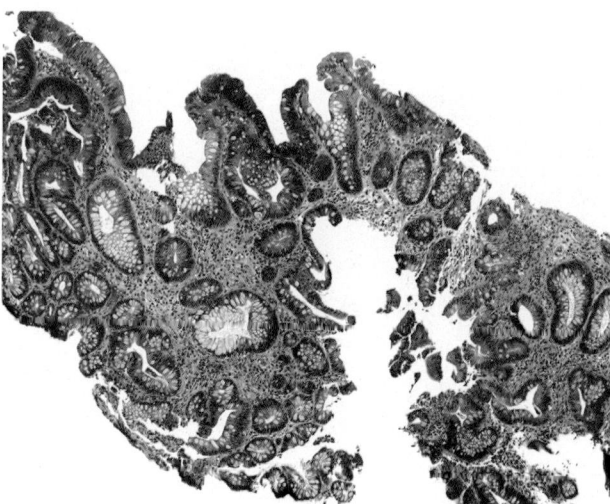

Figure 4-261. Low-grade dysplasia (LGD), IBD. As true for dysplasia at any site within the GI tract, dysplasia is a low-power diagnosis; it has abrupt transitions between normal and colon, and the atypia must involve the surface, as seen here.

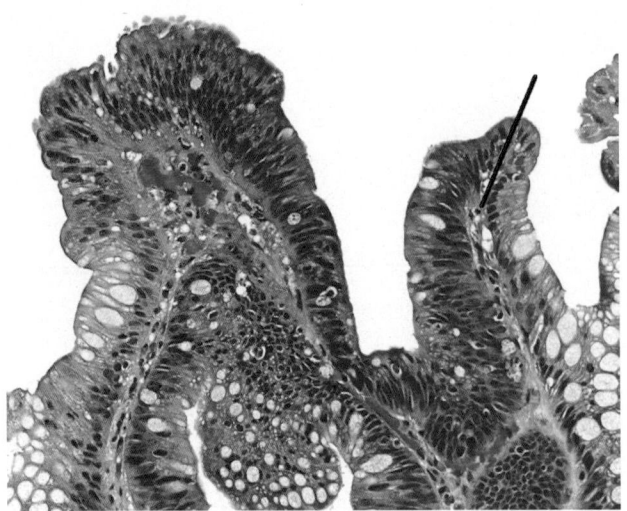

Figure 4-262. Low-grade dysplasia (LGD), IBD. Higher power of the previous figure. Note the abrupt transition between normal and colon (*line*). Dysplasia resembles a conventional tubular adenoma with columnar cells, pseudostratified nuclei, basophilia due to increased nuclear to cytoplasmic ratios, and hyperchromasia. In contrast to lesions that are indefinite for dysplasia, the atypia in this case is distinct and cannot be explained by inflammation or an adjoining erosion or ulcer.

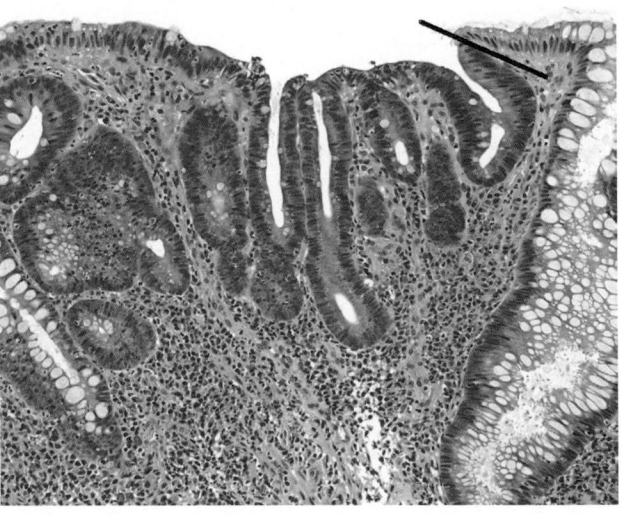

Figure 4-263. Low-grade dysplasia (LGD), IBD. Another low-power view of LGD. As is true for dysplasia at any site within the GI tract, the atypia is apparent at low power and is characterized by abrupt transitions between normal and atypia (*line*) and involves the surface.

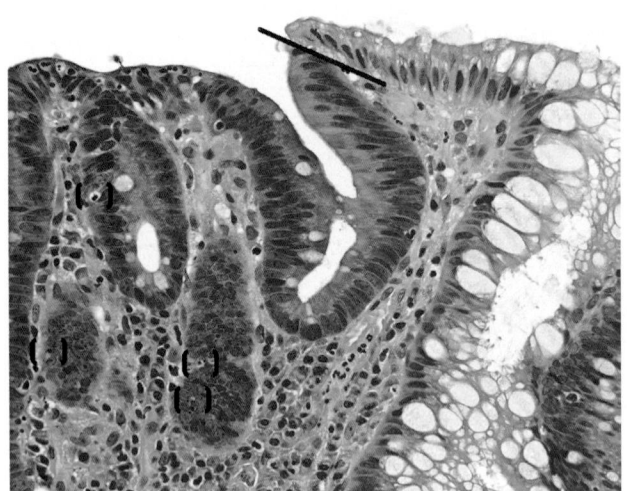

Figure 4-264. Low-grade dysplasia (LGD), IBD. Higher power of the previous figure. Note the abrupt transition between normal and dysplasia (*line*) and the prominent apoptotic bodies (*brackets*), supporting the LGD diagnosis.

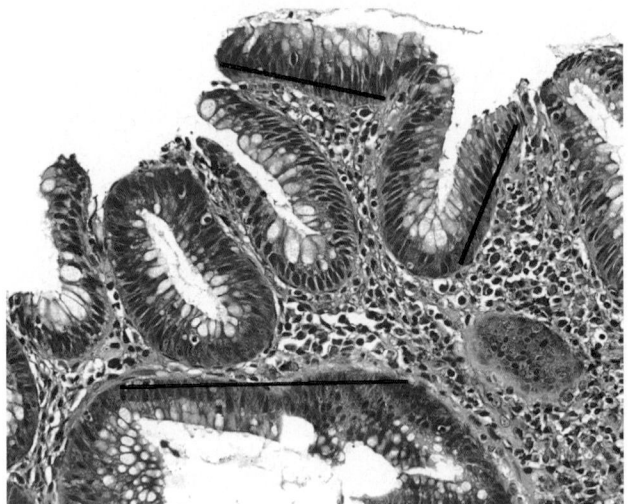

Figure 4-265. Low-grade dysplasia (LGD), IBD. This case is indistinguishable from the LGD seen in conventional tubular adenomas. This atypia is low grade because of the preserved nuclear polarity (*lines* drawn through the basal aspect of the cells capture all of the dysplastic nuclei).

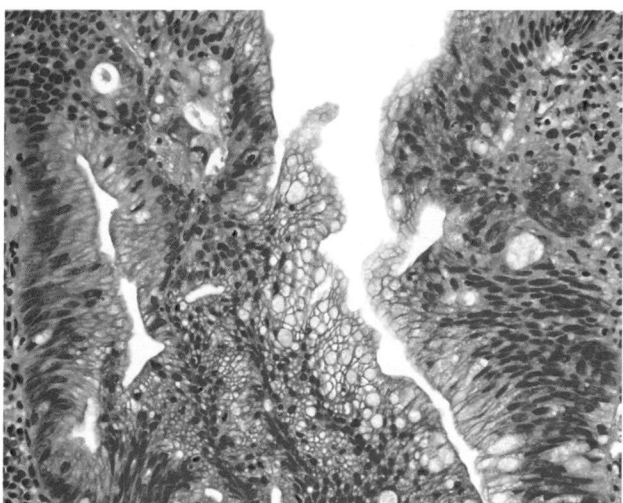

Figure 4-266. Low-grade dysplasia, IBD.

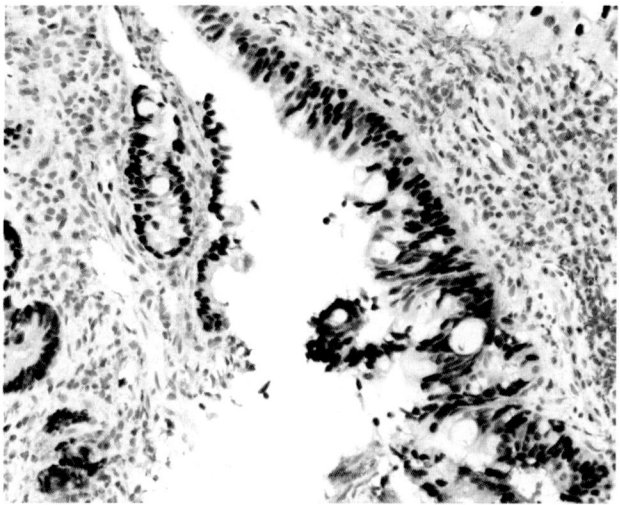

Figure 4-267. Low-grade dysplasia (LGD), IBD (p53). Dysplasia typically shows strong nuclear p53 immunoreactivity at the surface in the areas that are atypical on H&E, as seen here.

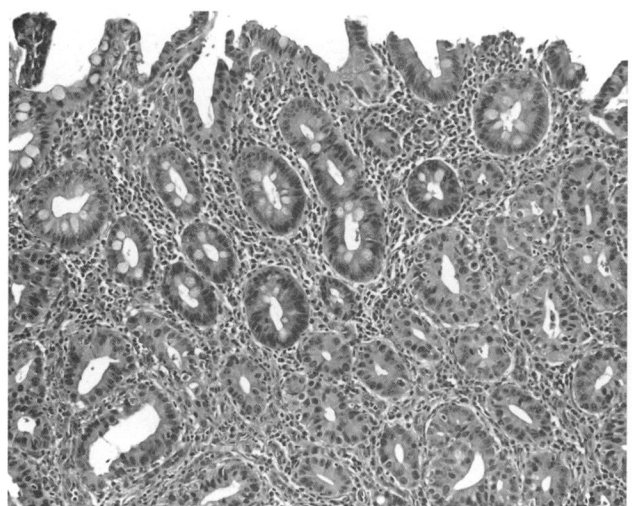

Figure 4-268. High-grade dysplasia (HGD), IBD. HGD in IBD requires only loss of nuclear polarity. This contrasts with the criteria for HGD in conventional adenomas, which requires both cytologic (loss of nuclear polarity) and architectural complexity (cribriforming) (compare with HGD in conventional adenomas [Figs. 4.31–4.36]).

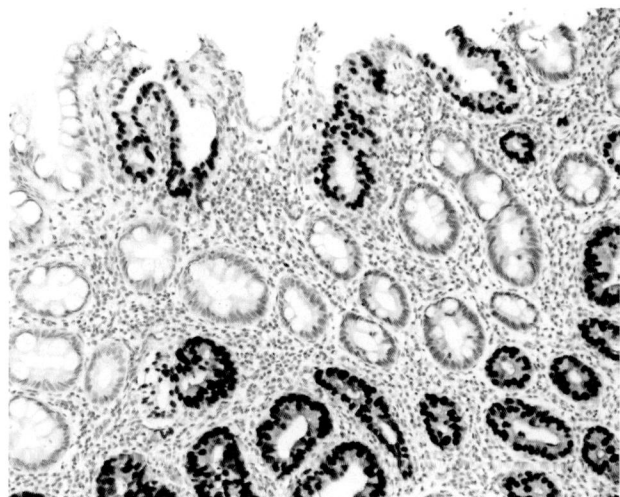

Figure 4-269. High-grade dysplasia (HGD), IBD (p53). Dysplasia typically shows strong nuclear p53 immunoreactivity at the surface in the areas that are atypical on H&E, as seen here.

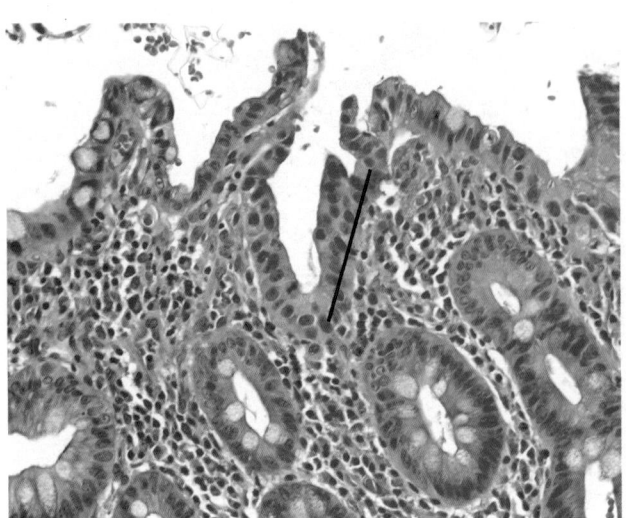

Figure 4-270. High-grade dysplasia (HGD), IBD. Higher power of the previous figure. Loss of nuclear polarity can be illustrated by drawing a *line* through the basal aspect of the cells and finding that at least half of the cells are not on the *line*, as seen here.

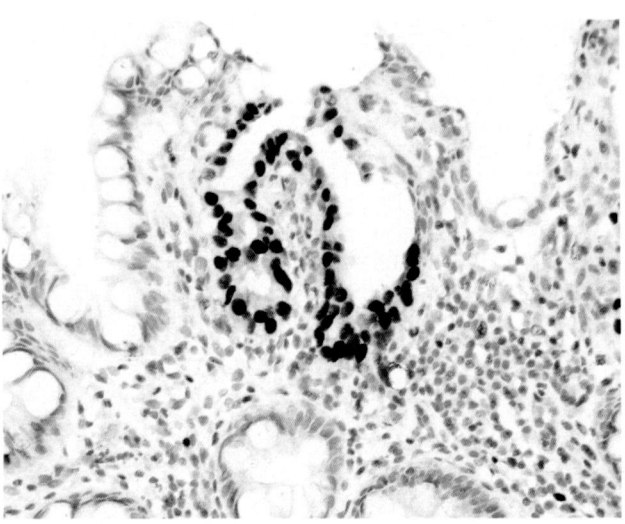

Figure 4-271. High-grade dysplasia (HGD), IBD (p53). The strong nuclear p53 immunoreactivity in the atypical cells seen on H&E supports the diagnosis of dysplasia, and the loss of polarity fulfills the criteria of HGD.

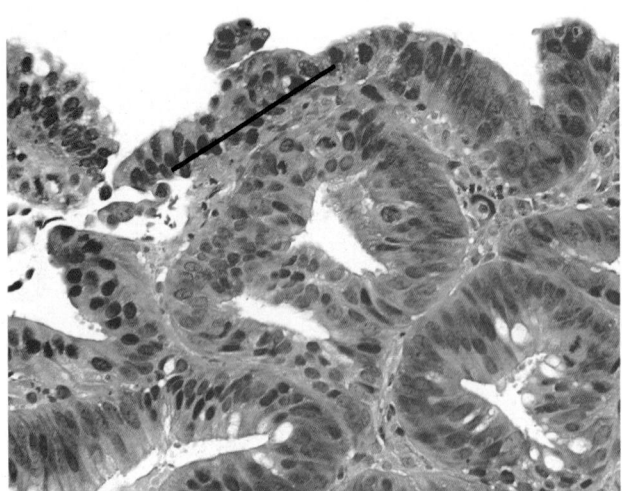

Figure 4-272. High-grade dysplasia (HGD), IBD. The *line* shows the loss of nuclear polarity, supporting the diagnosis of HGD.

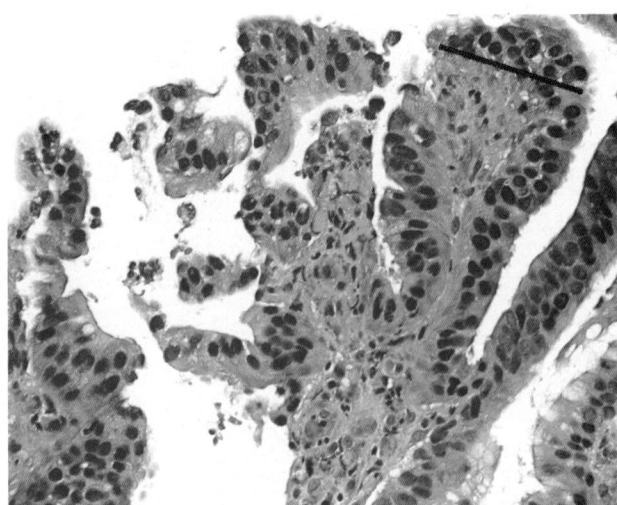

Figure 4-273. High-grade dysplasia (HGD), IBD. HGD can be focal and takes some time to evaluate, as in this case. The *line* shows the loss of nuclear polarity, supporting the diagnosis of HGD.

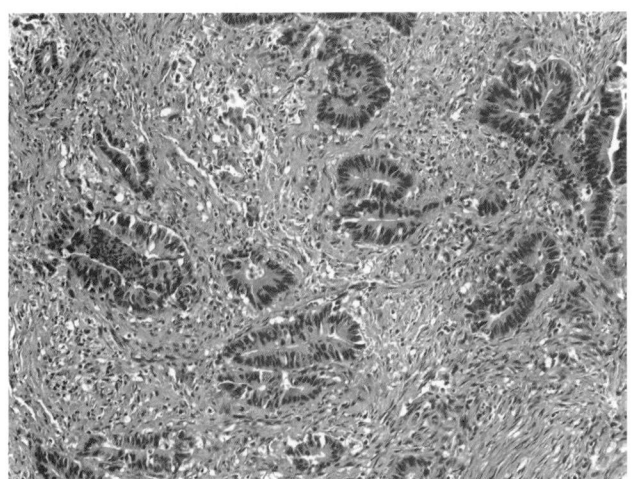

Figure 4-274. Invasive adenocarcinoma. Invasive adenocarcinoma refers to (at least) submucosal invasion and is signified by the presence of desmoplasia, as in this case. Desmoplasia imparts a *light blue* tint to the background lamina propria and submucosa and is best seen on low power. It is almost impossible to appreciate on 40×.

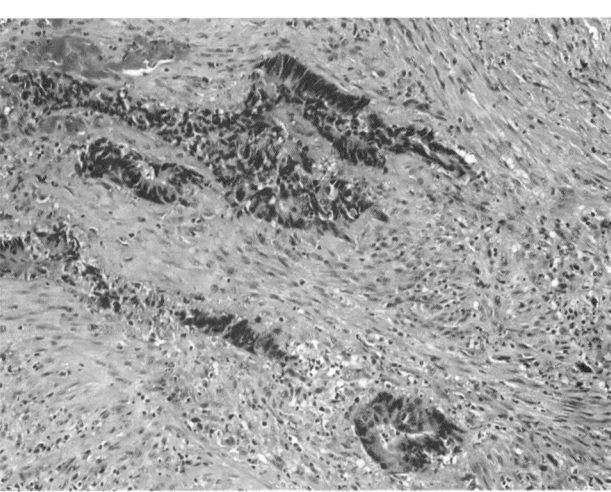

Figure 4-275. Invasive adenocarcinoma. This invasive case features desmoplasia and angulated neoplastic glands that lack investing lamina propria.

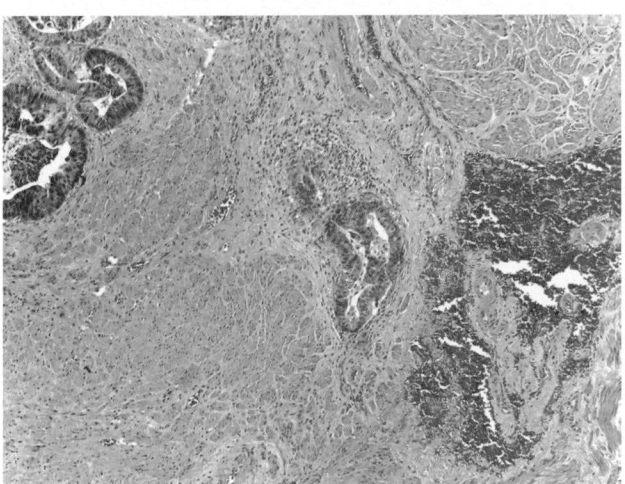

Figure 4-276. Invasive adenocarcinoma. This invasive case shows neoplastic glands in between large bundles of muscularis propria (center).

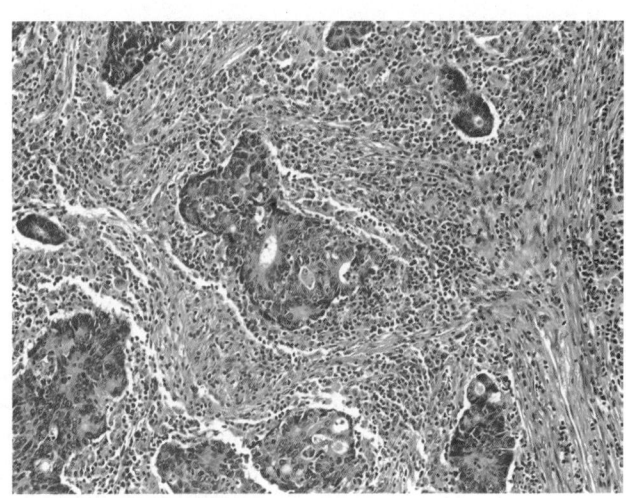

Figure 4-277. Invasive adenocarcinoma.

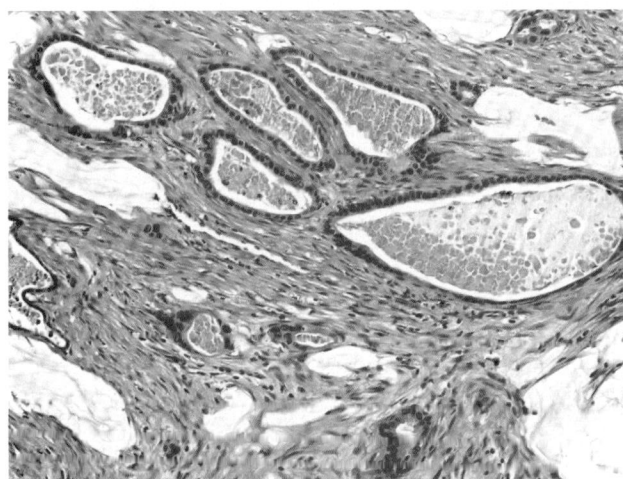

Figure 4-278. Invasive adenocarcinoma.

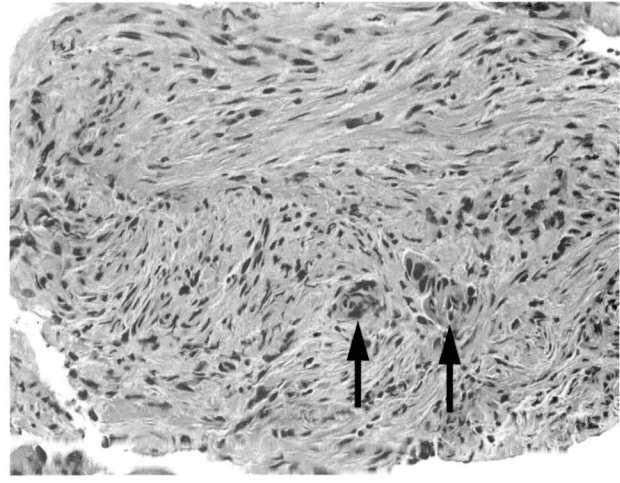

Figure 4-279. Invasive adenocarcinoma. Small angulated glands without lamina propria are seen (*arrows*) in a desmoplastic background. This carcinoma is at least pT1 because desmoplasia signifies at least submucosal invasion.

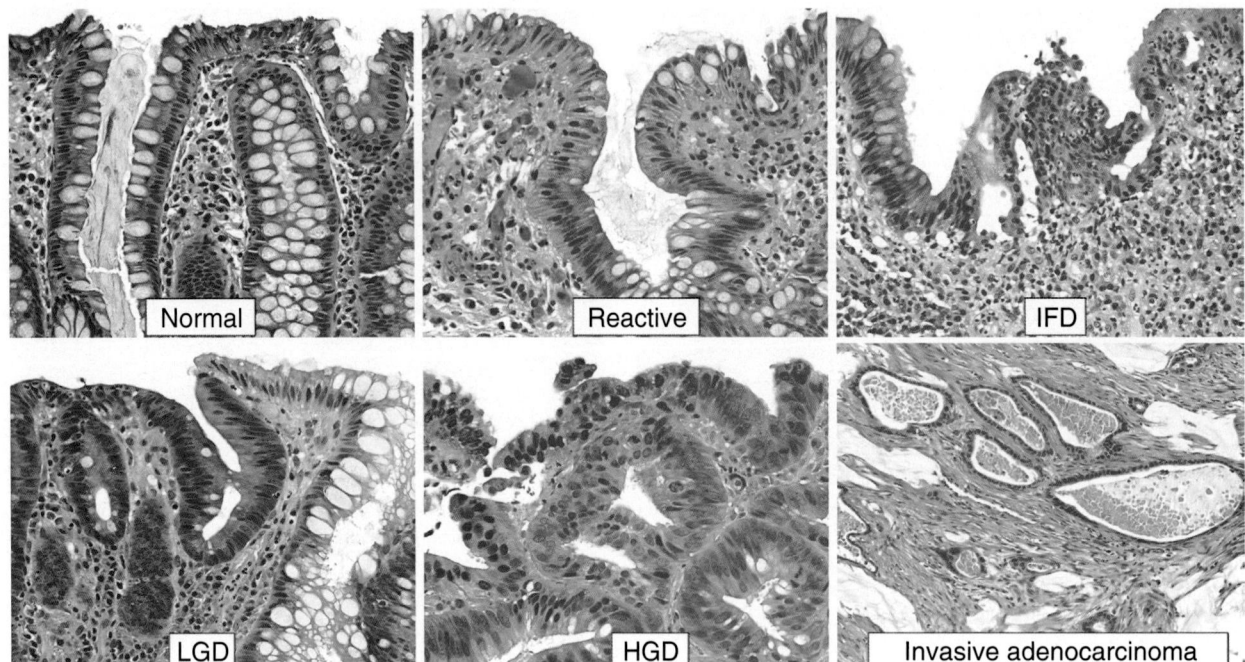

Figure 4-280. Composite illustration of the dysplasia categories in IBD. Normal colon: Normochromatic chromatin and small basally oriented nuclei that lack apoptotic bodies and mitotic figures. Reactive: Very mild atypia in proportion to the background inflammation or adjoining erosion or ulcer (not shown). Indefinite for dysplasia: Equivocal cases that are impossible to further classify. Common examples include atypia with florid inflammation, re-epithelialization of an eroded or ulcerated focus, a denuded surface, or concomitant CMV. Dysplasia is a low-power diagnosis with abrupt transitions and involves the surface. LGD: Retained nuclear polarity. HGD: Loss of nuclear polarity. Invasive adenocarcinoma: (At least) Submucosal invasion is signified by the presence of desmoplasia, infiltrating neoplastic glands, and an absence of lamina propria.

FAQ: Are there ancillary studies that can help categorize the atypia in IBD?

Answer: Sort of. Despite this simplified grading scheme, interobserver variability is moderate at best, even among GI subspecialized experts.[103-106] As a result, there has also been considerable interest in the development of biomarkers as diagnostic aides. Commonly discussed biomarkers include p53, Ki67, α-methylacyl-CoA racemase, aneuploidy, MSI, and the mucin-associated sialyl-Tn antigen (STn). At this time, these biomarkers are not sufficiently vetted for universal adoption in routine clinical practice. H&E, deeper sections, peer review, and a careful note are most reliably helpful for challenging cases; however, we occasionally perform p53 to support our H&E impressions. Beware: there are major pitfalls with the p53 immunohistochemical stain, outlined in the following list. Given these p53 complexities, for many this immunohistochemical stain is more of a headache than helpful, unless one has considerable experience with these limitations:

1. For unclear reasons, strong p53 immunolabeling can be seen in mucosa that is normal appearing on H&E. As a result, only evaluate the p53 immunohistochemical stain in atypical areas seen on H&E (H&E is the queen!).

2. Avoid overcalling p53 immunohistochemical reactivity by recognizing that the background mucosa normally shows a diffusely weak reactivity in the proliferative compartment (Figs. 4.247 and 4.248). For p53 to be reactive, the reactivity should be distinctly stronger than the background in the atypical focus seen originally on H&E (Figs. 4.266–4.271).

3. Some dysplasia completely lacks p53 immunoreactivity (the so-called p53 null phenotype defined by biallelic inactivation of the gene that completely silences it such that there is no p53 immunohistochemical detection). Accordingly, prominent atypia on H&E should not be disregarded simply because of p53 negativity (H&E is the queen!).

FAQ: What if the clinician wants to know if the dysplasia is colitis associated or sporadic?

Answer: Features favoring colitis-associated dysplasia include background mucosa with active chronic inflammatory injury; features favoring sporadic dysplasia (dysplasia that happened to be sampled in the course of surveillance) include a lack of background active chronic inflammatory injury in a patient over 50 years of age. See the following Sample Notes. However, based on the 2015 SCENIC guidelines, the issue today should be whether the lesion is endoscopically visible (and therefore endoscopically resectable) or invisible (nonresectable by endoscopy). If the dysplasia has distinct margins and endoscopic and histologic confirmation that it was completely removed and biopsies immediately adjacent to the resection site are free of dysplasia histologically, then the lesion should be fully resected via endoscopy regardless of whether it was colitis associated or sporadic. Identification of endoscopically invisible dysplasia should prompt discussion for surgical intervention, i.e., colectomy.

SAMPLE NOTE: Favor Colitis-Associated Dysplasia in a Patient With IBD

Colon, Polyp, Biopsy
• LGD arising in active chronic colitis, see Note

Note: The biopsy shows LGD. Based on the background active chronic colitis, colitis-associated dysplasia is favored. Regardless, both colitis-associated dysplasia and sporadic dysplasia are managed similarly: an endoscopically visible lesion can be endoscopically managed if it has distinct margins and endoscopic and histologic confirmation that it was completely removed and biopsies immediately adjacent to the resection site are free of dysplasia histologically. Negative for granulomata and viral cytopathic effect.

Reference:
Laine L, Kaltenbach T, Barkun A, et al. SCENIC international consensus statement on surveillance and management of dysplasia in inflammatory bowel disease. *Gastroenterology.* 2015;148:639.e628-651.e628.

SAMPLE NOTE: Favor Sporadic Dysplasia in a Patient With IBD

Colon, Polyp, Biopsy
• LGD arising in unremarkable colonic mucosa, see Note

Note: The biopsy shows LGD. Based on the background normal mucosa in a patient greater than 50 years of age, sporadic dysplasia (adenoma) is favored. Regardless, both sporadic dysplasia and colitis-associated dysplasia are managed similarly: an endoscopically visible lesion can be endoscopically managed if it has distinct margins and endoscopic and histologic confirmation that it was completely removed and biopsies immediately adjacent to the resection site are free of dysplasia histologically. Negative for granulomata and viral cytopathic effect.

Reference:
Laine L, Kaltenbach T, Barkun A, et al. SCENIC international consensus statement on surveillance and management of dysplasia in inflammatory bowel disease. *Gastroenterology.* 2015;148:639.e628-651.e628.

SAMPLE NOTE: Dysplasia in a Patient With IBD; Unclear If It Is Colitis Associated or Sporadic

Colon, Polyp, Biopsy
- LGD, see Note

Note: The biopsy shows LGD. There is no background mucosa to assess for potential background injury. Although there are no reliable histologic clues to definitively discern sporadic dysplasia versus colitis-associated dysplasia, both are managed similarly: an endoscopically visible lesion can be endoscopically managed if it has distinct margins endoscopic and histologic confirmation that it was completely removed and biopsies immediately adjacent to the resection site are free of dysplasia histologically. Negative for granulomata and viral cytopathic effect.

Reference:
Laine L, Kaltenbach T, Barkun A, et al. SCENIC international consensus statement on surveillance and management of dysplasia in inflammatory bowel disease. *Gastroenterology.* 2015;148:639. e628-651.e628.

PEARLS & PITFALLS: Filiform Polyps

Filiform polyps are nonneoplastic polyps that are almost exclusive to IBD, although rare reports describe them in the sporadic setting.[107-109] They are most commonly seen in the colon but can arise in the esophagus, stomach, and small bowel. They tend to cluster in areas of prior inflammation. Consequently, they are presumed postinflammatory in nature secondary to repeated cycles of ulceration and healing. Filiform polyps have a most peculiar macroscopic configuration that has been described as "wormlike" or "fingerlike" based on their long, slender gross appearance (Figs. 4.281, 4.282, and 4.286). Although they generally consist of only a handful per site, hundreds can coalesce into a gigantic tumor mass referred to as a giant filiform polyposis (Figs. 4.281 and 4.282). Histologically, the overlying, nondysplastic mucosa shows variable inflammation overlying a slender fibroconnective stalk consisting of fibrous tissue, vessels, lymphatics, nerves, and lymphoid aggregates (Figs. 4.283–4.290).

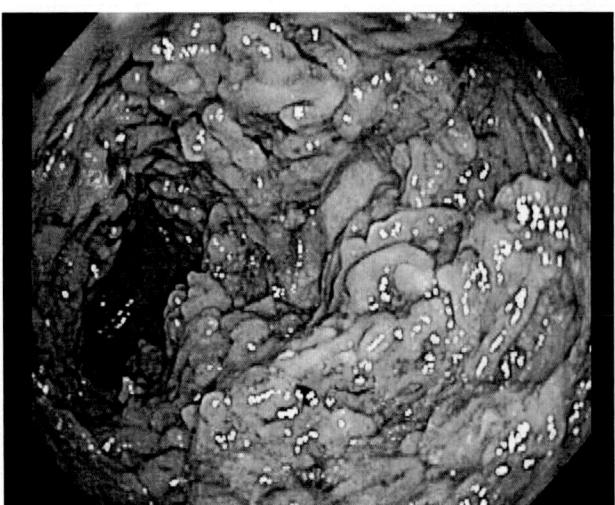

Figure 4-281. Giant filiform polyposis. This endoscopic image shows a coalescence of hundreds of filiform polyps forming a giant tumoral mass.

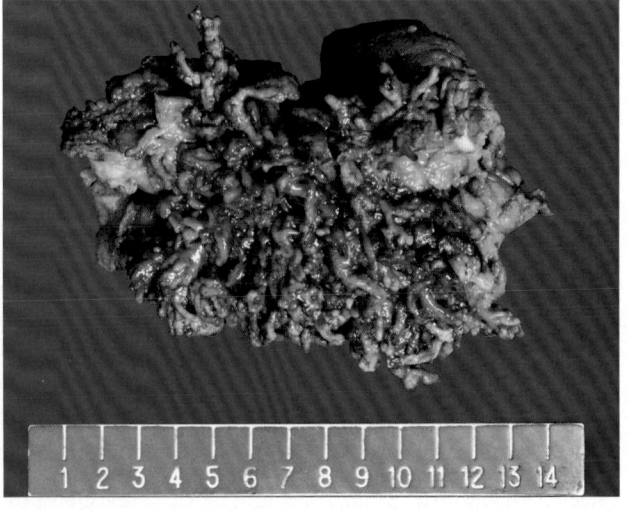

Figure 4-282. Giant filiform polyposis. Gross image of the previous figure. This mass had to be resected because it was causing obstruction.

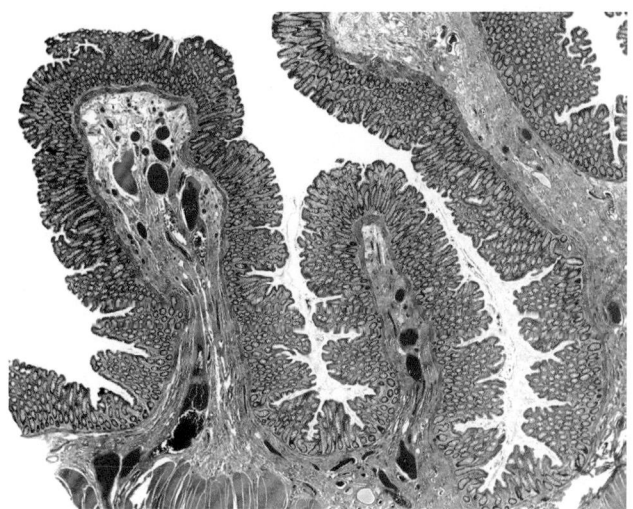

Figure 4-283. Giant filiform polyposis. Histology of the previous figure. The polyps consist of variably inflamed mucosa overlying fibrovascular cores.

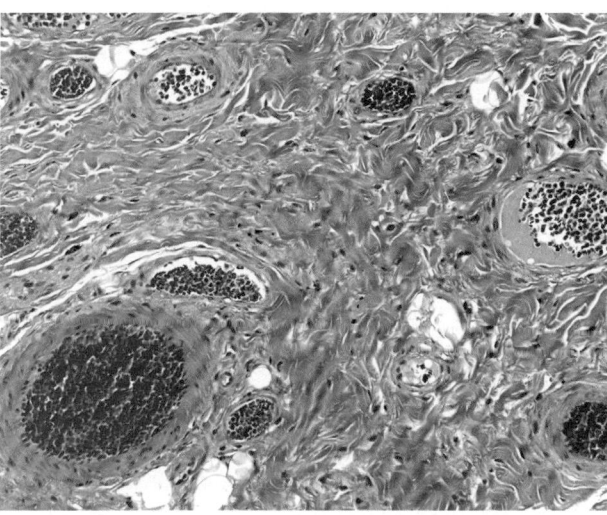

Figure 4-284. Giant filiform polyposis. Higher power of the previous figure showing the unremarkable fibrovascular cores. This patient had a long-standing history of Crohn disease. Filiform polyps are rarely seen outside of the setting of IBD.

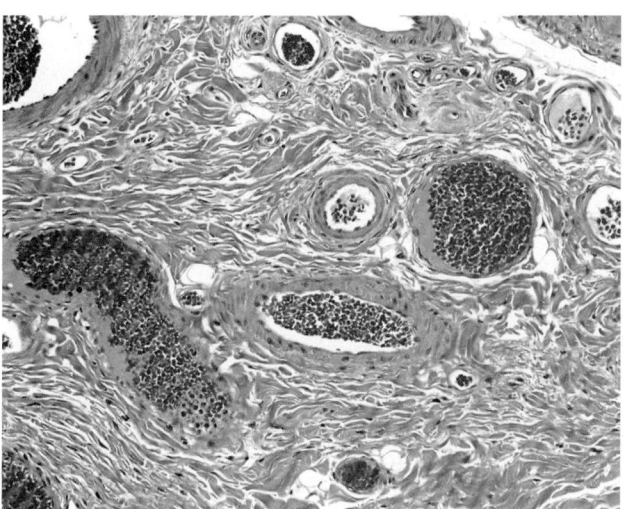

Figure 4-285. Giant filiform polyposis. A different view of the previous figure. Filiform polyps are invariably negative for dysplasia, but thorough sampling is suggested.

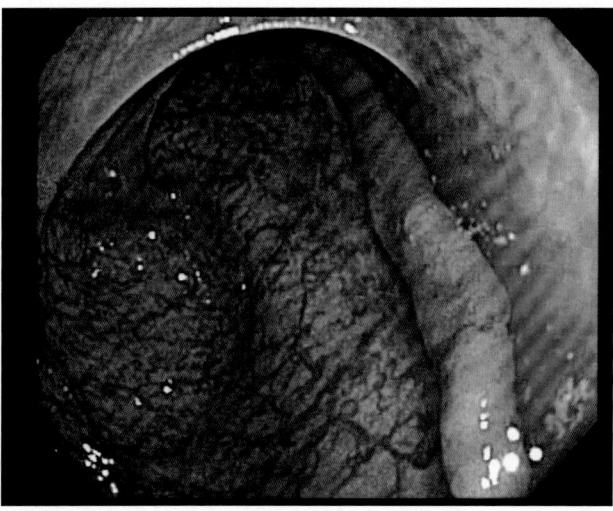

Figure 4-286. Filiform polyp. Endoscopic view of a different case. This patient also had a long-standing history of IBD. The filiform polyps typically appear similar to worms or fingers because of their long, slender form, as seen here.

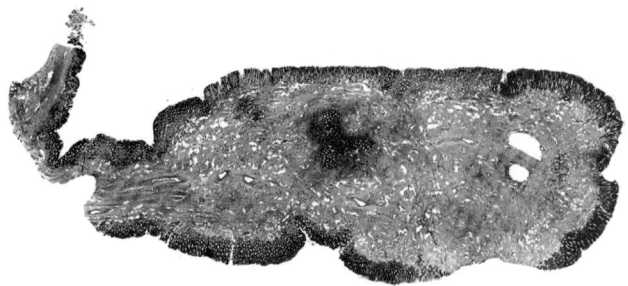

Figure 4-287. Filiform polyp. The histology of the previous figure shows a long, slender polyp consisting predominantly of a fibrovascular core.

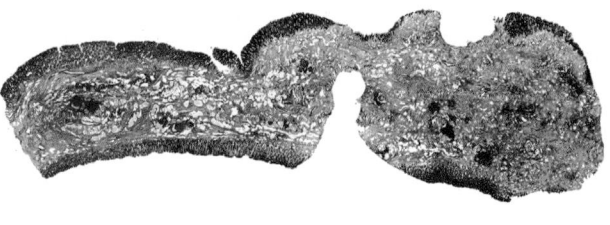

Figure 4-288. Filiform polyp. A separate polyp from the same patient.

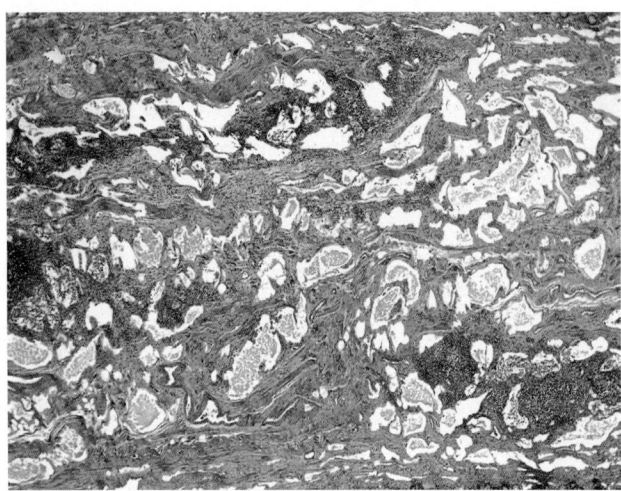

Figure 4-289. Filiform polyp. Higher power of the previous figure shows the fibroconnective stalk with fibrous tissue, lymphovascular spaces, and lymphoid aggregates.

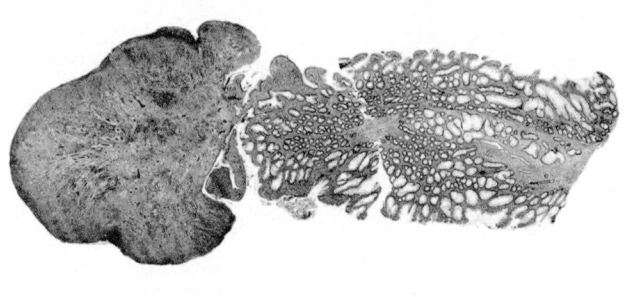

Figure 4-290. Filiform polyp.

PEARLS & PITFALLS: Serrated Epithelial Change (Hyperplastic Epithelial Change)

Serrated epithelial change (SEC; hyperplastic epithelial change) is a controversial, emerging concept in IBD. Interestingly, it was briefly mentioned in Riddell's 1983 seminal work on dysplasia in IBD,[102] but the literature trail since then has been sparse. It is an uncommon finding with an incidence of up to 3% of patients with IBD. It is endoscopically invisible and found histologically on tissue submitted as a nonpolypoid, random mucosal biopsy. Histologically, it appears as polypoid tissue with serrated architecture and cytoplasmic eosinophilia (Figs. 4.291–4.299). In our experience, the spectrum of changes is quite pronounced and ranges from a subtle surface serrated ruffling to something more overtly unnatural, inflamed, and bizarre. An uncontrolled study of 187 patients with IBD with at least one histologic finding of SEC, negative for typical features of dysplasia, and a mean disease duration of 16 years found that 13% had a prior history of dysplasia, 21% had synchronous or metachronous dysplasia or carcinoma, and location concordance was 68%.[110] Others have found similar results.[111-113] Until the concept is better defined, we comment on the finding in our reports and some of our clinicians follow as indefinite for dysplasia. See the following Sample Note. This finding can also be accompanied by conventional dysplasia, and, when present, the highest degree of dysplasia should be reported. Keep in mind that SEC is a contentious area and others have suggested that this change has no statistically significant risk of neoplasia after adjustment for prior conventional dysplasia.[114] Other similarly contentious areas on the IBD landscape include the hypermucinous variant of dysplasia and basal crypt dysplasia, both controversial entities not yet recognized by these authors based on the paucity of the available literature.

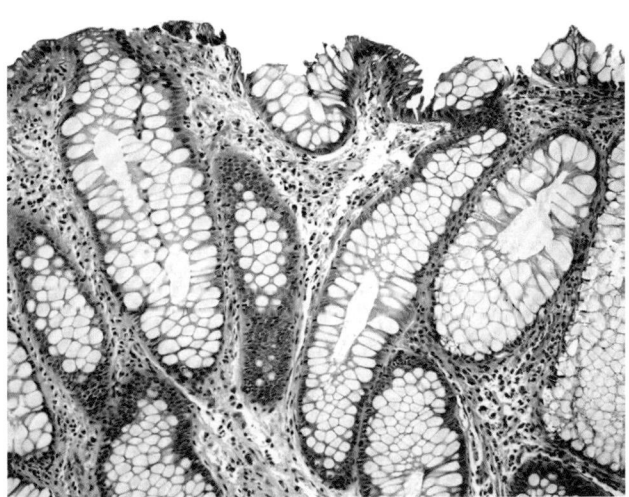

Figure 4-291. Serrated epithelial change (SEC), IBD. SEC is controversial, but some regard it as indefinite for dysplasia. SEC refers to endoscopically invisible (nonpolypoid) mucosa that histologically appears as polypoid tissue with serrated architecture, cytoplasmic eosinophilia, and variable inflammation. This biopsy, for example, looks like a goblet cell–rich hyperplastic polyp but was submitted as a flat biopsy from the transverse colon. Accordingly, it was classified as SEC.

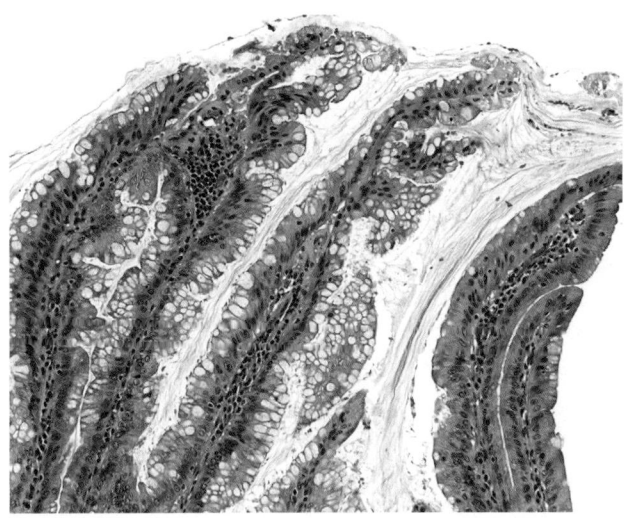

Figure 4-292. Serrated epithelial change (SEC), IBD. This example appears similar to the top of a microvesicular hyperplastic polyp (the crypt bases were narrow without serrations, not shown). However, this tissue was submitted as a random biopsy of nonpolypoid mucosa. Accordingly, it was classified as SEC. This patient was followed for decades with increasingly more prominent SEC seen; she eventually developed CRC. This case suggests following SEC as IFD is a reasonable approach.

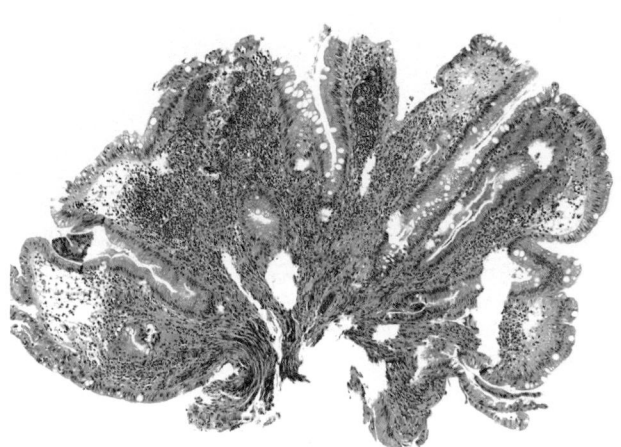

Figure 4-293. Serrated epithelial change (SEC), IBD. SEC often looks like an inflamed and architecturally distorted serrated polyp, as seen here.

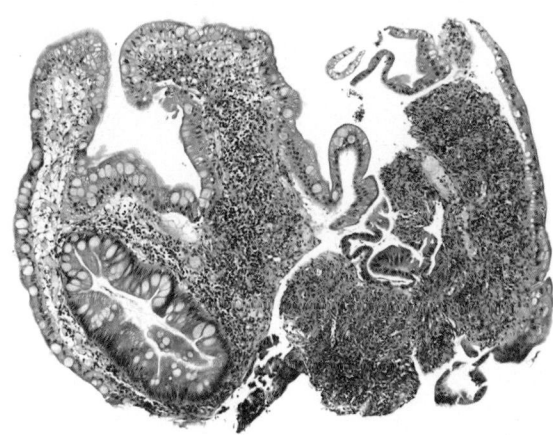

Figure 4-294. Serrated epithelial change (SEC), IBD. At this point, SEC is essentially only diagnosed in the setting of IBD.

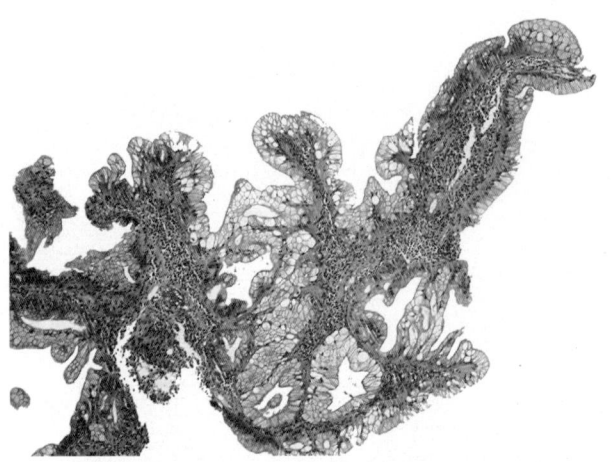

Figure 4-295. Serrated epithelial change (SEC), IBD. Many times, SEC looks like something that would never be found in nature with bizarre shapes, as in this case. This biopsy looks polypoid and as if it belongs in the serrated polyp family based on the undulated surface, frothy cytoplasm, and *pink* low-power look. However, this was an endoscopically invisible lesion and defies any of the current serrated polyp classifications. It appears similar to the Loch Ness monster or a snail with its head in the top right corner.

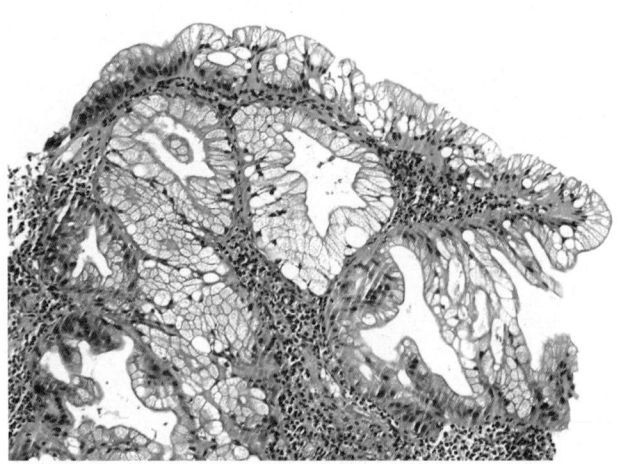

Figure 4-296. Serrated epithelial change, IBD.

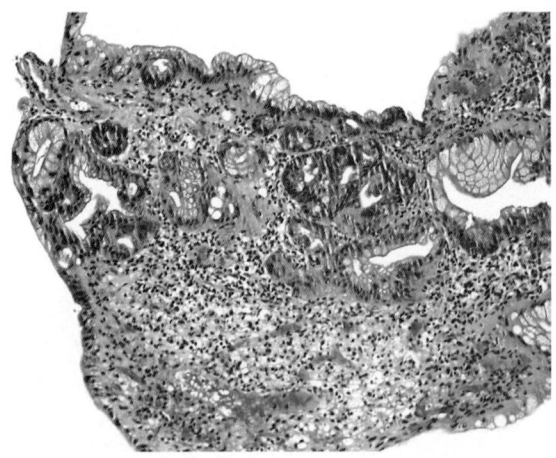

Figure 4-297. Serrated epithelial change, IBD.

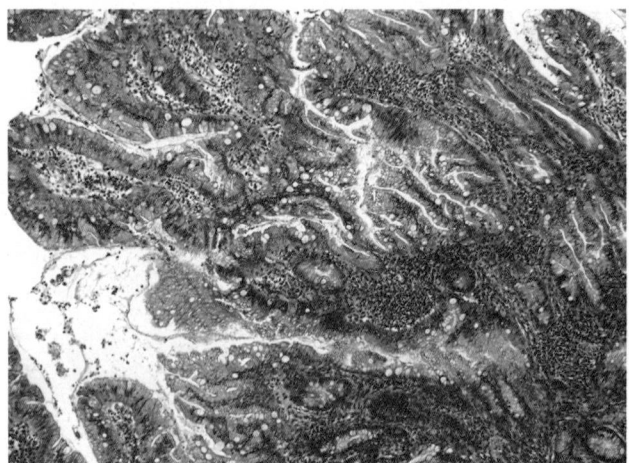

Figure 4-298. Serrated epithelial change (SEC), IBD. This case is follow-up from the case depicted in Fig. 4.292. After years of progressive SEC, the patient underwent a resection with extensive SEC seen, as depicted here.

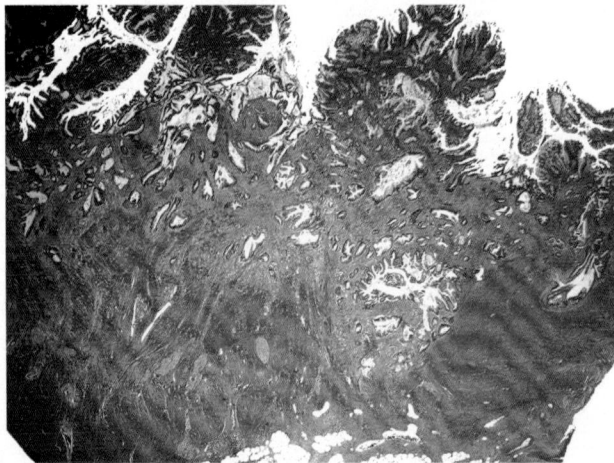

Figure 4-299. Adenocarcinoma arising in extensive SEC, IBD. A thorough sampling of the specimen found infiltrating glands into the muscularis propria with desmoplasia, resulting in the diagnosis of a pT2 CRC. This case emphasizes the importance of recognizing SEC and suggesting surveillance.

SAMPLE NOTE: Serrated Epithelial Change (Hyperplastic Epithelial Change)

Colon, Random Nonpolypoid Mucosa, Biopsy
- Inactive chronic colitis with SEC (hyperplastic epithelial change), see Note

Note: The clinical significance of SEC is unknown. Some regard it as equivalent to indefinite for dysplasia. Negative for granulomata, viral cytopathic effect, and conventional dysplasia.

References:
Johnson DH, Khanna S, Smyrk TC, et al. Detection rate and outcome of colonic serrated epithelial changes in patients with ulcerative colitis or Crohn's colitis. *Aliment Pharmacol Ther.* 2014;39:1408-1417.

Kilgore SP, Sigel JE, Goldblum JR. Hyperplastic-like mucosal change in Crohn's disease: an unusual form of dysplasia? *Mod Pathol.* 2000;13:797-801.

Parian A, Koh J, Limketkai BN, et al. Association between serrated epithelial changes and colorectal dysplasia in inflammatory bowel disease. *Gastrointest Endosc.* 2016;84:87.e81-95.e81.

Rubio CA, Rodensjö M. Flat serrated adenomas and flat tubular adenomas of the colorectal mucosa: differences in the pattern of cell proliferation. *Jpn J Cancer Res.* 1995;86:756-760.

KEY FEATURES: Dysplasia in IBD

- DALM and flat dysplasia are terms that should be abandoned by pathologists.
- Dysplasia can be managed endoscopically if it is endoscopically visible.
- Dysplasia is defined as an unequivocal neoplastic alteration of the colonic epithelium.
- Reactive epithelial change, negative for dysplasia = when the atypia is in proportion to the associated inflammation, a nearby erosion/ulceration, or CMV, for example.
- Indefinite for dysplasia = when the atypia cannot be explained by background inflammation, the surface epithelium is absent, or the atypia is not definitively dysplastic.
- LGD = retention of the nuclear polarity.
- HGD = high-grade cytologic atypia (loss of nuclear polarity); complex architecture (cribriforming) not required.
- SEC (hyperplastic epithelial change) is a controversial topic.
  - It is endoscopically invisible and submitted as a nonpolypoid, random mucosal biopsy.
  - Histologically, it appears as polypoid tissue with serrated architecture and cytoplasmic eosinophilia.
  - Some follow as indefinite for dysplasia.

The above approach is a practical one to the most common epithelial polyps, but there is so much more to the story! For more on mesenchymal polyps, see "Mesenchymal/Mesentary" chapter. For more on NETs, see "Small Intestine" chapter.

PEARLS & PITFALLS: Colorectal Neuroendocrine Tumors

Because most NETs arise in the small bowel, a thorough NET discussion is found in "Small Intestine" chapter. A few quick tips for colorectal NET are listed below (Figs. 4.300 and 4.301).

1. In the eighth edition of the AJCC, NETs are separately discussed in their own chapters according to site: ampulla of Vater, appendix, duodenum, pancreas, jejunum and ileum, stomach, and colorectum.

2. Among GI NETs, colonic NETs have the worst prognosis with a 5-year survival of 67%.[8] Most patients are symptomatic, and two-thirds of the patients have regional or distant metastasis at time of diagnosis. Radical surgery is the gold standard for most colonic NETs.

3. Among GI NETs, rectal NETs have the best prognosis with a 5-year survival of 96%.[8] Patients are generally asymptomatic, and the NET is usually found incidentally at time of screening colonoscopy. Only 4% of patients present with regional or distal metastasis. As a result, most small rectal NETs are treated with endoscopic mucosal resection.

4. Staging is based on size and depth of infiltration:

   pT1a: Tumor less than 1 cm in the greatest dimension

   pT1b: Tumor 1 to 2 cm in the greatest dimension

   pT2: Tumor invades the muscularis propria or is >2 cm with invasion of the lamina propria or submucosa

   pT3: Tumor invades through the muscularis propria into subserosal tissue without penetration of the overlying mucosa

   pT4: Tumor invades visceral peritoneum (serosa) or other organs or adjacent structures

5. As for all GI NETs, grading is based on a peak mitotic count per 10 high power fields with a minimum of 50 high power fields examined *and* peak Ki67 proliferation index and reported as a percentage of 500 to 2000 cells.

6. A panel IHC approach is suggested in the workup of NET, including AE1/3 (expected to be reactive), chromogranin and synaptophysin (usually at least one is reactive in well-differentiated NET), and Ki67 (required for WHO grading).

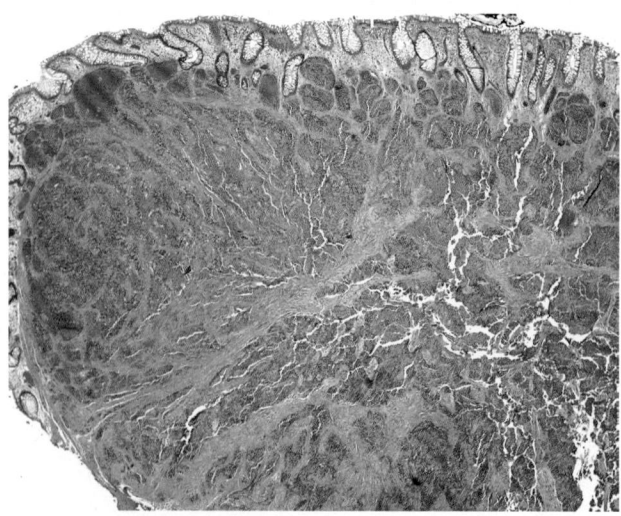

Figure 4-300. Well-differentiated WHO grade 1 neuroendocrine tumor (NET) (0 mitosis/10 HPF, less than 1% Ki67 proliferation index), involving the rectum. Among GI NETs, rectal NETs have the best prognosis. Most small rectal NETs are treated with endoscopic mucosal resection.

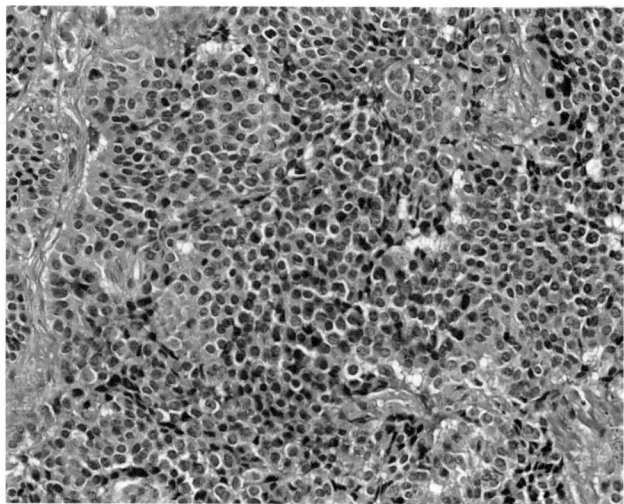

Figure 4-301. Well-differentiated WHO grade 1 NET (0 mitosis/10 HPF, less than 1% Ki67 proliferation index), involving the rectum. Higher power of the previous figure showing the typical nested architecture and salt-and-pepper chromatin of a NET. A panel IHC approach is suggested in the workup of NET, including AE1/3, chromogranin, synaptophysin, and Ki67 (not shown).

PEARLS & PITFALLS: Not a Colorectal NET (Figs. 302–304)

The above-mentioned case highlights the importance of maintaining a broad differential diagnosis, even in seemingly ordinary cases. This small rectal polyp was submitted from a surveillance colonoscopy in a 50-year-old woman with no significant past medical history. The contributor favored a NET but shared the case in consultation based on the astute concern that the lesion was nonreactive for neuroendocrine markers. Based on site and morphology, a NET is certainly a reasonable consideration, but be suspicious when the immunoprofile is not supportive of a NET. In this case, the psammomatous calcifications were suggestive of a gynecologic process and the PAX8 was reactive. The patient was subsequently found to have a uterine mass with histologic features identical to those in this lesion; both specimens were diagnosed as low-grade papillary serous adenocarcinomas.

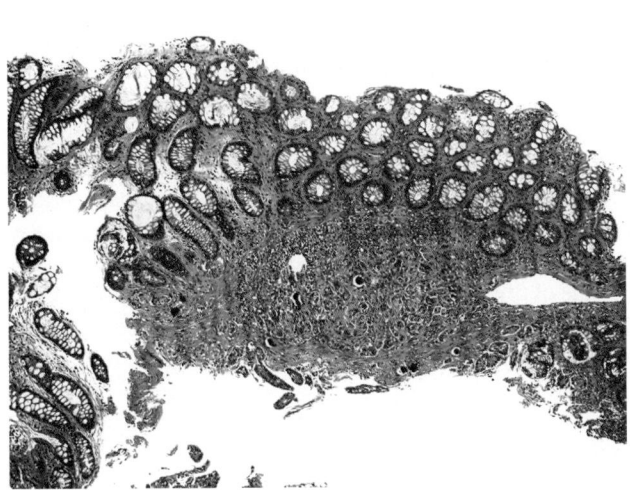

Figure 4-302. Not a rectal NET. This small rectal polyp was submitted from a surveillance colonoscopy in a 50-year-old woman with no significant past medical history.

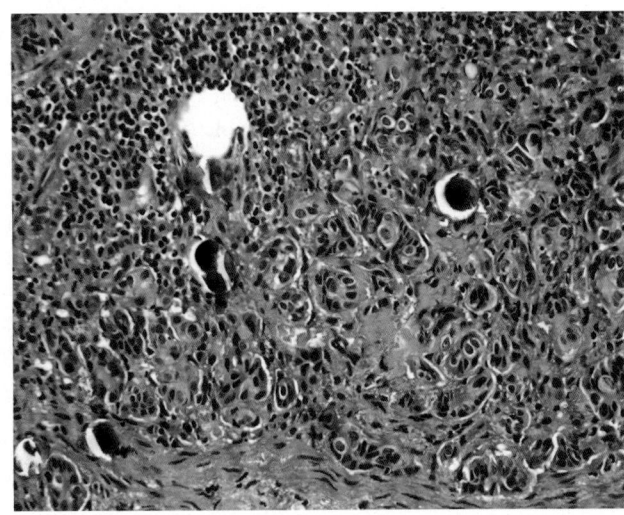

Figure 4-303. Not a rectal NET. Higher power of the previous figure. The initial pathologist favored that this lesion was a NET but shared the case in consultation based on the astute concern that the lesion was nonreactive for neuroendocrine markers.

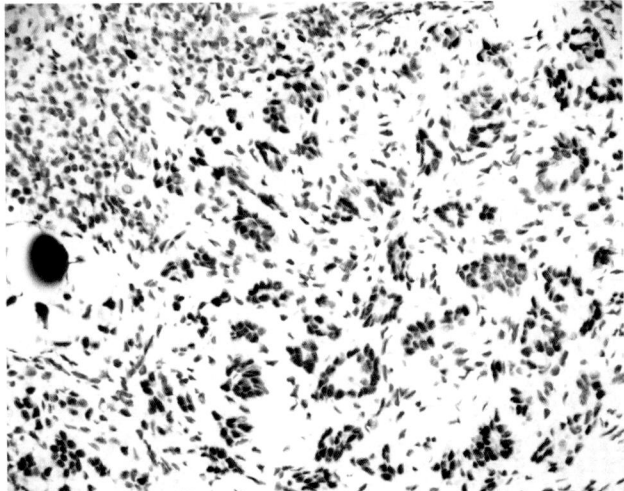

Figure 4-304. Not a rectal NET (PAX8). NET can be subjected to a panel IHC, including AE1/3, chromogranin, synaptophysin, and Ki67. Be suspicious if the supposed NET does not stain for either of the neuroendocrine markers chromogranin and synaptophysin. In this case, the psammomatous calcifications were suggestive of a gynecologic process, and the PAX8 was reactive. The patient was subsequently found to have a uterine mass identical to this lesion, both specimens were diagnosed as low-grade papillary serous adenocarcinomas.

ADENOCARCINOMA

APPROACH TO THE BIOPSY

For reporting purposes, the term invasive adenocarcinoma is reserved for cases with invasion beyond the muscularis mucosae into at least the submucosa and is staged as at least pT1 (Fig. 4.2). Although it is often technically difficult to sample the submucosa on mass-directed biopsies, identification of well-developed desmoplasia signifies at least submucosal invasion (Figs. 4.43–4.48, 4.185–4.189, and 4.274–4.279).[9] See also Pearls and Pitfalls: Controversies in Classifying Conventional Adenomas and Dysplasia Grading and Checklist: Approach to the Malignant Polyp, "Conventional Adenomatous Polyp" section. It is important to push beyond the H&E diagnosis of adenocarcinoma to appreciate other clinically relevant clues critical to guiding the next clinical steps. For example, if the adenocarcinoma arises in carpets of colonic conventional adenomas, then genetic predisposition syndromes, namely, FAP, would be an important consideration, in addition to a genetic counselor evaluation for the patient and family. If the adenocarcinoma arises in active chronic colitis, then IBD is an important consideration, as well as a careful examination of the remaining bowel to assess the background inflammatory disease and for possible synchronous or metachronous neoplasia. The morphologic approach to the most common precursors of colorectal adenocarcinoma has been discussed in the preceding sections, including for conventional adenomatous polyps, serrated polyps, select common syndromes, and IBD. In this section, a quick and dirty briefing on the three major underlying molecular pathways of carcinoma (chromosomal instability pathway, MSI pathway, and CIMP) and tips to ancillary testing is provided. This discussion is far from exhaustive and will likely be out of date by time of print based on intense research interests to develop improved predictive biomarkers and targeted therapies. Nevertheless, this section focuses on the most practical aspects of ancillary testing with emphasis on how the tests aid in classification, prognostication, and therapy.

MOLECULAR PATHWAYS 101

Chromosomal Instability Pathway

This pathway accounts for 75% of sporadic colorectal adenocarcinomas (CRC) as well as those that arise in FAP (Fig. 4.305). The chromosomal instability pathway is also termed the adenoma-carcinoma sequence and was conceptualized in 1990 by Fearon and Vogelstein.[115] This seminal work proposed that cancer was a nonrandom process that proceeded in a stepwise sequence with each major morphologic step due to specific genetic defects. In this pathway, normal mucosa first acquires inactivating mutations in the tumor suppressor *APC* followed by activating mutations of the *KRAS* proto-oncogene, resulting in a conventional TA. Next, mutations in *TP53*, *SMAD2*, and *SMAD4* are seen in step with the acquisition of HGD. Lastly, telomerase mutations, among others, are seen with the development of CRC. As a result, this pathway is characterized by gross chromosomal alterations, such as large-scale insertions, deletions, and duplications. The CRCs of this pathway are usually microsatellite stable (MSS) and CIMP negative.

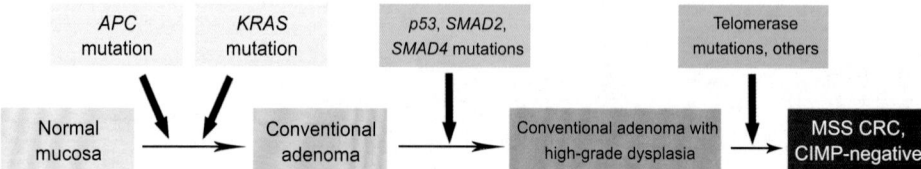

Figure 4-305. Chromosomal instability pathway. This pathway begins with *APC* and then *KRAS* mutations preceding the development of a conventional adenoma. Next, mutations in *TP53*, *SMAD2*, *SMAD4* (not necessarily in that order or all of those genes) accompany the acquisition of high-grade dysplasia. Last, mutations in the gene encoding for telomerase, among others, characterize the MSS, CIMP-negative CRC. This pathway is characterized by gross chromosomal alterations, such as large-scale insertions, deletions, and duplications.

Microsatellite Instability Pathway

The second CRC pathway is the MSI pathway, which accounts for 15% of sporadic CRC and those that arise in the setting of LS. The central defect of this pathway is a faulty MMR mechanism, which results in an increased mutation burden throughout the genome, particularly in microsatellites. MMR proteins include MLH1, PMS2, MSH2, MSH6, and EPCAM, with heterodimers forming between MLH1-PMS2 and MSH2-MSH6. Microsatellites are short tandem repeats that are particularly prone to mutations owing to their repetitive nature causing slippage on the DNA replication machinery. Regardless of whether the carcinoma is sporadic or syndromic, CRCs in this pathway are defined MMR defects that result in high levels of mutations in microsatellites (MSI-high). In contrast to MSI-low and MSS carcinomas, MSI-high carcinomas are typically right-sided and contain a mucinous, medullary, or poorly differentiated component; an expanding border; Crohn-like peritumoral response; and increased tumor infiltrating lymphocytes (Figs. 4.306–4.311). Patients with such tumors tend to present at a lower stage, have a better stage-specific prognosis, are less responsive to 5-fluorouracil and epidermal growth factor receptor (EGFR) targeted therapies (cetuximab and panitumumab), are more responsive to irinotecan, and may benefit from PD-1 immune checkpoint blockade therapies.[116,117]

Sporadic and syndromic MSI-high CRC differ in two important aspects: the mechanism of MMR inactivation and the precursor polyp (Table 4.8). Sporadic MSI-high CRC occurs through inactivation of the *MLH1* promoter via global hypermethylation (CIMP-high), and the precursor polyp is the SSA/P (Fig. 4.312). LS MSI-high CRC, in contrast, is due to MMR gene germline defects, and the precursor polyp is the conventional TA (Fig. 4.313). The diagnosis of LS is established by demonstrating the presence of deleterious MMR defects: (1) germline defects in the DNA MMR genes, *or* (2) germline methylation of the MLH1 promoter, *or* (3) inactivation of *MSH2* due to deletion of the 3′ exons of the *EPCAM (TACSTD1)* gene.

Universal screening for LS for all CRC has been broadly supported by the following major professional organizations: the US Multi-Society Task Force for CRC, the American College of Gastroenterology, American Society of Clinical Oncology, the National Comprehensive Cancer Network, the European Society of Medical Oncology, and the Evaluation of Genomic Applications in Practice and Prevention (a working group of the Centers for Disease Control).[51] The screening protocol at The Ohio State University is depicted in Fig. 4.314. Briefly, screening begins with a four-antibody panel of MMR protein IHC (MLH1, PMS1, MSH2, and MSH6); note that MSI-testing is an essentially equivalent screening tool preferred by some centers. If all MMRs are intact/present (or the CRC is MSI-low or MSS), then the CRC is likely sporadic and all subsequent LS screening is aborted. CRCs that are deficient in MLH1 (and its binding partner PMS2) could either be sporadic or syndromic and, therefore, require subsequent testing to identify patients with LS via *MLH1* promoter methylation studies; note that some centers prefer *BRAF* V600E mutational analysis as the next step. If *MLH1* promoter methylation is detected (or a *BRAF* V600E mutation is detected), then the CRC is likely sporadic and subsequent LS screening is aborted. If *MLH1* promoter methylation is absent (or a *BRAF* V600E mutation is absent), then the CRC is suspicious for LS. Loss of MSH2 (and its binding partner MSH6) or isolated loss of MSH6 or PMS2 is also suggestive of LS but does not require additional *MLH1* promoter methylation or *BRAF* V600E mutational analysis because these deficiencies are not seen in sporadic CRC. One important exception is that an isolated MSH6 loss can be seen in up to 20% of posttreatment MSS CRC.[118-121] Some have suggested that the MSH6 loss is due to treatment-related cell cycle inhibition based on low Ki67 proliferative indices.[121] Others have suggested treatment-related epigenetic changes or mutations.[118] Regardless, such cases should have the MMR IHC performed on the initial diagnostic material, if available, or MSI testing on the posttreatment biopsy.

For patients with a high probability of LS (for example, MLH1/PMS2 IHC deficient and absent *MLH1* promoter methylation, isolated MSH2 IHC deficient, isolated MSH6 IHC deficient, or MSH2/MSH6 IHC deficient), a genetic counselor evaluation and confirmatory germline genetic testing is offered. It is worthwhile to be familiar with the emerging concept of "Lynch-like syndrome." This refers to *sporadic* MSI-high CRC with unexplained MMR deficiency and for those with MLH1 MMR deficiencies, absent *MLH1* promoter methylation (or absent *BRAF* V600E mutational analysis), and absent germline defects in *MMR* or *EPCAM*. See also Pearls and Pitfalls: Lynch-Like Syndrome and MMR IHC Interpretation, Biomarker section (Table 4.8).

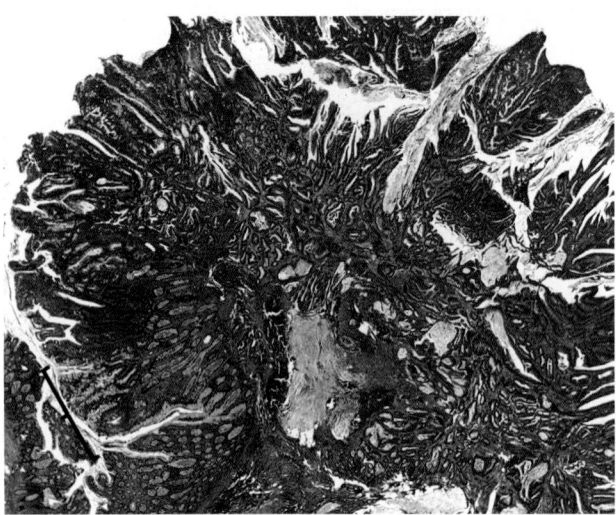

Figure 4-306. Clue to MSI-H CRC: Precursor serrated polyp. It is worthwhile to carefully examine CRC for the background precursor polyps. This case shows a tiny focus of a serrated polyp (*bracket*) along with dysplasia (right side of mass). The type of serrated polyp is not clear from this section, although it probably arose in an SSA/P based on the proximal colon location. The full resection specimen showed a T3 CRC (invasion not well demonstrated on this image). This right-sided CRC originated from a 79-year-old woman with sporadic MSI-H CRC (precursor serrated polyp, MLH1/PMS2 IHC deficiency, present *MLH1* promoter methylation).

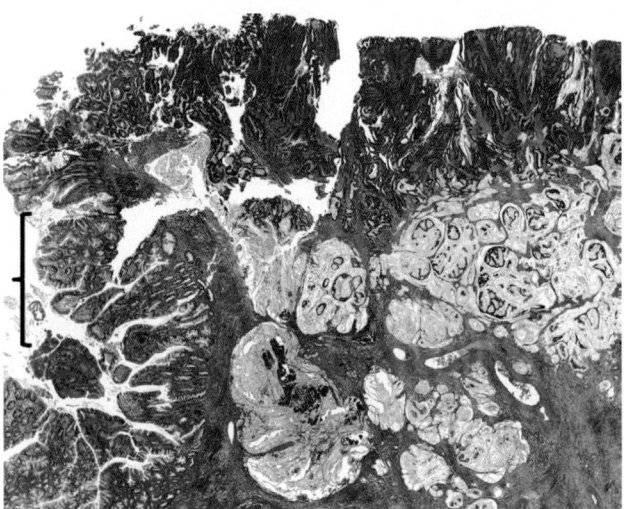

Figure 4-307. Clues to MSI-H CRC: Precursor serrated polyp and mucinous adenocarcinoma. This SSA/P is "caught in the act" of transitioning from a nondysplastic SSA (*bracket*) to dysplasia (top middle) to a mucinous carcinoma (center). Typical features of MSI-H CRC include a mucinous phenotype with expanding borders (not infiltrative) and a Crohn-like peritumoral response with peritumoral lymphoid aggregates and fibrosis, as seen here. This case originated from a 95-year-old man with sporadic MSI-H CRC (precursor serrated polyp, MLH1/PMS2 IHC deficiency, present *MLH1* promoter methylation).

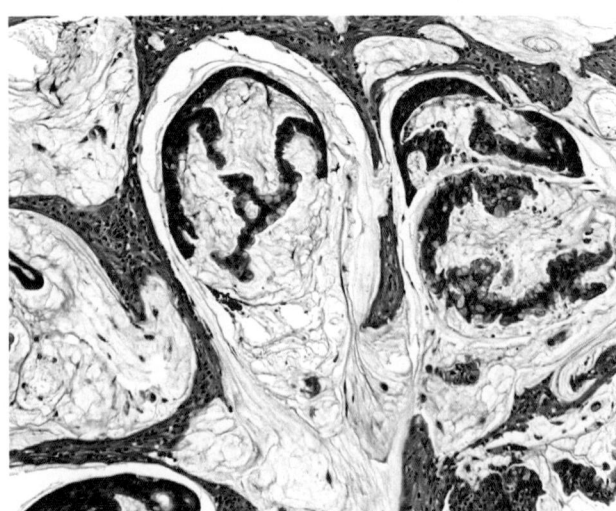

Figure 4-308. Clue to MSI-H CRC: Mucinous morphology. Higher power of the previous figure. A diagnosis of mucinous adenocarcinoma requires that at least 50% of the invasive tumor consists of mucin pools with suspended neoplastic glands, as seen here.

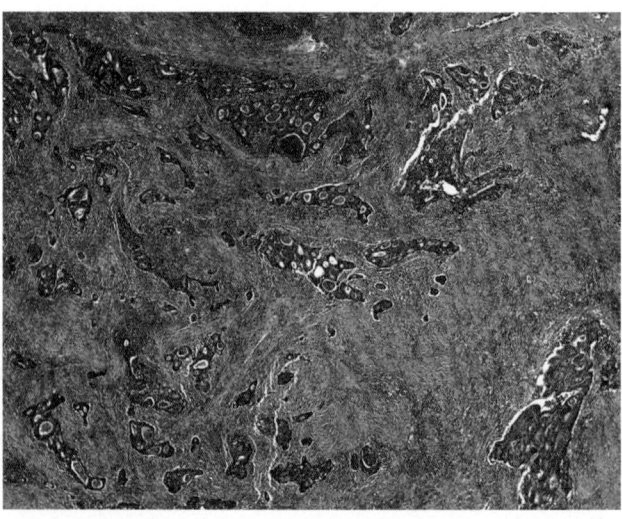

Figure 4-309. Clue to MSI-H CRC: Crohn-like peritumoral response. A Crohn-like peritumoral response refers to peritumoral lymphoid aggregates and fibrosis, as seen here.

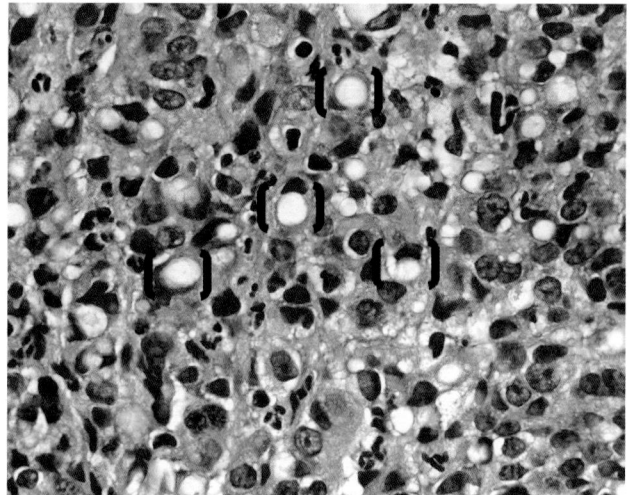

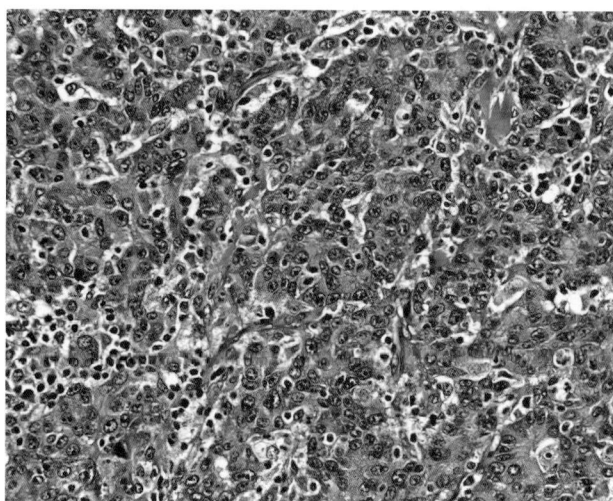

Figure 4-310. Clue to MSI-H CRC: A poorly differentiated morphology with signet ring cells. The *brackets* highlight the signet ring cells with their abundant round cytoplasm pushing the nucleus to the periphery of the cell, resembling a jewelry ring. A diagnosis of signet ring adenocarcinoma requires that at least 50% of the invasive tumor consists of signet ring cells, as seen here. This case originated from a 39-year-old man with Lynch syndrome, and the CRC showed the typical associations: the precursor polyp was a conventional adenoma, MSH2/MSH6 IHC deficient, and *MSH2* germline defect in a patient with a strong family history of CRC in young individuals.

Figure 4-311. Clue to MSI-H CRC: Medullary morphology. Medullary features refer to large neoplastic cells with prominent nucleoli, syncytial growth, abundant eosinophilic cytoplasm, and striking tumor infiltrating lymphocytes, as seen here. This case originated from an 18-year-old woman with Lynch syndrome, and the CRC showed the expected molecular signatures: MSH2/MSH6 IHC deficient, absent *MLH1* promoter methylation, and genetic confirmation of a *MSH2* germline defect in a patient with a strong family history of CRC in young individuals.

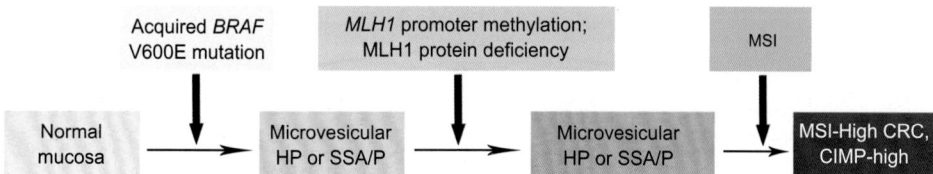

Figure 4-312. The microsatellite instable pathway (MSI): Sporadic. This pathway is characterized by an early acquired *BRAF* V600E mutation, resulting in a microvesicular hyperplastic polyp or sessile serrated adenoma/polyp. Next, *MLH1* promoter methylation occurs via global hypermethylation (CpG island methylator phenotype) resulting in *MLH1* gene inactivation, subsequent deficiencies in the MLH1 protein (and its binding partner PMS2), and cytologic dysplasia. Increasing MSI eventually leads to an MSI-high CRC, CIMP-high.

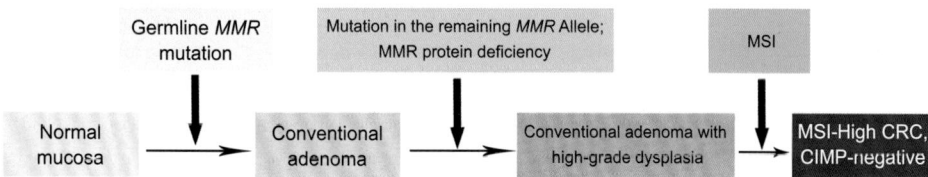

Figure 4-313. The microsatellite instable pathway (MSI): Lynch syndrome. Lynch syndrome is an autosomal dominantly inherited germline defect in a mismatch repair (MMR) gene, and the precursor lesion is the conventional adenoma. After mutation in the remaining MMR allele, MMR protein loss can be detected with MMR protein immunohistochemistry; this step is often accompanied by high-grade dysplasia. MMR deficiency results in MSI-high CRC independent of CIMP.

TABLE 4.8: Differentiating Sporadic Versus Syndromic Microsatellite Instability-High (MSI-H) Colorectal Carcinomas (CRC)

	Sporadic MSI-High CRC	Syndromic MSI-High CRC (Lynch Syndrome)
Precursor polyp	Sessile serrated adenoma/polyp	Tubular adenoma
MLH1/PMS2 MMR IHC deficiency	Present	Present; alternatively, can have MSH2 and MSH6 deficiencies, or isolated MSH6 or PMS2 deficiency
Mechanism of MLH1/PMS2 IHC loss	Methylation-related inactivation of *MLH1* promoter via CIMP	Germline defect
BRAF V600E mutation	Present	Absent
MLH1 promotion methylation	Present	Absent
CIMP	High	Negative

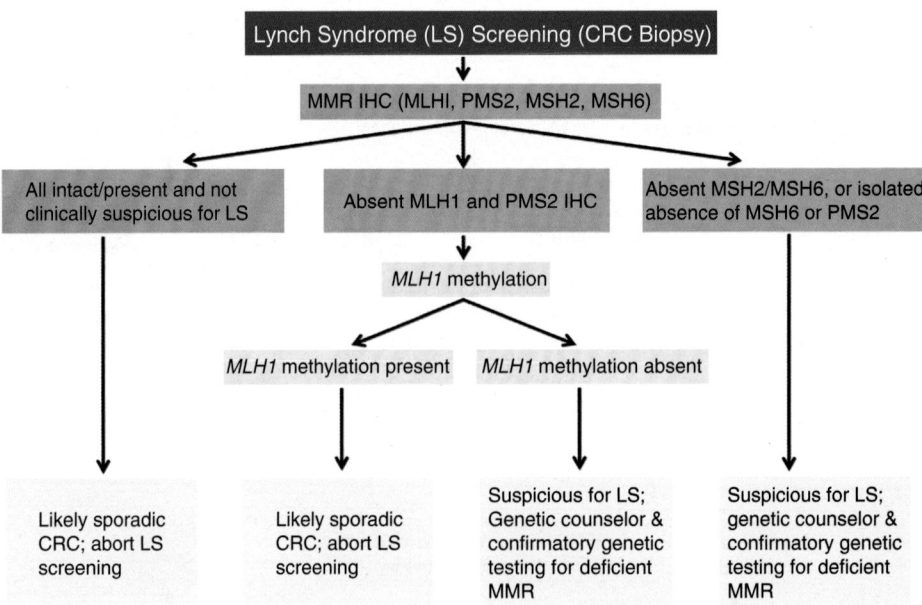

Figure 4-314. Method for universal screening for Lynch syndrome at OSU.

PEARLS & PITFALLS: Lynch-Like Syndrome

LS is an autosomal dominantly inherited germline defect in *MMR* that leads to CRC with MMR protein deficiencies, absent *MLH1* promoter methylation, absent *BRAF* V600E mutational analysis, MSI-high, and CIMP-negative (Fig. 4.313). In contrast, the term Lynch-like syndrome describes *sporadic* MSI-high CRC with unexplained MMR deficiencies. For those with MLH1 MMR deficiencies, absent *MLH1* promoter methylation and absent *BRAF* V600E mutations are seen. Germline *MMR* defects are absent. Because these CRCs are unassociated with heritable defects, many argue that the term Lynch-like syndrome should be abandoned because it implies a heritable defect with a high-risk of CRC that requires life-time surveillance. These proponents prefer the term sporadic MMR-deficient tumor to more accurately describe the genetic insults and to clearly distinguish them from LS. Possible explanations for their MMR deficiencies include the following[51,122-125]:

1. Misinterpretation of the MMR IHC
2. Biallelic somatic mutations in the MMR gene
3. An unidentified MMR gene germline mutation
4. An unidentified non-MMR gene germline mutation
5. Somatic mosaicism

CpG Island Methylator Phenotype

The third CRC pathway is the CIMP pathway, which underlies the serrated pathway of neoplasia. CpG islands are cytosine and guanine dinucleotides that serve as transcriptional regulatory elements that control gene expression via methylation. When the cytosines of the CpG islands are methylated, gene expression is inhibited via chromatin restriction that prevents engagement of the transcription machinery. This mechanism is termed epigenetic because it results in regulation of gene expression without genetic mutations. Although the CIMP pathway is a normal regulatory mechanism, many cancers manipulate this pathway toward growth promotion and apoptotic suppression. CRCs with widespread hypermethylation of CpG island loci are termed CIMP-high, in contrast to CIMP-low and CIMP-negative CRC. Specifically, the serrated pathway of neoplasia is characterized by an early *BRAF* mutation in the microvesicular hyperplastic polyp or SSA/P, followed by CIMP-mediated methylation and inactivation of the *MLH1* promoter, resulting in MLH1 and PMS2 loss, MSI, cytologic dysplasia, and, ultimately, MSI-high CRC, CIMP-high (Fig. 4.315, identical to the sporadic MSI pathway).

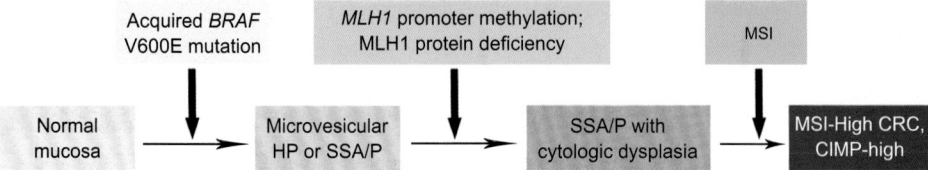

Figure 4-315. CpG island methylator phenotype; SSA/P. CIMP is the mechanism of the serrated pathway of neoplasia, and the precursor is the SSA/P. This is the same mechanism as that discussed in the sporadic MSI-high CRC (Fig. 4.305). This pathway is characterized by an early acquired *BRAF* V600E mutation, resulting in a microvesicular hyperplastic polyp or sessile serrated adenoma/polyp. Next, *MLH1* promoter methylation via global hypermethylation (CpG island methylator phenotype) results in *MLH1* gene inactivation, resultant deficiencies in the MLH1 protein (and its binding partner PMS2), and cytologic dysplasia. Increasing microsatellite instability eventually leads to an MSI-high CRC, CIMP-high.

FAQ: Where does the TSA fit on the existing CRC pathways?

Answer: The putative role of the TSA is less clear. TSAs are rare lesions in general, and, therefore, quality molecular studies validated from multiple groups are a bit more limited. Some have proposed that the TSA exists on its own pathway that is characterized by an early *KRAS* mutation in the goblet cell–rich hyperplastic polyp or TSA, followed by CIMP-low–mediated *MGMT* methylation, and, ultimately, MSS CRC (Fig. 4.316).[126-128]

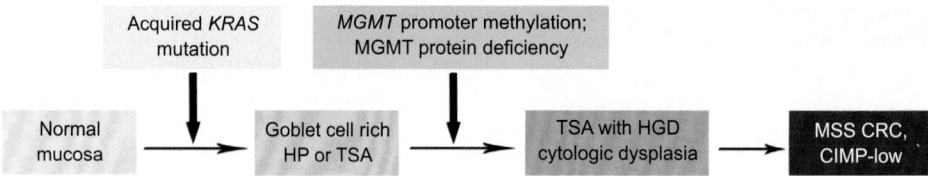

Figure 4-316. CpG island methylator phenotype (CIMP); TSA. Less is known about the TSA, but it is proposed to exist on its own CRC pathway. In this pathway, an early *KRAS* mutation in the goblet cell–rich hyperplastic polyp or TSA is followed by CIMP-low–mediated *MGMT* methylation and, ultimately, MSS CRC, CIMP-low.

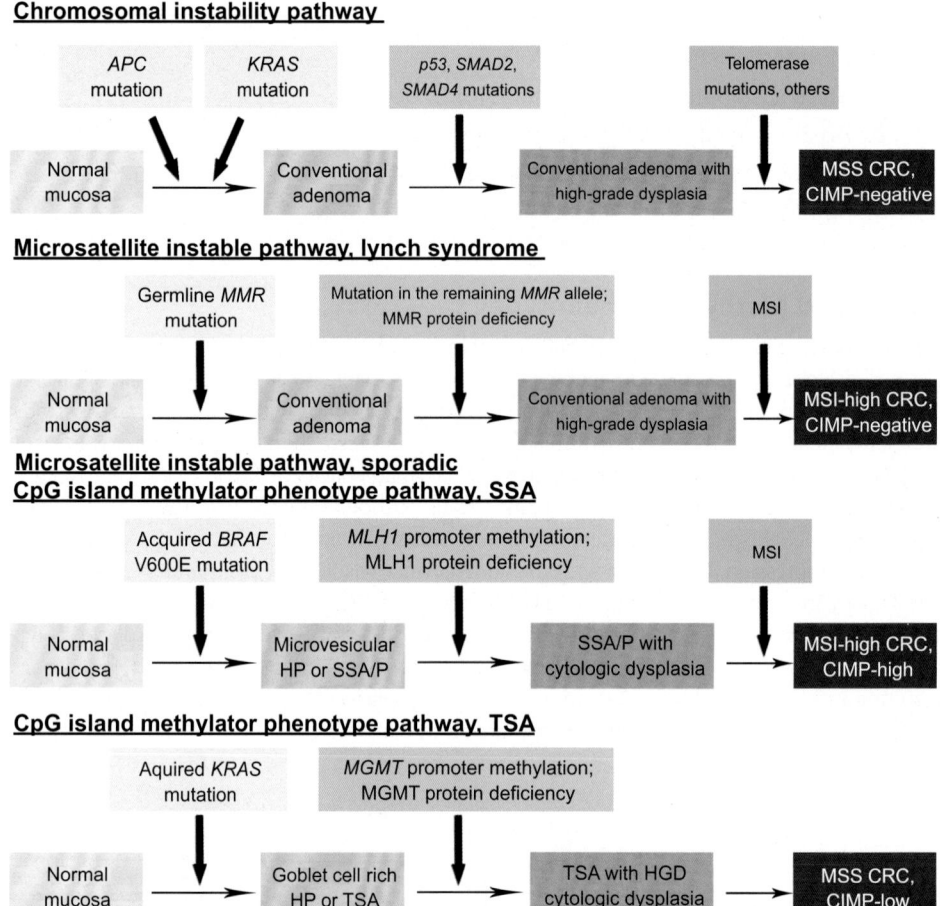

Figure 4-317. A composite image of the major molecular pathways of CRC.

See Fig. 4.317 for a side-by side comparison of the discussed CRC pathways.

BIOMARKER TESTING 101

A diagnosis of CRC can lead a stream of requested biomarker tests. This section is a quick and dirty summary of the most common requested tests.[129-134] Prognostic biomarkers are those that provide information on overall outcomes, whereas predictive biomarkers provide information on the expected response to a specific therapy. See also "Adenocarcinoma" section, "Lynch Syndrome" subsection, and MMR IHC Pearls and Pitfalls (Fig. 4.318; Table 4.9).

PEARLS & PITFALLS: Guidelines on Colorectal Carcinoma Biomarkers

In March 2017, an expert panel was assembled to provide evidence-based guidelines for the use of predictive biomarkers in colorectal cancer.[130] The panel represented a collaborative partnership between The American Society for Clinical Pathology, College of American Pathologists, Association for Molecular Pathology, and American Society of Clinical Oncology. Based on the review of more than 4,000 articles, the panel issued the following 21 guideline statements (Table 4.10).

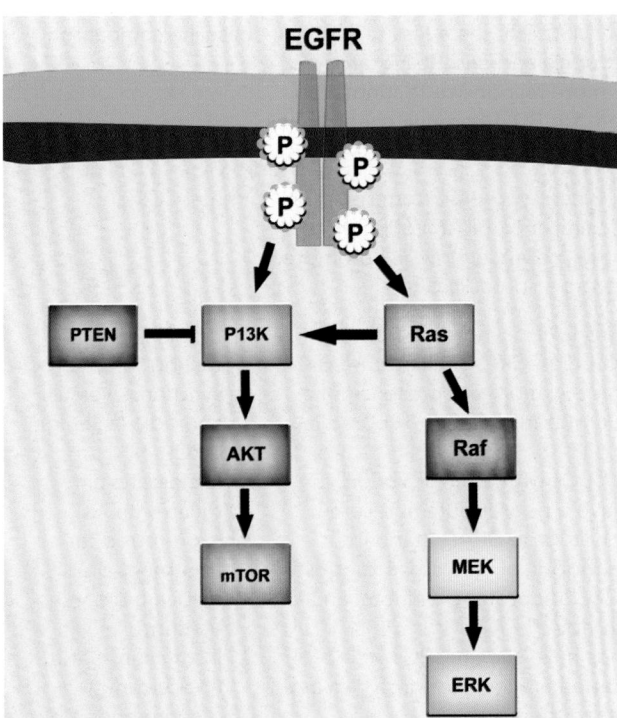

Figure 4-318. Schematic of the EGFR pathway. A super basic understanding of this pathway can decode the alphabet soup of requested molecular studies that follow a diagnosis of colorectal carcinoma. EGFR-based testing is, itself, no longer recommended because downstream activating mutations in *RAS/RAF/MEK/ERK* and the *PI3K/AKT/mTORC1* pathways can cause resistance to anti-EGFR–targeted therapies, regardless of the EGFR ligand status. Today, the major focus is on *RAS* testing in patients with metastatic CRC who are being considered for anti-EGFR–targeted therapies. Such patients benefit from anti-EGFR–based therapies only if the CRC has wild-type *KRAS*. This testing is best performed on the metastasis, if at all possible, and should include *KRAS* and *NRAS* (expanded or extended *RAS* panel). See also Table 4.9 for a complete list of biomarker testing and rationale.

TABLE 4.9: Approach to Select Colorectal Carcinoma Biomarkers

Biomarker	Function	Specimen of Choice
MMR IHC	Screening for Lynch syndrome and sporadic MSI-high CRC, similar to MSI testing; MSI-high CRCs have a better stage-specific prognosis than MSS CRCs, are less responsive to 5-fluorouracil and anti-EGFR targeted therapies, are more responsive to irinotecan, and may benefit from PD-1 immune checkpoint blockade therapies	Primary CRC
MSI PCR	Screening for Lynch syndrome and sporadic MSI-high CRC, similar to MMR testing; MSI-high CRCs have a better stage-specific prognosis than MSS CRCs, are less responsive to 5-fluorouracil and anti-EGFR targeted therapies, are more responsive to irinotecan, and may benefit for PD-1 immune checkpoint blockade therapies	Primary CRC with section of nonneoplastic tissue for baseline comparison
MLH1 promoter methylation	Differentiates Lynch syndrome from sporadic MSI-high CRC, similar to *BRAF* V600E mutations studies; the presence of *MLH1* promoter methylation favors a sporadic CRC	Primary CRC
BRAF V600E mutation	1. Differentiates Lynch syndrome from sporadic MSI-high CRC, similar to *MLH1* promoter methylation; the presence of a *BRAF* V600E mutation favors a sporadic CRC 2. Metastatic CRCs with a *BRAF V600E* mutation have a poorer outcome compared with wild-type *BRAF*, standard therapy is suboptimal, and some suggest FOLFIRINOX, 5-fluorouracil, irinotecan as first-line therapy.[130] 3. Some studies have shown CRCs with *BRAF* V600E mutation are less responsive to anti-EGFR targeted therapies	1. Primary CRC for testing of Lynch syndrome versus sporadic MSI-high CRC; 2. Metastatic or recurrent CRC is preferred for treatment-predictive biomarker testing; 3. Insufficient data, not currently recommended by 2017 Guidelines on CRC Biomarkers[130]
RAS mutation	*RAS* testing recommended in patients with metastatic CRC considered for anti-EGFR targeted therapies because this therapy benefits only patient with metastatic CRC and wild-type *KRAS* Testing should include *KRAS* and *NRAS* (expanded or extended *RAS* panel)	Metastatic or recurrent CRC is preferred for treatment-predictive biomarker testing
EGFR mutation	EGFR-based testing is no longer recommended because downstream mutations in RAS/RAF/MEK/ERK and the PI3K/AKT/mTORC1 pathways can cause resistance to anti-EGFR targeted therapies, regardless of the EGFR ligand status	No longer recommended

TABLE 4.9: Approach to Select Colorectal Carcinoma Biomarkers (Continued)

Biomarker	Function	Specimen of Choice
PIK3CA mutation	*PIK3CA* encodes for P13K, a protein with high oncogenic transformative activity. Some studies have shown CRCs with *PIK3CA* mutations are less responsive to anti-EGFR targeted therapies; some have shown patients with stage IV CRC with *PIK3CA* mutations have a poorer response and progression-free survival; some have found a survival advantage for posttreatment aspirin or COX-2 inhibitors in patients with *PIK3CA* mutations	Insufficient evidence; not currently recommended by 2017 Guidelines on CRC Biomarkers[130]
PTEN mutation or PTEN IHC	*PTEN* inhibits P13K such that *PTEN* loss as detected by IHC or FISH results in activation of the P13K pathway and less responsiveness to anti-EGFR targeted therapies	Insufficient evidence; not currently recommended by 2017 Guidelines on CRC Biomarkers[130]
HER2 amplification by IHC or FISH	CRC with HER2 amplification is less responsive to and linked to shorter progression-free survival on anti-EGFR-targeted therapies than HER2 nonamplified CRC, is a negative predictive biomarker for anti-EGFR antibody–targeted therapies in metastatic CRC; these patients may benefit from anti-HER2 inhibition (trastuzumab) with lapatinib or trastuzumab and pertuzumab. Note: Her2 scoring in CRC is different from that for gastroesophageal neoplasms	Insufficient evidence; not currently recommended by 2017 Guidelines on CRC Biomarkers[130]
PDL-1 IHC	MSI-high CRC may benefit from PD-1 immune checkpoint blockade therapies	Insufficient evidence; not currently recommended by 2017 Guidelines on CRC Biomarkers[130]

CRC, colorectal carcinoma; EGFR, epidermal growth factor receptor; IHC, immunohistochemistry; MMR, mismatch repair; MSI, microsatellite instability.

TABLE 4.10: Guidelines on Colorectal Carcinoma Biomarkers

Guideline Statement	Strength of Recommendation
1. *RAS* mutational testing recommended in patients with CRC considered for anti-EGFR therapy. Mutational analysis should include *KRAS* and *NRAS* codons 12 and 13 of exon 2, 59 and 61 of exon 3, and 117 and 146 of exon 4 (expanded or extended *RAS*)	Recommendation
2a. *BRAF* p.V600 [*BRAF* c.1799 (p.V600)] mutational analysis should be performed in CRC for prognostic stratification	Recommendation

(Continued)

TABLE 4.10: Guidelines on Colorectal Carcinoma Biomarkers   (Continued)

Guideline Statement	Strength of Recommendation
2b. *BRAF* p.V600 mutational analysis should be performed in MMR-deficient MLH1-deficient CRC to evaluate for Lynch syndrome: The presence of a *BRAF* mutation favors a sporadic CRC, and the absence suggests Lynch syndrome	Recommendation
3. Clinicians should order MMR testing in patients with CRC to identify patients at high risk for Lynch syndrome and/or prognostic stratification	Recommendation
4. There is insufficient evidence to recommend *BRAF* c.1799 p.V600 mutational status as a predictive biomarker for response to anti-EGFR inhibitors	No recommendation
5. There is insufficient evidence to recommend *PIK3CA* mutational analysis of CRC for therapy selection outside of a clinical trial. Retrospective studies have suggested improved survival with postoperative aspirin in patients with *PIK3CA* mutated CRC	No recommendation
6. There is insufficient evidence to recommend PTEN analysis in CRC for patients who are being considered for therapy selection outside of a clinical trial	No recommendation
7. Metastatic or recurrent CRCs are the preferred specimens for treatment-predictive biomarker testing. In their absence, primary tumor tissue is an acceptable alternative	Expert consensus opinion
8. Formalin-fixed, paraffin-embedded tissue is an acceptable specimen for CRC biomarker mutational testing. Use of other specimens (i.e., cytology specimens) will require additional adequate validation, as would any changes in tissue-processing protocols	Expert consensus opinion
9. Laboratories must use validated CRC molecular biomarker testing methods with sufficient performance characteristics for the intended clinical use. CRC molecular biomarker testing validation should follow accepted standards for clinical molecular diagnostics tests	Strong recommendation
10. Performance of molecular biomarker testing for CRC must be validated in accordance with best laboratory practices	Strong recommendation

TABLE 4.10: Guidelines on Colorectal Carcinoma Biomarkers   (Continued)

Guideline Statement	Strength of Recommendation
11. Laboratories must validate the performance of IHC testing for CRC molecular biomarkers in accordance with best laboratory practices	Strong recommendation
12. Laboratories must provide clinically appropriate turnaround times and optimal utilization of tissue specimens by using appropriate techniques for clinically relevant CRC molecular and IHC biomarkers	Expert consensus opinion
13. CRC molecular and IHC biomarker testing should be initiated in a timely fashion based on the clinical scenario and in accordance with institutionally accepted practices	Expert consensus opinion
14. Laboratories should establish policies to ensure efficient allocation and utilization of tissue for molecular testing, particularly in small specimens	Expert consensus opinion
15. Members of the patient's medical team, including pathologists, may initiate CRC molecular biomarker test orders in accordance with institutionally accepted practices	Expert consensus opinion
16. Laboratories that require send-out of tests for treatment-predictive biomarkers should process and send CRC specimens to reference molecular laboratories in a timely manner, with a benchmark of 90% of specimens sent out within 3 working days	Expert consensus opinion
17. Pathologists must evaluate candidate specimens for biomarker testing to ensure specimen adequacy, taking into account tissue quality, quantity, and malignant tumor cell fraction. Specimen adequacy findings should be documented in the patient report	Expert consensus opinion
18. Laboratories should use CRC molecular biomarker testing methods that are able to detect mutations in specimens with at least 5% mutant allele frequency, taking into account the analytical sensitivity of the assay (limit of detection or LOD) and tumor enrichment (i.e., microdissection). It is recommended that the operational minimal neoplastic carcinoma cell content tested should be set at least two times the assay's LOD	Expert consensus opinion

(Continued)

TABLE 4.10: Guidelines on Colorectal Carcinoma Biomarkers   (Continued)

Guideline Statement	Strength of Recommendation
19. CRC molecular biomarker results should be made available as promptly as feasible, both prognostic and predictive, with a benchmark of 90% of reports made available within 10 working days from date of receipt in the molecular diagnostics laboratory	Expert consensus opinion
20. CRC molecular biomarker testing reports should include results and interpretation readily understandable by oncologists and pathologists. Appropriate Human Genome Variation Society and Human Genome Organization nomenclature must be used in conjunction with any historical genetic designations.	Expert consensus opinion
21. Laboratories must incorporate CRC molecular biomarker testing methods into their overall laboratory quality improvement program, establishing appropriate quality improvement monitors as needed to ensure consistent performance in all steps of the testing and reporting process. In particular, laboratories performing CRC molecular biomarker testing must participate in formal proficiency testing programs, if available, or an alternative proficiency assurance activity	Strong recommendation

CRC, colorectal carcinoma; EGFR, epidermal growth factor receptor; IHC, immunohistochemistry; MMR, mismatch repair; PTEN, phosphatase and tensin homolog.

Mismatch Repair Immunohistochemistry

MMR IHC (or MSI testing) has been traditionally used to screen for LS in colorectal, endometrial, and small bowel carcinomas. A game-changing move occurred on May 23, 2017, when the US Food and Drug Administration (FDA) granted approval of Keytruda (pembrolizumab) to treat adult and pediatric patients with unresectable or metastatic solid tumors that are MMR deficient or MSI-H.[135] This approval was historic because, for the first time, the FDA approved a treatment based on a biomarker rather than the location of the primary malignancy, i.e., colon, breast, bladder, lung. As a result, MMR IHC (and MSI testing) is now broadly requested on a wide variety of malignancies in hopes of offering an effective therapy to patients. MMR IHC interpretation is usually straightforward, with most cases showing complete intact nuclear reactivity (Figs. 4.319–4.321) or complete absence/loss (Figs. 4.322–4.324). However, a small fraction of cases is difficult, and they need to be systematically approached for accurate evaluation. Below are handy tricks and tips to MMR IHC interpretation. This approach is similar for LS screening and for patients considered for immune checkpoint blockade inhibitor therapy, but important distinctions exist. See also "Programmed Death Receptor-1/Programmed Death Ligand-1" and "Cytotoxic T-Lymphocyte–Associated Antigen 4" sections.

1. The specimen of choice for LS screening is the initial biopsy over the colorectal resection specimen because a diagnosis of LS can alter surgical management. For example, a patient with LS would likely benefit from a complete or extended colectomy over a segmental resection based on the increased risk of synchronous and metachronous neoplasia in the remaining colorectum. Based on the increased risk of endometrial cancer, some women with LS opt for a tandem hysterectomy at the time of the colon resection.

2. For patients pending evaluation for immune checkpoint blockade inhibitor therapy, the resection specimen is preferred over the biopsy to offer the most accurate evaluation because the biomarkers can display significant tumor heterogeneity.[136] At time of writing, it is not yet clear if the primary tumor or the metastasis is the specimen of choice. This testing may become rapidly irrelevant because the correlation between PD-1 and PD-L1 expression with response seems suboptimal as indicated later for lung lesions. See also "Programmed Death Receptor-1/Programmed Death Ligand-1" and "Cytotoxic T-Lymphocyte–Associated Antigen 4" sections.

3. Testing for all four MMR proteins (MLH1, PMS2, MSH2, and MSH6) by IHC is recommended. To reduce costs, some centers use only a two-antibody MMR IHC approach with MSH6 and PMS2, but this approach can miss a (small) fraction of MMR-deficient cases.

4. The MMR IHC panel is performed on only one tumor slide from each distinct tumor. In the case of multiple CRCs, perform MMR IHC on each distinct tumor because a patient with LS could also have a synchronous sporadic CRC.[137]

5. Verify that internal controls worked by confirming intact/present MMR IHC reactivity in the background stromal and inflammatory cells adjacent to the tumor (compare working controls in Figs. 4.325 and 4.326 to failed controls in Figs. 4.327 and 4.328).

6. Evaluate the MMR IHC reactivity only in the invasive tumor, key point 1. MMR IHC reactivity in the background dysplasia can be misleading. For example, a patient with LS could show intact/present MMR IHC reactivity in the background adenoma and loss in the carcinoma.

7. Evaluate the MMR IHC reactivity in the invasive tumor, key point II. Tumor infiltrating lymphocytes serve as internal controls but can be distracting when interpreting the MMR IHC (Figs. 4.322–4.324). Avoid evaluating MMR IHC reactivity of the tumor based on the intervening infiltrating lymphocytes to avoid an incorrect interpretation. A careful review of the H&E in conjunction with the MMR IHC is most helpful in differentiating the tumor from the infiltrating lymphocytes.

8. A true intact/present MMR IHC should show diffuse nuclear reactivity comparable in intensity with the background internal controls. A speckled (Fig. 4.329), nucleolar, nuclear membrane, or cytoplasmic reactivity pattern is abnormal and should be reported as lost/absent. Nuclear reactivity weaker than the internal controls is scored as lost/absent (Figs. 4.330 and 4.331).

9. At The Ohio State University, a 5% cutoff is used for MMR IHC evaluation[122]: intact/present MMR IHC requires at least 5% of the tumor cells on the slide to have comparably strong nuclear reactivity as the internal controls (Figs. 4.332–4.335). This percentage is roughly determined by eye-ball estimates of the total tumor on the glass slide.

10. In ambiguous cases for which the positive control worked but the MMR IHC reactivity is around the 5% cutoff and/or weaker than the controls, repeat the MMR IHC. If the same result is seen, results can be reported as equivocal and repeat MMR IHC on the resection (or MSI testing on the current biopsy) is suggested.

11. One important tip is to remember that treatment can lead to weak MSH6 MMR reactivity in approximately 20% of MSS CRC (Figs. 4.336–4.338).[118-121] If the diminished reactivity is concerning, MMR IHC can be performed on the pretreatment biopsy, if available, or MSI testing performed on the posttreatment specimen.

12. Avoid reporting MMR IHC reactivity as positive, negative, weak, or diminished because these ambiguous terms can be misunderstood. Instead the terms present/intact or absent/lost are more precise.

13. Predictable deficiency patterns can be expected based on an understanding of MMR dimerization (Figs. 4.339 and 3.340). Because MLH1 dimerizes with PMS2, MLH1 deficiency usually results in PMS2 deficiency because PMS2 is too unstable in the absence of its stabilizing MLH1 binding partner. A similar rationale is applicable to the MSH2 and MSH6 dimerization. MSH2 deficiency usually results in MSH6 deficiency because MSH6 is too unstable in the absence of its stabilizing MSH2 binding partners. However, the reverse is not true. MLH1 and MSH2 remain present when PMS2 and MSH6 are deficient, respectively, because they can bind other stabilizing partners.

Based on this, some centers perform MMR evaluation with only PMS2 and MSH6, but this misses a small fraction of MMR-deficient cases. A four-panel MMR IHC with PMS2, MLH1, MSH2, and MSH6 is therefore recommended for MMR evaluation.

14. Because patients with LS can present with small bowel or endometrial cancer, it is worthwhile to perform MMR IHC on all small bowel carcinomas[138] and endometrial cancers,[139,140] in addition to all CRC. Beware, *BRAF* mutations are absent in extracolonic sporadic MSI-high neoplasms, such as endometrial cancer. In these settings, *MLH1* promoter methylation (or germline testing) is the only test that can distinguish LS from sporadic tumors.

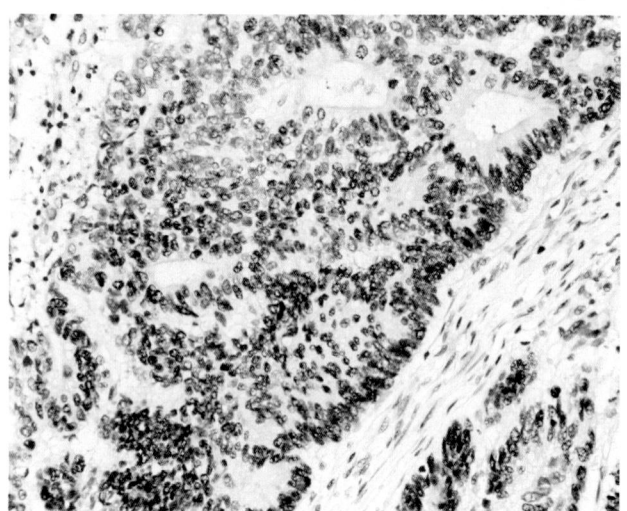

Figure 4-319. Intact/presence MMR IHC (MLH1). Intact/presence MMR IHC requires that at least 5% of the tumor cells show strong nuclear reactivity, as seen here.

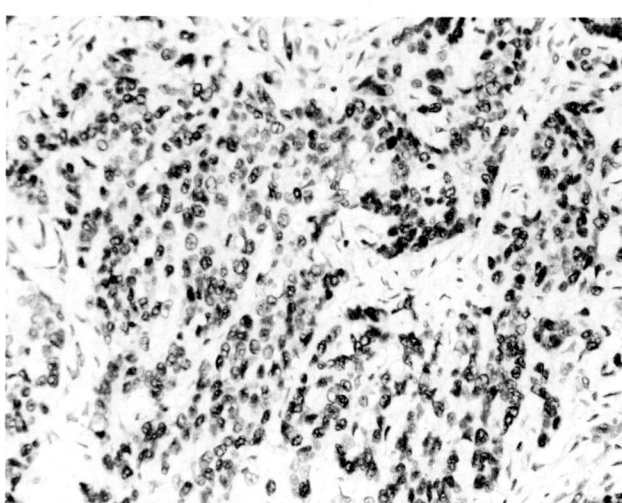

Figure 4-320. Intact/presence MMR IHC (MLH2). Verify that you are examining the MMR IHC reactivity in the tumor itself. MMR IHC reactivity in the background dysplasia or tumor infiltrating lymphocytes can be misleading and lead to a failed recognition of Lynch syndrome. For example, a patient with Lynch syndrome could show intact/present MMR IHC reactivity in the background adenoma and tumor infiltrating lymphocytes and loss in the carcinoma. The only reactivity that counts is in the carcinoma itself.

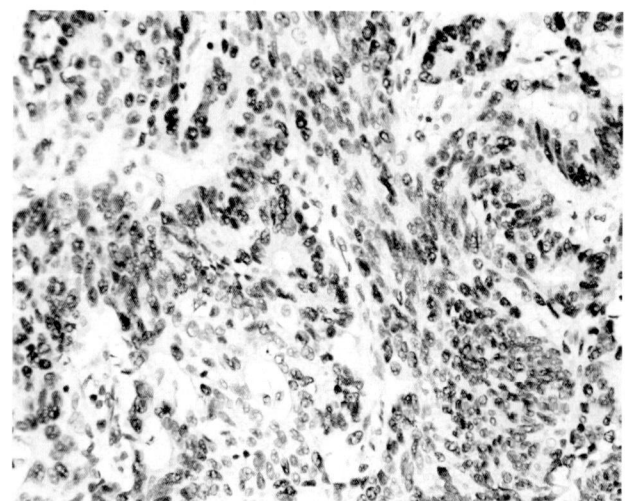

Figure 4-321. Intact/presence MMR IHC (MLH6). Universal CRC testing of all four MMR IHC (MLH1, PMS2, MSH2, and MSH6) on each distinct CRC, small bowel carcinoma, and endometrial carcinoma is recommended for thorough evaluation.

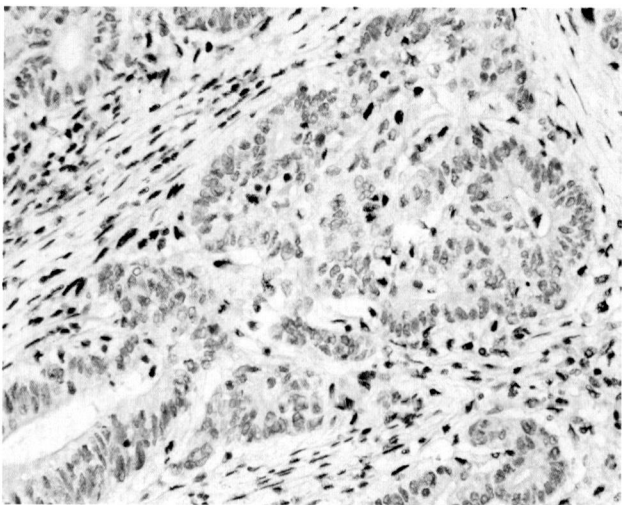

Figure 4-322. Absent/lost MMR IHC (MLH6). It is always important to evaluate MMR IHC reactivity with the H&E (Fig. 4.311). The nuclear reactivity seen here is from the intervening intraepithelial lymphocytes; the tumor cells are unequivocally negative.

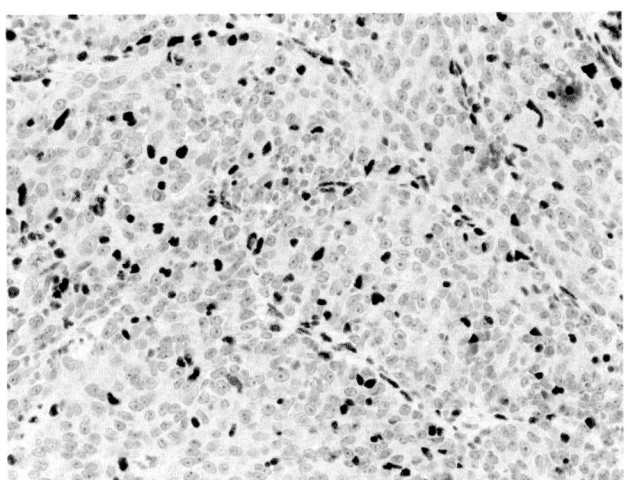

Figure 4-323. Absent/lost MMR IHC (MLH1). Avoid reporting MMR IHC reactivity with the ambiguous terms positive or negative. Instead, report them as intact/present or lost/absent to clearly report the MMR IHC reactivity.

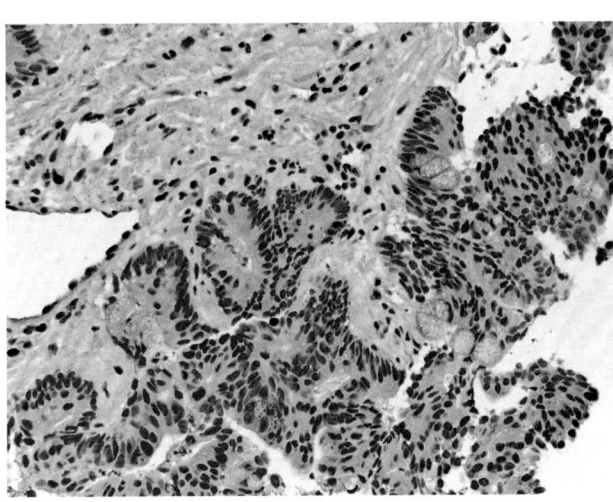

Figure 4-324. Absent/lost MMR IHC (MLH2). A diagnosis of absent/lost MMR IHC is straightforward when there is a complete absence of nuclear reactivity within the tumor, as seen here.

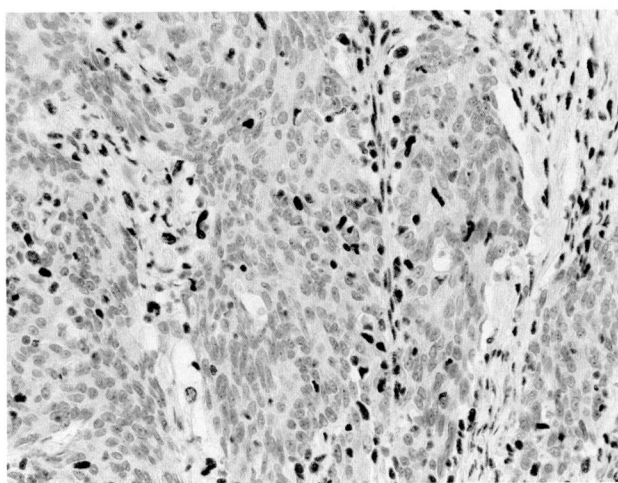

Figure 4-325. Intact internal controls (MSH2). The background stromal and inflammatory cells serve as internal controls and should show intact nuclear reactivity in properly stained sections, as seen here.

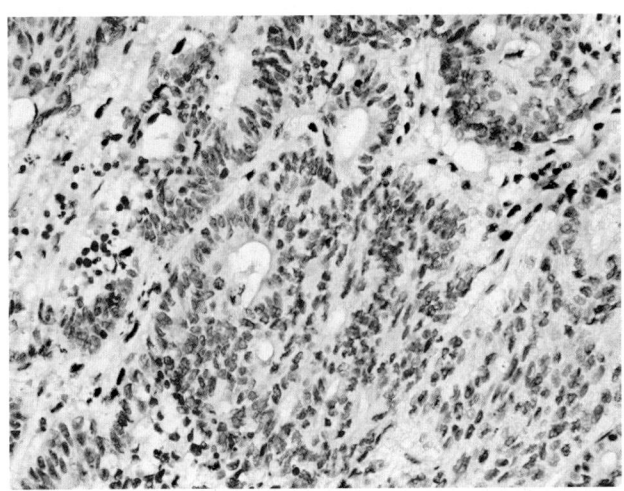

Figure 4-326. Intact internal controls (MSH6). The intensity of the nuclear reactivity of the internal controls (stromal and inflammatory cells) provides a baseline to evaluate the tumor cells. Present/intact MMR IHC reactivity should be at least as strong as the internal controls.

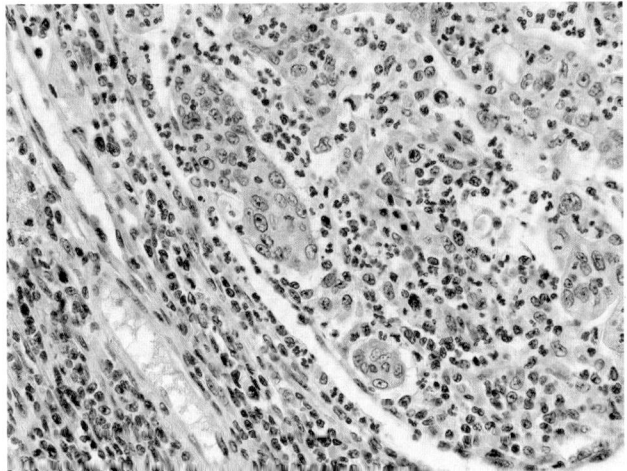

Figure 4-327. Failed internal controls (MSH1). If the background internal controls did not work, as seen here, the IHC must be repeated. (Glass slide courtesy of Dr. Wei Chen [OSU].)

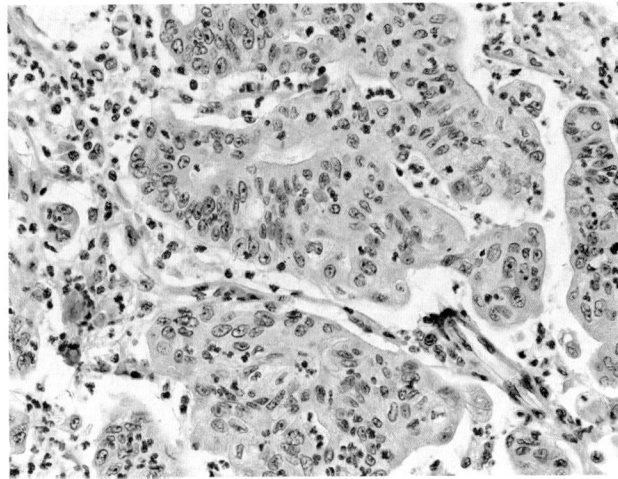

Figure 4-328. Failed internal controls (PMS2). As seen here, an absence of staining in the background stromal and inflammatory cells signifies failed internal controls and requires repeat IHC. (Glass slide courtesy of Dr. Wei Chen [OSU].)

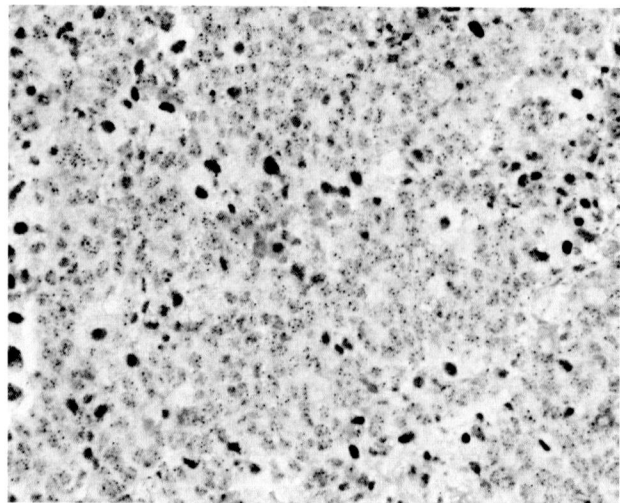

Figure 4-329. Absent/lost MMR IHC (MLH1). Remember that only strong nuclear reactivity within the tumor counts. Speckled (as seen here), nucleolar, nuclear membrane, or cytoplasmic reactivity pattern should be reported as lost/absent. (Photomicrograph courtesy of Dr. Lysandra Voltaggio [JHMI].)

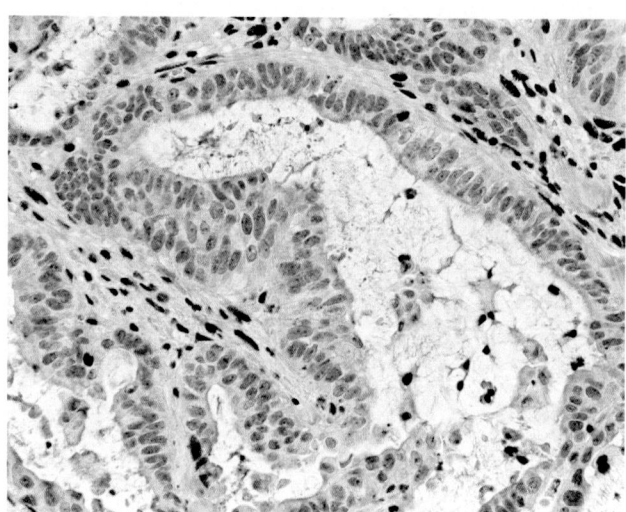

Figure 4-330. Absent/lost MMR IHC (MSH2). A true intact/present MMR IHC should show diffuse nuclear reactivity comparable in intensity with the background internal controls. As seen here, the very weak nuclear MSH2 reactivity pattern is weaker than the controls and, therefore, does not count. (Glass slide courtesy of Dr. Wei Chen [OSU].)

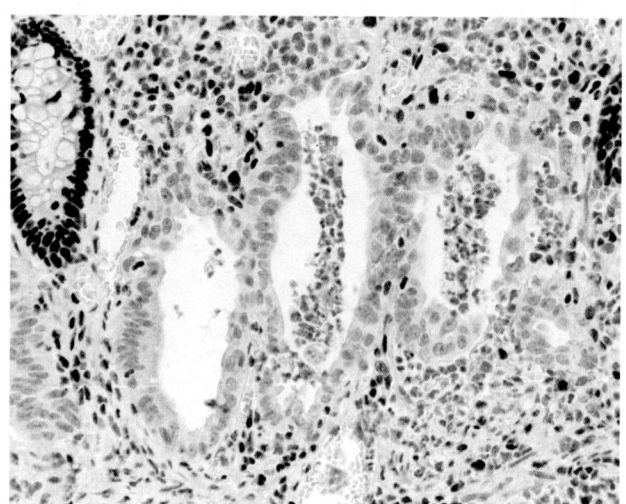

Figure 4-331. Absent/lost MMR IHC (MLH1). Nuclear reactivity weaker than the internal controls, as seen here, does not count and is interpreted as absent/lost. (Glass slide courtesy of Dr. Wei Chen [OSU].)

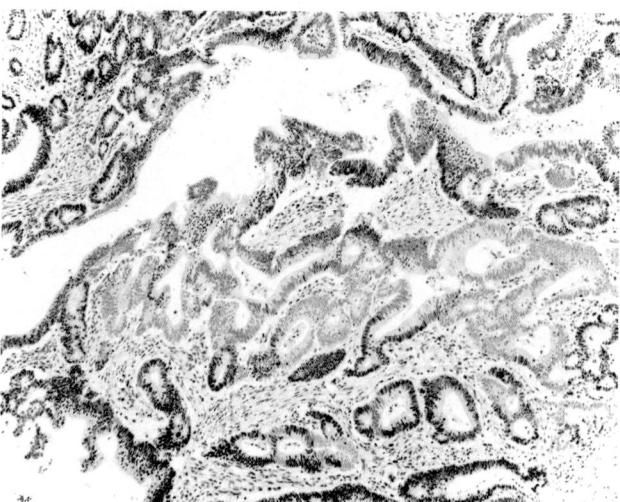

Figure 4-332. Present/intact MMR IHC, heterogenous pattern (PMS2). We use a 5% cutoff for MMR IHC evaluation. Even though this case shows heterogeneous IHC reactivity, it is intact/present because more than 5% of the tumor cells display comparably strong nuclear reactivity as the internal controls. (Glass slide courtesy of Dr. Wei Chen [OSU].)

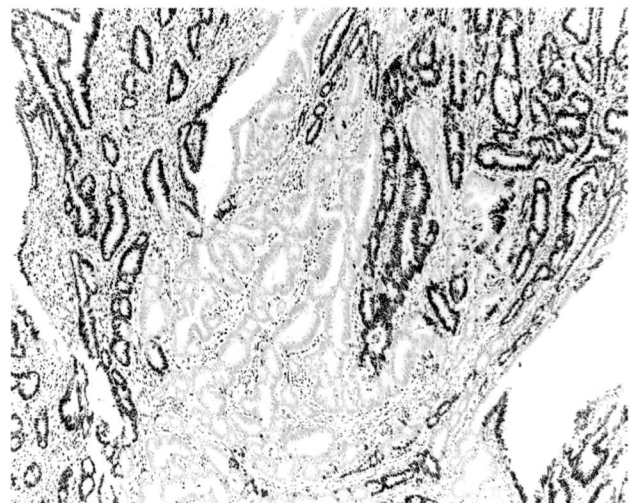

Figure 4-333. Present/intact MMR IHC, heterogenous pattern (MLH1). We do not include the "heterogenous" descriptor in the report. The significance of this staining pattern is not well understood, but it is reported as present/intact because more than 5% of the tumor has strong nuclear reactivity. One could imagine that if a biopsy was in the area of complete loss, it would be reported as absent/lost, emphasizing the importance of subsequent testing before diagnosing Lynch syndrome (genetic counselor evaluation, *MLH1* promoter methylation studies, genetic confirmation of germline mutations, and so on). (Glass slide courtesy of Dr. Wei Chen [OSU].)

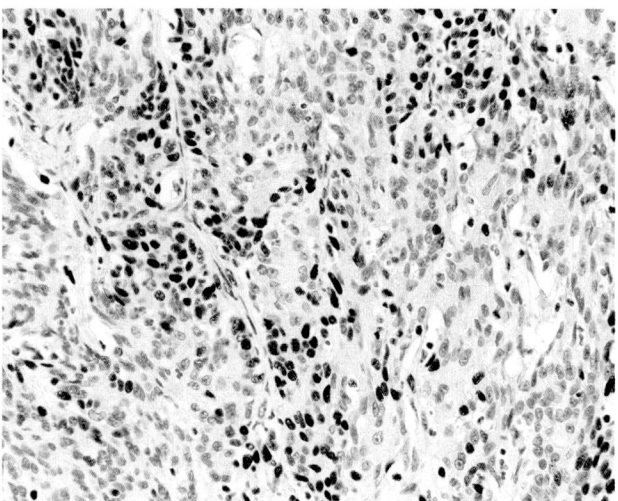

Figure 4-334. Present/intact MMR IHC, heterogenous pattern (MSH2). Because more than 5% of the tumor has strong nuclear reactivity, it is reported as present/intact. We do not report the percentage of tumor reactivity. (Glass slide courtesy of Dr. Wei Chen [OSU].)

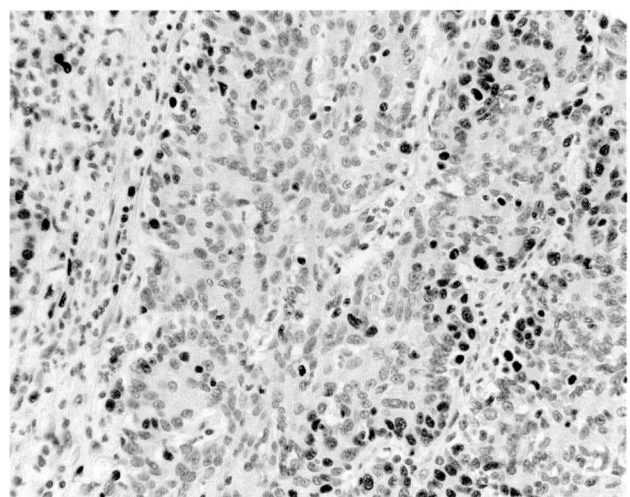

Figure 4-335. Present/intact MMR IHC, heterogenous pattern (MLH1). Even though the immunoreactivity is patchy, it is reported as present/intact because more than 5% of the tumor has strong nuclear reactivity comparable with the internal controls. (Glass slide courtesy of Dr. Wei Chen [OSU].)

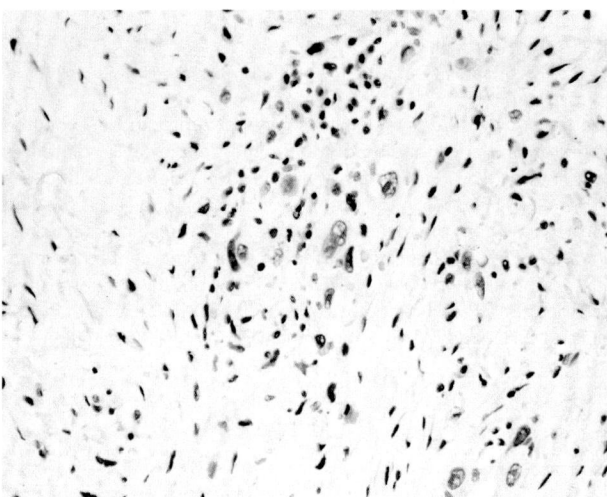

Figure 4-336. Present/intact MMR IHC, status post therapy (MSH6). MSH6 MMR IHC is notorious for showing a weak pattern after chemoradiation therapy.[118] Even though the reactivity is weak, it is approximately as strong as the internal controls and more than 5% of the tumor shows reactivity. Accordingly, this pattern is classified as present/intact. (Glass slide courtesy of Dr. Wei Chen [OSU].)

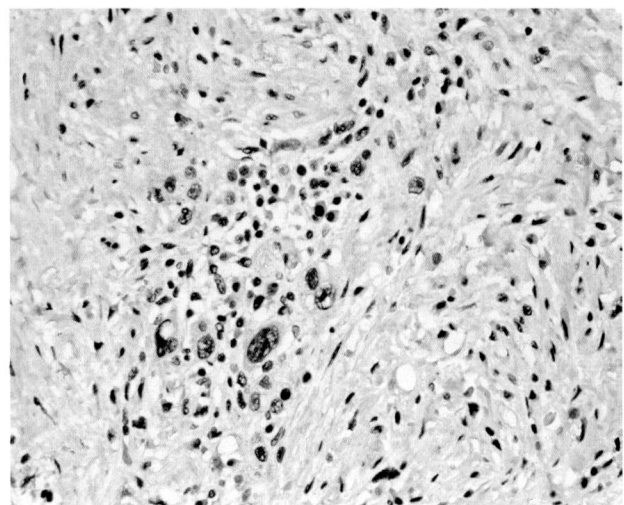

Figure 4-337. Present/intact MMR IHC, status post therapy (MSH6). General knowledge of this pitfall resolves most of the challenging IHC cases. If the diminished reactivity is concerning, MMR IHC can be performed on the pretreatment biopsy, if available. (Glass slide courtesy of Dr. Wei Chen [OSU].)

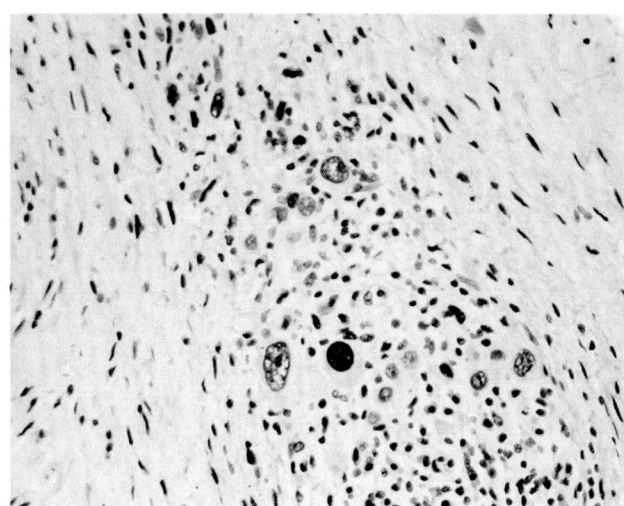

Figure 4-338. Present/intact MMR IHC, status post therapy (MSH6). (Glass slide courtesy of Dr. Wei Chen [OSU].)

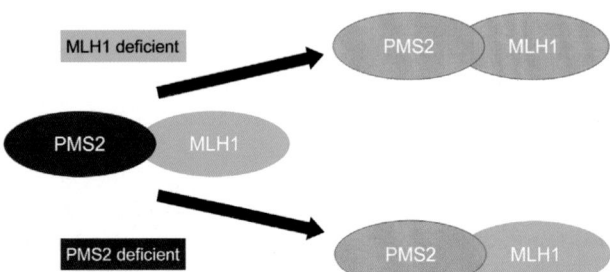

Figure 4-339. Predictable deficiency patterns can be expected based on an understanding of MMR dimerization. MLH1 dimerizes with PMS2. MLH1 deficiency results in PMS2 deficiency because PMS2 is too unstable in the absence of its stabilizing MLH1 binding partner. However, the reverse is not true. MLH1 remains intact/present when PMS2 is deficient. Based on this, some centers perform MMR evaluation with only PMS2 and MSH6, but this misses a small fraction of MMR-deficient cases. A four-panel MMR IHC with PMS2, MLH1, MSH2, and MSH6 is recommended for MMR evaluation.

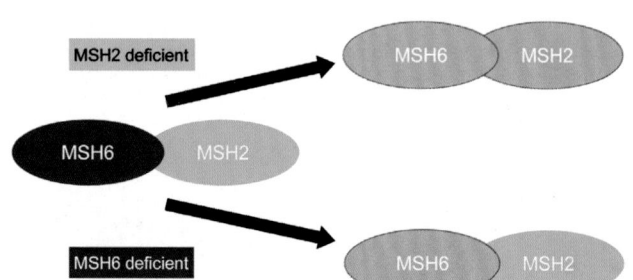

Figure 4-340. Predictable deficiency patterns can be expected based on an understanding of MMR dimerization. MSH2 dimerizes with MSH6. MSH2 deficiency results in MSH6 deficiency because MSH6 is too unstable in the absence of its stabilizing MSH2 binding partner. However, the reverse is not true. MSH2 remains intact/present when MSH6 is deficient. Based on this, some centers perform MMR evaluation with only PMS2 and MSH6, but this misses a small fraction of MMR-deficient cases. A four-panel MMR IHC with PMS2, MLH1, MSH2, and MSH6 is recommended for MMR evaluation.

FAQ: What is the preferred approach for gastroenterologists who request MMR IHC on a TA to rule out LS?

Answer: MMR IHC screening is intended as a screening tool for adenocarcinomas. Its utility on noninvasive precursor lesions can be misleading. With such requests, it is reasonable to perform the MMR IHC and include a note that, although loss/absence of MMR IHC is suggestive of LS (Fig. 4.341), intact/present MMR IHC in a noninvasive lesion cannot exclude LS.

FAQ: What is the preferred approach for gastroenterologists who request MMR IHC on an SSA/P to rule out LS?

Answer: The precursor lesion in LS is the tubular adenoma. There is no utility in performing MMR IHC on an SSA/P to evaluate for LS.

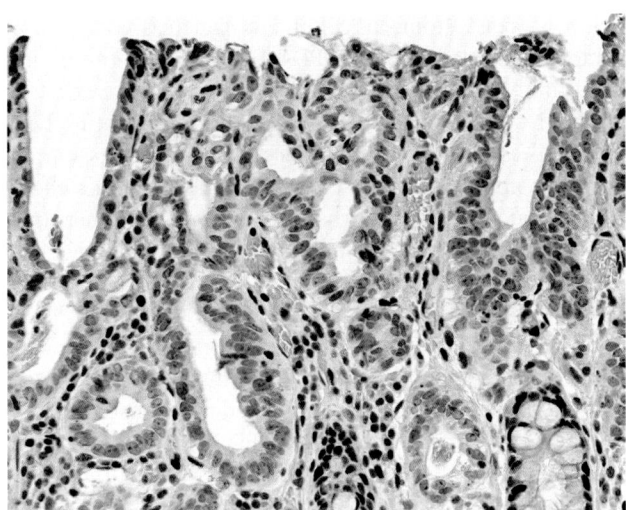

Figure 4-341. Absent/loss MMR IHC (MSH2). MMR IHC screening is intended as a screening tool for adenocarcinomas, but occasionally requests are submitted for adenomas with the goal of helping direct potential surveillance or surgery. We generally honor such requests with the disclaimer that, although loss/absence of MMR IHC is suggestive of Lynch syndrome, as seen here, intact/present MMR IHC in a noninvasive lesion cannot exclude Lynch syndrome. Further studies are always required before diagnosing Lynch syndrome (genetic counselor evaluation, *MLH1* promoter methylation studies, genetic confirmation of germline mutations, and so on). (Glass slide courtesy of Dr. Wei Chen [OSU].)

Immune Surveillance Pathways

At the time of writing, there are two immune surveillance pathways important to understanding cancer therapy: the programmed death receptor-1/programmed death ligand-1 (PD-1/PD-L1) and the cytotoxic T-lymphocyte–associated antigen 4 (CTLA-4) signaling pathways. You cannot wave a stick without hitting an abstract, paper, or lecture related to these pathways because they have revolutionized oncologic therapies. These pathways are normal, regulatory mechanisms that shut down the immune system to prevent immune hyperactivity and autoimmune diseases. Tumors that subvert these normal mechanisms have a survival advantage because they can "hide" from the immune system by shutting down their ability to recognize and destroy the tumors. Treatments that target these pathways by "unmasking" the tumors and restoring the immune system's antitumor function can lead to oncologic cures in some cases. Keep in mind that this area of medicine is in rapid evolution as more is learned about the complex web of immune surveillance pathways, novel medications, emerging drug targets, combination therapies, tumor microenvironments, and so on. This section focuses on the practical aspects of the two most common pathways encountered by pathologists in routine practice. See also "Cytotoxic T-Lymphocyte–Associated Antigen 4" section.

Programmed Death Receptor-1/Programmed Death Ligand-1

The PD-1/PD-L1 pathway is involved in immune checkpoint surveillance that regulates T-lymphocyte activation (Fig. 4.342). PD-1 is a cell surface receptor found on activated T lymphocytes, B lymphocytes, monocytes, and natural killer cells. When PD-1 binds its ligand PD-L1, the result is inhibition of the T-cell-mediated immune response. PD-L1 is broadly expressed on T lymphocytes, B lymphocytes, dendritic cells, macrophages, epithelial cells, and endothelial cells and functions in normal homeostatic mechanisms to suppress T-cell activation. It is the molecule that helps prevent the body's immune system from attacking the body's epithelial cells! PD-L1 is also expressed by some tumors as a survival mechanism to subvert immune system recognition and destruction. In essence, PD-L1 hides the tumor from the immune system so that the tumor can continue to proliferate. PD-L1 protein expression has been identified in lymphoma, lung cancer, glioblastoma, melanoma, and cancers of the kidney, breast, stomach, colon, and pancreas, among others.[136] Monoclonal antibody therapies that block PD-1 or PD-L1 unmask the tumor and restore the immune system's antitumor function and are effective in a wide variety of tumors. Tumors that are particularly responsive are those with both (1) infiltrating lymphocytes with high PD-1 receptor expression and (2) high PD-L1 ligand expression. As expected for a therapy that restores the immune systems effector function, the side effects are related to immune hyperreactivity, such as rash, diarrhea, pneumonitis, and hepatitis. Essentially, anti-PD-L1/PD-1 drugs create iatrogenic autoimmunity. Treatment of these side effects includes drug cessation or concomitant immunosuppression.

To identify which patients might benefit from anti-PD-1/PD-L1 therapy, PD-1/PD-L1 testing can be performed. An important side note includes a recent report that some patients with squamous carcinoma of the lung benefited from nivolumab (Opdivo) despite negative PD-L1 tumor expression.[141] Based on this work, the US FDA approved nivolumab (Opdivo) for non–small cell lung cancer (NSCLC), regardless of the tumor's PD-L1 expression status. As a result, some patients are treated with nivolumab without PD-1/PD-L1 tumor testing. Determination of the PD-L1 expression status can be accomplished with IHC, flow cytometry, enzyme-linked immunosorbent assay, or real-time quantitative polymerase chain reaction. In addition, fluorescence in situ hybridization (FISH) probe targeting the *PD-L1* gene has been proposed as a surrogate marker for PD-L1 expression and is used in some centers. This discussion will focus on PD-L1 IHC testing because it is relatively easily incorporated into laboratories, it can be performed on formalin-fixed paraffin-embedded tissue blocks, most surgical pathologists are familiar with general IHC interpretation, and it offers the advantage of direct visualization of the tumor. Below are the basics of PD-L1 IHC interpretation.

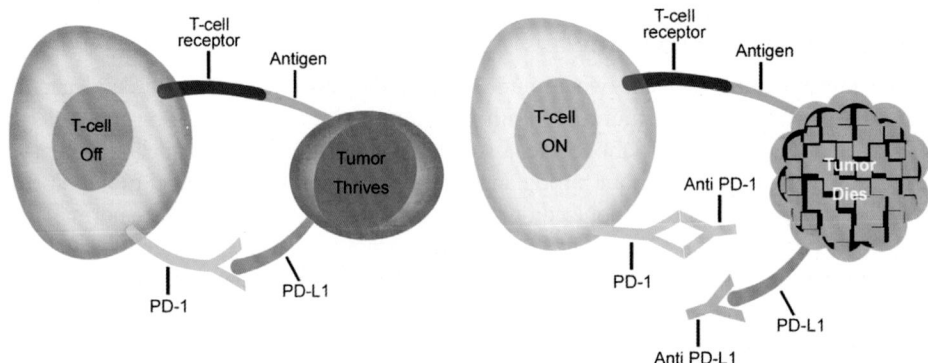

Figure 4-342. An illustration of the PD-1/PD-L1 pathway. PD-1 is a cell surface receptor found on activated T lymphocytes, and its ligand PD-L1 is expressed on inflammatory cells and epithelial cells. The binding of PD-1 to PDL-1 results in suppression of T-cell activation and is an important, normal mechanism to prevent autoimmune diseases. PD-L1 is also expressed by some tumors as a survival mechanism to subvert immune system recognition and destruction. In essence, PD-L1 hides the tumor from the immune system so that the tumor can continue to proliferate (*left panel*). Monoclonal antibodies that block PD-1 or PD-L1 unmask the tumor and restore the immune system's antitumor function, allowing the tumor to be recognized and destroyed by the immune system (*right panel*).

Tissue Preparation for PD-L1 IHC

1. The resection specimen is preferred over a biopsy to offer the most accurate evaluation because the biomarkers can display significant tumor heterogeneity.[136] At the time of writing, it is not yet clear if the primary tumor or the metastasis should be the specimen of choice.
2. The global standard tissue source is the formalin-fixed paraffin-embedded tissue block, although testing can also be performed on cell blocks, smears, and fluids, assuming sufficient tumor is present.

3. There are no official guidelines on cold-ischemia time, but it is reasonable to minimize this interval between tissue procurement and initiation of fixation. Tissue with excessive cold-ischemia times may be unreliable and should be interpreted with caution.

4. There are no official guidelines on formalin fixation times, but 6 to 48 hours of fixation is recommended for biopsies and 24 to 28 hours of fixation is recommended for resections.[142] Tissue with suboptimal fixation times may be unreliable and should be interpreted with caution.

5. The preferred fixative is 10% neutral buffered formalin (4% formaldehyde) with at least 10 times the volume of the tissue specimen.

6. Tissue samples should be cut at 3 to 5 μm and stained within 2 months to minimize artifacts.

7. Tissue blocks should be less than 3 years old for IHC testing. Blocks greater than 5 years old may have unreliable IHC reactivity and should be interpreted with caution.

8. Decalcified specimens are subject to harsh acidic agents that can destroy antigenicity and lead to inaccurate IHC reactivity patterns. As a result, IHC on decalcified specimens should be avoided, when possible. If there are no other reasonable tissue specimens, the request can be honored but should be reported with the disclaimer that the IHC has not been validated for these specimens.

PD-L1 IHC Interpretation

1. Ensure that the positive control worked. There is no official recommendation on the ideal tissue to serve as a positive control, but many use tonsil, which shows membranous staining in the crypt epithelium, lymphocytes, and macrophages (Figs. 4.343–4.345). Infiltrating lymphocytes and macrophages can serve as internal controls.

2. The reactivity patterns are scored as follows:

   0 = No staining (Figs. 4.346–4.348)

   1+ = weak staining visible only at 40× (Figs. 4.349–4.351)

   2+ = moderate staining seen at 10× (Figs. 4.352–4.354)

   3+ staining = strong staining visible at 2× (Figs. 4.355–4.357).

   See Fig. 4.358 for a side-by-side comparison of the PD-L1 IHC reactivity patterns for kit 22C3.

3. Verify that the background has a score of 0. If the background is 1+ or greater, the IHC should be disregarded and repeated.

4. Necrotic and normal tissue often shows PD-L1 IHC reactivity and are excluded from the IHC interpretation (Figs. 4.359–4.361).

5. There are several kits available for PD-L1 IHC testing. It is critical to report the specific kit used because interpretation guidelines vary (Table 4.11). See Sample Note: PD-L1 Reporting.

   a. PD-L1 IHC requires that sufficient tumor be present. At least 50 cells are required for the SP142 kit, and at least 100 cells are required for the 28-8, SP263, and 22C3 kits.

   b. Positive staining for the 28-8, 22C3, SP263, and 73-10 kits require completely or partly circumferential plasma membrane staining of any intensity. The reactivity patterns must be distinct from those of the cytoplasm; cytoplasmic reactivity is disregarded. In contrast, positive staining for the SP263 kit includes either membrane or cytoplasmic staining of any intensity; linear or granular staining is regarded as positive.

   c. For the SP142 kit, both the immune cells and the tumor cells are included in the evaluation. For the remaining kits, the PD-L1 IHC reactivity is evaluated only in the tumor.

   d. Positive staining:

      i. The 28-8 and 73-10 kits require at least 1% of tumor cell reactivity.

      ii. The SP263 kit requires at least 25% of tumor cell reactivity.

      iii. The 22C3 kit requires at least 50% of tumor cell reactivity.

      iv. Any reactivity in the SP142 kit is considered positive.

6. The PD-L1 scoring involves examining all *viable* tumor present on one IHC slide. It is reported as an overall percentage of PD-L1 IHC reactivity in the viable tumor, or the tumor proportion score (TPS). Beware that the reactivity can be patchy, so it is important to carefully assess all tumor on the IHC slide and report the overall average tumor reactivity as a percentage.

7. Beware that the tumor edges can be difficult to interpret. Recall, normal tissue is expected to have PD-L1 IHC reactivity. Tumor edges in close approximation to the normal tissue can be easily misinterpreted (Figs. 4.362–4.364). In these cases, it is best to compare the IHC reactivity in conjunction with the H&E to ensure that only the tumor reactivity is recorded.

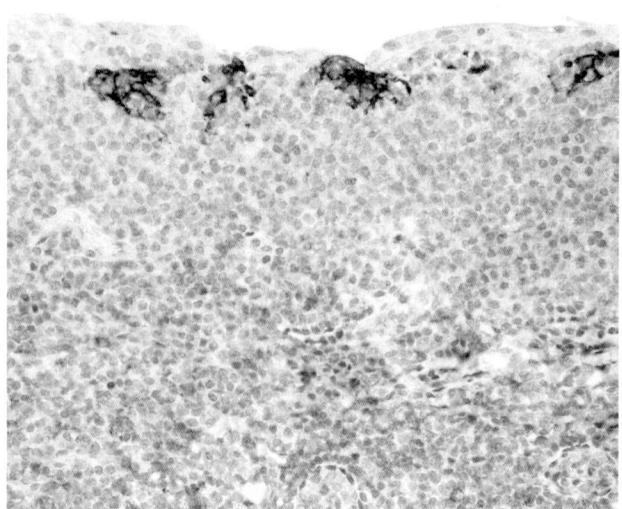

Figure 4-343. PD-L1 IHC positive control, 22C3 kit. Every PD-L1 IHC evaluation starts with ensuring the positive control worked. Most use tonsil as the positive control, and this tissue shows membranous staining in the crypt epithelium, lymphocytes, and macrophages, as seen here.

Figure 4-344. PD-L1 IHC positive control, 22C3 kit. The background lymphocytes and macrophages serve as internal controls in the patient tissue.

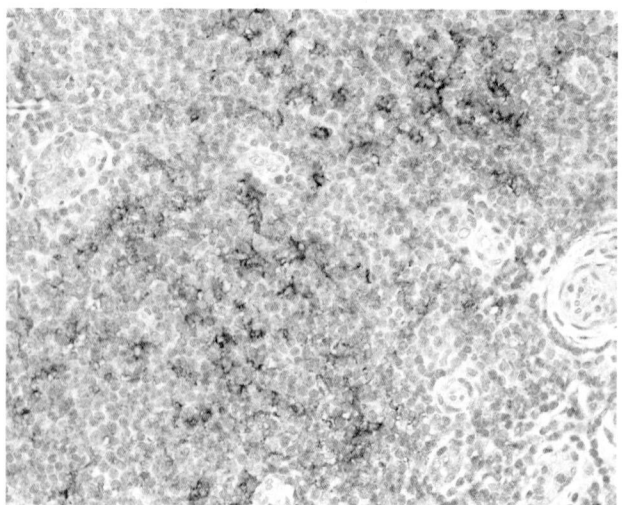
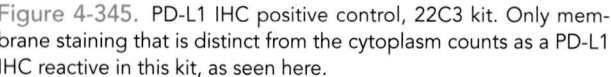
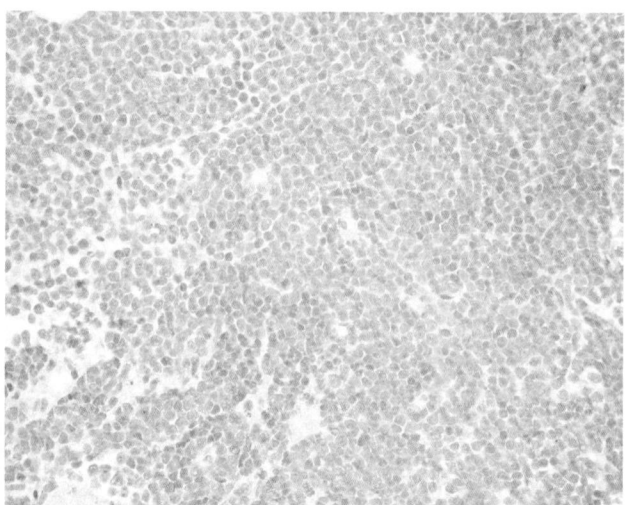

Figure 4-345. PD-L1 IHC positive control, 22C3 kit. Only membrane staining that is distinct from the cytoplasm counts as a PD-L1 IHC reactive in this kit, as seen here.

Figure 4-346. PD-L1 IHC score = 0, 22C3 kit. For this kit, a score of 0 requires an absence of membrane staining in the viable tumor.

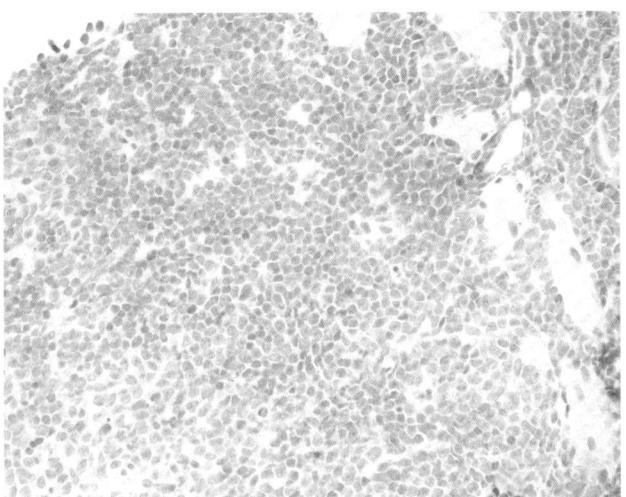

Figure 4-347. PD-L1 IHC score = 0, 22C3 kit. Only membranous staining in the viable tumor counts as reactive for this kit. Nonspecific staining in the cytoplasm, in the necrotic debris, and in the normal tissue is scored as 0.

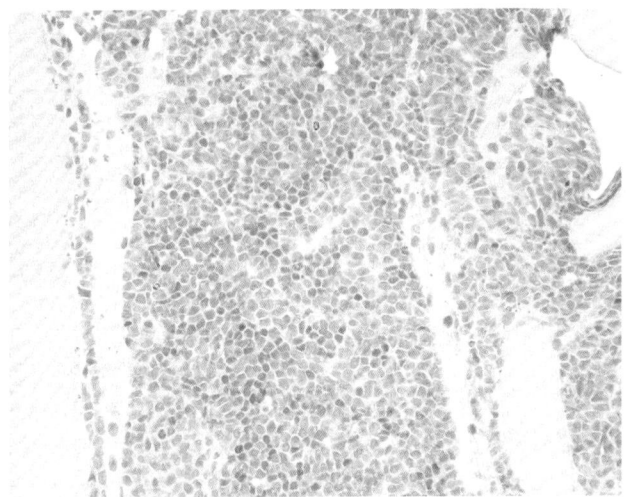

Figure 4-348. PD-L1 IHC score = 0, 22C3 kit.

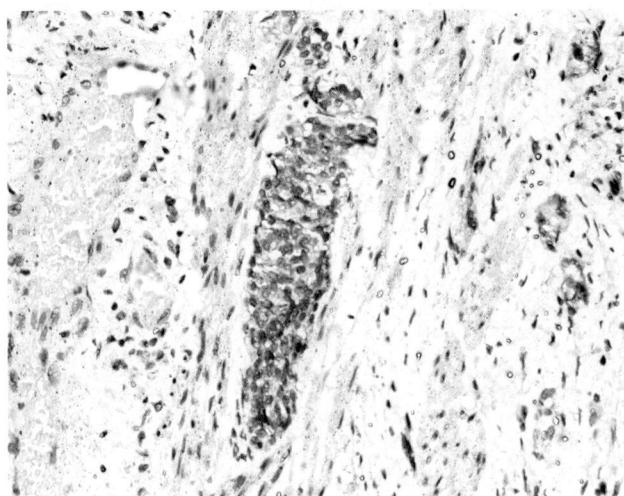

Figure 4-349. PD-L1 IHC score = 1+, 22C3 kit. A score of 1+ refers to weak membranous reactivity in viable tumor cells that is only discernable at 40×, as seen here.

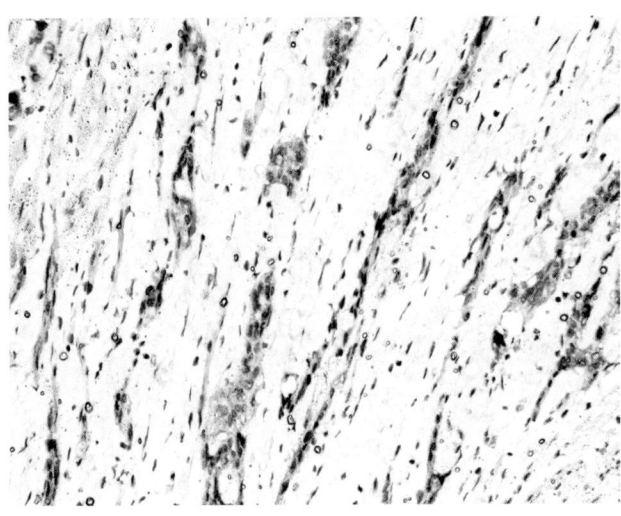

Figure 4-350. PD-L1 IHC score = 1+, 22C3 kit. Recall, only membranous staining in the viable tumor counts as reactive for this kit.

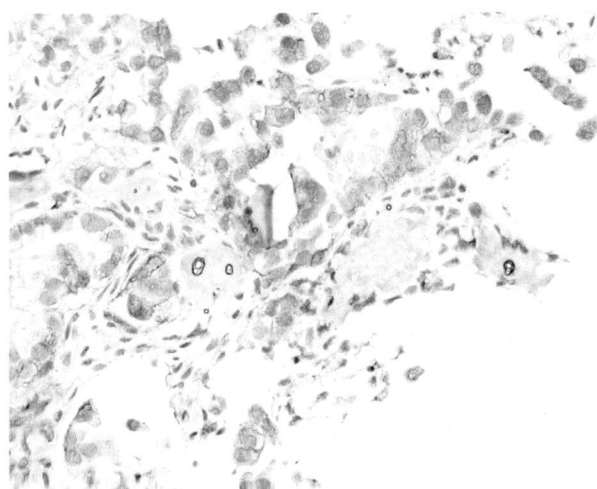

Figure 4-351. PD-L1 IHC score = 1+, 22C3 kit.

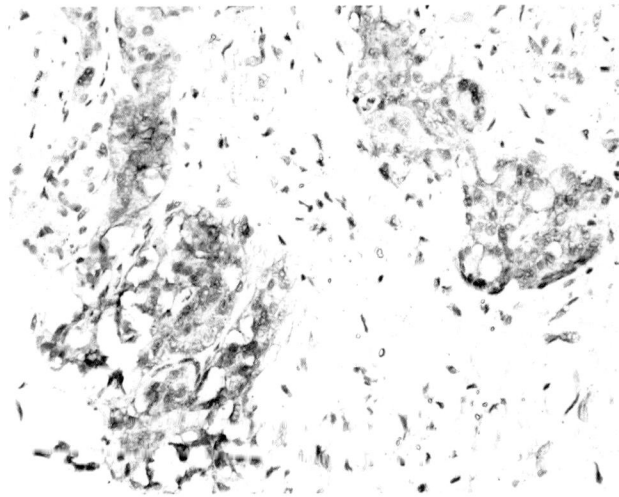

Figure 4-352. PD-L1 IHC score = 2+, 22C3 kit. A score of 2+ refers to moderate membranous reactivity in viable tumor cells that is discernable at 10×. This example is at 40× for comparison purposes.

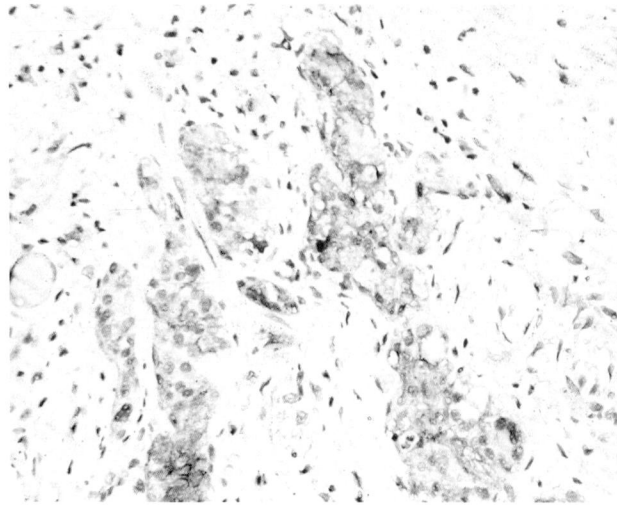

Figure 4-353. PD-L1 IHC score = 2+, 22C3 kit.

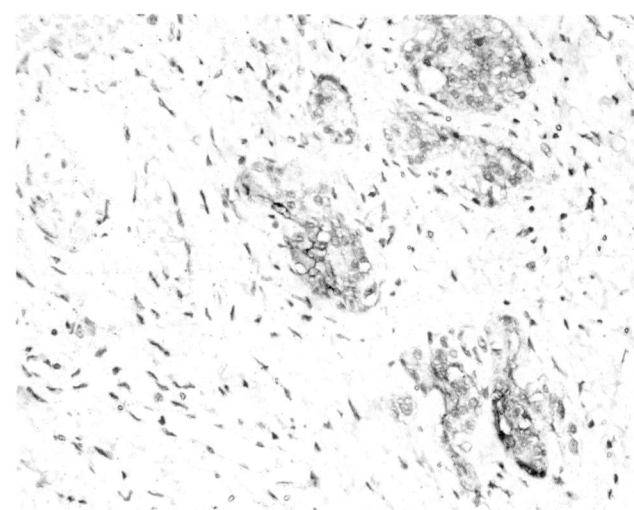

Figure 4-354. PD-L1 IHC score = 2+, 22C3 kit.

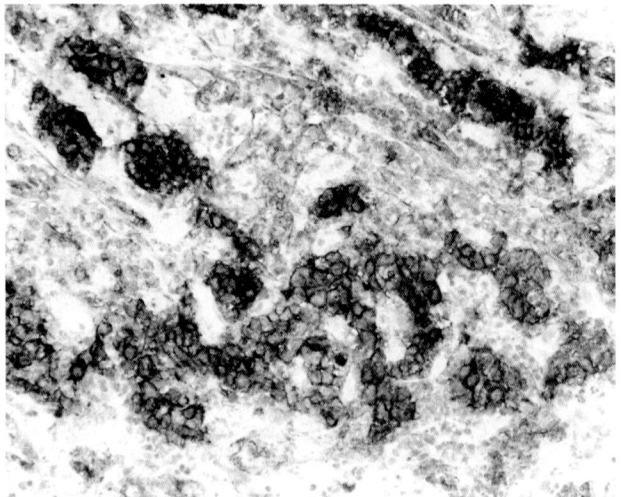

Figure 4-355. PD-L1 IHC score = 3+, 22C3 kit. A score of 3+ refers to strong membranous reactivity in viable tumor cells that is discernable at 2×. This example is at 40× for comparison purposes.

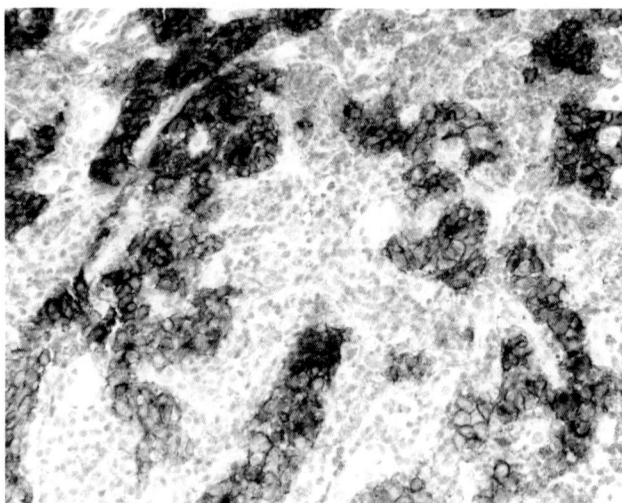

Figure 4-356. PD-L1 IHC score = 3+, 22C3 kit.

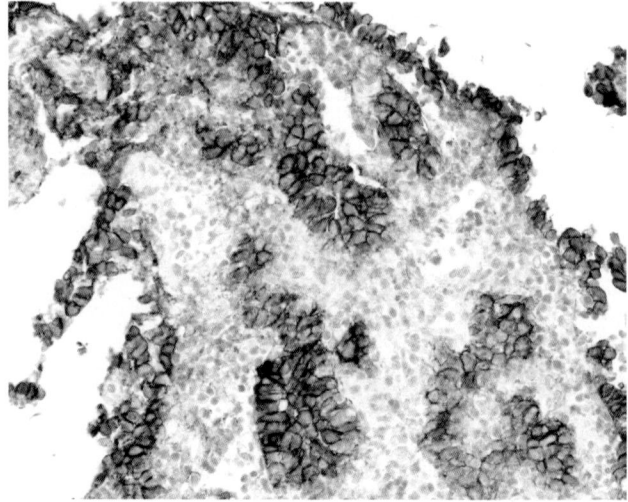

Figure 4-357. PD-L1 IHC score = 3+, 22C3 kit.

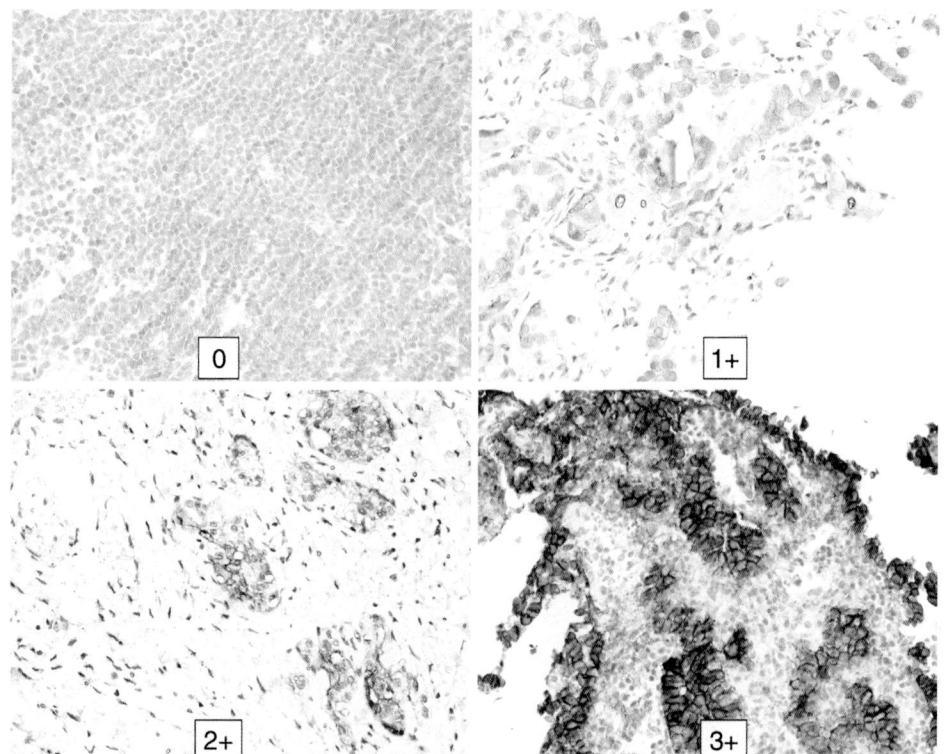

Figure 4-358. A composite of PD-L1 IHC reactivity patterns for kit 22C3. For this kit, a score of 0 requires an absence of membrane staining in the viable tumor, and only membranous staining in the viable tumor counts as reactive. A score of 1+ refers to weak membranous reactivity in viable tumor that is only discernable at 40×. A score of 2+ refers to moderate membranous reactivity in viable tumor that is discernable at 10×. A score of 3+ refers to strong membranous reactivity in viable tumor that is discernable at 2×. These examples are at 40× for comparison purposes.

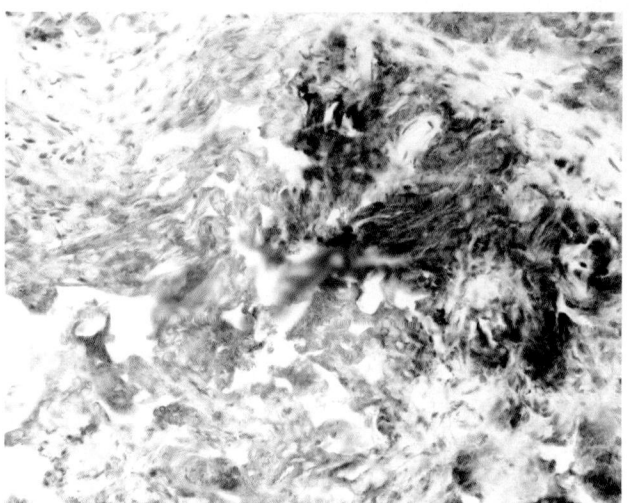

Figure 4-359. PD-L1 IHC score = 0, 22C3 kit. Although this focus would be visible at 2×, it is entirely disregarded because it is necrotic. Necrotic debris and normal tissue can be PD-L1 IHC reactive, but only membranous staining in viable tumor is scored; this case is scored as 0 based on the absence of membranous staining in the viable tumor.

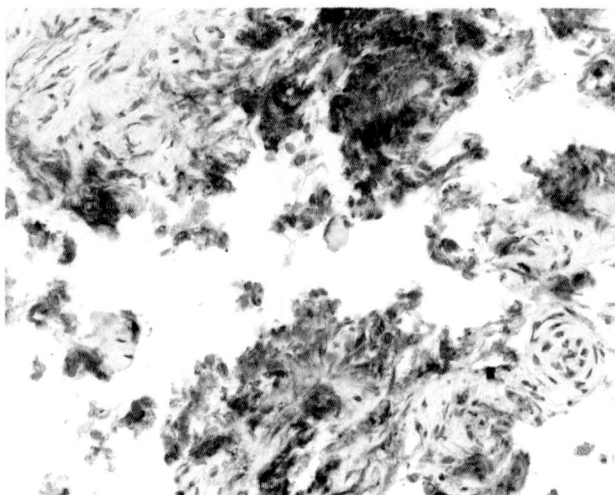

Figure 4-360. PD-L1 IHC score = 0, 22C3 kit. Similar to the previous figure.

TABLE 4.11: PDL1

Drug	PD-L1 Clone Kit	Minimum Required Viable Tumor Cells	Evaluable Cells	Reactivity Pattern Required for Positive Score	Criteria for Positive IHC Reactivity	Reporting Categories
Nivolumab	28-8	100	Tumor Only	Complete circumferential or partial plasma membrane staining only	≥1% tumor cells	None (<1%), ≥1%, ≥5%, ≥10%
Avelumab	73-10	100	Tumor Only	Complete circumferential or partial plasma membrane staining only	≥1% tumor cells	• Expression <1% • Expression ≥1%
Durvalumab	SP263	100	Tumor Only	Membrane and/or cytoplasmic	≥25% tumor cells	For durvalumab <25% Expression ≥25% Expression For nivolumab Expression <1% Expression ≥1% to <5% Expression ≥5% to <10% Expression ≥10%
Pembrolizumab	22C3	100	Tumor Only	Complete circumferential or partial plasma membrane staining only	≥50% tumor cells	None (<1%), low (1–49%), or high (≥50%)
Atezolizumab	SP142	50	Tumor and Immune Cells	Complete circumferential or partial plasma membrane staining only	Any	• Tumor cell expression ≥50% • Immune cell expression ≥10% (and tumor cell expression <50%) • Tumor cell expression <50%, Immune cell expression <10% • Expression status Tumor cell % (<1%, ≥1%, ≥5%,≥50%) Immune cell % (<1%, >1%, >5%,>10%)

IHC, immunohistochemistry.

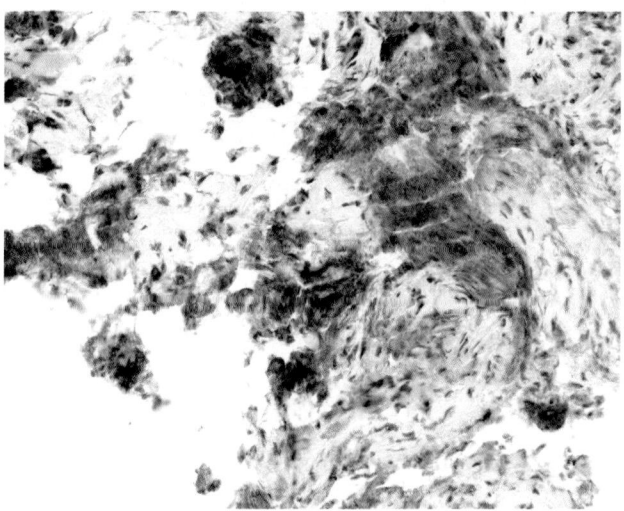

Figure 4-361. PD-L1 IHC score = 0, 22C3 kit. Similar to the previous figure.

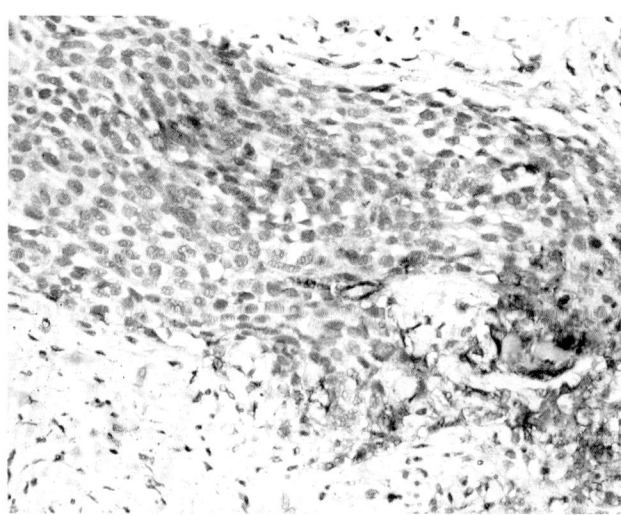

Figure 4-362. PD-L1 IHC score = 0, 22C3 kit. Even though PD-L1 membranous reactivity is seen here, the reactivity is only in the macrophages at the edge of the tumor. The tumor itself is negative. Such cases can be easy to inaccurately report as reactive, but remember that only membranous staining in the viable tumor is scored as reactive; this case is scored as 0 based on the absence of membranous staining in the viable tumor.

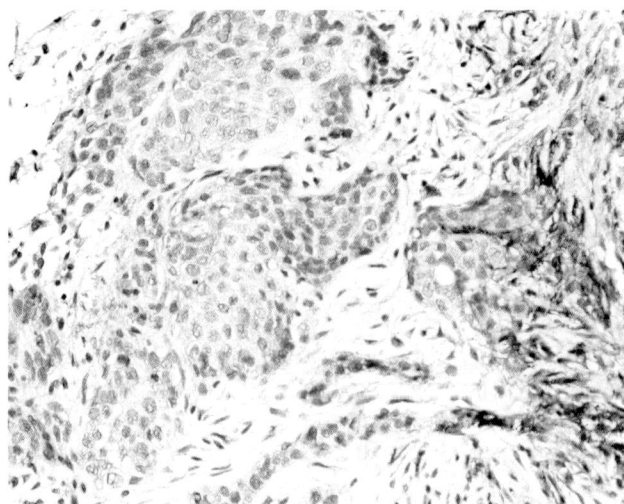

Figure 4-363. PD-L1 IHC score = 0, 22C3 kit. Similar to the previous figure.

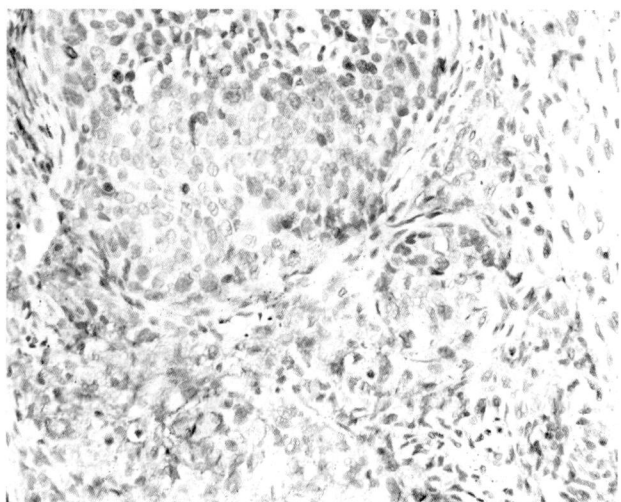

Figure 4-364. PD-L1 IHC score = 0, 22C3 kit. Similar to the previous figure.

PEARLS & PITFALLS: Decoding Monoclonal Antibody Nomenclature

The names of pharmaceutical medications often seem like a foreign language. If these dizzyingly complicated names trigger a headache, here are helpful clues from Dr. John Barone's On-Line Guide[143] (Fig. 4.365). Monoclonal antibodies are named by combining a nonsense prefix + Antibody Target + Antibody Source and end with "-mab" for monoclonal antibody.[143] For example, nivolumab has a nonsense prefix of "nivo," antibody target "li" = immune modulating, antibody source "u" = human, and ends with "mab" because it is a monoclonal antibody.

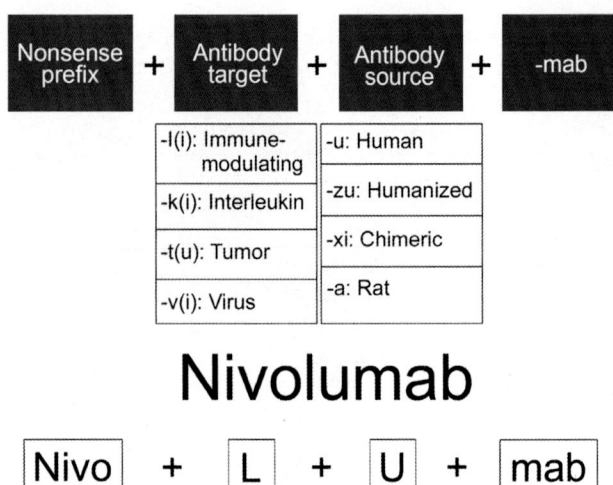

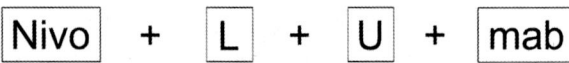

Figure 4-365. Deciphering monoclonal antibody nomenclature by Dr. John Barone, MD.[143] Monoclonal antibodies are named by combining a nonsense prefix + Antibody Target + Antibody Source and end with "-mab" for monoclonal antibody. For example, nivolumab has a nonsense prefix of "nivo", antibody target "li" = immune-modulating, antibody source "u" = human, and ends with "mab" because it is a monoclonal antibody.

SAMPLE NOTE: PD-L1 Reporting

PD-L1 IHC 22C3 pharmDx[a] Result

Expression Level
Positive for high PD-L1 expression (TPS greater than or equal to 50%)

Tumor proportion score (TPS)[a]: >95%

Comments to Treating Physician
Pembrolizumab is indicated for treatment of patients with metastatic NSCLC whose tumors have high PD-L1 expression (TPS greater than or equal to 50%) as determined by an FDA-approved test, with no *EGFR* or *ALK* genomic tumor aberrations and no prior systemic chemotherapy treatment of metastatic NSCLC. Pembrolizumab is also indicated for the treatment of patients with metastatic NSCLC whose tumors express PD-L1 (TPS greater than or equal to 1%) as determined by an FDA-approved test, with disease progression on or after platinum-containing chemotherapy. Patients with *EGFR* or *ALK* genomic tumor aberrations should have disease progression on FDA-approved therapy for these aberrations before receiving pembrolizumab.

PD-L1 IHC serves as a complementary diagnostic in regards to other PD-L1/PD-1-targeted therapies (e.g., nivolumab, atezolizumab, durvalumab).

[a]PD-L1 IHC 22C3 pharmDx is an FDA-approved companion diagnostic for pembrolizumab performed on Dako Autostainer Link 48. Positivity is scored only in viable tumor cells with membrane staining (partial or complete) of greater than or equal to 1+ intensity. The TPS is estimated by manual quantification of PD-L1 positivity. Certain tissue processing factors such as decalcification, formalin fixation time outside an acceptable range (4 to 168 hours), and prolonged time to fixation can affect PD-L1 staining/expression levels, and results should be interpreted with caution in such instances. In addition, tissue from older (greater than 5 years) formalin-fixed paraffin-embedded blocks may lose PD-L1 immunoreactivity. This assay is not validated for decalcified specimens.

Cytotoxic T-Lymphocyte–Associated Antigen 4

CTLA-4 is the other major immune surveillance pathway important for oncologic therapies. It shares important similarities with PD-1/PDL-1, including that both enhance immune-mediated tumor destruction.[144] CTLA-4 is expressed on activated and regulatory T cells (Fig. 4.366). Once bound to its ligand B7, T-cell activation is suppressed. Tumors that express the B7 ligand can engage CTLA-4 and lead to suppress the immune system's ability to recognize and destroy the tumor. In essence, the CTLA-4/B7 pathway hides the tumor from the immune system so that the tumor can continue to proliferate. B7 ligand expression occurs in melanoma and cancers of the prostate, ovary, esophagus, stomach, pancreas, colorectum, urothelial, among others.[145] Anti-CTLA-4 therapies bind and block CTLA-4's suppressive effects on the immune system, thereby unmasking the tumor and restoring immune system–mediated tumor destruction. The anti-CTLA-4 drug ipilimumab was the first FDA-approved immune checkpoint blockade agent. Similar to anti-PD-1/PD-L1 therapies, anti-CTLA-4 therapies also have the side effect of immune hyperreactivity symptoms. See also "Colon" chapter, "Chronic Colitis" section, *Atlas of GI Pathology: A Pattern Based Approach to Non-Neoplastic Biopsies*. Anti-CTLA-4 based therapies have not enjoyed as much attention as PD-1/PD-L1 therapies. This is, in part, because CTLA-4 and B7 are widely expressed and, consequently, are not useful biomarkers to identify which patients would benefit from anti-CTLA-4 therapy. In addition, anti-CTLA-4 therapies have been limited by toxicity,[145] which appears to be more pronounced than that seen with PD-1/PD-L1 therapies.

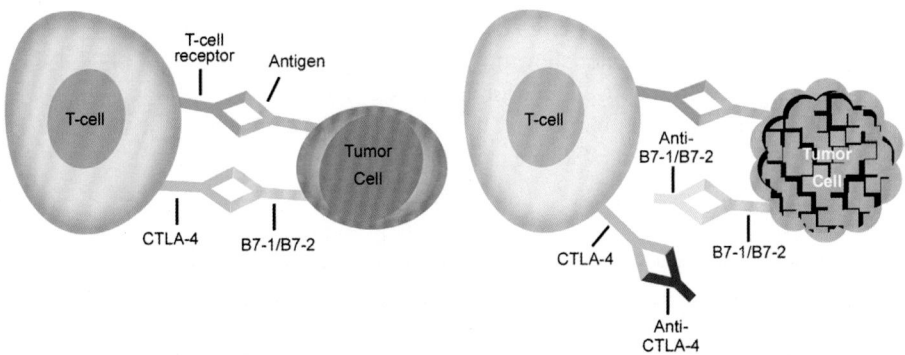

Figure 4-366. Cytotoxic T-lymphocyte–associated antigen 4. CTLA-4 is expressed on activated and regulatory T cells. Once bound to its ligand B7, T-cell activation is suppressed. Tumors that express the B7 ligand can engage CTLA-4 and lead to suppress the immune system's ability to recognize and destroy the tumor. Anti-CTLA-4 therapies bind and block CTLA4's suppressive effects on the immune system, thereby unmasking the tumor and restoring immune system–mediated tumor destruction.

Her2 in Colorectal Carcinoma

The human epidermal growth factor receptor 2 gene (*HER2*) is overexpressed in a variety of neoplasms, and its detection can be evaluated with IHC and FISH. Its role as a therapeutic target with the anti-Her2 agent trastuzumab (Herceptin) is well known in breast and gastric carcinomas. See also "Stomach" chapter, "*Her2*" section. More recently, the 2016 HERACLES trial reported combination trastuzumab and lapatinib benefited patients with treatment refractory, *KRAS* wild-type, *HER2*-amplified metastatic CRC.[133,134] Although this biomarker test was not recommended by the 2017 Guidelines on Colorectal Carcinoma Biomarkers,[129] requests for *HER2* on CRC are encountered with some regularity. It is important to be aware that the *HER2* IHC interpretation guidelines in the colorectum are markedly different from the gastric guidelines (Table 4.12). See the following helpful tips:

1. Eligible patients include patients with *KRAS* wild-type, *HER2*-amplified metastatic CRC.
2. The specimen of choice is the metastasis, although the test has concordance between primary and metastatic tumor sites.[134] There are no official recommendations on biopsy or resection serving as the tissue of choice.
3. The VENTANA 4B5 antibody was selected as the preferred HER2 antibody and is processed according to manufacturer's instructions.[134]
4. At the time of writing, there are no official guidelines on optimized cold ischemia time or formalin fixation times.
5. Evaluate the IHC reactivity in all viable tumor present on the IHC slide.
6. The reactivity patterns are scored as follows:
   0 = No staining or staining in less than 10% of cells
   1+ = Faint, barely perceptible staining in more than 10% of cells in a segmental or granular pattern
   2+ = Weak to moderate staining in more than 10% cells in a circumferential, basolateral, or lateral pattern
   3+ staining = Intense staining in more than 10% of cells in a circumferential, basolateral, or lateral pattern
   See also "Stomach" chapter, "Her2" section for grading Her2 IHC immunoreactivity.
7. Negative staining includes the cases with 0, 1+, or 2+ in <50%, or 3+ in ≤10% of tumor.[134] These patients are not eligible for anti-Her2 therapy.
8. Equivocal staining includes cases with 2+ in ≥50% of tumor. These cases require a repeat IHC. If >50% are confirmed 2+, then proceed to FISH. Patients with amplified *HER2* are eligible for anti-HER2 therapy.
9. Positive staining is defined as follows[134]:
   a. 3+ in >10% or <50% of tumor. These cases require confirmation with repeat IHC. Cases with >10% of tumor showing 3+ on the repeat IHC proceed to FISH. Patients with amplified *HER2* are eligible for anti-HER2 therapy.
   b. 3+ in ≥50% of viable tumor cells. These cases require confirmation with repeat IHC. Patients with amplified *HER2* are eligible for anti-HER2 therapy.

TABLE 4.12: Overview of Her2 Immunohistochemistry Stain for Colorectal Carcinoma

IHC Staining	Interpretation	Next Step	Eligible for Anti-Her2 Therapy
0	Negative	Done	No
1+	Negative	Done	No
2+ in <50%	Negative	Done	No
2+ in ≥50% of tumor	Equivocal	Repeat IHC; proceed to FISH if >50% are confirmed 2+	Yes, for patients with FISH-amplified HER2
3+ in ≤10% of tumor	Negative	Done	No
3+ in >10% or <50% of tumor	Positive	Repeat IHC; proceed to FISH if >10% are confirmed 3+	Yes, for patients with FISH-amplified HER2
3+ in ≥50% of tumor	Positive	Repeat IHC	Yes

NEAR MISS

BEWARE THE SUBOPTIMAL BIOPSY

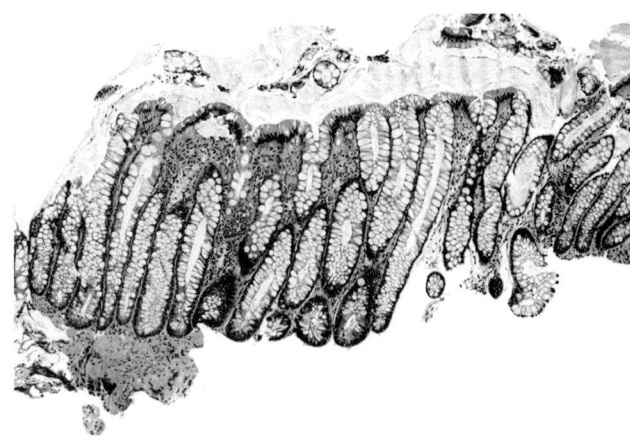

Figure 4-367. A suboptimal biopsy. This biopsy would be easy to dismiss as normal under any circumstance.

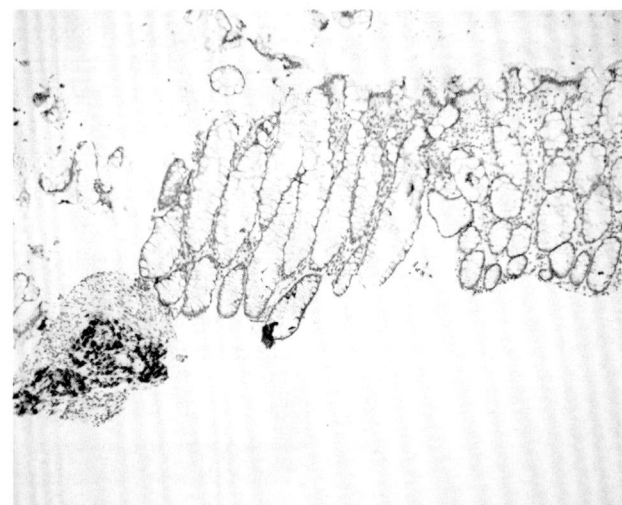

Figure 4-368. A suboptimal biopsy (GATA3). Based on the history of urothelial carcinoma and that this biopsy was submitted as an irregular, rectal ulceration, deeper sections and a GATA3 were ordered. The GATA3 highlights the tiny focus of urothelial carcinoma.

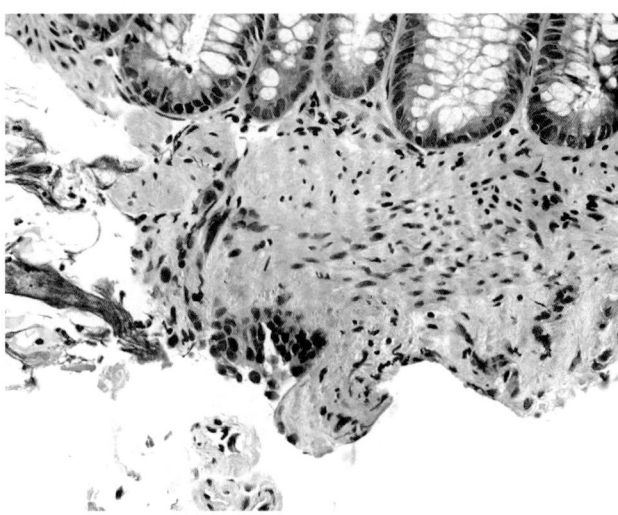

Figure 4-369. A suboptimal biopsy. Higher power of the previous figure. Looking back at the original H&E, this focus is just plain missable. It could easily have been dismissed as a crushed crypt base, but the worrisome history and clinical impression were keys to keep working up the case.

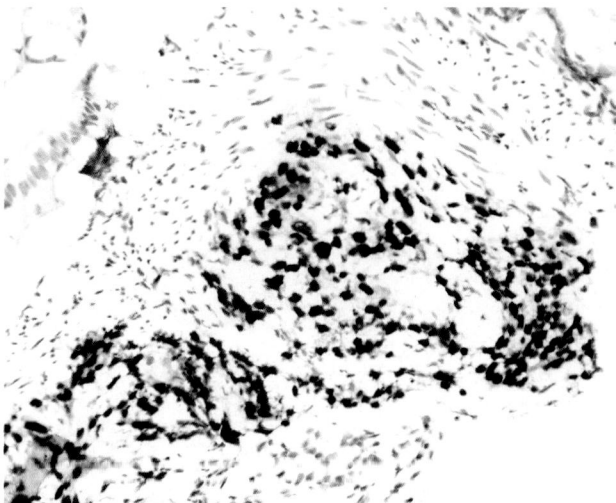

Figure 4-370. A suboptimal biopsy (GATA3). Take every clue you can get! Read the requisition and prior pathology reports, look at every piece of tissue on the slide, and remember it is OK to get deepers or a confirmatory IHC. The best diagnosis is worth the wait.

Sneaky malignancies in suboptimal biopsies with crush and cautery artifact are the makings of a perfect disaster. The aforementioned biopsy has a small focus of urothelial carcinoma, which was almost entirely missable on the initial sections (Figs. 4.367–4.370). Had no history been available, this focus could easily have been dismissed as a crushed crypt base. This case highlights the importance of looking at every little piece of the biopsy with a bit of suspicion and looking twice if there are red flags. It can be easy for our eyes to dismiss tissue edges, crushed tissue, cauterized fragments, and tissue burritos (areas where the tissue folds on itself), but take all the clues available and do not leave any potential clue on the slide—look at every piece of the biopsy! This biopsy was from a patient with a history of urothelial carcinoma and was submitted as an irregular, rectal ulceration. These red flags triggered deeper sections and additional immunohistochemical stains, which ultimately led to the diagnosis of urothelial carcinoma involving the rectum. Another important lesson is that it is OK to take some time to pursue deeper sections or request additional tissue—it is not fun, but it is OK. The justice system and QA reconciliation forms are filled with doctors who wish they could go back in time and order deeper sections or write a more careful note requesting additional tissue. Do not be that guy! It is OK to take time for the best diagnosis, which will guide optimal therapy and outcomes. In this case, we suspected the small atypical focus would have been exhausted on deeper sections, in which case we were prepared to sign out the case as "minute focus of atypical cells, rebiopsy suggested, if clinically feasible." Most of the time, a repeat biopsy with decent lesional tissue can lead to a solid diagnosis and additional material for ancillary testing. If the area sampled is indeed malignant, it is likely amenable to repeat sampling. Also, avoid using the term metastatic urothelial carcinoma, for example, because there is a possibility that the neoplasm involves the bowel through direct extension.

PEARLS & PITFALLS: Suboptimal Biopsies

- As simple as it sounds, make it a habit to look at every piece of the biopsy.
- Look twice if you are so lucky as to have a red flag, such as a history of malignancy or a clinical impression of a mass or thickened fold.
- Look three times if the clinician calls and is concerned about a missed diagnoses. Do not be insulted, we are all on the same team and all want the best diagnosis.
- Do not be afraid to take some time to order deeper sections or ancillary stains or request additional tissue.

EXTRACOLONIC NEOPLASMS INVOLVING THE COLON

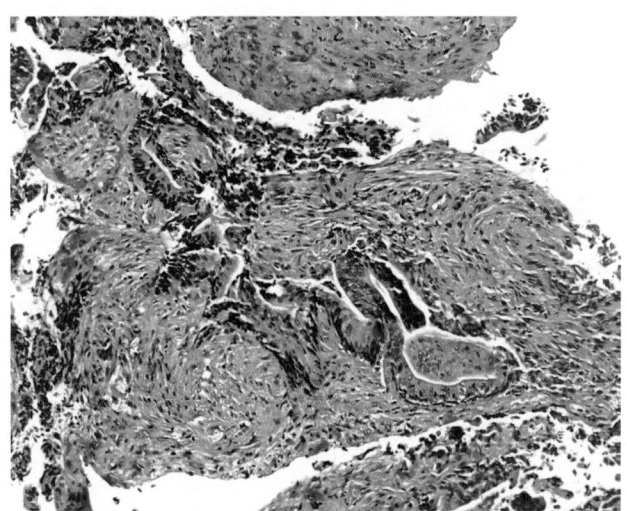

Figure 4-371. Endometrial adenocarcinoma. Extracolonic neoplasms involving the bowel can perfectly simulate primary GI malignancies. This biopsy was submitted as a colon mass and was initially misdiagnosed as colorectal adenocarcinoma cancer. Although it is true that the angulated glands and backdrop of desmoplasia are in keeping with a diagnosis of adenocarcinoma, this morphology is not specific to the colorectum. The patient had a history of endometrial adenocarcinoma and this material was morphologically and immunophenotypically consistent with endometrial adenocarcinoma (IHC not shown).

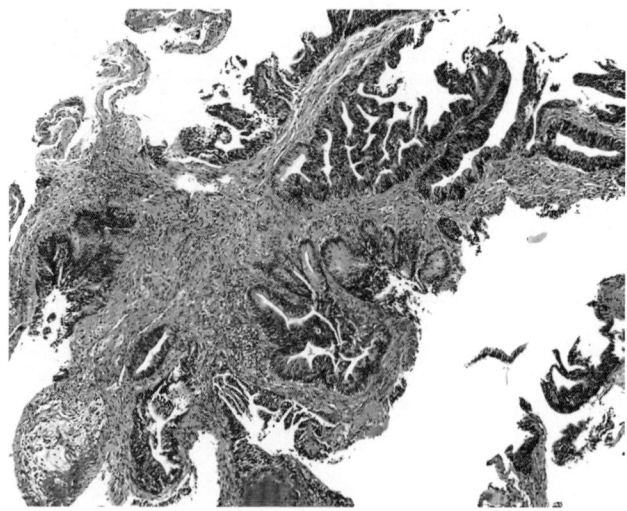

Figure 4-372. Endometrial adenocarcinoma. Another patient with a colon mass. The complex architecture and desmoplasia are consistent with adenocarcinoma but are nonspecific to site of primary.

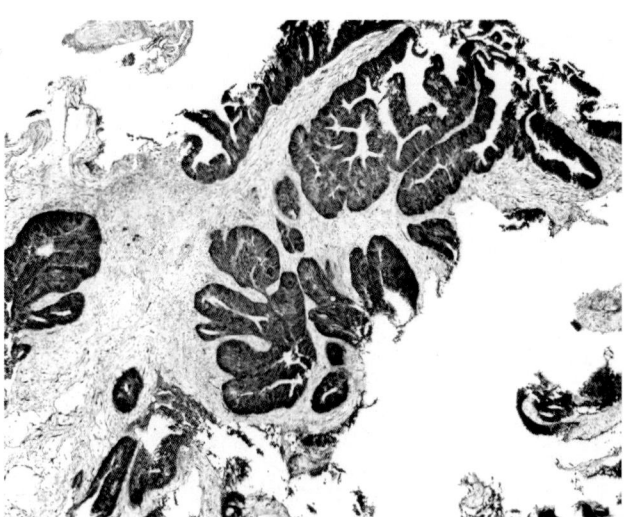

Figure 4-373. Endometrial adenocarcinoma (CK7). Based on a noted history of endometrial adenocarcinoma, this case was compared with the known primary and was morphologically similar. Furthermore, the CK7 and P16 (not shown) were strong and diffuse and CK20 and CDX2 (not shown) were nonreactive, in keeping with a diagnosis of endometrial adenocarcinoma.

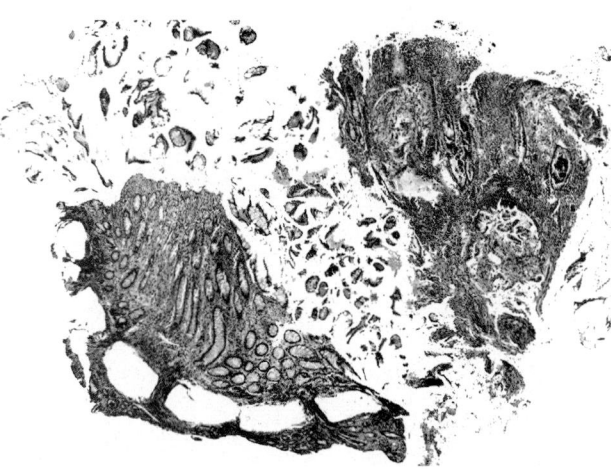

Figure 4-374. Pancreatic adenocarcinoma involving the colon. This case was submitted as a transverse colon mass. It is a real-life example of terrible histology and happens in every laboratory. It looks like the tissue exploded in the middle of the field, leaving hundreds of tiny pieces of cauterized tissue across the slide. Despite these difficulties, pathologists are still expected to yield a clinically useful diagnosis.

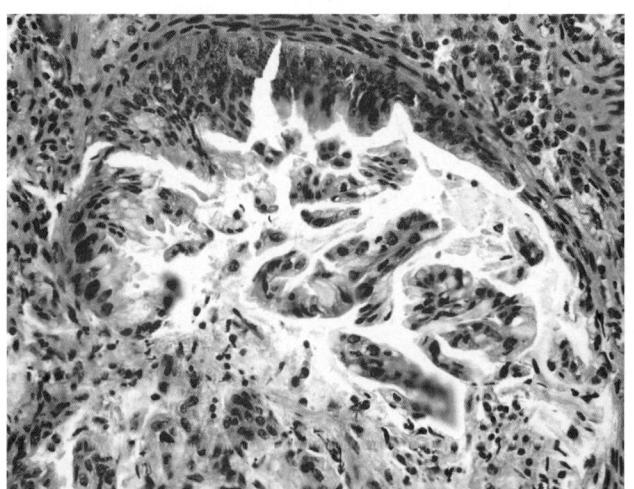

Figure 4-375. Pancreatic adenocarcinoma involving the colon. Higher power of the previous figure shows a cribriform gland. Although this was the only complex gland, it does appear neoplastic. It lacks the typical luminal necrosis seen with CRC, and the nuclei appear a bit blander with no obvious apoptosis, mitotic figures, or pleomorphism. The requisition also specified that the patient had a pancreatic mass, prompting further investigation.

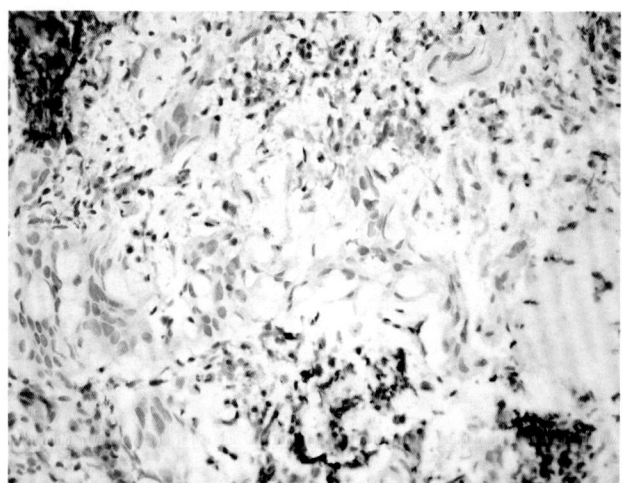

Figure 4-376. Pancreatic adenocarcinoma involving the colon (DPC4/SMAD4). Based on the atypical morphology and the presence of a pancreatic mass, a DPC4 IHC was performed and was negative in the neoplastic cells, supporting a diagnosis of "adenocarcinoma involving the colon, favor pancreatobiliary primary." The pancreatic mass was resected and showed identical morphology in a background of extensive pancreatic ductal intraepithelial neoplasia. This case highlights the importance of not assuming every colon mass is a colorectal primary.

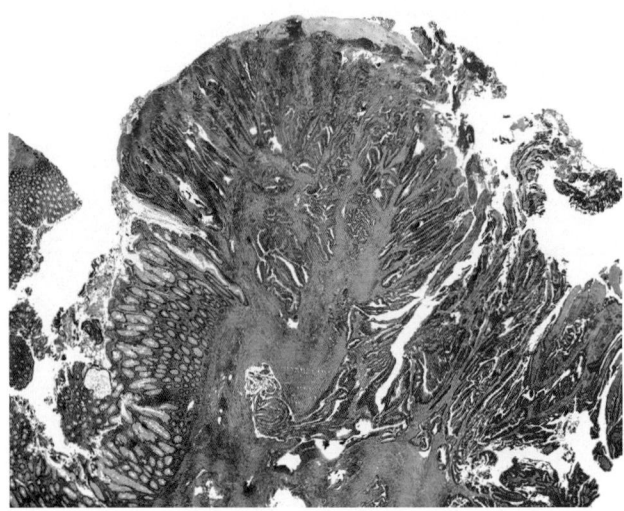

Figure 4-377. Endometrial adenocarcinoma involving the colon. This colonic mass was initially misdiagnosed as a moderately differentiated colorectal adenocarcinoma. The background mucosal colonization perfectly simulates dysplasia.

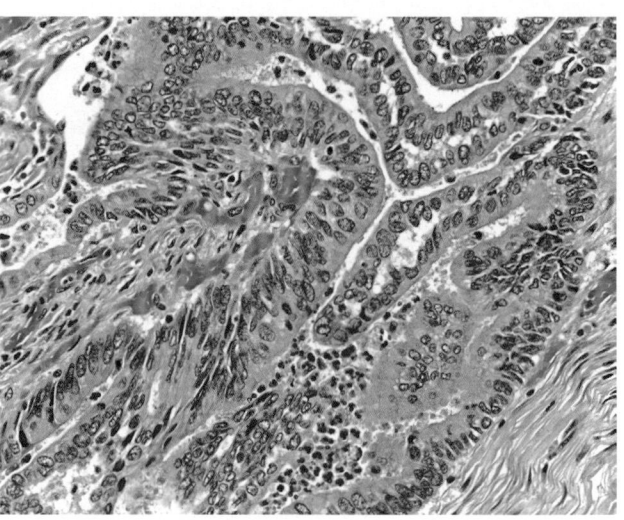

Figure 4-378. Endometrial adenocarcinoma involving the colon. Higher power of the previous figure. Keep in mind that gynecologic and genitourinary primaries are notorious for simulating primary GI neoplasms when they involve the bowel.

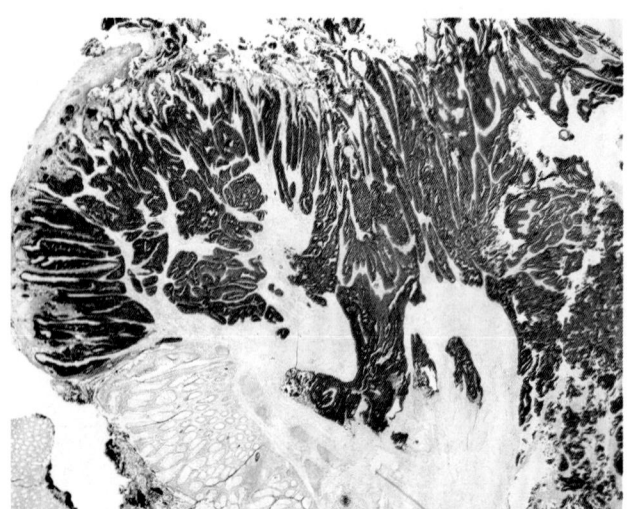

Figure 4-379. Endometrial adenocarcinoma (P16) involving the colon. Based on the history of an endometrial adenocarcinoma, this case was worked up and found to be P16 and CK7 (not shown) reactive and negative for CK20 and CDX2, in keeping with a diagnosis of endometrial adenocarcinoma.

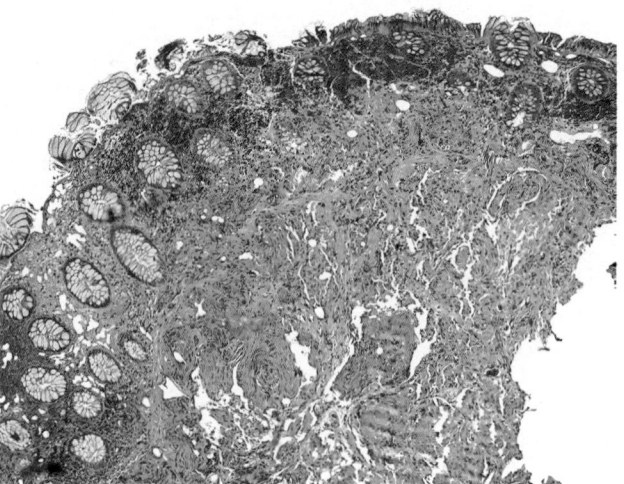

Figure 4-380. Prostate adenocarcinoma involving the colon. This small rectal polyp had been initially misdiagnosed as a carcinoid tumor. The terribly smooshed and cauterized mucosa only make this case more difficult.

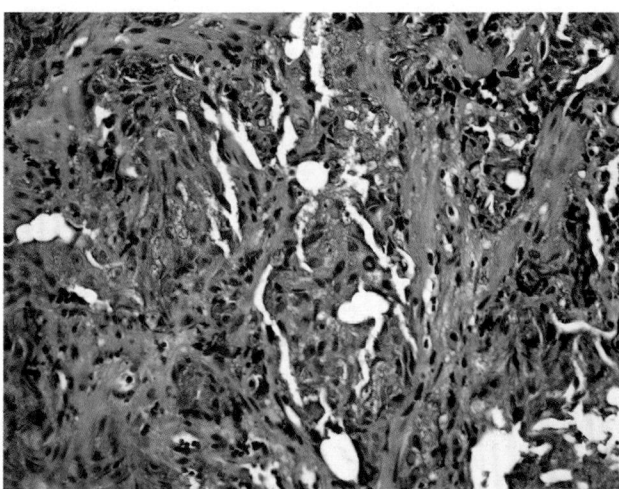

Figure 4-381. Prostate adenocarcinoma involving the colon. Higher power of the previous figure. The patient was an 89-year-old man. This author has come to reflexively consider prostate cancer in a rectal lesion from a patient of this demographic. The NKX3.1 was diffusely positive, confirming the earlier diagnosis (not shown). NKX3.1 is the marker of choice for these authors because PSA can be negative following hormonal therapy.

The above-mentioned cases originate from five unique patients. Several of these cases were originally misdiagnosed as primary CRCs, but each case is an example of mucosal colonization by an extracolonic neoplasm simulating CRC (Figs. 4.371–4.381). Mucosal colonization involves the extracolonic neoplasm growing into the bowel wall and extending to the mucosal surface. It can be indistinguishable from dysplasia/adenoma. Usually, the presence of a precursor polyp or associated dysplasia serves as evidence of a primary tumor, whereas mucosal colonization is a perfect mimic of dysplasia and can erroneously suggest a primary neoplasm to those not familiar with this phenomenon.[146] The wrong diagnosis can lead to potentially the wrong chemotherapy, the wrong surgery, a bad clinical outcome, and a lawsuit. Our advice is to realize that, although these cases are the minority of colorectal masses, it is prudent to maintain a low threshold to consider metastasis or direct invasion from elsewhere. Genitourinary and gynecologic primaries are notorious for crawling over to the colorectum, particularly to the rectum, but any process can similarly involve the bowel. Primary small bowel carcinomas are extraordinarily rare, and more often small intestinal carcinomas are metastasis/direct invasion from elsewhere.[146] Our advice is to keep it simple. The top-line diagnosis is adenocarcinoma, not colorectal adenocarcinoma and not small bowel adenocarcinoma. If there are red flags, such as a history of endometrial cancer or prostate cancer, have a low threshold to write a careful note or pursue additional immunohistochemical stains to confirm the site of the primary. Also, avoid using the term metastatic endometrial carcinoma, for example, if there is a possibility that the neoplasm involves the bowel through direct extension.

SAMPLE NOTE: Adenocarcinoma Involving the Small Bowel

Small Bowel, Mass, Biopsy
- Adenocarcinoma, See Note

Note: Primary small bowel adenocarcinomas are extraordinarily rare outside of the setting of LS or FAP. In this case, it may be worthwhile to correlate with imaging studies to evaluate for other potential primary sites (colon, gynecologic tract [for woman], genitourinary tract, for example). MMR proteins are all intact/present by IHC (MLH1, PMS2, MSH2, and MSH6)

Reference:
Estrella JS, Wu TT, Rashid A, et al. Mucosal colonization by metastatic carcinoma in the gastrointestinal tract: a potential mimic of primary neoplasia. *Am J Surg Pathol.* 2011;35:563-572.

ENDOMETRIOSIS

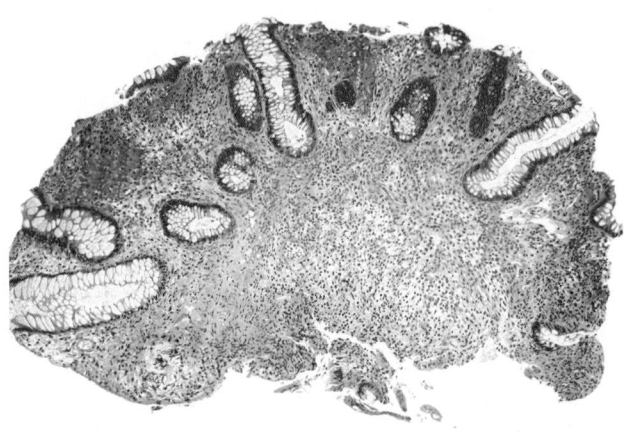

Figure 4-382. Endometriosis involving the colon. Endometriosis is a benign diagnosis but occasionally raises concerns for malignancy or IBD, especially in suboptimal biopsies. This biopsy is challenging because only the stromal component is seen on the initial sections.

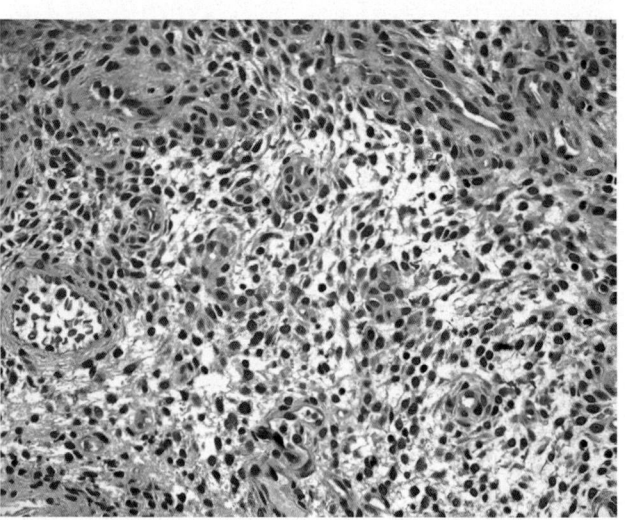

Figure 4-383. Endometriosis involving the colon. Higher power of the previous figure. Occasionally, these cases are misdiagnosed as a spindle cell sarcoma.

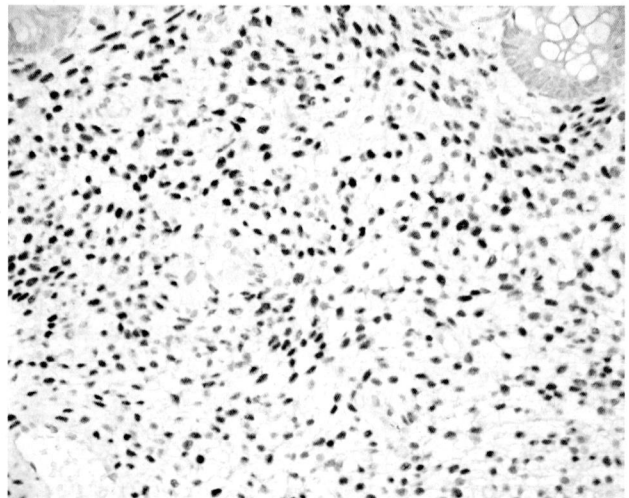

Figure 4-384. Endometriosis involving the colon (ER). Deeper sections and confirmatory ER, PR (not shown), CD10 (not shown) can be reassuring, especially if the patient is a young woman with a history of endometriosis. A single endometrial gland appeared on the deeper sections (not shown).

Up to 37% of women with endometriosis have bowel involvement.[147] The majority involve the rectum (73%), but 20% involve the sigmoid, 7% involve the ileum, and a portion involve the appendix (our experience).[147] Endometriosis can clinically manifest as abdominal pain, bloody diarrhea, strictures, obstruction, perforation, or a mass and, thereby, can raise clinical concerns for IBD, diverticular disease, appendicitis, or malignancy.[147-152] A histologic diagnosis of endometriosis requires two of these three features outside of the uterus: endometrial glands, endometrial stroma, or hemorrhage. Although endometriosis harbors mutations that have been associated with malignant neoplasms, it is benign and not uncommon.[153] However, it occasionally is misdiagnosed as a malignancy or IBD, particularly in mangled, crushed, or otherwise suboptimal biopsies. Biopsies with only the endometrial stromal component can also raise concerns for a sarcoma (Figs. 4.382–4.384). A tiny focus of haphazard endometrial glands in a specimen designated as a mass can simulate adenocarcinoma, particularly if the overlying reactive epithelial changes are misinterpreted as adenomatous. Similarly, the dense, sometimes inflamed, endometrial stroma can occasionally raise concerns for IBD. In general, a low threshold to consider endometriosis is generally a good idea, with deeper sections and confirmatory ER, PR, and CD10 immunohistochemical stains reassuring.

SNEAKY DIAGNOSES WITH INFLAMMATORY INFILTRATES
Sexually Transmitted Infectious Proctitis

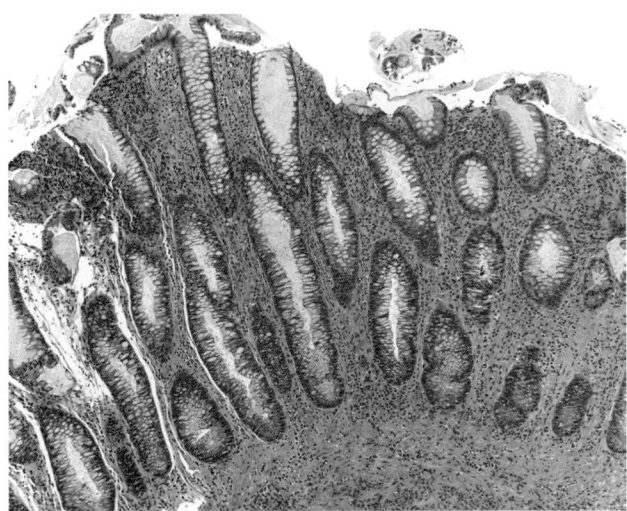

Figure 4-385. Sexually transmitted infectious (STI) colitis. STI colitis is caused by syphilis and/or lymphogranuloma venereum (LGV). It most commonly raises concerns for malignancy and IBD. Histologically, it typically shows intense infiltrate of *submucosal* plasma cells and a lack of architectural distortion and eosinophilia, as seen here in this confirmed case of syphilitic and LGV colitis. Both STI colitis and IBD show prominent *mucosal* plasma cells (not shown).

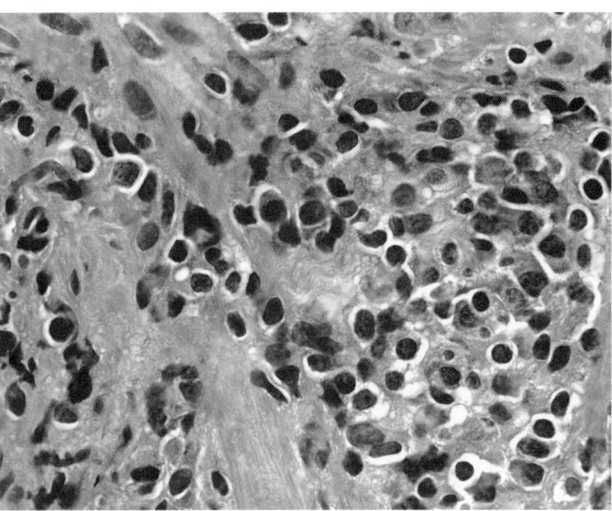

Figure 4-386. STI colitis. On high power, note the prominent plasma cells in the submucosa. IBD, in contrast, shows lymphocytes, histiocytes, and eosinophils in the submucosa (Fig. 4.388). This case highlights that both syphilis and LGV must be clinically tested, because either infection alone in isolation or in combination can lead to the identical morphology, and treatment of both is required to resolve the symptoms and prevent the onward transmission of the infections.

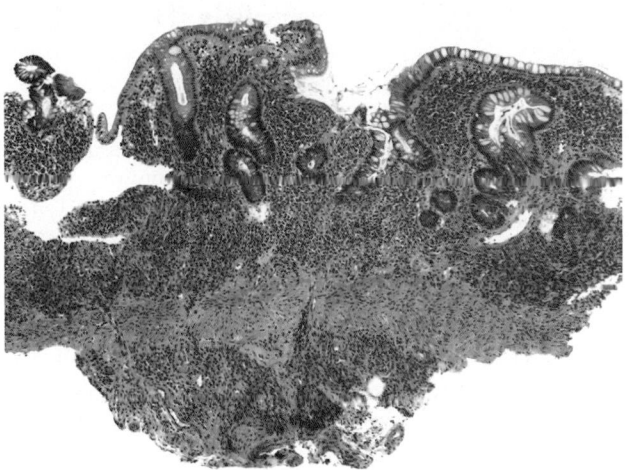

Figure 4-387. Inflammatory bowel disease (IBD). In contrast to STI colitis (see Fig. 4.385), note that IBD is characterized by prominent architectural distortion, as seen here. Note the abnormal crypt configurations, basal lymphoplasmacytosis, crypt shortfall, and crypt dropout.

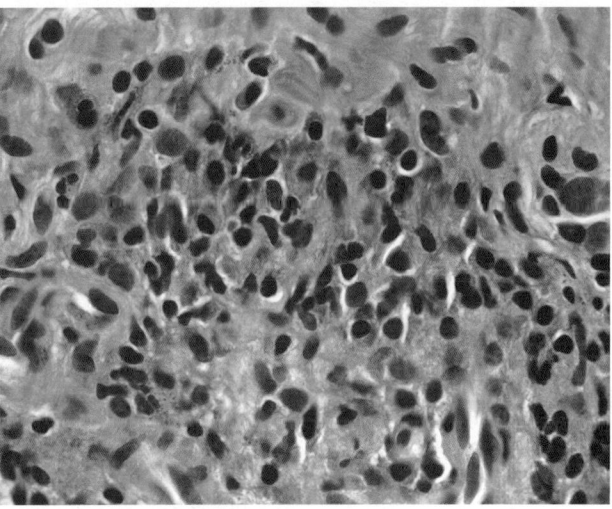

Figure 4-388. Inflammatory bowel disease (IBD). In contrast to STI colitis (see Fig. 4.386), note that IBD is characterized by submucosal inflammation rich in lymphocytes, histiocytes, and eosinophils. The mucosa in IBD also tends to have more eosinophils than that in STI colitis (not shown).

Syphilitic and lymphogranuloma venereum (LGV) proctocolitis are collectively referred to as sexually transmitted infectious (STI) proctocolitis. STI colitis is discussed in this section because it can simulate malignancy, as well as IBD.[154] A common clue to the diagnosis is a history of an HIV positive man who has sex with men (MSM). Patients typically present with anal bleeding, anal pain, and tenesmus.[154-156] Endoscopically, STI proctitis can present as ulcerations, nodules, polyps, and masses. Overlapping histologic features with IBD included active chronic colitis, skip lesions, aphthoid lesions, granulomata, foreign body giant cells, fibrosis, Paneth cell metaplasia, and lymphoid aggregates.[156] Features favoring STI colitis include the presence of an intense infiltrate of *submucosal* plasma cells and a lack of architectural distortion and eosinophilia (compare the typical features of STI colitis [Figs. 4.385 and 4.386] with the typical findings of IBD [Figs. 4.387 and 4.388]). If the specimen is labeled mass and consists of intense lymphoplasmacytic inflammation, consider STI colitis, CMV colitis, and a hematolymphoid evaluation. Beware that most cases prospectively lack the helpful clinical red flags of HIV and MSM status, emphasizing that a familiarity with the typical morphology is critical. See also *Atlas of GI Pathology: A Pattern Based Approach to Non-Neoplastic Biopsies.*

KEY FEATURES: Syphilitic or LGV Proctocolitis Pattern

- Both are curable mimics of malignancy and IBD
- Cause: Syphilitic and/or LGV infections
- Cure: Antibiotics
- Confirmatory studies: Clinical tests; routine studies available to pathologists are insufficiently sensitive for confirmation
- Red flags: HIV+ men who have sex with men (MSM)

FAQ: Are there any ancillary studies to confirm syphilitic and LGV infections?

Answer: At this time, clinical tests provide the best means to establish this diagnosis (detailed in the following Sample Note). Silver stains and *Treponema pallidum* immunohistochemical stains are too insensitive to confirm or exclude syphilitic infections, and there are no routine commercially available LGV studies available for the pathologist.[154]

SAMPLE NOTE: Syphilitic or LGV Proctocolitis (HIV+ MSM History Provided)

Rectum, Mass, Biopsy
- Rectal mucosa with intense lymphohistiocytic infiltrate and copious submucosal plasma cells.
- Negative for architectural changes and eosinophilia.
- A CMV immunohistochemical stain is negative.
- Deeper sections examined; a hematopathology evaluation to follow in an addendum.

Note: The history of an HIV+ man who has sex with men with a rectal mass is noted. The above-mentioned findings are reminiscent of so-called STI colitis of the sort caused by syphilitic and/or LGV infections. Clinical serologies provide the best means to establish this diagnosis. It is important to evaluate for both organisms, as either organism in isolation or combination can lead to identical morphology and symptoms. Syphilis: serum rapid plasma reagin (RPR), RPR titer, and a *Treponema*-specific serology such as fluorescent treponemal antibody; lymphogranuloma venereum: rectal swab collected in the absence of lubricant for *Chlamydia trachomatis* nucleic acid probe test or culture and LGV PCR.

References:
Arnold CA, Limketkai BN, Illei PB, Montgomery E, Voltaggio L. Syphilitic and lymphogranuloma venereum (LGV) proctocolitis: clues to a frequently missed diagnosis. *Am J Surg Pathol.* 2013;37(1):38-46.
Arnold CA, Roth R, Arsenescu R, et al. Sexually transmitted infectious colitis vs inflammatory bowel disease: distinguishing features from a case-controlled study. *Am J Clin Pathol.* 2015;144:771-781.

SAMPLE NOTE: Syphilitic or LGV Proctocolitis (No History Provided)

Rectum, Mass, Biopsy

- Rectal mucosa with intense lymphohistiocytic infiltrate and copious submucosal plasma cells.
- Negative for architectural changes and eosinophilia.
- A CMV immunohistochemical stain is negative.
- Deeper sections examined; a hematopathology evaluation to follow in an addendum.

Note: The above-mentioned findings are reminiscent of so-called STI colitis of the sort caused by syphilitic and or LGV infections. Clinical serologies provide the best means to establish this diagnosis. It is important to evaluate for both organisms, as either organism in isolation or combination can lead to identical morphology and symptoms. Syphilis: serum RPR, RPR titer, and a treponemal specific serology such as fluorescent treponemal antibody; lymphogranuloma venereum: rectal swab collected in the absence of lubricant for *Chlamydia trachomatis* nucleic acid probe test or culture and LGV PCR.

References:

Arnold CA, Limketkai BN, Illei PB, Montgomery E, Voltaggio L. Syphilitic and lymphogranuloma venereum (LGV) proctocolitis: clues to a frequently missed diagnosis. *Am J Surg Pathol.* 2013;37(1):38-46.

Arnold CA, Roth R, Arsenescu R, et al. Sexually transmitted infectious colitis vs inflammatory bowel disease: distinguishing features from a case-controlled study. *Am J Clin Pathol.* 2015;144:771-781.

Malignant Hematolymphoid Processes

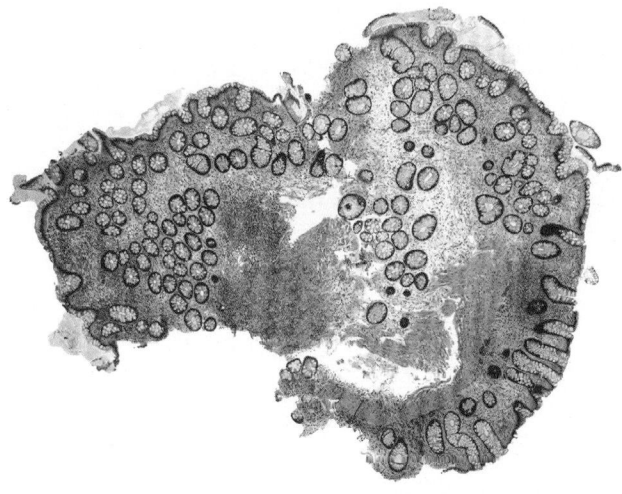

Figure 4-389. EBV-associated lymphoproliferative disorder involving the colon. This case would be very easy to dismiss as benign lymphoid aggregates on a busy sign-out day. Thank goodness this case came with an important clinical clue of "history of bone marrow transplantation" on the requisition, which prompted very careful examination of these seemingly innocuous lymphoid aggregates.

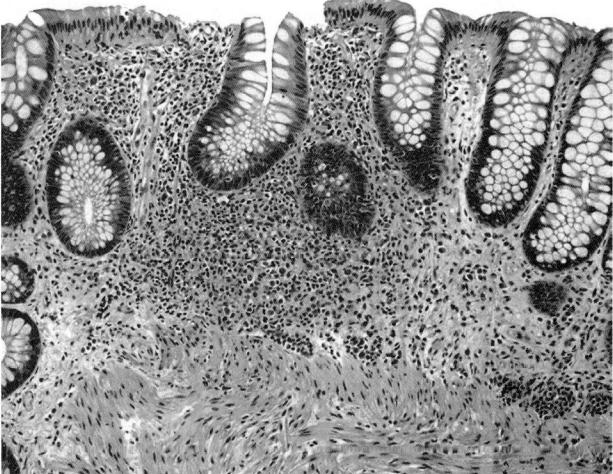

Figure 4-390. EBV-associated lymphoproliferative disorder involving the colon. Higher power of the previous figure.

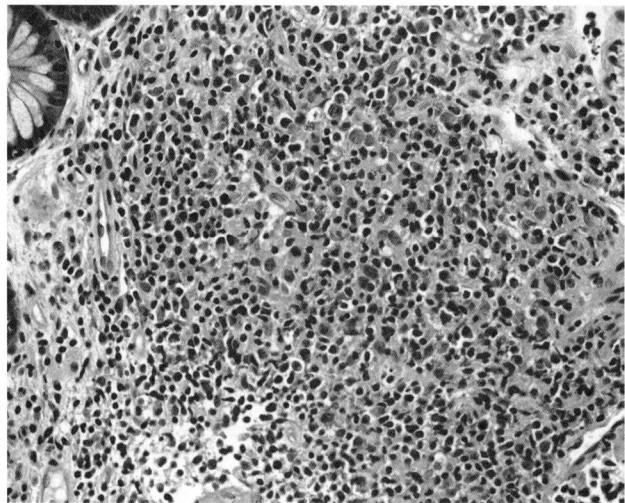

Figure 4-391. EBV-associated lymphoproliferative disorder involving the colon. Higher power of the previous figure. These lymphoid aggregates displayed strong EBV reactivity (not shown), supporting the earlier diagnosis.

Hematolymphoid malignancies are historically challenging to recognize in the GI tract because of the overlap between benign and malignant lymphoproliferative processes. Lymphoid aggregates, in particular, represent treacherous areas where it is wise to have a low threshold to share with a colleague with hematolymphoid expertise. Figs. 4.389–4.391 show a seemingly innocuous lymphoid aggregate that was ultimately signed out as an EBV-associated lymphoproliferative disorder in a patient with a history of a bone marrow transplant (EBV not shown). The bottom-line is that it is important to always consider the possibility of a hematolymphoid malignancy, especially if there is a history of a hematolymphoid malignancy or bone marrow transplant.

PEARLS & PITFALLS: Features That Trigger Additional Hematolymphoid Evaluation

Red flags to consider additional workup include the following:
1. A specimen designated as a mass with lymphoid infiltrates
2. Monotonous lymphoid infiltrates
3. Pleomorphic lymphoid infiltrates
4. Infiltrates that lack germinal centers or tingle-body macrophages
5. Lymphoid infiltrates that appear to destroy surrounding structures
6. Patients with a history of a hematolymphoid malignancy
7. Patients with a history of a bone marrow transplant

Merkel Cell Carcinoma

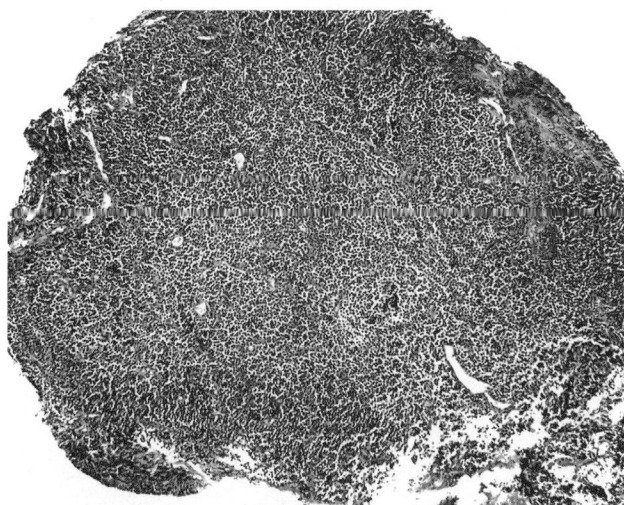

Figure 4-392. Metastatic Merkel cell carcinoma involving the colon. Generally good advice is to be a bit wary of lymphoid aggregates. This case was submitted as a polyp and appears as a lymphoid aggregate at low power but represents metastatic Meckel cell carcinoma.

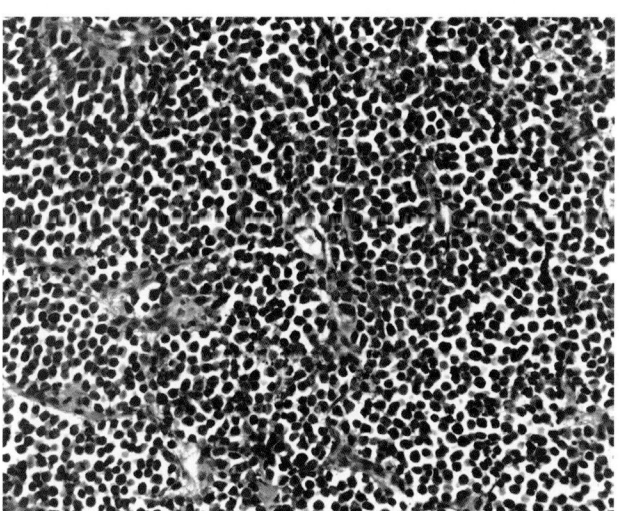

Figure 4-393. Metastatic Merkel cell carcinoma involving the colon. Every polyp is worth a quick glance at 40× for unusual features that might trigger additional workup.

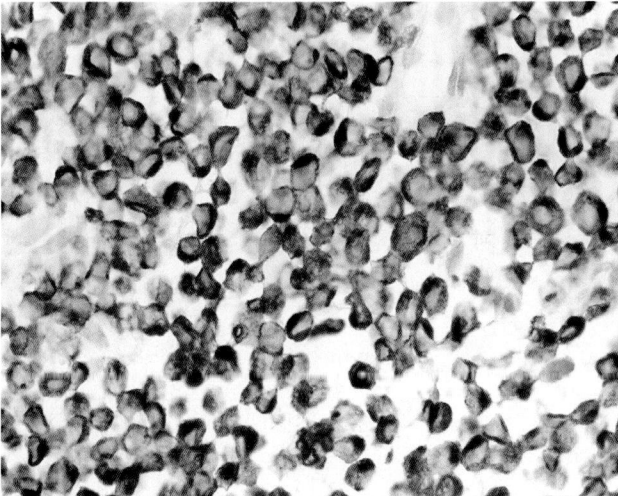

Figure 4-394. Metastatic Merkel cell carcinoma involving the colon (CK20). The morphology of this case was not especially alarming, but given the provided history of Merkel cell carcinoma, this case was approached with caution. The CK20 shows dotlike reactivity, confirming the earlier diagnosis.

In general, be a bit wary of supposed lymphoid aggregates. The earlier case was submitted as a polyp and appears as a lymphoid aggregate at low power but represents metastatic Merkel cell carcinoma (Figs. 4.392–4.394). Every polyp, even seemingly "good-old-lymphoid-aggregates," are worth a quick glance at 40× for unusual features that might trigger additional workup.

OTHER "FORGET ME NOTS"
Spirochetosis

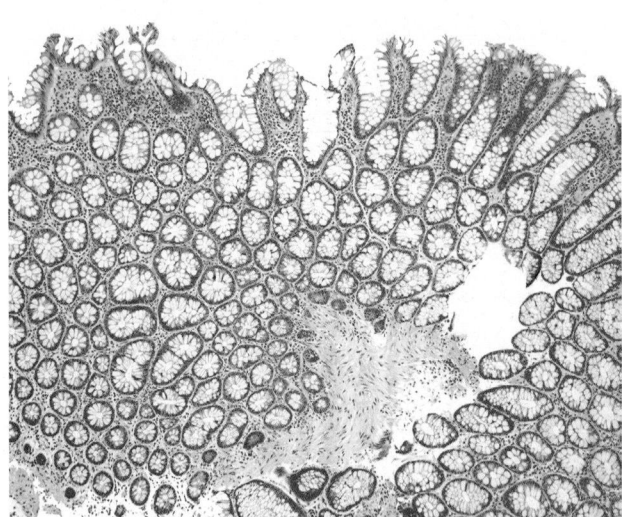

Figure 4-395. Hyperplastic polyp, goblet cell–rich type, with spirochetosis. This small rectal polyp is easy to blow off as a hyperplastic polyp, but it also has spirochetosis. This case emphasizes the importance of looking for the second (or third or fourth) diagnosis that exists a little beyond the first obvious diagnosis.

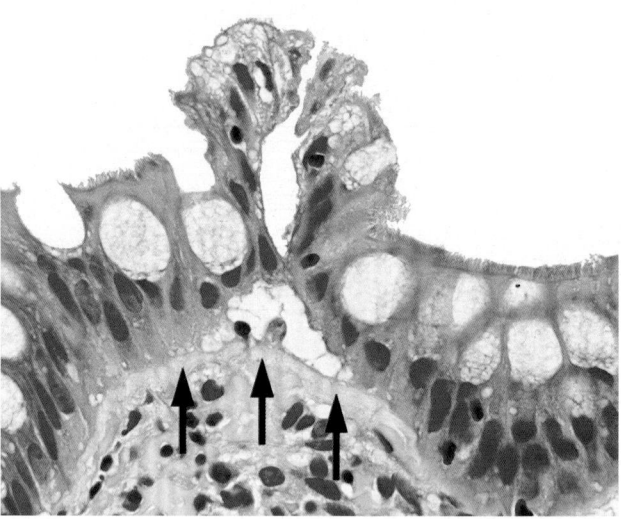

Figure 4-396. Hyperplastic polyp, goblet cell–rich type, with spirochetosis. Most infections are asymptomatic, but some cases are associated with antibiotic-responsive diarrhea and abdominal pain. These spiraled bacteria impart a fuzzy, basophilic border to the surface epithelium on H&E, which is best seen on intermediate power (*arrows*).

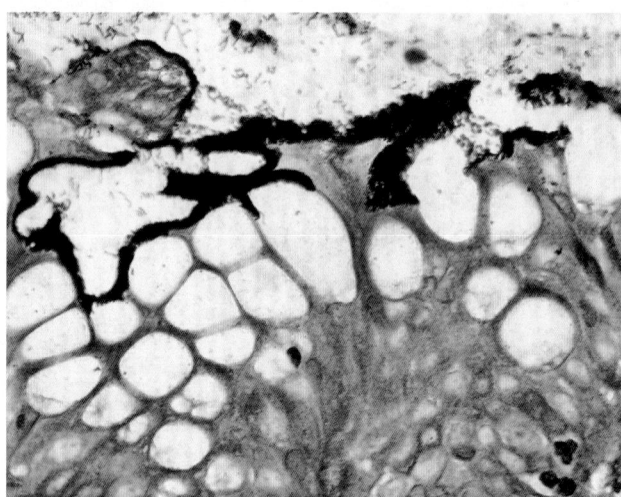

Figure 4-397. Hyperplastic polyp, goblet cell–rich type with spirochetosis (Warthin-Starry). Spirochetosis is transmitted via fecal oral contamination. Its presence does not indicate sexual activity or abuse. The *Brachyspira* organisms cross-react with the *Treponema pallidum* immunohistochemical stains, and their presence can also be confirmed with silver impregnation stains, such as the Warthin-Starry special stain, as seen here.

Polyps are fun specimens because their diagnoses usually can be made with a quick low-power peek, but beware of sneaky diagnoses that can lurk in the shadows of these seemingly simple specimens. In this example, spirochetosis can be seen at higher power (Figs. 4.395–4.397). In a recent Japanese study of more than 5,200 consecutive colorectal biopsies, spirochetosis was identified in 5.5% of HIV-positive patients and 1.7% of HIV-negative patients.[157] Rates can climb to more than 50% in developing regions and among MSM.[158-161] Spirochetosis is caused by *Brachyspira* species, and, although it was originally linked to HIV-positive MSM, it has since been identified in a broader demographic that includes patients with IBD and immunocompetent children and adults.[161,162] Spirochetosis is transmitted via fecal oral contamination; its presence does not indicate sexual activity or abuse. Most infections are asymptomatic, but some cases are associated with antibiotic responsive diarrhea and abdominal pain. These spiraled bacteria impart a fuzzy, basophilic border to the surface epithelium on H&E. The most common diagnostic pitfall to avoid is misdiagnosing a thick section of normal surface epithelium with heavy mucin for spirochetosis. A handy tip is that true spirochetosis should be visible at 10×. A 40× view of almost any bowel surface epithelium with thick mucin will appear similar to spirochetosis. In worrisome cases, a thin recut or confirmatory stain is worthwhile. The *Brachyspira* organisms cross-react with the *Treponema pallidum* immunohistochemical stains, and their presence can also be confirmed with silver impregnation stains, such as the Warthin-Starry special stain.[163,164] Other sneaky diagnoses important to consider in all cases include parasites (Figs. 4.398 and 4.399), medications (Figs. 4.400 and 4.401), CMV, malignancy, vasculitis, common variable immunodeficiency, autoimmune enteropathy, and colchicine toxicity. Avoid missing these challenging diagnoses by making a quick 40× view of every polyp a routine practice. See also *Atlas of GI Pathology: A Pattern Based Approach to Non-Neoplastic Biopsies.*

KEY FEATURES: Spirochetosis

- Spirochetosis is caused by *Brachyspira* species.
- It was originally associated with HIV-positive MSM but can be seen in immunocompetent children and adults.
- It is transmitted via fecal oral contamination.
- H&E: Spiraled bacteria impart a fuzzy, basophilic border to the surface epithelium.
- Confirmatory stains: *Treponema pallidum* immunohistochemical stains (organisms cross-react with *Treponema*) and silver stains.

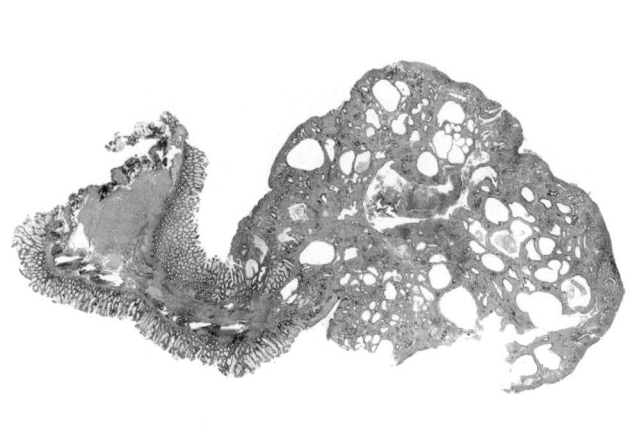

Figure 4-398. Enterobius vermicularis in a juvenile polyp. Another example of sneaky diagnoses in seemingly bland polyps.

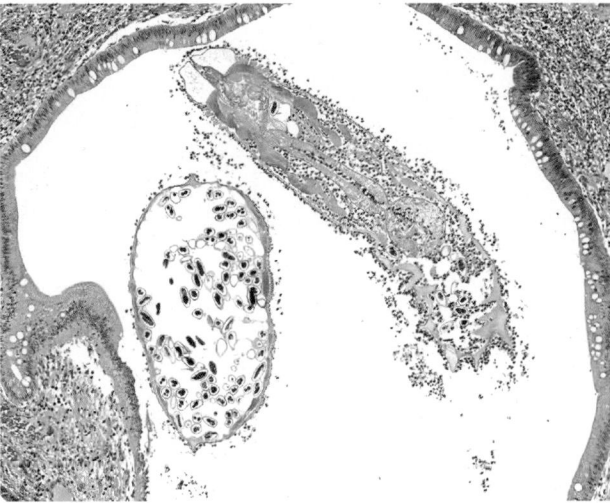

Figure 4-399. Enterobius vermicularis in a juvenile polyp. This juvenile polyp harbors *Enterobius vermicularis* (within the crypt lumen). These organisms are also called pinworms. Characteristically they have bipolar prominences (similar to spikes), as seen here (*arrows*). The second (nonobvious diagnosis) is always the hardest. (Case courtesy of Dr. Geok Chin Tan [Nationwide Children's Hospital].)

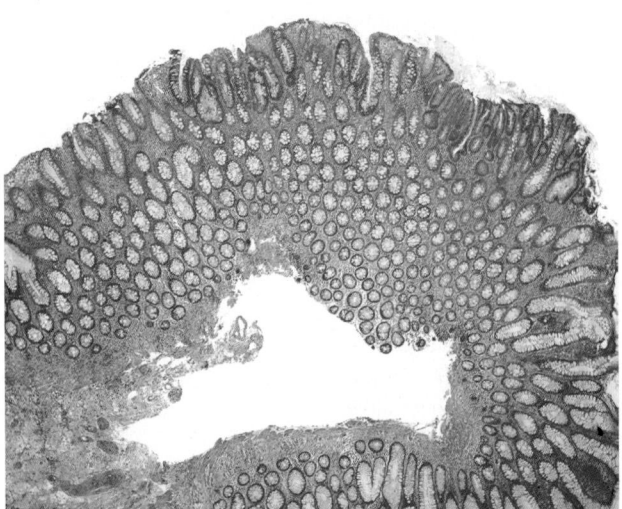

Figure 4-400. TA with sevelamer crystal. After making the obvious diagnosis of TA, make sure to carefully examine the background tissue for other important diagnosis. This case also features sevelamer crystals on the rightmost aspect of the polyp.

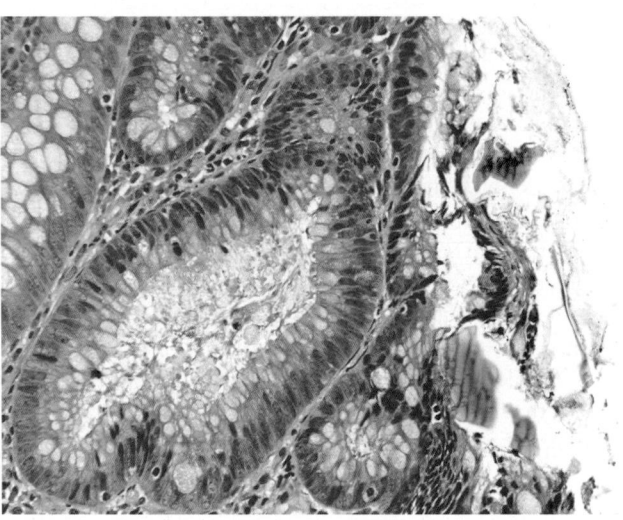

Figure 4-401. TA with sevelamer crystal. Higher power of the previous figure. Typical features of sevelamer include its crystal shape, "fish-scale" texture, and two-toned coloration with a *bright pink* center and *yellow* edges, as seen here. For more on medication resins, see also *Atlas of GI Pathology: A Pattern Based Approach to Non-Neoplastic Biopsies.*

Amyloid

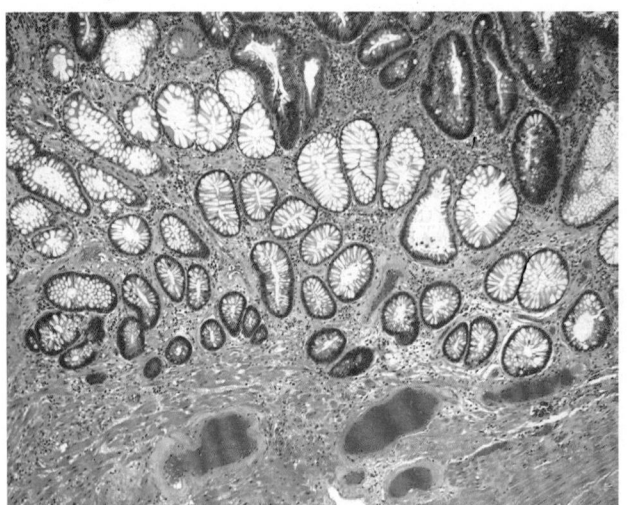

Figure 4-402. Amyloidosis involving a TA. The large submucosal vessels are involved by amyloid, which appears smooth and eosinophilic on H&E.

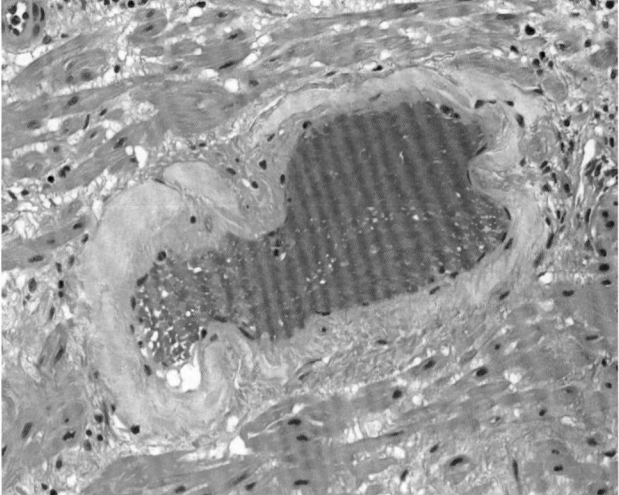

Figure 4-403. Amyloidosis involving a TA. Higher power of the previous figure shows the characteristic amyloid deposition of the large submucosal vessels. Similar changes were seen in the small mucosal vessels.

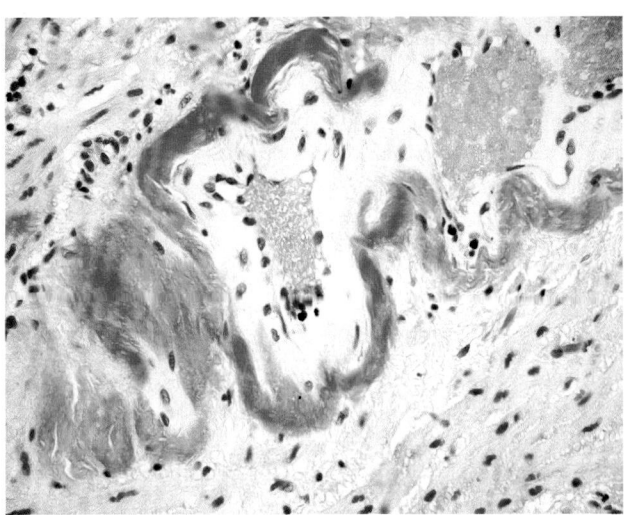

Figure 4-404. Amyloidosis involving a TA (Congo red). The Congo red stain was confirmatory: The amyloid was *bright orange* under direct light and apple green under polarized light (not shown). This diagnosis ultimately led to the detection of a previously unrecognized plasma cell neoplasm. Make sure to look at the vessels in every case!

Do not forget to always look at the vessels! Almost every GI biopsy has vessels, and it is worthwhile to have a habit of examining them. The earlier case is more than just a TA. The vessels are involved by amyloid, which appears smooth and eosinophilic on H&E, bright orange under direct light on Congo red, and apple green under polarized light on Congo red (not shown) (Figs. 4.402–4.404). The patient had a subsequent workup that revealed a plasma cell neoplasm. Other important diagnoses that can be seen by routine examination of the vessels include vasculitides, CMV infection, lymphovascular space invasion, fungal infections, and more. See also *Atlas of GI Pathology: A Pattern Based Approach to Non-Neoplastic Biopsies.*

References

1. Eidelman S, Lagunoff D. The morphology of the normal human rectal biopsy. *Hum Pathol.* 1972;3(3):389-401.
2. Carr NJ, Mahajan H, Tan KL, Hawkins NJ, Ward RL. Serrated and non-serrated polyps of the colorectum: their prevalence in an unselected case series and correlation of BRAF mutation analysis with the diagnosis of sessile serrated adenoma. *J Clin Pathol.* 2009;62(6):516-518.
3. Hamilton SR, Bosman F, Boffetta P, et al. Carcinoma of the colon and rectum. In: Bosman FT, Carneiro F, Hruban RH, Theise ND, eds. *WHO Classification of Tumours of the Digestive System.* Switzerland: Stylus Publishing; 2010:134-146.
4. Lieberman DA, Rex DK, Winawer SJ, Giardiello FM, Johnson DA, Levin TR. Guidelines for colonoscopy surveillance after screening and polypectomy: a consensus update by the US Multi-Society Task Force on colorectal cancer. *Gastroenterology.* 2012;143(3):844-857.
5. Fenoglio CM, Kaye GI, Lane N. Distribution of human colonic lymphatics in normal, hyperplastic, and adenomatous tissue. Its relationship to metastasis from small carcinomas in pedunculated adenomas, with two case reports. *Gastroenterology.* 1973;64(1):51-66.
6. Fogt F, Zimmerman RL, Ross HM, Daly T, Gausas RE. Identification of lymphatic vessels in malignant, adenomatous and normal colonic mucosa using the novel immunostain D2-40. *Oncol Rep.* 2004;11(1):47-50.
7. Robert ME. The malignant colon polyp: diagnosis and therapeutic recommendations. *Clin Gastroenterol Hepatol.* 2007;5(6):662-667.
8. *American Joint Committee on Cancer Staging Manual.* 8th ed. Switzerland: Springer International Publishing; 2017.
9. Luscher LD, Niemann TH, Lucas JG, Kurokawa AM, Frankel WL. Large colorectal adenomas. An approach to pathologic evaluation. *Am J Clin Pathol.* 2001;116(3):336-340.

10. *Protocol for the Examination of Specimens From Patients With Primary Carcinoma of the Colon and Rectum.* 2016. http://www.cap.org/ShowProperty?nodePath=/UCMCon/Contribution%20 Folders/WebContent/pdf/cp-colon-16protocol-3400.pdf. Accessed December 31, 2016.

11. Griggs RK, Novelli MR, Sanders DS, et al. Challenging diagnostic issues in adenomatous polyps with epithelial misplacement in bowel cancer screening: 5 years' experience of the Bowel Cancer Screening Programme Expert Board. *Histopathology.* 2016;70(3):466-472.

12. Muto T, Bussey HJ, Morson BC. Pseudo-carcinomatous invasion in adenomatous polyps of the colon and rectum. *J Clin Pathol.* 1973;26(1):25-31.

13. Muto T, Bussey HJ, Morson BC. The evolution of cancer of the colon and rectum. *Cancer.* 1975;36(6):2251-2270.

14. Panarelli NC, Somarathna T, Samowitz WS, et al. Diagnostic challenges caused by endoscopic biopsy of colonic polyps: a systematic evaluation of epithelial misplacement with review of problematic polyps from the bowel cancer screening program, United Kingdom. *Am J Surg Pathol.* 2016;40(8):1075-1083.

15. Lin J, Goldblum JR, Bennett AE, Bronner MP, Liu X. Composite intestinal adenoma-microcarcinoid. *Am J Surg Pathol.* 2012;36(2):292-295.

16. Salaria SN, Abu Alfa AK, Alsaigh NY, Montgomery E, Arnold CA. Composite intestinal adenoma-microcarcinoid clues to diagnosing an under-recognised mimic of invasive adenocarcinoma. *J Clin Pathol.* 2013;66(4):302-306.

17. Mills SE, Allen MS, Cohen AR. Small-cell undifferentiated carcinoma of the colon. A clinicopathological study of five cases and their association with colonic adenomas. *Am J Surg Pathol.* 1983;7(7):643-651.

18. Vortmeyer AO, Lubensky IA, Merino MJ, et al. Concordance of genetic alterations in poorly differentiated colorectal neuroendocrine carcinomas and associated adenocarcinomas. *J Natl Cancer Inst.* 1997;89(19):1448-1453.

19. Nash JW, Niemann T, Marsh WL, Frankel WL. To step or not to step: an approach to clinically diagnosed polyps with no initial pathologic finding. *Am J Clin Pathol.* 2002;117(3):419-423.

20. Wu ML, Dry SM, Lassman CR. Deeper examination of negative colorectal biopsies. *Am J Clin Pathol.* 2002;117(3):424-428.

21. Warnecke M, Engel UH, Bernstein I, Mogensen AM, Holck S. Biopsies of colorectal clinical polyps–emergence of diagnostic information on deeper levels. *Pathol Res Pract.* 2009;205(4):231-240.

22. Snover DC, Ahnen DJ, Burt RW, et al. *Serrated Polyps of the Colon and Rectum and Serrated Polyposis.* Lyon, France: IARC Press; 2010.

23. Limketkai BN, Lam-Himlin D, Arnold MA, Arnold CA. The cutting edge of serrated polyps: a practical guide to approaching and managing serrated colon polyps. *Gastrointest Endosc.* 2013;77(3):360-375.

24. Torlakovic E, Skovlund E, Snover DC, Torlakovic G, Nesland JM. Morphologic reappraisal of serrated colorectal polyps. *Am J Surg Pathol.* 2003;27(1):65-81.

25. Rex DK, Ahnen DJ, Baron JA, et al. Serrated lesions of the colorectum: review and recommendations from an expert panel. *Am J Gastroenterol.* 2012;107(9):1315-1329.

26. Torlakovic E, Snover DC. Serrated adenomatous polyposis in humans. *Gastroenterology.* 1996;110(3):748-755.

27. Agaimy A, Stoehr R, Vieth M, Hartmann A. Benign serrated colorectal fibroblastic polyps/intramucosal perineuriomas are true mixed epithelial-stromal polyps (hybrid hyperplastic polyp/mucosal perineurioma) with frequent BRAF mutations. *Am J Surg Pathol.* 2010;34(11):1663-1671.

28. Groisman G, Amar M, Alona M. Early colonic perineurioma: a report of 11 cases. *Int J Surg Pathol.* 2010;18(4):292-297.

29. Pai RK, Mojtahed A, Rouse RV, et al. Histologic and molecular analyses of colonic perineurial-like proliferations in serrated polyps: perineurial-like stromal proliferations are seen in sessile serrated adenomas. *Am J Surg Pathol.* 2011;35(9):1373-1380.

30. Groisman GM, Hershkovitz D, Vieth M, Sabo E. Colonic perineuriomas with and without crypt serration: a comparative study. *Am J Surg Pathol.* 2013;37(5):745-751.

31. Longacre TA, Fenoglio-Preiser CM. Mixed hyperplastic adenomatous polyps/serrated adenomas. A distinct form of colorectal neoplasia. *Am J Surg Pathol.* 1990;14(6):524-537.

32. Bettington ML, Walker NI, Rosty C, et al. A clinicopathological and molecular analysis of 200 traditional serrated adenomas. *Mod Pathol.* 2015;28(3):414-427.

33. Torlakovic EE, Gomez JD, Driman DK, et al. Sessile serrated adenoma (SSA) vs. traditional serrated adenoma (TSA). *Am J Surg Pathol.* 2008;32(1):21-29.

34. Kalimuthu SN, Chelliah A, Chetty R. From traditional serrated adenoma to tubulovillous adenoma and beyond. *World J Gastrointest Oncol.* 2016;8(12):805-809.

35. Chetty R. Traditional serrated adenoma (TSA): morphological questions, queries and quandaries. *J Clin Pathol.* 2016;69(1):6-11.

36. Yantiss RK, Oh KY, Chen YT, Redston M, Odze RD. Filiform serrated adenomas: a clinicopathologic and immunophenotypic study of 18 cases. *Am J Surg Pathol.* 2007;31(8):1238-1245.

37. Wiland HO, Shadrach B, Allende D, et al. Morphologic and molecular characterization of traditional serrated adenomas of the distal colon and rectum. *Am J Surg Pathol.* 2014;38(9):1290-1297.

38. Hafezi-Bakhtiari S, Wang LM, Colling R, Serra S, Chetty R. Histological overlap between colorectal villous/tubulovillous and traditional serrated adenomas. *Histopathology.* 2015;66(2):308-313.

39. Väyrynen SA, Väyrynen JP, Klintrup K, Mäkelä J, Tuomisto A, Mäkinen MJ. Ectopic crypt foci in conventional and serrated colorectal polyps. *J Clin Pathol.* 2016;69(12):1063-1069.

40. Chetty R, Hafezi-Bakhtiari S, Serra S, Colling R, Wang LM. Traditional serrated adenomas (TSAs) admixed with other serrated (so-called precursor) polyps and conventional adenomas: a frequent occurrence. *J Clin Pathol.* 2015;68(4):270-273.

41. Bettington M, Walker N, Rosty C, et al. Serrated tubulovillous adenoma of the large intestine. *Histopathology.* 2016;68(4):578-587.

42. Goldstein NS. Small colonic microsatellite unstable adenocarcinomas and high-grade epithelial dysplasias in sessile serrated adenoma polypectomy specimens: a study of eight cases. *Am J Clin Pathol.* 2006;125(1):132-145.

43. Giardiello FB, R W, Jarvinen J, OfferhausG. *Familial Adenomatous Polyposis.* 4th ed. 2010.

44. Morreau H, Riddell R, Aretz S. *MUTYH-Associated Polyposis.* 4th ed. Lyon, France: IARC Press; 2010.

45. Rosty C, Buchanan DD, Walsh MD, et al. Phenotype and polyp landscape in serrated polyposis syndrome: a series of 100 patients from genetics clinics. *Am J Surg Pathol.* 2012;36(6):876-882.

46. Rosty C, Walsh MD, Walters RJ, et al. Multiplicity and molecular heterogeneity of colorectal carcinomas in individuals with serrated polyposis. *Am J Surg Pathol.* 2013;37(3):434-442.

47. Crowder CD, Sweet K, Lehman A, Frankel WL. Serrated polyposis is an underdiagnosed and unclear syndrome: the surgical pathologist has a role in improving detection. *Am J Surg Pathol.* 2012;36(8):1178-1185.

48. Offerhaus G, Howe J. *Juvenile Polyposis.* 4th ed. Lyon, France: IARC; 2010.

49. Campos FG, Figueiredo MN, Martinez CA. Colorectal cancer risk in hamartomatous polyposis syndromes. *World J Gastrointest Surg.* 2015;7(3):25-32.

50. Offerhaus G, Billaud M, Gruber SB. *Peutz-Jeghers Syndrome.* 4th ed. Lyon, France: IARC; 2010.

51. Pai RK. A practical approach to the evaluation of gastrointestinal tract carcinomas for Lynch syndrome. *Am J Surg Pathol.* 2016;40(4):e17-e34.

52. Lam-Himlin D, Arnold CA, DePetris G. Gastric polyps and polyposis syndromes. *Diagn Histopathol.* 2014;20:1-11.

53. Seshadri D, Karagiorgos N, Hyser MJ. A case of Cronkhite-Canada syndrome and a review of gastrointestinal polyposis syndromes. *Gastroenterol Hepatol (N Y).* 2012;8(3):197-201.

54. Hampel H, Frankel WL, Martin E, et al. Feasibility of screening for Lynch syndrome among patients with colorectal cancer. *J Clin Oncol.* 2008;26(35):5783-5788.

55. Lynch HT, Snyder CL, Shaw TG, Heinen CD, Hitchins MP. Milestones of Lynch syndrome: 1895-2015. *Nat Rev Cancer.* 2015;15(3):181-194.

56. Umar A, Boland CR, Terdiman JP, et al. Revised Bethesda Guidelines for hereditary nonpolyposis colorectal cancer (Lynch syndrome) and microsatellite instability. *J Natl Cancer Inst.* 2004;96(4):261-268.

57. Syngal S, Brand RE, Church JM, et al. ACG clinical guideline: genetic testing and management of hereditary gastrointestinal cancer syndromes. *Am J Gastroenterol.* 2015;110(2):223-262; quiz 263.

58. Natarajan N, Watson P, Silva-Lopez E, Lynch HT. Comparison of extended colectomy and limited resection in patients with Lynch syndrome. *Dis Colon Rectum.* 2010;53(1):77-82.

59. Lynch HT, Lynch PM, Harris RE. Minimal genetic findings and their cancer control implications. A family with the cancer family syndrome. *J Am Med Assoc.* 1978;240(6):535-538.

60. Schmeler KM, Lynch HT, Chen LM, et al. Prophylactic surgery to reduce the risk of gynecologic cancers in the Lynch syndrome. *N Engl J Med*. 2006;354(3):261-269.

61. Watson P, Vasen HF, Mecklin JP, et al. The risk of extra-colonic, extra-endometrial cancer in the Lynch syndrome. *Int J Cancer*. 2008;123(2):444-449.

62. Stoffel EM, Mangu PB, Gruber SB, et al. Hereditary colorectal cancer syndromes: American Society of Clinical Oncology Clinical Practice Guideline endorsement of the familial risk-colorectal cancer: European Society for Medical Oncology Clinical Practice Guidelines. *J Clin Oncol*. 2015;33(2):209-217.

63. Wood LD, Salaria SN, Cruise MW, Giardiello FM, Montgomery EA. Upper GI tract lesions in familial adenomatous polyposis (FAP): enrichment of pyloric gland adenomas and other gastric and duodenal neoplasms. *Am J Surg Pathol*. 2014;38(3):389-393.

64. Wimmer K, Rosenbaum T, Messiaen L. Connections between constitutional mismatch repair deficiency syndrome and neurofibromatosis type 1. *Clin Genet*. 2017;91(4):507-519.

65. Al-Tassan N, Chmiel NH, Maynard J, et al. Inherited variants of MYH associated with somatic G: C-->T:A mutations in colorectal tumorsInherited variants of MYH associated with somatic G: C-->T:A mutations in colorectal tumorsInherited variants of MYH associated with somatic G: C-->T:A mutations in colorectal tumors. *Nat Genet*. 2002;30(2):227-232.

66. Jones N, Vogt S, Nielsen M, et al. Increased colorectal cancer incidence in obligate carriers of heterozygous mutations in MUTYH. *Gastroenterology*. 2009;137(2):489-494, 494.e1; quiz 725-726.

67. Boparai KS, Mathus-Vliegen EM, Koornstra JJ, et al. Increased colorectal cancer risk during follow-up in patients with hyperplastic polyposis syndrome: a multicentre cohort study. *Gut*. 2010;59(8):1094-1100.

68. Boparai KS, Reitsma JB, Lemmens V, et al. Increased colorectal cancer risk in first-degree relatives of patients with hyperplastic polyposis syndrome. *Gut*. 2010;59(9):1222-1225.

69. Hui VW, Steinhagen E, Levy RA, et al. Utilization of colonoscopy and pathology reports for identifying patients meeting the world health organization criteria for serrated polyposis syndrome. *Dis Colon Rectum*. 2014;57(7):846-850.

70. Shaco-Levy R, Jasperson KW, Martin K, et al. Morphologic characterization of hamartomatous gastrointestinal polyps in Cowden syndrome, Peutz-Jeghers syndrome, and juvenile polyposis syndrome. *Hum Pathol*. 2016;49:39-48.

71. Lam-Himlin D, Park JY, Cornish TC, Shi C, Montgomery E. Morphologic characterization of syndromic gastric polyps. *Am J Surg Pathol*. 2010;34(11):1656-1662.

72. Burkart AL, Sheridan T, Lewin M, Fenton H, Ali NJ, Montgomery E. Do sporadic Peutz-Jeghers polyps exist? Experience of a large teaching hospital. *Am J Surg Pathol*. 2007;31(8):1209-1214.

73. Tse JY, Wu S, Shinagare SA, et al. Peutz-Jeghers syndrome: a critical look at colonic Peutz-Jeghers polyps. *Mod Pathol*. 2013;26(9):1235-1240.

74. Nelen MR, Padberg GW, Peeters EA, et al. Localization of the gene for Cowden disease to chromosome 10q22-23. *Nat Genet*. 1996;13(1):114-116.

75. Pilarski R, Burt R, Kohlman W, Pho L, Shannon KM, Swisher E. Cowden syndrome and the PTEN hamartoma tumor syndrome: systematic review and revised diagnostic criteria. *J Natl Cancer Inst*. 2013;105(21):1607-1616.

76. Shaco-Levy R, Jasperson KW, Martin K, et al. Gastrointestinal polyposis in Cowden syndrome. *J Clin Gastroenterol*. 2016;51(7):e60-e67.

77. Daniel ES, Ludwig SL, Lewin KJ, Ruprecht RM, Rajacich GM, Schwabe AD. The Cronkhite-Canada Syndrome. An analysis of clinical and pathologic features and therapy in 55 patients. *Medicine (Baltimore)*. 1982;61(5):293-309.

78. Bettington M, Brown IS, Kumarasinghe MP, de Boer B, Bettington A, Rosty C. The challenging diagnosis of Cronkhite-Canada syndrome in the upper gastrointestinal tract: a series of 7 cases with clinical follow up. *Am J Surg Pathol*. 2014;38(2):215-223.

79. Sweetser S, Ahlquist DA, Osborn NK, et al. Clinicopathologic features and treatment outcomes in Cronkhite-Canada syndrome: support for autoimmunity. *Dig Dis Sci*. 2012;57(2):496-502.

80. Fan RY, Wang XW, Xue LJ, An R, Sheng JQ. Cronkhite-Canada syndrome polyps infiltrated with IgG4-positive plasma cells. *World J Clin Cases*. 2016;4(8):248-252.

81. De Petris G, Chen L, Pasha SF, Ruff KC. Cronkhite-Canada syndrome diagnosis in the absence of gastrointestinal polyps: a case report. *Int J Surg Pathol*. 2013;21(6):627-631.

82. Burke AP, Sobin LH. The pathology of Cronkhite-Canada polyps. A comparison to juvenile polyposis. *Am J Surg Pathol.* 1989;13(11):940-946.

83. Yamakawa K, Yoshino T, Watanabe K, et al. Effectiveness of cyclosporine as a treatment for steroid-resistant Cronkhite-Canada syndrome; two case reports. *BMC Gastroenterol.* 2016;16(1):123.

84. Gillen CD, Walmsley RS, Prior P, Andrews HA, Allan RN. Ulcerative colitis and Crohn's disease: a comparison of the colorectal cancer risk in extensive colitis. *Gut.* 1994;35(11):1590-1592.

85. Farraye FA, Odze RD, Eaden J, Itzkowitz SH. AGA technical review on the diagnosis and management of colorectal neoplasia in inflammatory bowel disease. *Gastroenterology.* 2010;138(2):746-774, 774.e1-774.e4; quiz e12-e13.

86. Canavan C, Abrams KR, Mayberry J. Meta-analysis: colorectal and small bowel cancer risk in patients with Crohn's disease. *Aliment Pharmacol Ther.* 2006;23(8):1097-1104.

87. Bernstein CN, Blanchard JF, Kliewer E, Wajda A. Cancer risk in patients with inflammatory bowel disease: a population-based study. *Cancer.* 2001;91(4):854-862.

88. Duricova D. What can we learn from epidemiological studies in inflammatory bowel disease? *Dig Dis.* 2017;35(1-2):69-73.

89. Sharan R, Schoen RE. Cancer in inflammatory bowel disease. An evidence-based analysis and guide for physicians and patients. *Gastroenterol Clin North Am.* 2002;31(1):237-254.

90. Eaden JA, Abrams KR, Mayberry JF. The risk of colorectal cancer in ulcerative colitis: a meta-analysis. *Gut.* 2001;48(4):526-535.

91. Harpaz N, Talbot IC. Colorectal cancer in idiopathic inflammatory bowel disease. *Semin Diagn Pathol.* 1996;13(4):339-357.

92. Ekbom A, Helmick C, Zack M, Adami HO. Increased risk of large-bowel cancer in Crohn's disease with colonic involvement. *Lancet.* 1990;336(8711):357-359.

93. Kornfeld D, Ekbom A, Ihre T. Is there an excess risk for colorectal cancer in patients with ulcerative colitis and concomitant primary sclerosing cholangitis? A population based study. *Gut.* 1997;41(4):522-525.

94. Broomé U, Löfberg R, Veress B, Eriksson LS. Primary sclerosing cholangitis and ulcerative colitis: evidence for increased neoplastic potential. *Hepatology.* 1995;22(5):1404-1408.

95. Farraye FA, Odze RD, Eaden J, et al. AGA medical position statement on the diagnosis and management of colorectal neoplasia in inflammatory bowel disease. *Gastroenterology.* 2010;138(2):738-745.

96. Rubin CE, Haggitt RC, Burmer GC, et al. DNA aneuploidy in colonic biopsies predicts future development of dysplasia in ulcerative colitis. *Gastroenterology.* 1992;103(5):1611-1620.

97. Laine L, Kaltenbach T, Barkun A, et al. SCENIC international consensus statement on surveillance and management of dysplasia in inflammatory bowel disease. *Gastroenterology.* 2015;148(3):639.e628-651.e628.

98. Kappelman MD, Farkas DK, Long MD, et al. Risk of cancer in patients with inflammatory bowel diseases: a nationwide population-based cohort study with 30 years of follow-up evaluation. *Clin Gastroenterol Hepatol.* 2014;12(2):265.e261-273.e261.

99. Kruis W, Nguyen PG, Morgenstern J. Promises and dangers of combination therapy. *Dig Dis.* 2017,35(1-2):56-60.

100. Deepak P, Sifuentes H, Sherid M, Stobaugh D, Sadozai Y, Ehrenpreis ED. T-cell non-Hodgkin's lymphomas reported to the FDA AERS with tumor necrosis factor-alpha (TNF-α) inhibitors: results of the REFURBISH study. *Am J Gastroenterol.* 2013;108(1):99-105.

101. Parakkal D, Sifuentes H, Semer R, Ehrenpreis ED. Hepatosplenic T-cell lymphoma in patients receiving TNF-α inhibitor therapy: expanding the groups at risk. *Eur J Gastroenterol Hepatol.* 2011;23(12):1150-1156.

102. Riddell RH, Goldman H, Ransohoff DF, et al. Dysplasia in inflammatory bowel disease: standardized classification with provisional clinical applications. *Hum Pathol.* 1983;14(11):931-968.

103. Odze RD, Goldblum J, Noffsinger A, Alsaigh N, Rybicki LA, Fogt F. Interobserver variability in the diagnosis of ulcerative colitis-associated dysplasia by telepathology. *Mod Pathol.* 2002;15(4):379-386.

104. Odze RD, Tomaszewski JE, Furth EE, et al. Variability in the diagnosis of dysplasia in ulcerative colitis by dynamic telepathology. *Oncol Rep.* 2006;16(5):1123-1129.

105. Dixon MF, Brown LJ, Gilmour HM, et al. Observer variation in the assessment of dysplasia in ulcerative colitis. *Histopathology.* 1988;13(4):385-397.

106. Eaden J, Abrams K, McKay H, Denley H, Mayberry J. Inter-observer variation between general and specialist gastrointestinal pathologists when grading dysplasia in ulcerative colitis. *J Pathol.* 2001;194(2):152-157.

107. Ponte R, Mastracci L, Di Domenico S, et al. Giant Filiform polyposis not associated with inflammatory bowel disease: a case report. *Viszeralmedizin.* 2015;31(1):58-60.

108. Boulagnon C, Jazeron JF, Diaz-Cives A, Ehrhard F, Bouché O, Diebold MD. Filiform polyposis: a benign entity? Case report and literature review. *Pathol Res Pract.* 2014;210(3):189-193.

109. Kim HS, Lee KY, Kim YW. Filiform polyposis associated with sigmoid diverticulitis in a patient without inflammatory bowel disease. *J Crohns Colitis.* 2010;4(6):671-673.

110. Parian A, Koh J, Limketkai BN, et al. Association between serrated epithelial changes and colorectal dysplasia in inflammatory bowel disease. *Gastrointest Endosc.* 2016;84(1):87.e81-95.e81.

111. Kilgore SP, Sigel JE, Goldblum JR. Hyperplastic-like mucosal change in Crohn's disease: an unusual form of dysplasia? *Mod Pathol.* 2000;13(7):797-801.

112. Johnson DH, Khanna S, Smyrk TC, et al. Detection rate and outcome of colonic serrated epithelial changes in patients with ulcerative colitis or Crohn's colitis. *Aliment Pharmacol Ther.* 2014;39(12):1408-1417.

113. Rubio CA, Rodensjö M. Flat serrated adenomas and flat tubular adenomas of the colorectal mucosa: differences in the pattern of cell proliferation. *Jpn J Cancer Res.* 1995;86(8):756-760.

114. Polydorides AD, Harpaz N. Serrated lesions in inflammatory bowel disease. *Gastrointest Endosc.* 2017;85(2):461.

115. Fearon ER, Vogelstein B. A genetic model for colorectal tumorigenesis. *Cell.* 1990;61(5):759-767.

116. Le DT, Uram JN, Wang H, et al. PD-1 Blockade in tumors with mismatch-repair deficiency. *N Engl J Med.* 2015;372(26):2509-2520.

117. Lin AY, Lin E. Programmed death 1 blockade, an Achilles heel for MMR-deficient tumors? *J Hematol Oncol.* 2015;8:124.

118. Bao F, Panarelli NC, Rennert H, Sherr DL, Yantiss RK. Neoadjuvant therapy induces loss of MSH6 expression in colorectal carcinoma. *Am J Surg Pathol.* 2010;34(12):1798-1804.

119. Radu OM, Nikiforova MN, Farkas LM, Krasinskas AM. Challenging cases encountered in colorectal cancer screening for Lynch syndrome reveal novel findings: nucleolar MSH6 staining and impact of prior chemoradiation therapy. *Hum Pathol.* 2011;42(9):1247-1258.

120. Hartman DJ, Brand RE, Hu H, et al. Lynch syndrome-associated colorectal carcinoma: frequent involvement of the left colon and rectum and late-onset presentation supports a universal screening approach. *Hum Pathol.* 2013;44(11):2518-2528.

121. Kuan SF, Ren B, Brand R, Dudley B, Pai RK. Neoadjuvant therapy in microsatellite stable colorectal carcinoma induces concomitant loss of MSH6 and Ki67 expression. *Hum Pathol.* 2017;63:33-39.

122. Chen W, Swanson BJ, Frankel WL. Molecular genetics of microsatellite-unstable colorectal cancer for pathologists. *Diagn Pathol.* 2017;12(1):24.

123. Rodríguez-Soler M, Pérez-Carbonell L, Guarinos C, et al. Risk of cancer in cases of suspected lynch syndrome without germline mutation. *Gastroenterology.* 2013;144(5):926.e921-932. e921; quiz e913-e924.

124. Liccardo R, De Rosa M, Izzo P, Duraturo F. Novel implications in molecular diagnosis of Lynch syndrome. *Gastroenterol Res Pract.* 2017;2017:2595098.

125. Mensenkamp AR, Vogelaar IP, van Zelst-Stams WA, et al. Somatic mutations in MLH1 and MSH2 are a frequent cause of mismatch-repair deficiency in Lynch syndrome-like tumors. *Gastroenterology.* 2014;146(3):643.e648-646.e648.

126. Bettington M, Walker N, Clouston A, Brown I, Leggett B, Whitehall V. The serrated pathway to colorectal carcinoma: current concepts and challenges. *Histopathology.* 2013;62(3):367-386.

127. O'Brien MJ, Zhao Q, Yang S. Colorectal serrated pathway cancers and precursors. *Histopathology.* 2015;66(1):49-65.

128. Noffsinger AE. Serrated polyps and colorectal cancer: new pathway to malignancy. *Annu Rev Pathol.* 2009;4:343-364.

129. Das V, Kalita J, Pal M. Predictive and prognostic biomarkers in colorectal cancer: a systematic review of recent advances and challenges. *Biomed Pharmacother.* 2017;87:8-19.

130. Sepulveda AR, Hamilton SR, Allegra CJ, et al. Molecular biomarkers for the evaluation of colorectal cancer: guideline summary from the American Society for Clinical Pathology, College of

American Pathologists, Association for Molecular Pathology, and American Society of Clinical Oncology. *J Oncol Pract*. 2017;13(5):333-337.

131. Yantiss RK, Samowitz WS. Molecular pathology of gastrointestinal cancer. *Surg Pathol Clin*. 2012;5(4):821-842.

132. Loree JM, Kopetz S, Raghav KP. Current companion diagnostics in advanced colorectal cancer; getting a bigger and better piece of the pie. *J Gastrointest Oncol*. 2017;8(1):199-212.

133. Sartore-Bianchi A, Trusolino L, Martino C, et al. Dual-targeted therapy with trastuzumab and lapatinib in treatment-refractory, KRAS codon 12/13 wild-type, HER2-positive metastatic colorectal cancer (HERACLES): a proof-of-concept, multicentre, open-label, phase 2 trial. *Lancet Oncol*. 2016;17(6):738-746.

134. Valtorta E, Martino C, Sartore-Bianchi A, et al. Assessment of a HER2 scoring system for colorectal cancer: results from a validation study. *Mod Pathol*. 2015;28(11):1481-1491.

135. *FDA approves first cancer treatment for any solid tumor with a specific genetic feature*. https://www.fda.gov/NewsEvents/Newsroom/PressAnnouncements/ucm560167.htm?source=govdelivery-&utm_medium=email&utm_source=govdelivery. Accessed June 7, 2017.

136. Guan J, Lim KS, Mekhail T, Chang CC. Programmed death ligand-1 (PD-L1) expression in the programmed death receptor-1 (PD-1)/PD-L1 blockade: a key player against various cancers. *Arch Pathol Lab Med*. 2017;141(6):851-861.

137. Roth RM, Haraldsdottir S, Hampel H, Arnold CA, Frankel WL. Discordant mismatch repair protein immunoreactivity in Lynch syndrome-associated neoplasms: a recommendation for screening synchronous/metachronous neoplasms. *Am J Clin Pathol*. 2016;146(1):50-56.

138. Xia M, Singhi AD, Dudley B, Brand R, Nikiforova M, Pai RK. Small bowel adenocarcinoma frequently exhibits lynch syndrome-associated mismatch repair protein deficiency but does not harbor sporadic MLH1 deficiency. *Appl Immunohistochem Mol Morphol*. 2016;25(6):399-406.

139. Mills AM, Sloan EA, Thomas M, et al. Clinicopathologic comparison of Lynch syndrome-associated and "Lynch-like" endometrial carcinomas identified on universal screening using mismatch repair protein immunohistochemistry. *Am J Surg Pathol*. 2016;40(2):155-165.

140. Mills AM, Liou S, Ford JM, Berek JS, Pai RK, Longacre TA. Lynch syndrome screening should be considered for all patients with newly diagnosed endometrial cancer. *Am J Surg Pathol*. 2014;38(11):1501-1509.

141. Brahmer J, Reckamp KL, Baas P, et al. Nivolumab versus docetaxel in advanced squamous-cell non-small-cell lung cancer. *N Engl J Med*. 2015;373(2):123-135.

142. Tsao MS, Kerr KM, Dacic S, Yatabe Y, Hirsch FR. International Association for the Study of Lung Cancer atlas of PD-L1 immunohistochemistry testing in lung cancer. https://www.iaslc.org/sites/default/files/wysiwyg-assets/pd-l1_atlas_book_lo-res.pdf. Accessed June 6, 2017.

143. Barone J. http://www.baronerocks.com/index.php/mnemonics/mnemonics-pharmacology. Accessed June 7, 2017.

144. Hodi FS, O'Day SJ, McDermott DF, et al. Improved survival with ipilimumab in patients with metastatic melanoma. *N Engl J Med*. 2010;363(8):711-723.

145. Mahoney KM, Rennert PD, Freeman GJ. Combination cancer immunotherapy and new immunomodulatory targets. *Nat Rev Drug Discov*. 2015;14(8):561-584.

146. Estrella JS, Wu TT, Rashid A, Abraham SC. Mucosal colonization by metastatic carcinoma in the gastrointestinal tract: a potential mimic of primary neoplasia. *Am J Surg Pathol*. 2011;35(4):563-572.

147. Jiang W, Roma AA, Lai K, Carver P, Xiao SY, Liu X. Endometriosis involving the mucosa of the intestinal tract: a clinicopathologic study of 15 cases. *Mod Pathol*. 2013;26(9):1270-1278.

148. Yantiss RK, Clement PB, Young RH. Endometriosis of the intestinal tract: a study of 44 cases of a disease that may cause diverse challenges in clinical and pathologic evaluation. *Am J Surg Pathol*. 2001;25(4):445-454.

149. Rowland R, Langman JM. Endometriosis of the large bowel: a report of 11 cases. *Pathology*. 1989;21(4):259-265.

150. Tong YL, Chen Y, Zhu SY. Ileocecal endometriosis and a diagnosis dilemma: a case report and literature review. *World J Gastroenterol*. 2013;19(23):3707-3710.

151. Dong C, Ngu WS, Wakefield SE. Endometriosis masquerading as Crohn's disease in a patient with acute small bowel obstruction. *BMJ Case Rep*. 2015;2015.

152. Yildirim S, Nursal TZ, Tarim A, Torer N, Bal N, Yildirim T. Colonic obstruction due to rectal endometriosis: report of a case. *Turk J Gastroenterol*. 2005;16(1):48-51.

153. Anglesio MS, Papadopoulos N, Ayhan A, et al. Cancer-associated mutations in endometriosis without cancer. *N Engl J Med.* 2017;376(19):1835-1848.

154. Arnold CA, Limketkai BN, Illei PB, Montgomery E, Voltaggio L. Syphilitic and lymphogranu-loma venereum (LGV) proctocolitis: clues to a frequently missed diagnosis. *Am J Surg Pathol.* 2013;37(1):38-46.

155. Arnold CA, Bhaijee F, Lam-Himlin D. Fifty shades of chronic colitis: non-infectious imposters of inflammatory bowel disease. *Diagn Histopathol.* 2015;21(7):276-282.

156. Arnold CA, Roth R, Arsenescu R, et al. Sexually transmitted infectious colitis vs inflamma-tory bowel disease: distinguishing features from a case-controlled study. *Am J Clin Pathol.* 2015;144(5):771-781.

157. Tateishi Y, Takahashi M, Horiguchi S, et al. Clinicopathologic study of intestinal spirochetosis in Japan with special reference to human immunodeficiency virus infection status and species types: analysis of 5265 consecutive colorectal biopsies. *BMC Infect Dis.* 2015;15:13.

158. Teglbjaerg PS. Intestinal spirochaetosis. *Curr Top Pathol.* 1990;81:247-256.

159. McMillan A, Lee FD. Sigmoidoscopic and microscopic appearance of the rectal mucosa in homosexual men. *Gut.* 1981;22(12):1035-1041.

160. Cooper C, Cotton DW, Hudson MJ, Kirkham N, Wilmott FE. Rectal spirochaetosis in homosexual men: characterisation of the organism and pathophysiology. *Genitourin Med.* 1986;62(1):47-52.

161. Tsinganou E, Gebbers JO. Human intestinal spirochetosis—a review. *Ger Med Sci.* 2010;8:Doc01.

162. Koteish A, Kannangai R, Abraham SC, Torbenson M. Colonic spirochetosis in children and adults. *Am J Clin Pathol.* 2003;120(6):828-832.

163. Ogata S, Shimizu K, Oda T, Tominaga S, Nakanishi K. Immunohistochemical detection of human intestinal spirochetosis. *Hum Pathol.* 2016;58:128-133.

164. Ruiz SJ, Procop GW. Cross-reactivity of anti-Treponema immunohistochemistry with non-Trepo-nema spirochetes: a simple call for caution. *Arch Pathol Lab Med.* 2016;140(10):1021-1022.

CHAPTER OUTLINE

THE UNREMARKABLE ANUS

An understanding of the anal anatomy is important for correct staging and therapy (Figs. 5.1–5.6). In general terms, the anus is approximately 3 to 5 cm in length in the average adult, and it is interposed between the distal rectum and proximal perianal skin. The anus is derived from the fusion of the endodermal hindgut and ectodermal proctodeum at the dentate line. For most adults, the dentate line separates the upper two-thirds of the anal canal from the lower third. This landmark is clinically important because lymphatics proximal to the dentate line drain to the inferior mesenteric lymph nodes, whereas

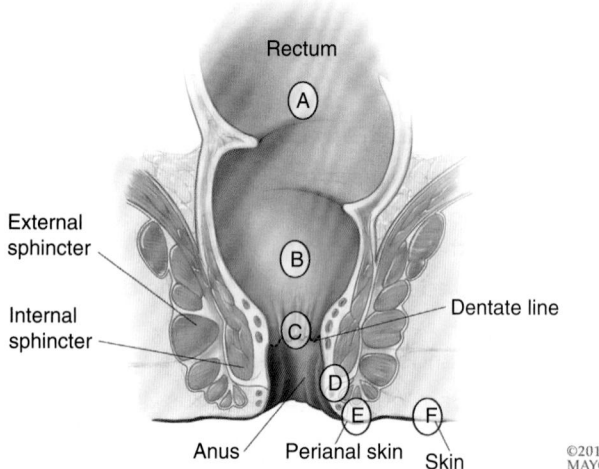

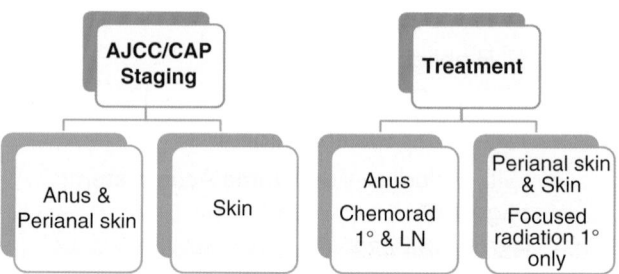

Figure 5-1. Anatomy of the anus, cartoon. The anus is interpositioned between the distal rectum and proximal perianal skin. The dentate line is an anatomic landmark that divides the upper two-thirds of the anus from the lower one-third. A: Neoplasms that arise above the anus are classified as rectal primaries. B–D: Neoplasms that originate in the anal canal that cannot be completely visualized with gentle retraction of the buttocks are classified as anal primaries. E: Neoplasms that arise within 5.0 cm of the anus that can be entirely visualized with gentle retraction of the buttocks are classified as perianal skin primaries. F: Skin neoplasms more than 5.0 cm distal to the anus are classified as skin primaries.

Figure 5-2. Correct anatomic designation is critical for staging and treatment, cartoon. Left Panel: Anal and perianal skin cancers are staged in the 2017 AJCC and CAP; skin cancers are separately staged. *Right panels*: For treatment purposes, perianal skin and skin cancers are treated similarly with focused irradiation without inclusion of regional lymph node groups, whereas anal cancers are treated with chemoradiation and the radiation targets the primary neoplasm and regional node groups.

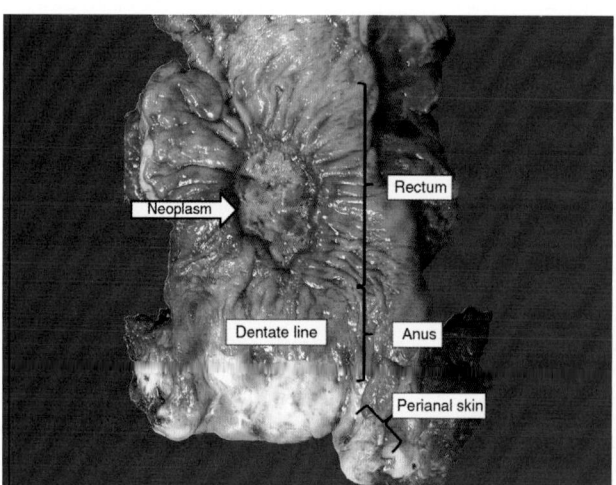

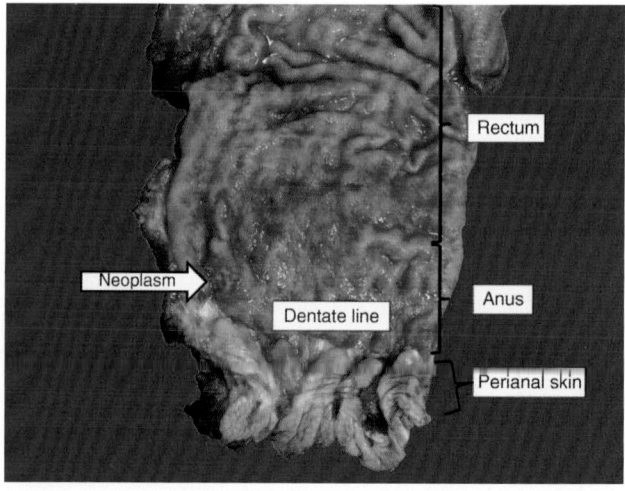

Figure 5-3. Rectal primary, colorectal and anal resection. Neoplasms that arise above the anus are classified as rectal primaries (*arrow*) and staged with colorectal primaries. The specimen was clinically designated a rectal cancer.

Figure 5-4. Anal primary, anal resection. Neoplasms that originate in the anal canal that cannot be completely visualized with gentle retraction of the buttocks are classified as anal primaries. The neoplasm in this case (*arrow*) is near the dentate line. Anal and perianal skin cancers are staged together based on size in the 2017 AJCC and CAP.

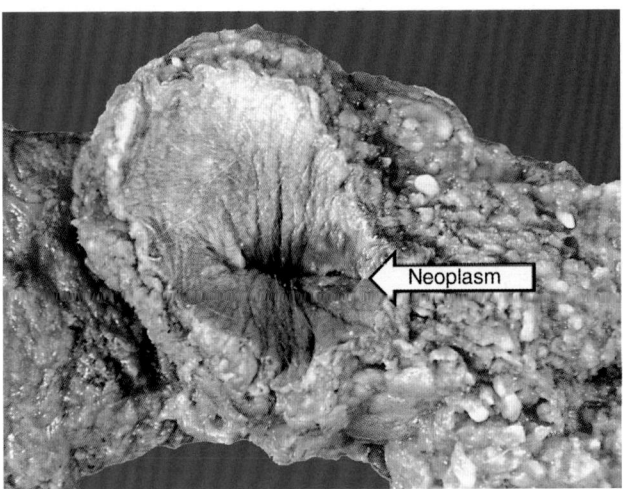

Figure 5-5. Perianal skin primary, anal resection, intact. Neoplasms (*arrow*) that arise within 5.0 cm of the anus that can be entirely visualized with gentle retraction of the buttocks are classified as perianal skin primaries. Neoplasms that involve the skin more than 5.0 cm from the anus are staged separately as skin tumors. For treatment purposes, perianal skin and skin cancers are treated similarly with focused irradiation without inclusion of regional lymph node groups.

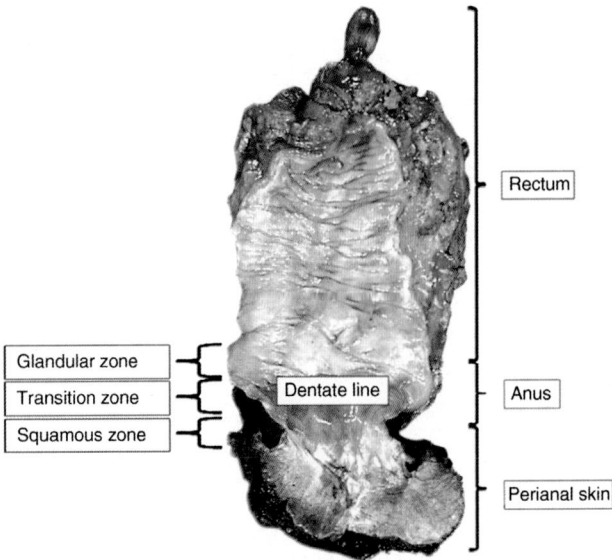

Figure 5-6. Perianal skin primary, anal resection, longitudinal section of the previous figure. The anus is subdivided into three zones based on the type of mucosa present: the glandular zone, the anal transition zone, and the squamous zone. The perianal skin consists of nonkeratinizing squamous mucosa with appendages.

lymphatics distal to the dentate line drain to the internal iliac and inguinal nodes. The dentate line is grossly defined by the undulating anal mucosal columns with their papillae and sinuses; the latter structures become obscured with age. Three of the anal columns are prominent and are called "anal cushions" (left lateral, right posterior, and right anterior columns). The anal cushions are normal structures that function in anal closure. They contain branches of the superior rectal artery and vein, and their slippage from the anchoring connective tissue results in "hemorrhoids" (see "Nondysplastic Polyps" section). Ganglion cells and interstitial cells of Cajal are generally absent (or markedly decreased) in the anus.

Like the rest of the tubular gastrointestinal (GI) tract, the anus consists of a mucosa (epithelium, lamina propria, muscularis mucosae), submucosa, and external muscle layer (Fig. 5.7). The anus can be subdivided into three zones based on the type of mucosa present (Fig. 5.8). The most proximal zone is the glandular zone: it consists exclusively of colorectal-lined mucosa and appears grossly tan (Figs. 5.6 and 5.9–5.14). Next, the anal transition zone (ATZ) spans uninterrupted colorectal mucosa above and uninterrupted squamous mucosa below; it appears grossly brown-pink. The ATZ mucosa is 4 to 9 cell layers of small, squamoid cells that appear variably flat, cuboidal, columnar, or polygonal (Figs. 5.15–5.21). A familiarity with the normal ATZ morphology is important to avoid overcalling dysplasia. Although the ATZ is normally cellular and a bit dark, histologically unremarkable ATZ lacks cells with coarse nuclear chromatin, irregular nuclear borders, prominent nucleoli, and abundant mitoses that would be expected in dysplasia. See also "HPV-Associated Neoplasms" section. Anal ducts are seen near the dentate line, and they are lined by epithelium similar to that of the ATZ mucosa (Figs. 5.8 and 5.22–5.30). Anal ducts transmit secretions from the anal glands to the luminal surface of the anus, and they can be identified anywhere along their course to the mucosa. They occasionally raise concerns for adenocarcinoma to those not familiar with their characteristic morphology. Clues to their benignity include their lobular architecture, absence of desmoplasia, and bland cytology that lacks prominent mitotic figures and pleomorphism. Scattered goblet cells can be seen. The most distal zone is the squamous zone. It consists exclusively of nonkeratinizing squamous-lined mucosa devoid of appendages, such as sweat glands, sebaceous glands, apocrine glands, and hair follicles (Figs. 5.31–5.36) and appears grossly gray-white. Normal squamous epithelium can have abundant, clear cytoplasm with vague nuclear halos (Figs. 5.32–5.36), raising concerns for dysplasia. Helpful features of a reactive (not dysplastic) change include the lack of hyperchromasia,

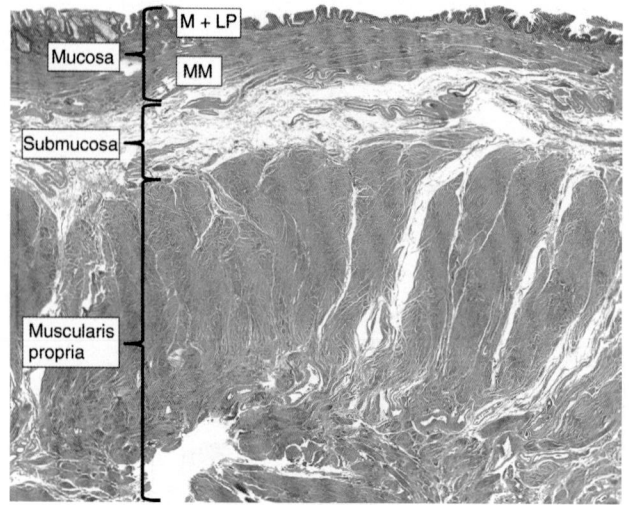

Figure 5-7. The layers of the anus. Like the rest of the tubular GI tract, the anus consists of three layers: a mucosa (epithelium, lamina propria, muscularis mucosae), submucosa, and external muscle layer. The internal sphincter is a continuation of the muscularis propria of the rectum; it is composed of smooth muscle and is under involuntary control. The external most muscle is the external sphincter; it consists of skeletal muscle and is under voluntary control (not shown). The anal longitudinal muscle sits between the internal and external anal sphincter and is composed of a combination of smooth and skeletal muscle (not shown).

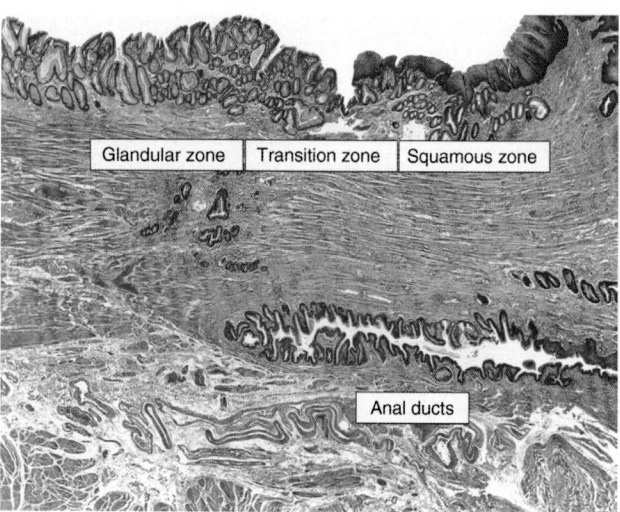

Figure 5-8. The mucosal zones of the anus. The anus is divided into three zones based on the type of mucosa present. The most proximal zone is the glandular zone: it consists exclusively of colorectal-lined mucosa. Next, the anal transition zone (ATZ) spans uninterrupted colorectal mucosa above and uninterrupted squamous mucosa below. Anal ducts are lined by epithelium similar to the ATZ mucosa. The most distal zone is the squamous zone: it consists of nonkeratinizing squamous-lined mucosa devoid of appendages. The perianal skin (not shown) consists of nonkeratinizing squamous mucosa with appendages.

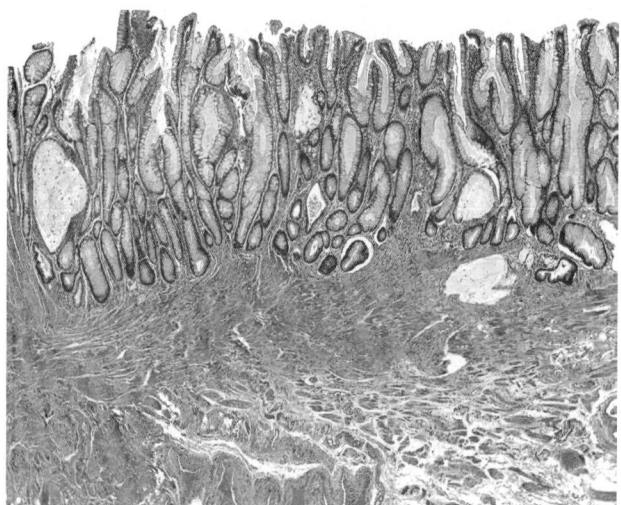

Figure 5-9. Proximal (glandular) zone. The most proximal zone is histologically identical to the rectum. This glandular mucosa is normally a bit more distorted than that of the colon, as seen here with the variably sized and positioned glands.

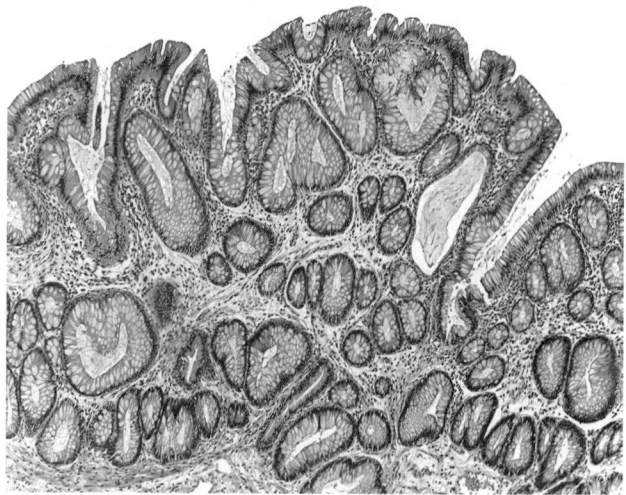

Figure 5-10. Proximal (glandular) zone. Higher power shows the slightly disordered look to the anal glandular zone. This appearance is normal and is not a feature of chronic injury.

irregular nuclear contours ("raisinoid" nuclei), and binucleate cells (compare with Figs. 5.91–5.130). The squamous mucocutaneous junction is formed from the merging of the squamous zone with the perianal skin; the latter consists of nonkeratinizing squamous mucosa with associated appendages (Figs. 5.37–5.43). The perianal skin is grossly wrinkled with hair and histologically indistinguishable from skin at other sites. The lengths of these zones vary from person to person and with age. See Fig. 5.44 for a side-by-side comparison of all thee mucosal zones of the anus and the perianal skin. The external aspect of the anus is encased in thick muscle bundles. The internal sphincter is a continuation of the muscularis propria of the rectum. Accordingly, it is composed of smooth

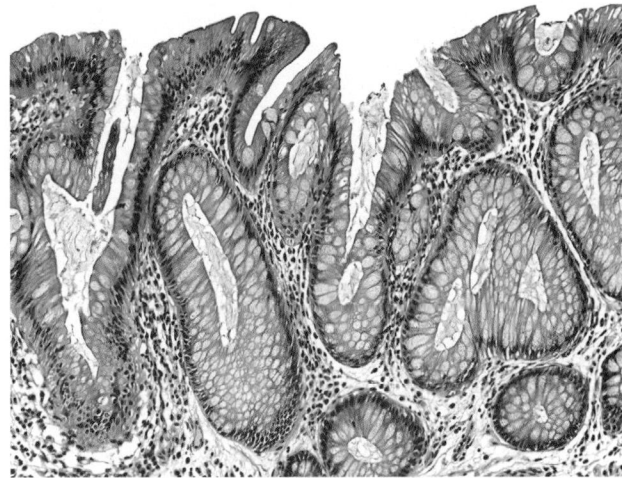

Figure 5-11. Proximal (glandular) zone.

Figure 5-12. Proximal (glandular) zone.

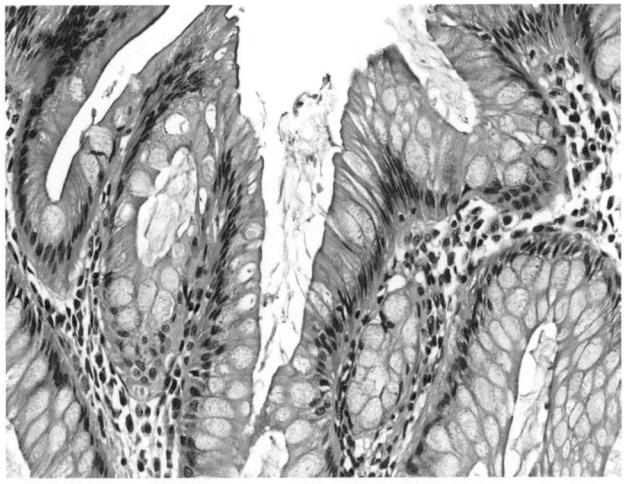

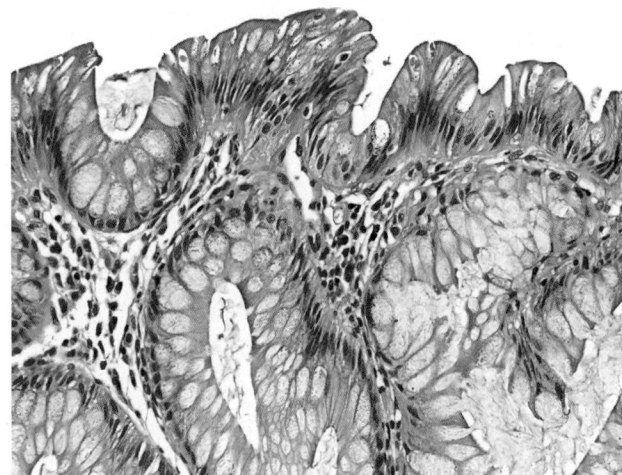

Figure 5-13. Proximal (glandular) zone. Highest power shows the expected small, bland nuclei and abundant cytoplasm of the unremarkable glandular zone.

Figure 5-14. Proximal (glandular) zone.

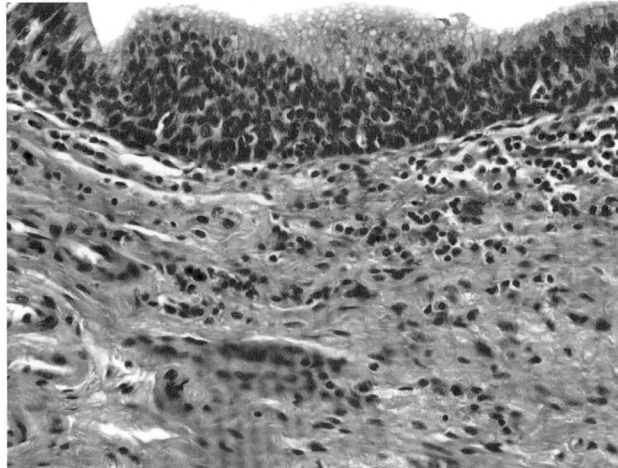

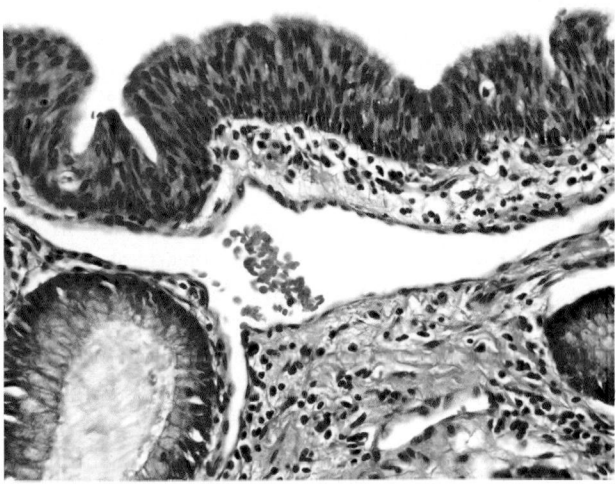

Figure 5-15. Anal transition zone (ATZ). The ATZ is positioned between the proximal glandular zone and the distal squamous zone. The ATZ mucosa is composed of 4–9 cell layers of small, squamoid cells that appear variably flat, cuboidal, columnar, or polygonal, as seen here.

Figure 5-16. Anal transition zone (ATZ). The ATZ is normally cellular and a bit dark. It occasionally raises concerns for dysplasia, but the normal ATZ lacks cells with coarse chromatin, irregular nuclear borders, prominent nucleoli, and abundant mitoses that would be expected in dysplasia. See also "HPV-Associated Neoplasms" section.

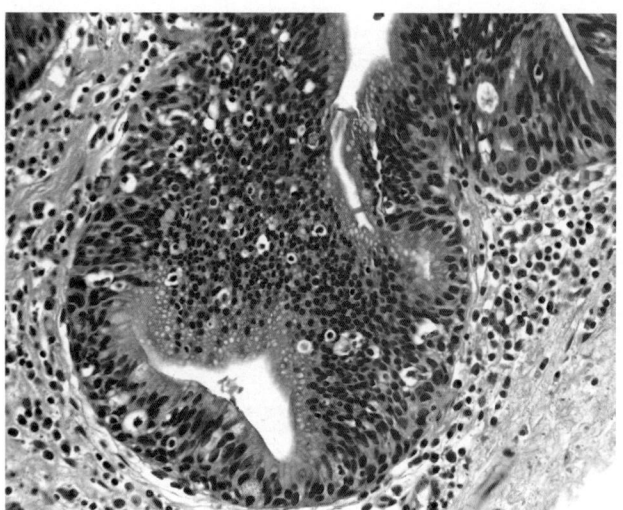

Figure 5-17. Anal transition zone (ATZ). This ATZ appears vaguely cribriforming but represents folds of nondysplastic mucosa. Note the smooth, normochromatic chromatin characteristic of histologically unremarkable ATZ.

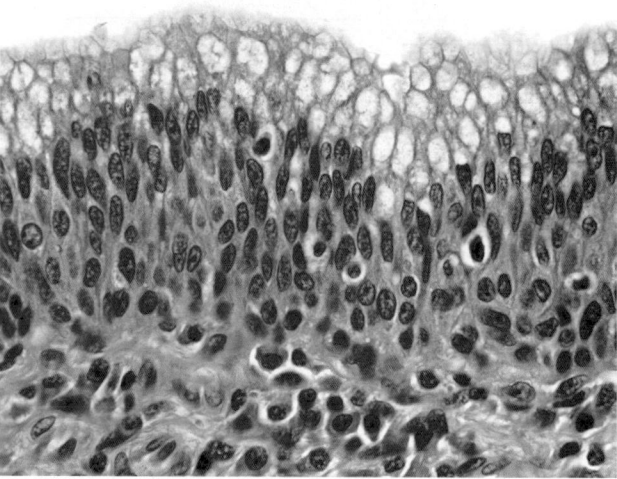

Figure 5-18. Anal transition zone (ATZ). On higher power, the normal ATZ consists of small cells with an orderly arrangement. The normochromatic chromatin is lighter than that of the subjacent plasma cells, and the nuclei display regular nuclear borders and inconspicuous nucleoli, and mitotic figures are not prominent.

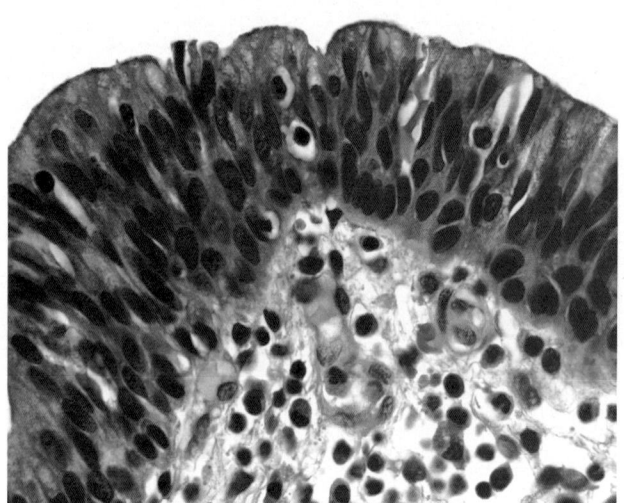

Figure 5-19. Anal transition zone (ATZ). Although this is a thick and dark section, note that the chromatin of the ATZ is lighter than that of the subjacent plasma cells, an important clue that this focus represents histologically unremarkable ATZ, negative for dysplasia.

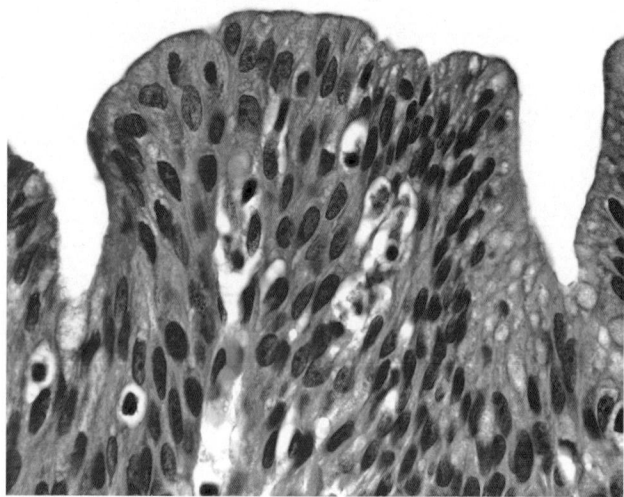

Figure 5-20. Anal transition zone (ATZ). In challenging cases of histologically unremarkable ATZ versus high-grade squamous intraepithelial lesion (HSIL) a p16 can be helpful (negative in normal ATZ, positive in HSIL; see also "HPV-Associated Neoplasms" section).

muscle and is under involuntary control. The external most muscle is the external sphincter. It consists of skeletal muscle and is under voluntary control. The anal longitudinal muscle sits between the internal and external anal sphincter and is composed of a combination of smooth and skeletal muscle.[1] It is involved in sphincter contraction, bridging the internal and external sphincter both spatially and functionally.

Most malignancies involving the anus and perianal skin are squamous cell carcinomas, discussed in detail in the subsequent sections. Correct classification of tumors as anal versus perianal versus skin cancers is important for staging and therapy. Technically, the anal canal begins at the point where the rectum enters the puborectalis sling at the apex of the anal sphincter complex and terminates at the squamous mucocutaneous junction. According to the 2017 American Joint Committee on Cancer (AJCC), neoplasms that originate in the anal canal that cannot be completely visualized with gentle retraction of

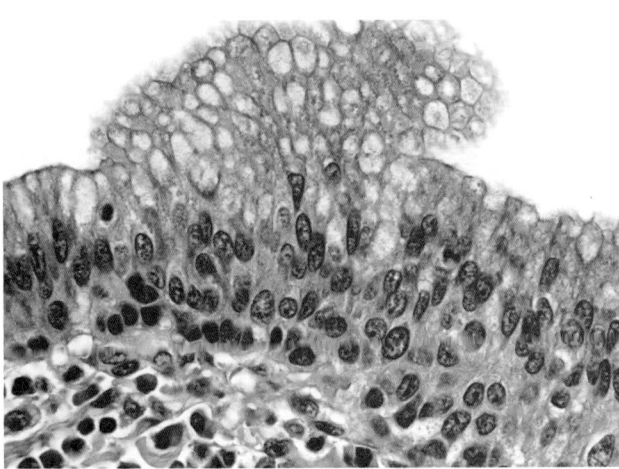

Figure 5-21. Anal transition zone.

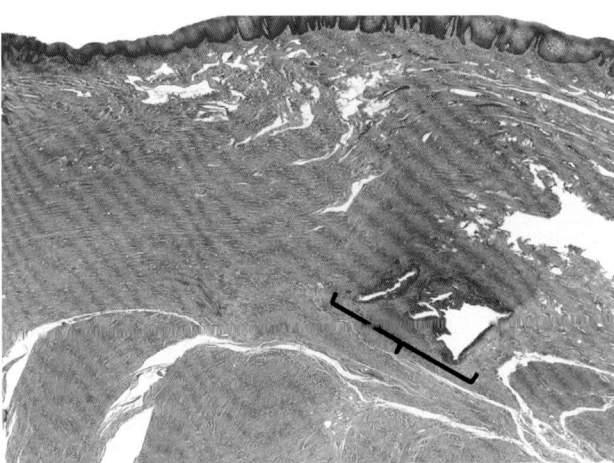

Figure 5-22. Anal ducts. Anal ducts (*bracket*) are seen in the region of the dentate line anywhere along their course from or to the mucosa. Clues to their benignity include their lobular architecture, absence of desmoplasia, and bland cytology that lacks prominent mitotic figures and pleomorphism.

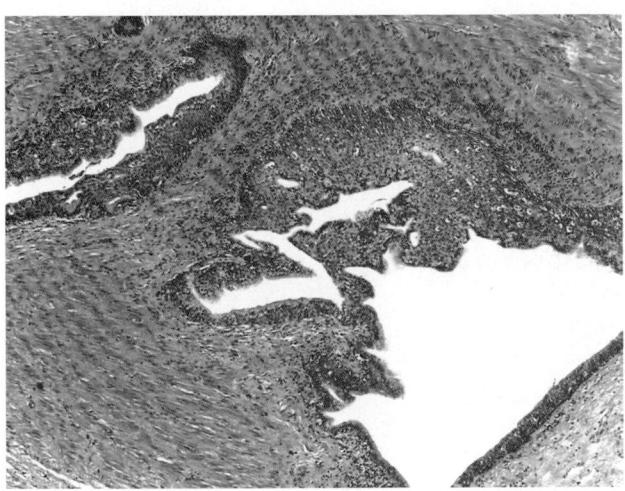

Figure 5-23. Anal ducts. Higher power of the previous figure. Note their typical lobular architecture and absence of desmoplasia.

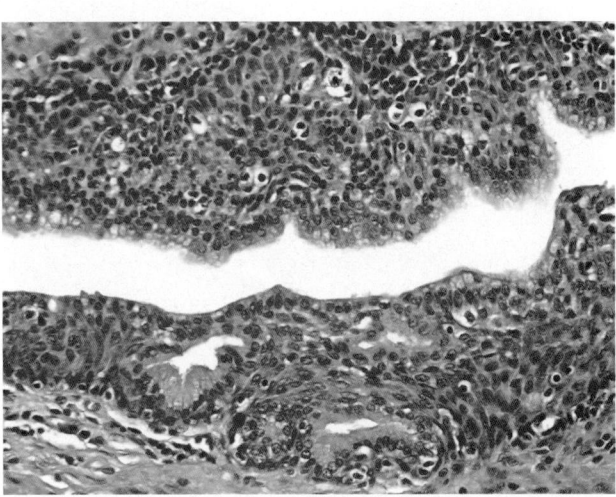

Figure 5-24. Anal ducts. Highest power of the previous figure. Anal ducts are lined by epithelium similar to that in the ATZ mucosa. Note their typical bland cytology that lacks prominent mitotic figures and pleomorphism.

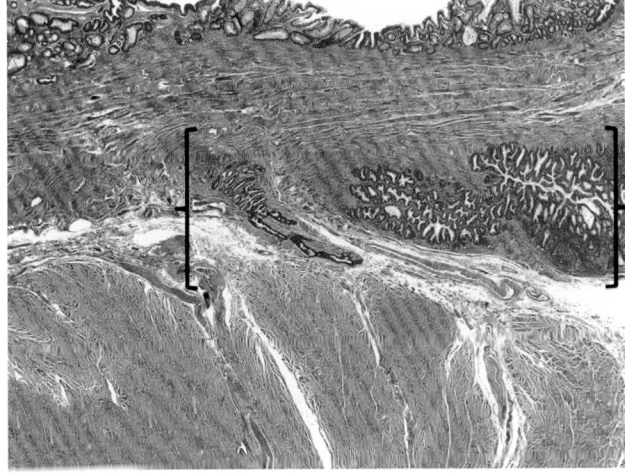

Figure 5-25. Anal ducts (*brackets*). Note their typical lobular architecture and absence of desmoplasia as they traverse the muscularis mucosae in their course to the luminal surface.

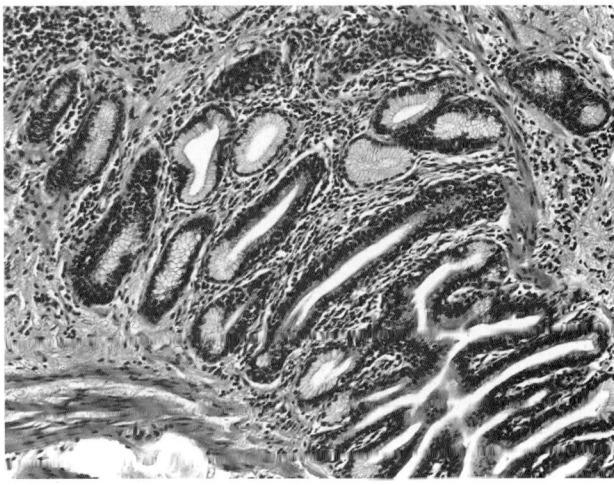

Figure 5-26. Anal ducts. Higher power of the previous figure.

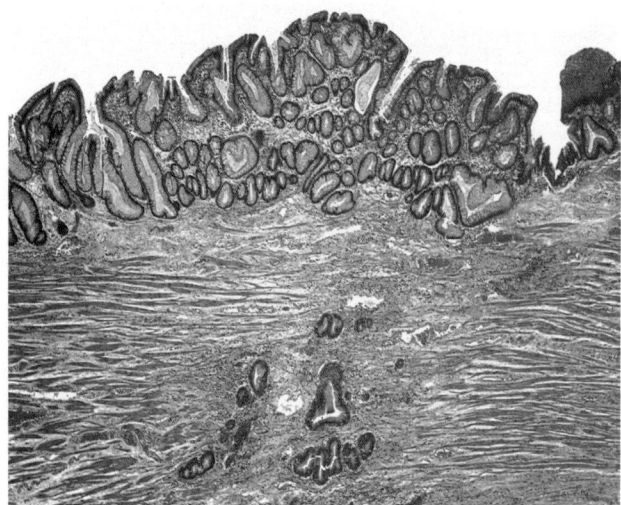

Figure 5-27. Anal ducts.

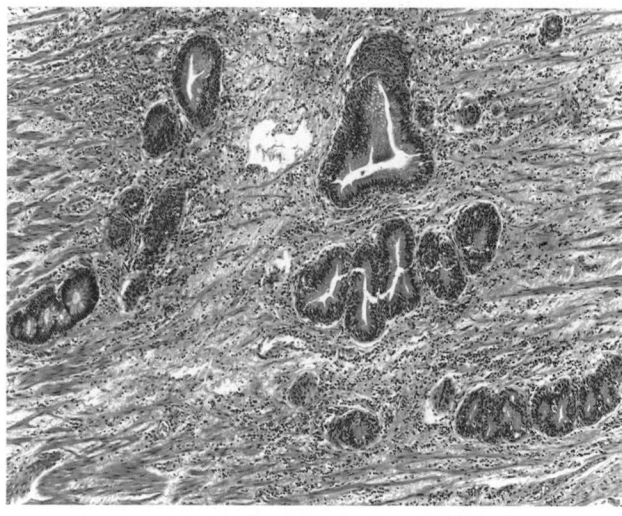

Figure 5-28. Anal ducts. Higher power of the previous figure.

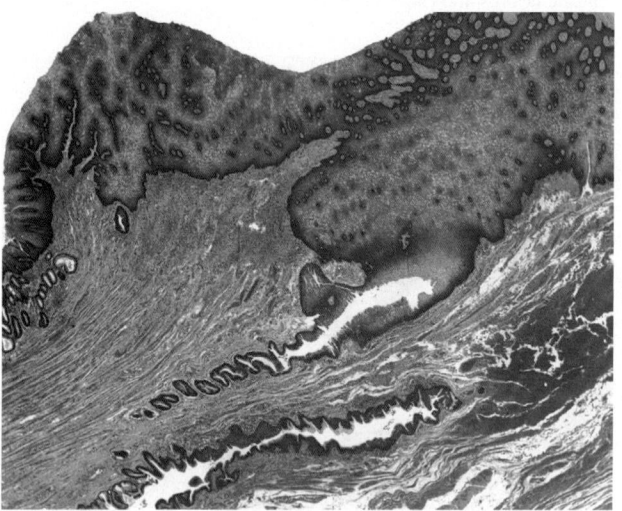

Figure 5-29. Anal ducts. In this rare example, the anal ducts are seen piercing the muscularis mucosae and connecting to the surface.

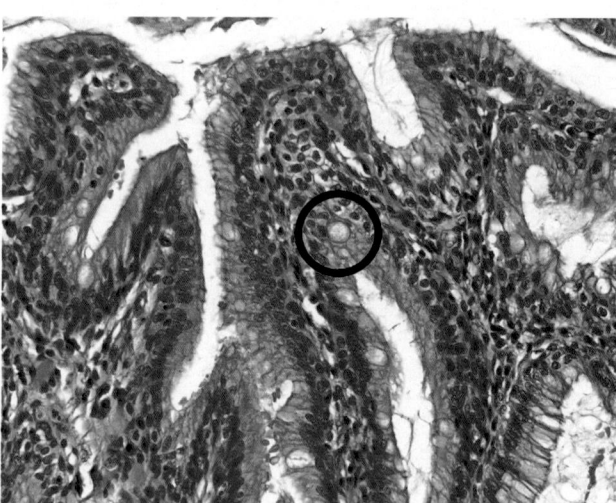

Figure 5-30. Anal ducts. Higher power of the previous figure. Goblet cells can occasionally be seen (*circle*).

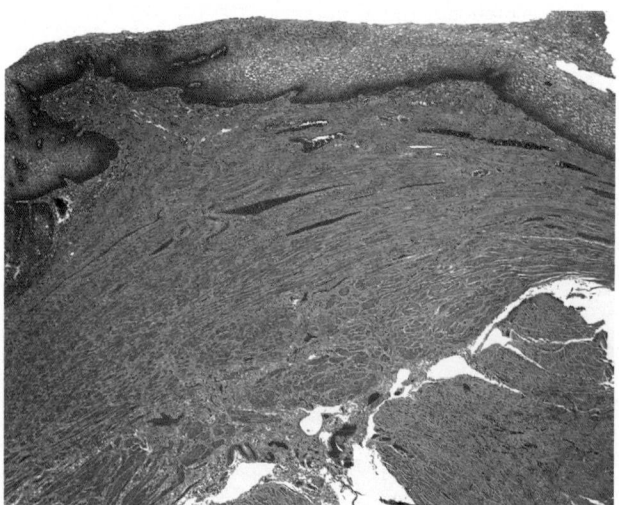

Figure 5-31. Distal (squamous) zone. The most distal zone is the squamous zone. It consists exclusively of nonkeratinizing squamous-lined mucosa devoid of appendages, such as sweat glands, sebaceous glands, apocrine glands, and hair follicles, as seen here.

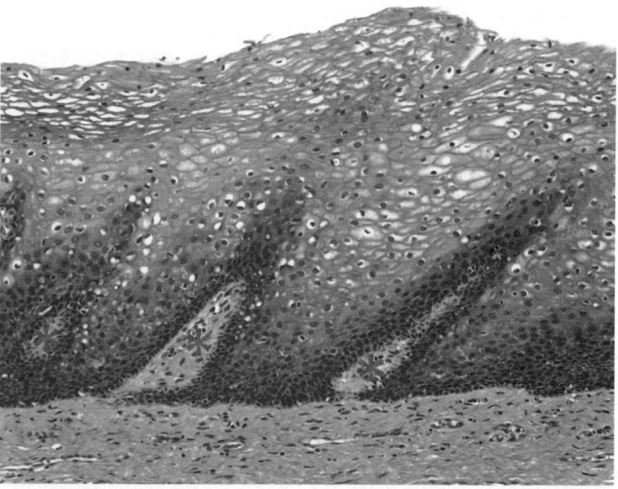

Figure 5-32. Distal (squamous) zone. Higher power of the previous figure. Note the undulating basal papilla (*asterisks*) that defines the interface of the deepest aspect of the epithelium and the lamina propria. An understanding of this boundary is important for dysplasia grading in "HPV-Associated Neoplasms" section.

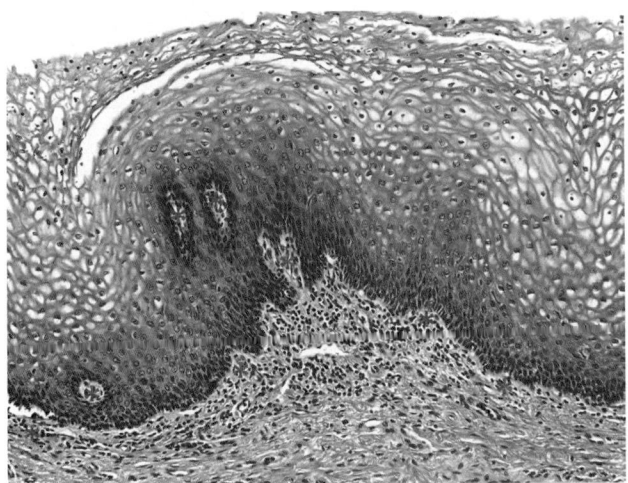

Figure 5-33. Distal (squamous) zone. Normal squamous epithelium can have abundant, clear cytoplasm with vague nuclear halos, raising concerns for dysplasia. Helpful features of a reactive (not dysplastic) change include the lack of nuclei with hyperchromatic, irregular nuclear contours (raisinoid nuclei), and binucleation, as seen here (compare with and see also Figs. 5.37–5.73). *Asterisks* define the interface of the deepest aspect of the epithelium and the lamina propria.

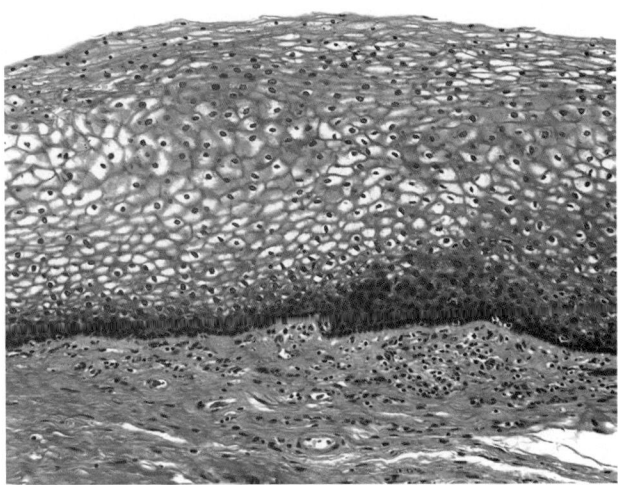

Figure 5-34. Distal (squamous) zone.

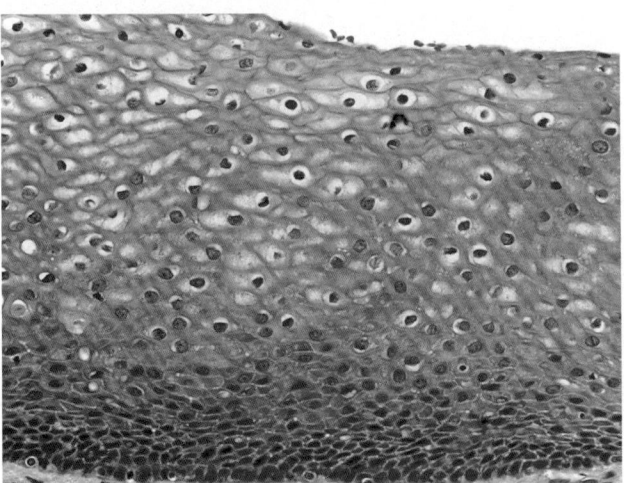

Figure 5-35. Distal (squamous) zone.

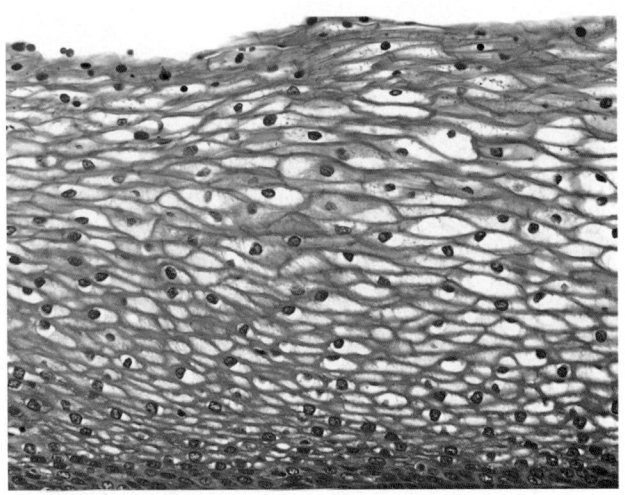

Figure 5-36. Distal (squamous) zone.

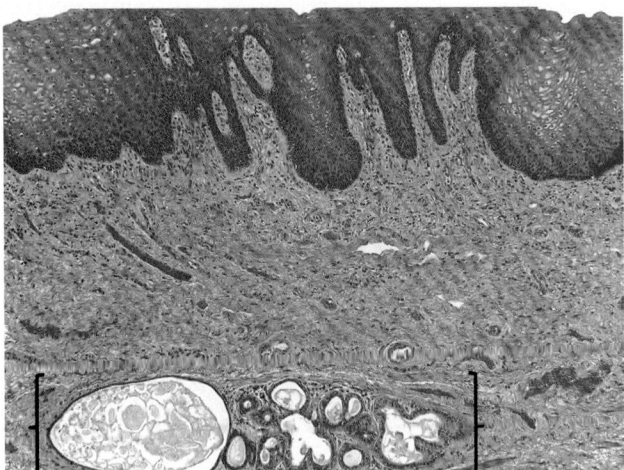

Figure 5-37. Perianal skin. The perianal skin contains skin appendages (*brackets*), which distinguish it from the anal distal squamous zone that lacks appendages.

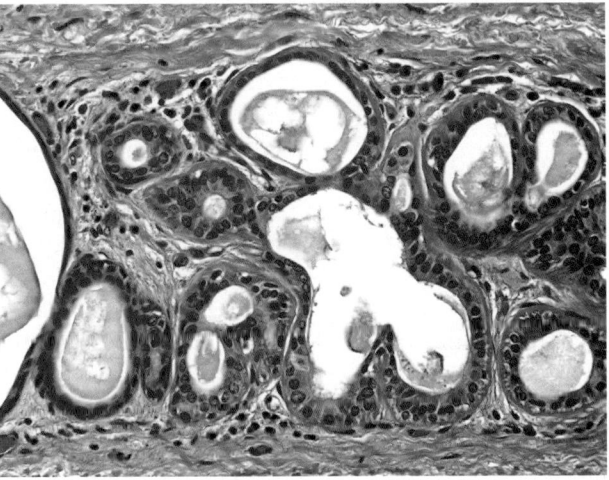

Figure 5-38. Perianal skin. Higher power of the previous figure shows a lobular collection of eccrine appendages. Eccrine glands (sweat glands) function in thermoregulation.

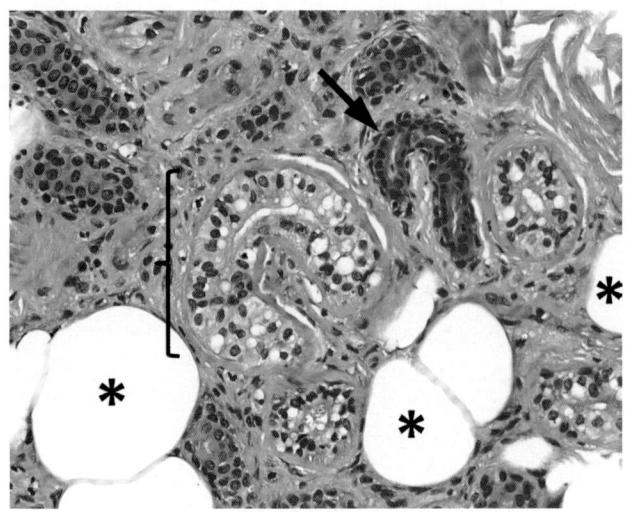

Figure 5-39. Perianal skin. The typical configuration of eccrine structures includes a combination of eccrine glands (*bracket*, abundant pale cytoplasm), eccrine ducts (*arrow*, darker cytoplasm, smaller cell), and admixed fat (*asterisks*).

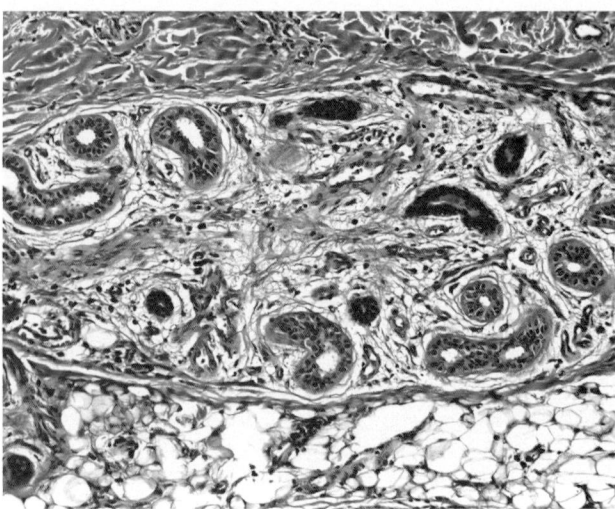

Figure 5-40. Perianal skin with eccrine glands and ducts.

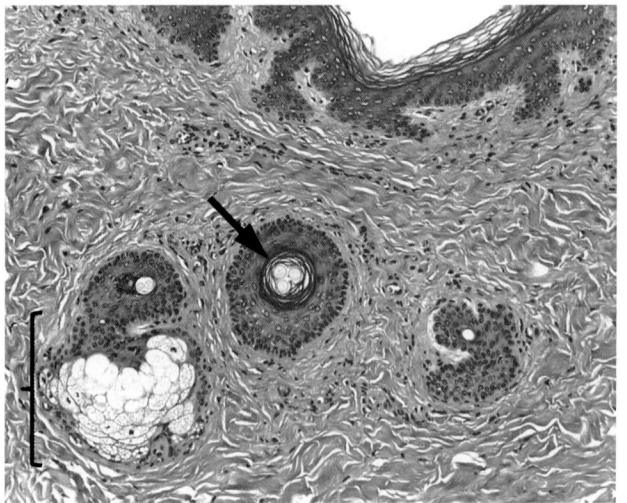

Figure 5-41. Perianal skin with a sebaceous gland and hair. Sebaceous glands (*bracket*) express their lipid-rich secretions into their adjoining hair follicle (*arrow*).

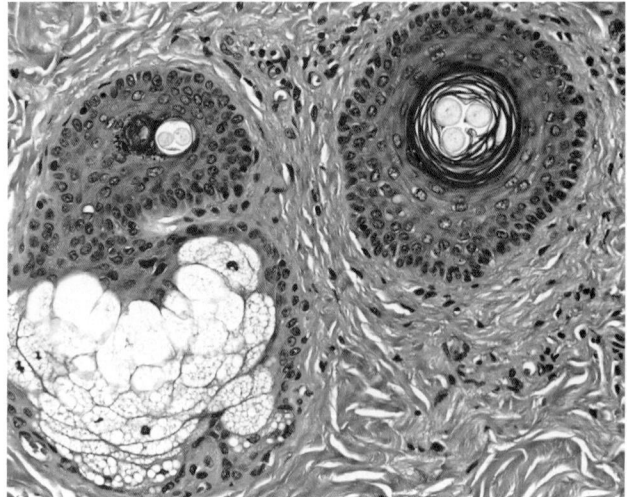

Figure 5-42. Perianal skin with a sebaceous gland and hair. Higher power of the previous figure. A sebaceous gland is composed of a lobular collection of sebocytes that display prominent, vacuolated cytoplasm and cuboidal nuclei, as seen here.

the buttocks are classified "anal cancers."[2] Neoplasms that arise at or distal to the squamous mucocutaneous junction within 5.0 cm of the anus that can be entirely visualized with gentle retraction of the buttocks are classified "perianal cancers," which are associated with a better prognosis than anal cancer.[3] "Skin cancers" refer to skin neoplasms that are more than 5.0 cm distal to the anus. Clearly, these landmarks are impossible to discern by the pathologist. As such, relying on the surgeon's in vivo impressions is key to accurate staging as anal, perianal, or skin cancer. Handy fact alert!: the new 2017 AJCC and College of American Pathologists (CAP) both lump the staging of anal and perianal cancers together based on size:

pT1 Neoplasm ≤2 cm
pT2 Neoplasm >2 cm but ≤5 cm
pT3 Neoplasm >5 cm
pT4 Neoplasm of any size invading adjacent organ(s), such as vagina, urethra, or bladder[2,4]

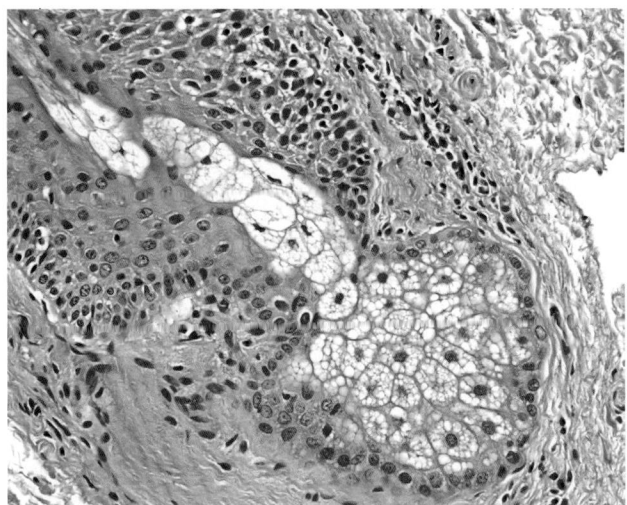

Figure 5-43. Perianal skin with a sebaceous gland. Because peri-anal skin cannot be distinguished from that at any other cutaneous site, it is important to rely on the clinician's anatomic designation for staging perianal and skin cancers. Recall that perianal skin cancers are staged with anal cancers but are treated like skin cancers, assuming they are not deeply invasive.

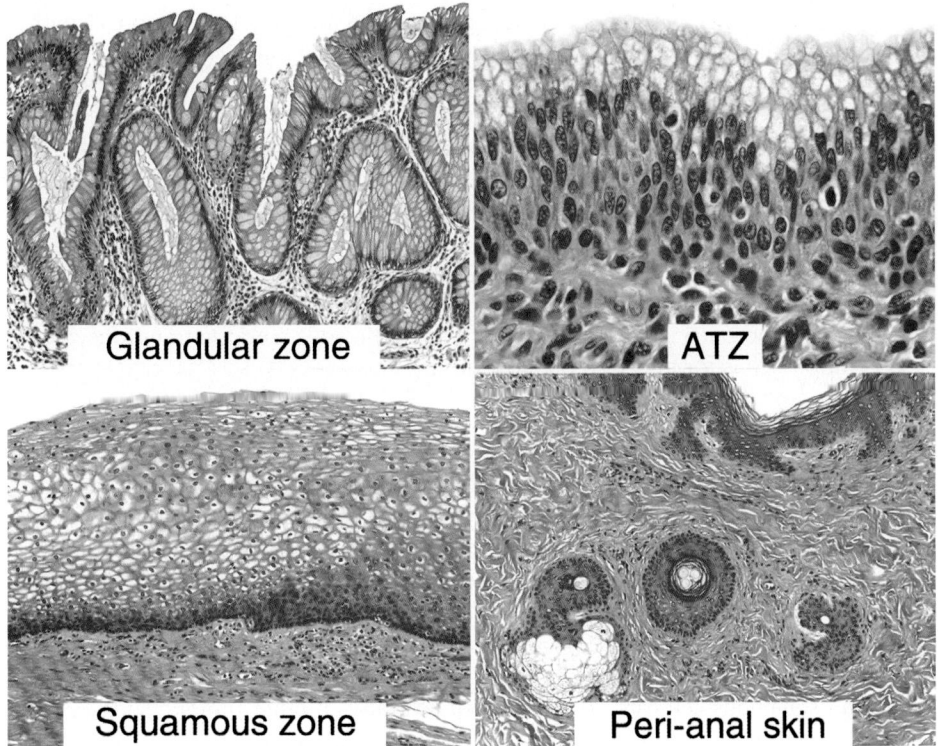

Figure 5-44. Anal zone composite. The anus can be subdivided into three zones based on the type of mucosa present. The most proximal zone is the glandular zone, and it consists exclusively of colorectal-lined-type mucosa. Next, the anal transition zone (ATZ) spans uninterrupted colorectal-type mucosa above and uninterrupted squamous mucosa below. The most distal zone is the squamous zone. It consists exclusively of nonkeratinizing squamous-lined mucosa devoid of appendages, such as sweat glands, sebaceous glands, apocrine glands, and hair follicles. The perianal skin is distinguished from the anal squamous zone by the presence of skin appendages.

Direct invasion of the perianal skin, subcutaneous tissue, sphincter muscle, or rectal wall is not classified as pT4. Neoplasms involving the skin more than 5.0 cm distal to the anus are staged as skin cancers. This staging scheme does not apply to anal melanoma (not staged in AJCC), well-differentiated neuroendocrine tumor (not staged in AJCC), lymphoma (consider lymphoma staging), and sarcoma, including gastrointestinal stromal tumor (GIST; consider sarcoma staging).[2] Anal cancers are rarely resected because they are usually successfully treated with a combination of chemotherapy and radiation therapy. Irradiation of anal cancers targets the primary neoplasm and regional node groups. In contrast, tumors designated perianal and skin cancers are treated with focused irradiation without inclusion of regional lymph node groups, assuming there is no deep invasion. Deep invasion of perianal and skin neoplasms warrants additional irradiation of regional lymph node groups.

PEARLS & PITFALLS: Lower Anterior Resections, Abdominoperineal Resections, and Transanal Versus Transcoccygeal Excision

Here are a few descriptions of common abbreviations of surgical procedures involving the rectum and anus.

1. Lower anterior resections (LARs) are a type of surgical resection for patients with a malignancy involving the upper two-thirds of the rectum. In this procedure, the malignancy is removed along with the rectum and regional lymph nodes. LARs are preferred over abdominoperineal resections (APRs) because the anal sphincter remains intact, and the patient maintains normal bowel function.

2. Abdominoperineal resections (APRs) are a type of surgical resection for patients with a malignancy close to or involving the anus, with regional lymph node excision indicated. In this procedure, the malignancy is removed along with the rectum, anus (including anal sphincter), and regional lymph nodes. Because the anal sphincter is sacrificed, there is a loss of normal bowel function, a permanent colostomy, and a significant quality of life adjustment for the patient.

3. Limited sphincter-sparing procedures are offered to a subset of patients with malignancies close to the anus. Such patients either have a low-stage lesion, negative lymph node involvement by ultrasonography, and a well-differentiated morphology, *or* are unable to tolerate an LAR or APR. The transanal approach is for tumors very close to the anus, and the transcoccygeal approach is for tumors a bit closer to the rectum.

Anal lesions comprise less than 1% of GI specimens. Although they are infrequent, or maybe because they are infrequent, they can be challenging. The anus is an especially interesting site because theoretically any benign or malignant process that involves the adjacent GI tract or skin can invade the anus. For example, rectal tumors can dip down and involve the anus, and cutaneous processes can extend upward into the anus. Developmental cysts and gastric, prostatic, and breast heterotopias can present as anal polyps or masses. The anus can serve as a primary site for melanoma, GIST, Kaposi sarcoma, and squamous cell carcinomas, as well as a host of other tumors, such as Paget disease, basal cell carcinoma (BCC), granular cell tumors, leiomyomas, and hematolymphoid lesions. Keep in mind that metastasis can also involve the anus and genital tract lesions can spread directly to the anus. As a result of these varied processes, it is important to maintain a broad differential diagnosis and careful approach. Below is a practical approach to the most common anal specimens. See also "Colon" and "Mesenchymal Lesions" chapters.

NONDYSPLASTIC POLYPS

HEMORRHOIDS

Although hemorrhoids are not neoplastic, they are featured in this chapter because they are the most common anal specimen encountered and they can contain or mimic neoplasms. They are associated with fiber-poor diets, obesity, portal hypertension, and pregnancy. Common symptoms include anal discomfort, bleeding, pruritus, and pain. Recall, the three anal cushions are derived from three anal columns (left lateral, right posterior, and right anterior columns). They are physiologic structures important for continence via closure of the anus and contain branches of the superior rectal artery and vein (hemorrhoidal plexus). With age and chronic constipation, the anchoring connective tissue within these cushions erodes and results in slippage or prolapse of the anal cushions (hemorrhoids). Hemorrhoids above the dentate line involve the superior hemorrhoidal plexus and are termed "internal hemorrhoids." These are painless and result in bright red blood per rectum. The degree of prolapse of internal hemorrhoids determines the clinical classification[5]:

Grade I: No prolapse; only prominent blood vascularity
Grade II: Prolapse upon bowel movements or straining with spontaneous reduction
Grade III: Prolapse upon bowel movements or straining, require manual reduction
Grade IV: Irreducible prolapse

Hemorrhoids below the dentate line involve the inferior hemorrhoidal plexus and are termed "external hemorrhoids." These can be painful, particularly when thrombosed. There is no grading scheme for external hemorrhoids. Treatment is initially conservative for smaller hemorrhoids with high-fiber diets, increased fluid intake, topical creams, stool softeners, sitz baths, and increased exercise. Patients who fail conservative therapy are eligible for banding procedures, sclerotherapy, or surgical excision. Typical histologic findings include engorged vascular spaces encased in prominent fibroconnective tissue (Figs. 5.45–5.54). Organizing thrombi are common, and overlying ulceration can be seen. The overlying mucosa can be columnar, ATZ, and/or squamous. Make sure to carefully examine the mucosa for other pathology, such as dysplasia, colitis, amyloidosis, and malignancy.

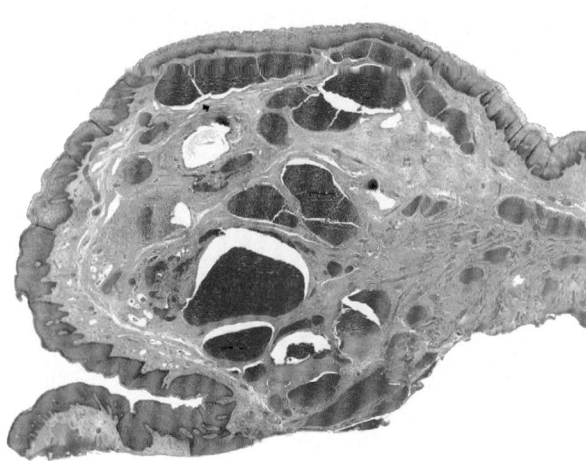

Figure 5-45. Hemorrhoid. Hemorrhoids are the most common anal specimen encountered in most practices. Their typical 1X morphology shows a nodular specimen with prominent vasculature and intervening connective tissue, as seen here.

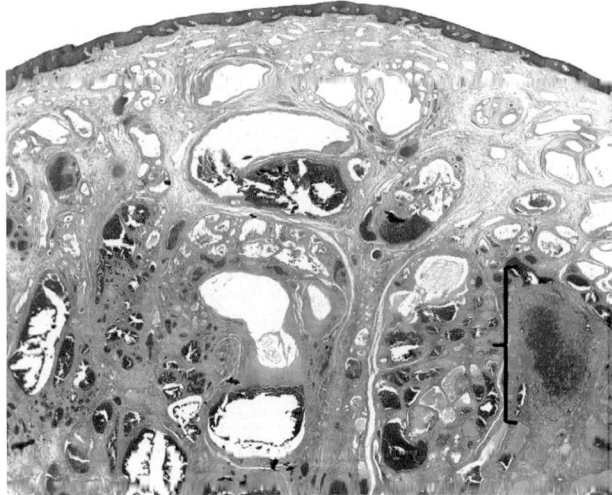

Figure 5-46. Hemorrhoid with organizing thrombus. The occasionally extreme pain associated with thrombosed hemorrhoids (*bracket*) is a common indication for their removal.

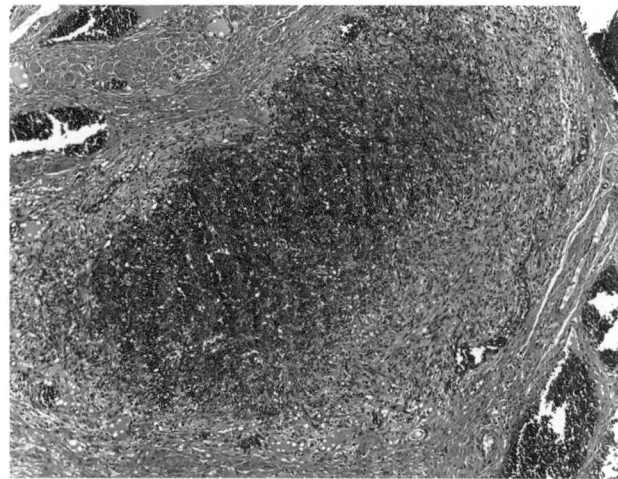

Figure 5-47. Hemorrhoid with organizing thrombus. Higher power of the previous figure. The organizing thrombus has central hemorrhage with organizing myofibroblasts.

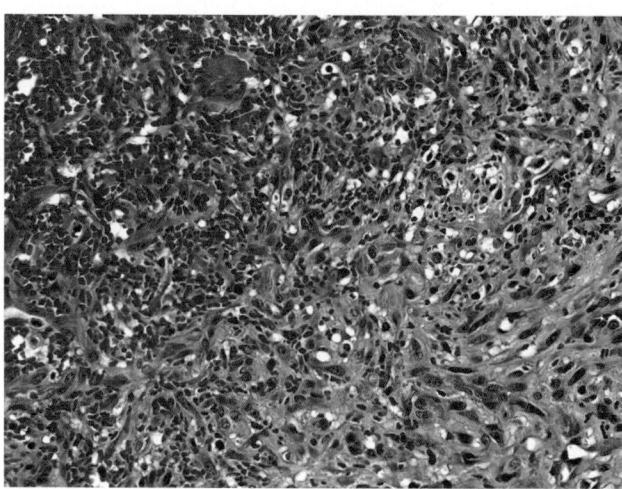

Figure 5-48. Hemorrhoid with organizing thrombus. Higher power of the previous figure. Although this focus is visually busy, the cellularity is within normal for an organizing thrombus and no atypia is seen.

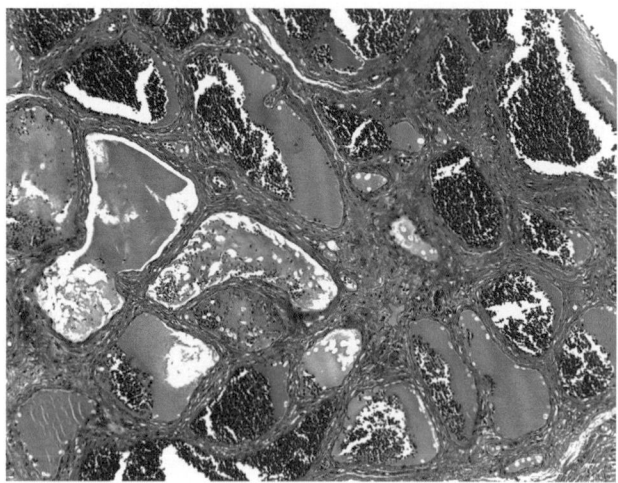

Figure 5-49. Hemorrhoid. On higher power, note that the vascular spaces have no muscular wall, as would be expected for veins and arteries. These vascular spaces are referred to as a "hemorrhoidal plexus" that derive from branches of the superior rectal artery and vein.

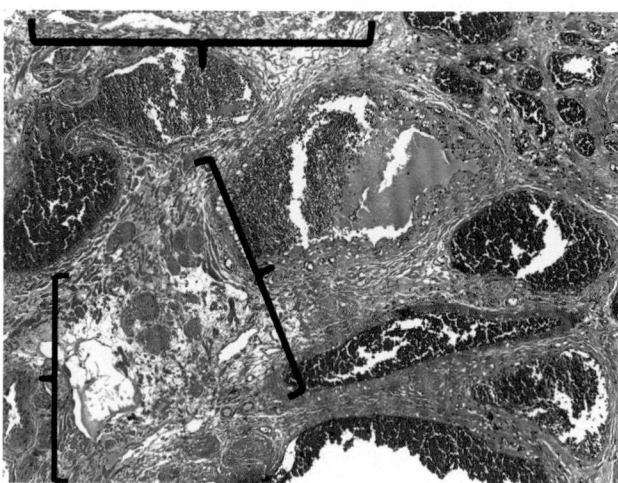

Figure 5-50. Hemorrhoid. Junior trainees often mistakenly consider hemorrhoids as simply engorged vasculature, but they consist of prolapsed vasculature and fibroconnective tissue (*brackets*) from the anal cushions.

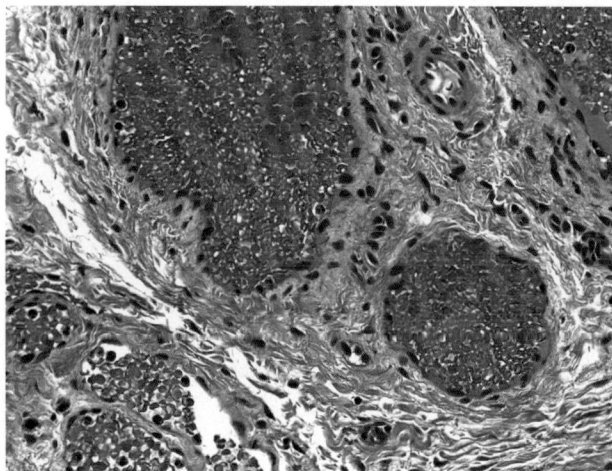

Figure 5-51. Hemorrhoid. High power shows the bland endothelial lining of a hemorrhoid.

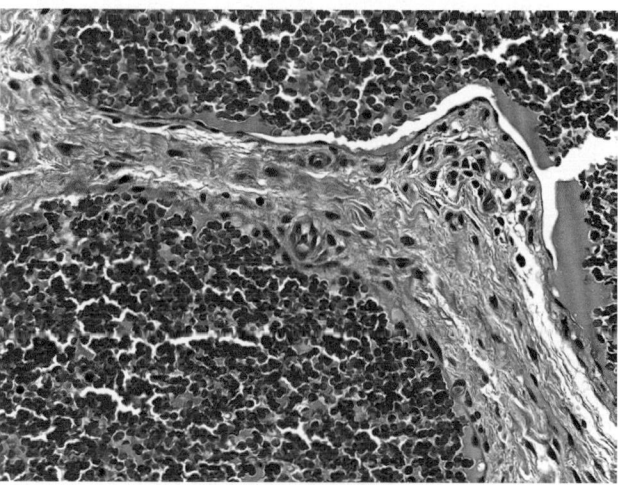

Figure 5-52. Hemorrhoid. High power shows the bland endothelial lining of a hemorrhoid.

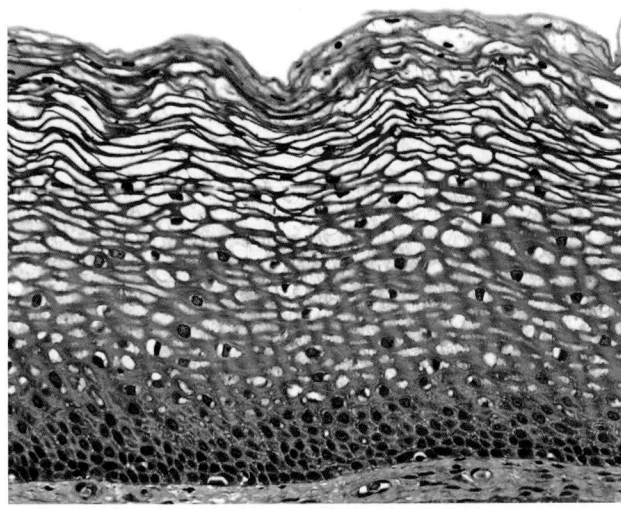

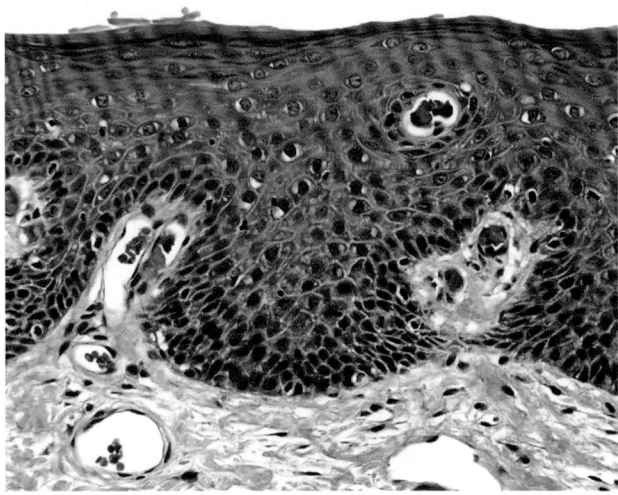

Figure 5-53. Unremarkable overlying squamous mucosa in a hemorrhoid. The overlying mucosa can be columnar, ATZ, and or squamous. Make sure to carefully examine the mucosa for other pathology, such as dysplasia, colitis, or malignancy.

Figure 5-54. Unremarkable overlying squamous mucosa in a hemorrhoid.

KEY FEATURES: Hemorrhoids

- This condition is associated with fiber-poor diets, obesity, portal hypertension, and pregnancy.
- Common symptoms include anal discomfort, bleeding, pruritus, and pain.
- A hemorrhoid is a **prolapsed anal cushion resulting from erosion of anchoring connective tissue.**
- Internal hemorrhoids are above the dentate line, are painless, result in bright red blood per rectum, and are clinically graded based on degree of prolapse.
- External hemorrhoids are below the dentate line and painful.
- Treatment is conservative versus excision.
- **Histology shows engorged vascular spaces encased in prominent fibroconnective tissue, organizing thrombi, and ulceration.**
- **Carefully examine the entire specimen for sneaky, additional diagnoses.**

FIBROEPITHELIAL POLYPS

Anal polyps comprise less than 1% of all GI specimens, and many of these polyps are benign fibroepithelial polyps (FEPs).[6] Anal FEPs are also known as hypertrophied papillae or anal skin tags and are analogous to cutaneous skin tags at any other site. They are an acquired hypertrophy secondary to prior damage, such as ulceration, fissure, fistula, trauma, or surgery. FEPs are asymptomatic when small but can cause discomfort and interfere with hygiene as they enlarge. They are rarely described as masslike,[7] and resection is curative in all cases. Their diagnosis can generally be suggested at scanning magnification based on their characteristic polypoid appearance with prominent fibroconnective tissue (Figs. 5.55–5.57). On closer inspection, they consist of bland fibroconnective tissue with variable inflammation, myxoid degeneration, and collagenization (Figs. 5.58–5.64). Delicate, small vessels and mast cells are common. Up to 70% to 80% of FEPs feature occasional reactive, binucleate myofibroblasts or fibroblasts,[8,9] which should not raise concerns for malignancy. The overlying anal mucosa shows mild acanthosis (epidermal thickening) of the nonkeratinizing squamous epithelium and is free of dysplasia.

Clinically presumed FEPs overlap in appearance with a variety of other diagnoses. A few of the most common mimics are discussed in the following text. The polyp in polypoid squamous dysplasia consists of dysplastic epithelium, whereas the polyp in FEP consists of

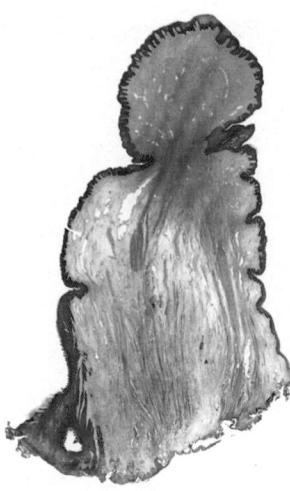

Figure 5-55. Fibroepithelial polyp (FEP). FEPs are an acquired hypertrophy secondary to prior damage and generally present as polyps. The polyp is due to the prominent core of fibroconnective tissue, as seen here.

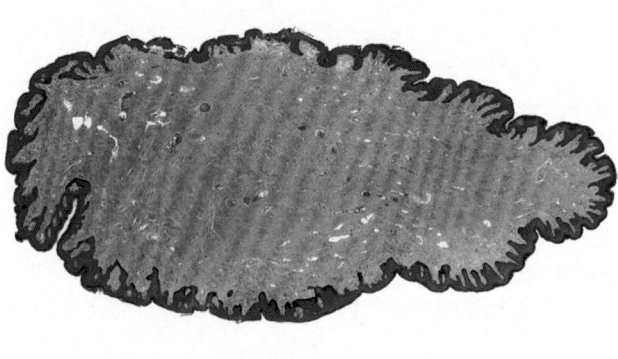

Figure 5-56. Fibroepithelial polyp. The diagnosis can generally be suggested at scanning magnification based on the characteristic polypoid appearance with prominent fibroconnective tissue, as seen here.

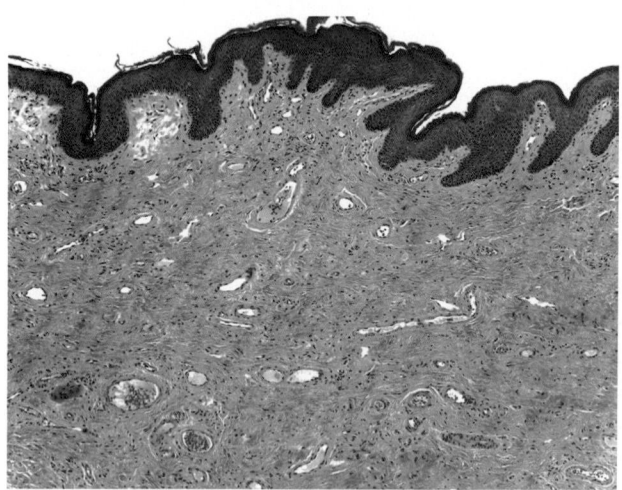

Figure 5-57. Fibroepithelial polyp. Characteristically, FEPs feature evenly spaced, delicate, small vessels with prominent fibroconnective tissue and unremarkable overlying squamous epithelium.

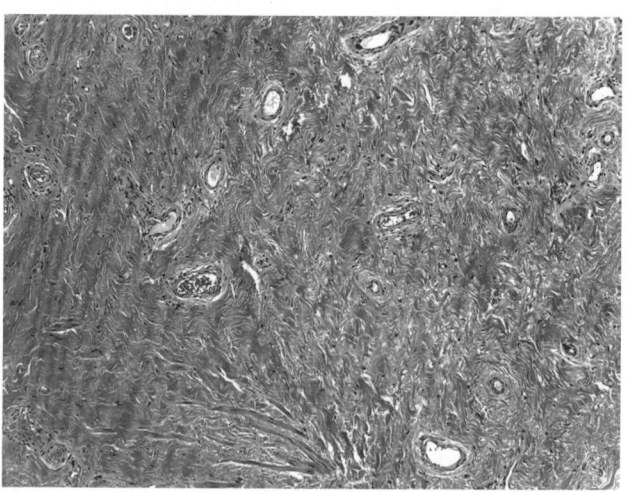

Figure 5-58. Fibroepithelial polyp. Another example of an FEP with a prominent core of dense collagenization and delicate, small vessels.

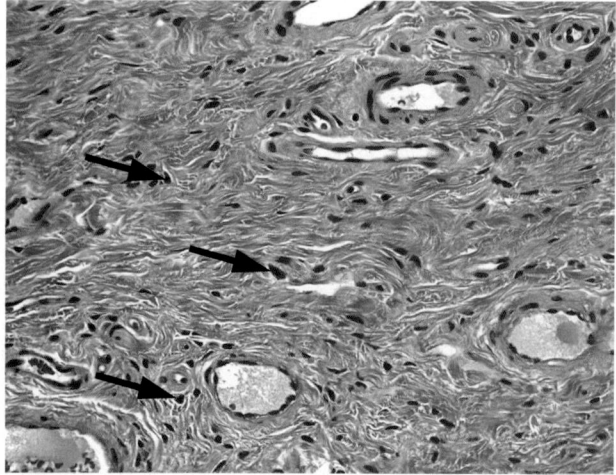

Figure 5-59. Fibroepithelial polyp. Higher power shows the bland endothelial lining of the small vessels. Scattered mast cells are common (arrows).

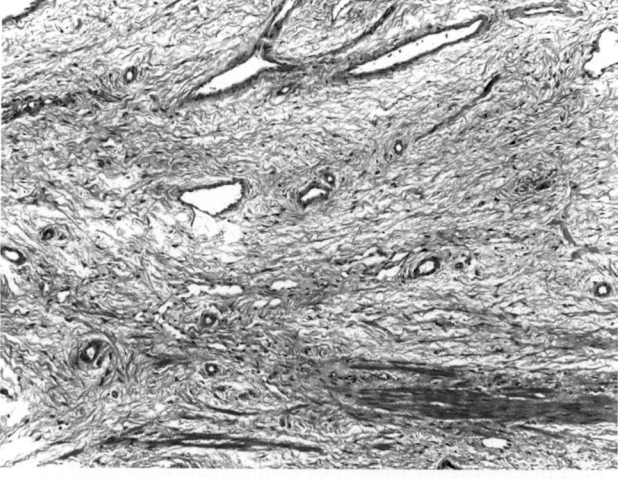

Figure 5-60. Fibroepithelial polyp. Myxoid degeneration is commonly seen, which imparts a pale, edematous appearance to the stroma, as seen here.

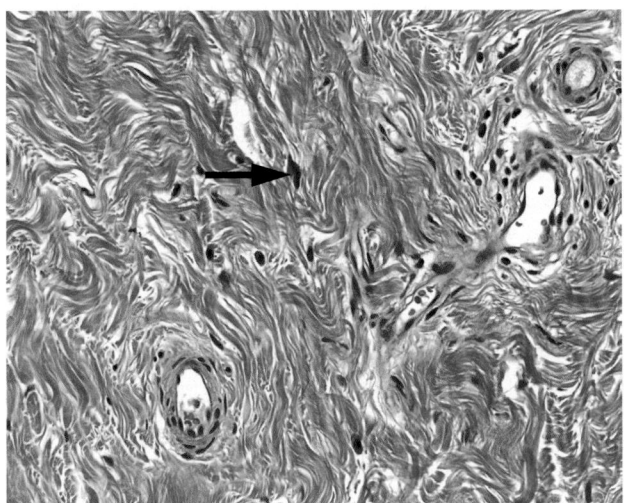

Figure 5-61. Fibroepithelial polyp. Most FEPs feature occasional reactive myofibroblasts or fibroblasts, as seen here (*arrow*). Dense collagenization with delicate vessels and mast cells are seen in the background.

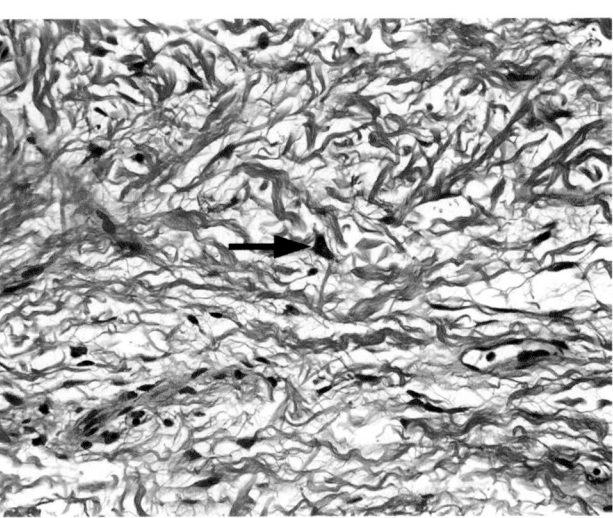

Figure 5-62. Fibroepithelial polyp. The atypical reactive myofibroblasts or fibroblasts occasionally appear binucleate (*arrow*). They are benign and commonly seen in FEP.

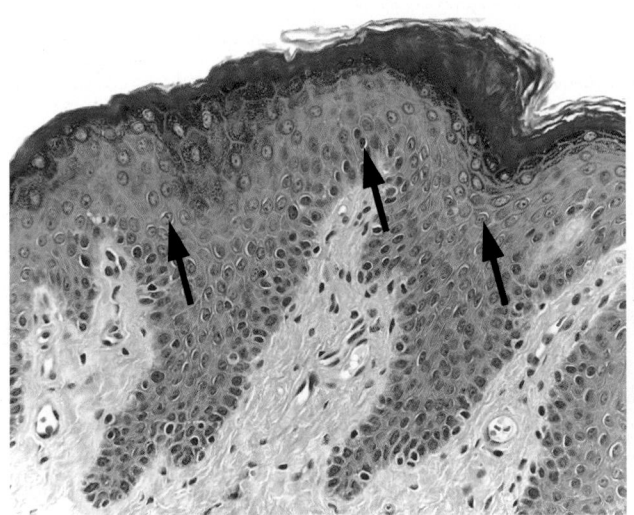

Figure 5-63. FEP with vague perinuclear halos, negative for dysplasia. One important pitfall is to be aware of the occasional fake perinuclear halos (*arrows*) that can be seen in FEP or normal squamous epithelium that could lead to a misdiagnosis of dysplasia

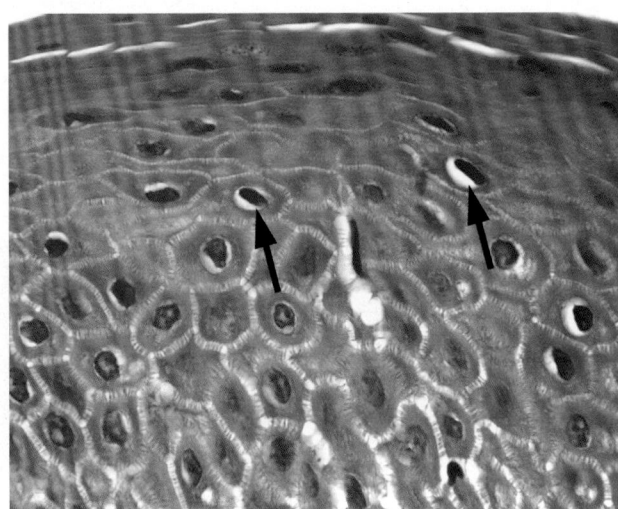

Figure 5-64. FEP with fake perinuclear halos, negative for dysplasia. Although FEPs can have fake perinuclear halos (*arrows*), their nuclei lack hyperchromatic chromatin, irregular nuclear contours (raisinoid nuclei), and binucleate cells required for a diagnosis of squamous dysplasia (Figs. 5.91–5.130).

abundant fibroconnective tissue and the overlying squamous epithelium lacks dysplasia. The polyp in hemorrhoids consists of prominent, ectatic, and engorged vessels embedded in abundant connective tissue (Fig. 5.45). In contrast, FEPs have delicate, small vessels. Theoretically, any benign or malignant process can present as a polyp. Clinically presumed "anal FEPs" can simulate schistosomiasis,[10] fibrous histiocytoma,[11] syphilis, or lymphogranuloma venereum (*Chlamydia* sp.) infections, melanoma, and malignancy, among others. As a result, careful inspection is worthwhile, even (or especially!) in these seemingly uninspiring specimens.

PEARLS & PITFALLS: Avoid Overcalling Reactive Changes in FEPs as Dysplasia

Up to 40% of anal polyps diagnosed as "condyloma acuminatum" were reclassified as normal or FEP in one recent series,[12] underscoring the difficulty in accurately diagnosing these routine specimens. One important pitfall is the occasional fake perinuclear halo seen in the squamous epithelium of an FEP and normal squamous epithelium that can raise concerns for squamous dysplasia (Figs. 5.63 and 5.64). Although FEP can have fake perinuclear halos, the cells are small and their nuclei lack hyperchromatic chromatin, irregular nuclear contours (raisinoid nuclei), and binucleation required for a diagnosis of squamous dysplasia (Figs. 5.65 and 5.91–5.130). This is a clinically important distinction because of the social implications and divergent clinical management. Although FEP is benign, cured by resection, and requires no further follow-up, squamous dysplasia implies a sexually transmitted disease (human papillomavirus, HPV) and requires clinical follow-up. For challenging cases, some advocate a Ki67 (limited to the deepest two to three layers of basal keratinocytes in normal and FEPs) and p16 (entirely negative in normal and FEPs).[12] See also "HPV-Associated Neoplasms" section.

KEY FEATURES: FEP

- FEPs are analogous to cutaneous skin tags at any other site.
- They are an **acquired hypertrophy** secondary to prior damage.
- They are usually small but can be masslike.
- Polyps consist of **bland fibroconnective tissue with small vessels and are covered by nondysplastic squamous epithelium.**
- Clinically presumed FEPs can mimic a variety of benign or malignant processes.

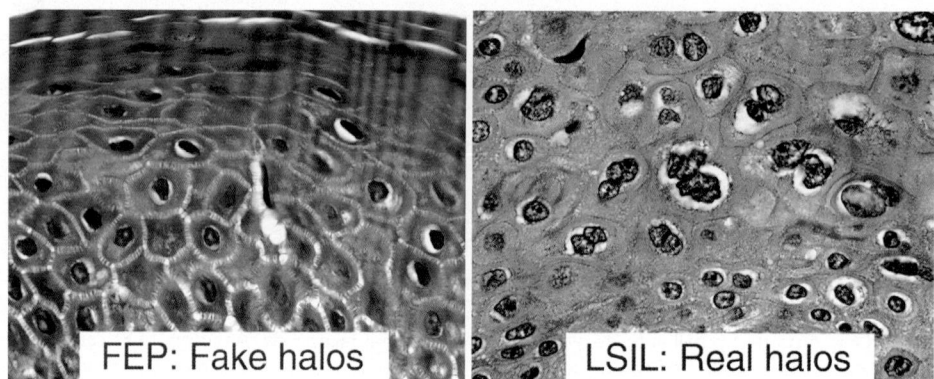

Figure 5-65. FEP fake perinuclear halo versus LSIL real halo composite. FEP and normal squamous epithelium can have fake perinuclear halos that sometimes lead to the incorrect diagnosis of LSIL. Note that the nuclei in FEP, in contrast to those associated with the real halos of LSIL, are small and lack hyperchromatic chromatin, irregular nuclear contours (raisinoid nuclei), and binucleate cells. See also Figs. 5.91–5.130.

INFLAMMATORY CLOACOGENIC POLYP

Mucosal prolapse can occur anywhere along the tubular GI tract, resulting in the formation of polyps, but the nomenclature varies by site. Mucosal prolapse of the rectum is clinically referred to as "solitary rectal ulcer syndrome" (SRUS), and the identical process in the anus is termed "inflammatory cloacogenic polyp" (ICP). Keep in mind SRUS is a clinical diagnosis. The term is misleading because the lesions can be multiple (not just solitary), polypoid (not just ulcerated), and the identical morphology can be seen anywhere along the tubular GI tract. See Sample Note SRUS. Alternatively, the phrases "polypoid mucosal prolapse" or "mucosal prolapse polyp" can be used as a general diagnostic term to describe prolapse at any site. Mucosal prolapse in the rectum and anus is a result of fecal firmness, intraluminal pressures, and constipation-related straining. Conservative management includes a high-fiber diet with increased fluid intake. Surgical resection is an option for symptomatic, larger lesions or those that are clinically concerning for a deeper malignant process. Prolapse is characterized by the ingrowth of thick muscle bundles that can mechanically "squeeze" the ensnarled epithelium and is often accompanied by variable inflammation, ulceration, and reactive epithelial change (Figs. 5.66–5.70). In contrast to rectal prolapse, by definition, ICP must feature some bit of squamous epithelium, although it is typically only focal and, instead, usually dominated by glandular epithelium. Prolapse can simulate invasive carcinoma when the glands are displaced into the submucosa or between muscle bundles or when the mechanical stress of the misplaced glands results in gland rupture and extruded mucin (see also "Epithelial Misplacement" section, "Colon" chapter). Helpful clues of prolapse include its lobular glandular architecture surrounded by lamina propria, hemosiderin-laden macrophages, and a lack of desmoplasia. An awareness of these typical morphologic features, deeper sections, and sharing with a colleague is reassuring in challenging cases. Beware that prolapse can also overlie a deeper, malignant process, and some such cases require a carefully crafted note. See Sample Note Prolapse in a Specimen Designated "Mass."

See also discussion on prolapse in "Colon" chapter "Serrated Polyp" section, FAQ on the importance of site and size for serrated polyp classification, and "Conventional Adenoma" section, "Epithelial Misplacement as a Mimic of Invasion" subsection.

SAMPLE NOTE: SRUS

Rectum, SRUS, Biopsy

- Fragments of mucosal prolapse (clinically solitary rectal ulcer syndrome, SRUS)

SAMPLE NOTE: Prolapse in a Specimen Designated "Mass"

Anus, Mass, Biopsy

- Fragments of mucosal prolapse with unremarkable squamous epithelium, see Note
- Deeper sections examined

Note: The clinical impression of a mass is noted. The biopsies show prominent mucosal prolapse involving the anus (inflammatory cloacogenic polyp, ICP). Deeper sections examined. Although ICP can present as a mass lesion, it can also overlie a deeper process. In this case, repeat (deeper) sampling is a consideration, if the lesion remains clinically concerning.

KEY FEATURES: ICP
- **SRUS** is a *clinical* diagnosis and refers to mucosal **prolapse of the rectum.**
- **ICP** refers to mucosal **prolapse of the anus** and must include at least some squamous epithelium.
- **Polypoid mucosal prolapse** is a general phrase to describe mucosal prolapse at any site.
- Prolapse is characterized by lobular glandular architecture, smooth muscle ingrowth, variable inflammation, ulceration, and reactive epithelial change.
- **Prolapse can also overlie a deeper, malignant process.**

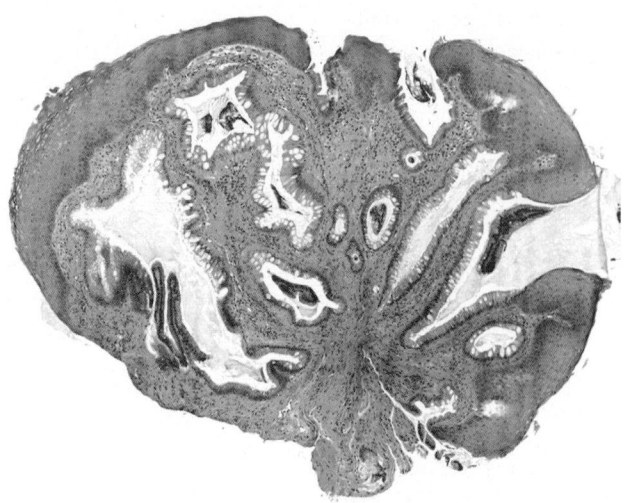

Figure 5-66. Inflammatory cloacogenic polyp (ICP). ICP refers to mucosal prolapse of the anus and requires at least a bit of squamous epithelium. This example is unusual because it contains substantial squamous epithelium; ICPs usually are dominated by glandular mucosa.

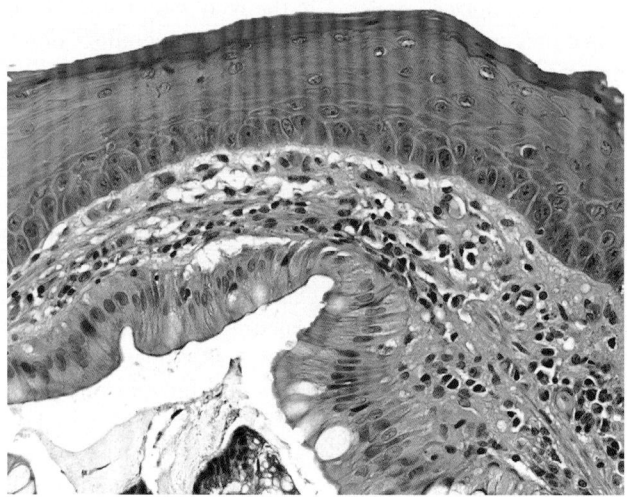

Figure 5-67. Inflammatory cloacogenic polyp. Higher power of the previous figure shows mild hyperkeratosis of the squamous epithelium. Mucosal prolapse of the rectum is clinically referred to as solitary rectal ulcer syndrome (SRUS). Polypoid mucosal prolapse can be used as a general diagnostic term to describe mucosal prolapse at any site.

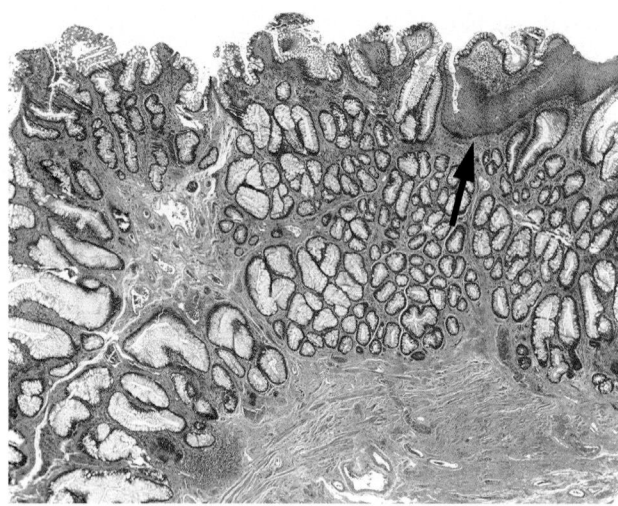

Figure 5-68. Inflammatory cloacogenic polyp. Prolapse is characterized by the ingrowth of thick muscle bundles that mechanically "squeeze" the ensnarled epithelium and is often accompanied by variable inflammation, ulceration, and reactive epithelial change. By definition, ICP must feature some bit of squamous epithelium (arrow), although it is typically only focal and, instead, usually dominated by glandular epithelium, as seen here.

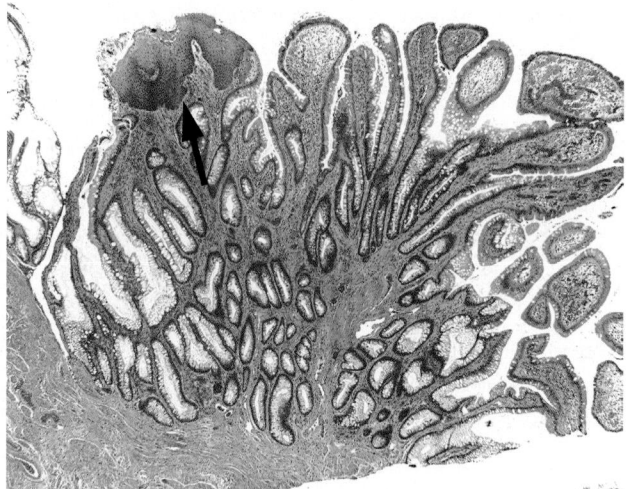

Figure 5-69. Inflammatory cloacogenic polyp. An arrow highlights the squamous epithelium. The prominent smooth muscle ingrowth and mechanically compressed crypt bases are easily seen on low power.

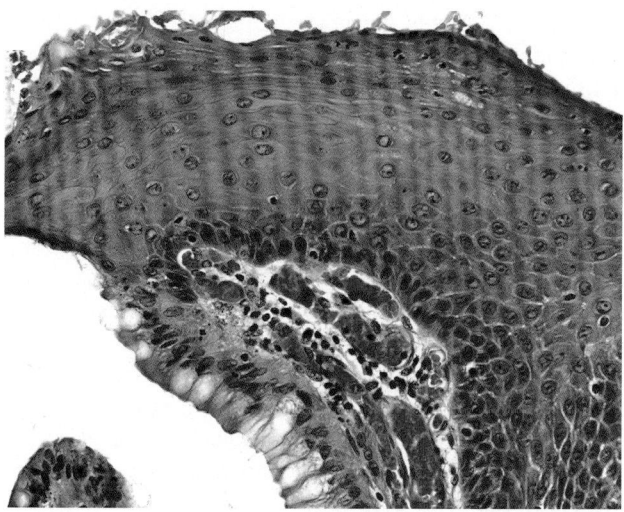

Figure 5-70. Inflammatory cloacogenic polyp. Higher power of the previous figure shows mild acute inflammation of the squamous epithelium.

HIDRADENOMA PAPILLIFERUM

Hidradenoma papilliferum is a benign neoplasm derived from anogenital mammarylike glands and predominantly seen in women. Anal lesions typically present as small, well-circumscribed nodules or ulcerations. Excision is curative, and no further management is needed. Histologically, most cases of hidradenoma papilliferum have a papillary architecture that is easily appreciated on low and intermediate power (Figs. 5.71–5.74). High power shows a double layer of epithelium lining the papilla overlying the fibrous stroma (Figs. 5.75 and 5.76), similar to normal breast tissue. In a 2016 study of 264 anogenital cases, the authors reported that these lesions can display changes that mirror findings seen in benign breast, such as columnar cell change, sclerosing adenosislike changes, and atypical and usual ductal hyperplasia.[13] For reporting purposes, the simple diagnosis of hidradenoma papilliferum is sufficient. More recently, mutations in *PI3K-AKT* and *MAPK* signaling pathways have been identified.[14] Hidradenoma papilliferum is unassociated with HPV.[14,15]

KEY FEATURES: Hidradenoma Papilliferum
- This is a benign neoplasm derived from anogenital mammarylike glands.
- It **predominantly affects women.**
- Small, well-circumscribed nodules or ulcerations are seen.
- It has a **papillary architecture, a double-layer of epithelium lining the papilla overlying the fibrous stroma**
- Lesions can display changes that mirror findings seen in benign breast, such as columnar cell changes and sclerosing adenosislike changes.
- A simple diagnosis of hidradenoma papilliferum is sufficient.
- *PI3K-AKT* and *MAPK* **mutations have been identified.**

HPV-ASSOCIATED NEOPLASMS

OVERVIEW

HPV infections drive most neoplastic squamous proliferations in the anus. Low-risk subtypes (HPV types 6, 11, 40, 42, 43, 44, 54, 61, 70, 72, and 81) are associated with transient infections, low-grade squamous intraepithelial lesion (LSIL), and a low-risk of squamous cancer.[7] High-risk HPV subtypes (HPV types 16, 18, 31, 33, 35, 39, 45, 50, 51, 53, 56, 58, 59, and 68) are associated with a high risk of high-grade squamous intraepithelial lesion (HSIL) and squamous cancer.[3] HPV-related diagnostic nomenclature has evolved rapidly in step with an improved understanding of its biology and malignant potential. Unfortunately, the expanding terminology has resulted in biologically equivalent lesions diagnosed by a variety of terms based on site (anus, genitourinary, gynecologic, or skin) and by the subspecialty interests and habits of the pathologist (GI, Genitourinary, Gynecologic, or Dermatopathology). For example, low-grade lesions have been termed mild dysplasia, condyloma acuminatum, grade 1 *anal* intraepithelial lesion (AIN 1), grade 1 *perianus* intraepithelial lesion (PAIN 1), grade 1 *penile* intraepithelial lesion (PeIN 1), grade 1 *cervical* intraepithelial lesion (CIN 1), grade 1 *vulvar* intraepithelial lesion (VIN 1), or grade 1 *vagina* intraepithelial lesion (VaIN 1). Analogously, moderate dysplasia has been termed AIN 2, PeIN 2, CIN 2, or VIN 2, and severe dysplasia has been termed carcinoma in situ, AIN 3, PeIN 3, CIN 3, and VIN 3. The term "Bowen disease" is applied to cutaneous sites and used synonymously with carcinoma in situ. Game-changing consensus recommendations were issued in October 2012 by the CAP and the American Society for Colposcopy and Cervical Pathology.[16] This work was a collaborative effort between 35 participating organizations and representation from surgical pathologists, GI pathologists, gynecologic pathologists, dermatopathologists, gynecologists, gynecologic oncologists, dermatologists, surgeons, and infectious disease experts. These recommendations were termed *Lower Anogenital Squamous Terminology Standardization Project for HPV-Associated Lesions (LAST)*, and they provide a single grading scheme to harmonize reporting of HPV-associated neoplasia in the lower anogenital tract. The consensus statement overhauls the HPV nomenclature to minimize diagnostic variability, institute reporting that better reflects HPV biology, and helps ensure proper management through standardized reporting of biologically equivalent lesions. Select highlights from the consensus document are outlined in the following text.[16]

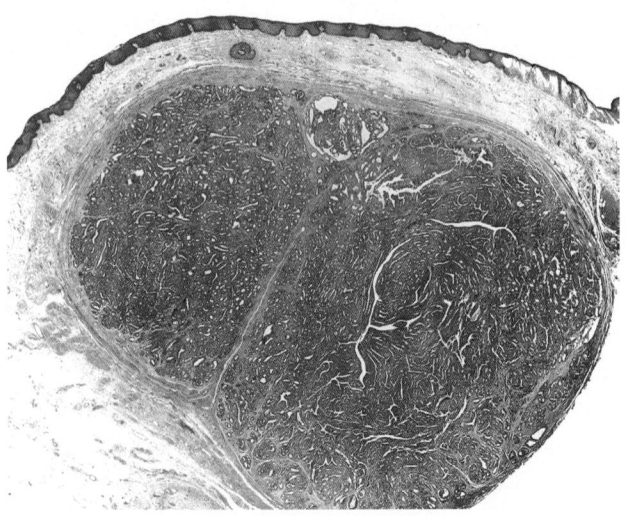

Figure 5-71. Hidradenoma papilliferum. Anal lesions typically present as small, well-circumscribed nodules, and a papillary architecture can be seen at low power.

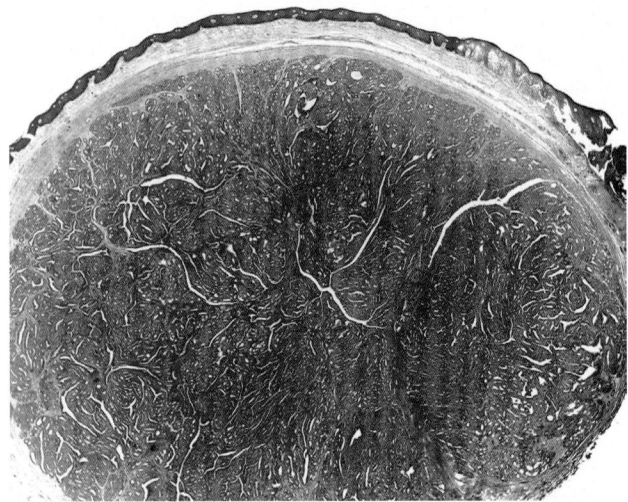

Figure 5-72. Hidradenoma papilliferum. Hidradenoma papilliferum is a benign neoplasm derived from anogenital mammarylike glands and predominantly seen in women.

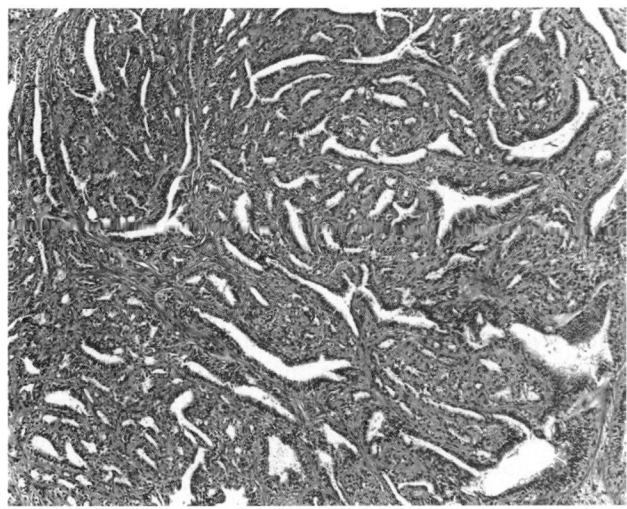

Figure 5-73. Hidradenoma papilliferum. The individual papillae are more easily seen on intermediate power.

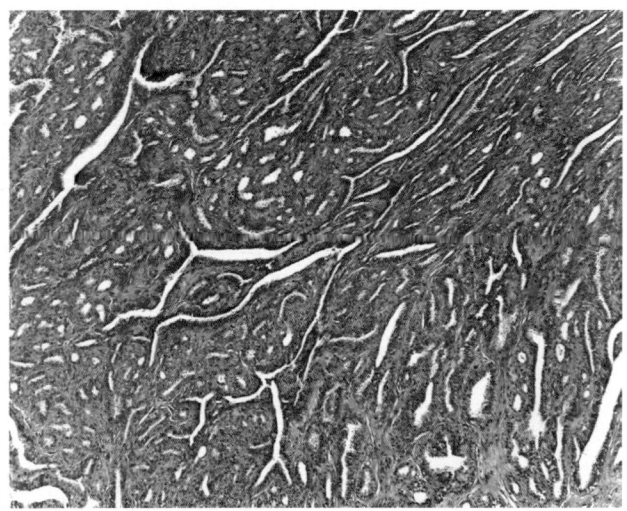

Figure 5-74. Hidradenoma papilliferum. Mutations in *PI3K-AKT* and *MAPK* signaling pathways have been identified in some cases of hidradenoma papilliferum.

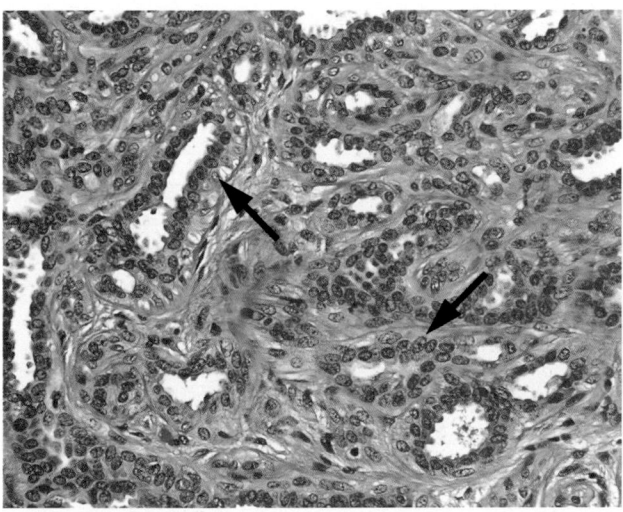

Figure 5-75. Hidradenoma papilliferum. The highest power shows a double layer of epithelium lining the papillae overlying the fibrous stroma (*arrows*).

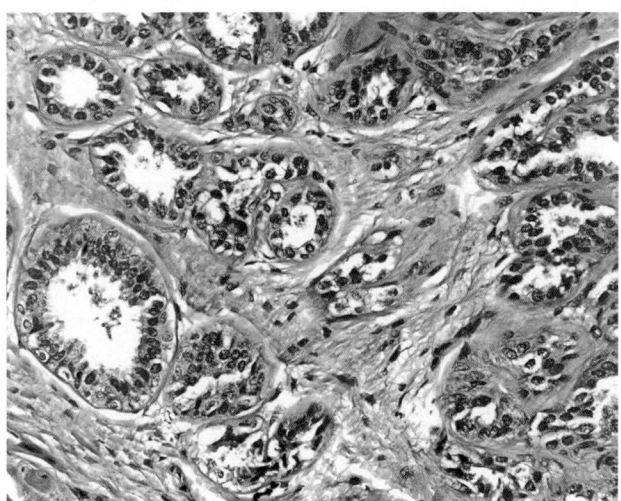

Figure 5-76. Hidradenoma papilliferum.

LAST HIGHLIGHTS

Uniform Grading Scheme

LAST introduces a single grading system that is applicable to all lower anogenital sites, including the anus, perianus, penis, cervix, vulva, and vagina. This provides for uniform reporting while simplifying the diagnostic process in anatomic sites difficult to discern, i.e., it can be difficult for clinicians (and almost impossible for pathologists) to accurately distinguish the vulva, perianus, and anus.

Two-Tiered System

Noninvasive HPV-associated squamous dysplasia of the lower anogenital tract are now classified by a two-tiered system. LSIL (formerly "-IN 1") and HSIL (formerly "-IN 2" and "-IN 3"). This two-tiered system offers several advantages. It better reflects the current understanding that low-grade lesions are typically self-limited and high-grade lesions harbor an increased risk of malignant transformation. It also eliminates the poor interobserver agreement of the -IN 2 category, many of which progress to -IN 3. Lastly, it harmonizes the grading systems for surgical pathology and cytology.[17] Based on the messy historical nomenclature, a further qualification of the diagnosis with -IN in parentheses is suggested, whereby -IN refers to intraepithelial neoplasia terminology of the particular site, such as AIN for anus, VIN for vulva, and CIN for cervix. This is particularly important in the cervix because CIN 2 is managed conservatively in young women to protect reproductive health. See Sample Note LAST LSIL and HSIL reporting.

LSIL, Including Condyloma Acuminatum

LSIL (formerly -IN 1) is synonymously referred to as "koilocytic change," which consists of increased nuclear to cytoplasmic ratios, binucleation, perinuclear halos/cavities, hyperchromatic chromatin, and irregular nuclear contours similar to the shape of a raisin (Figs. 5.77–5.82). In LSIL, mitotic figures (Figs. 5.83–5.90) are confined to the lower one-third of the epithelium and the epithelium matures in the top two-thirds of the epithelium (Figs. 5.91–5.102). Condyloma acuminatum is a type of LSIL that presents as a nodule or polyp and has a papillary architecture (Figs. 5.103–5.105). Based on the 2012 LAST guidelines, condyloma acuminatum is subsumed under the LSIL category and should be reported as LSIL (formerly condyloma acuminatum).[16] Most LSILs are transient and associated with a low risk of malignant transformation. See Sample Note LAST LSIL, Condyloma Acuminatum reporting.

See Fig. 5.173 for a side-by-side comparison of normal, LSIL, HSIL, and invasive squamous cell carcinoma.

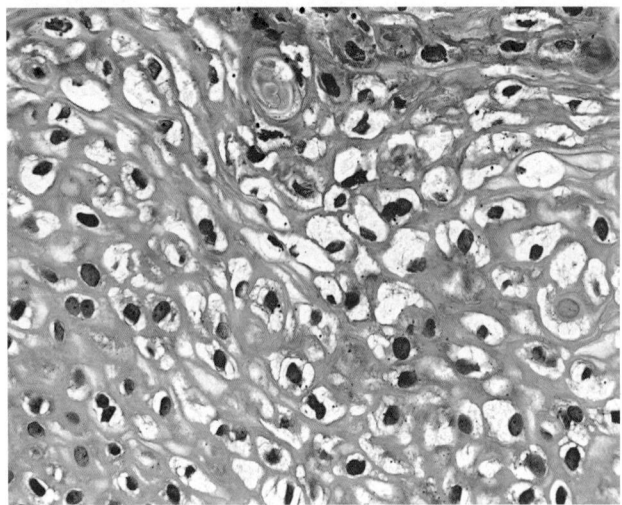

Figure 5-77. Koilocytes. LSIL (formerly -IN 1) is synonymously referred to as koilocytic (or koilocytotic) change, which consists of increased nuclear to cytoplasmic ratios, binucleation, perinuclear halos, hyperchromatic chromatin, and irregular nuclear contours similar to the shape of a raisin, as seen here.

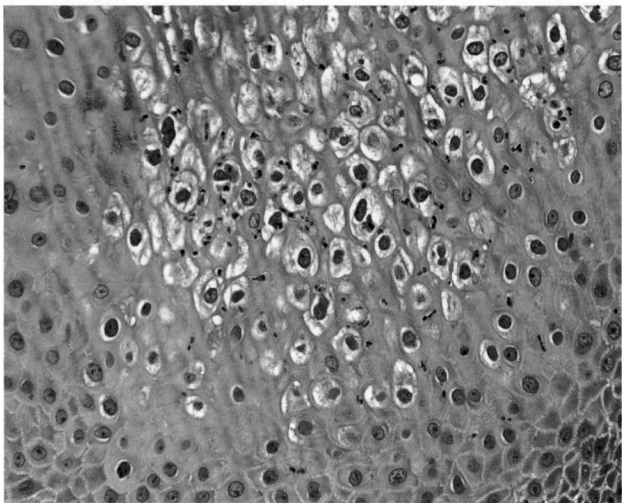

Figure 5-78. Koilocytes.

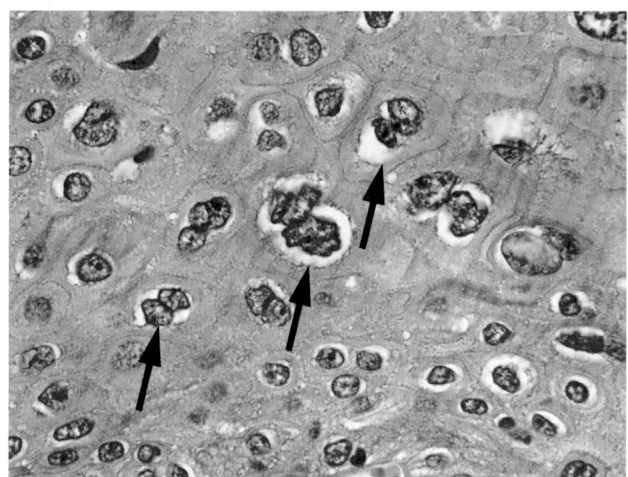

Figure 5-79. Koilocytes (*arrows*). Under oil immersion, note the koilocyte's binucleation, perinuclear halos, hyperchromatic chromatin, and irregular nuclear contours. These changes are often referred to as raisinoid based on the similarity to a raisin.

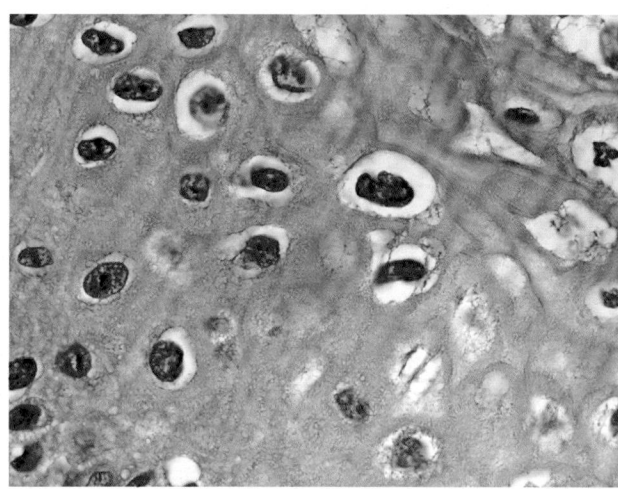

Figure 5-80. Koilocytes.

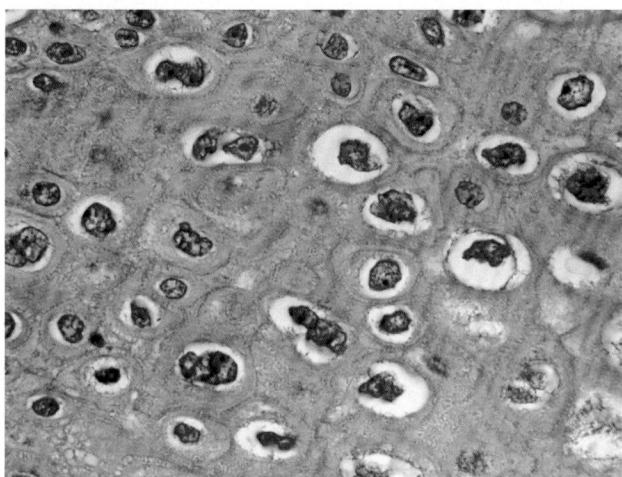

Figure 5-81. Koilocytes.

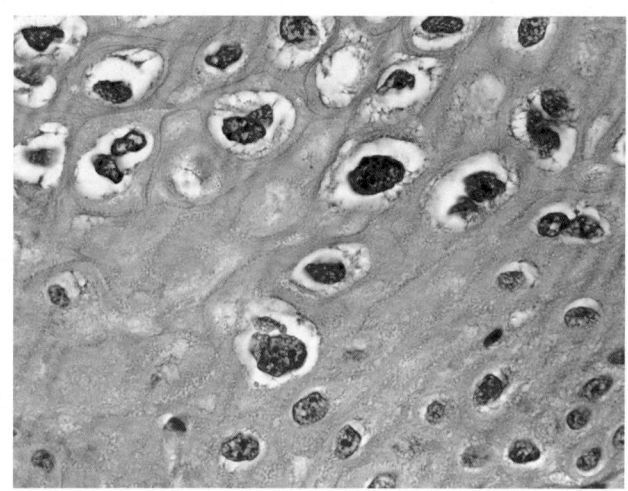

Figure 5-82. Koilocytes.

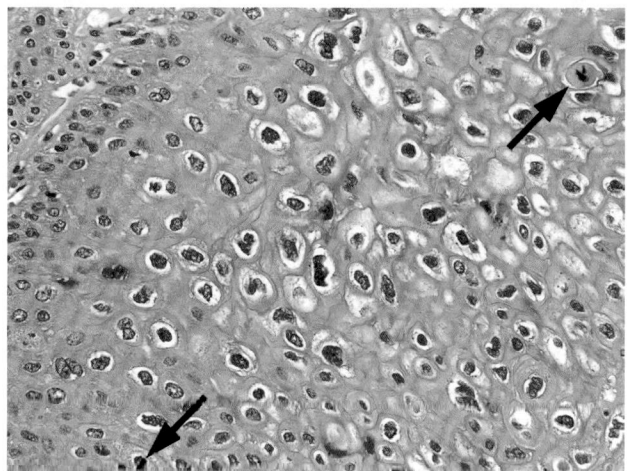

Figure 5-83. Mitotic figures (*arrows*). It is critical to be able to identify mitotic figures to accurately grade dysplasia. Mitotic figures represent cells in the process of dividing. The nuclei lack the usual rounded shape and, instead, appear as various sharply defined geometric structures in the center of the cell, as seen here. The precise shape varies depending on the stage of chromosomes during condensation, replication, and division.

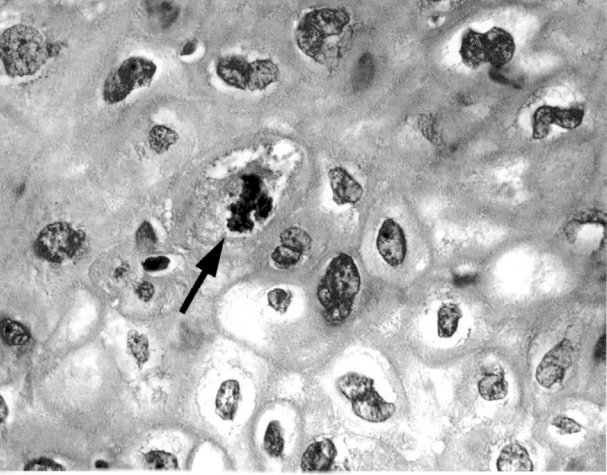

Figure 5-84. Mitotic figure (*arrow*). This mitotic figure appears tripolar with three distinct endpoints. It is considered an abnormal mitotic figure because normal mitotic figures are bipolar. Compare with the next image.

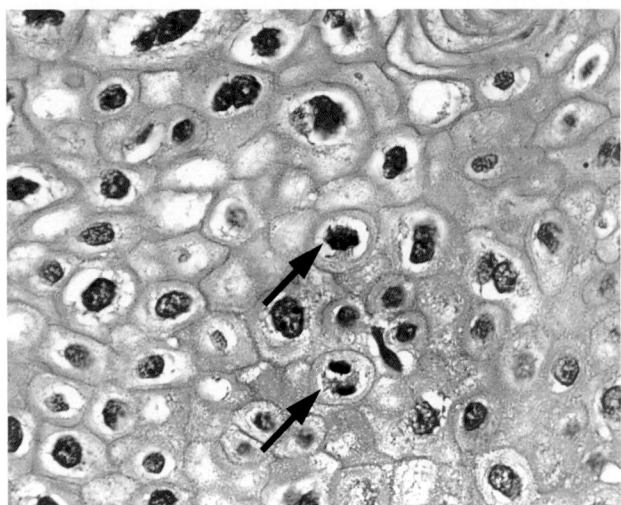

Figure 5-85. Mitotic figures (*arrows*). Both mitotic figures are of the usual type. The top mitotic figure shows the chromosomes arranged in an orderly fashion along the middle of the cell (metaphase), and the lower mitotic figure shows the chromosomes in a bipolar configuration (anaphase) as the nuclei are further along in mitoses and approaching the point of cellular division into two cells.

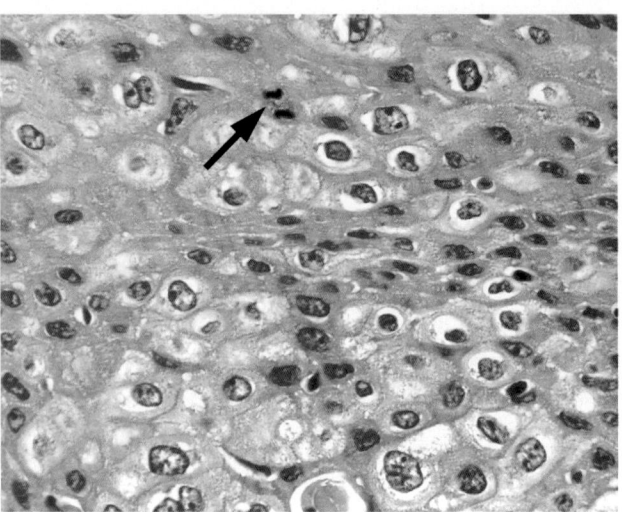

Figure 5-86. Mitotic figure (*arrow*).

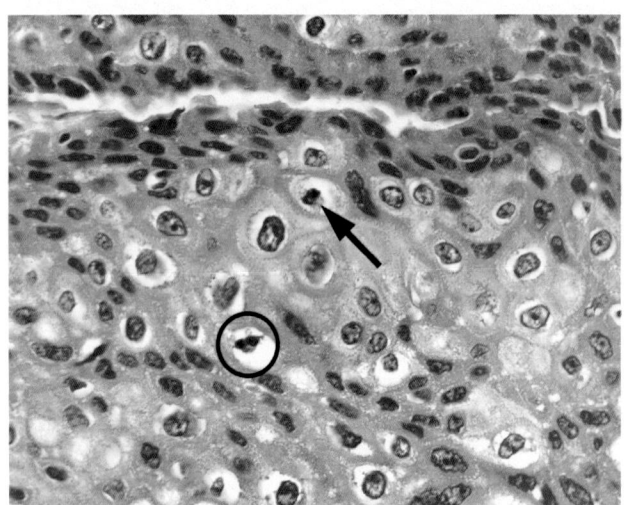

Figure 5-87. Mitotic figures. This normal mitotic figure (*arrow*) contrasts with the degenerating debris (*circle*). In this example of degenerating debris, the focus approximates the size of something that might have been a cell at one point but no longer retains the usual cellular detail of an intact cell with a clear nucleus, cytoplasm, and expected cellular outline (compare with the neighboring, intact cells). Common mimics of mitotic figures include apoptotic bodies (tiny bits of irregular nuclear debris), inflammatory cells, and degenerating debris.

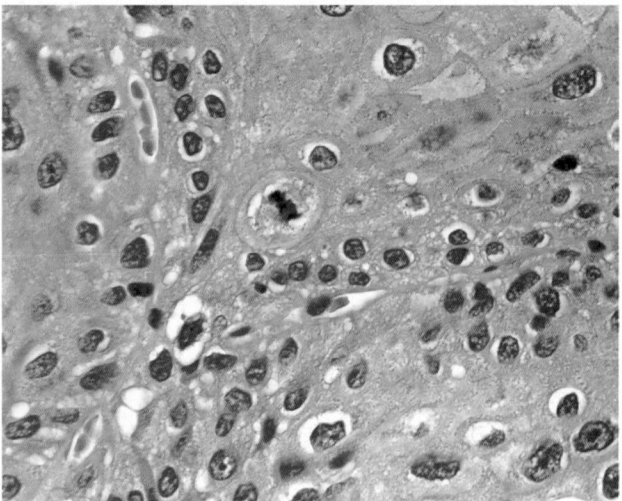

Figure 5-88. Mitotic figure.

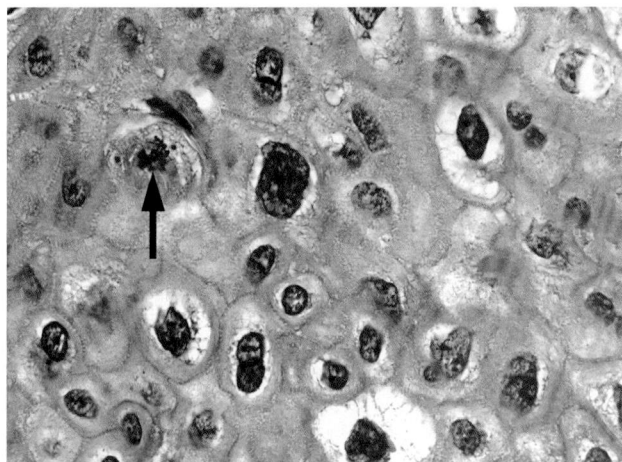

Figure 5-89. Mitotic figure (*arrow*).

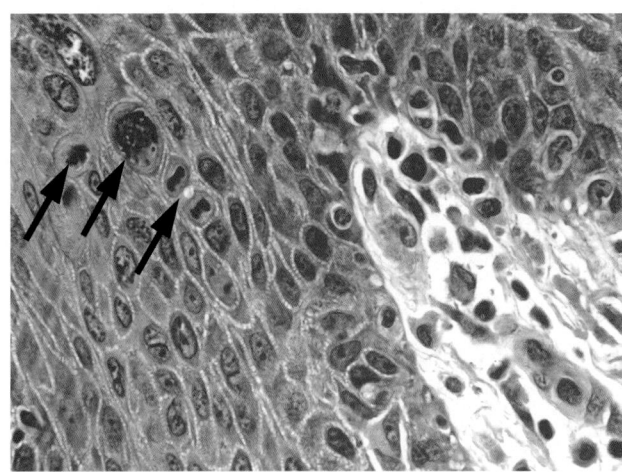

Figure 5-90. Mitotic figure (*arrows*).

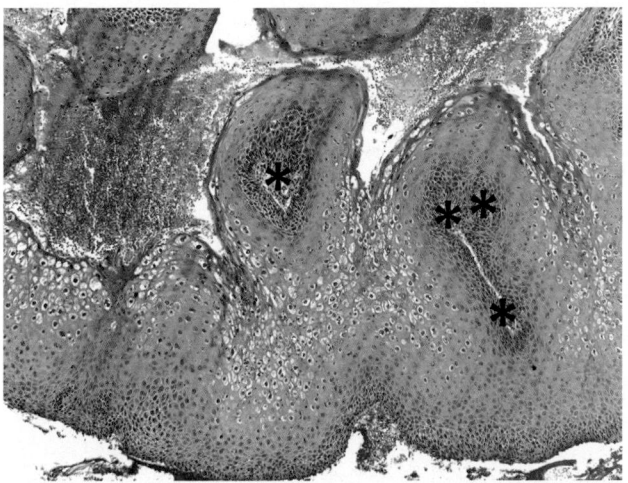

Figure 5-91. Low-grade squamous intraepithelial neoplasia (LSIL). A papillary configuration is seen from this magnification, which aligns with the clinical impression of "anal warts." *Asterisks* highlight the papillary cores. Recall, epithelium surrounding these cores is the deepest aspect of the epithelium, although it can appear toward the top of the tissue section in tangential sections, such as this.

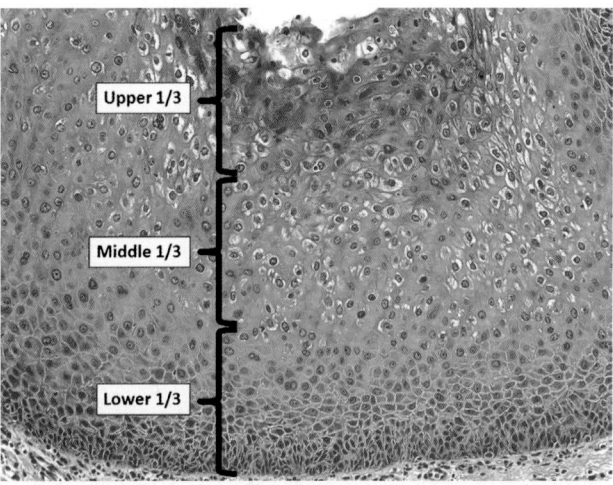

Figure 5-92. Low-grade squamous intraepithelial lesion. In this example, note that the numerous koilocytes are in the upper two-thirds of the epithelium (*brackets*). Characteristic features of koilocytes include increased nuclear to cytoplasmic ratios, binucleation, perinuclear halos, hyperchromatic chromatin, and irregular nuclear contours similar to the shape of a raisin. The immature squamous epithelium is confined to the lower third of the epithelial thickness (*bracket*), satisfying the criteria for LSIL.

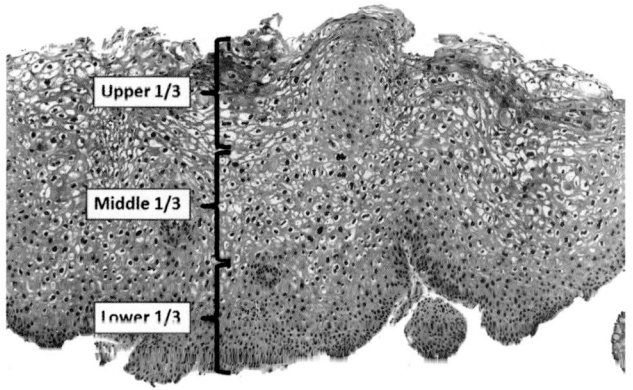

Figure 5-93. Low-grade squamous intraepithelial lesion. Another well orientated LSIL with prominent koilocytes and mature epithelium in the upper two-thirds of the epithelial thickness (*brackets*). Mitoses (not shown) in LSIL are in the lower third of the epithelial.

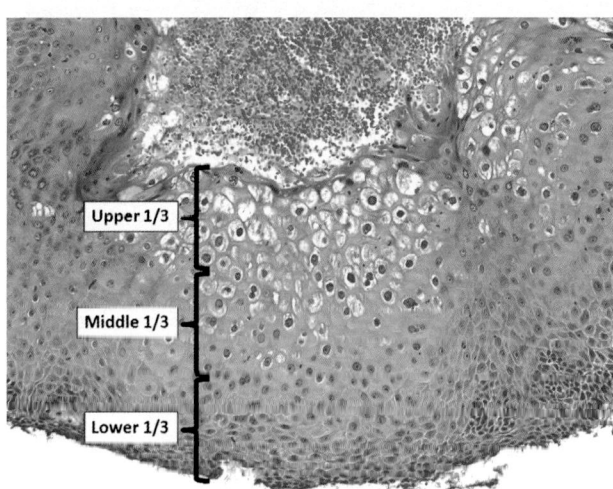

Figure 5-94. Low-grade squamous intraepithelial lesion.

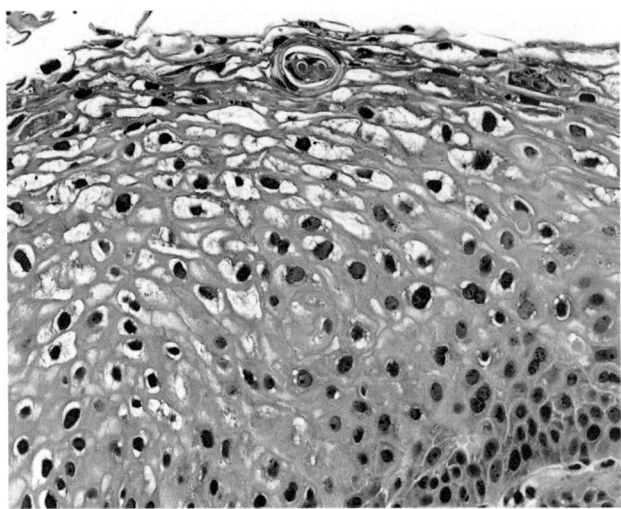

Figure 5-95. Low-grade squamous intraepithelial lesion.

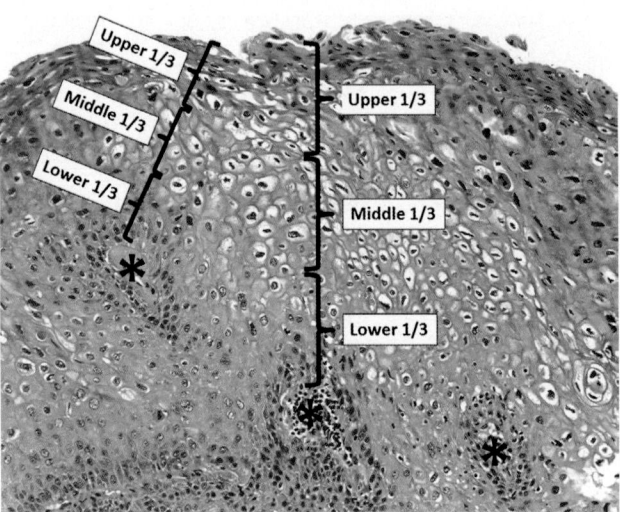

Figure 5-96. Low-grade squamous intraepithelial lesion. Although the previous cases are easy to orient because the tissue is perfectly embedded, real-life cases are often tangentially embedded such that the tissue is a bit twisted, as in this case. It is critical to recognize that the epithelium surrounding the papilla (*asterisks*) is the deepest aspect of the epithelium and to adjust your bearings for lower, middle, and upper thirds of the epithelial thickness accordingly, as illustrated here.

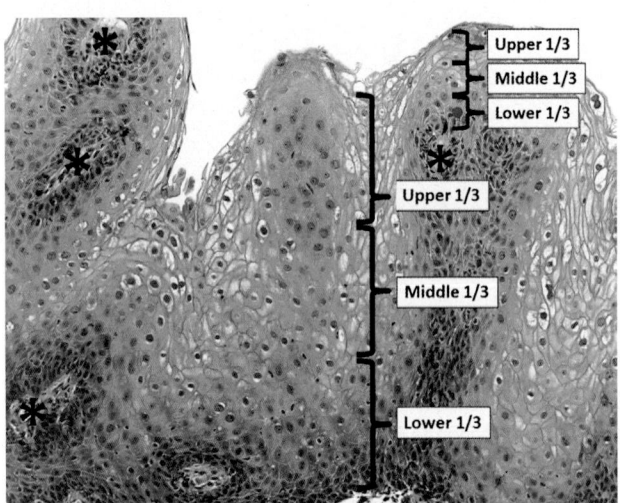

Figure 5-97. Low-grade squamous intraepithelial lesion. This case emphasizes that proper assignment of the lower, middle, and upper thirds of the epithelial thickness is critical for dysplasia grading in the anus. This case had been misdiagnosed as HSIL based on the presence of the mitotic figure at the *red dot*. Although the *dot* is in the top portion of the tissue, this tissue is tangentially embedded. The papilla (*asterisks*) is the reference point for the tissue base at this focus, and the lower, middle, upper third compartments must be adjusted accordingly to this reference point (*brackets*). Even though the *dot* is in the top of the tissue, the *dot* is within the lower third of the epithelial thickness for this focus, justifying the revised diagnosis of LSIL.

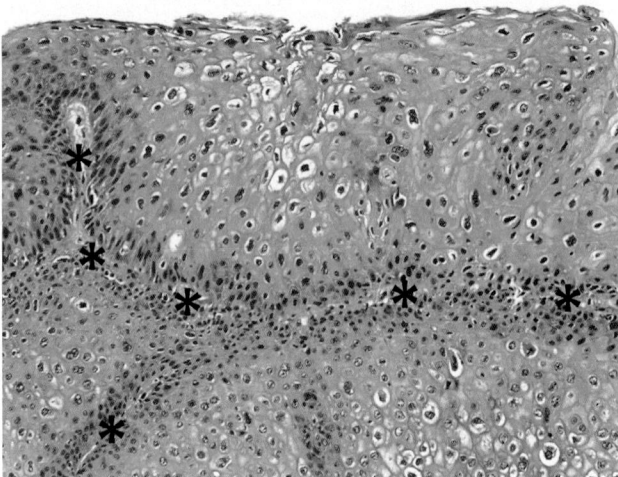

Figure 5-98. Low-grade squamous intraepithelial lesion. The papilla (*asterisks*) is the reference point for the tissue base at this focus, and the lower, middle, upper third compartments must be adjusted accordingly to this reference point.

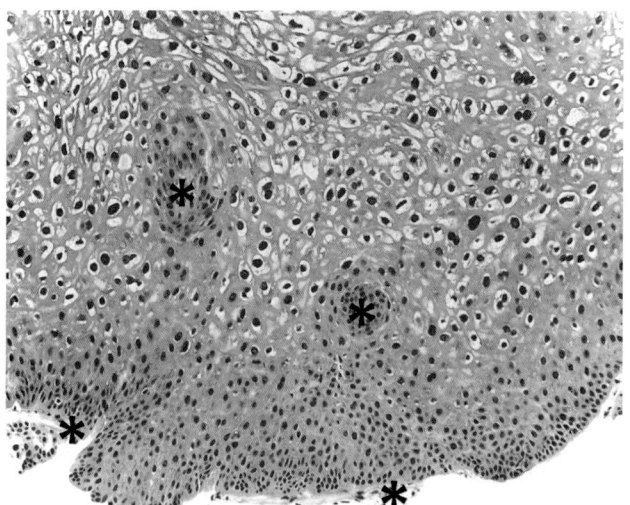

Figure 5-99. Low-grade squamous intraepithelial lesion. Prominent koilocytes and mature epithelium in the upper two-thirds of the epithelial thickness justify the LSIL diagnosis. The papilla (*asterisks*) is the reference point for the tissue base at this focus, and the lower, middle, upper third compartments must be adjusted accordingly to this reference point.

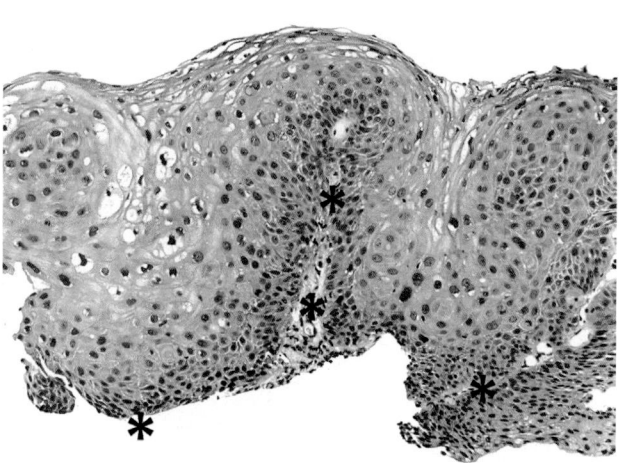

Figure 5-100. Low-grade squamous intraepithelial lesion. The papilla (*asterisks*) is the reference point for the tissue base at this focus, and the lower, middle, upper third compartments must be adjusted accordingly to this reference point.

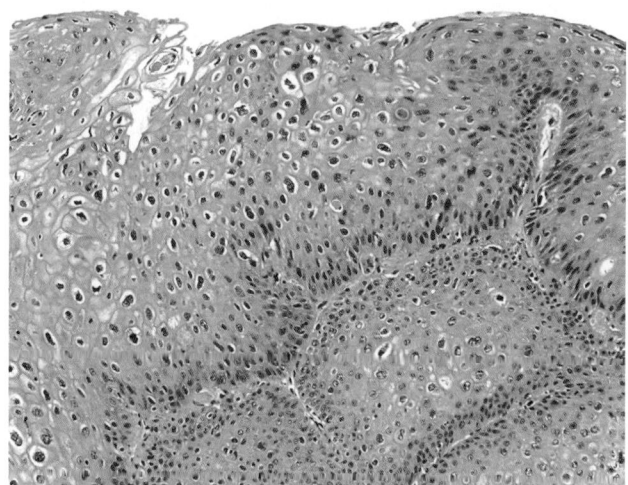

Figure 5-101. Low-grade squamous intraepithelial lesion. Recall, the term condyloma acuminatum is now obsolete. This is a type of LSIL that presents as a nodule or polyp. Based on the 2012 LAST guidelines, condyloma acuminatum is subsumed under the LSIL category and should be reported as LSIL (formerly condyloma acuminatum).

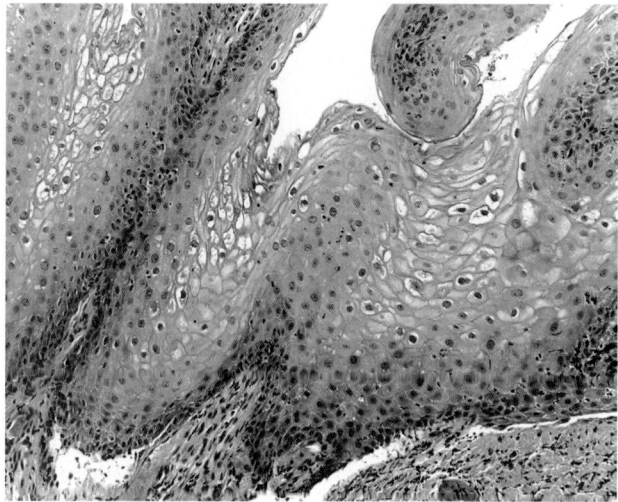

Figure 5-102. Low-grade squamous intraepithelial lesion. Most LSIL is transient and associated with a low risk of malignant transformation.

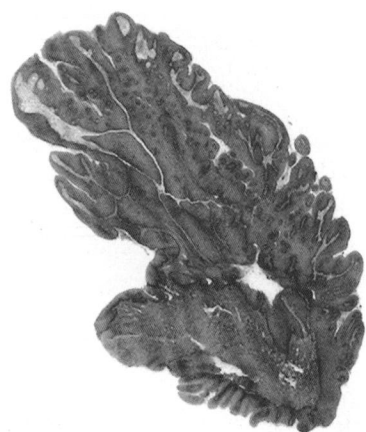

Figure 5-103. Low-grade squamous intraepithelial lesion (formerly condyloma acuminatum). Condyloma acuminatum is now subsumed under the LSIL category. It has identical histology to the previous LSIL examples but has a more papillary 1X appearance and clinically presents as a nodule, polyp, or anal warts.

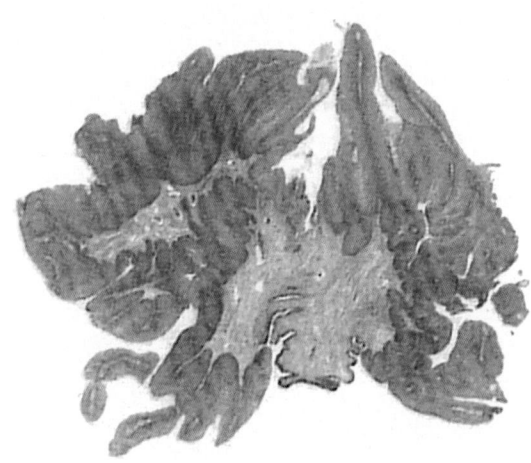

Figure 5-104. Low-grade squamous intraepithelial lesion (formerly condyloma acuminatum). Such cases can be signed out with both terms Because clinicians are less familiar with the LAST recommendations, i.e., LSIL (formerly condyloma acuminatum).

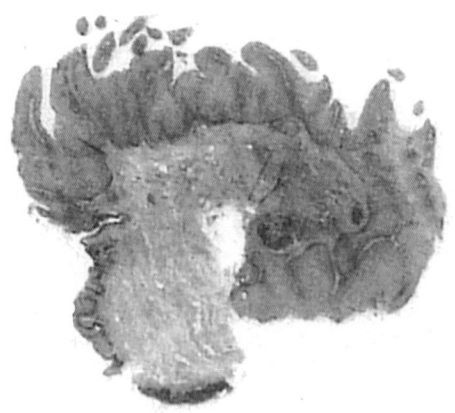

Figure 5-105. Low-grade squamous intraepithelial lesion (formerly condyloma acuminatum).

PEARLS & PITFALLS: Mitotic Figures

The ability to identify mitotic figures is fundamental to pathology and essential for grading dysplasia in the lower anogenital tract. It is so fundamental that an explanation is virtually always omitted in textbooks with the assumption that the reader understands this essential skill, which is usually the case. These pearls and pitfalls are for those trainees who have not yet acquired the mitotic figure hunting skill. Mitotic figures represent cells in the process of dividing. They can be seen in normal and inflamed tissue and do not, by themselves, signify neoplasia. The nucleus of a cell in the process of dividing lacks the usual round shape and, instead, appears as various sharply defined geometric structures in the center of the cell (Figs. 5.83–5.90). The precise shape of the mitotic figure varies depending on the stage of chromosomal condensation, replication, and division. Atypical mitotic figures include those that are tripolar or quadripolar (instead of bipolar) (Fig. 5.84), X-shaped, or with scattered chromatin similar to the stars in the night sky, circular contours, or bizarre shapes. Atypical mitotic figures are more often seen in neoplasms than in nonneoplastic lesions. Mimics of mitotic figures include apoptotic bodies (tiny bits of irregular nuclear debris), inflammatory cells, and degenerating debris (Fig. 5.87).

FAQ (Tangential Sections, Where is the True Bottom?): Because knowing the lower, middle, and upper thirds is important for dysplasia grading, what are tips to approaching tangential sections?

Answer: Proper assessment of the lower, middle, and upper thirds of the epithelial thickness is critical for dysplasia grading in the anus. Although perfectly embedded tissue is easy to orient (Figs. 5.91–5.95 and 5.106), real-life cases are often tangentially embedded such that the tissue is a bit twisted (Figs. 5.96–5.102 and 5.107). It is critical to recognize that the epithelium surrounding the papilla (asterisks in Fig. 5.107) is the deepest aspect of the epithelium and to adjust your bearings for the lower, middle, and upper thirds of the epithelial thickness accordingly (Fig. 5.97). If adjustments are not made, a seemingly "high" mitosis in the top portion of tangentially embedded tissue that is near a papilla can lead to an overcall of HSIL and inappropriate management that places all involved in medicolegal jeopardy. See Fig. 5.97 for a real-life example.

SAMPLE NOTE: LAST Recommendations for LSIL Reporting

Anus, Biopsy

- Low-grade squamous intraepithelial neoplasia (LSIL) (formerly "AIN 1")

SAMPLE NOTE: "Condyloma Acuminatum" Reporting

Anus, Polyp, Biopsy

- Low-grade squamous intraepithelial neoplasia (LSIL) (formerly condyloma acuminatum)

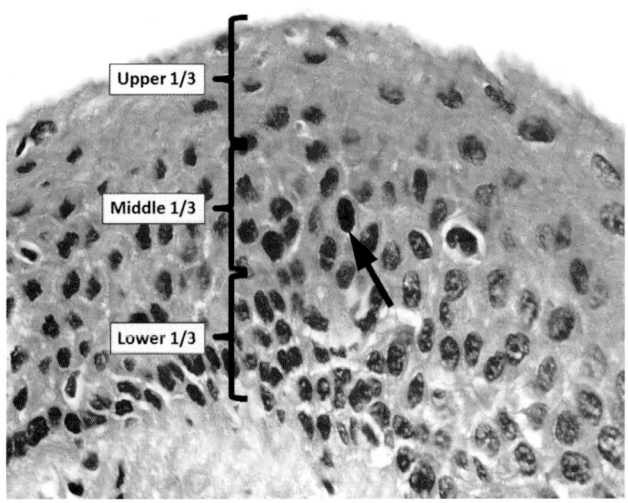

Figure 5-106. High-grade squamous intraepithelial neoplasia (HSIL, AIN2). HSIL (AIN2) is defined by atypia and mitoses (*arrow*) in the lower two-thirds and maturity of the upper third of the epithelium (*brackets*).

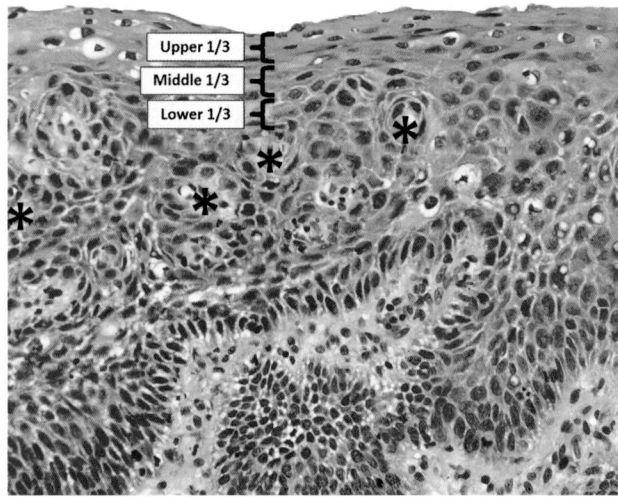

Figure 5-107. High-grade squamous intraepithelial lesion(AIN2). Although the above case is easy to orient because the tissue is perfectly embedded, this is a real-life case that is partially tangentially embedded. Recall that the epithelium surrounding the papilla (*asterisks*) is the deepest aspect of the epithelium and to adjust your bearings for lower, middle, and upper thirds of the epithelial thickness accordingly (*brackets*), as illustrated here.

HSIL

HSIL (formerly -IN 2 and -IN 3) is defined by mitotic figures in the superficial two-thirds of the epithelium. The cytologic features in HSIL are more atypical than those in LSIL, with a lack of maturity of the epithelium in the middle (-IN 2, Figs. 5.106–5.119) or upper third (-IN 3, Figs. 5.120–5.130) of the epithelium, loss of nuclear polarity, anisonucleosis, and increased nuclear to cytoplasmic ratios and hyperchromasia. Prominent mitoses and abnormal mitotic figures are more common in HSIL. For cases of HSIL, we additionally include a line diagnosis regarding the presence or absence of invasion and margin status. See Sample Note LAST HSIL reporting.

See Fig. 5.173 for a side-by-side comparison of normal, LSIL, HSIL, and invasive squamous cell carcinoma.

FAQ (Hyperkeratosis, Where is the True Top?): Because knowing the lower, middle, and upper thirds is important for dysplasia grading, what are tips to approaching specimens with prominent hyperkeratosis?

Answer: Proper assessment of the lower, middle, and upper thirds of the epithelial thickness is critical for dysplasia grading in the anus. Hyperkeratosis (abnormal keratinization) can complicate assessment of locating the true top of the specimen (Figs. 5.131–5.134). The true top is the most superficial epithelium with discernable nuclei to allow for evaluation of atypia and mitotic figure assessment. The true top is not the most superficial hyperkeratotic layer because this zone contains no discernable nuclear detail and, consequently, cannot be evaluated for atypia and mitotic figure assessment.

SAMPLE NOTE: LAST Recommendations for HSIL Reporting

Anus, Biopsy

- High-grade squamous intraepithelial neoplasia (HSIL) (formerly "AIN 2")
- Negative for invasion
- Margins uninvolved

FAQ: How can one classify dysplastic lesions with discordant morphology and mitotic figures, i.e., an LSIL with a high mitotic index or a HSIL with a low mitotic index?

Answer: Unfortunately, there are no official recommendations to cite for this practical question. Most of the time, this issue resolves itself by looking at the entirety of the tissue with a clearly high mitotic index and atypia in the middle and upper portion of the tissue justifying a HSIL designation, for example. For the rare case for which the tissue is limited and a decision must be rendered on a tiny bit of tissue with discordant morphology and mitotic figure location, we prioritize morphology. For example, if the lesion morphologically looks like LSIL but there is a single mitotic figure in the middle or upper third, we classify the lesion as an LSIL. Alternatively, if the morphology shows atypia in the middle or upper third and only low mitoses are found, we classify this lesion as a HSIL. If sufficient tissue is present, p16 immunohistochemistry (IHC) is worthwhile in such borderline cases, with a negative p16 favoring LSIL and diffuse, blocklike p16 reactivity favoring a diagnosis of HSIL. See the following p16 discussion.

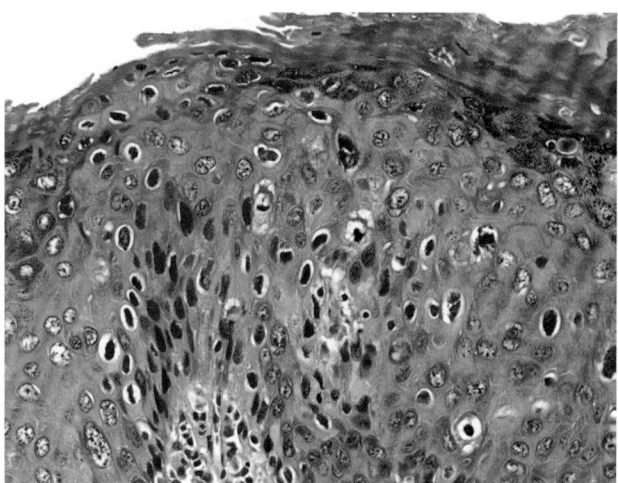

Figure 5-108. High-grade squamous intraepithelial lesion (AIN2). The atypia in the lower two-thirds, mitotic figure in the middle of the epithelium (*arrow*), and maturity of the upper third of the epithelium support a diagnosis of HSIL (AIN2).

Figure 5-109. High-grade squamous intraepithelial lesion (AIN2). The HSIL category lumps together the previous AIN2 and AIN3 categories. For reporting purposes, a diagnosis of HSIL is followed by a further qualification as AIN2 or AIN3 in parentheses for clarity.

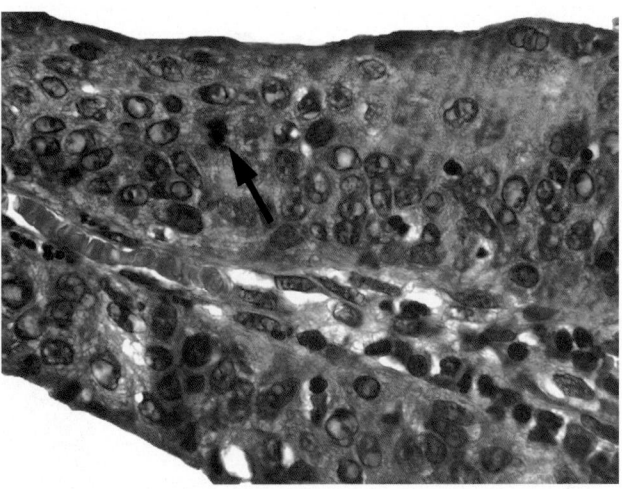

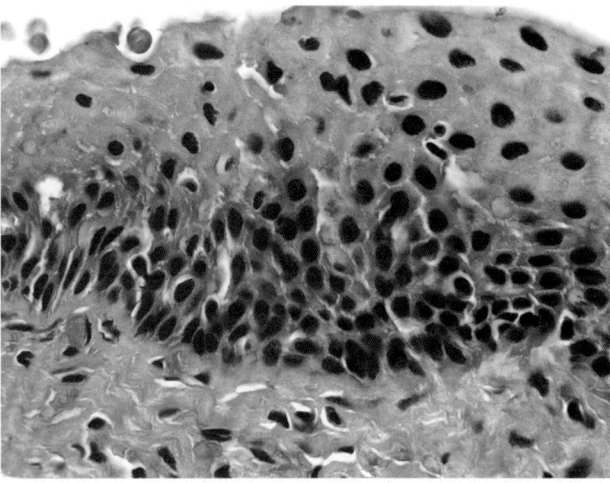

Figure 5-110. High-grade squamous intraepithelial lesion (AIN2). The atypia and mitotic figure in the middle of the epithelium (*arrow*) support a diagnosis of HSIL (AIN2).

Figure 5-111. High-grade squamous intraepithelial lesion (AIN2). Even though no mitotic figures are seen, the atypia in the lower two-thirds and maturity of the upper third of the epithelium support a diagnosis of HSIL (AIN2).

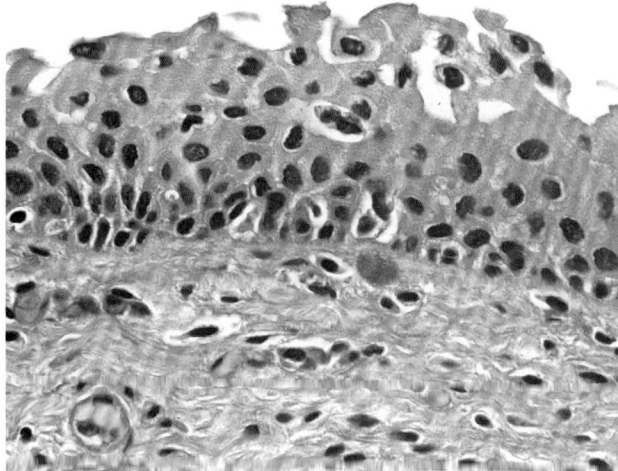

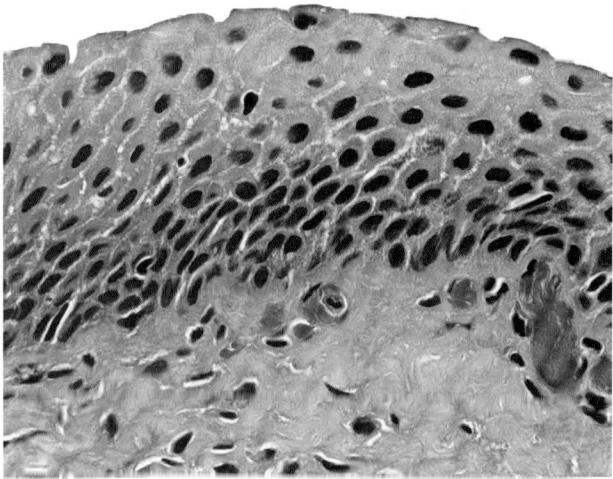

Figure 5-112. High-grade squamous intraepithelial lesion (AIN2). In comparison with those of LSIL, the cytologic features in HSIL are more atypical in terms of more striking anisonucleosis, increased nuclear to cytoplasmic ratios, and hyperchromasia.

Figure 5-113. High-grade squamous intraepithelial lesion (AIN2). Prominent mitoses and abnormal mitotic figures are more common in HSIL but are not required for the diagnosis.

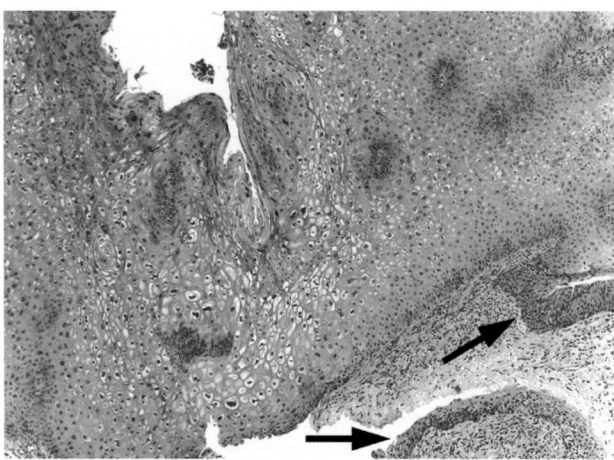

Figure 5-114. High-grade squamous intraepithelial lesion (AIN2). Beware that HSIL can be difficult to identify in a pile of LSIL, as seen in this case. LSIL can dominate the visual field and contains larger cells that easily obscure the small focus of HSIL (*arrows*), but the latter diagnosis will drive the prognosis and treatment and is critical to recognize. Take your time with squamous dysplasia, it can be subtle.

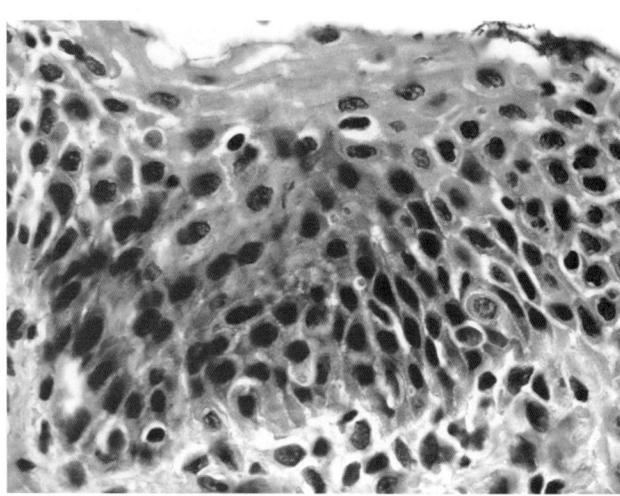

Figure 5-115. High-grade squamous intraepithelial lesion (AIN2). Higher power of the previous figure. For cases of HSIL, we additionally include a line diagnosis regarding the presence or absence of invasion and margin status. See Sample Note "LAST Recommendations for HSIL reporting."

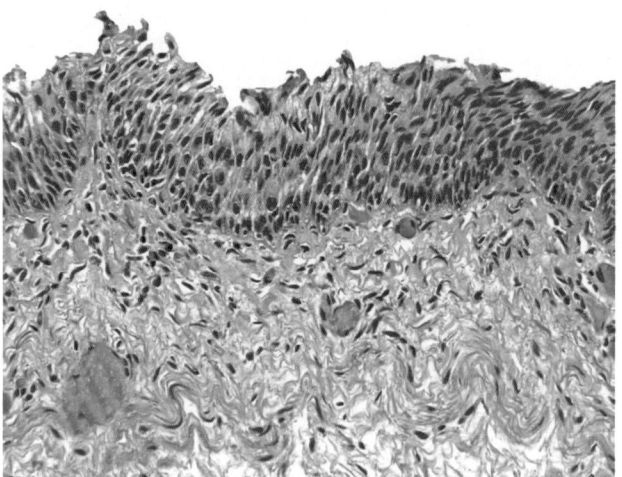

Figure 5-116. High-grade squamous intraepithelial lesion (AIN2). Beware that HSIL can be difficult to identify in a heavily cauterized or crushed focus. In such cases, p16 can be helpful to discern HSIL from atypia secondary to cautery and crush artifact.

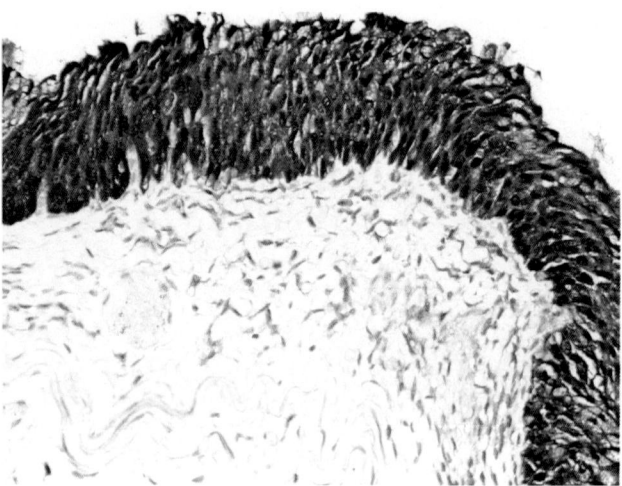

Figure 5-117. High-grade squamous intraepithelial lesion (AIN2), p16. A p16 shows diffuse nuclear and cytoplasmic reactivity, supporting a diagnosis of HSIL (AIN2).

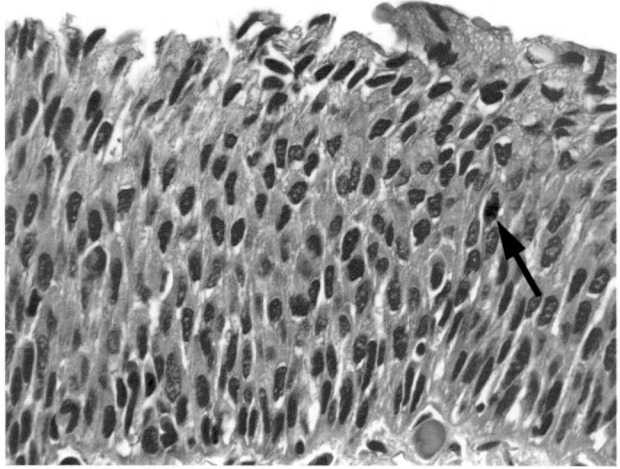

Figure 5-118. High-grade squamous intraepithelial lesion (AIN2). Although this field is a bit cauterized, a midlevel mitosis (*arrow*) is seen concerning for HSIL (AIN2).

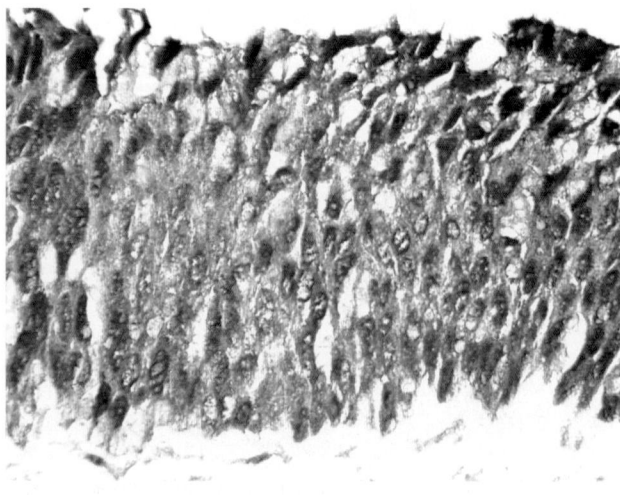

Figure 5-119. High-grade squamous intraepithelial lesion (AIN2), p16. A p16 shows diffuse nuclear and cytoplasmic reactivity, supporting a diagnosis of HSIL (AIN2).

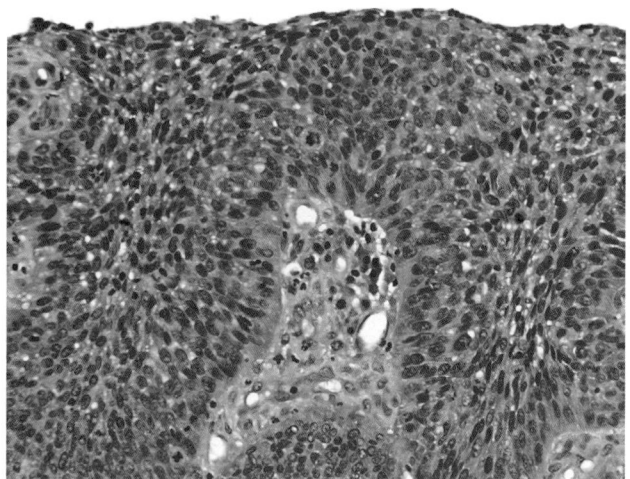

Figure 5-120. High-grade squamous intraepithelial lesion (AIN3). A well-orientated case like this is rarely a diagnostic challenge. Full-thickness and overt atypia support the diagnosis of HSIL (AIN3).

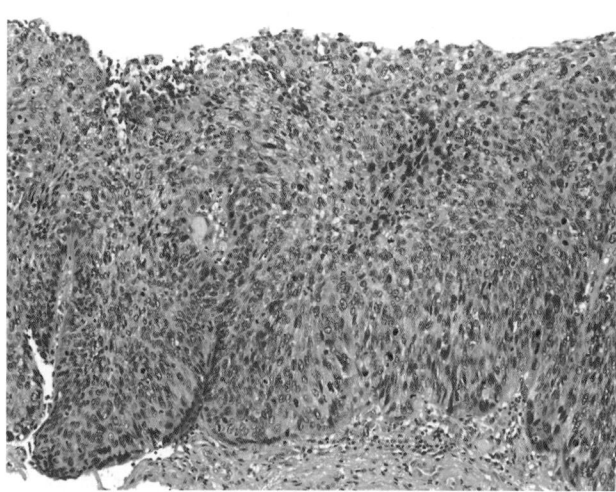

Figure 5-121. High-grade squamous intraepithelial lesion (AIN3). Compared with HSIL (AIN2), HSIL (AIN3) shows more striking anisonucleosis, increased nuclear to cytoplasmic ratios, and hyperchromasia.

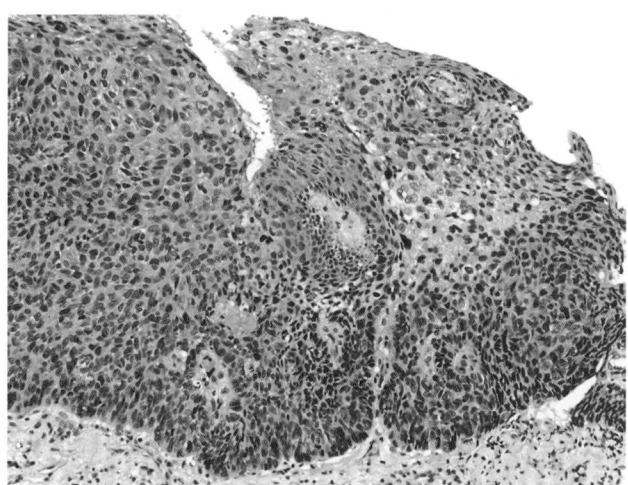

Figure 5-122. High-grade squamous intraepithelial lesion (AIN3). Generally speaking, there is less emphasis in distinguishing HSIL (AIN2) from HSIL (AIN3) because both are followed similarly in the anus. In contrast, HSIL (CIN2) in the cervix is sometimes treated more conservatively to protect fertility (cervical competence) in young women.

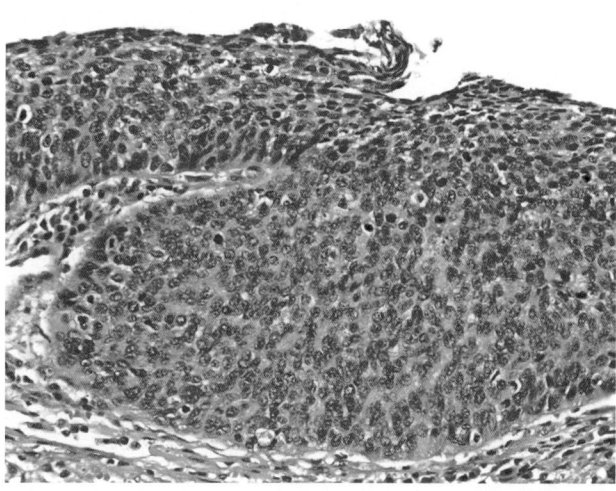

Figure 5-123. High-grade squamous intraepithelial lesion (AIN3).

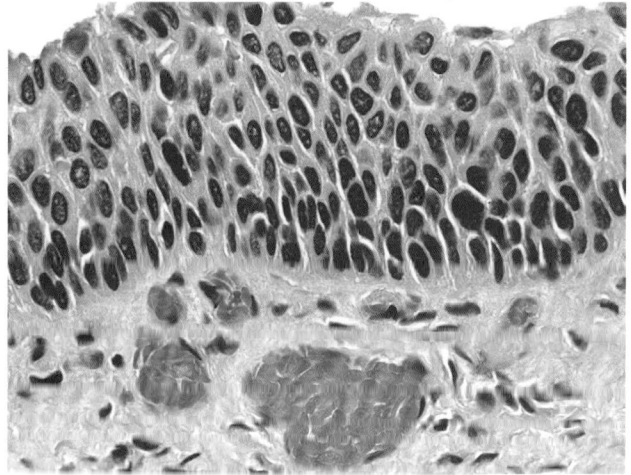

Figure 5-124. High-grade squamous intraepithelial lesion (AIN3). HSIL (AIN3) is defined by full-thickness atypia.

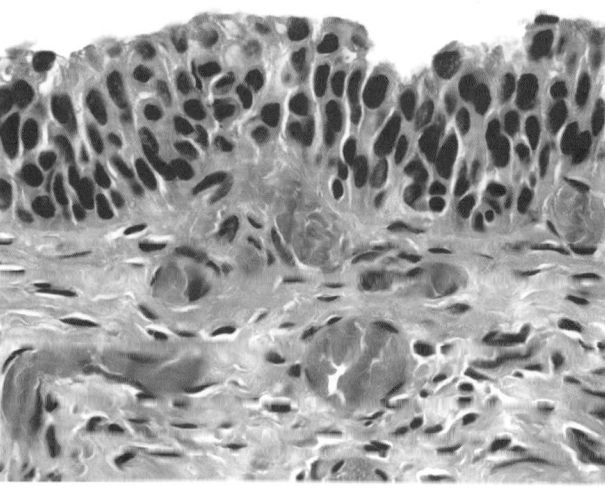

Figure 5-125. High-grade squamous intraepithelial lesion (AIN3).

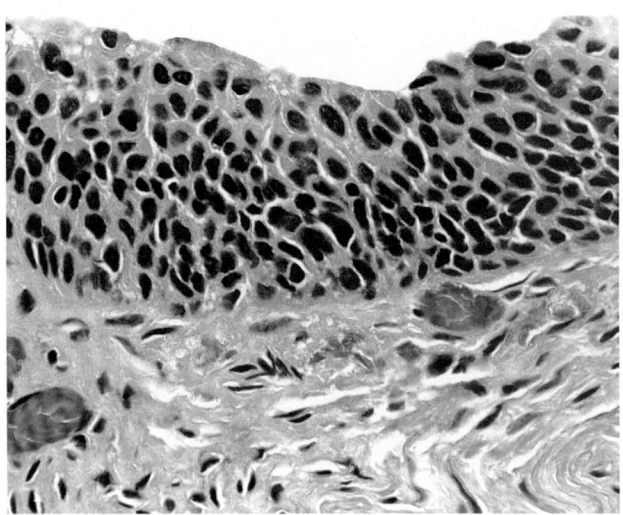

Figure 5-126. High-grade squamous intraepithelial lesion (AIN3).

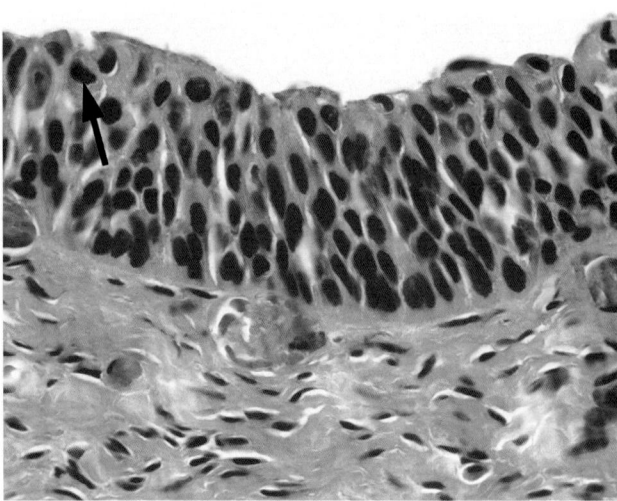

Figure 5-127. High-grade squamous intraepithelial lesion (AIN3). Mitotic figures are not required for a diagnosis of HSIL but can be encountered in the upper third of the epithelium in AIN3 (*arrow*).

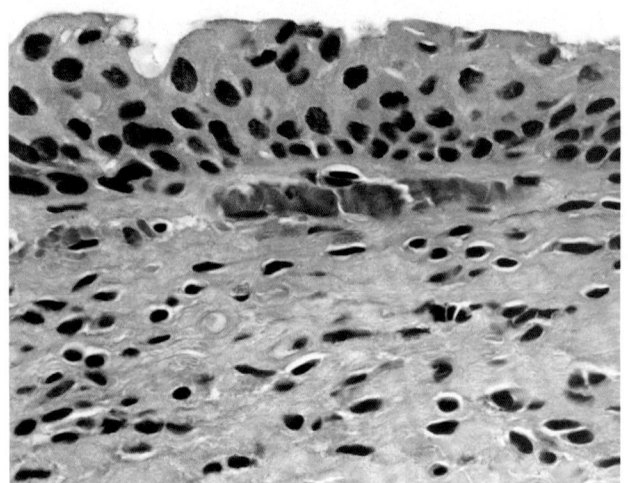

Figure 5-128. High-grade squamous intraepithelial lesion (AIN3).

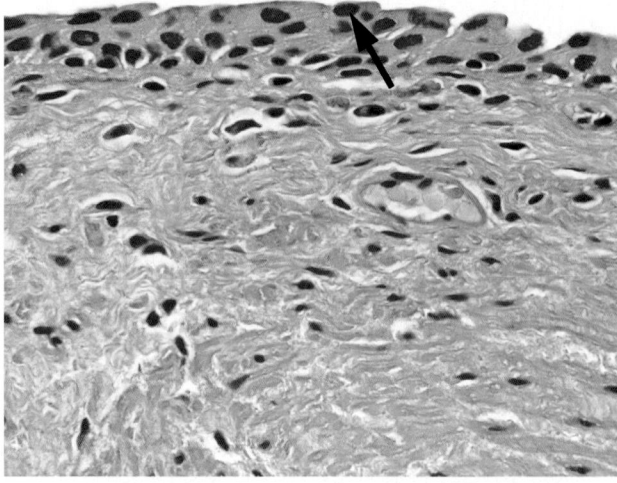

Figure 5-129. High-grade squamous intraepithelial lesion (AIN3). Beware, HSIL is easy to miss when it is only a few cells thick. Make sure to take your time with these cases. This focus shows full-thickness atypia, supporting a diagnosis of HSIL (AIN3). The mitotic figure in the upper third of the epithelium (*arrow*) supports the diagnosis.

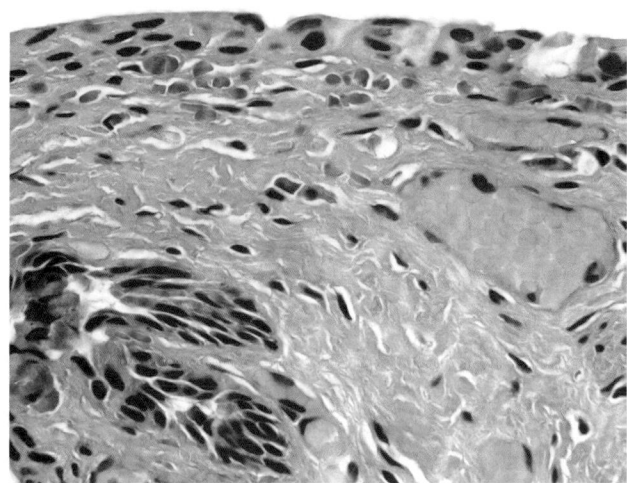

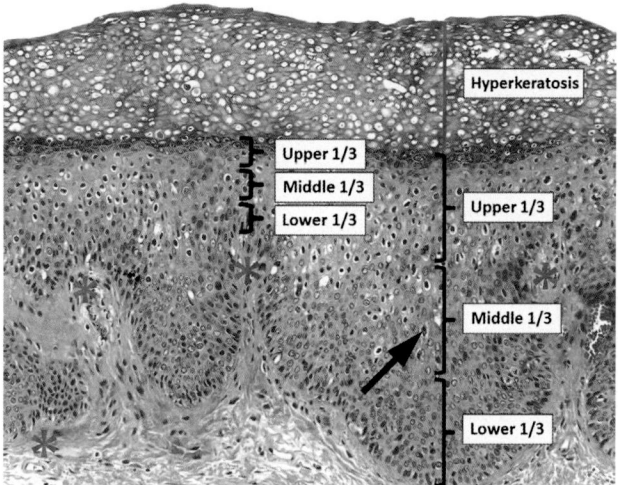

Figure 5-130. High-grade squamous intraepithelial lesion (AIN3). Even though this focus is only a few cells thick, the full-thickness atypia supports a diagnosis of HSIL (AIN3). Mitotic figures are not required for the diagnosis, although when found in the upper third of the epithelium, they support an HSIL diagnosis.

Figure 5-131. High-grade squamous intraepithelial lesion (AIN2) with hyperkeratosis. Hyperkeratosis refers to abnormal keratinization (*red bracket*). The true top is the most superficial epithelium with discernable nuclei to allow for evaluation of atypia and mitotic figure assessment. The true top is not the most superficial orthokeratotic layer because this zone contains no nuclei and, consequently, cannot be evaluated for atypia and mitotic figures. The *arrow* highlights a midlevel mitosis, supporting the diagnosis of HSIL (AIN2). *Asterisks* define the true bottom of the tissue (*asterisks*).

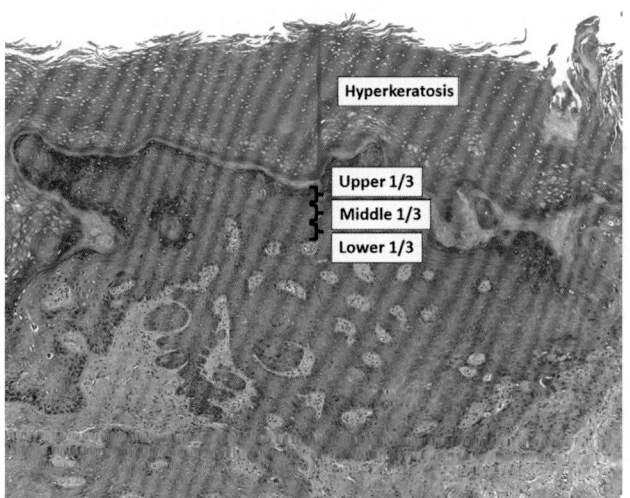

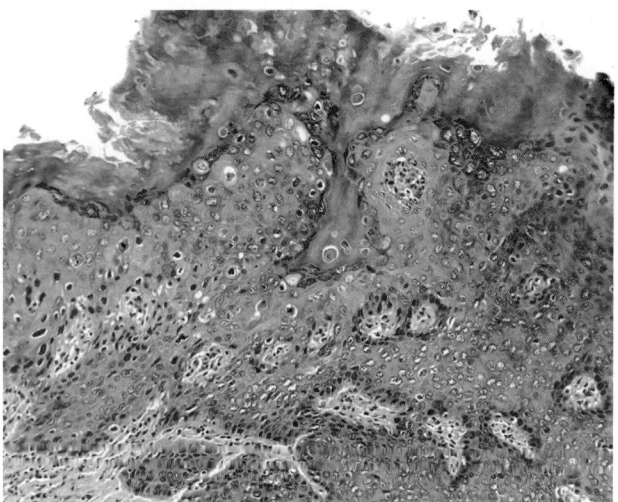

Figure 5-132. Squamous cell carcinoma (not shown) with hyperkeratosis. The true top is not the most superficial hyperkeratotic layer (*bracket*) because this zone contains no nuclei and, consequently, cannot be evaluated for atypia and mitotic figure assessment. In other sections, this lesion showed a well-differentiated invasive squamous cell carcinoma.

Figure 5-133. HSIL (AIN2) with hyperkeratosis. Disregard the hyperkeratosis for defining the true top of the lesion. A midlevel mitosis supports the diagnosis of HSIL (AIN2).

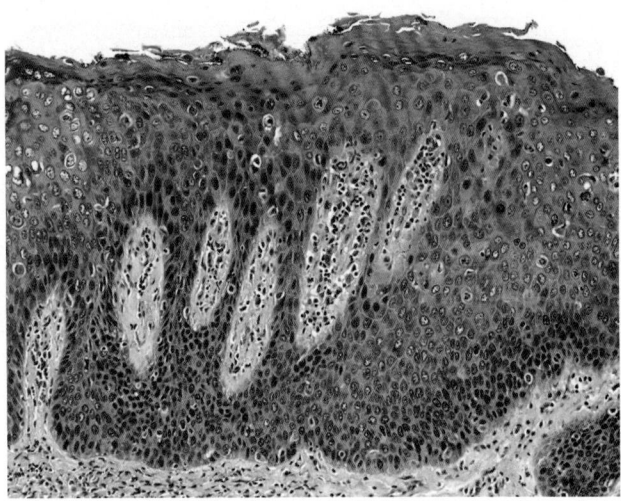

Figure 5-134. HSIL (AIN2) with hyperkeratosis. Disregard the hyperkeratosis for defining the true top of the lesion.

BIOMARKERS

LAST includes recommendations for the use of biomarkers as diagnostic aides. After identifying almost 2,300 relevant articles, p16 was named the only recommended biomarker based on its ability to act as a surrogate marker for HPV-16, to predict which patients are at higher risk for malignant transformation, and to reduce interobserver variability in the assessment of the -IN 2 category. P16 is a cyclin-dependent kinase inhibitor encoded by the tumor suppressor *CDKN2A*. It can be broadly applied as an adjunct test to all lower anogenital sites in a similar fashion.[16] p16 is recommended in two narrowly defined contexts: (1) when the diagnostic issue is HSIL versus a HSIL mimic, such as immature squamous epithelium, reactive epithelial change, atrophy, and tangential sections, *or* (2) when there is a discrepancy between the cytology and surgical biopsy to ensure that a small focus of HSIL was not overlooked in the surgical specimen. Prior high-risk cytologic interpretations that trigger p16 on the non-HSIL surgical specimen include HSIL, ASC-H, ASC-US/HPV-16+, or AGC (NOS). For example, p16 is indicated in the case of a cytology diagnosis of HSIL that is followed by a non-HSIL diagnosis on the corresponding or subsequent biopsy. ProEX C and Ki67 were also studied and found to lack sufficient literature support, either alone or in combination with other potential biomarkers.

PEARLS & PITFALLS: p16 IHC Is Not a Magic Bullet

Although accurate evaluation of p16 is critical to guide clinical management, it is a difficult IHC to interpret. The following are the need-to-know tips of the p16 IHC.

1. Avoid ordering p16 up front on all cases. It should only be ordered in two narrowly defined contexts:

   a. when the diagnostic issue is HSIL versus a HSIL mimic *or*

   b. when there is a discrepancy between the cytology and surgical biopsy

2. Reactive p16 immunoreactivity requires diffuse, block immunolabeling that highlights the nucleus and cytoplasm of the basal layer and at least the continuous one-third of the epithelial thickness in the atypical foci seen on hematoxylin-eosin (H&E) (Figs. 5.135–5.144). Full-thickness reactivity is not required for positive p16 immunolabeling (Figs. 5.139–5.144). Nonreactive p16 can be entirely negative, focal, patchy, or only cytoplasmic (Figs. 5.145–5.152).

3. The H&E morphology is the priority. A positive p16 supports a diagnosis of HSIL only if the case satisfies the morphologic criteria for HSIL on the H&E

(Figs. 5.135–5.144). Similarly, in general, avoid ordering p16 in the non-HSIL differential diagnoses. P16 is notoriously unreliable in these settings and could display potentially misleading results that could lead to clinical overmanagement (Figs. 5.153 and 5.154).

4. Avoid ordering p16 when the differential diagnosis is unequivocally -IN 2 versus -IN 3 on H&E because both are regarded as HSIL. For unclear reasons, a small subset of overt HSIL is p16 nonreactive. Avoid ordering p16 on unequivocal HSIL on H&E to avoid incorrectly downgrading a HSIL lesion, resulting in clinical undertreatment.

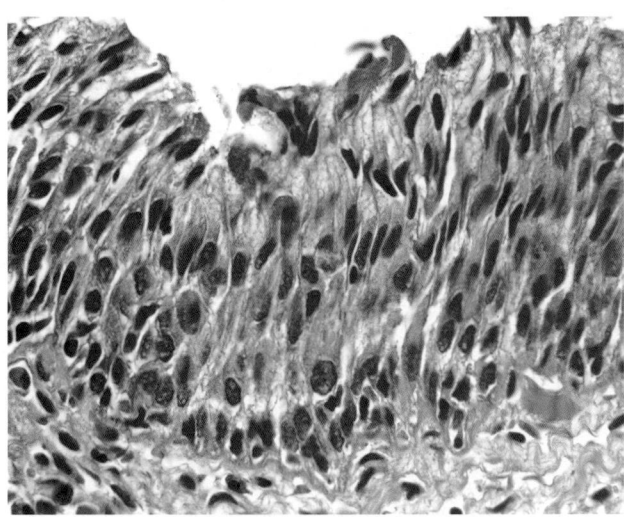

Figure 5-135. High-grade squamous intraepithelial lesion (AIN2). P16 is a handy tool when the diagnostic issue is HSIL versus a HSIL mimic. This focus is cauterized, and the differential diagnosis was HSIL (AIN2) versus cauterized ATZ.

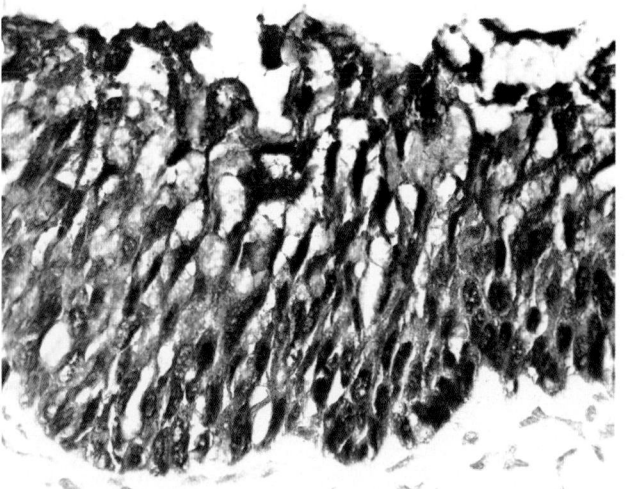

Figure 5-136. HSIL (AIN2), p16 reactive. The corresponding p16 is reactive, supporting the diagnosis of HSIL (AIN2). Reactive p16 immunoreactivity requires diffuse, block immunolabeling that highlights the nuclei and cytoplasm of the basal layer and at least the continuous one-third of the epithelial thickness in the atypical foci seen on H&E.

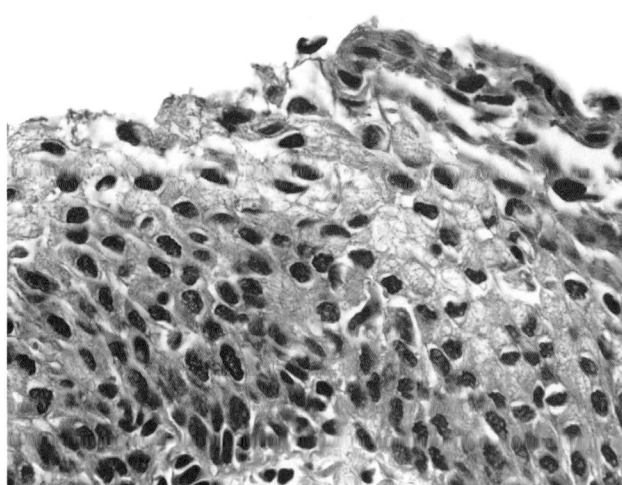

Figure 5-137. High-grade squamous intraepithelial lesion (AIN2). P16 is a tricky immunostain to accurately evaluate. It can be reactive in LSIL and nonreactive in HSIL. Consequently, it should be ordered only when the diagnostic issue is HSIL versus a HSIL mimic or when there is a discrepancy between the cytology and surgical biopsy to avoid inappropriate subsequent management.

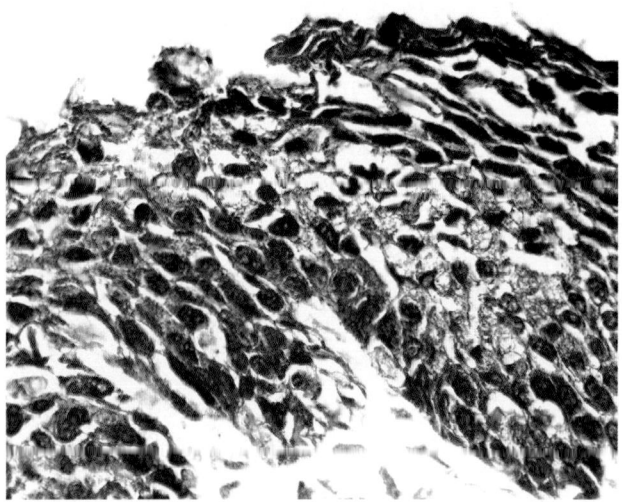

Figure 5-138. HSIL (AIN2), p16 reactive. Remember that the H&E morphology is the priority. A positive p16 supports a diagnosis of HSIL only if the case satisfies the morphologic criteria for HSIL on the H&E, as in this case.

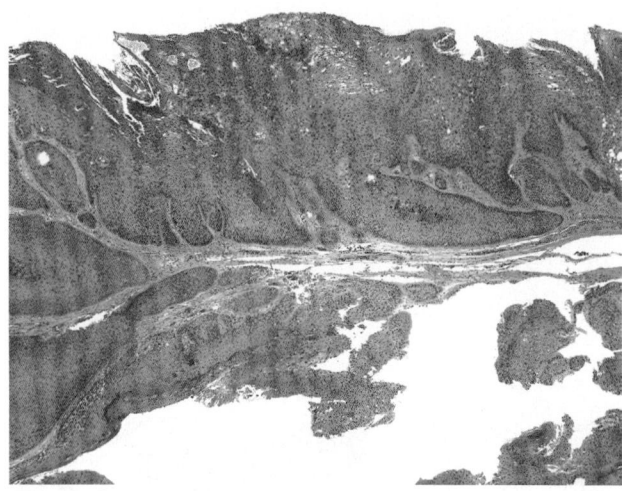

Figure 5-139. High-grade squamous intraepithelial lesion (AIN2).

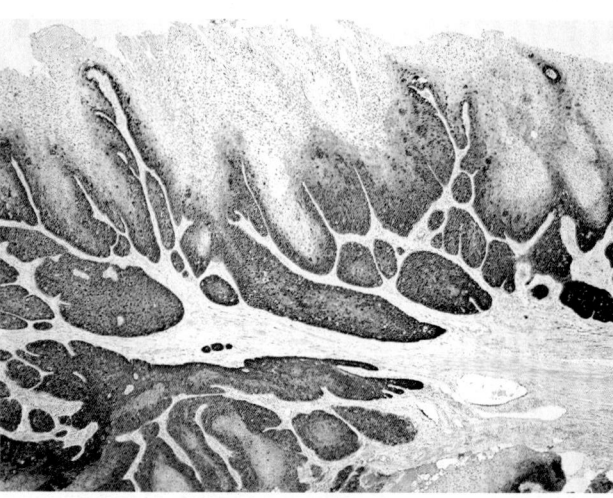

Figure 5-140. HSIL (AIN2), p16 reactive. Reactive p16 immunoreactivity requires diffuse, blocklike immunolabeling of the basal layer and at least the continuous one-third of the epithelial thickness. Full-thickness reactivity is not required for positive p16 immunolabeling.

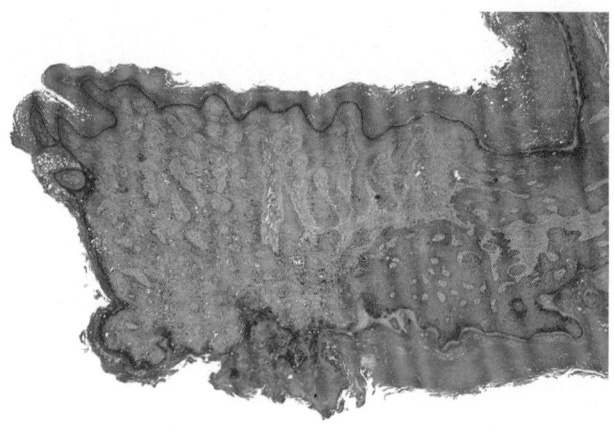

Figure 5-141. High-grade squamous intraepithelial lesion (AIN2).

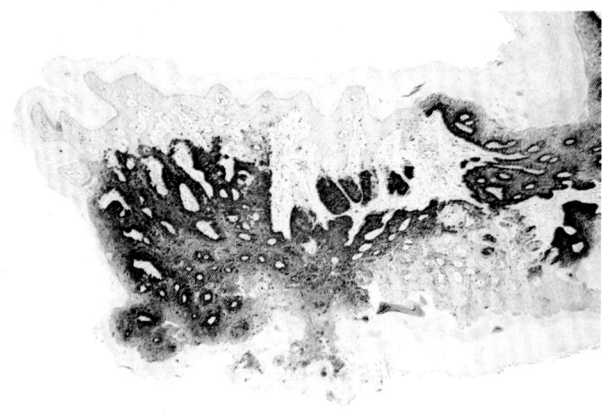

Figure 5-142. HSIL (AIN2), p16 reactive. Full-thickness reactivity is not required for positive p16 immunolabeling.

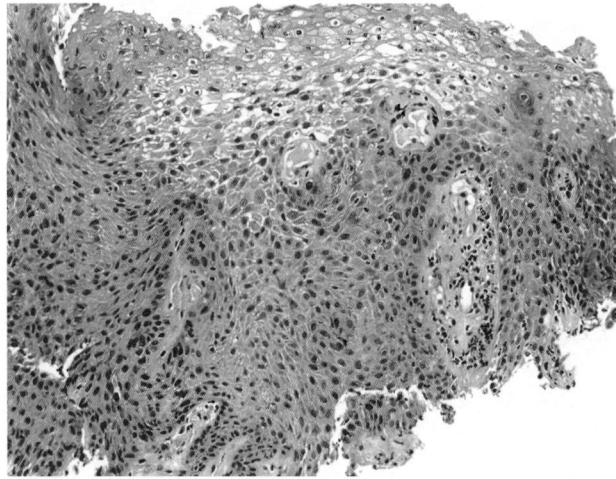

Figure 5-143. High-grade squamous intraepithelial lesion (AIN2). A subset of HSIL is p16 nonreactive. Avoid ordering p16 on unequivocal HSIL on H&E to avoid incorrectly downgrading a HSIL lesion, resulting in clinical undertreatment.

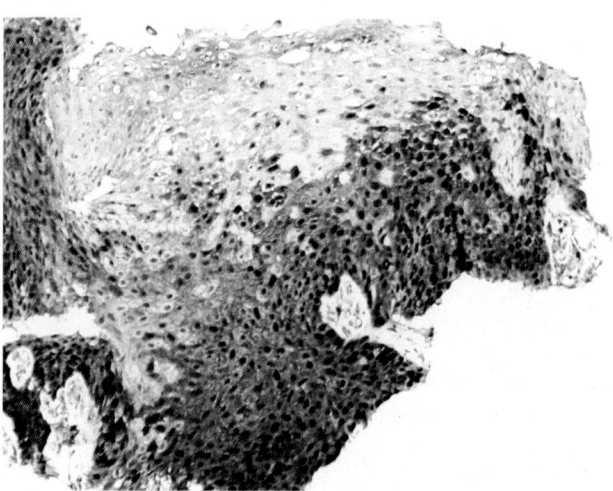

Figure 5-144. HSIL (AIN2), p16 reactive. Reactive p16 immunoreactivity requires diffuse, blocklike immunolabeling of the basal layer and at least the continuous one-third of the epithelial thickness. Full-thickness reactivity is not required for positive p16 immunolabeling.

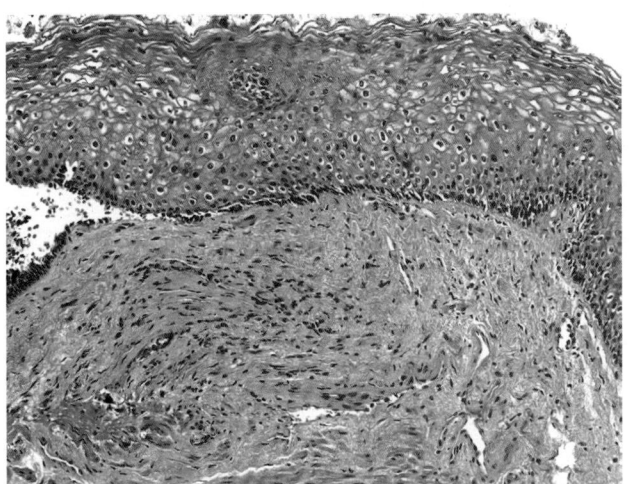

Figure 5-145. Low-grade squamous intraepithelial lesion.

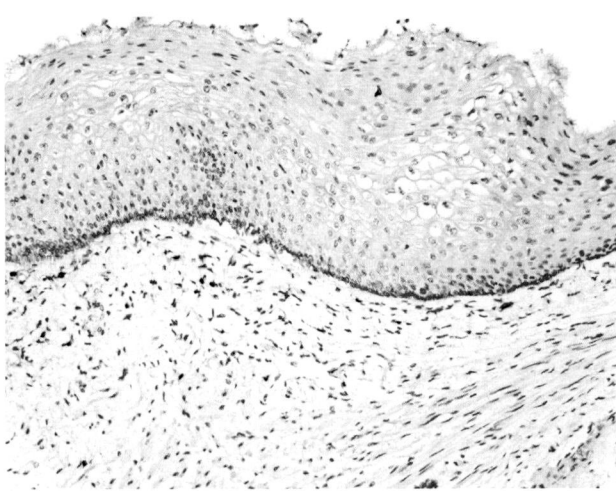

Figure 5-146. LSIL, p16 nonreactive. Nonreactive p16 can be entirely negative, as in this case, focal, patchy, or only cytoplasmic.

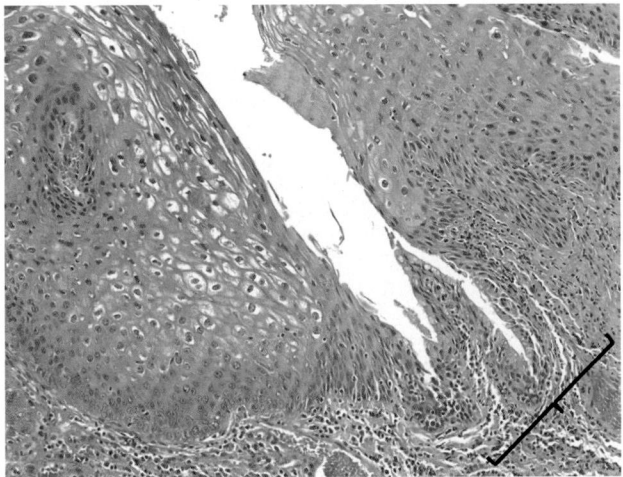

Figure 5-147. Low-grade squamous intraepithelial lesion. A p16 was ordered to assess the atypical focus (bracket) because the differential diagnosis was between normal ATZ and HSIL. The neighboring epithelium shows classic LSIL features.

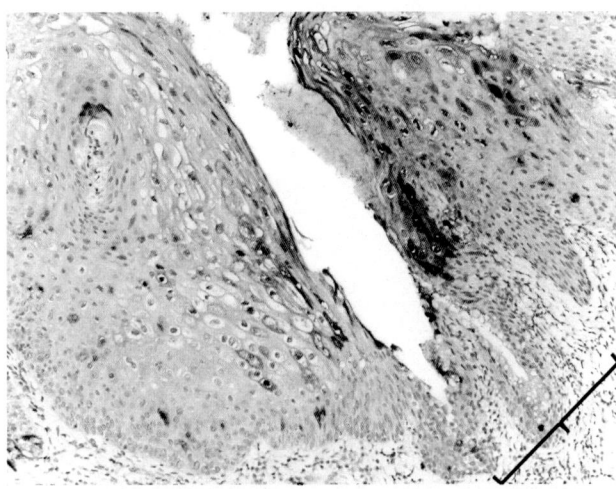

Figure 5-148. LSIL, p16 nonreactive. The atypical focus (bracket) is p16 negative, supporting the diagnosis of normal ATZ rather than a focus of HSIL. The limited staining present is within the spectrum for negative. Nonreactive p16 can be entirely negative, focal, patchy (as in this case), or only cytoplasmic. The diagnosis of LSIL was rendered based on the adjacent epithelium that shows classic LSIL features on H&E.

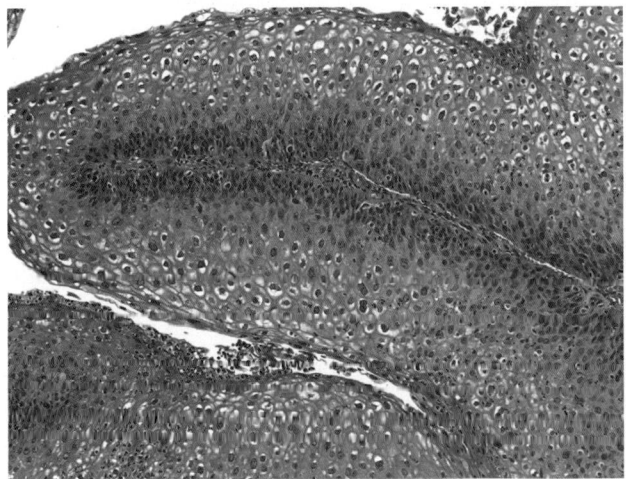

Figure 5-149. Low-grade squamous intraepithelial lesion.

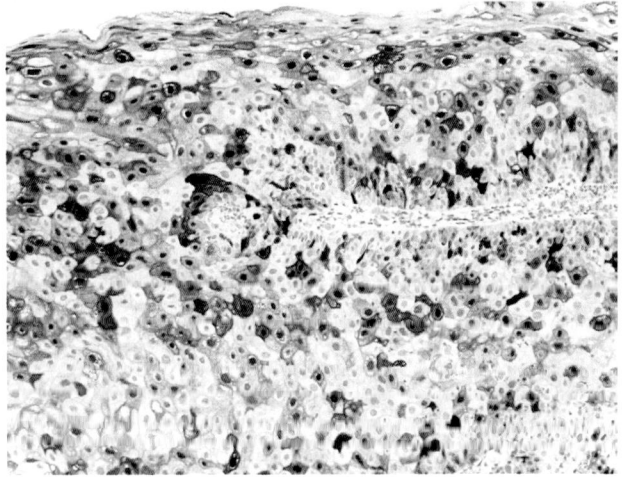

Figure 5-150. LSIL, p16 nonreactive. Although this is quite a bit of staining, it is in a patchy, checkerboard pattern and, therefore, negative/nonreactive. Nonreactive p16 can be entirely negative, focal, patchy (as in this case), or only cytoplasmic.

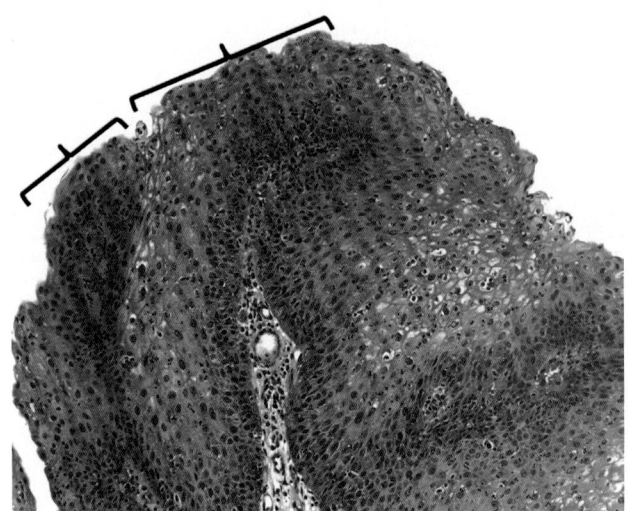

Figure 5-151. Low-grade squamous intraepithelial lesion. P16 was ordered in this inflamed epithelium because the differential diagnosis was focal HSIL (AIN2) (*brackets*) versus inflamed LSIL with tangential sections.

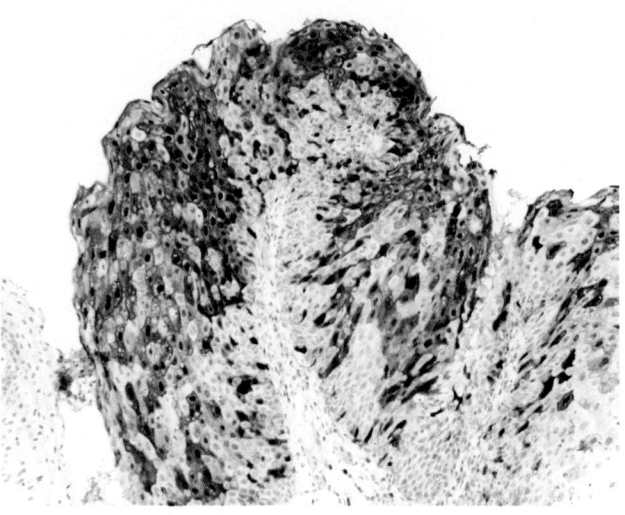

Figure 5-152. LSIL, p16 nonreactive. Although this is quite a bit of staining, the basal epithelium is entirely negative and, therefore, the p16 is negative/nonreactive, supporting a diagnosis of LSIL. P16 immunoreactivity requires diffuse, block immunolabeling that highlights the nuclei and cytoplasm of the basal layer and at least the continuous one-third of the epithelial thickness in the atypical foci seen on H&E.

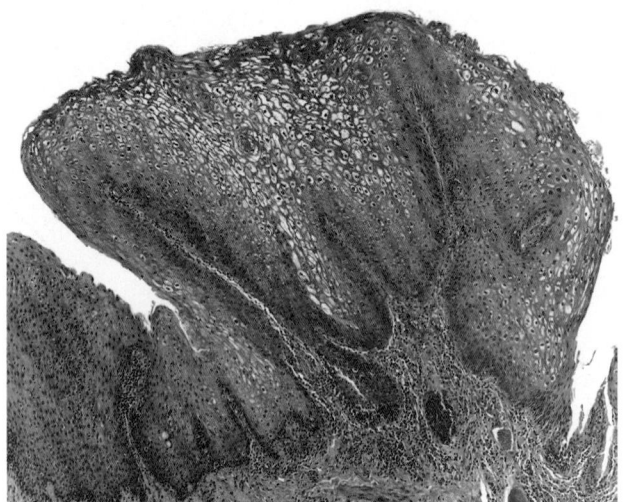

Figure 5-153. Low-grade squamous intraepithelial lesion. P16 was ordered to evaluate another field on this specimen where the differential diagnosis was LSIL versus HSIL (AIN2) (not shown).

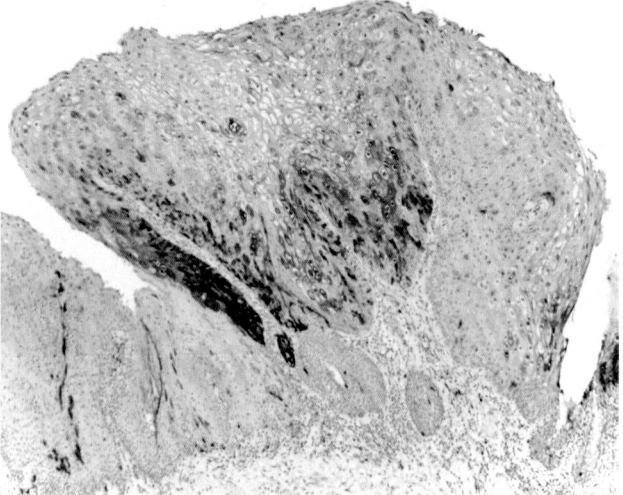

Figure 5-154. LSIL, p16 nonreactive. P16 shows focal reactivity in this example of unequivocal LSIL on H&E. Recall, p16 immunoreactivity requires immunoreactivity in atypical foci seen on H&E. If the H&E is unequivocal LSIL, as in this case, the p16 should not be ordered or should be entirely disregarded (if ordered to evaluate another focus of HSIL vs. a non-HSIL diagnosis).

Squamous Cell Carcinoma

Epidemiology

Squamous cell carcinoma of the anus is the most common malignancy of the anus (but it is still uncommon), affecting <1 per 100,000 patients.[3] Risk factors include HPV infection, female sex, anal receptive sex, tobacco smoking, urban setting, chronic infections or fistulas, and immunosuppression, including HIV. EGFR overexpression has been identified in a subset, which may suggest a role for anti-EGFR-based therapy.[18,19]

Superficially Invasive Versus Invasive

Squamous cell carcinoma is classified as superficially invasive (SISCCA) or invasive (without the "superficial" qualifier) based on the extent of invasion and margin status.

SISCCA defines a subset of patients eligible for conservative, local excision. The following SISCCA criteria for the anus and perianus were chosen to parallel the criteria for the cervix and allow for uniform reporting in the lower anogenital tract: depth ≤3 mm, horizontal spread ≤7 mm, and completely excised. Invasive squamous cell carcinoma, in contrast, is defined by depth >3 mm and horizontal spread >7 mm (Fig. 5.155). See "Measurement Tips" section. At this time, the presence or absence of lymphovascular invasion does not affect the classification of SISCCA in the anus and perianus.[16] In contrast, SISCCA in the penis requires the absence of lymphovascular space invasion. If the invasive component is present at the margins or tissue edges, the lesion may be incompletely excised and should be reported as such. For incompletely excised invasion less than or equal to the required dimensions of SISCCA (SISCCA = depth ≤3 mm and horizontal spread ≤7 mm), report as "*at least* superficially invasive squamous carcinoma". For invasion that exceeds the required dimensions of SISCAA (SISCAA = depth ≤3 mm and horizontal spread ≤7 mm), report as "invasive squamous carcinoma." See "Measurement Tips" section.

MEASUREMENT TIPS

Measuring the size of invasive lesions is almost as enjoyable as counting eosinophils in the esophagus, but it is important for accurate reporting and to ensure proper clinical management. Here are some handy measurement tips. The three measurements needed for assessing squamous invasion in anal specimens are the depth of invasion, the horizontal spread of invasion, and the tumor thickness. Keep in mind, anal SISCCA requires a depth ≤3 mm, a horizontal spread ≤7 mm, and complete excision. Invasion beyond these measurements is best termed invasive squamous cell carcinoma without the superficial qualifier; these cases are generally not amenable to local therapy. Below are helpful tips adapted from the 2012 LAST Consensus Recommendations.[16]

Depth of Invasion: This measurement is from the nearest discernable nonneoplastic epidermal-dermal (epithelial/subepithelial) junction to the deepest point of invasion.

Tumor Thickness: If the tumor is keratinizing, the thickness is measured from the granular cell layer to the deepest point of invasion. If the epithelium is not keratinized or is ulcerated, the thickness is measured from the surface of the tumor or ulcerated tumor to the deepest point of invasion.

Horizontal Spread of Invasion: This measurement spans the widest dimension of the invasion and is perpendicular to the depth of invasion.

Histology

Histologically, invasion (Figs. 5.156–5.172) is denoted by infiltrating individual neoplastic cells or nests of cells beyond the basement membrane in a desmoplastic background. The invading cells often display "reverse maturity," whereby they appear more eosinophilic, large, and mature than the overlying epithelium. Invasive squamous cell carcinoma can be extremely well differentiated, making it a challenging diagnosis. Helpful clues to invasion include invasion into the lymphovascular spaces, nerves, and surrounding tissues. Background dysplasia may be present but is not a prerequisite for a diagnosis of invasion. The histologic patterns of squamous cell carcinoma vary between patients and within individual tumors. Subtypes include the large cell keratinizing, large cell nonkeratinizing, basaloid (peripheral palisading, retraction artifact, and central eosinophilic necrosis), adenoid cysticlike pattern of basaloid, and mucoepidermoid carcinoma subtypes.[3,20-22] At this point, there are no clear associations between the morphologic patterns, HPV tumor types, and outcomes. Moreover, there is poor reproducibility in subclassification between pathologists. As a result, the 2010 WHO recommends reporting a top-line diagnosis of squamous cell carcinoma and reserving the morphologic description or subtype in the note.[3]

See Fig. 5.173 for a side-by-side comparison of normal, LSIL, HSIL, and invasive squamous cell carcinoma.

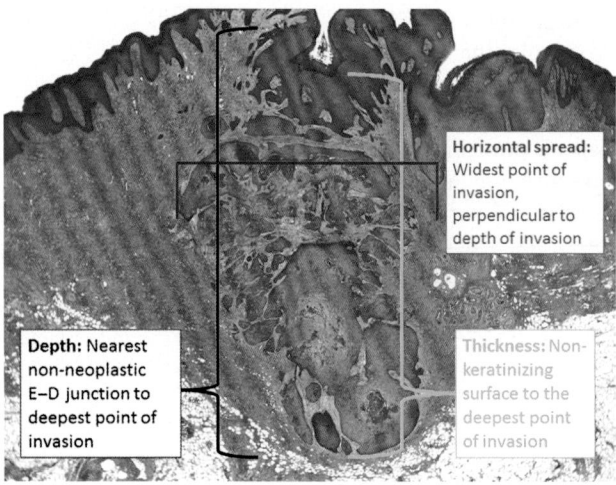

Horizontal spread: Widest point of invasion, perpendicular to depth of invasion

Depth: Nearest non-neoplastic E–D junction to deepest point of invasion

Thickness: Non-keratinizing surface to the deepest point of invasion

Figure 5-155. Superficially invasive squamous cell carcinoma (SISCCA). The SISCCA criteria for the anus and perianus include depth ≤3 mm (*bracket*), horizontal spread ≤7 mm (*bracket*), and complete excision. This case features the invasion on only this one slide. At this time, lymphovascular invasion does not affect the classification of SISCCA in the anus and perianus.

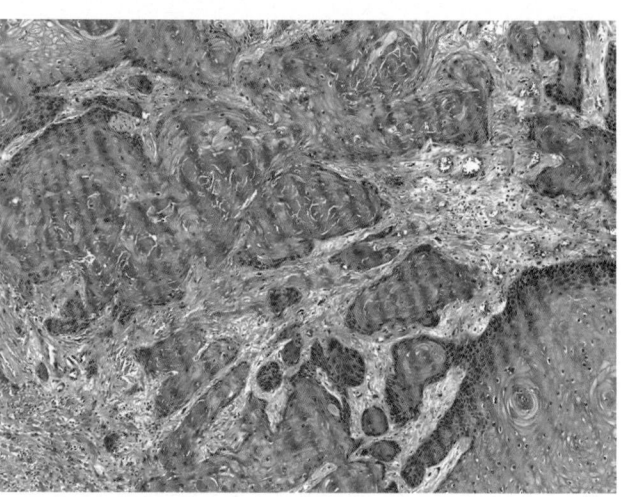

Figure 5-156. Invasive squamous cell carcinoma (ISCCA). ISCCA is denoted by infiltrating individual neoplastic cells or nests of cells beyond the basement membrane in a desmoplastic background, as seen here.

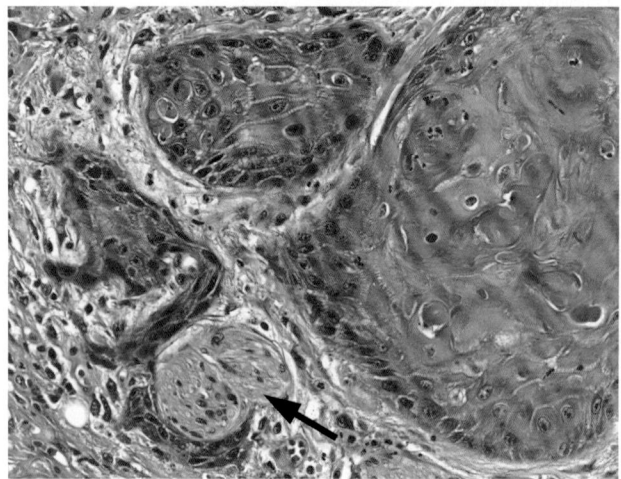

Figure 5-157. Invasive squamous cell carcinoma. ISCCA can be extremely well differentiated, making it a challenge to diagnose. The presence of perineural invasion is a helpful clue to ISCCA (*arrow*).

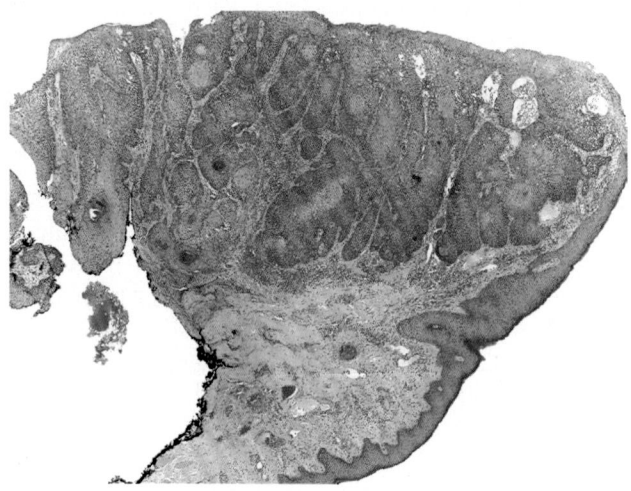

Figure 5-158. Invasive squamous cell carcinoma. Other helpful clues to ISCCA include the specimen designation as a mass with deeply infiltrative nests of neoplastic cells, as seen here.

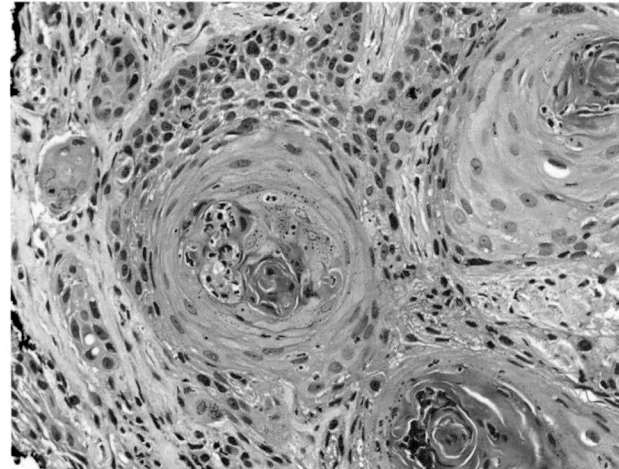

Figure 5-159. Invasive squamous cell carcinoma. Higher power shows nests of keratinizing epithelium in a desmoplastic background.

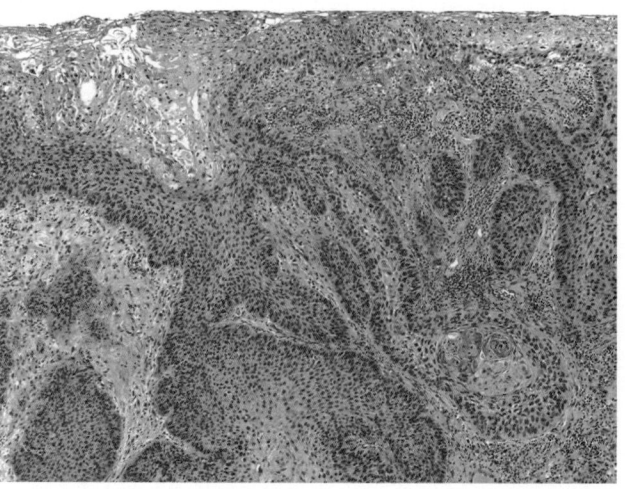

Figure 5-160. Invasive squamous cell carcinoma. The deeply infiltrative nests in a desmoplastic background are clues to ISCCA.

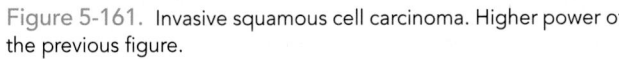

Figure 5-161. Invasive squamous cell carcinoma. Higher power of the previous figure.

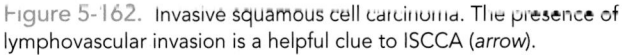

Figure 5-162. Invasive squamous cell carcinoma. The presence of lymphovascular invasion is a helpful clue to ISCCA (*arrow*).

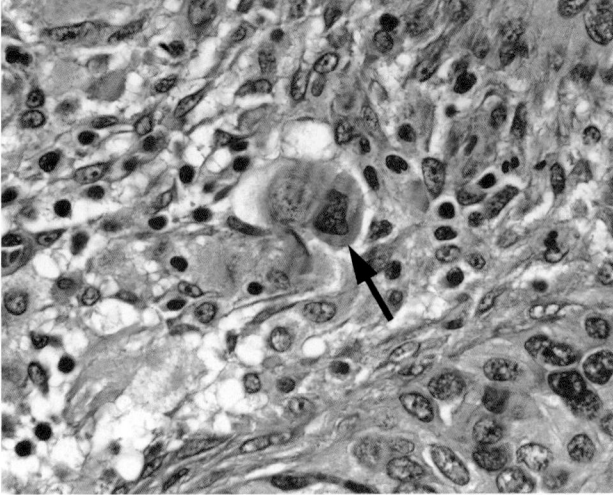

Figure 5-163. Invasive squamous cell carcinoma. The invading cells often display reverse maturity, whereby they appear more eosinophilic, large, and mature than the overlying epithelium (*arrow*).

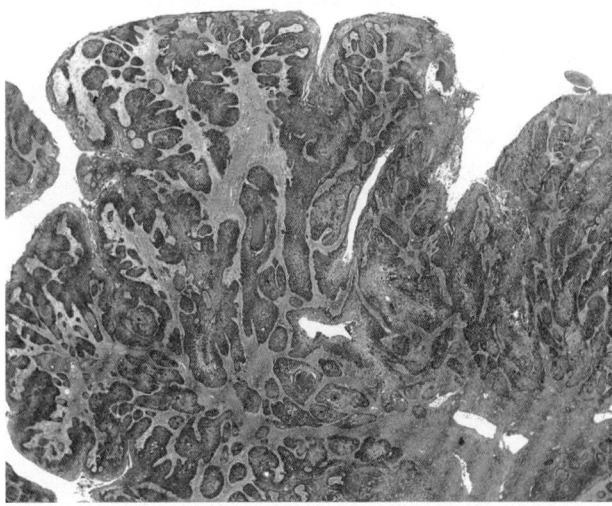

Figure 5-164. Invasive squamous cell carcinoma. The complex architecture of the keratinizing squamous cells is suggestive of ISCCA at low power.

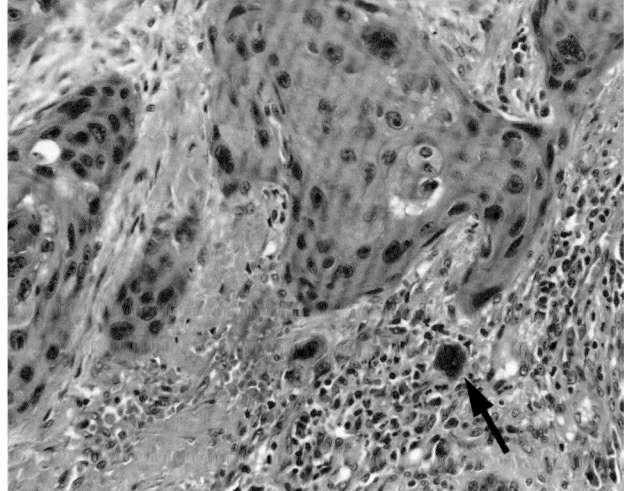

Figure 5-165. Invasive squamous cell carcinoma. Higher power of the previous figure. Individual invading cells are highlighted by an *arrow*.

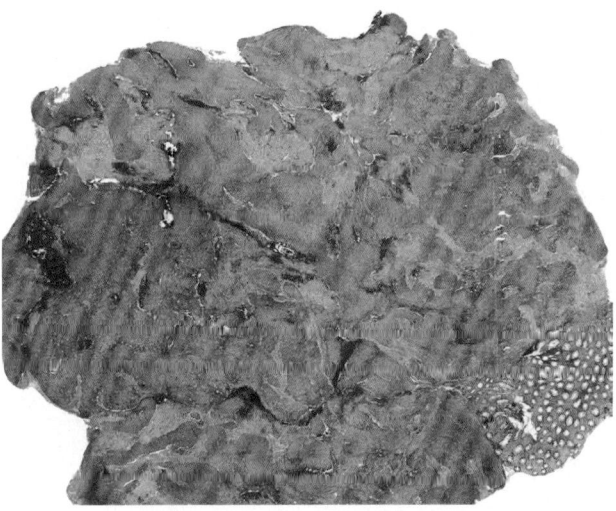

Figure 5-166. Basaloid SCCA. Although the 2010 WHO recommends avoiding subclassifying squamous cell carcinomas, this case displays the typical features of ISCCA with basaloid squamous features, features best seen on higher power.

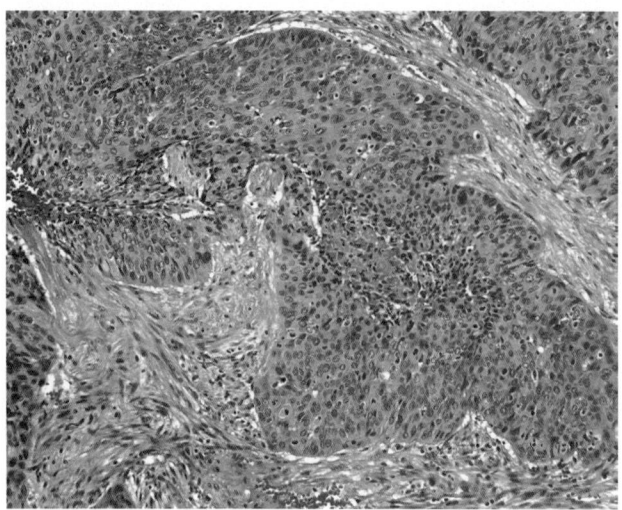

Figure 5-167. Basaloid SCCA. Higher power of the previous figure shows infiltrative nests with central necrosis in a desmoplastic background. As typical for basaloid squamous differentiation, note that the neoplastic cells lack keratinization, and central necrosis is present.

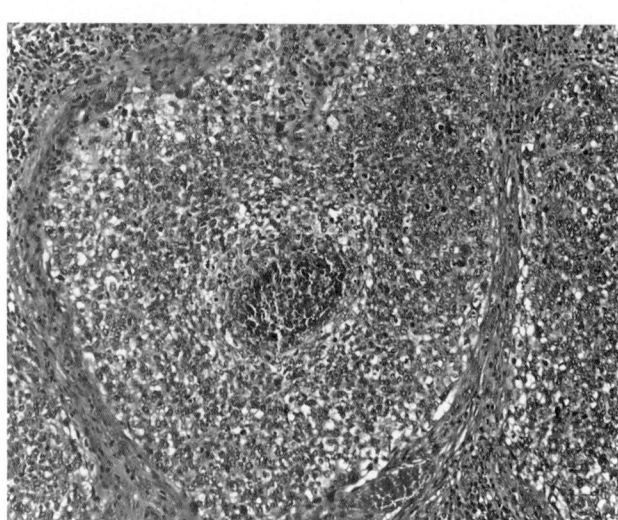

Figure 5-168. Basaloid SCCA. Typical features of basaloid squamous differentiation include central necrosis, vague nuclear palisading at the periphery, and primitive-appearing cells lacking abundant cytoplasm and keratinization.

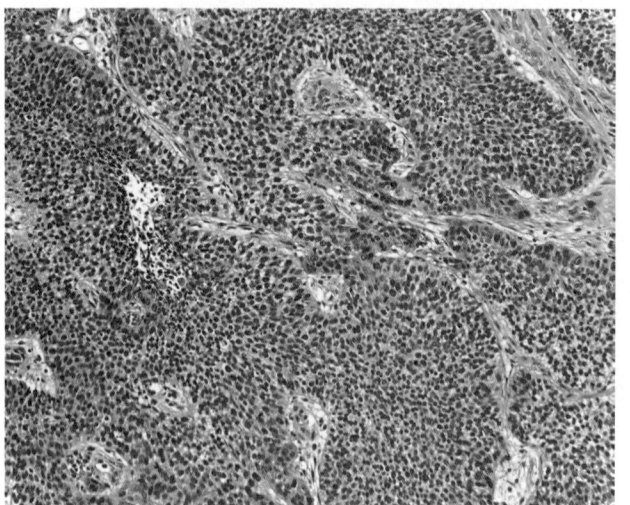

Figure 5-169. Basaloid SCCA. The lesional cells are small with vague nuclear palisading at the periphery, and scant cytoplasm is present without keratinization.

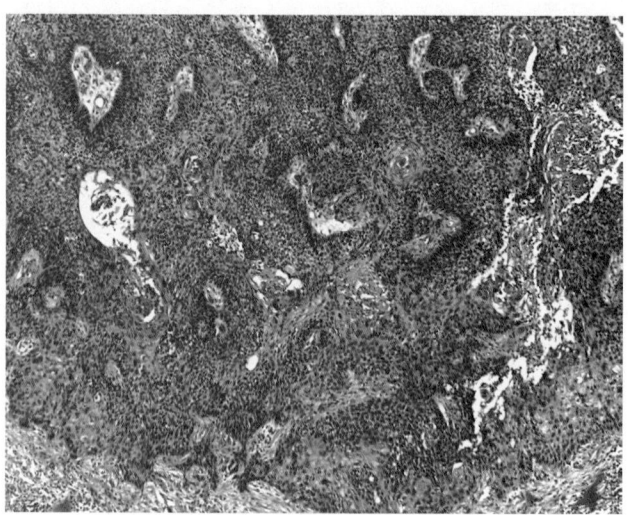

Figure 5-170. Basaloid SCCA. Basaloid squamous lesions appear dark on lower power because they lack keratinization and the lesional cells have only scant cytoplasm.

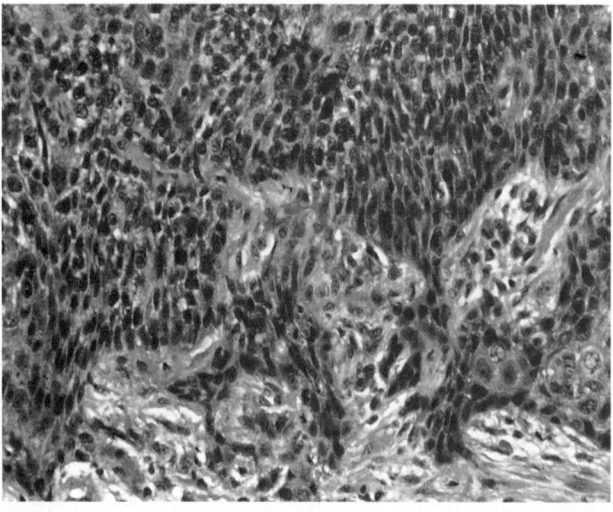

Figure 5-171. Basaloid SCCA. Higher power of the previous figure shows vague nuclear palisading at the periphery.

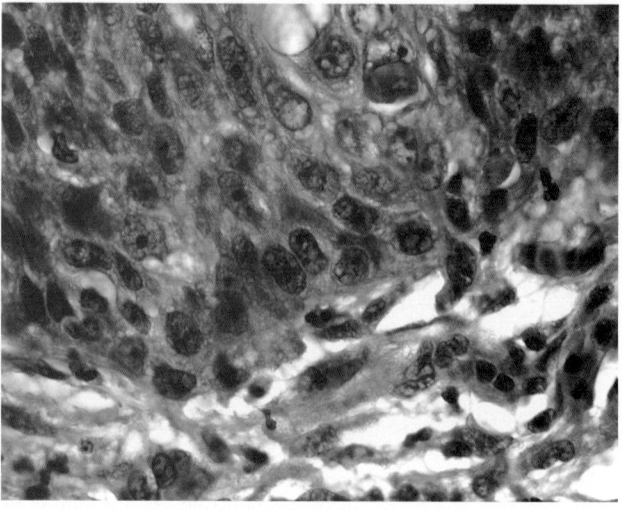

Figure 5-172. Basaloid SCCA. Higher power of the previous figure.

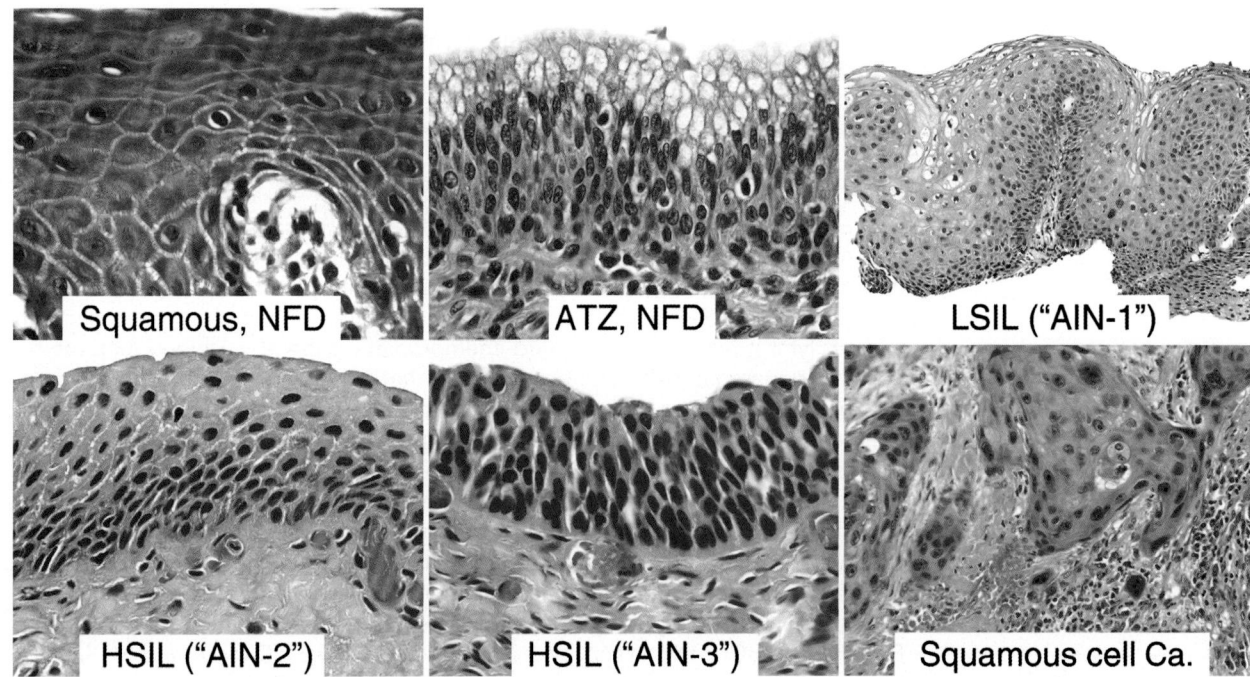

Figure 5-173. Composite of normal and neoplasia. Normal squamous mucosa can have fake perinuclear halos, but lacks hyperchromatic, irregular nuclear membranes, and prominent mitoses seen in dysplasia. ATZ normally is a bit cellular with normochromatic chromatin and an orderly array of cell layers. LSIL is characterized by koilocytes and mitoses in the lower third of the epithelium, and the atypia matures in the upper two-thirds. HSIL (AIN2) is characterized by atypia and mitoses in the middle third, and the atypia matures in the upper third. HSIL (AIN3) is characterized by full-thickness atypia and mitoses in the upper third. Invasive squamous cell carcinoma displays infiltrating nests of neoplastic cells in a desmoplastic background and reverse maturity.

CHECKLIST: Squamous Cell Carcinoma Reporting of a Biopsy Specimen

☐ Specify unifocal or multifocal invasion

☐ Size of each tumor

☐ Depth of invasion for each tumor

☐ Widest point of horizontal invasion for each tumor

☐ Margin status

☐ Presence or absence of lymphovascular invasion

☐ Presence of background pathology, such as squamous dysplasia

PEARLS & PITFALLS: The Term "Cloacogenic Carcinoma" Is Obsolete, as Is "Condyloma Acuminatum"

Cloacogenic carcinoma is an outdated term that referred to a type of squamous cell carcinoma with basaloid- or transitional-type differentiation of presumed ATZ origination. Typical histologic features include a nested architecture of small neoplastic cells lacking intercellular bridges and prominent necrosis, mitotic figures, and nuclear palisading at the periphery of the lesion.[23] The 2010 WHO recommends reporting a top-line diagnosis of squamous cell carcinoma without subclassifying the morphologic type.[3] Consequently, the term cloacogenic carcinoma is no longer in use. Similarly, the term condyloma acuminatum has been retired in place of an LSIL designation according to the 2012 LAST recommendations.[16]

FAQ: What are tips to correctly subclassify basaloid squamous cell carcinoma and distinguish it from BCC?

Answer: Based on a lack of clinical significance of the squamous carcinoma subtypes and poor reproducibility in subclassification between pathologists, the 2010 WHO recommends reporting a top-line diagnosis of squamous cell carcinoma and avoiding subclassification.[3] It is clinically important to distinguish basaloid squamous cell carcinoma from BCC because the former is an aggressive neoplasm with metastatic potential that is treated with chemoradiation, resection, and lymph node dissection. In contrast, BCC is treated with conservative resection without lymph node dissection and chemoradiation therapy. Unique features of basaloid squamous cell carcinoma include that it is HPV related, it often has a background of LSIL or HSIL, and it usually arises in the anal canal. Histologically, the neoplastic cells display more pleomorphism, mitoses (often atypical), and necrosis (Figs. 5.166–5.172). In contrast to basaloid squamous cell carcinoma, BCC is extremely rare in the anus; when present, it usually originates in the perianal skin. BCC displays lower-grade histology with a lack of prominent and atypical mitoses, pleomorphism, and necrosis (Figs. 5.174–5.186). Characteristically, BCC has retraction artifact around the neoplasm's edge and the small nuclei display nuclear palisading along the neoplasm's periphery. For difficult cases, diffuse Ber-EP4 and BCL2 IHC reactivity favor BCC and diffuse CDKN2A and SOX2 IHC reactivity favor basaloid squamous cell carcinoma (Table 5.1).[24]

See Fig. 5.187 for a side-by-side comparison of basaloid squamous cell carcinoma and BCC.

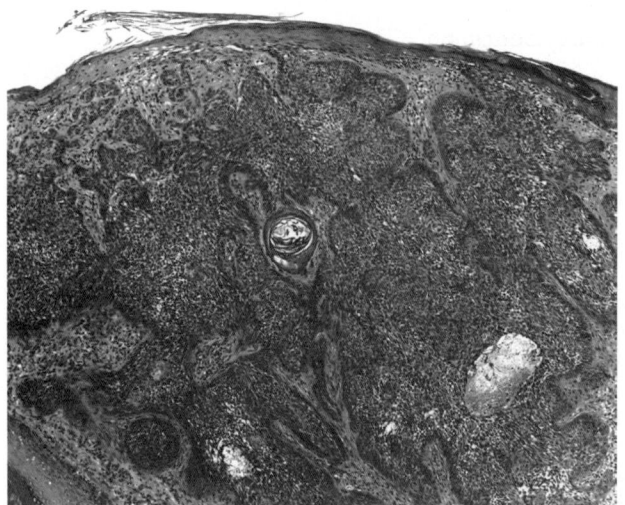

Figure 5-174. Basal cell carcinoma (BCC). BCC appears *blue* at low power because the cells have scanty cytoplasm.

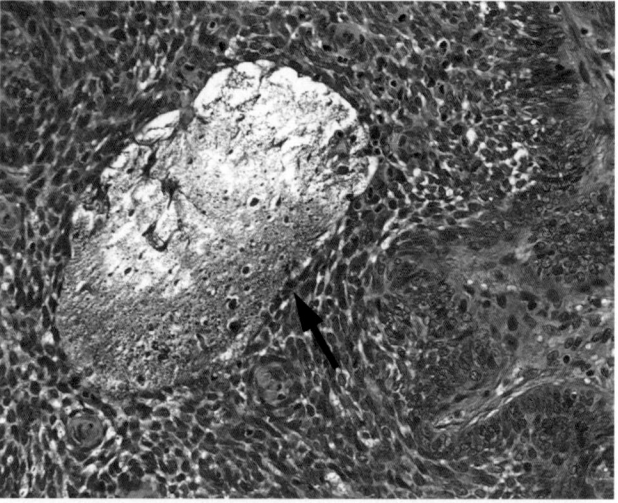

Figure 5-175. Basal cell carcinoma. Mucin deposition is common in BCC (*arrow*).

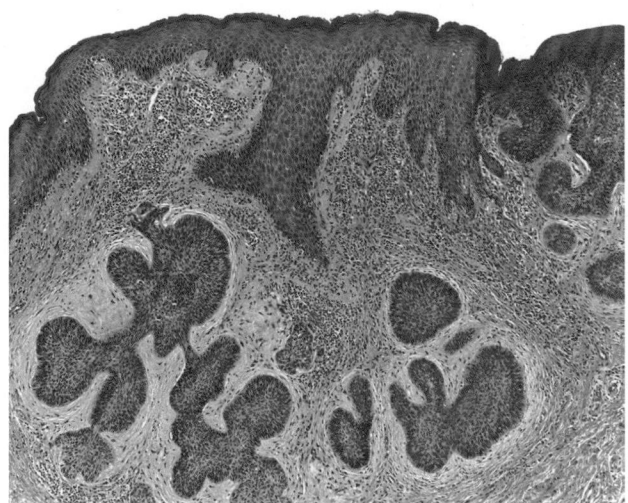

Figure 5-176. Basal cell carcinoma. BCC usually has a neater low power impression compared with basaloid SCCA owing its low-grade features, crisp nuclear palisading at the periphery, and *light blue* hue to the stroma surrounding the neoplasm, as seen here.

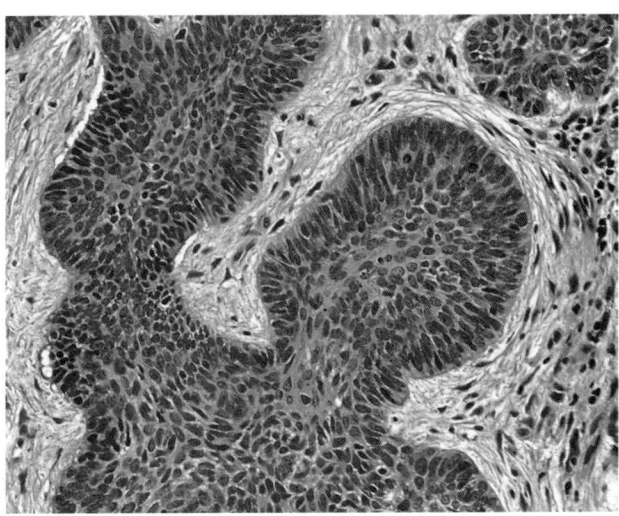

Figure 5-177. Basal cell carcinoma. Higher power of the previous figure shows low-grade nuclear features, crisp nuclear palisading at the periphery, and *light blue* hue to the stroma surrounding the neoplasm.

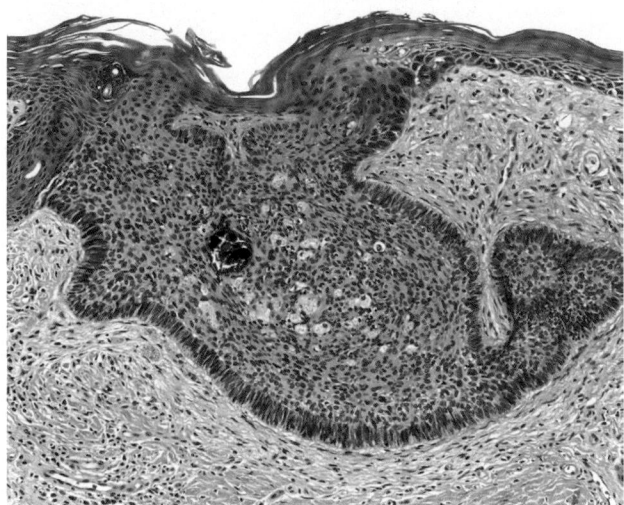

Figure 5-178. Basal cell carcinoma. This BCC connects to the overlying epidermis and has an intralesional calcification.

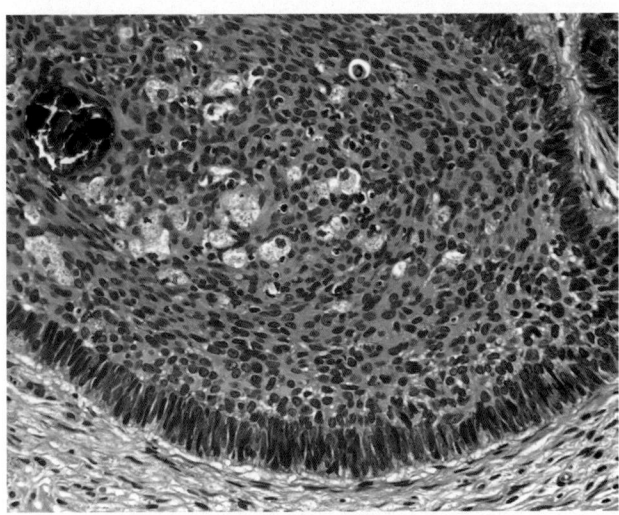

Figure 5-179. Basal cell carcinoma. Higher power of the previous figure shows the crisp nuclear palisading at the periphery.

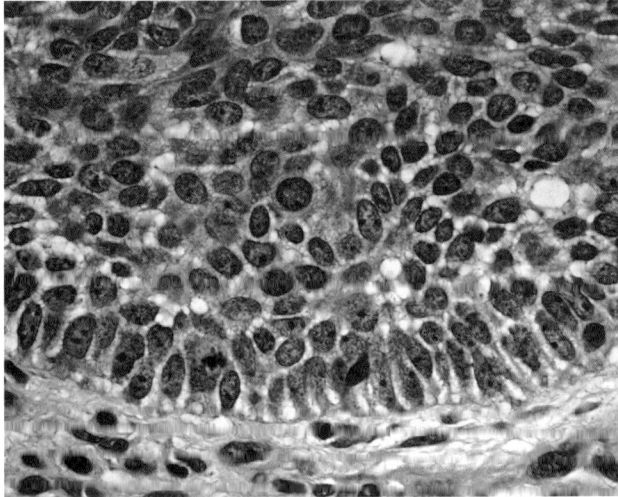

Figure 5-180. Basal cell carcinoma. Low-grade features are seen with nuclear palisading at the periphery.

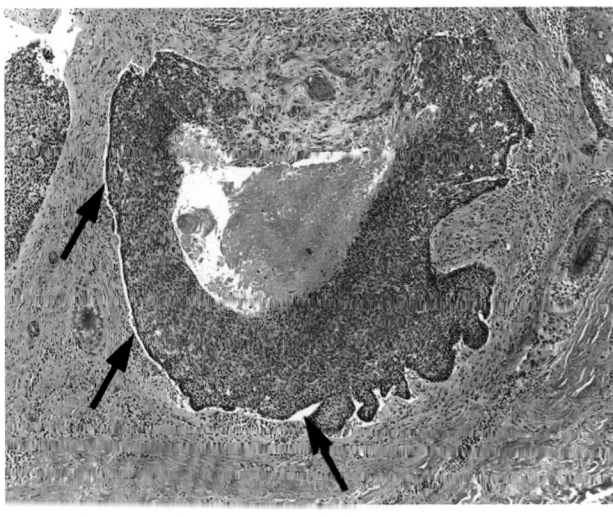

Figure 5-181. Basal cell carcinoma. This case features a peripheral cleft, or retraction artifact (*arrows*).

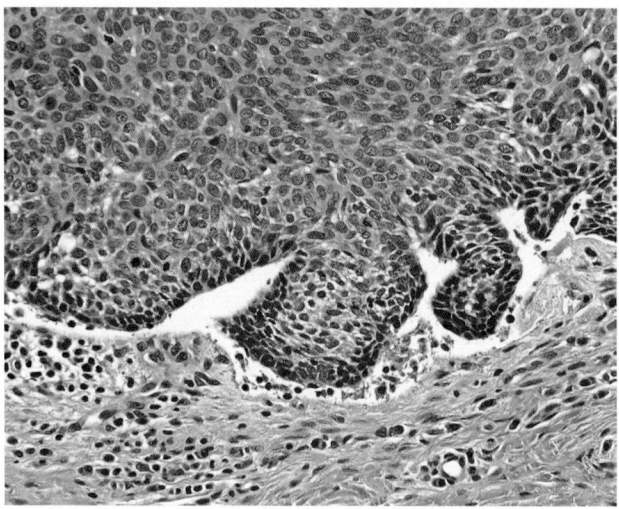

Figure 5-182. Basal cell carcinoma. Higher power of the previous figure emphasizes the peripheral cleft, or retraction artifact.

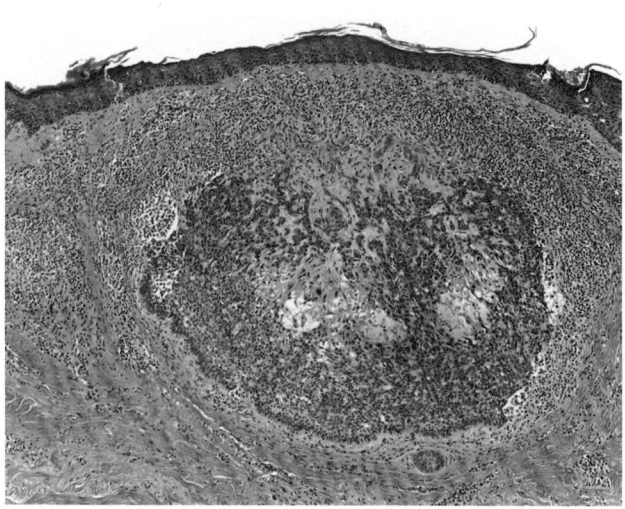

Figure 5-183. Basal cell carcinoma.

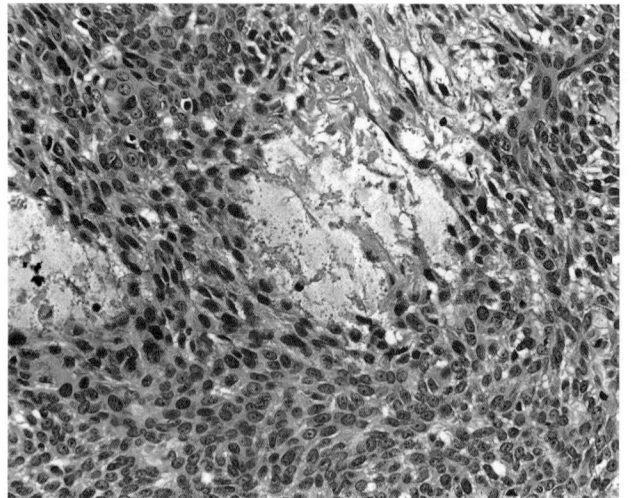

Figure 5-184. Basal cell carcinoma. Mucin deposition is common to BCC.

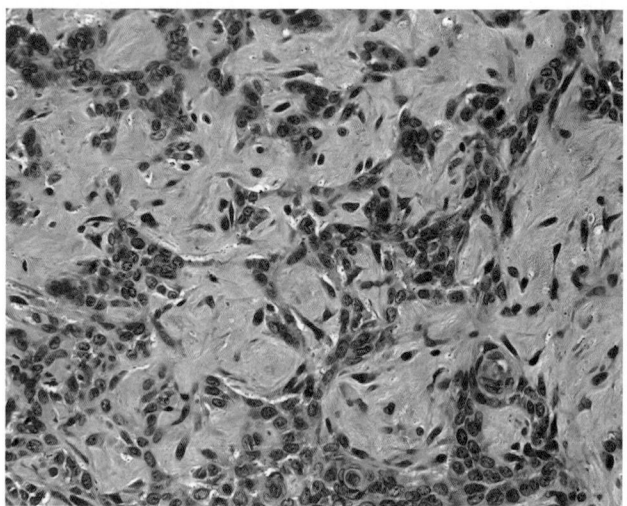

Figure 5-185. Basal cell carcinoma. The stroma in BCC also appears *blue*, as seen here.

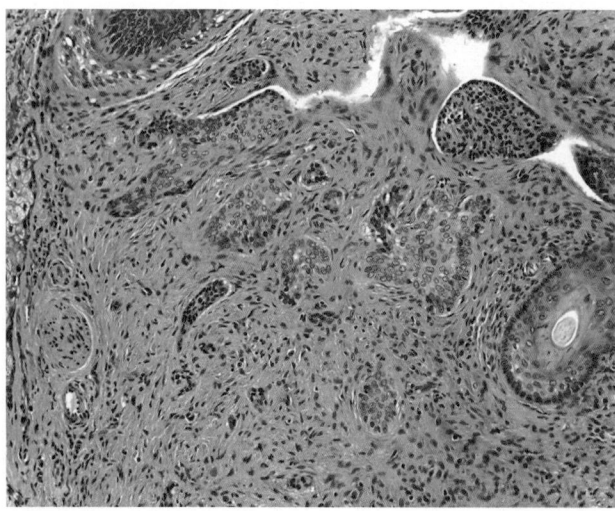

Figure 5-186. Basal cell carcinoma. BCC can feature small nests of glands, as seen here.

TABLE 5.1: Distinguishing Features of Basaloid Squamous Cell Carcinoma (SCCA) and Basal Cell Carcinoma (BCC)

	Basaloid SCCA	BCC
Treatment	Aggressive	Conservative
Origin	Anal canal	Perianal skin
HPV related	Yes	No
Background LSIL/HSIL	Common	No
Prominent mitoses, necrosis	Yes	No
Retraction artifact	No	Yes
Peripheral nuclear palisading	Vague	Crisp
Cytologic atypia	High grade	Low grade
IHC reactivity	CDKN2A, SOX2	Ber-EP4, BCL2

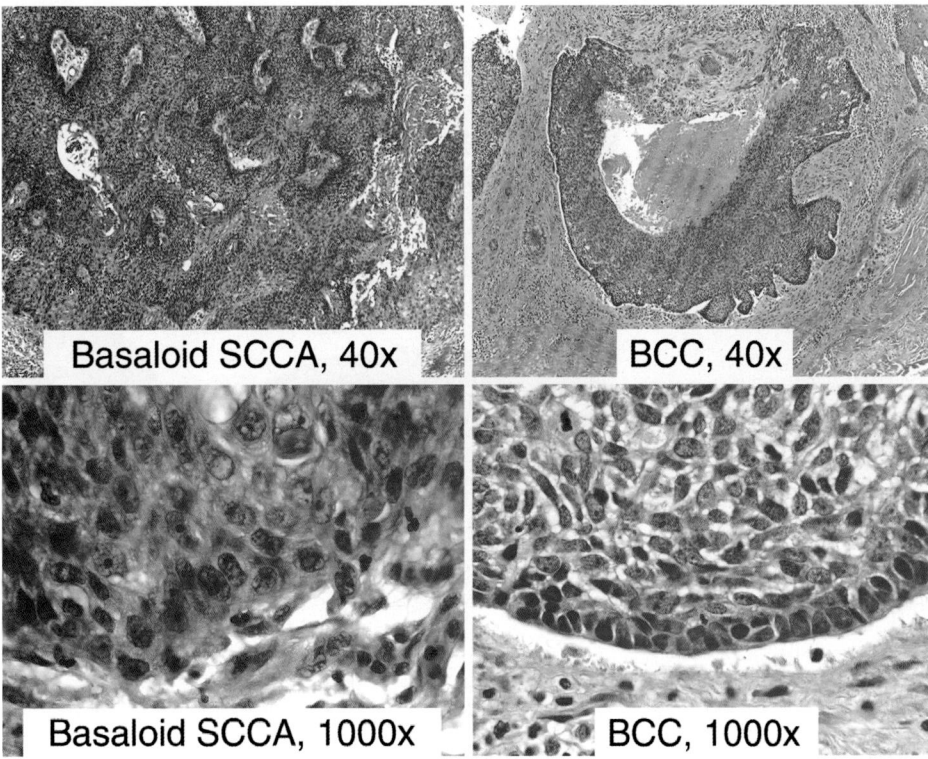

Basaloid SCCA, 40x   BCC, 40x

Basaloid SCCA, 1000x   BCC, 1000x

Figure 5-187. Basaloid SCCA versus BCC composite. Unique features of basaloid SCCA include that the neoplastic cells display more pleomorphism, mitoses (often atypical), and necrosis. In contrast to basaloid squamous cell carcinoma, BCC displays lower-grade histology and a lack of prominent and atypical mitoses, pleomorphism, and necrosis. Characteristically, BCC has retraction artifact around the neoplasm edges and the small nuclei display crisp nuclear palisading along the neoplasm's periphery.

Invasion Mimics

Dysplasia extension into the adjoining anal glands or into the colorectal glands is within the spectrum of squamous intraepithelial lesion (SIL) and not evidence of invasion (Figs. 5.188 and 5.189). This is analogous to the cervix, where dysplasia extension into the endocervical glands is within the spectrum of SIL and not indicative of invasion. Other mimics of invasion include reactive myofibroblasts following chemoradiation treatment

(Figs. 5.190–5.195) and pseudoepitheliomatous hyperplasia (Figs. 5.196 and 5.197). Reactive myofibroblasts can demonstrate alarming atypia worrisome for malignancy, particularly in patients who had a prior malignancy that was treated with chemoradiation. Atypical myofibroblasts are large cells with large nuclei and often prominent nucleoli. Other helpful clues to radiation atypia include a backdrop of fibrosis and hyalinization, a lack of desmoplasia surrounding the atypical myofibroblasts, and damaged, hyalinized vessels. Although the atypical myofibroblasts are large, they are normochromatic (their chromatin is as dark as that in the neighboring nonneoplastic cells). Other reassuring features include their normal nuclear to cytoplasmic ratios and cytokeratin nonreactivity. In such cases, a cytomegalovirus (CMV) immunostain is worthwhile. Pseudoepitheliomatous hyperplasia can similarly simulate invasive squamous cell carcinoma. It is a benign reactive response and most commonly associated with granular cell tumors, trauma, chronic inflammation, or infections. Characteristic histology includes hyperplastic squamous epithelium that has a nodular growth pattern that pushes down into the lamina propria, mimicking invasive well-differentiated squamous cell carcinoma. Reassuring features of benignity include that the reactive cells do not extend beyond the inciting agent (granular cell tumor or infection) and that the atypia is in proportion to the inciting agent (granular cell tumor, infection, inflammation, for example). Deeper sections and sharing with a colleague are often worthwhile.

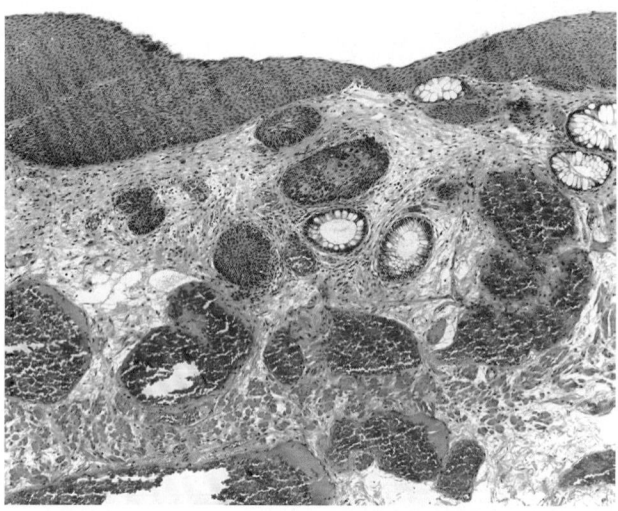

Figure 5-188. SIL extension is not invasion. The nests of SIL adjoining the colonic glands and undermining the squamous epithelium are within the spectrum of noninvasive SIL and are not evidence of invasion. This is analogous to the cervix, where dysplasia extension into the endocervical glands is within the spectrum of SIL.

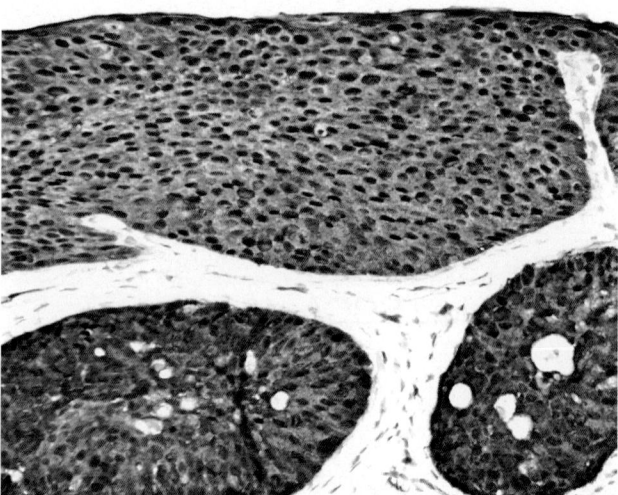

Figure 5-189. SIL extension is not invasion.

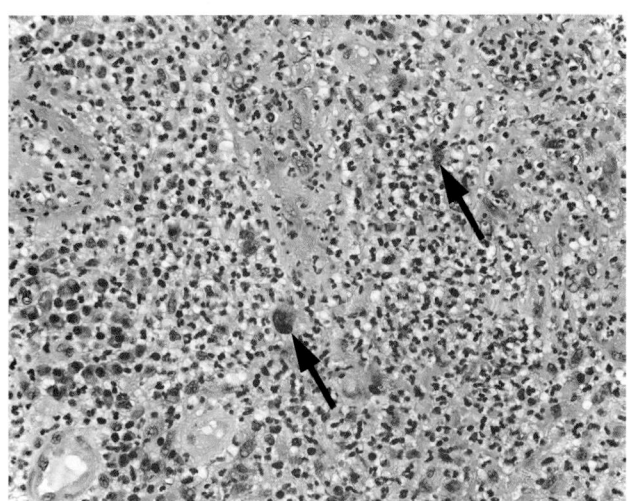

Figure 5-190. Radiation atypia. Reactive myofibroblasts (*arrows*) following chemoradiation treatment can have striking atypia worrisome for malignancy. This patient had a history of anal squamous cell carcinoma with an ulcerative mass identified after chemoradiation therapy.

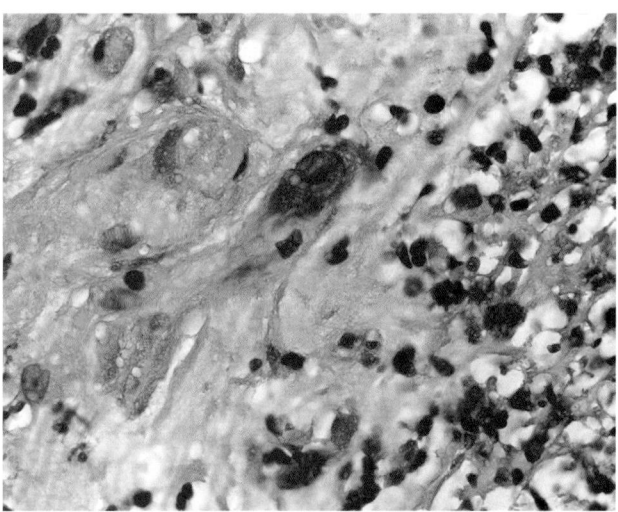

Figure 5-191. Radiation atypia. Higher power of the previous figure. The entire submitted mass consisted of ulceration, abscess, and scattered atypical myofibroblasts with large nuclei and prominent nucleoli. In such cases, a cytokeratin and CMV are worthwhile; both were nonreactive in this case.

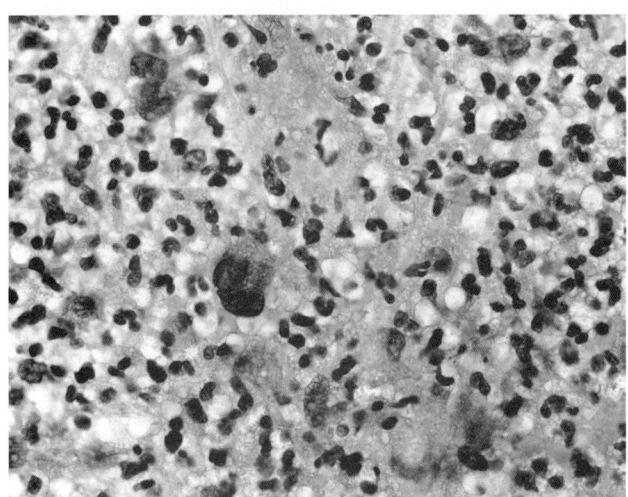

Figure 5-192. Radiation atypia. Higher power of the previous figure. Reassuring features of benignity include the cells' normal nuclear to cytoplasmic ratios and cytokeratin nonreactivity (not shown).

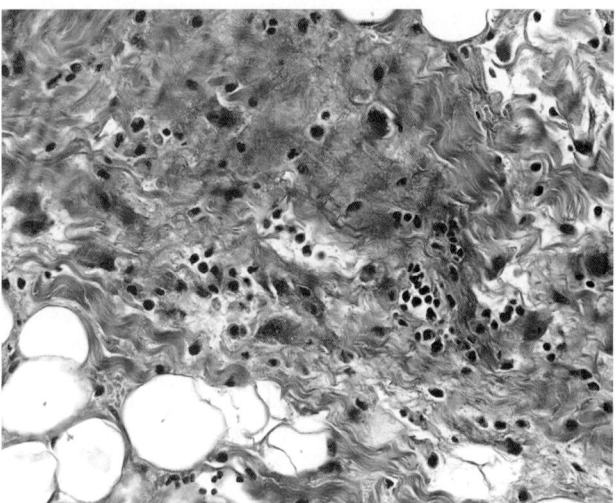

Figure 5-193. Radiation atypia. Other helpful clues to radiation atypia include a backdrop of fibrosis and hyalinization and a lack of desmoplasia surrounding the atypical myofibroblasts, as seen here. Damaged, hyalinized vessels are also common features of radiation injury (not shown).

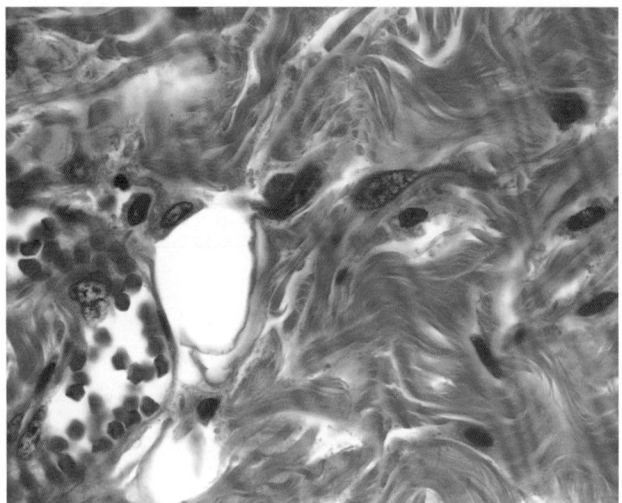

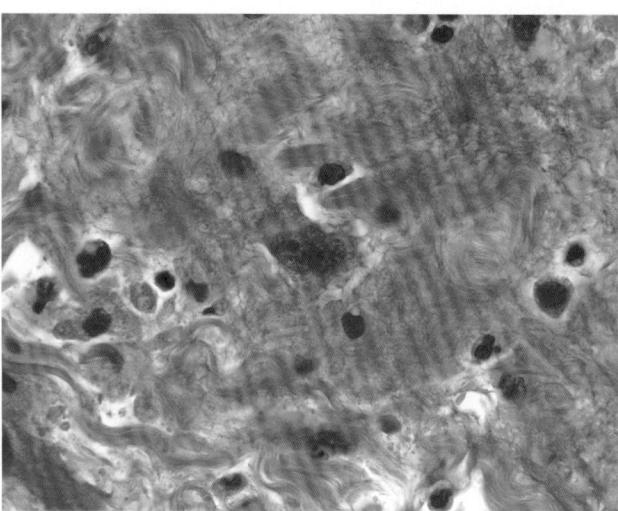

Figure 5-194. Radiation atypia. Higher power of the previous figure. Note that, although the atypical myofibroblasts are large, they have normal chromasia (their chromatin is as dark as the neighboring nonneoplastic cells).

Figure 5-195. Radiation atypia.

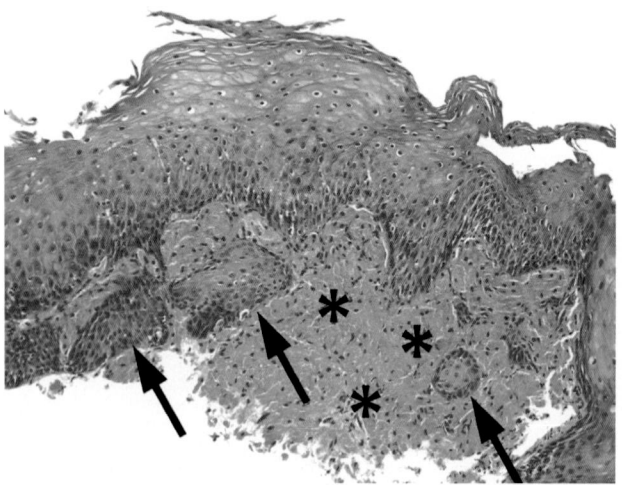

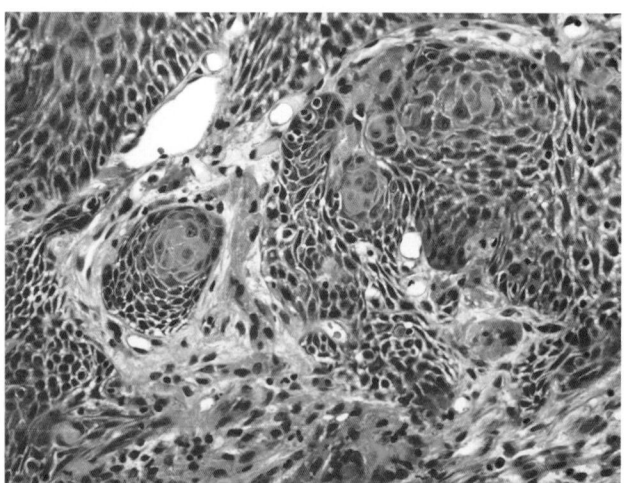

Figure 5-196. **Pseudoepitheliomatous hyperplasia (PEH) and granular cell tumor.** PEH can also simulate malignancy but is a benign, reactive response commonly associated with granular cell tumors (as in this case, *asterisks*), trauma, chronic inflammation, and infections. Characteristic histology includes hyperplastic squamous epithelium that has a nodular growth pattern that pushes down into the lamina propria (*arrows*).

Figure 5-197. PEH and granular cell tumor (not shown). Reassuring features of benignity include that the reactive cells do not extend beyond the inciting agent (granular cell tumor or infection) and that the atypia is in proportion to the inciting agent. This case had been diagnosed as an invasive squamous cell carcinoma. Other sections showed an adjoining granular cell tumor, and the diagnosis was revised to granular cell tumor with marked PEH.

VERRUCOUS CARCINOMA AND GIANT CONDYLOMA (BUSCHKE-LOWENSTEIN TUMOR)

Verrucous carcinoma is a well-differentiated variant of squamous cell carcinoma. It is slow growing, is locally destructive, and has a negligible risk of metastasis. It is composed of prominent endophytic projections with broad, pushing borders (Figs. 5.198–5.209), as is typical of verrucous carcinoma at other sites. The cell layers are orderly with marked parakeratosis ("church-spire" pattern), intraepithelial microabscesses, and enlarged spinous cells (keratinocytes with prominent intracellular bridges in the superficial epithelium). Koilocytes are absent, and mitoses are rare and confined to the basal layer. Lymphoplasmacytic inflammation at the epidermal-dermal junction is common. Because their characteristic architecture is crucial to the diagnosis and they lack dysplasia and koilocytic change, their diagnosis is best reserved for the thoroughly sampled resection specimen to avoid an unsampled typical (and more aggressive) invasive squamous cell carcinoma.

Verrucous carcinoma is synonymously termed giant condyloma (Buschke-Lowenstein tumor) in the 2010 WHO Classification of Tumours of the Digestive System,[3] AJCC eighth edition,[2] and the 2017 CAP Tumor Template for the Anus,[4] but this terminology is contentious as is the role of HPV in verrucous carcinoma. Although earlier work implicated that a subset of verrucous carcinomas were associated with HPV 6 and 11,[3,25] more recent studies suggest they are unassociated.[26-30] As a result, some advocate that verrucous carcinoma should be distinguished from the giant condyloma (Buschke-Lowenstein) based on disparate histology, etiology, and HPV associations. Giant condyloma (Buschke-Lowenstein) is a benign diagnosis associated with low-risk HPV subtypes 6 and 11. It histologically is characterized by papillary architecture and LSIL with prominent koilocytes (Figs. 5.210–5.219). In contrast to verrucous carcinoma, it has less prominent parakeratosis and intraepithelial microabscesses, it lacks endophytic pushing borders, and mitotic figures are a bit easier to identify. Both verrucous carcinoma and giant condyloma (Buschke-Lowenstein) lack marked atypia. If identified, thorough sampling, if not complete submission, should be pursued to evaluate for invasion/classic squamous cell carcinoma. Lesions with invasion or metastasis in the background of marked atypia are best classified as invasive squamous cell carcinoma, which may result in resection, lymph node dissection, and chemoradiation.

See Fig. 5.220 for a side-by-side comparison of verrucous carcinoma and giant condyloma (Buschke-Lowenstein tumor).

KEY FEATURES: HPV-Associated Neoplasms

- LAST provides **a single grading scheme** for grading HPV-associated squamous proliferations at **all lower anogenital sites.**
- It is a *two-tiered* system: **LSIL (formerly -IN 1)** or **HSIL (formerly -IN 2 and -IN 3).**
- **LSIL** shows koilocytotic change, and mitotic figures are confined to the lower one-third of the epithelium.
- **Condyloma acuminatum** is by definition a papillary proliferation with LSIL and should be reported as **LSIL, formerly condyloma acuminatum.**
- **HSIL** is defined by mitotic figures in the superficial two-thirds of the epithelium, marked nuclear atypia, and shows strong p16 reactivity.
- **SISCCA** of the anus and perianus requires invasion with a depth ≤3 mm, horizontal spread ≤7 mm, and complete excision.
- **Avoid subclassification of squamous cell carcinoma variants in the top line.**
- **p16 is the only recommended biomarker** in lower anogenital sites.
- **Order** p16 only in two specific contexts:
  - when the diagnostic issue is HSIL versus an HSIL mimic *or*
  - when there is a discrepancy between the cytology and surgical biopsy
- **Avoid ordering** p16 in these contexts:
  - Routine, up front for all cases
  - In the non-HSIL differential diagnoses
  - When the differential is unequivocally -IN 2 versus -IN 3
- **Positive p16 immunoreactivity requires diffuse, block immunolabeling that highlights the nucleus and cytoplasm of the basal layer and at least the contiguous one-third of the epithelial thickness in the atypical foci seen on H&E.**
- A positive p16 supports a diagnosis of HSIL only if the case satisfies the morphologic criteria for HSIL on the H&E.
- **Verrucous carcinoma** is a **well-differentiated variant of squamous cell carcinoma** that is locally destructive with a negligible risk of metastasis; it is characterized by prominent endophytic projections, **pushing borders**, church-spire parakeratosis, intraepithelial microabscesses, and lymphoplasmacytic inflammation, and **dysplasia and koilocytes are absent**; it is **unassociated with HPV.**
- **Giant condyloma** (Buschke-Lowenstein tumor) is a **benign diagnosis** associated with **low-risk HPV subtypes 6 and 11**; it is characterized by **papillary architecture and presence of koilocytic change**; the older literature lumps verrucous carcinoma and giant condyloma together, but these lesions should be distinguished based on disparate morphology and etiology.

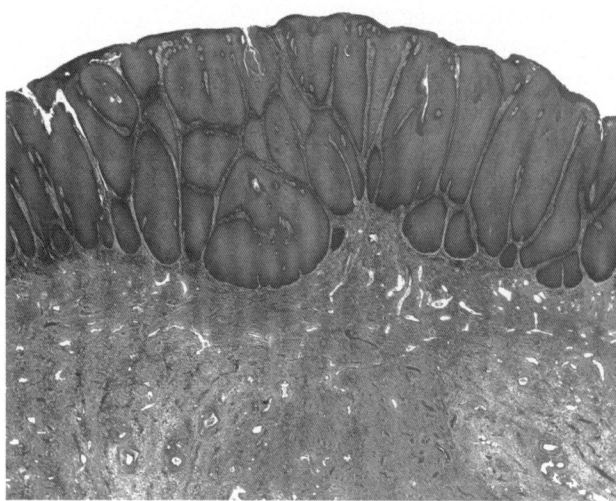

Figure 5-198. Verrucous carcinoma. Typical of verrucous carcinoma at other sites, it is composed of prominent endophytic projections with broad, pushing borders, as seen here.

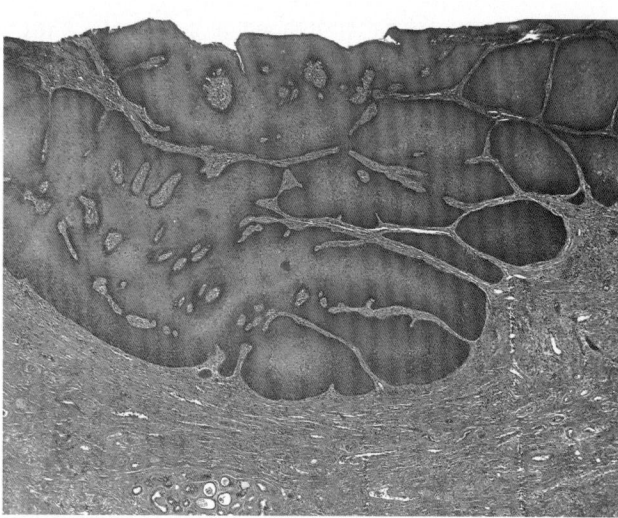

Figure 5-199. Verrucous carcinoma. Verrucous carcinoma is a well-differentiated variant of squamous cell carcinoma. It is slow growing, is locally destructive, and has a negligible risk of metastasis.

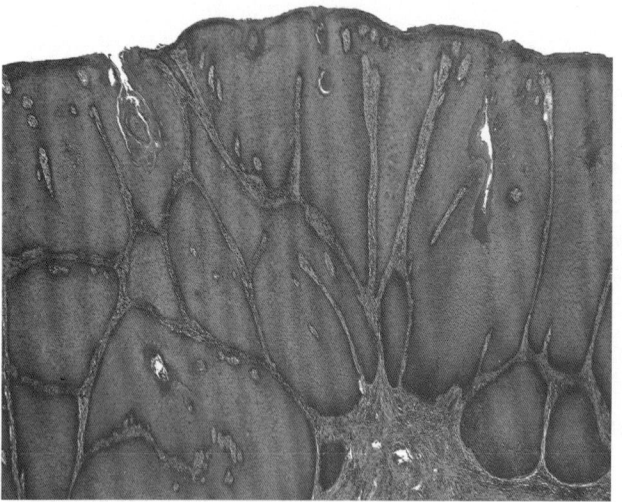

Figure 5-200. Verrucous carcinoma. Because recognizing the characteristic architecture is crucial to the diagnosis and invasion can be excluded only after extensive sampling, this diagnosis is best reserved for the thoroughly sampled resection specimen.

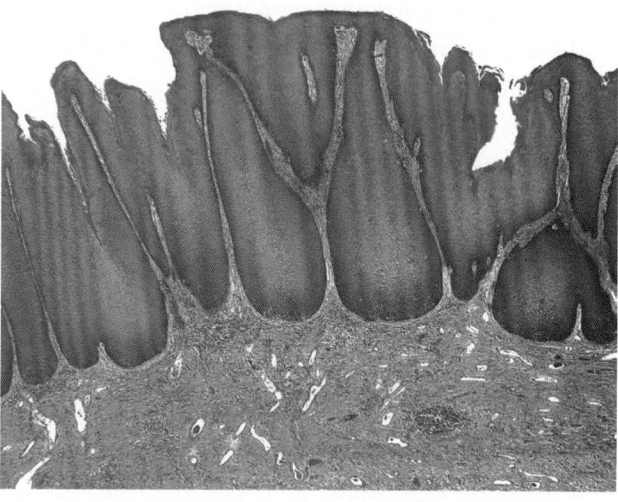

Figure 5-201. Verrucous carcinoma. Avoid diagnosing verrucous carcinoma on a biopsy specimen, unless the entire lesion was excised and histologically examined.

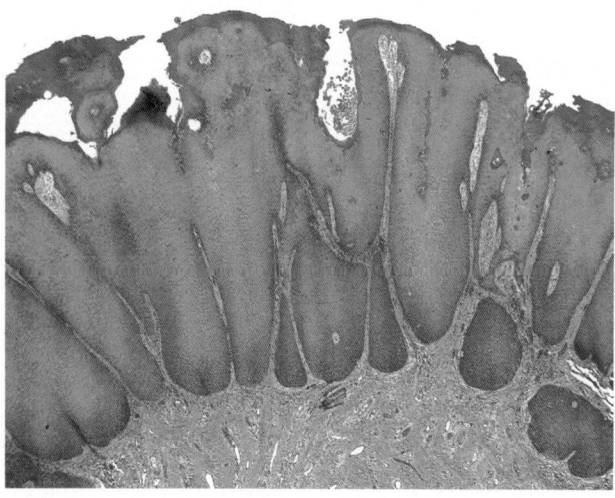

Figure 5-202. Verrucous carcinoma.

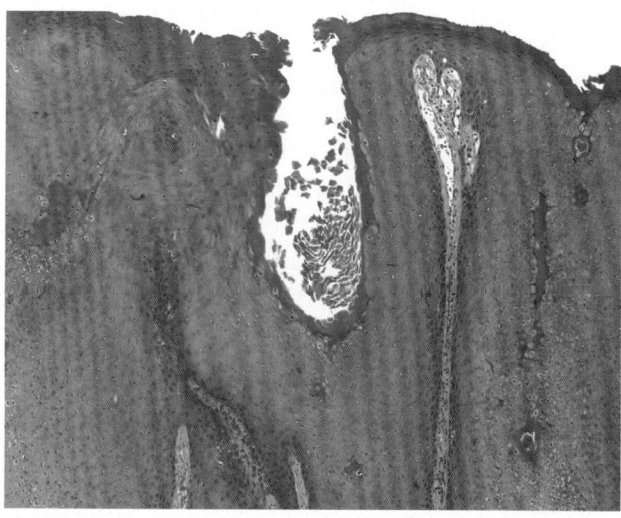

Figure 5-203. Verrucous carcinoma. Marked parakeratosis (abnormal keratinization with nuclei) is common in verrucous carcinoma.

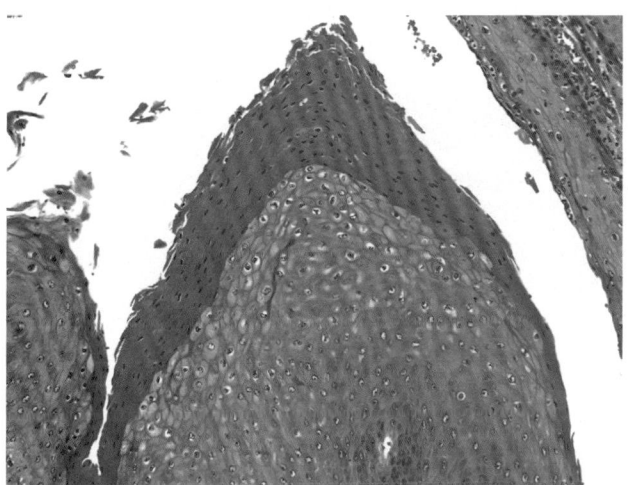

Figure 5-204. Verrucous carcinoma. The marked parakeratosis is often described as a church-spire pattern, with piled parakeratosis cascading from peaks of squamous epithelium, similar to a church spire.

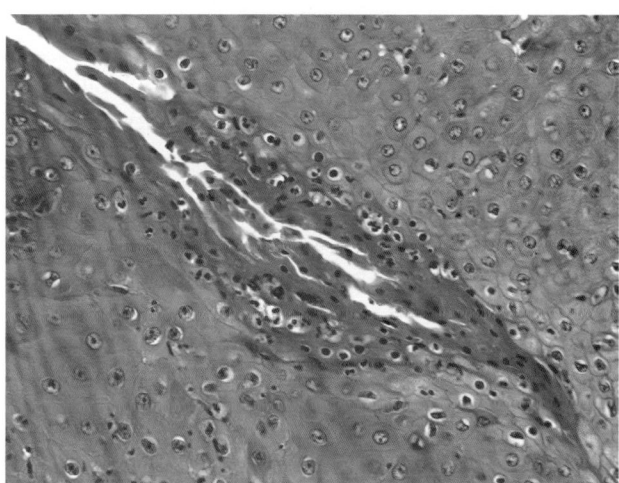

Figure 5-205. Verrucous carcinoma. Intraepithelial microabscesses are common in verrucous carcinoma, as seen here.

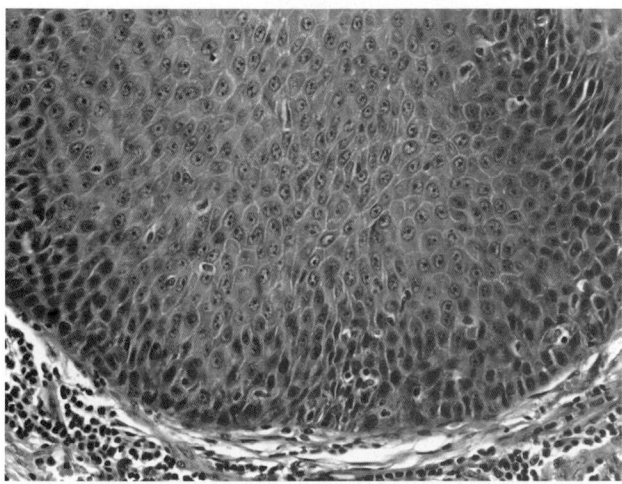

Figure 5-206. Verrucous carcinoma. A dense lymphoplasmacytic infiltrate is often seen at the epidermal-dermal junction in verrucous carcinoma.

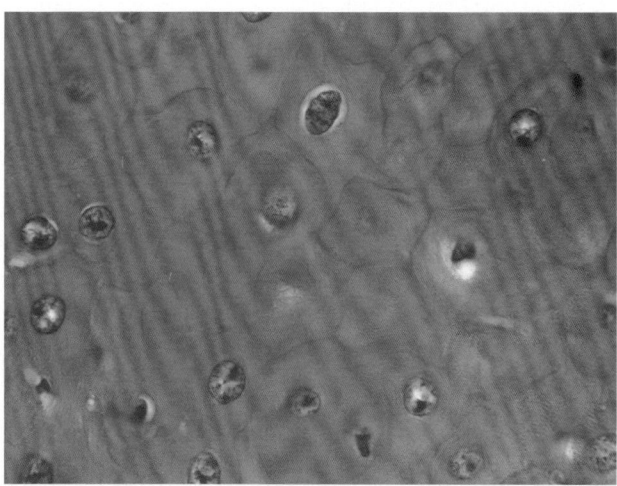

Figure 5-207. Verrucous carcinoma. Koilocytes and atypia are absent in verrucous carcinoma. The occasional perinuclear cleft, as seen here, is within the spectrum of normal. True koilocytes are large with hyperchromatic, irregular nuclear contours (raisinoid nuclei) and binucleate cells.

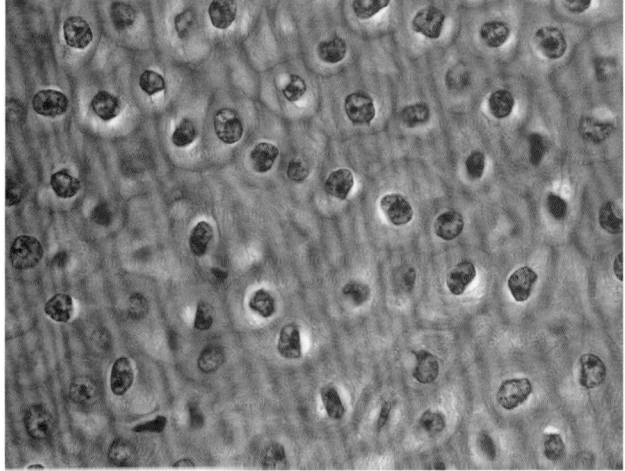

Figure 5-208. Verrucous carcinoma. Koilocytes and atypia are absent in verrucous carcinoma. Mitoses are rare and confined to the basal layer (not shown).

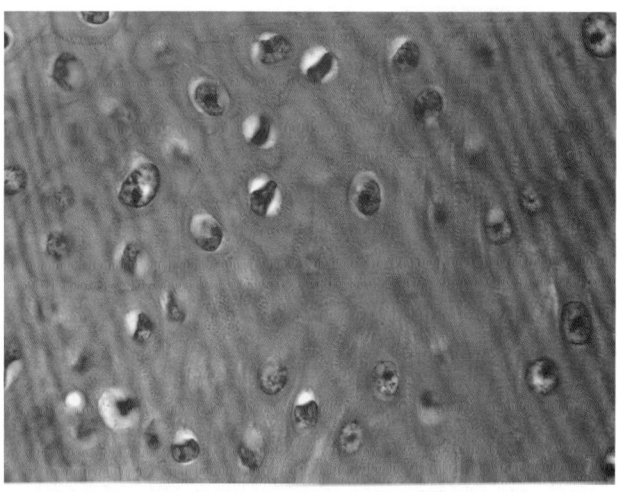

Figure 5-209. Verrucous carcinoma.

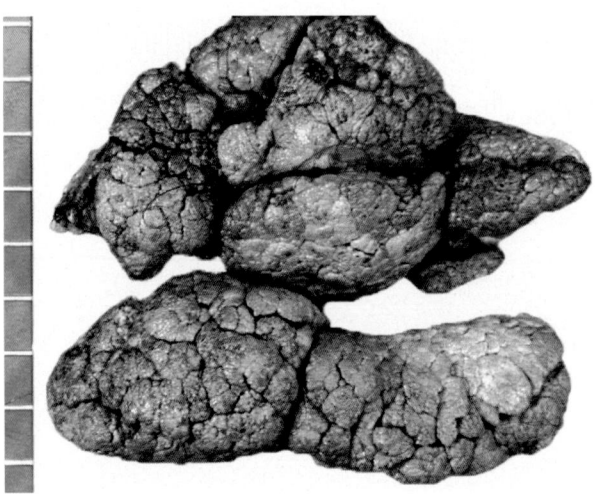

Figure 5-210. Giant condyloma (Buschke-Lowenstein tumor). Giant condyloma are usually large resection specimens, as seen here.

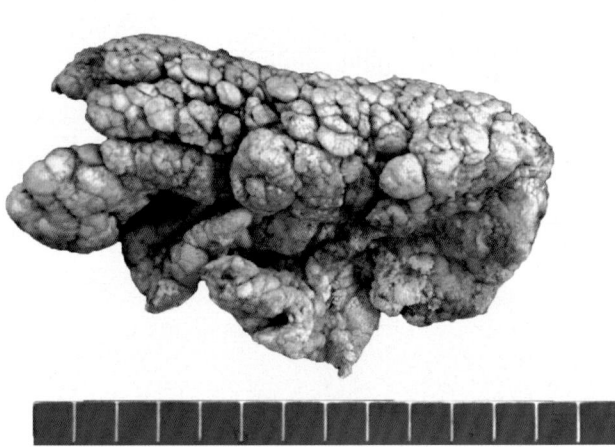

Figure 5-211. Giant condyloma (Buschke-Lowenstein tumor). They are associated with low-risk HPV subtypes 6 and 11 and display prominent LSIL/koilocytic change.

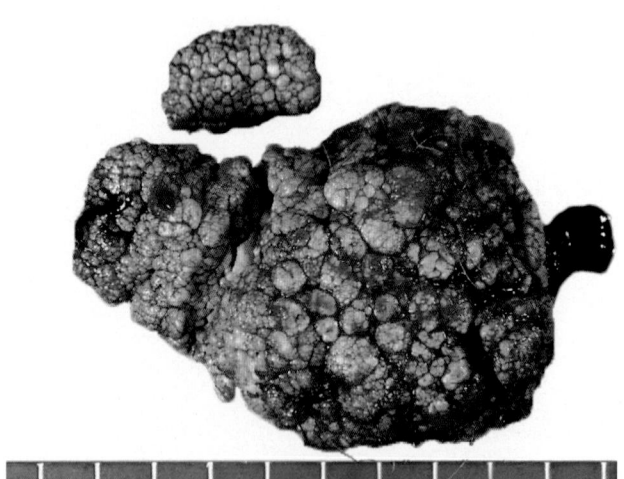

Figure 5-212. Giant condyloma (Buschke-Lowenstein tumor).

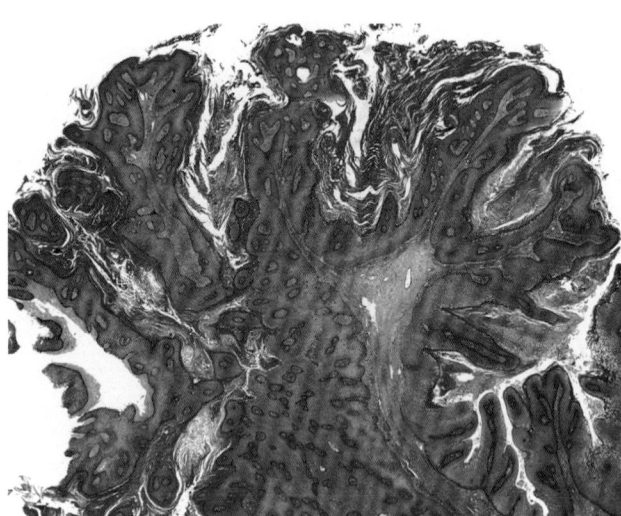

Figure 5-213. Giant condyloma (Buschke-Lowenstein tumor). Histologically, prominent papillary architecture is seen with an absence of an endophytic, pushing border; the latter feature is more common to verrucous carcinoma.

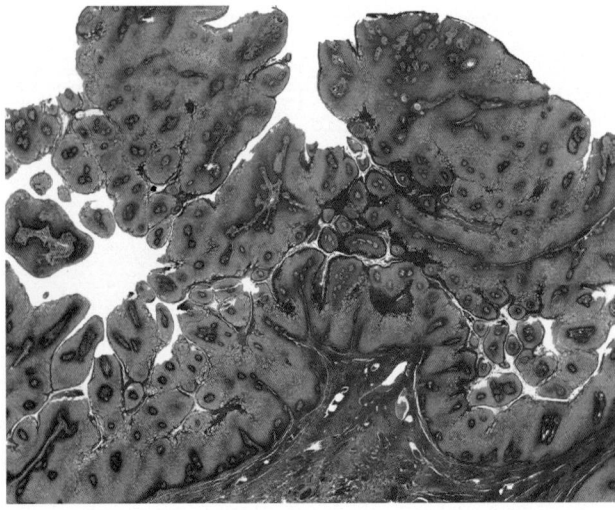

Figure 5-214. Giant condyloma (Buschke-Lowenstein tumor).

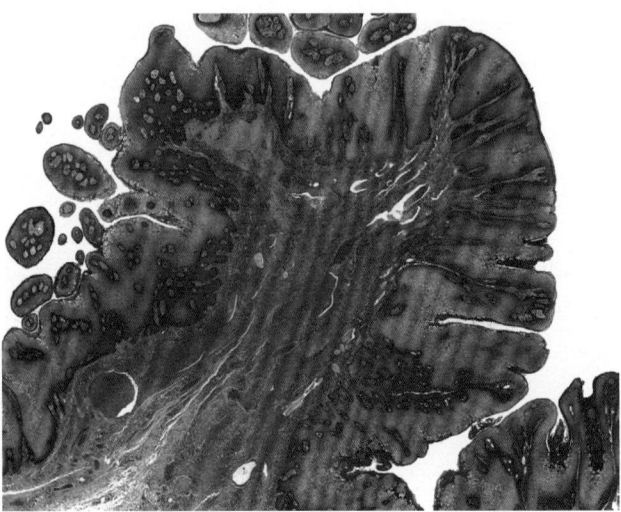

Figure 5-215. Giant condyloma (Buschke-Lowenstein tumor).

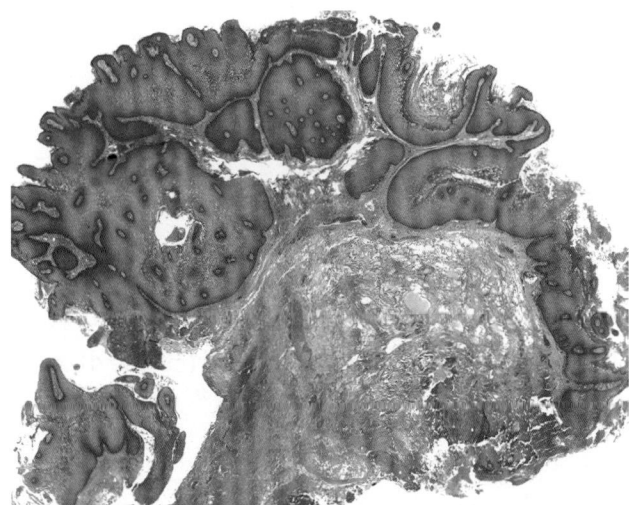

Figure 5-216. Giant condyloma (Buschke-Lowenstein tumor).

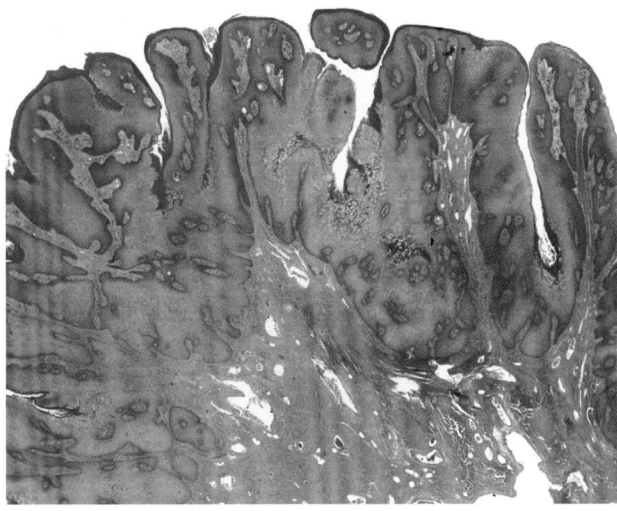

Figure 5-217. Giant condyloma (Buschke-Lowenstein tumor).

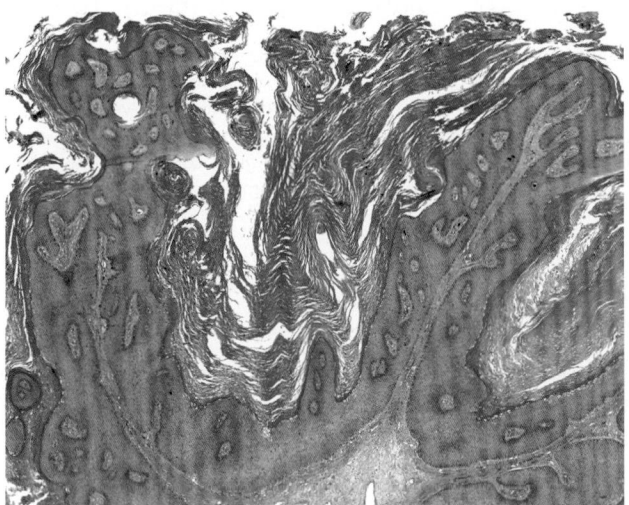

Figure 5-218. Giant condyloma (Buschke-Lowenstein tumor). Variable parakeratosis can be seen.

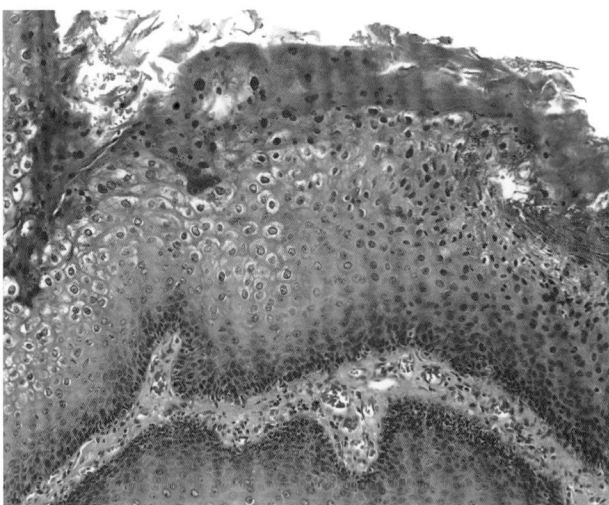

Figure 5-219. Giant condyloma (Buschke-Lowenstein tumor). A defining feature of giant condyloma, which is not seen in verrucous carcinoma, is the presence of prominent koilocytes (LSIL). Any degree of atypia in giant condyloma or verrucous carcinoma should prompt thorough sampling to evaluate for the presence of invasion. If invasion is found, the lesion is best classified as invasive squamous cell carcinoma.

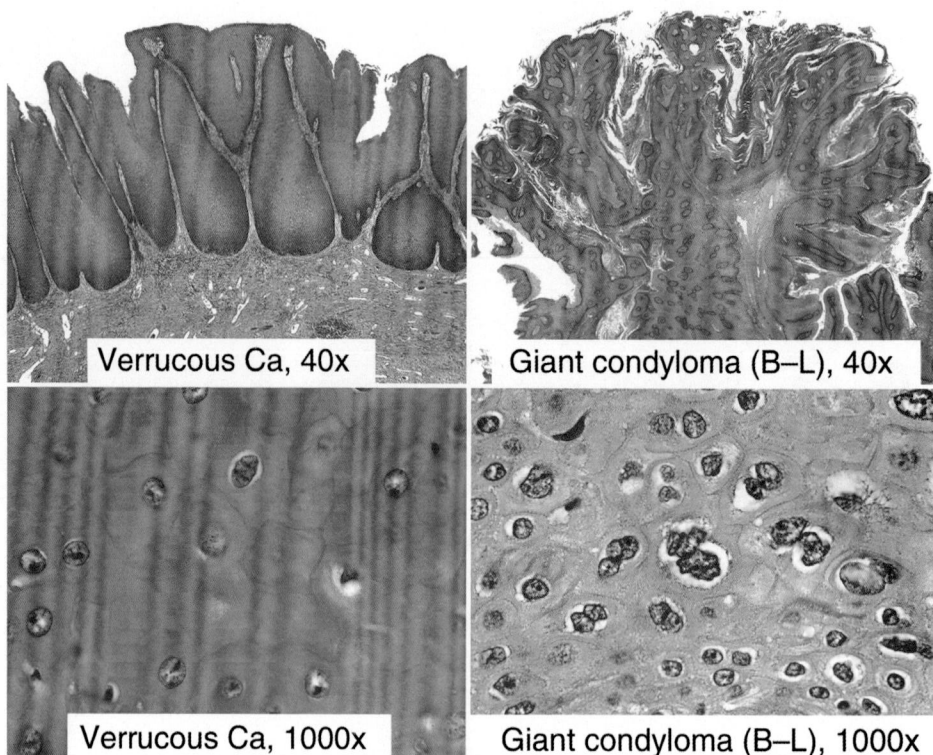

Figure 5-220. Verrucous carcinoma versus giant condyloma (Buschke-Lowenstein tumor). At 40X, verrucous carcinoma has prominent endophytic projections with broad, pushing borders, and giant condyloma (Buschke-Lowenstein tumor) has a prominent papillary architecture. At 1000X, verrucous carcinoma lacks koilocytes, but koilocytes are a defining feature of giant condyloma (Buschke-Lowenstein tumor). Atypia and invasion are absent in both verrucous carcinoma and giant condyloma (Buschke-Lowenstein tumor); if seen, the lesion is best classified as an invasive squamous cell carcinoma.

ADENOCARCINOMA

Adenocarcinoma accounts for only 4% of anal neoplasms. It can generally be subclassified based on site of involvement as (1) direct invasion or metastasis from elsewhere (most commonly direct invasion from an adjacent colorectal primary), (2) anal duct adenocarcinomas, or (3) adenocarcinoma arising in fistulous disease. In general, distal rectal, anal, and perianal adenocarcinomas require abdominal perineal excisions with or without chemotherapy. Adenocarcinomas are staged similarly to squamous cell carcinomas of this site, and patients have a worse stage for stage prognosis than those with squamous cell carcinoma.[2]

METASTASIS OR DIRECT INVASION

Most adenocarcinomas involving the anus are an extension of a colorectal adenocarcinoma. They are morphologically, immunophenotypically, and biologically identical to the usual colorectal adenocarcinomas, as discussed extensively in "Colon" chapter, "Adenocarcinoma" section (Figs. 5.221–5.226). Based on close proximity, genitourinary and gynecologic sites are important considerations for malignancies involving the anus. Often a review of imaging studies and the intraoperative impressions along with a pertinent immunohistochemical panel can help resolve most diagnostic issues. The remaining challenging cases are managed with a carefully crafted note describing the diagnostic considerations and suggesting clinical consideration of other potential sites of primary. See Sample Note ADC.

ANAL DUCT CARCINOMA

Anal duct carcinoma (ADC) (also termed anal gland carcinoma) involves malignant transformation of the anal ducts. It is unassociated with HPV and accounts for up to 10% of anal malignancies.[31] Its occurrence may become more common with the expected decrease in HPV-related neoplasia due to the HPV vaccine. Some have suggested its poor prognosis is due to delayed presentation and symptomology overlap with other benign conditions, such as bleeding, painful hemorrhoids. In the small series available, ADC is more common in older men and is treated by excision with or without radiation. Recurrence and distant metastasis have been described. Histologically, the typical features of adenocarcinoma are seen with angulated, neoplastic glands in a desmoplastic background without surface involvement (Figs. 5.227–5.233).[32] The individual cells are cuboidal, with a high nuclear to cytoplasmic ratio and prominent nucleoli. Mucin pools and Pagetoid extension into the overlying squamous mucosa can be seen. The overlying squamous epithelium is usually unremarkable, and p16 and HPV in situ hybridization are negative.[32,33] Some examples do show Pagetoid extension into the overlying squamous epithelium.[32] Normal anal ducts show immunoreactivity for the myoepithelial and basal cell markers CK5/6 and p53, whereas both are lost in ADC.[33,34] Demonstration of the tumor in continuity with the anal glands is helpful but not always possible, as the tumor grows and destroys local structures. ADC glands generally have less luminal necrosis than colorectal carcinomas, smaller cuboidal nuclei, and a disparate immunoprofile (ADC = CK7+, CK20−, CDX2−; colorectal carcinoma = usually, but not always, CK7−, CK20+, CDX2+). Before diagnosing ADC, it is critical to exclude metastasis and direct invasion by a review of the imaging studies, thorough immunohistochemical workup, and a careful note. See Sample Note ADC.

See Fig. 5.234 for a side-by-side comparison of ADC and colorectal carcinoma.

SAMPLE NOTE: ADC

Anus, Mass, APR

- Moderately differentiated adenocarcinoma, 1.0 cm, underlying unremarkable squamous epithelium
- Adenocarcinoma limited to the submucosa
- Negative for lymphovascular and perineural invasion
- Fifteen negative lymph nodes (0/15)
- All margins uninvolved

Note: The aforementioned resection specimen shows a moderately differentiated adenocarcinoma in association with anal ducts. The electronic record has been reviewed, and, per report, this neoplasm radiologically represents an isolated anal lesion in a patient with an unremarkable medical history. The immunoprofile demonstrates that the lesional cells are reactive for CK7 and nonreactive for CK20, CDX2, prostate cancer marker NKX3.1, and breast and genitourinary marker GATA3. Overall, the morphology, immunophenotype, and history are in keeping with an ADC, assuming that metastasis and direct invasion have been clinically excluded. This neoplasm is morphologically and immunophenotypically indistinguishable from a wide variety of nonanal primary neoplasms (breast, colorectal, upper GI tract, pancreatobiliary, and genitourinary and gynecologic tract neoplasms, among others). Careful correlation with the medical history, imaging studies, and physical examination have been suggested to ensure that this lesion does not represent metastasis or direct invasion from elsewhere.

KEY FEATURES: ADC

- ADC is **unassociated with HPV.**
- Most patients present with **painful anal bleeding.**
- Angulated, neoplastic glands lined by cuboidal cells are present; mucin pools and Pagetoid extension into the overlying squamous mucosa can be seen; the overlying squamous epithelium is otherwise unremarkable.
- ADC is **CK7+, CK20−, CDX2−.**
- **It is critical to exclude metastasis and direct invasion.**

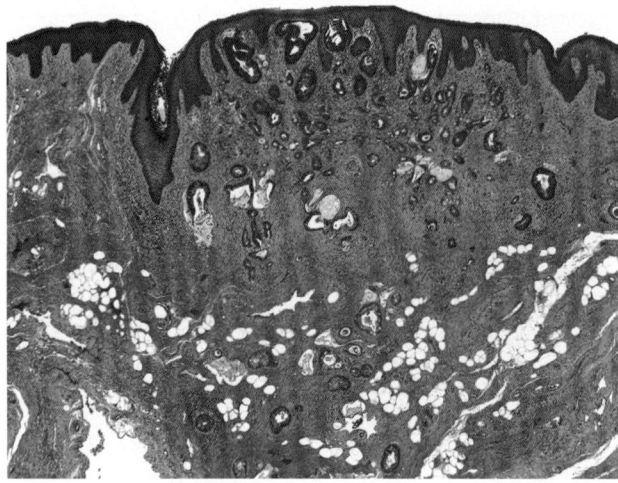

Figure 5-221. Adenocarcinoma, extension from known colorectal primary. Most adenocarcinomas involving the anus are extensions of colorectal adenocarcinomas. As seen here, these types of adenocarcinomas are morphologically, immunophenotypically, and biologically identical to the usual colorectal adenocarcinomas.

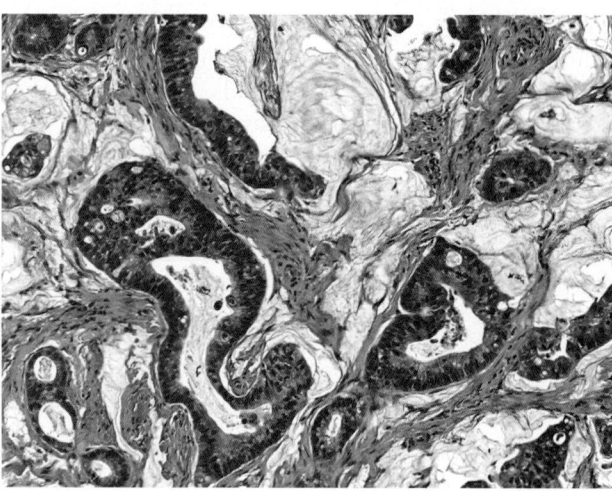

Figure 5-222. Adenocarcinoma, extension from known colorectal primary. Higher power of the previous figure shows neoplastic glands admixed in extruded mucin. Before considering a primary anal adenocarcinoma, it is critical to exclude direct invasion or metastasis from elsewhere because primary anal adenocarcinomas are uncommon.

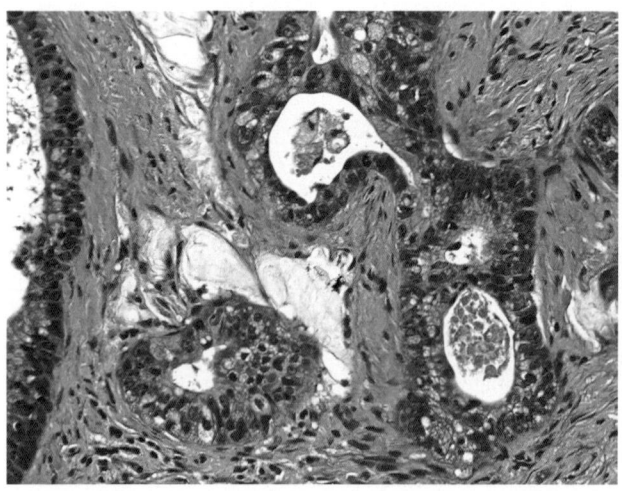

Figure 5-223. Adenocarcinoma, extension from known colorectal primary. Higher power of the previous figure shows cribriforming necrosis and scattered goblet cells.

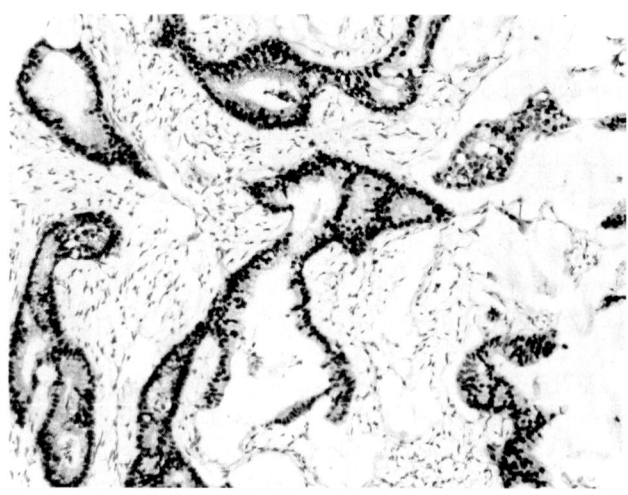

Figure 5-224. Adenocarcinoma, extension from known colorectal primary, CDX2. The patient had a known low rectal adenocarcinoma that grossly extended into the anus. Strong CDX2 immunoreactivity is in keeping with a tubular GI tract primary.

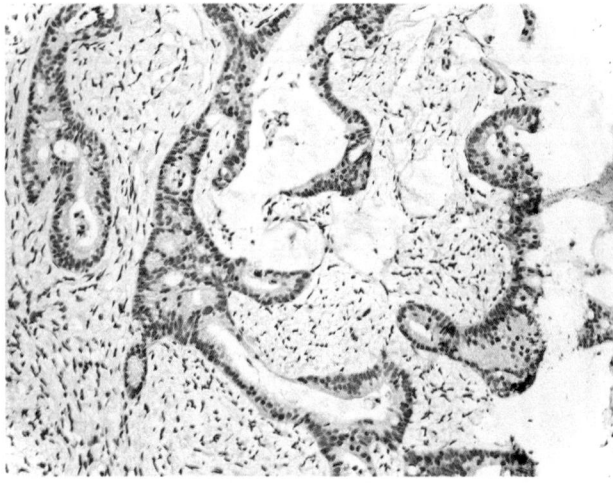

Figure 5-225. Adenocarcinoma, extension from known colorectal primary, CK7. Most colorectal primaries are CK7 nonreactive.

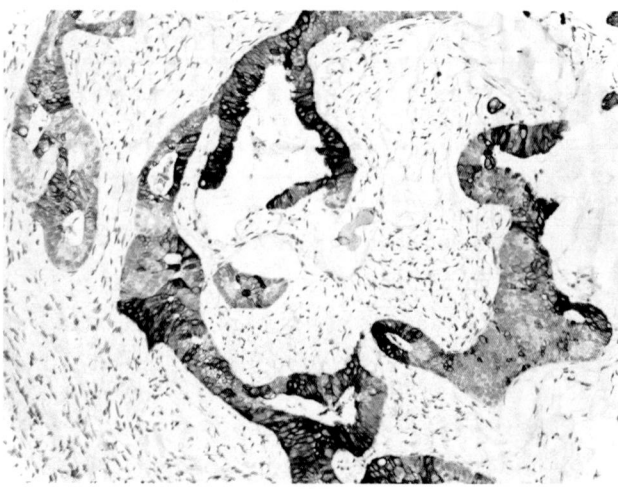

Figure 5-226. Adenocarcinoma, extension from known colorectal primary, CK20. Most colorectal primaries are CK20 reactive.

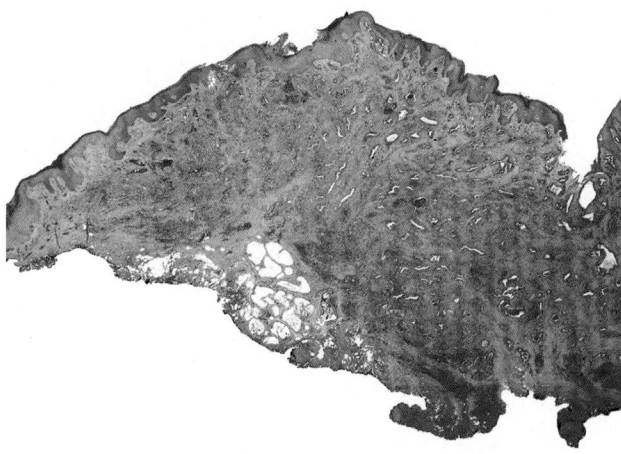

Figure 5-227. Anal duct carcinoma (ADC). ADC involves malignant transformation of the anal ducts/glands. It is unassociated with HPV and is more common in older men.

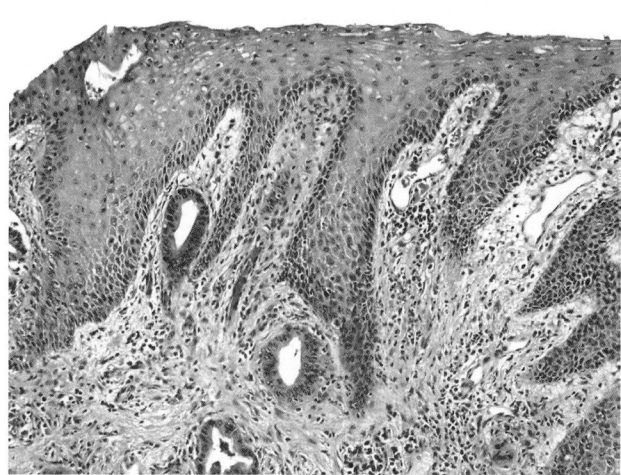

Figure 5-228. Anal duct carcinoma. Histologically, the typical features of adenocarcinoma are seen with angulated, neoplastic glands in a desmoplastic background. The overlying squamous epithelium is otherwise unremarkable, and p16 and HPV in situ hybridization are negative.

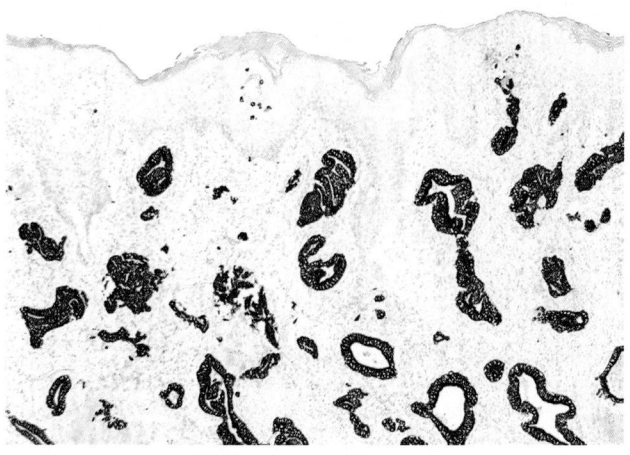

Figure 5-229. Anal duct carcinoma, CK7. Their immunoprofile reflects the immunoprofile of anal ducts (CK7 reactive, CK20/CDX2 nonreactive, not shown).

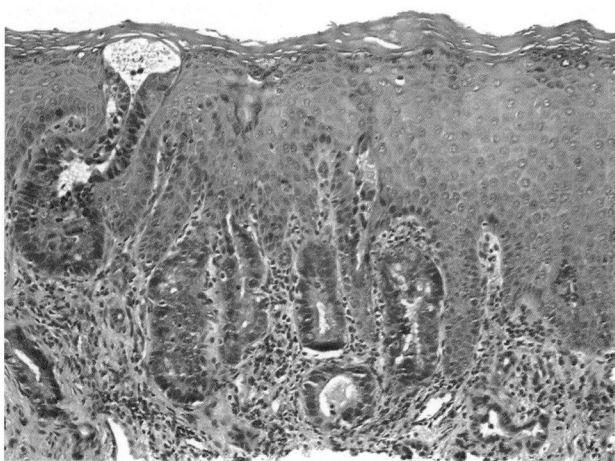

Figure 5-230. Anal duct carcinoma. The individual cells are cuboidal with a high nuclear to cytoplasmic ratio and prominent nucleoli. Mucin pools and Pagetoid extension into the overlying squamous mucosa can be seen (not shown).

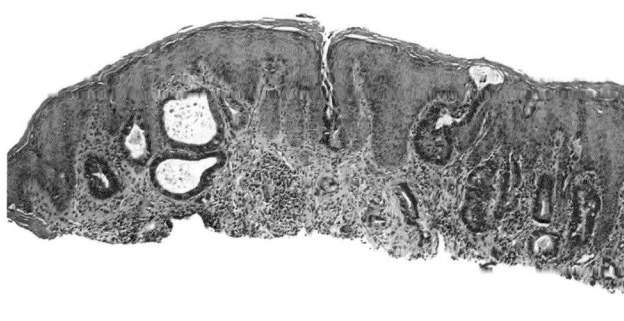

Figure 5-231. Anal duct carcinoma. Demonstration of the tumor in continuity with the anal glands is helpful, but this is rarely seen as the tumor more often destroys local structures.

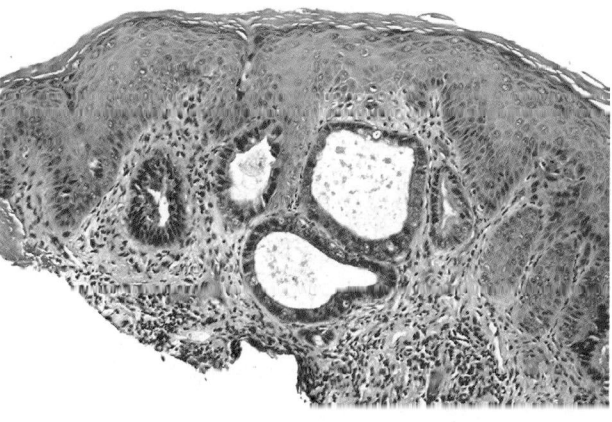

Figure 5-232. Anal duct carcinoma. Before diagnosing ADC, it is critical to exclude metastasis and direct invasion by a review of the imaging studies and thorough immunohistochemical workup and to provide a careful note that conveys the need to clinically exclude spread from another site.

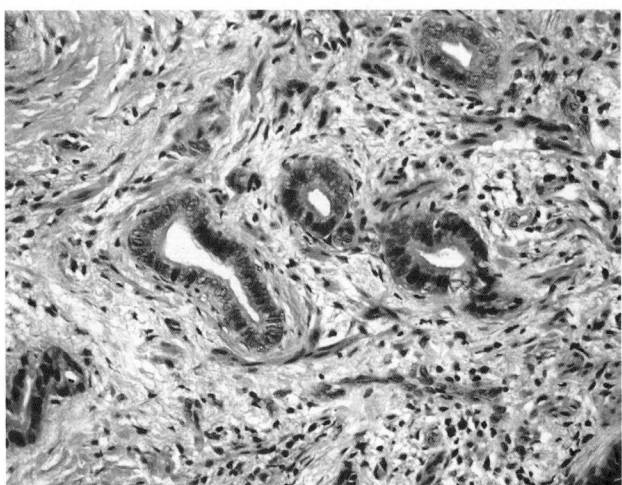

Figure 5-233. Anal duct carcinoma. ADC is treated by excision with or without radiation. Recurrence and distant metastasis have been described.

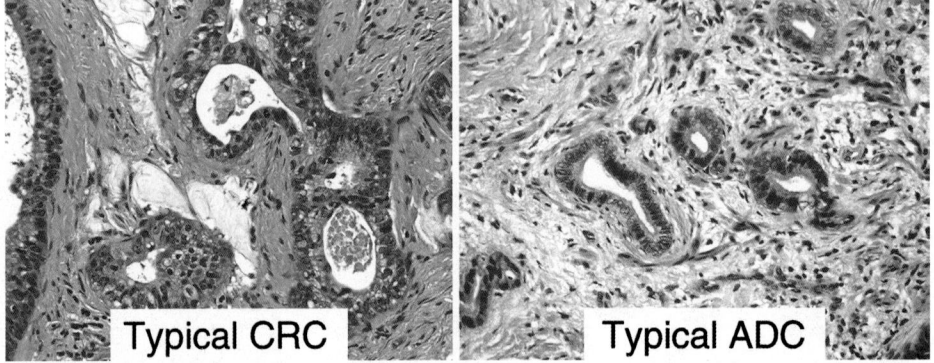

Figure 5-234. Colorectal adenocarcinoma versus ADC composite. The glands of ADC generally have less luminal necrosis than those of colorectal carcinomas, smaller-cuboidal nuclei, and a disparate immunoprofile (colorectal carcinoma = usually, but not always, CK7–, CK20+, CDX2+) (anal ducts CK7+, CK20–, CDX2–).

ADENOCARCINOMA ARISING IN FISTULOUS DISEASE

A subset of anal adenocarcinomas arises in patients with a history of long-standing anal fistula (Figs. 5.235–5.238). These patients often have a history of Crohn disease or previous surgical procedure or both. Those adenocarcinomas associated with Crohn disease can feature epithelioid granulomata.

EXTRAMAMMARY PAGET DISEASE

Extramammary Paget disease is an extremely high-yield topic for Board preparation(!) and also important for real-life sign-out. It represents a precursor to adenocarcinoma (adenocarcinoma in situ) and is unassociated with HPV. It can theoretically occur at any squamous-lined site with apocrine glands, such as the axilla, eyelids, or external ear canal, but is most commonly found in the anogenital tract (vulva, penis, scrotum, anus, perianus). Clinically, it presents as a slow-growing, erythematous plaque. Histologically, the squamous epithelium is infiltrated by large neoplastic cells with abundant pale cytoplasm, vesicular chromatin, and prominent nucleoli (Figs. 5.239–5.248). These cells sometimes appear signet ring in shape. Anal Paget disease is staged in AJCC and CAP.[4,35] This is *not* a H&E diagnosis. A small immunohistochemical workup is important to exclude melanoma and to determine which type of anal Paget disease is present to assess for the risk of an underlying malignancy. Anal Paget disease is divided equally into two groups.

1. Primary Paget disease: About half of patients with an anal Paget disease pattern have primary Paget disease with no underlying malignancy. This type is an intraepithelial adenocarcinoma with sweat duct differentiation.[3] Noninvasive forms can be treated conservatively with wide local excision.[2] The immunoprofile of this type reflects its derivation from the apocrine glands (CK7+, CK20−, and reactive for the apocrine marker GCDFP) and is identical to the immunoprofile of mammary Paget.[3,36,37] The cytoplasmic mucin can be highlighted with a mucicarmine or PAS special stain.

2. Secondary Paget disease: The remaining half of patients whose biopsies show a neoplasm with the pattern of anal Paget disease have secondary Paget disease that is secondary to an underlying synchronous or metachronous malignancy. Colorectal primary adenocarcinomas are the most common, but neoplasms of the endometrium, endocervix, bladder, urethra, and prostate that "colonize" the squamous anal epithelium have been described. The immunoprofile of this type reflects the typical immunoprofile of the underlying malignancy, i.e., colorectal adenocarcinoma (CK7−, CK20+, and are nonreactive for the apocrine marker GCDFP) or urothelial carcinoma (CK7+, CK20+, GCDFP−, GATA3+).[36-38] The cytoplasmic mucin can be highlighted with a mucicarmine or PAS special stain.

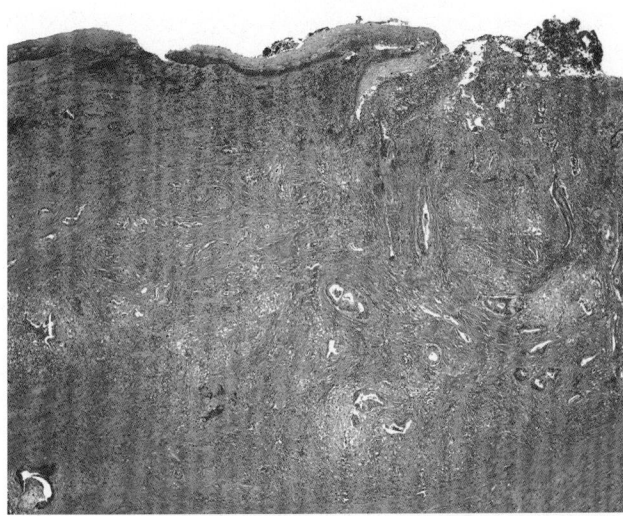

Figure 5-235. Adenocarcinoma in long-standing anal fistula. Patients with long-standing anal fistulas are at increased risk for adenocarcinoma.

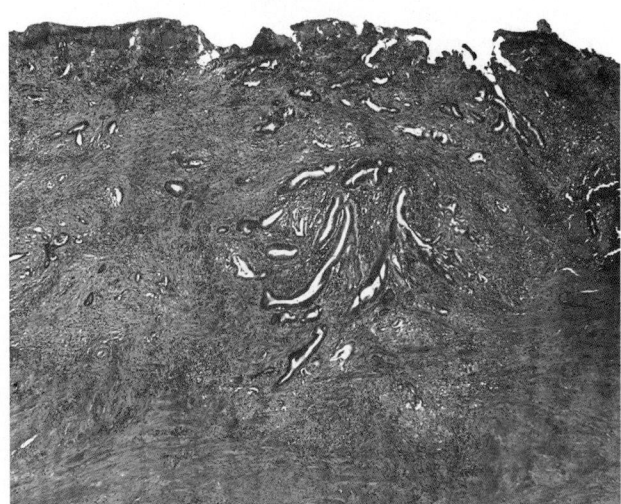

Figure 5-236. Adenocarcinoma in long-standing anal fistula. Such patients often have a history of Crohn disease, previous surgical procedure, or both.

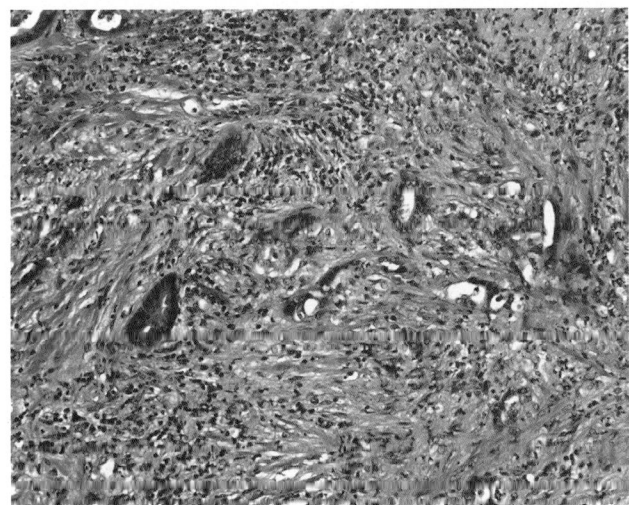

Figure 5-237. Adenocarcinoma in long-standing anal fistula. The adenocarcinomas demonstrate the usual features of adenocarcinoma, such as angulated, neoplastic glands in a desmoplastic background, as seen here.

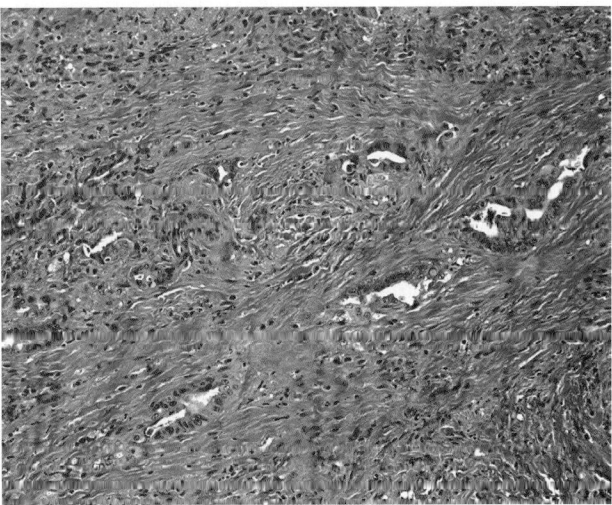

Figure 5-238. Adenocarcinoma in long-standing anal fistula.

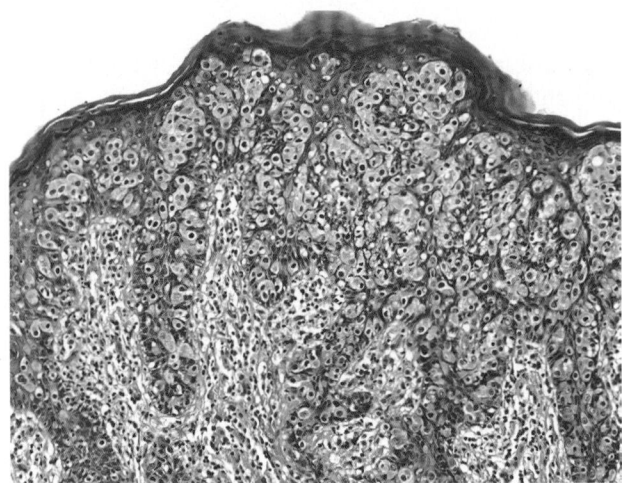

Figure 5-239. Anal Paget disease. Paget disease consists of squamous epithelium infiltrated by large neoplastic cells with abundant pale cytoplasm, vesicular chromatin, and prominent nucleoli.

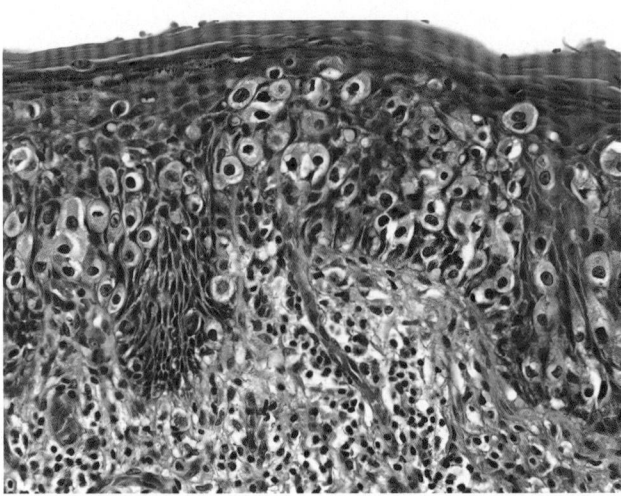

Figure 5-240. Anal Paget disease. Paget disease represents a precursor to adenocarcinoma (adenocarcinoma in situ) and is unassociated with HPV.

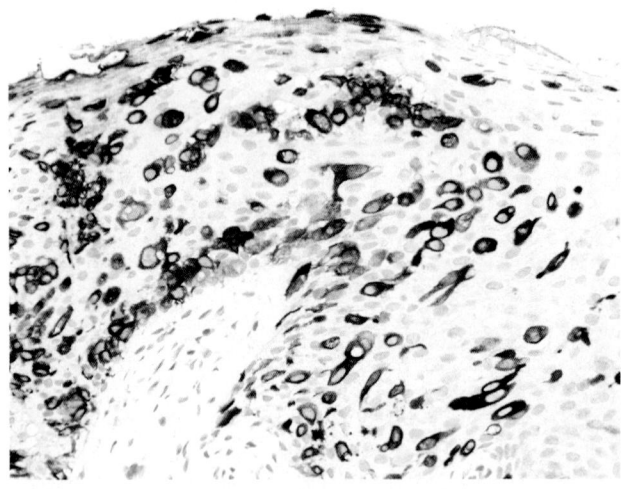

Figure 5-241. Anal Paget disease, CK7. The diagnosis of Paget disease is *not* an H&E diagnosis. An immunohistochemical workup is important to exclude melanoma and to determine which type of anal Paget disease is present to assess for the risk of an underlying malignancy. This case displayed the following immunophenotype: CK7+ (shown), CK20–, CDX2–, and GCDFP+, in keeping with an apocrine origin. The apocrine form of Paget disease is unassociated with an underlying malignancy.

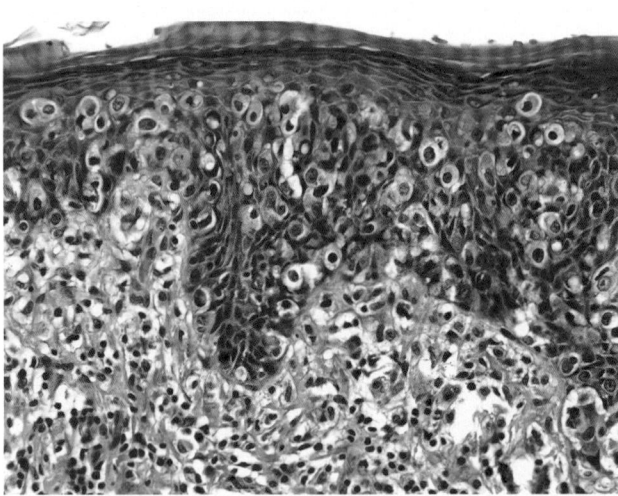

Figure 5-242. Anal Paget disease. This case displayed the following immunophenotype (CK7–, CK20+, CDX2+, and GCDFP–), suggesting the form of Paget disease associated with an underlying malignancy. In these cases, the immunoprofile reflects the typical immunoprofile of the underlying malignancy, i.e., colorectal adenocarcinoma in this case.

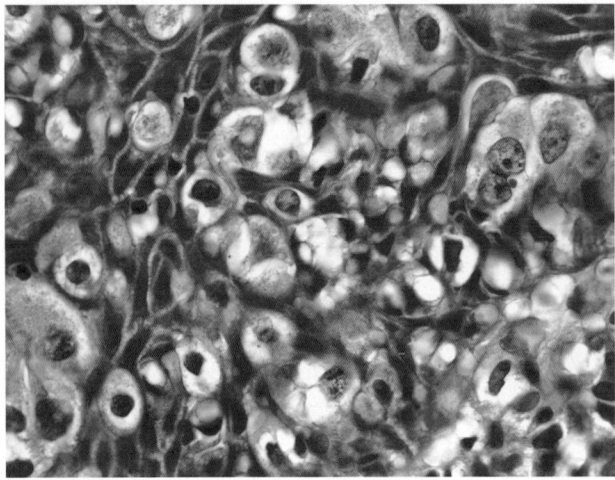

Figure 5-243. Anal Paget disease. Higher power of the previous figure shows the marked atypia of the neoplastic cells.

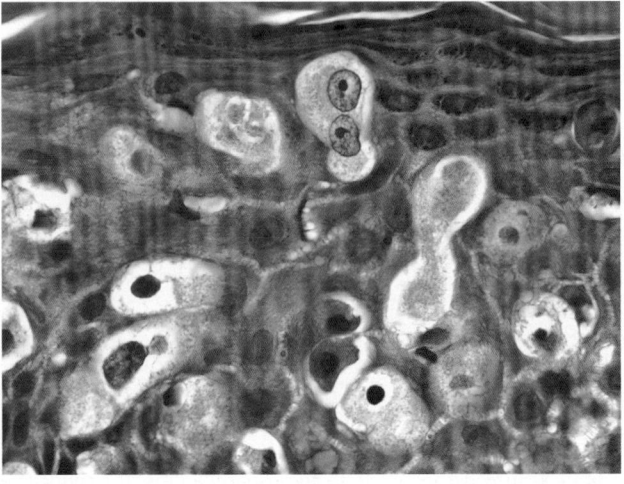

Figure 5-244. Anal Paget disease. The neoplastic cells display nuclearmegaly and prominent nucleoli.

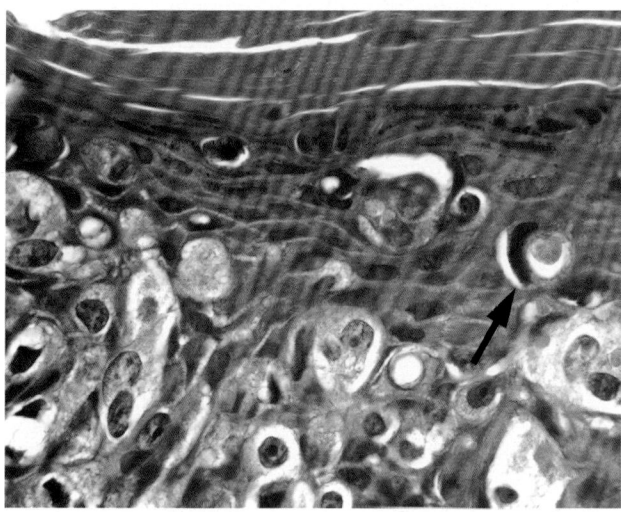

Figure 5-245. Anal Paget disease. Occasional cells that simulate signet ring are seen (*arrow*).

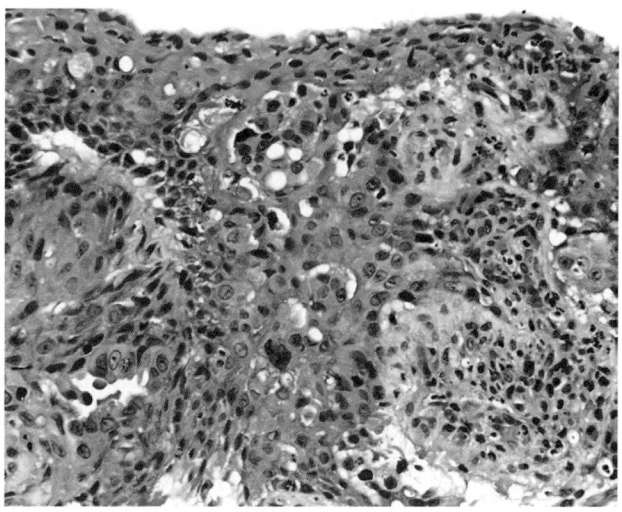

Figure 5-246. Anal Paget disease. Clinically, it presents as a slow-growing, erythematous plaque.

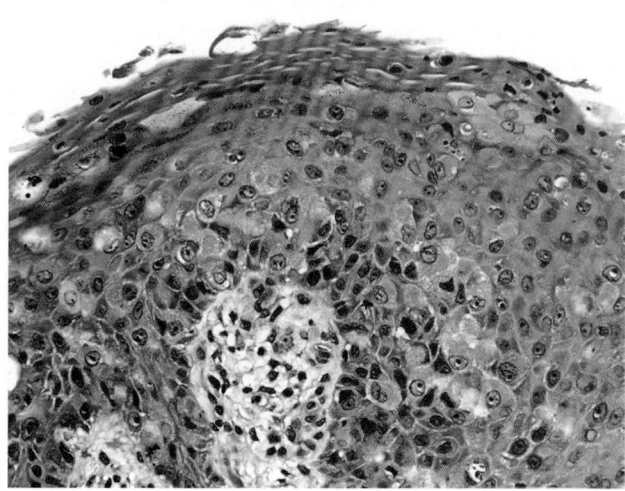

Figure 5-247. Anal Paget disease. Anal Paget disease is staged in AJCC and CAP.

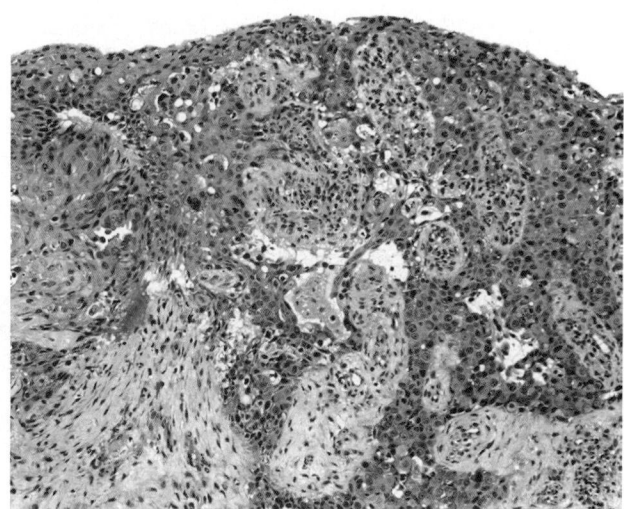

Figure 5-248. Anal Paget disease.

SAMPLE NOTE: Anal Paget Disease

Anus, Plaque, Biopsy

- Extramammary Paget disease, see Note
- Margins uninvolved
- Negative for an invasive component
- Background squamous mucosa with nondiagnostic findings

Note: The electronic record has been reviewed, and the unremarkable clinical history is noted.

There are two forms of extramammary Paget disease: a primary apocrine type and a form that is associated with an underlying synchronous or metachronous malignancy. The immunoprofile (GCDFP−, CK7−, CK20+, CDX2+) suggests the latter. Careful correlation with imaging studies and physical examination to assess for the site of potential primary is suggested (colorectal favored).

FAQ: How does extramammary differ from mammary Paget disease?

Answer: Paget disease of the breast is almost always associated with an underlying breast malignancy and displays the following immunoprofile: CK7+, CK20−, CDX2−, GCDFP+. In contrast, only 50% of patients with extramammary Paget disease of the anus have an associated underlying malignancy.[3] Those with an underlying malignancy typically display the immunoprofile of the primary and are GCDFP nonreactive, and those without an underlying malignancy display the same immunoprofile as mammary Paget (CK7+, CK20−, CDX2−, GCDFP+). Please do not go to your board examination without memorizing these factoids!

PEARLS & PITFALLS: Fake Paget Disease

Beware that normal squamous epithelium can feature cells with perinuclear clefts that can simulate Paget disease (Figs. 5.249–5.254). These normal cells, however, lack the atypia, nucleomegaly, prominent nucleoli characteristic of true Paget disease and are negative for CK7, CK20, and GCDFP. See Fig. 5.255 for a side-by-side comparison of fake and true Paget cells.

KEY FEATURES: Extramammary Paget Disease

- It represents a precursor to adenocarcinoma in cases that show sweat duct differentiation.
- It is unassociated with HPV.
- Clinically, it presents as a slow-growing, erythematous plaque.
- Histologically, the **squamous epithelium is infiltrated by large neoplastic cells with abundant pale cytoplasm, vesicular chromatin, and prominent nucleoli.**
- **A small immunohistochemical workup is important to exclude melanoma** and to determine which type of anal Paget disease is present.
- Anal Paget disease is subclassified into two groups:
  - **Half of anal Paget disease is associated with an underlying malignancy** and display the immunoprofile of the primary and are **GCDFP−.**
  - The other half of patients with anal Paget disease have **no underlying malignancy and display the following immunoprofile: CK7+, CK20−, and GCDFP+ (identical to mammary Paget).**
- Although mammary Paget disease is almost always associated with an underlying breast malignancy (and is CK7+, CK20−, CDX2−, GCDFP+), **only 50% of patients with anal Paget disease have an associated underlying malignancy.**

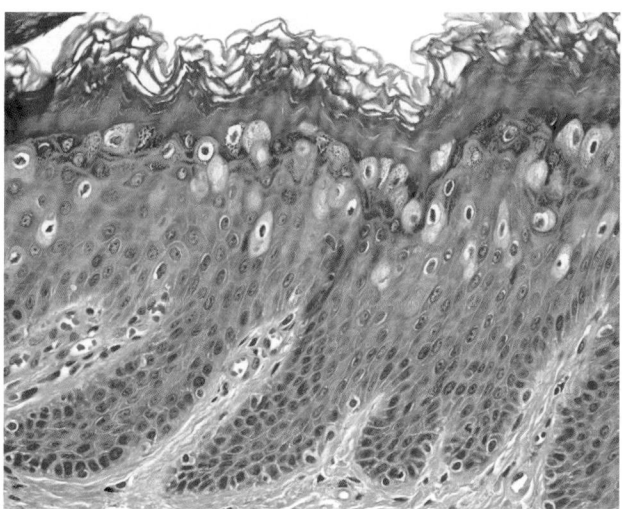

Figure 5-249. Fake Paget disease. Beware that normal squamous epithelium can feature cells with perinuclear clefts that can simulate Paget disease, as seen here.

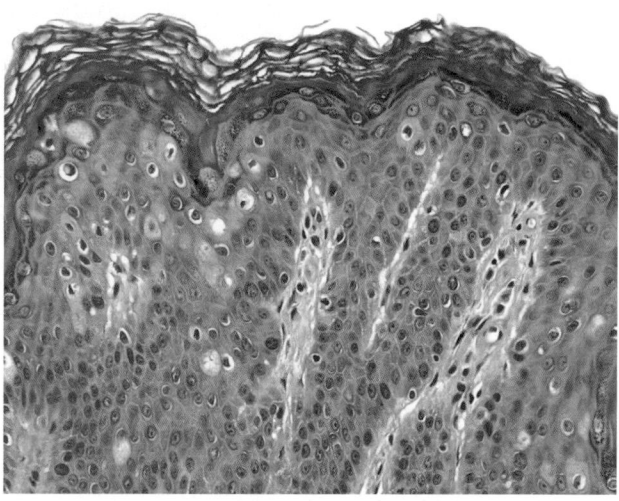

Figure 5-250. Fake Paget disease. These normal cells lack the requisite atypia, nuclear, and prominent nucleoli characteristic of true Paget disease.

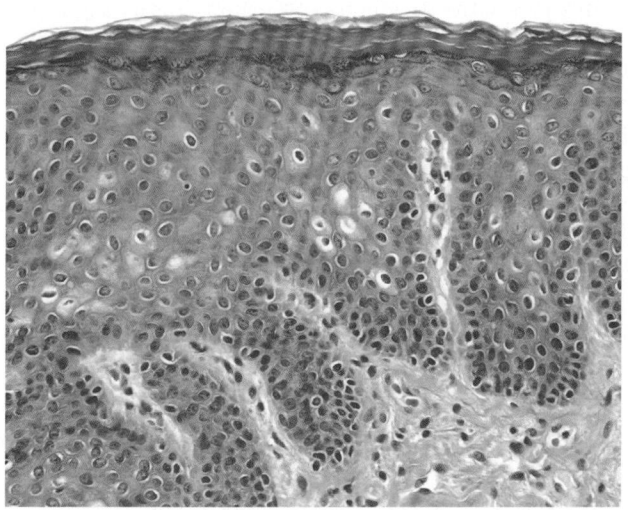

Figure 5-251. Fake Paget disease. These normal cells are negative for CK7 and CK20, supporting that these cells are not neoplastic cells of Paget disease.

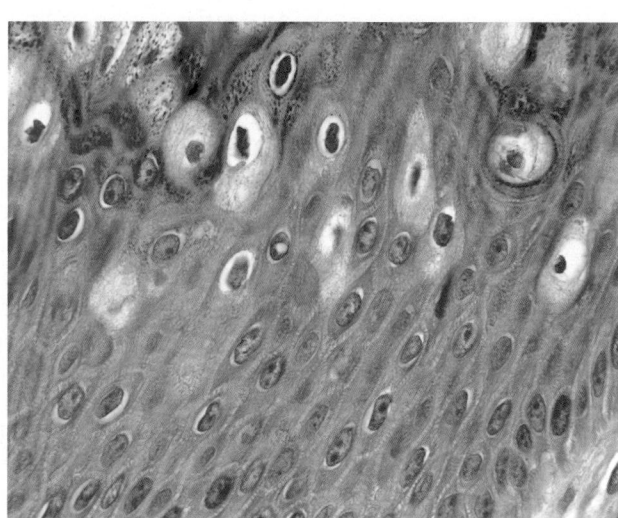

Figure 5-252. Fake Paget disease. These normal cells are bland.

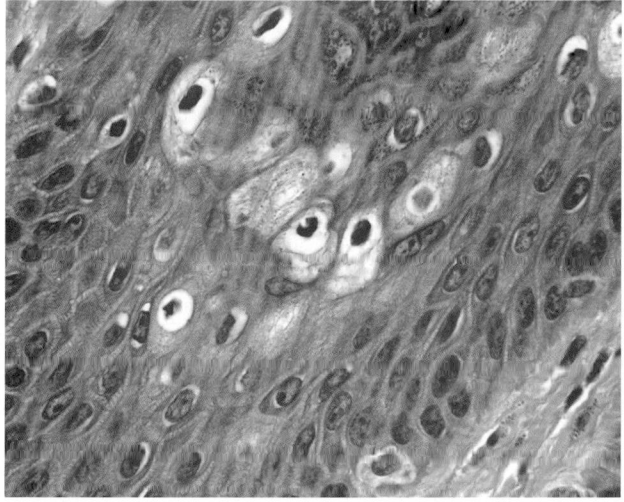

Figure 5-253. Fake Paget disease.

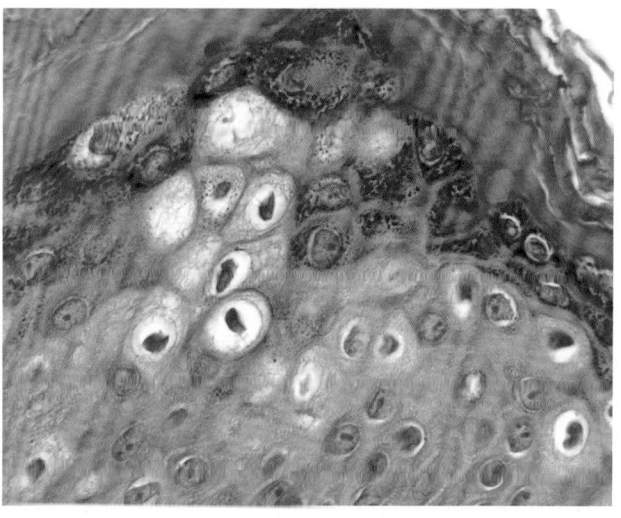

Figure 5-254. Fake Paget disease.

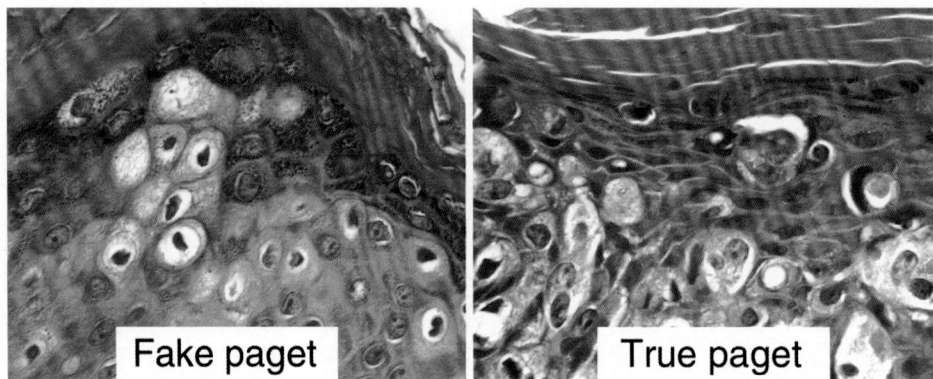

Figure 5-255. Fake Paget versus true Paget disease. Normal squamous epithelium can feature cells with perinuclear clefts that can simulate Paget disease, but these normal cells lack the atypia, nucleomegaly, and prominent nucleoli characteristic of true Paget disease and are negative for CK7, CK20, and GCDFP (not shown).

MALIGNANT MELANOMA

Anal melanoma arises from melanocytes in the squamous epithelium. It is an aggressive neoplasm with a 5-year survival of 19.8%.[39] It comprises up to 23.8% of all mucosal melanomas and up to 3% of all anal neoplasms.[3,39] In a study of more than 84,000 cases of cutaneous and noncutaneous melanoma, mucosal melanoma was more common in women and African-American and Hispanic patients.[39] Most patients present with anal bleeding and have a polypoid or fungating mass.[40] Again, site of involvement is key in directing management. About 91.5% of cutaneous melanomas are treated with surgery alone, whereas patients with mucosal melanomas are less likely to be treated with surgery alone (56.4%) and more likely to receive additional radiation (19.3%). In contrast to cutaneous melanoma, which is caused by UV light exposure and associated with *BRAF* mutations, anal melanoma is not linked to UV light exposure and more often has *KIT* mutations. KIT is a transmembrane tyrosine kinase receptor that promotes growth activating pathways when bound to its ligand or mutated. As a result, KIT inhibitory therapies may be beneficial for a subset of patients with metastatic melanoma and *KIT* mutations.[41,42]

The histology of anal melanoma is similar to melanoma at any other site with solid, nested, or fascicular architecture of epithelioid, plasmacytoid, or spindled neoplastic cells (Figs. 5.256–5.265).[40] Pleomorphism is generally prominent and mitoses are usually frequent. Melanotic pigment is a clue when present, but up to 30% of anal melanomas are amelanotic. A primary diagnosis of malignant melanoma is rarely an H&E diagnosis owing to the morphologic overlap with a wide variety of lesions. The following is a suggested immunohistochemical panel approach for such cases. Melanoma can histologically mimic extramammary Paget disease, but the S100 protein–reactive, cytokeratin-nonreactive immunolabeling profile of melanoma distinguishes it from Paget disease (S100 protein nonreactive, cytokeratin reactive). Beware that up to 75% of anal melanoma display CD117 reactivity, and these cases should not be confused for a GIST (Fig. 5.265).[40,43] In these cases the panel approach is reassuring, with anal melanomas usually displaying strong reactivity for multiple melanoma markers and reactivity with only one of the GIST makers (CD117). Similarly, beware that focal cytokeratin expression can be seen in up to 10% of anal melanoma, which should not result in an interpretation of carcinoma.[40] Again the panel approach is helpful, with anal melanomas displaying strong reactivity for multiple melanoma markers and only focal cytokeratin expression.

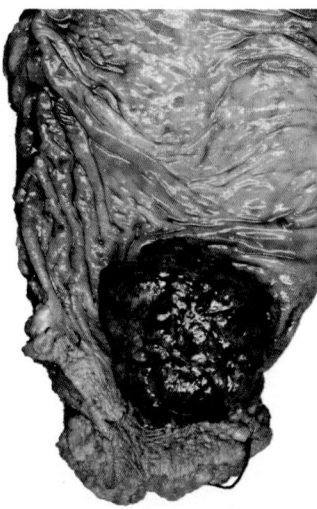

Figure 5-256. Melanoma. This melanoma presented as a large, pigmented anal mass. (Photo courtesy of Laura G. Pastrián MD, "La Paz" University Hospital, Madrid, Spain, @DraEosina.)

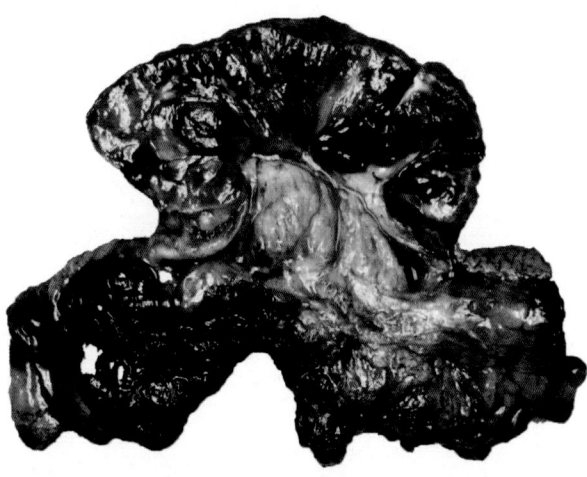

Figure 5-257. Melanoma. Cross section of the case in the previous figure. (Photo courtesy of Laura G. Pastrián MD, "La Paz" University Hospital, Madrid, Spain, @DraEosina.)

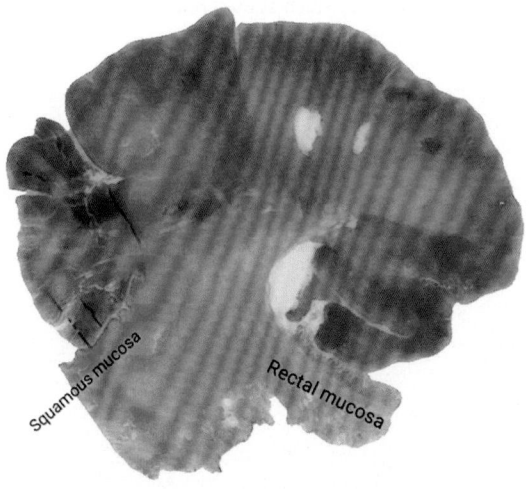

Figure 5-258. Melanoma. The neoplasm is based at the squamo-columnar junction, as seen here. (Photo courtesy of Laura G. Pastrián MD, "La Paz" University Hospital, Madrid, Spain, @DraEosina.)

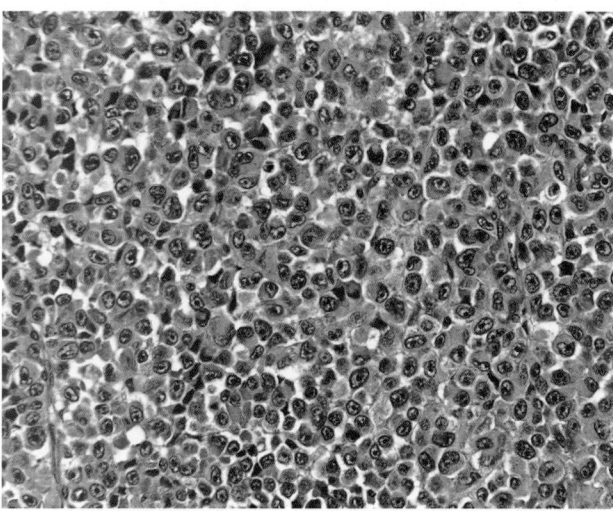

Figure 5-259. Melanoma. The histology of anal melanoma is similar to that of melanoma at any other site, with solid, nested, or fascicular architecture of epithelioid (as seen here), plasmacytoid, or spindled neoplastic cells.

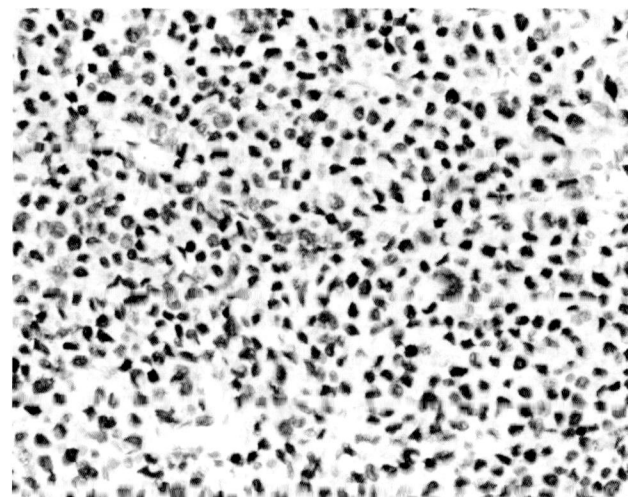

Figure 5-260. Melanoma, SOX10. A variety of melanoma markers is available and includes SOX10 (shown here), S100 protein, MiTF, tyrosinase, HMB-45, and MELAN-A.

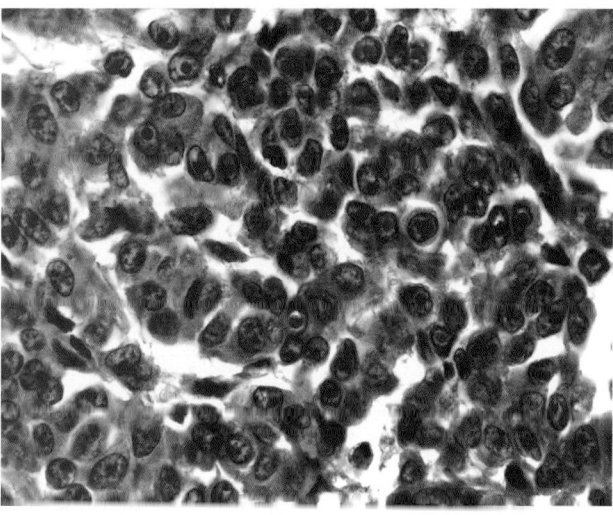

Figure 5-261. Melanoma. Melanoma can display a variety of morphologies. Typical features include prominent nucleoli, as seen here.

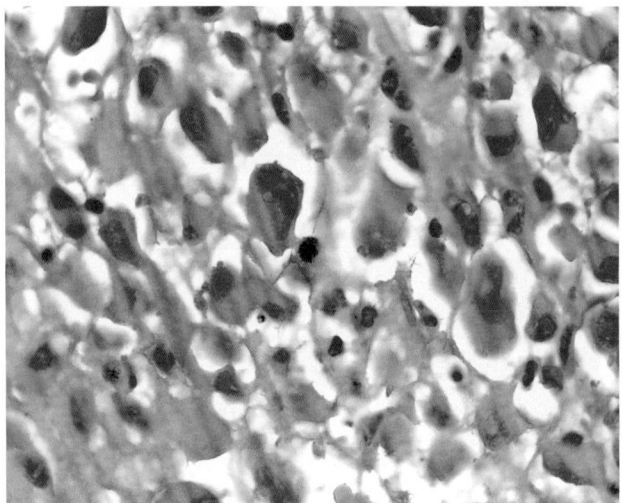

Figure 5-262. Melanoma. This melanoma shows plasmacytoid morphology with prominent nucleoli and scattered melanin pigment. Up to 30% of anal melanoma are amelanotic.

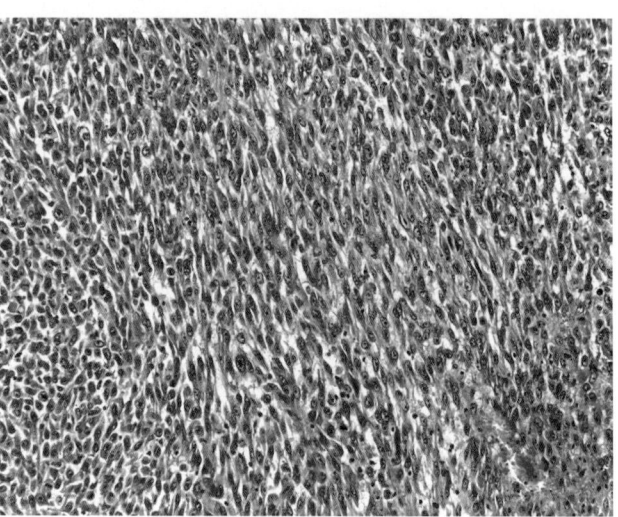

Figure 5-263. Melanoma. Melanoma can also bear a spindled morphology. Beware that up to 75% of anal melanoma display CD117 reactivity, and these cases should not be confused for a GIST. In addition, focal cytokeratin expression can be seen in up to 10% of anal melanomas, which should not result in a diagnosis of sarcomatoid carcinoma.

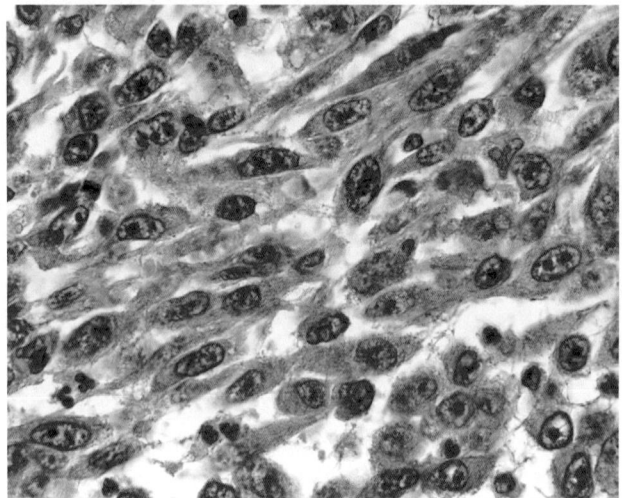

Figure 5-264. Melanoma. Higher power of the previous figure. Anal melanoma is not linked to UV light exposure and more often has *KIT* mutations. In contrast to cutaneous melanomas, mucosal melanomas are more commonly treated with surgery and radiation.

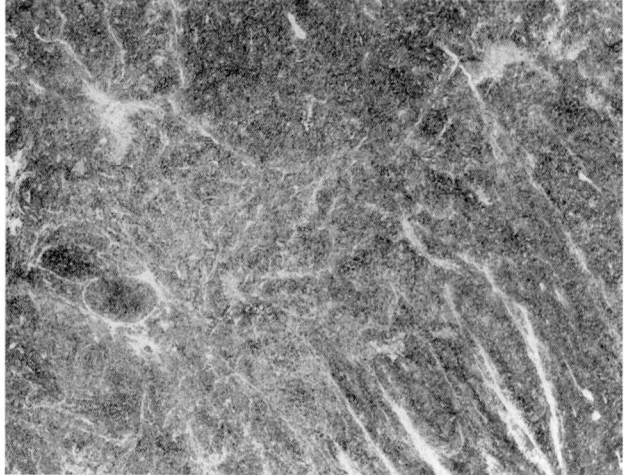

Figure 5-265. Melanoma, CD117. Up to 75% of anal melanoma display CD117 reactivity, and these cases should not be confused for GISTs. A panel immunohistochemical approach is recommended in the primary diagnosis of melanoma (melanoma commonly displays CD117 reactivity in addition to other melanoma makers; GIST is never diffusely reactive for melanoma markers but often is reactive for other GIST markers, such as DOG1 and CD34).

CHECKLIST: Anal Melanoma Immunohistochemical Panel Approach

☐ Two melanoma markers S100 protein, SOX10

☐ S100 also evaluates for neural processes, such as a schwannoma

☐ AE1/3 to evaluate for a sarcomatoid carcinoma (focal reactivity can be seen in melanoma)

☐ CD117 and DOG1 to evaluate for a GIST (strong CD117 is common in anal melanoma)

☐ Smooth muscle actin and desmin to evaluate for a smooth muscle tumor

CHECKLIST: Anal Melanoma AJCC Staging

Per the AJCC, eighth edition (2017), there is no staging system of mucosal malignant melanoma of the rectum or anus.[35] For these specimens, follow this checklist approach to include the usual pertinent negatives. Cutaneous melanoma is staged under "Melanoma of the Skin" in the AJCC, eighth edition.

☐ Size
☐ Depth of infiltration
☐ Margins
☐ Lymphovascular invasion
☐ Perineural invasion
☐ Lymph node assessment
☐ Background findings (melanoma in situ)

KEY FEATURES: Malignant Melanoma

- Most cutaneous melanomas are treated with **surgery alone.**
- Mucosal melanomas are more commonly treated with **surgery and radiation.**
- Anal melanoma is **not linked to UV light exposure** and more often **has *KIT* mutations.**
- **KIT inhibitory therapies can be beneficial for patients with metastatic melanoma and *KIT* mutations.**
- The histology of anal melanoma is similar to that of melanoma at any other site with solid, nested, or fascicular architecture of epithelioid, plasmacytoid, or spindled neoplastic cells.
- **Up to 30% of anal melanoma are amelanotic.**
- Melanoma can **histologically mimic extramammary Paget disease.**
- **A primary diagnosis of malignant melanoma is rarely an H&E only diagnosis;** an immunohistochemical panel approach is suggested to confirm melanoma and exclude its mimics.
- **Anal melanoma commonly shows CD117 strong reactivity and sometimes displays focal cytokeratin reactivity.**
- **There is no AJCC staging system of mucosal malignant melanoma of the rectum or anus;** cutaneous melanoma is staged under Melanoma of the Skin in the AJCC, eighth edition.

NEAR MISS

BEYOND THE FIRST DIAGNOSIS

The "Near Miss" section emphasizes the importance of seeing beyond the first, obvious diagnosis by working through real-life examples. The above-mentioned example is a mass excision from a patient with a history of widely metastatic malignant melanoma and a rectal mass extending into the anus. Although the initial sections look compatible with the known diagnoses, note the lower-grade spindle cells at the periphery of the lesion (Figs. 5.266–5.268). Before assuming that these spindle cells are myofibroblasts laying down a desmoplastic background or assuming that they are a spindle melanoma, consider the possibility that they could represent a second neoplasm. A panel approach to melanoma was pursued that demonstrated that the high-grade pleomorphic cells are melanoma (S100 protein+, SOX10+, MiTF+) metastatic to a GIST (S100 protein-, SOX10-, MiTF-; CD117+, DOG1+, CD34+) (Figs. 5.269 and 5.270).

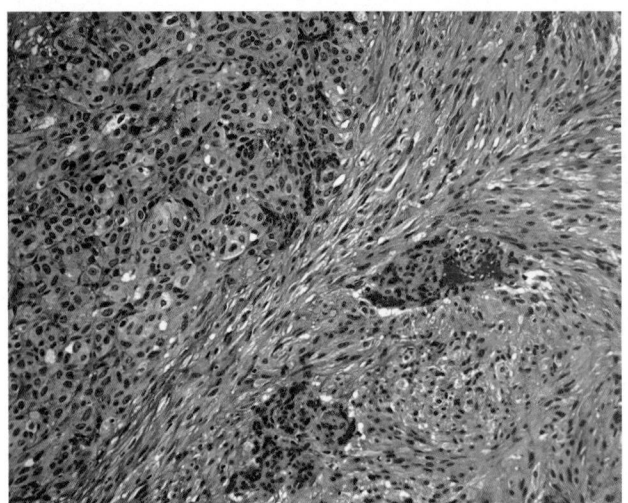

Figure 5-266. Beyond the first diagnosis. The section is from a rectal/anal mass from a patient with a history of widely metastatic malignant melanoma. The initial sections look compatible with the known diagnoses.

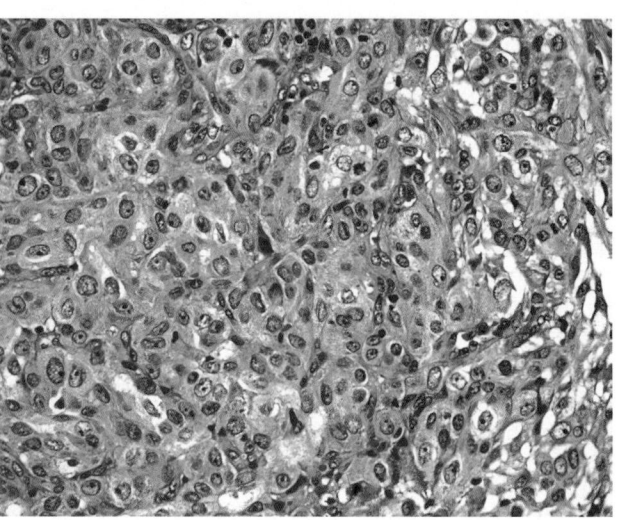

Figure 5-267. Beyond the first diagnosis. Higher power of the previous figure shows the typical features of melanoma with a nested architecture of pleomorphic cells and prominent mitotic figures.

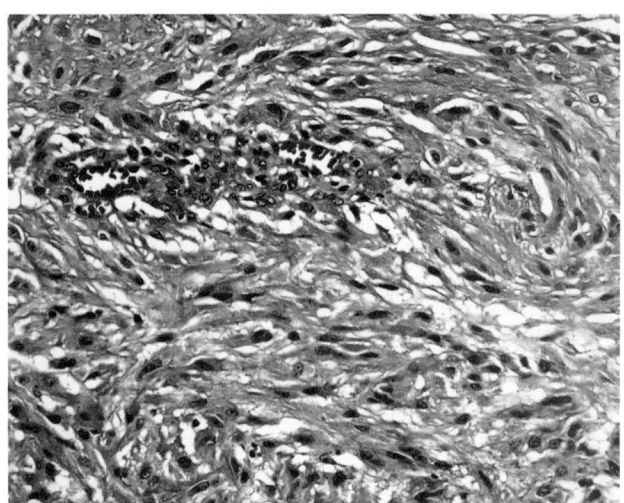

Figure 5-268. Beyond the first diagnosis. Adjacent to the obvious melanoma are lower-grade spindle cells. They are too cellular and cohesive for myofibroblasts laying down a desmoplastic background, and yet they are quite bland compared with the neighboring melanoma. Note the absence of pleomorphism and mitotic figures. In such a case, it is best to consider the possibility that they could represent a second neoplasm.

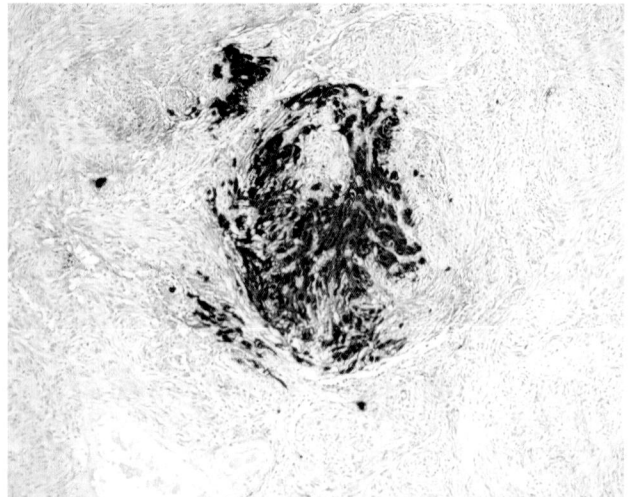

Figure 5-269. Beyond the first diagnosis, S100 protein. An S100 protein (shown), SOX10, and MiTF highlighted the pleomorphic component, confirming a diagnosis of metastatic malignant melanoma.

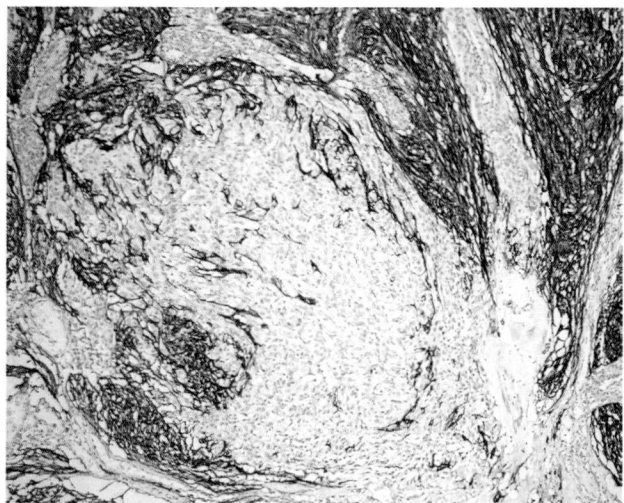

Figure 5-270. Beyond the first diagnosis, DOG1. The low-grade spindle population was a GIST (S100 protein–, SOX10–, MiTF–; CD117+, DOG1+ [shown], CD34+). This case represented a metastatic melanoma to a GIST and emphasizes the importance of always looking beyond the first, obvious diagnosis.

UNEXPECTED FINDINGS IN A HEMORRHOID

Hemorrhoid specimens are common and seemingly unexciting, but they require as much time and attention as any other specimen. Diagnostic features of hemorrhoids include prominent ectatic, engorged vessels embedded in fibroconnective tissue (Figs. 5.45–5.54). Additional "bonus" findings include luminal parasites or medications, dysplasia of the surface squamous (Figs. 5.271–5.275) or colonic epithelium, colitis, amyloidosis, viral cytopathic effect, fungal infections, and sneaky malignancies, among others.

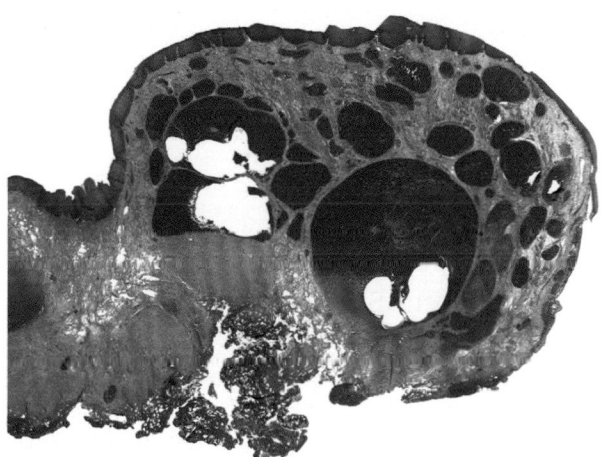

Figure 5-271. Unexpected findings in a hemorrhoid. The "routine specimens" are often the most challenging because they may contain unexpected findings that take a bit more effort to locate than findings in the ordinary oncologic resection. Diagnostic features of hemorrhoids include prominent ectatic, engorged vessels embedded in fibroconnective tissue (Figs. 5.45–5.54), as seen here.

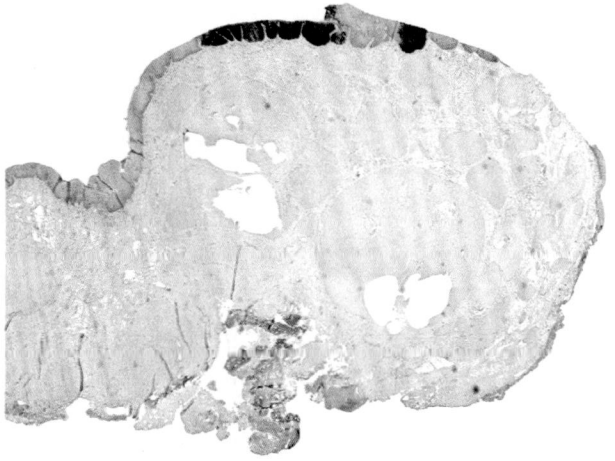

Figure 5-272. Unexpected findings in a hemorrhoid, p16. Make sure to carefully inspect all tissue in these seemingly uninspiring specimens. The overlying mucosa may contain squamous epithelium (check for dysplasia) or glandular epithelium (check for dysplasia and colitis). This case features an unexpected focus of HSIL (AIN2) highlighted by the p16.

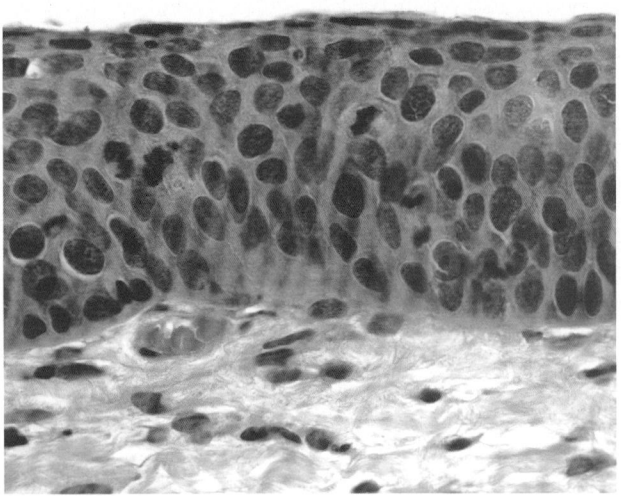

Figure 5-273. Unexpected findings in a hemorrhoid. Higher power shows the diagnostic features of HSIL (AIN2).

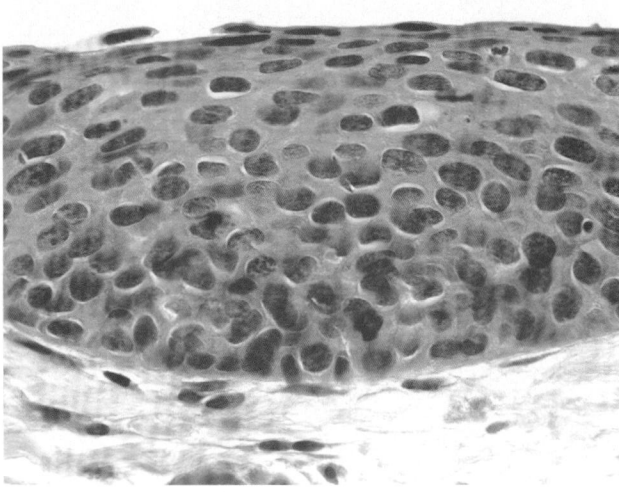

Figure 5-274. Unexpected findings in a hemorrhoid. Hemorrhoid specimens are common, and the prominent vessels can be distracting to other important diagnoses. Take whatever time it requires to carefully assess all aspects of the tissue to ensure proper patient management.

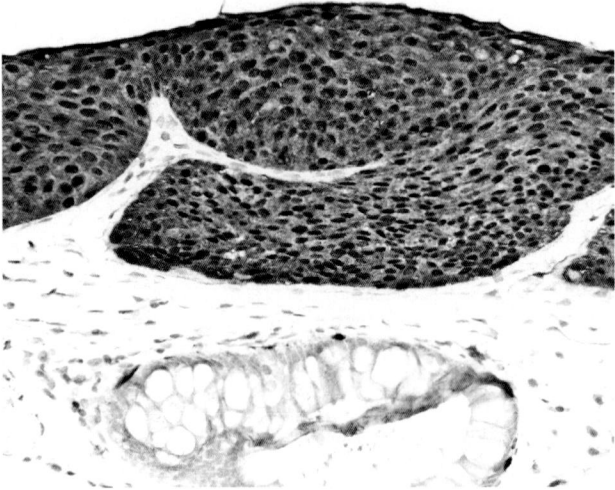

Figure 5-275. Unexpected findings in a hemorrhoid, p16. Other potential bonus findings in hemorrhoid specimens include amyloidosis, viral cytopathic effect, fungal infections, and sneaky malignancies, among others.

PAPILLARY ENDOTHELIAL HYPERPLASIA

Papillary endothelial hyperplasia (PEH) (also known as Masson tumor) is a benign endothelial hyperplasia in response to tissue damage. It is important to recognize this tumor because it can present as a mass and mimic angiosarcoma. PEH has been widely described in the lung, digits, orbit, mandible, tongue, salivary glands, penis, breast, bladder, small intestine, stomach, and vulva and is occasionally encountered within thrombosed hemorrhoids, where it was in fact first described years ago by Masson![44] Typical histologic features of PEH include delicate papilla and anastomosing cords of endothelial hyperplasia surrounding hyaline cores (Figs. 5.276–5.285).[45-47] Hemorrhage and necrosis can occasionally be seen. In contrast to angiosarcoma, distinguishing features of PEH include its well-defined borders and a lack of atypia, mitoses, solid growth, and infiltration or dissection of adjoining tissues.[45] The endothelium can be highlighted with vascular markers CD34 and CD31,[48] but these stains are rarely necessary with familiarity of the characteristic features.

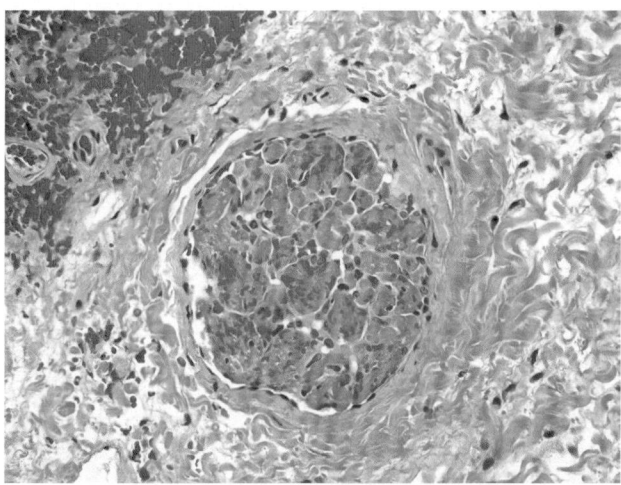

Figure 5-276. Papillary endothelial hyperplasia (PEH). PEH is a benign endothelial hyperplasia in response to organizing thrombi. It has been widely described in a variety of sites and is occasionally seen in thrombosed hemorrhoids, as in this case.

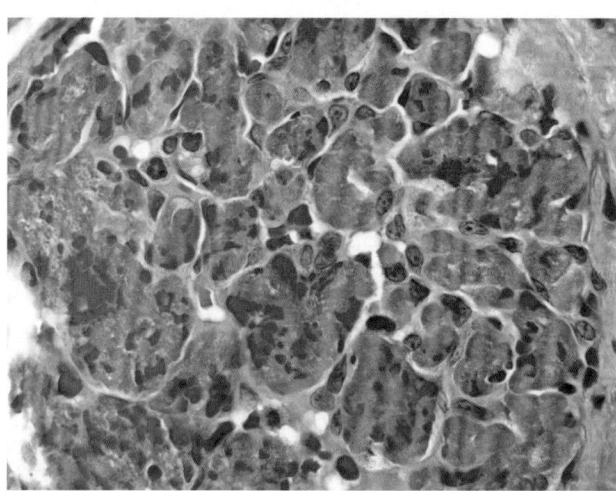

Figure 5-277. Papillary endothelial hyperplasia. Higher power of the previous figure. Typical histologic features of benign PEH include delicate papillae and anastomosing cords of endothelial hyperplasia surrounding hyaline cores.

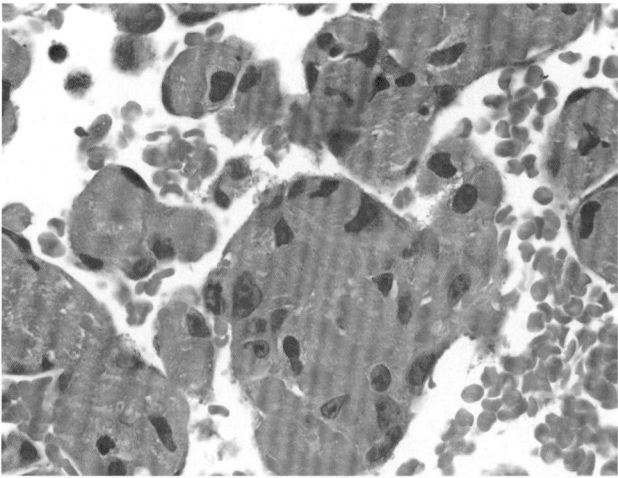

Figure 5-278. Papillary endothelial hyperplasia. It is important to recognize PEH because it can mimic angiosarcoma. Clues to PEH include its background hemorrhoid with thrombosis, well-defined borders, and a lack of atypia, mitoses, solid growth, and infiltration or dissection of adjoining tissues. The last features are more common with angiosarcoma. PEH instead shows cores of fibrin covered by a monolayer of endothelial cells.

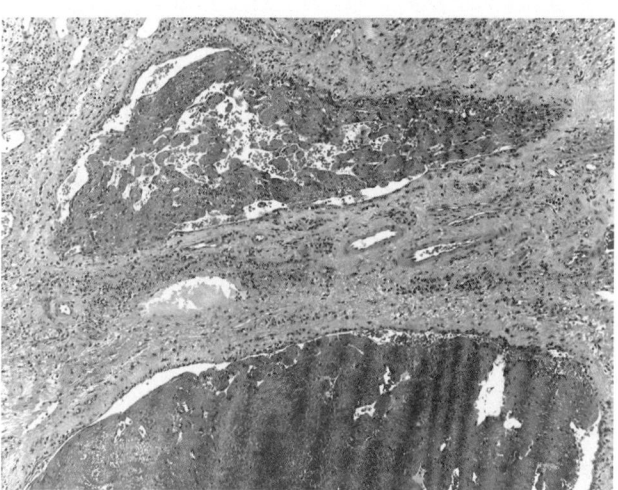

Figure 5-279. Papillary endothelial hyperplasia. A thrombosed vascular space is the typical backdrop of PEH.

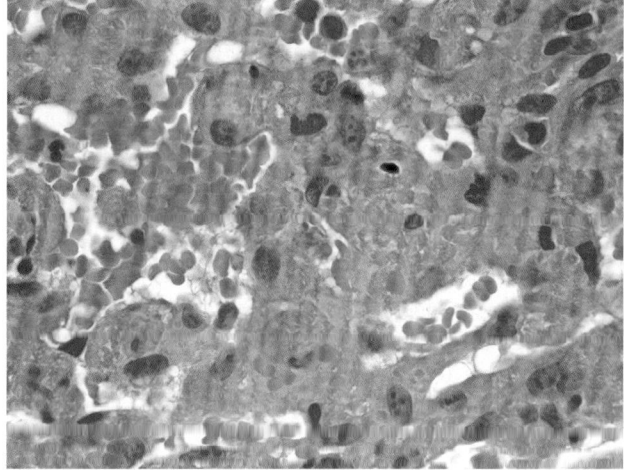

Figure 5-280. Papillary endothelial hyperplasia. Higher power of the previous figure.

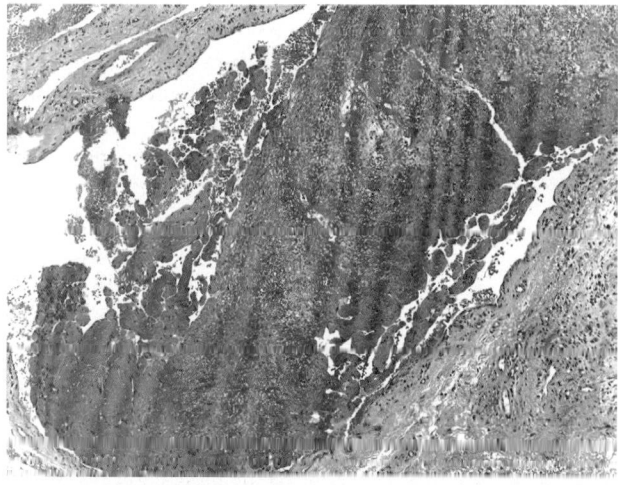

Figure 5-281. Papillary endothelial hyperplasia. PEH is typically found at the periphery of a thrombosed vessel, as seen here.

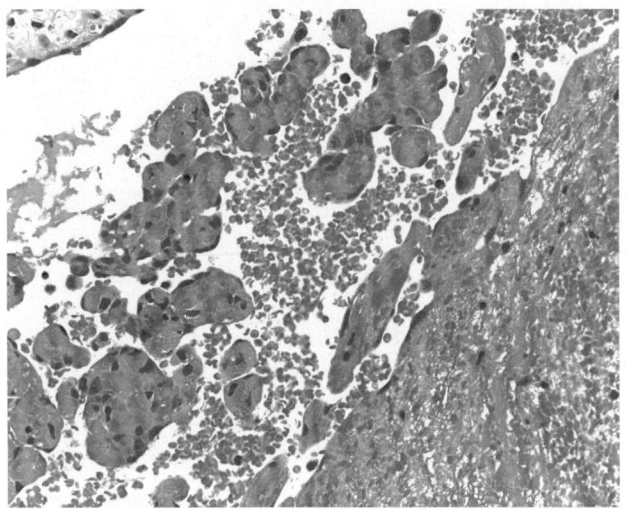

Figure 5-282. Papillary endothelial hyperplasia. Higher power of the previous figure. Its lobular architecture with well-defined borders is a clue to its benign nature.

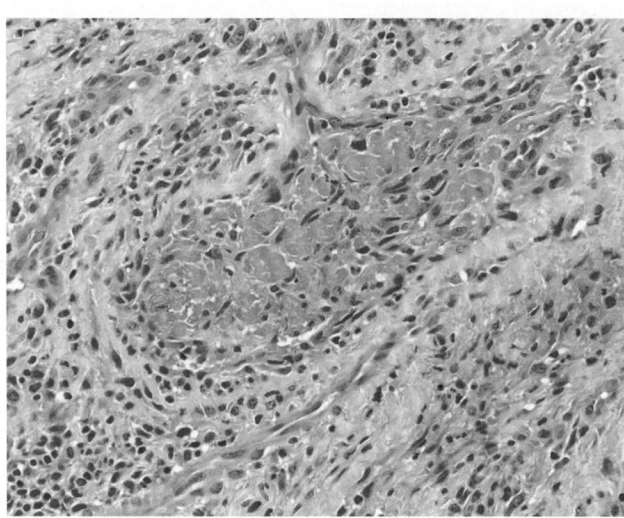

Figure 5-283. Papillary endothelial hyperplasia. PEH is also known as Masson tumor.

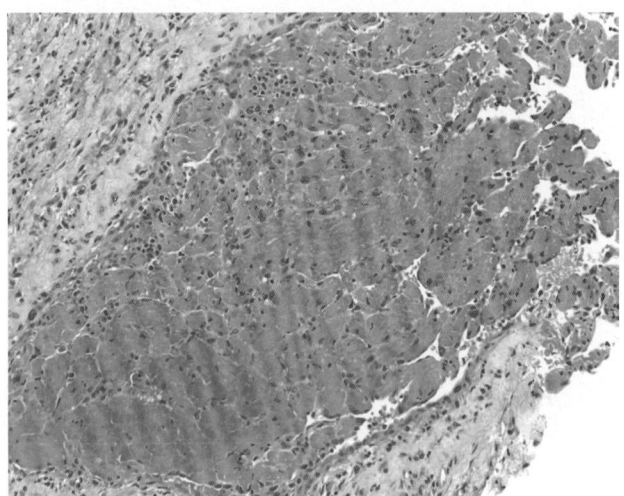

Figure 5-284. Papillary endothelial hyperplasia.

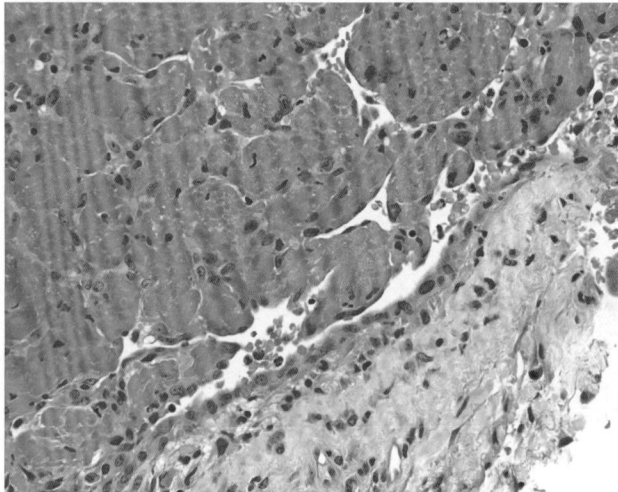

Figure 5-285. Papillary endothelial hyperplasia. PEH is typically found at the periphery of a thrombosed vessel, as seen here.

EPSTEIN-BARR VIRUS MUCOCUTANEOUS ULCER

Epstein-Barr virus mucocutaneous ulcer (EBV MCU) is an isolated lesion seen in the skin, oral cavity, or GI tract in patients with a history of iatrogenic or age-related immunosuppression. It is a self-limited lesion with an indolent course that responds well to conservative management, such as decreased immunosuppression. It is presumed to be caused by transient immunosuppression that facilitates the EBV-induced mucocutaneous ulcer. The case presented here is from a patient with a history of bone marrow transplantation who presented with a painful anal ulcer. Histologically, a heavy polymorphous infiltrate is seen admixed with large B-cell blasts with Reed-Sternberg–like appearance, necrosis, and ulceration (Figs. 5.286–5.291).[49,50] The B cells label with CD30 and EBER and appear in a background of prominent, small T cells. Clonal immunoglobulin heavy chain gene rearrangements are seen in up to 39%, and clonal T-cell patterns are seen in up to 31%.[50] As a result, an evaluation from a pathologist with hematopathology expertise is worthwhile in these wildly atypical morphologic cases in precarious patients. The differential diagnosis is the more clinically aggressive posttransplant lymphoproliferative disease. Distinguishing features of EBV MCU include its presentation as an isolated ulcer (not a mass) and the absence of circulating EBV DNA in the peripheral blood. Correct classification is important because EBV MCU responds to conservative therapy, whereas posttransplant lymphoprolif-erative disease often requires chemotherapy. In the small series available, the ulcers resolved over a period of weeks with no EBV MCU–related fatalities.[49,50] A CMV immunohistochem-ical stain is suggested in all cases based on the intense lymphoid infiltrate.

KEY FEATURES: EBV MCU

- It is associated with iatrogenic or age-related **immunosuppression.**
- It is a **self-limited lesion with an indolent course** that responds well to conservative management.
- Histologically, **a heavy polymorphous infiltrate is seen admixed with large B-cell blasts with Reed-Sternberg–like appearance.**
- The B cells label with CD30 and **EBER.**
- **Clonal** immunoglobulin heavy chain gene rearrangements clonal T-cell patterns are seen.
- **An evaluation from a pathologist with hematopathology expertise is worthwhile.**
- **A CMV immunohistochemical** stain is suggested in all cases.

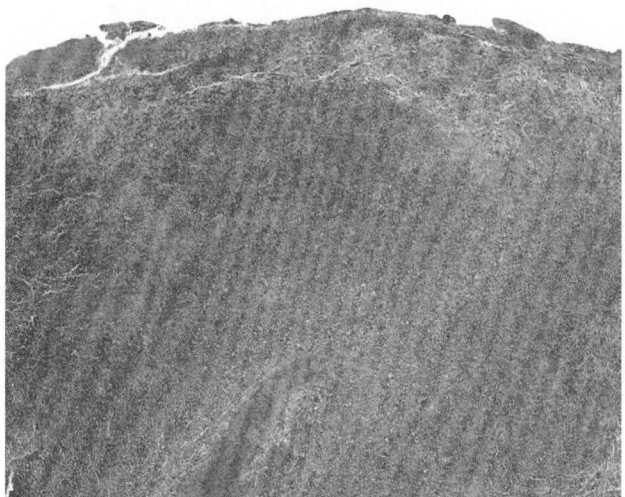

Figure 5-286. EBV mucocutaneous ulcer (EBV MCU). EBV MCU shows an intense inflammatory infiltrate. Its cause is presumed to reflect transient immunosuppression that facilitates the EBV-induced mucocutaneous ulcer. It is a self-limited lesion with an indolent course that responds well to conservative management.

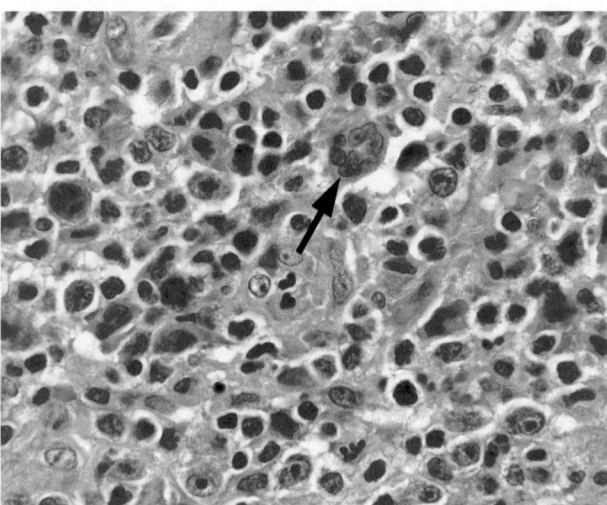

Figure 5-287. EBV mucocutaneous ulcer. On higher power, a heavy polymorphous infiltrate is seen admixed with large B-cell blasts with a Reed-Sternberg–like appearance (*arrow*), necrosis, and ulceration. The B cells label with CD30 and EBER and appear in a background of prominent, small T cells. Prominent mitoses are seen.

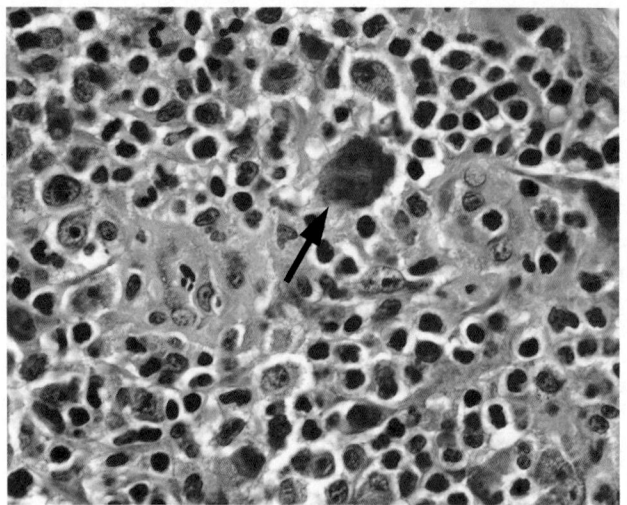

Figure 5-288. EBV mucocutaneous ulcer. The *arrow* highlights a characteristic Reed-Sternberg–like cell (*arrow*). Clonal immunoglobulin heavy chain gene rearrangements are seen in up to 39%, and clonal T-cell patterns are seen in up to 31%.[50] As a result, an evaluation from a pathologist with hematopathology expertise is worthwhile.

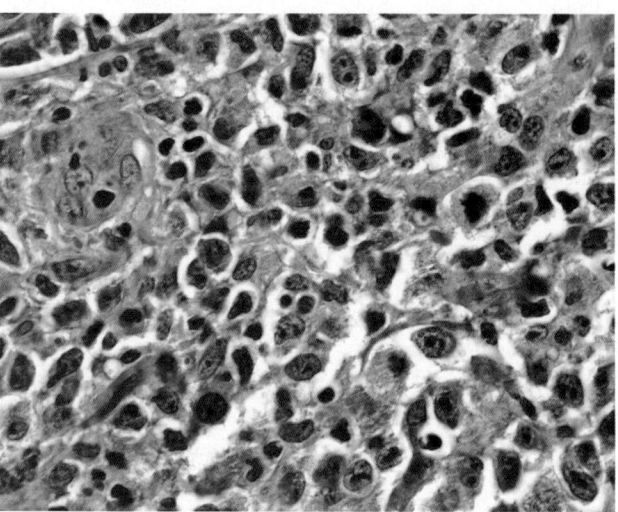

Figure 5-289. EBV mucocutaneous ulcer. Prominent mitoses are seen. The differential diagnosis is the more clinically aggressive posttransplant lymphoproliferative disease. Distinguishing features of EBV MCU include its presentation as an isolated ulcer (not a mass) and the absence of circulating EBV DNA in the peripheral blood.

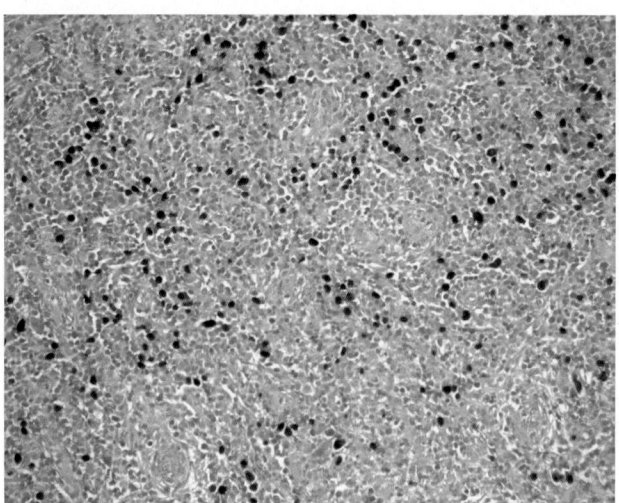

Figure 5-290. EBV mucocutaneous ulcer, EBER. EBER and CD30 (not shown) highlight the B cells.

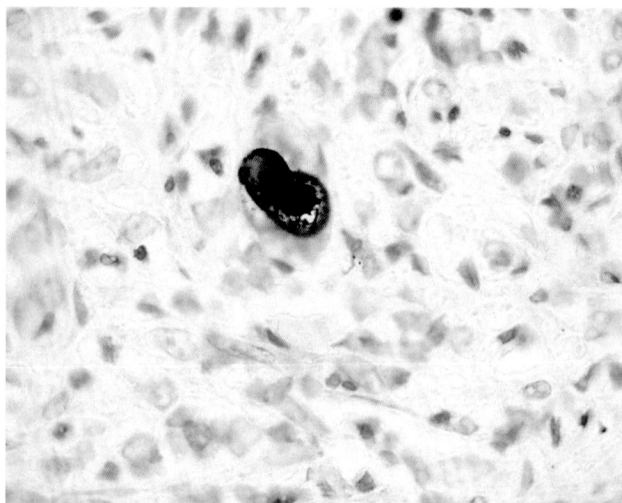

Figure 5-291. EBV mucocutaneous ulcer, CMV. A rare CMV immunolabeled cell was seen. EBV MCU is an isolated lesion seen in patients with a history of iatrogenic or age-related immunosuppression. Because the patients are immunosuppressed and CMV can result in a similar morphology, a CMV IHC is suggested in all cases.

SYPHILITIC AND LYMPHOGRANULOMA VENEREUM PROCTOCOLITIS (STI PROCTITIS)

Syphilitic and lymphogranuloma venereum (LGV) proctocolitis were discussed in the "Near Miss" section of the "Colon" chapter and are briefly mentioned here because they can also be seen in anal specimens submitted as clinically worrisome ulcers or masses. Recall, common clues to the diagnosis include a history of HIV-positive men who have sex with men (MSM), and these men typically present with anal bleeding, anal pain, and tenesmus.[51-53] Beware that most cases prospectively lack the helpful clinical red flags of HIV and MSM status, emphasizing that a familiarity with the typical morphology is critical. Endoscopically, STI proctocolitis can present as ulcerations, nodules, polyps, and masses. Histologically, an intense bandlike plasma cell infiltrate is seen at the squamous epithelium-lamina propria interface with variable granulomata and fibrosis (Figs. 5.292–5.299). The overlying squamous epithelium is usually unremarkable, but keep in mind that these patients may have multiple concomitant processes. For example, because STI colitis is sexually transmitted, by definition, these patients are at risk for multiple sexually transmitted infections and, therefore, STI colitis can also be accompanied by HPV-associated neoplasia, HPV, and so on. As a result, it is important to thoroughly evaluate the overlying epithelium for dysplasia in a case of STI colitis. Similarly, it is important to examine the lamina propria and submucosa for potential STI colitis in cases of LSIL and HSIL lesions. Silver stains and *Treponema pallidum* immunohistochemical stains are too insensitive to confirm or exclude syphilitic infections, and there are no routine commercially available LGV studies available for the pathologist. As a result, clinical tests provide the best means to establish this diagnosis (syphilis: serum rapid plasma reagin, rapid plasma reagin titer, and a *Treponema*-specific serology, such as fluorescent treponemal antibody; lymphogranuloma venereum: rectal swab collected in the absence of lubricant for *Chlamydia trachomatis* nucleic acid probe test or culture and LGV polymerase chain reaction).[51,54] In general, specimens with intense plasma cell infiltrates should include consideration of STI colitis, CMV, and a hematolymphoid evaluation. See also "Near Miss" section, "Colon" chapter, and *Atlas of GI Pathology: A Pattern Based Approach to Non-Neoplastic Biopsies*.

SAMPLE NOTE: STI Proctitis

Anus, Mass, Biopsy

- Squamous mucosa with intense plasma cell–rich inflammation, see Note.

Note: The history of a rectal mass is noted. The biopsy findings have been associated with syphilitic and/or LGV infections. In such cases, clinical studies provide the best means of evaluation. It would be important to evaluate for both because identical histologic features can be seen with either agent either in isolation or in combination. A CMV immunostain is negative. Deeper sections examined. A hematopathology workup was noncontributory. If the lesion remains concerning, repeat sampling is a consideration.

Syphilis: Serum RPR, RPR titer, and a treponemal-specific serology.

LGV: Rectal swab collected in the absence of lubricant for C. trachomatis *nucleic acid probe test, indirect immunofluorescence, culture, or LGV PCR.*

Reference:
Arnold CA, Limketkai BN, Illei PB, Montgomery E, Voltaggio L. *Am J Surg Pathol.* 2013;37(1):38-46.

KEY FEATURES: STI Proctitis
- Syphilitic and LGV proctocolitis can be seen in anal specimens submitted as clinically worrisome ulcers or masses
- Common clues to the diagnosis include a history of **HIV-positive men who have sex with men (MSM).**
- **Most cases prospectively lack the helpful clinical red flags of HIV and MSM status.**
- Endoscopically, STI proctocolitis can present as **ulcerations, nodules, polyps, and masses.**
- Histologically, an **intense bandlike plasma cell infiltrate is seen at the squamous epithelium-lamina propria interface with variable granulomata and fibrosis.**
- **Clinical tests provide the best means to establish this diagnosis.**
- Also consider concomitant **HPV-associated neoplasia, CMV, and a hematolymphoid** evaluation.

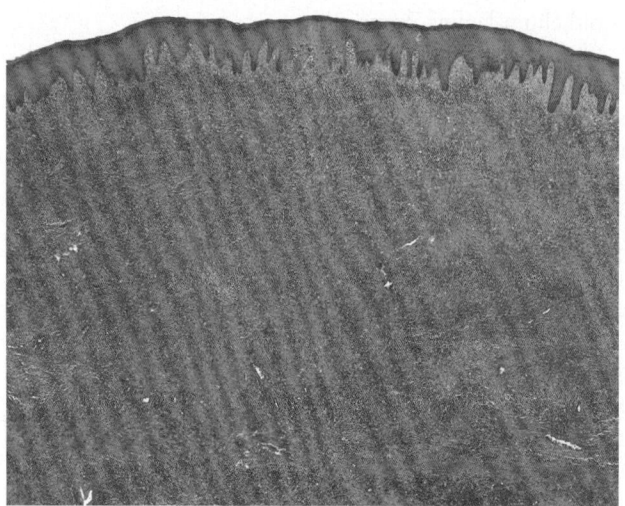

Figure 5-292. Syphilitic and lymphogranuloma venereum (LGV) proctocolitis (STI proctitis). This specimen was designated a clinically worrisome anal mass. An intense bandlike infiltrate is seen.

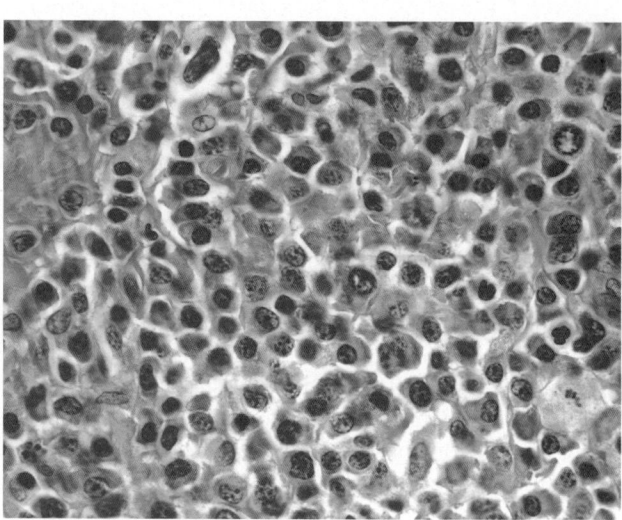

Figure 5-293. STI proctitis. Higher power of the previous figure shows prominent plasma cells.

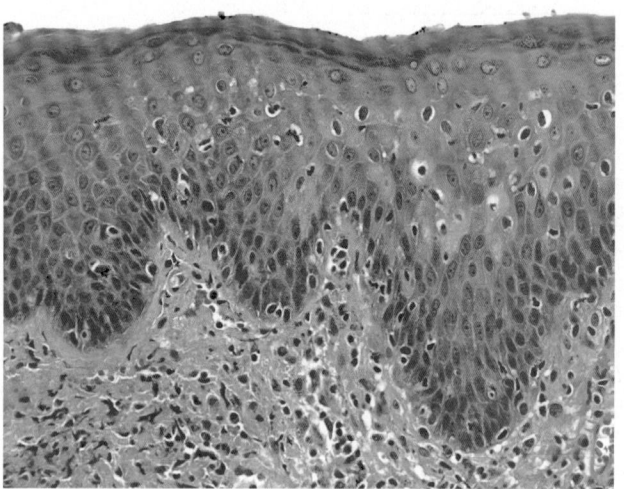

Figure 5-294. STI proctitis. The squamous epithelium is unremarkable. The patient was found to have HIV, syphilis, and LGV. The mass resolved with pertinent antibiotic therapy.

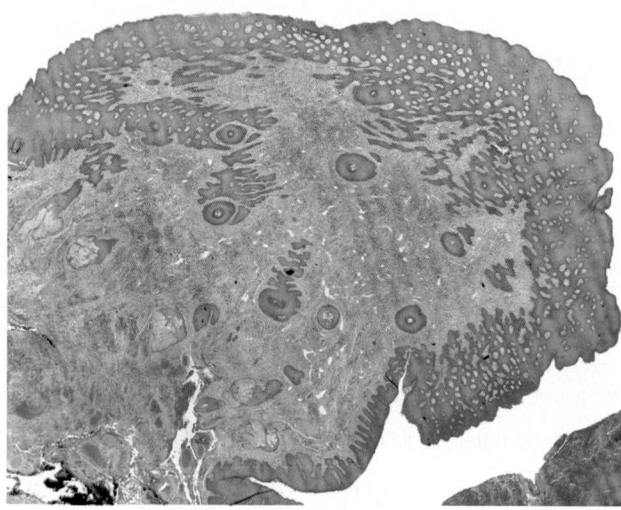

Figure 5-295. STI proctitis. This case from a different patient was also designated as a clinically worrisome mass. Common clues to the diagnosis include a history of HIV positivity MSM (men who have sex with men) behavior, but most cases prospectively lack this information, emphasizing that a familiarity with the typical morphology is critical.

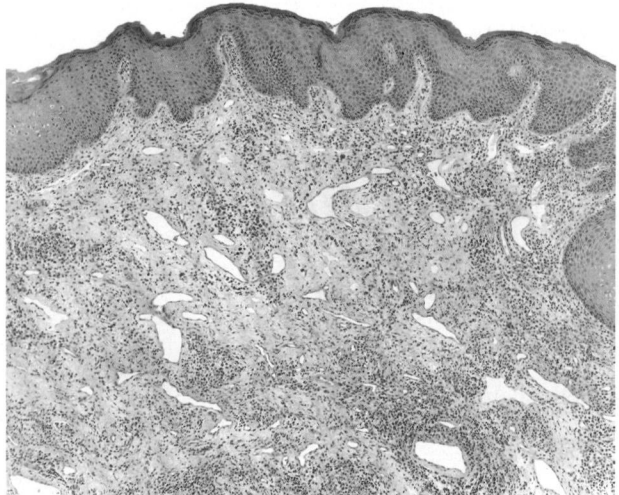

Figure 5-296. STI proctitis. Endoscopically, STI proctocolitis can present as ulcerations, nodules, polyps, and masses.

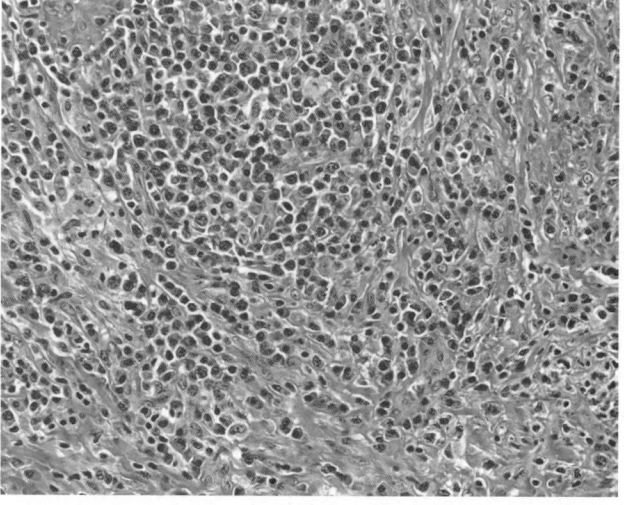

Figure 5-297. STI proctitis. Histologically, an intense bandlike plasma cell infiltrate is seen with variable granulomata and fibrosis.

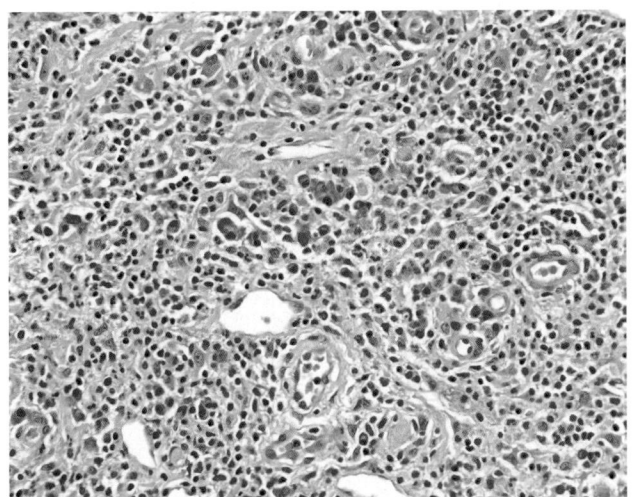

Figure 5-298. STI proctitis. In general, specimens with intense plasma cell infiltrates should prompt consideration of STI colitis, CMV, and adding a hematolymphoid evaluation.

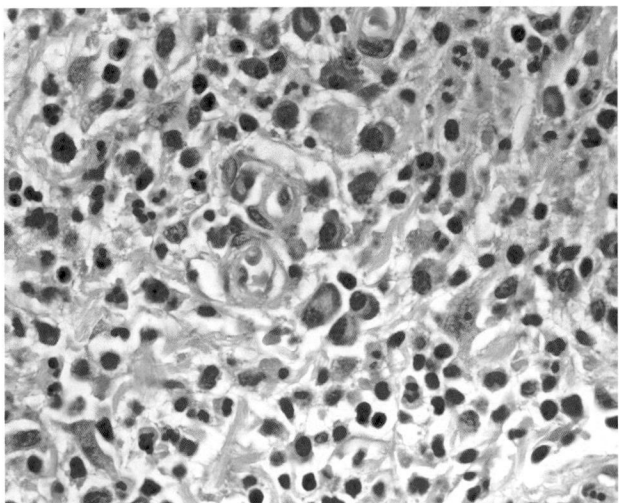

Figure 5-299. STI proctitis. Silver stains and *Treponema pallidum* immunohistochemical stains are too insensitive to confirm or exclude syphilitic infections, and there are no routine commercially available LGV studies available for the pathologist. As a result, clinical tests provide the best means to establish this diagnosis.

UNEXPECTED HERPES SIMPLEX VIRUS

This case features an anal ulcer with no viral cytopathic effect on the initial sections, but herpes simplex virus (HSV) was demonstrated on the HSV immunostain and deeper sections (Figs. 5.300–5.303). When an anal ulcer is encountered, CMV and HSV immunostains are worthwhile. CMV viral cytopathic effect is most commonly seen at the ulcer base, with the involved stromal and endothelial cells showing cytomegalic changes (huge cells), nuclear viral inclusions similar to an owl's eye, red-granular cytoplasmic inclusions, and chromatin smudging. The HSV viral cytopathic effect is most commonly seen at the ulcer edge, with the involved squamous epithelium displaying Multinucleation, nuclear Molding, and chromatin Margination (so-called 3 M's of HSV viral cytopathic effect).

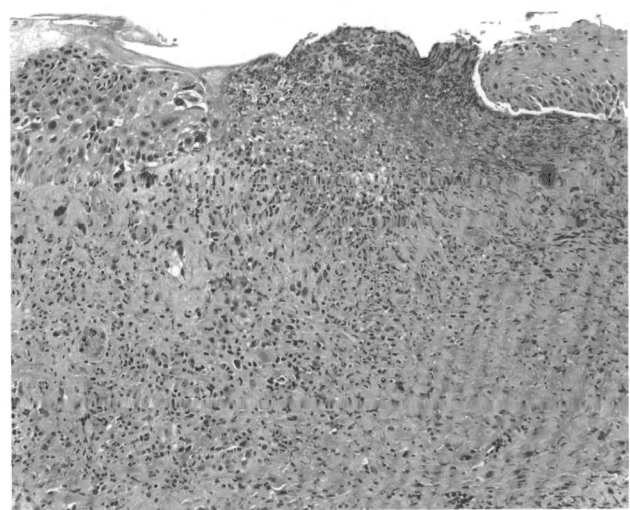

Figure 5-300. Herpes simplex virus. This case features an anal ulcer with no viral cytopathic effect on the initial H&E sections.

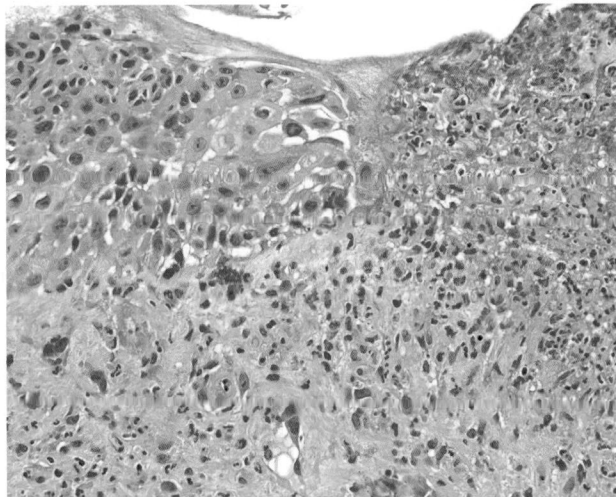

Figure 5-301. Herpes simplex virus. A prudent practice is to order CMV, HSV on anal ulcers.

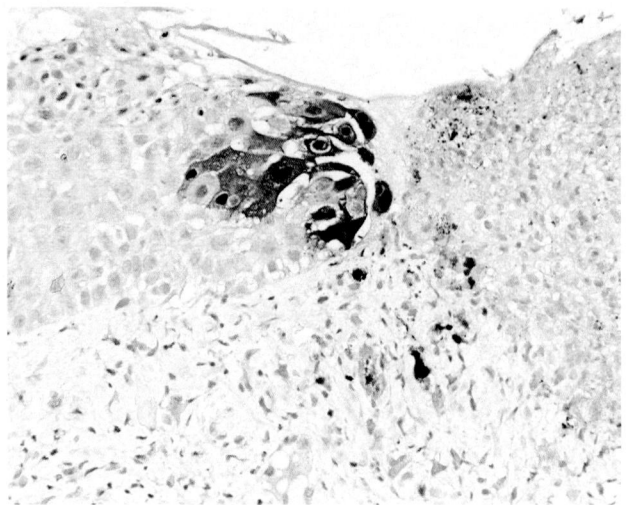

Figure 5-302. Herpes simplex virus, HSV IHC. Although HSV was not seen on the initial sections, a HSV immunostain was reactive.

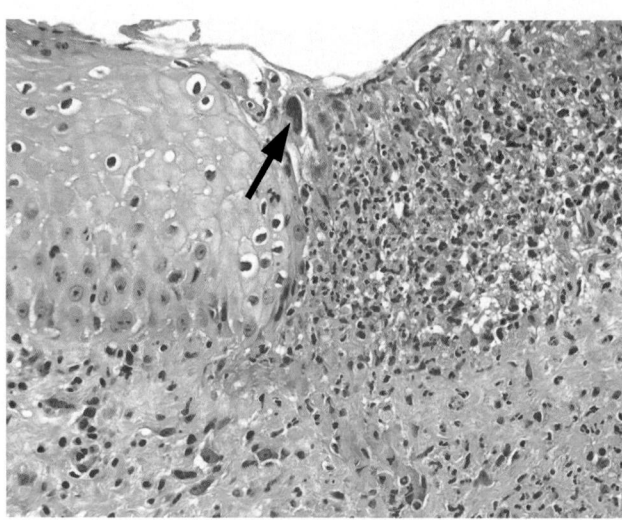

Figure 5-303. Herpes simplex virus. Deeper sections show atypical changes suspicious for HSV (*arrow*), such as focal hyperchromasia and multinucleation in the squamous epithelium adjoining the ulcer.

References

1. Macchi V, Porzionato A, Stecco C, Vigato E, Parenti A, De Caro R. Histo-topographic study of the longitudinal anal muscle. *Clin Anat.* 2008;21(5):447-452.

2. Welton ML, Steele S, Goodman K, et al. *American Joint Committee on Cancer.* 8th ed. Chicago, Illinois: Springer Nature; 2017:275-284.

3. Welton M, Lambert R, Bosman F. Tumours of the anal canal. In: Bosman F, Carneiro F, Hruban R, Theise N, eds. *WHO Classification of Tumours of the Digestive Tract.* 4th ed. Lyon, France: International Agency for Research on Cancer; 2010:185-193.

4. Sanjay K, Chanjuan S, David DK, et al. *Protocol for the Examination of Specimens from Patients with Carcinoma of the Anus.* 2017; http://www.cap.org/ShowProperty?nodePath=/UCMCon/Contribution%20Folders/WebContent/pdf/cp-anus-17protocol-4000.pdf. Accessed July 14, 2017.

5. Banov L, Knoepp LF, Erdman LH, Alia RT. Management of hemorrhoidal disease. *J S C Med Assoc.* 1985;81(7):398-401.

6. Bettington B, Brown I. Polyps and polypoid lesions of the anus. 2014;20(1):38-45.

7. Yilmaz B, Coban S, Usküdar O, Unverdi H, Aktaş B, Yüksel O. Giant fibroepithelial polyp of the anus. *Turk J Gastroenterol.* 2011;22(6):651-652.

8. Groisman GM, Polak-Charcon S. Fibroepithelial polyps of the anus: a histologic, immunohistochemical, and ultrastructural study, including comparison with the normal anal subepithelial layer. *Am J Surg Pathol.* 1998;22(1):70-76.

9. Groisman GM, Amar M, Polak-Charcon S. Multinucleated stromal cells of the anal mucosa: a common finding. *Histopathology.* 2000;36(3):224-228.

10. Gholam P, Autschbach F, Hartschuh W. Schistosomiasis in an HIV-positive patient presenting as an anal fissure and giant anal polyp. *Arch Dermatol.* 2008;144(7):950-952.

11. AbdullGaffar B, Abdulrahim M, Ghazi E. Benign fibrous histiocytoma presenting as anal canal polyp: first case report. *Ann Diagn Pathol.* 2013;17(5):464-465.

12. Pirog EC, Quint KD, Yantiss RK. P16/CDKN2A and Ki-67 enhance the detection of anal intraepithelial neoplasia and condyloma and correlate with human papillomavirus detection by polymerase chain reaction. *Am J Surg Pathol.* 2010;34(10):1449-1455.

13. Konstantinova AM, Michal M, Kacerovska D, et al. Hidradenoma papilliferum: a clinicopathologic study of 264 tumors from 261 patients, with emphasis on mammary-type alterations. *Am J Dermatopathol.* 2016;38(8):598-607.

14. Pfarr N, Sinn HP, Klauschen F, et al. Mutations in genes encoding PI3K-AKT and MAPK signaling define anogenital papillary hidradenoma. *Genes Chromosomes Cancer.* 2016;55(2):113-119.

15. Kazakov DV, Nemcova J, Mikyskova I, Belousova IE, Vazmitel M, Michal M. Human papillomavirus in lesions of anogenital mammary-like glands. *Int J Gynecol Pathol.* 2007;26(4):475-480.

16. Darragh TM, Colgan TJ, Cox JT, et al. The lower anogenital squamous terminology standardization Project for HPV-associated lesions: background and consensus recommendations from the College of American Pathologists and the American Society for Colposcopy and Cervical Pathology. *Arch Pathol Lab Med.* 2012;136(10):1266-1297.

17. Stoler MH, Vichnin MD, Ferenczy A, et al. The accuracy of colposcopic biopsy: analyses from the placebo arm of the Gardasil clinical trials. *Int J Cancer.* 2011;128(6):1354-1362.

18. Alvarez G, Perry A, Tan BR, Wang HL. Expression of epidermal growth factor receptor in squamous cell carcinomas of the anal canal is independent of gene amplification. *Mod Pathol.* 2006;19(7):942-949.

19. Walker F, Abramowitz L, Benabderrahmane D, et al. Growth factor receptor expression in anal squamous lesions: modifications associated with oncogenic human papillomavirus and human immunodeficiency virus. *Hum Pathol.* 2009;40(11):1517-1527.

20. Graham RP, Arnold CA, Naini BV, Lam-Himlin DM. Basaloid squamous cell carcinoma of the anus revisited. *Am J Surg Pathol.* 2016;40(3):354-360.

21. Kondo R, Hanamura N, Kobayashi M, Seki T, Adachi W, Ishii K. Mucoepidermoid carcinoma of the anal canal: an immunohistochemical study. *J Gastroenterol.* 2001;36(7):508-514.

22. Chetty R, Serra S, Hsieh E. Basaloid squamous carcinoma of the anal canal with an adenoid cystic pattern: histologic and immunohistochemical reappraisal of an unusual variant. *Am J Surg Pathol.* 2005;29(12):1668-1672.

23. Shia J. An update on tumors of the anal canal. *Arch Pathol Lab Med.* 2010;134(11):1601-1611.

24. Patil DT, Goldblum JR, Billings SD. Clinicopathological analysis of basal cell carcinoma of the anal region and its distinction from basaloid squamous cell carcinoma. *Mod Pathol.* 2013;26(10):1382-1389.

25. Rubin MA, Kleter B, Zhou M, et al. Detection and typing of human papillomavirus DNA in penile carcinoma: evidence for multiple independent pathways of penile carcinogenesis. *Am J Pathol.* 2001;159(4):1211-1218.

26. Zidar N, Langner C, Odar K, et al. Anal verrucous carcinoma is not related to infection with human papillomaviruses and should be distinguished from giant condyloma (Buschke-Löwenstein tumour). *Histopathology.* 2017;70(6):938-945.

27. del Pino M, Bleeker MC, Quint WG, Snijders PJ, Meijer CJ, Steenbergen RD. Comprehensive analysis of human papillomavirus prevalence and the potential role of low-risk types in verrucous carcinoma. *Mod Pathol.* 2012;25(10):1354-1363.

28. Odar K, Kocjan BJ, Hošnjak L, Gale N, Poljak M, Zidar N. Verrucous carcinoma of the head and neck - not a human papillomavirus-related tumour? *J Cell Mol Med.* 2014;18(4):635-645.

29. Patel KR, Chernock RD, Zhang TR, Wang X, El-Mofty SK, Lewis JS. Verrucous carcinomas of the head and neck, including those with associated squamous cell carcinoma, lack transcriptionally active high-risk human papillomavirus. *Hum Pathol.* 2013;44(11):2385-2392.

30. Stokes A, Guerra E, Bible J, et al. Human papillomavirus detection in dysplastic and malignant oral verrucous lesions. *J Clin Pathol.* 2012;65(3):283-286.

31. Basik M, Rodriguez-Bigas MA, Penetrante R, Petrelli NJ. Prognosis and recurrence patterns of anal adenocarcinoma. *Am J Surg.* 1995;169(2):233-237.

32. Meriden Z, Montgomery EA. Anal duct carcinoma: a report of 5 cases. *Hum Pathol.* 2012;43(2):216-220.

33. Lisovsky M, Patel K, Cymes K, Chase D, Bhuiya T, Morgenstern N. Immunophenotypic characterization of anal gland carcinoma: loss of p63 and cytokeratin 5/6. *Arch Pathol Lab Med.* 2007;131(8):1304-1311.

34. Carpenter JB, Rennels MA. Immunophenotypic characteristics of anal gland carcinoma. *Arch Pathol Lab Med.* 2008;132(10):1547-1548.

35. *American Joint Committee on Cancer Staging Manual.* 8th ed. Switzerland: Springer International Publishing; 2017.

36. Goldblum JR, Hart WR. Perianal Paget's disease: a histologic and immunohistochemical study of 11 cases with and without associated rectal adenocarcinoma. *Am J Surg Pathol.* 1998;22(2):170-179.

37. Yang EJ, Kong CS, Longacre TA. Vulvar and anal intraepithelial neoplasia: terminology, diagnosis, and ancillary studies. *Adv Anat Pathol.* 2017;21(3):136-150.

38. Goldblum JR, Hart WR. Vulvar Paget's disease: a clinicopathologic and immunohistochemical study of 19 cases. *Am J Surg Pathol*. 1997;21(10):1178-1187.

39. Chang AE, Karnell LH, Menck HR. The National Cancer Data Base report on cutaneous and noncutaneous melanoma: a summary of 84,836 cases from the past decade. The American College of Surgeons Commission on Cancer and the American Cancer Society. *Cancer*. 1998;83(8):1664-1678.

40. Tariq MU, Ud Din N, Ud Din NF, Fatima S, Ahmad Z. Malignant melanoma of anorectal region: a clinicopathologic study of 61 cases. *Ann Diagn Pathol*. 2014;18(5):275-281.

41. Guo J, Si L, Kong Y, et al. Phase II, open-label, single-arm trial of imatinib mesylate in patients with metastatic melanoma harboring c-Kit mutation or amplification. *J Clin Oncol*. 2011;29(21):2904-2909.

42. Carvajal RD, Antonescu CR, Wolchok JD, et al. KIT as a therapeutic target in metastatic melanoma. *J Am Med Assoc*. 2011;305(22):2327-2334.

43. Chute DJ, Cousar JB, Mills SE. Anorectal malignant melanoma: morphologic and immunohistochemical features. *Am J Clin Pathol*. 2006;126(1):93-100.

44. Masson P. Hemangioendotheliome vegetant intravasculaire. *Bull Soc Anat Paris*. 1923;93:517-523.

45. Branton PA, Lininger R, Tavassoli FA. Papillary endothelial hyperplasia of the breast: the great impostor for angiosarcoma: a clinicopathologic review of 17 cases. *Int J Surg Pathol*. 2003;11(2):83-87.

46. Tavora F, Montgomery E, Epstein JI. A series of vascular tumors and tumorlike lesions of the bladder. *Am J Surg Pathol*. 2008;32(8):1213-1219.

47. Lane Z, Epstein JI. Pseudocarcinomatous epithelial hyperplasia in the bladder unassociated with prior irradiation or chemotherapy. *Am J Surg Pathol*. 2008;32(1):92-97.

48. Akdur NC, Donmez M, Gozel S, Ustun H, Hucumenoglu S. Intravascular papillary endothelial hyperplasia: histomorphological and immunohistochemical features. *Diagn Pathol*. 2013;8:167.

49. Hart M, Thakral B, Yohe S, et al. EBV-positive mucocutaneous ulcer in organ transplant recipients: a localized indolent posttransplant lymphoproliferative disorder. *Am J Surg Pathol*. 2014;38(11):1522-1529.

50. Dojcinov SD, Venkataraman G, Raffeld M, Pittaluga S, Jaffe ES. EBV positive mucocutaneous ulcer–a study of 26 cases associated with various sources of immunosuppression. *Am J Surg Pathol*. 2010;34(3):405-417.

51. Arnold CA, Limketkai BN, Illei PB, Montgomery E, Voltaggio L. Syphilitic and lymphogranuloma venereum (LGV) proctocolitis: clues to a frequently missed diagnosis. *Am J Surg Pathol*. 2013;37(1):38-46.

52. Arnold CA, Bhaijee F, Lam-Himlin D. Fifty shades of chronic colitis: non-infectious imposters of inflammatory bowel disease. *Diagn Histopathol*. 2015;21(7):276-282.

53. Arnold CA, Roth R, Arsenescu R, et al. Sexually transmitted infectious colitis vs inflammatory bowel disease: distinguishing features from a case-controlled study. *Am J Clin Pathol*. 2015;144(5):771-781.

54. Gopal P, Shah RB. Primary anal canal syphilis in men: the clinicopathologic spectrum of an easily overlooked diagnosis. *Arch Pathol Lab Med*. 2015;139(9):1156-1160.

MESENCHYMAL LESIONS

CHAPTER OUTLINE

THE LAYOUT OF THE REAL ESTATE

Although we have mentioned several mesenchymal lesions in "Esophagus," "Stomach," the "Small Bowel," "Colon," and "Anus" chapters, it is important to present a concept of gastrointestinal tract mesenchymal lesions because they can be handled in a logical fashion with attention to a few principles. The key idea is that many of the tumors are nearly always encountered in a certain layer of the tubular gastrointestinal tract and many are found predominantly or even exclusively (based on data to date) in a specific layer (mucosa, submucosa, muscularis propria, serosa) or anatomic location. Figs. 6.1–6.4 show some of the tumors found in each of the layers and each of the sites. The anus is not shown, but we have pointed out anal granular cell tumors and melanomas in "Anus" chapter. Knowing which tumors arise in which layer can really help with differential diagnosis. For example, both

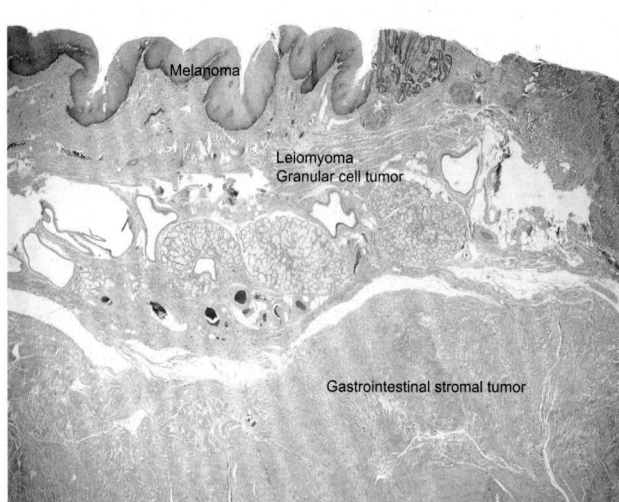

Figure 6-1. Esophagus, favored sites for select spindle cell/mesenchymal lesions. Melanoma is not a mesenchymal lesion, but it can show a spindle cell phenotype and mimic a sarcoma. Leiomyomas can arise in association with either the muscularis mucosae or muscularis propria, but in biopsies, most lesions are found associated with the muscularis mucosae.

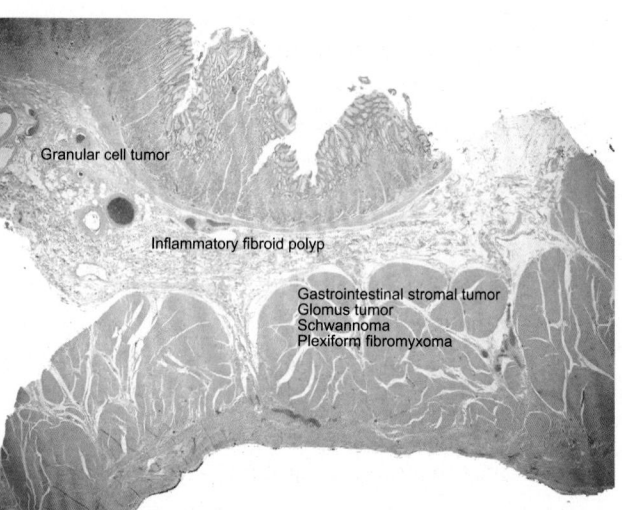

Figure 6-2. Stomach, favored sites for select spindle cell/mesenchymal lesions. Remember also that some spindle cell lesions that are found in the stomach are metastases from sarcomatoid carcinomas that originated in other sites (the kidney and lung). The most common primary lesion encountered in the muscularis propria is gastrointestinal stromal tumor, but knowing the other options is important when assessing a case.

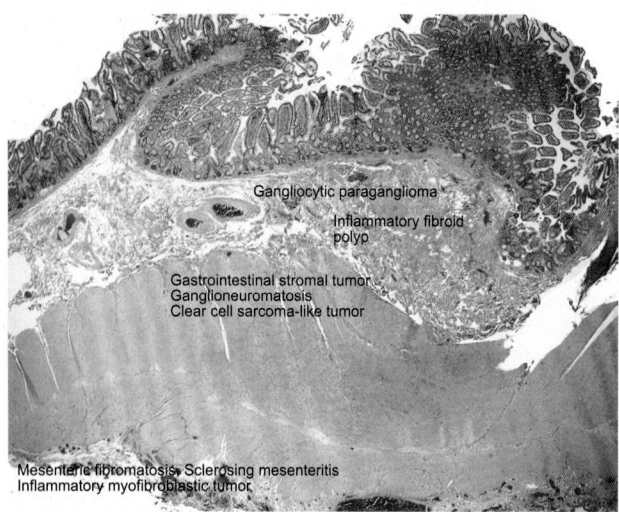

Figure 6-3. Small intestine, favored sites for select spindle cell/mesenchymal lesions. Note that the mesenteric lesions can be associated with other parts of the gastrointestinal tract, but the small bowel mesentery is the site for most of them, probably because the small intestine has the most mesentery.

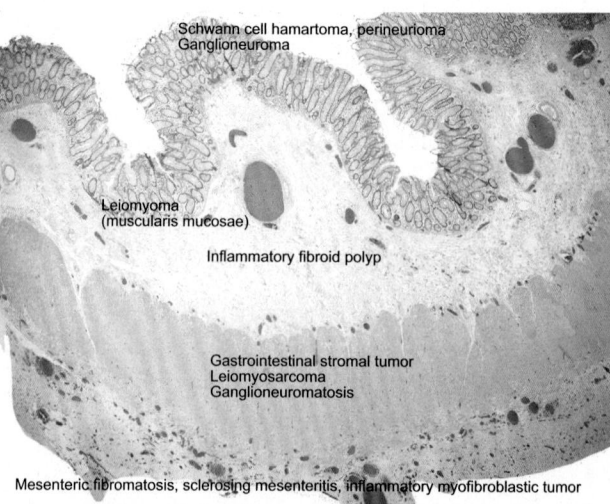

Figure 6-4. Colon, favored sites for select spindle cell/mesenchymal lesions. The lamina propria of the colon is the usual home for several types of mesenchymal polyps with nerve sheath, neural, or perineurial differentiation.

inflammatory fibroid polyp and inflammatory myofibroblastic tumor feature inflammatory cells, but inflammatory fibroid polyps are centered in the submucosa and inflammatory myofibroblastic tumors generally arise in the mesentery. Glomus tumor is essentially always in the muscularis propria and usually in the stomach. Gastrointestinal tract schwannomas have the same story—they arise in the muscularis propria, nearly always in the stomach. As we discuss each lesion, we will point out the favored layer and, in some cases, how knowing about it can be a clue to avoid mishaps.

IMMUNOLABELING COMMENTS

FAQ: When encountering a spindle cell lesion, should vimentin be included in my immunolabeling panel?

Answer: No, never. First and foremost, **never** order a vimentin on a lesion that may be a mesenchymal lesion of the gastrointestinal tract. For that matter, do not order a vimentin to address a mesenchymal lesion in any organ system. There is no value to it and it may waste the last bit of tissue that could have been used to actually make a diagnosis. When confronted with a tiny sample of a mystery lesion, get help before wasting 1 ng of tissue on a vimentin stain! In the earliest years of immunolabeling, some regarded vimentin as a test that could be used to demonstrate that the tissue was sufficiently well preserved to be amenable to immunolabeling, but this is rather a weak logic. There are almost always internal controls in tissues to help address general tissue integrity issues.

IMMUNOLABELING

Learning to choose a smart immunolabeling panel takes some time and effort and experience. The diagnostic panel should be driven by the morphology rather than a shotgun panel. Choosing a careful panel is less of an issue in resections other than that a shotgun approach wastes money and can result in positive tests that shed heat rather than light on the diagnostic considerations. The real issue is in small biopsies, which are our daily reality. When confronted with a spindle cell lesion, there are frequently diagnostic clues on H&E that obviate the need for any immunolabeling at all. However, some lesions can only be classified initially as malignant neoplasm or, in the most humbling cases, as neoplasm or, at the worst, abnormal. However, there are lots of clues. For example, if a gastrointestinal tract spindle cell lesion has prominent nuclear pleomorphism, it is probably not a gastrointestinal stromal tumor (GIST) (with occasional exceptions as with everything).

When confronted with a small sample of an overtly malignant neoplasm that could be anything, it is never terrible to begin with a CD20 (the vast majority of lymphomas that appear overtly malignant on biopsies and have spindle cells are diffuse large B cell lymphomas), an S100 protein (for spindle cell melanoma), and a pankeratin for sarcomatoid carcinoma. Do not waste tissue beginning with special subsets of keratins such as CK20, CK7, and p40 if it is unclear whether the lesion is a carcinoma or something else. Get a batch of unstained sections up front in case you need to order additional stains. This is to avoid wasting tissue when the block is being trimmed. If a spindle cell lesion is not overtly atypical, cellular, and has monotonous nuclei, then begin with stains to address GIST. If the morphology is characteristic, the CD117 is enough to confirm your interpretation. If there is anything odd, consider congeners. Table 6.1 addresses several tumor types and immunolabeling considerations for lesions of the stomach, small intestine, and colon.

TABLE 6.1: Summary of Gastrointestinal Tract Mesenchymal Tumors by Location and Layer

Site	Layer	Likely Choices	Immunostains to Consider	Pitfall Alerts
Stomach	Mucosa	Upper portion of inflammatory fibroid polyp Malignant GIST invading mucosa Nerve sheath tumors Granular cell tumor (upper portion)	CD34 CD117 DOG1 S100 protein	• CD117 and CD34 react with Kaposi sarcoma • Adenocarcinomas often express DOG1 • Melanomas often express CD117
	Submucosa	Inflammatory fibroid polyp GIST	CD34 CD117, DOG1	
	Muscularis propria	GIST Glomus tumor Schwannoma Plexiform fibromyxoma Smooth muscle tumors	CD117, DOG1 S100 protein Smooth muscle actin Desmin	Glomus tumors can show synaptophysin staining but lack chromogranin and keratin
	Serosa	Mesenteric fibromatosis, inflammatory myofibroblastic IgG4-related fibrosclerosing disease	β-Catenin ALK IgG4	β-Catenin staining must be nuclear to confirm fibromatosis
Small intestine	Mucosa	Gangliocytic paraganglioma GIST invading the mucosa	Chromogranin, synaptophysin, S100 protein, CD117, DOG1	
	Submucosa	Inflammatory fibroid polyp Gangliocytic paraganglioma GIST	CD34 Chromogranin, synaptophysin, S100 protein, CD117, DOG1	
	Muscularis propria	GIST Clear cell sarcoma–like tumor Smooth muscle tumors	CD117, DOG1, S100 protein Desmin	Clear cell sarcoma–like tumors can express synaptophysin but lack chromogranin labeling and keratin expression
	Serosa	Mesenteric fibromatosis Inflammatory myofibroblastic tumor IgG4-related fibrosclerosing disease Calcifying fibrous tumor Sclerosing mesenteritis	β-Catenin ALK IgG4 ROS1	Sampling error is a factor in needle biopsies; ileal well differentiated neuroendocrine (carcinoid) tumors often invoke a striking fibroinflammatory response

TABLE 6.1: Summary of Gastrointestinal Tract Mesenchymal Tumors by Location and Layer   (Continued)

Site	Layer	Likely Choices	Immunostains to Consider	Pitfall Alerts
Colon	Mucosa	Nerve sheath tumors (perineurioma, Schwann cell hamartoma, epithelioid nerve sheath tumor, ganglioneuroma) Granular cell tumor Leiomyomas associated with muscularis mucosae	S100 protein, EMA, Glut1, Muc1	Leiomyomas in this site are easy to diagnose on H&E and usually do not require immunolabeling to recognize
	Submucosa	Inflammatory fibroid polyp	CD34	
	Muscularis propria	GIST Smooth muscle tumors	CD117, DOG1 Desmin	
	Serosa	Mesenteric fibromatosis, inflammatory myofibroblastic IgG4-related fibrosclerosing disease Calcifying fibrous tumor Sclerosing mesenteritis	β-Catenin ALK IgG4	

MESENTERIC LESIONS

Mesenteric lesions can be tricky on needle biopsies, which are frequent, but many can be solved with a little thought and a few immunostains. Mesenteric fibromatosis is easy to diagnose with attention to a few H&E principles and attention to some pitfalls. Remember that lots of people have adhesions and remember that they can result in an interpretation of mesenteric fibromatosis (Fig. 6.5). It is important to learn whether a needle biopsy is from a mass.

MESENTERIC FIBROMATOSIS

Mesenteric fibromatosis usually presents as a slowly growing mass that involves the small bowel mesentery or the retroperitoneum. The theory is that it might be triggered by scarring in susceptible persons. It is relatively common. Mesenteric fibromatosis in patients with Gardner syndrome, essentially a form of familial adenomatous polyposis (FAP), is more likely to recur than sporadic mesenteric fibromatosis. Gardner syndrome is associated with an 8% to 12% incidence of developing fibromatosis. The incidence of fibromatosis overall is on the order of 2.4 to 4.3 new cases per million inhabitants per annum, at least in Scandinavia.[1]

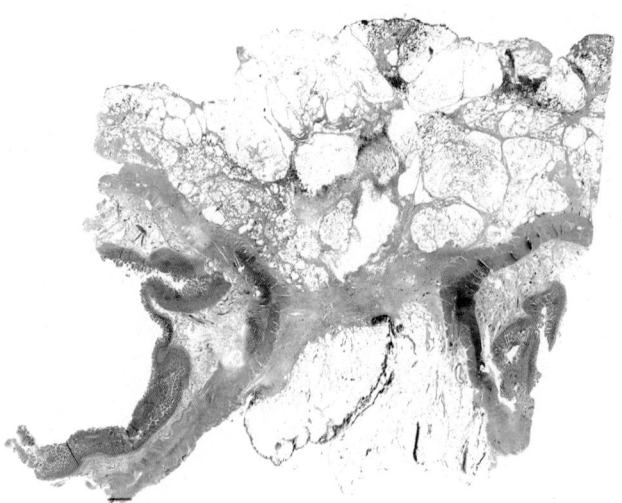

Figure 6-5. Adhesion between two loops of the small intestine. There is fat necrosis in the fat in the center of the field and a dense adhesion connecting two loops of the obstructed bowel that were resected. It is easy to imagine how a needle biopsy could sample the thick nonneoplastic band of scar tissue that forms the adhesion.

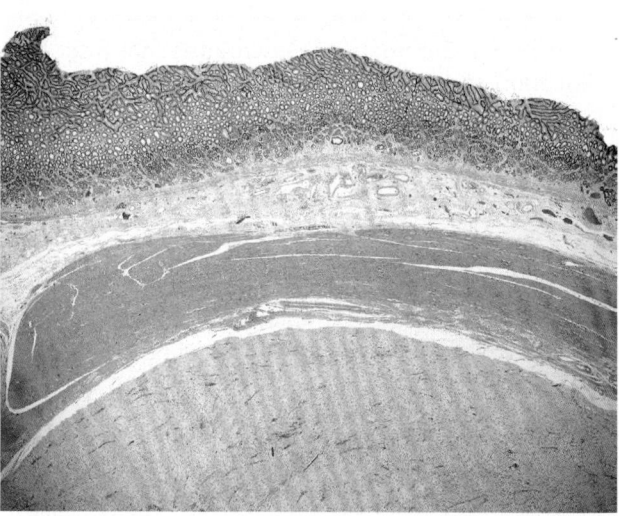

Figure 6-6. Mesenteric fibromatosis. There is a pale rose–colored spindle cell lesion in the mesentery at the bottom of the image. Compare the color of the lesion (pale rose) to the muscularis propria above it (*bright pink*). Note also that there is a uniform density of cells in the fibromatosis. Note also that even at this low magnification, it is easy to spot small capillaries in the lesion brcause the lesion is so pale.

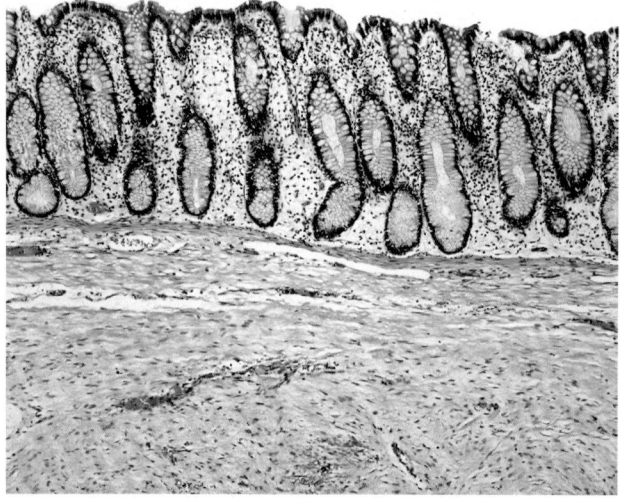

Figure 6-7. Mesenteric fibromatosis. It is unusual for fibromatoses to extend into the submucosa and mucosa, but this one is seen in the colonic submucosa, where it has a pale appearance and capillaries that pop out.

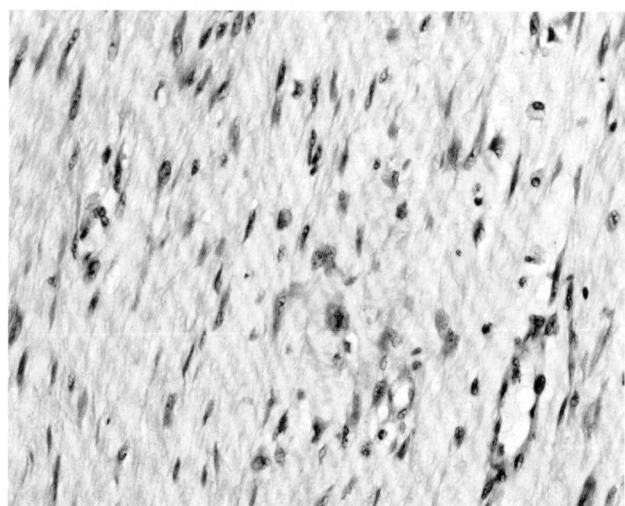

Figure 6-8. Mesenteric fibromatosis. Compare the nuclei in the lesion to those in the capillary at the right. They are paler. The one in the center has a delicate round nucleolus, a typical feature of fibromatosis, whether mesenteric or involving the soft tissues.

In FAP patients, fibromatosis typically arises through biallelic (germline then somatic) inactivation of the *APC* gene, whereas tumors in non-FAP patients occur through either somatic biallelic *APC* inactivation or somatic mutation of a single *CTNNB1* (the gene that encodes for β catenin) allele. FAP patients have a >850-fold increased risk of developing fibromatoses (desmoid tumors), typically intra-abdominal lesions.[2] That's impressive!

Not surprisingly, mesenteric fibromatoses involve the mesentery. However, they often infiltrate into the muscularis propria but seldom into the submucosa or mucosa, so they are not encountered on mucosal biopsies. They are usually received as resected lesions that have resulted in obstruction. Microscopically, the tumor usually has infiltrative margins, but do not let a well-demarcated gross appearance push you to change your mind about the diagnosis. The tumor cells consist of spindled fibroblasts separated by abundant collagen (Figs. 6.6–6.18). The cells are usually very evenly dispersed through the lesion with about the same density of cells present everywhere. The pale tumor cells and collagen are

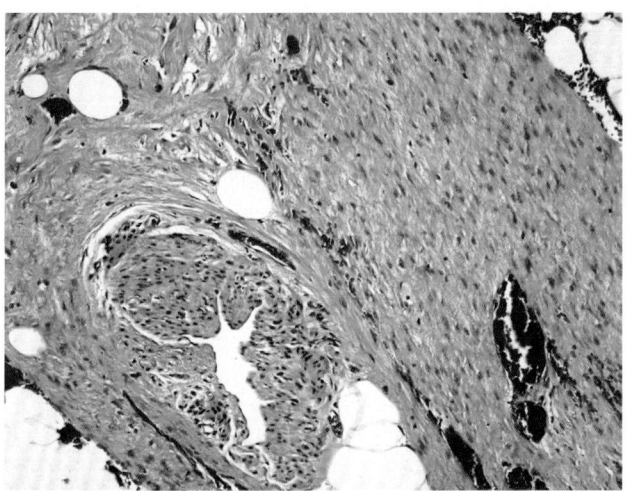

Figure 6-9. Mesenteric fibromatosis. This mesenteric fibromatosis has encased a small muscular artery. Note the uniform distribution of the nuclei at the right of the image. This sample is from a needle biopsy.

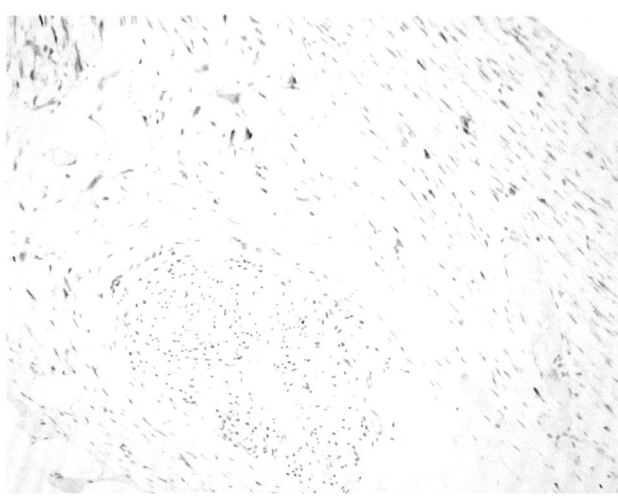

Figure 6-10. Mesenteric fibromatosis. This is a β-catenin stain. In this example, quite a few nuclei label and the nuclei in the endothelial cells do not. Do not expect to see labeling in every nucleus to confirm a morphologic impression of mesenteric fibromatosis and be sure to check that the vascular endothelial cell nuclei are unstained. Endothelial cytoplasmic labeling is acceptable.

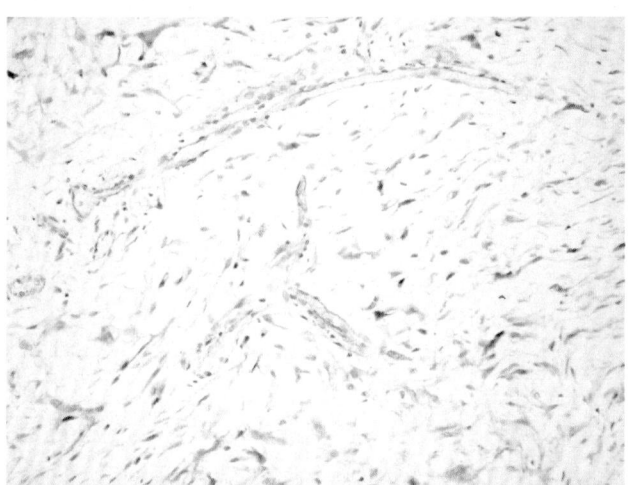

Figure 6-11. Mesenteric fibromatosis. Although the endothelial cell nuclei are unlabeled, scattered lesional nuclei are reactive with a β-catenin immunostain. This pattern confirms a morphologic diagnosis of mesenteric fibromatosis.

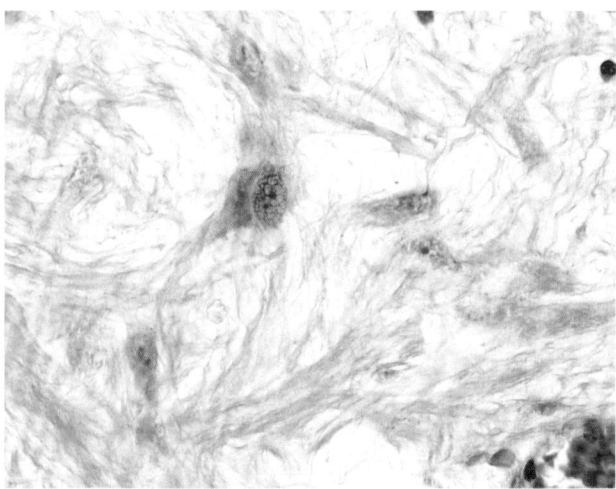

Figure 6-12. Mesenteric fibromatosis. This very high magnification image shows the cytologic features of mesenteric fibromatosis. The cells have produced collagen, which relatively evenly separates them, but the cells are myofibroblastic and thus there is amphophilic cytoplasm (containing a touch of eosin and a touch of hematoxylin all mixed to give a *pale blue* blush to the pinkish cytoplasm), the color of myofibroblasts. Each cell has delicate nuclear chromatin and a dainty round nucleolus and stellate cytoplasm.

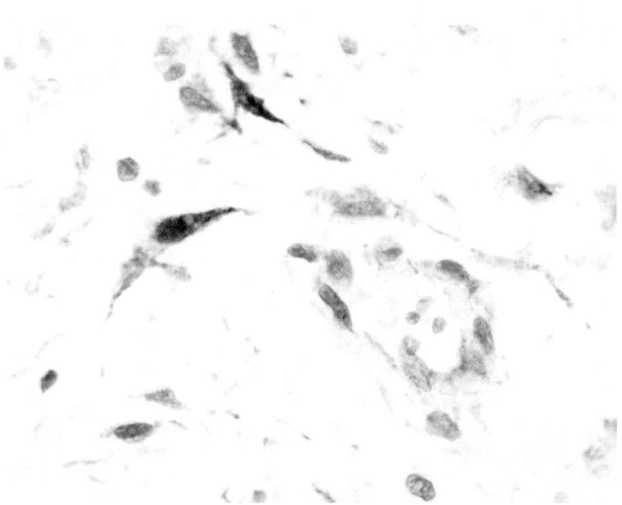

Figure 6-13. Mesenteric fibromatosis. This very high magnification of a β-catenin stain shows that some of the lesional myofibroblastic cell nuclei are labeled but none of the endothelial cell nuclei are stained.

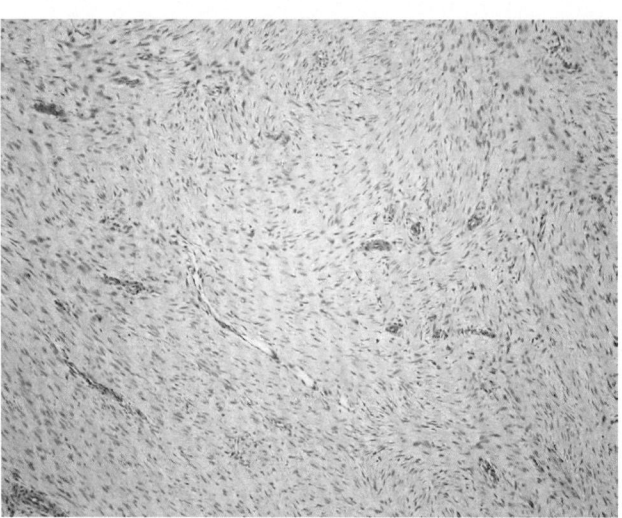

Figure 6-14. Mesenteric fibromatosis. This image shows the key features of mesenteric fibromatosis. The cellularity is uniform throughout the tumor, and the tumor is pale on hematoxylin and eosin staining. Small capillaries and other vessels are easy to see because the adjoining tumor cells are pale.

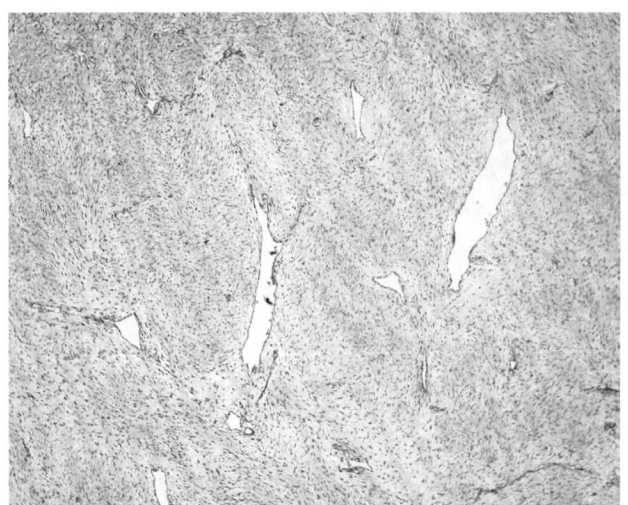

Figure 6-15. Mesenteric fibromatosis. This pattern of gaping vessels is very typical of mesenteric fibromatosis.

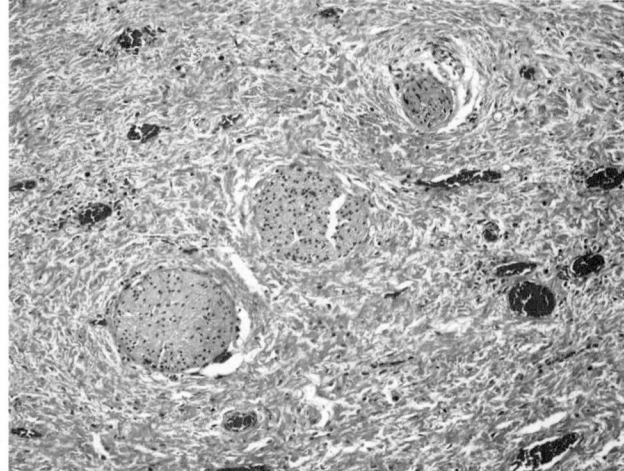

Figure 6-16. Mesenteric fibromatosis. This sclerotic portion of a mesenteric fibromatosis has encased small nerves. Note in this image and others of mesenteric fibromatosis that there are very few inflammatory cells associated with the lesion.

organized in parallel arrays. Sometimes, keloidlike collagen and hyalinization obscure the original pattern of the tumor. The vascular patterns are a clue to the diagnosis (Figs. 6.8, 6.14, 6.15, and 6.17). The vessels, though thin-walled, pop out at scanning magnification because the lesional cells are very pale. The nuclei of the tumor cells are much lighter than those of the endothelial cells. In addition, the smooth muscle cytoplasm in vessel walls is pinker than that of the surrounding myofibroblastic tumor cells. Mitotic figures are infrequent, but their presence is not anything to be concerned about. Mesenteric examples often have a storiform pattern similar to that of nodular fasciitis in the soft tissue of the extremities, even featuring extravasated erythrocytes—do not diagnose nodular fasciitis in the case of a large mesenteric lesion. Because fibromatoses are myofibroblastic, the pitfall is that they express actin but usually not desmin or CD34. An important caveat concerning mesenteric fibromatosis is that these tumors frequently need to be distinguished from GISTs. Although their features are readily distinguishable on routine H&E stained slides,

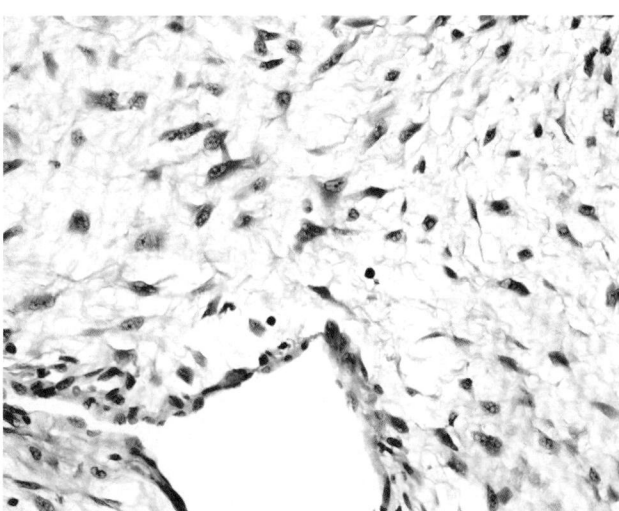

Figure 6-17. Mesenteric fibromatosis. This high magnification image shows the stellate cytoplasm of the tumoral myofibroblastic cells to advantage. In more heavily collagenized zones of fibromatoses, the stellate cytoplasm is harder to see but can be found in looser zones of the tumor.

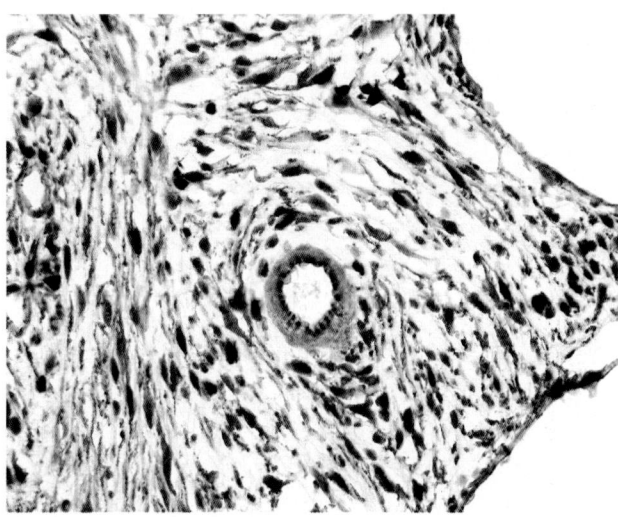

Figure 6-18. Mesenteric fibromatosis. This overstained β-catenin preparation can still be used to confirm the diagnosis because the nuclei of the endothelial cells of the capillary in the center are unstained even though the luminal cytoplasm is strongly reactive.

sometimes fibromatoses show expression of KIT, especially if antigen retrieval is heavy.[3] β-Catenin immunostaining can be helpful (Figs. 6.10, 6.11, 6.13, and 6.18) because, at least among the lesions in the differential diagnosis, nuclear staining is only seen in desmoids,[4,5] but this stain can be difficult to use and some colleagues prefer not to use it. If you choose to use it, it is important to pay close attention to internal controls; the nuclei of endothelial cells in the lesion should be negative even though there can be endothelial cytoplasmic staining.

SCLEROSING MESENTERITIS

Sclerosing mesenteritis has been described using a lot of confusing names, and it is easy to misinterpret as IgG4-related fibrosclerosing disease, but if careful criteria are used, it can usually be separated because it looks like glorified fat necrosis and makes a mass! This condition has been termed mesenteric panniculitis, retractile mesenteritis, liposclerotic mesenteritis, mesenteric Weber Christian disease, xanthogranulomatous mesenteritis, mesenteric lipogranuloma, systemic nodular panniculitis, inflammatory pseudotumor, and mesenteric lipodystrophy. It most commonly affects the small bowel mesentery, presenting as an isolated large mass although some patients (about 20%) have multiple lesions. It is assumed to reflect a reparative response although the stimulus is a mystery; prior trauma/surgery is usually not reported.

As discussed earlier, the appearance is that of glorified fat necrosis—tumors consist of fibrous bands infiltrating and encasing fat lobules with an associated variable sprinkling of inflammatory cells, typically lymphocytes, plasma cells, and eosinophils (Figs. 6.19–6.22). Sometimes there are even prominent IgG4-reactive plasma cells, and a lymphocytic phlebitis pattern can be seen, but the storiform fibrosis characteristic of IgG4-related fibrosclerosing disease is absent.[6] If there is an abscess to explain the nasty reactive-appearing mass, then the lesion is not sclerosing mesenteritis. In contrast to the IgG4-related sclerosing disorders, usually sclerosing mesenteritis does not respond to steroids and is less likely to display prominent IgG4 labeling.

Two similar lesions are so called reactive nodular fibrous pseudotumor (Figs. 6.23–6.26),[7] which lacks the prominent fat necrosis and heterotopic mesenteric ossification (Figs. 6.27 and 6.28),[8] which is presumably a reactive lesion that ossifies. Splitting hairs about classifying them is not important—they are all benign and do not tend to recur.

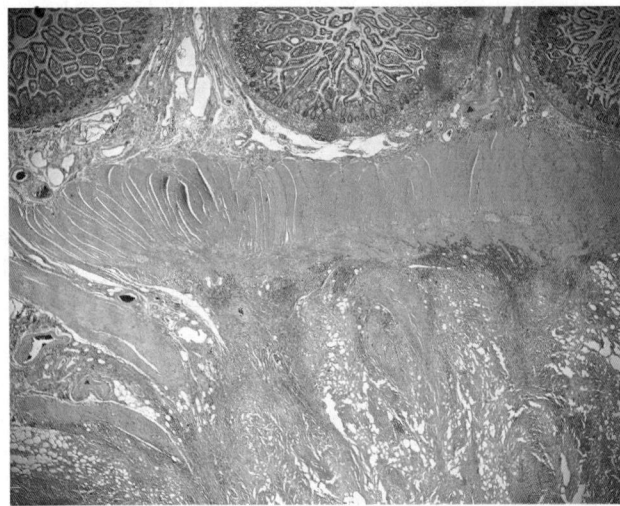

Figure 6-19. Sclerosing mesenteritis. Although there are lymphoid aggregates cuffing this process in the small bowel mesentery, the main event is fat necrosis.

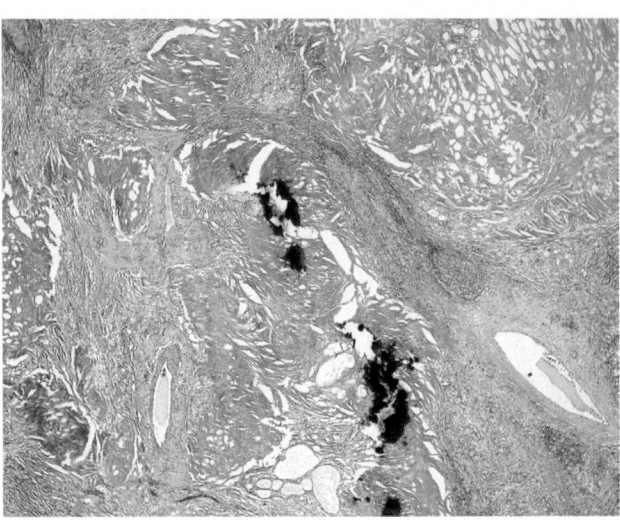

Figure 6-20. Sclerosing mesenteritis. There is a bit of inflammation and scarring and a lot of fat necrosis and not much else. This example has areas of calcification just to make the image pretty.

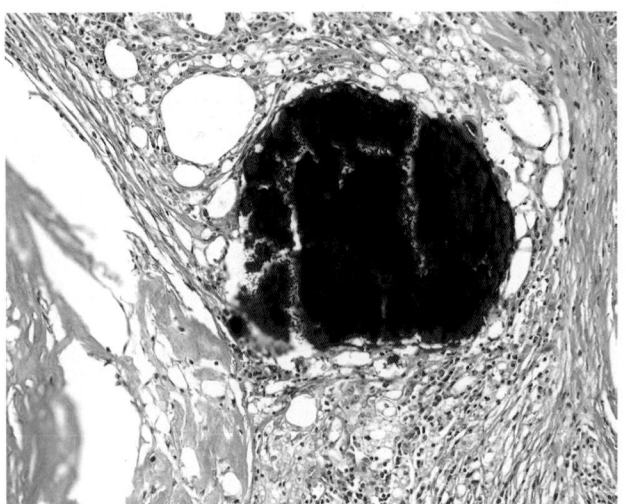

Figure 6-21. Sclerosing mesenteritis. There is calcification and a lot of fat necrosis and some background chronic inflammation.

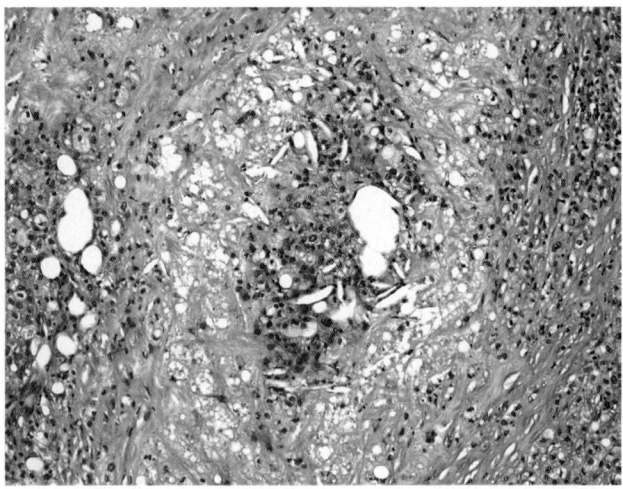

Figure 6-22. Sclerosing mesenteritis. This area contains fat necrosis and inflammation that includes histiocytes. There are cholesterol clefts as well.

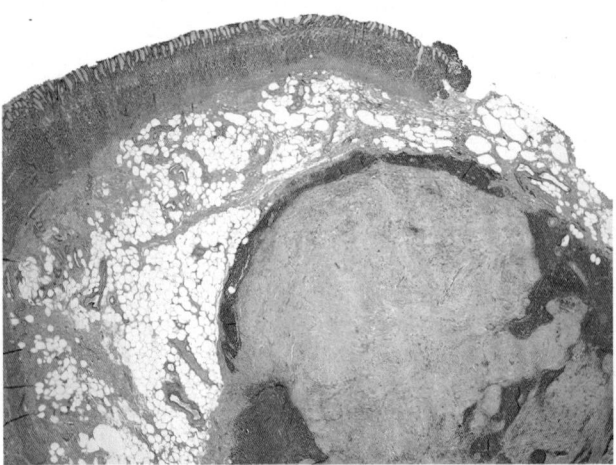

Figure 6-23. Reactive nodular fibrous pseudotumor. This sclerotic lesion is surrounded by lymphoid cells and itself is very hypocellular. It is like sclerosing mesenteritis but without fat necrosis.

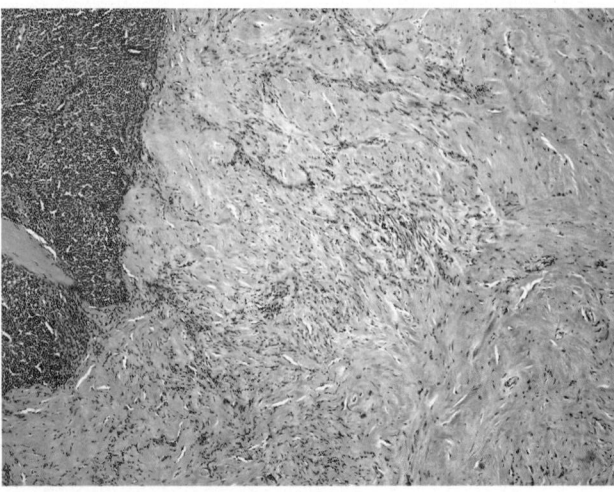

Figure 6-24. Reactive nodular fibrous pseudotumor. The process is sclerotic and not particularly cellular.

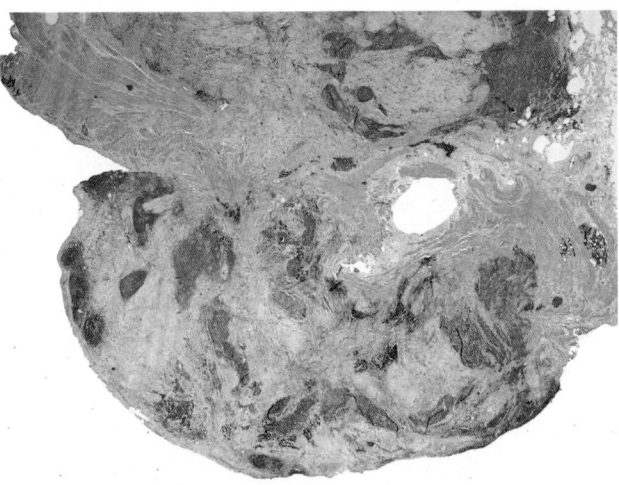

Figure 6-25. Reactive nodular fibrous pseudotumor. Note that the lesion has extended from the serosa to the submucosa.

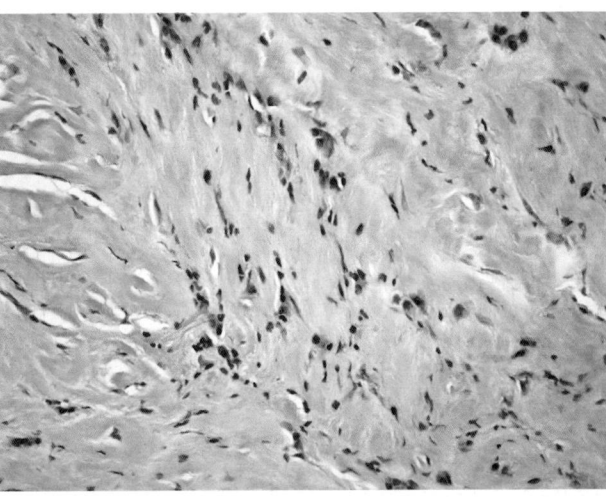

Figure 6-26. Reactive nodular fibrous pseudotumor. The process displays very bland cytologic features.

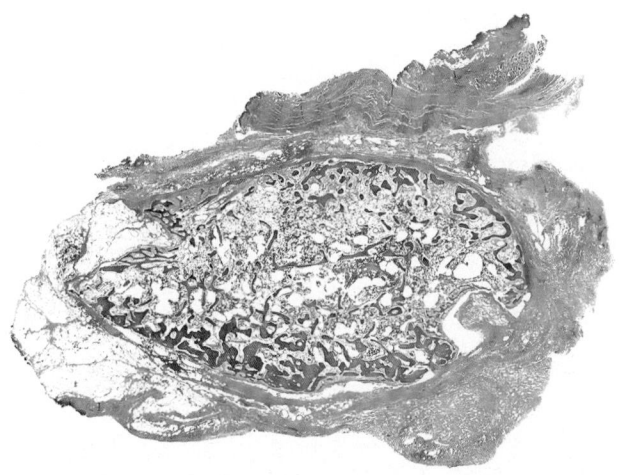

Figure 6-27. Heterotopic mesenteric ossification. This benign lesion must have had very interesting imaging characteristics. It is analogous to myositis ossificans. It is not clear what the stimulus is for such a lesion.

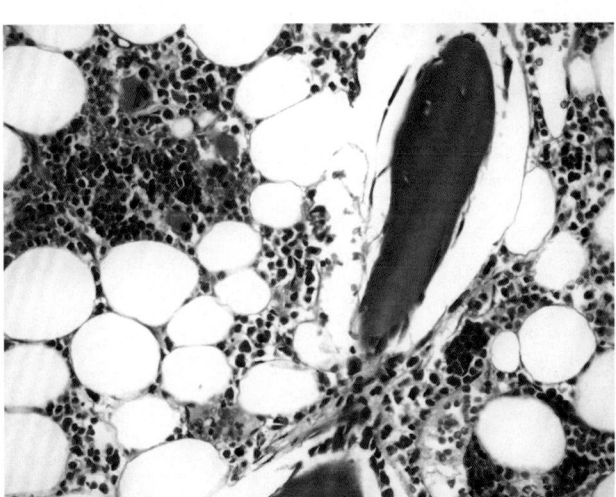

Figure 6-28. Heterotopic mesenteric ossification. This example even contains bone marrow elements.

INFLAMMATORY MYOFIBROBLASTIC TUMOR

These tumors are usually situated in the mesentery and can be solitary or multinodular (about a third) and can attain large sizes. The tumors consist of myofibroblasts and fibroblasts in fascicles (Figs. 6.29–6.38). Sometimes there is a vague storiform appearance, but the lesions are not nearly as sclerotic as IgG4-related disease, as discussed later in this section. Nuclear pleomorphism can be moderate and nucleoli are often prominent, but mitoses are infrequently seen. There is a variable but often striking inflammatory infiltrate, predominantly plasmacytic but with some lymphocytes, and occasionally neutrophils or eosinophils as well. Fibrosis and calcification are sometimes present. These tumors often express smooth muscle actin (SMA) because they are myofibroblastic and many examples express cytokeratin, especially where there is submesothelial extension. Anaplastic lymphoma kinase (ALK) protein expression has been detected in about 60% of cases by immunolabeling, usually corresponding to ALK gene rearrangements by fluorescence in situ hybridization (FISH), and ALK negative cases, especially in children, often have ROS1 gene rearrangements; immunolabeling is available to test for the latter rearrangement.[9] Finding either alteration can be exploited for both diagnosis and targeted therapy. The tumors

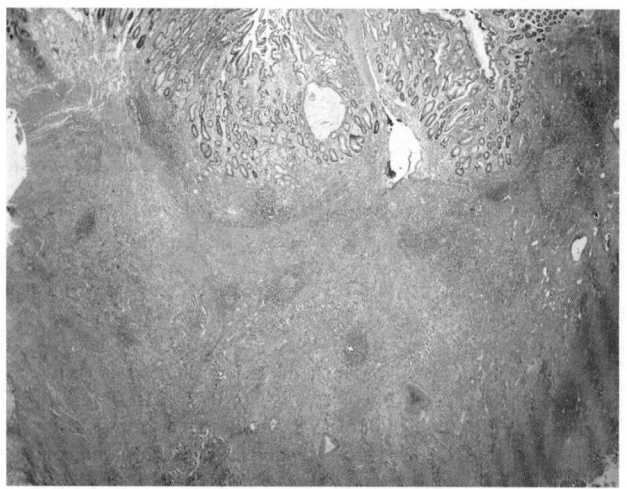

Figure 6-29. Inflammatory myofibroblastic tumor. This example is in the gastric mesentery although the process is most common in the small bowel mesentery. Lymphoid aggregates cuff an inflammatory cell–rich cellular process that has extended into the muscularis propria and submucosa.

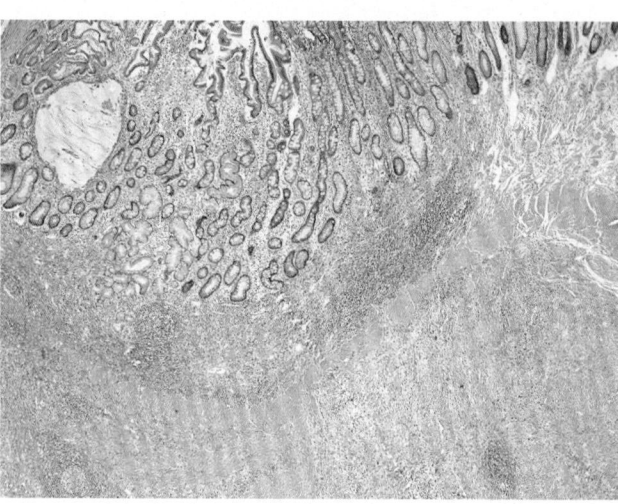

Figure 6-30. Inflammatory myofibroblastic tumor. The tumor at the bottom of the field is full of inflammatory cells. The overlying gastric mucosa has intestinal metaplasia.

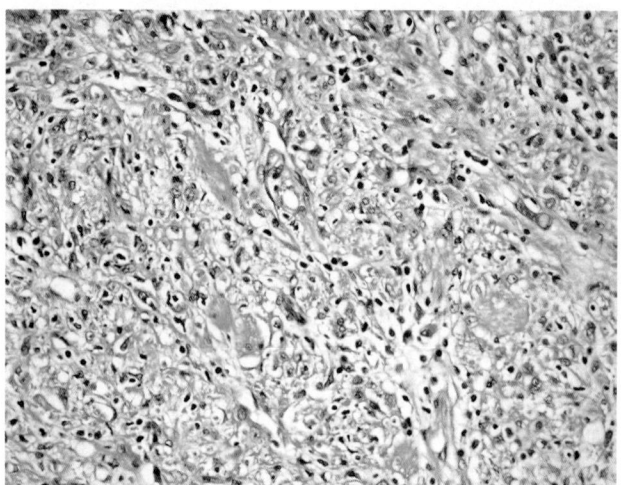

Figure 6-31. Inflammatory myofibroblastic tumor. The tumor consists of myofibroblastic cells in a cellular background with prominent lymphoplasmacytic cells. Fat necrosis is not a feature.

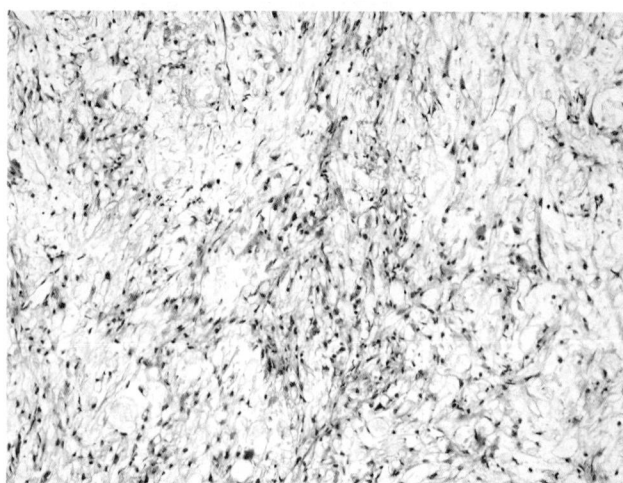

Figure 6-32. Inflammatory myofibroblastic tumor. This example has a looser more myxoid appearance than the lesion shown in Fig. 6.31 but still has the inflammatory background and myofibroblastic cells with stellate cytoplasm.

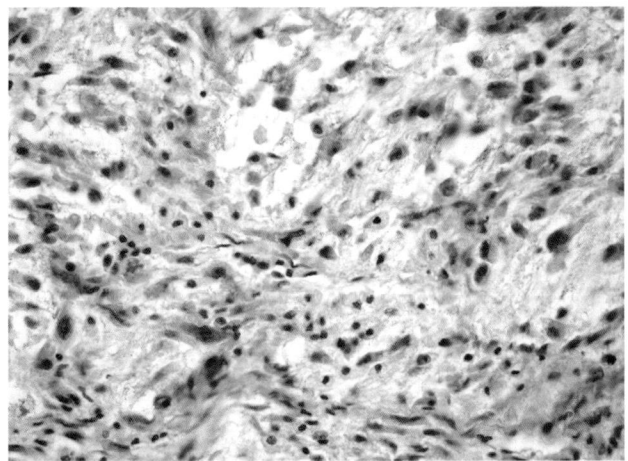

Figure 6-33. Inflammatory myofibroblastic tumor. This is a higher magnification of the lesion depicted in Fig. 6.32. Several of the cells have perfectly round macronucleoli, a characteristic feature of inflammatory myofibroblastic tumor.

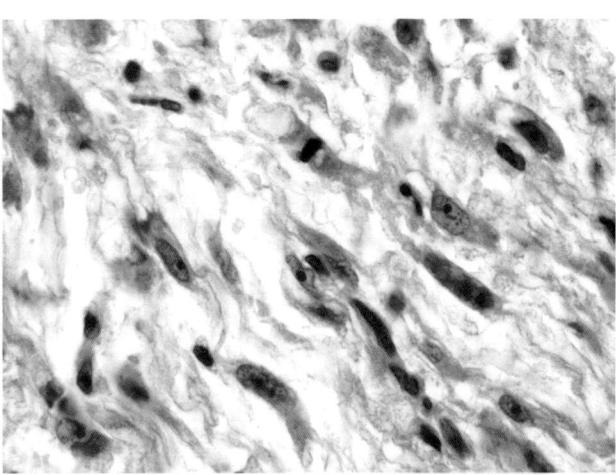

Figure 6-34. Inflammatory myofibroblastic tumor. This is a very high magnification image of the lesion seen in Figs. 6.32 and 6.33. The macronucleoli are seen to full advantage. Note the color of the cells' cytoplasm—not quite pink like smooth muscle but more metachromatic (not quite eosinophilic nor basophilic) in keeping with myofibroblastic differentiation.

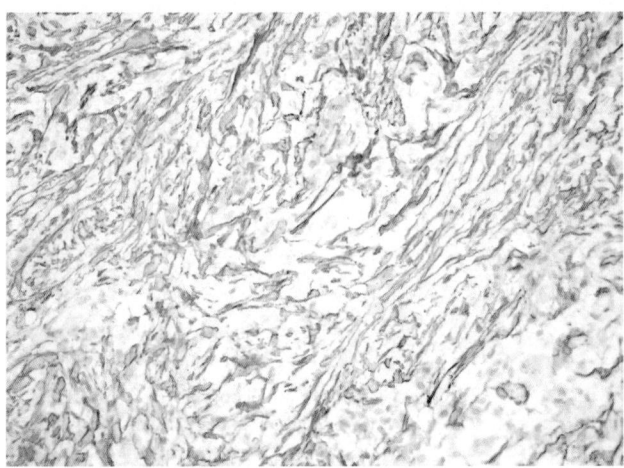

Figure 6-35. Inflammatory myofibroblastic tumor. This smooth muscle actin stain highlights the stellate contours of the cells' cytoplasm, a feature of myofibroblastic differentiation. Not all inflammatory myofibroblastic tumors have such prominent actin expression.

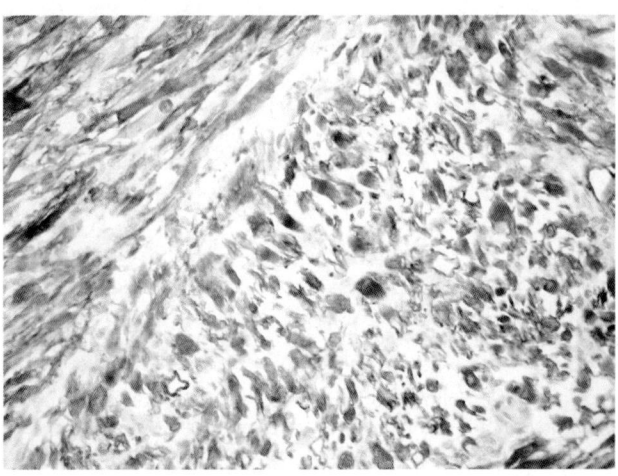

Figure 6-36. Inflammatory myofibroblastic tumor. This ALK stain shows strong cytoplasmic labeling.

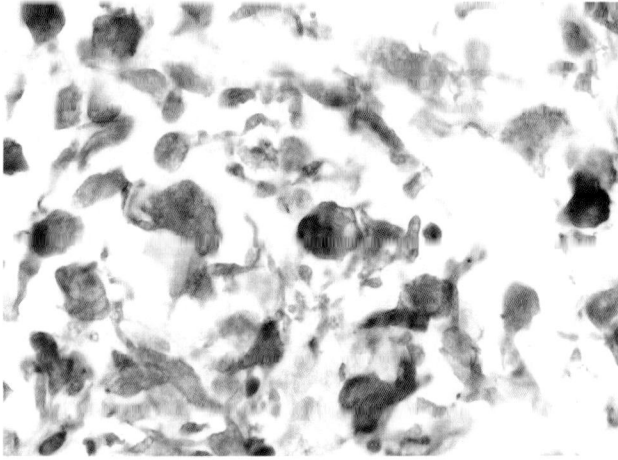

Figure 6-37. Inflammatory myofibroblastic tumor. This ALK stain highlights cytoplasmic processes extending in all directions (stellate appearance).

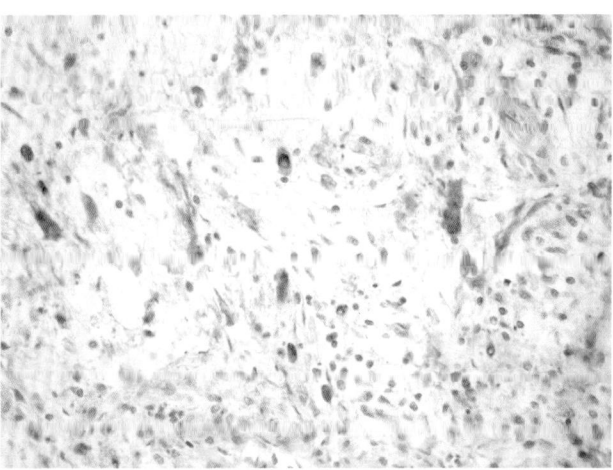

Figure 6-38. Inflammatory myofibroblastic tumor. This is an ALK stain from a myxoid area of an inflammatory myofibroblastic tumor.

invade adjacent viscera; occasional examples metastasize and are aggressive, but most are treated surgically and have indolent behavior. A pitfall is that these tumors often have a prominent infiltration of IgG4-labeled plasma cells, but they lack the vascular changes seen in IgG4-related fibrosclerosing disease.[10,11] Additionally, they can have the same altered ratio of IgG4 to total IgG-labeled plasma cells (which is another reason not to waste time doing IgG as well as IgG4 labeling).

Inflammatory myofibroblastic tumors are more cellular than sclerosing mesenteritis in general. Furthermore, an aggressive overtly malignant subset has been described and termed epithelioid inflammatory myofibroblastic sarcoma[12] (Figs. 6.39–6.46). This subset has two peculiar patterns of ALK immunolabeling with a rim of staining around the nuclear membrane or a perinuclear pattern (Figs. 6.42, 6.45, and 6.46). Both inflammatory myofibroblastic tumor (low grade) and epithelioid inflammatory fibroblastic sarcoma (high grade) are important to separate from other neoplasms because their *ALK* or *ROS1* mutations are targetable with crizotinib and newer related inhibitors.[13,14] Unfortunately, often there is an initial response to these tyrosine kinase inhibitors that vanishes after a certain point.

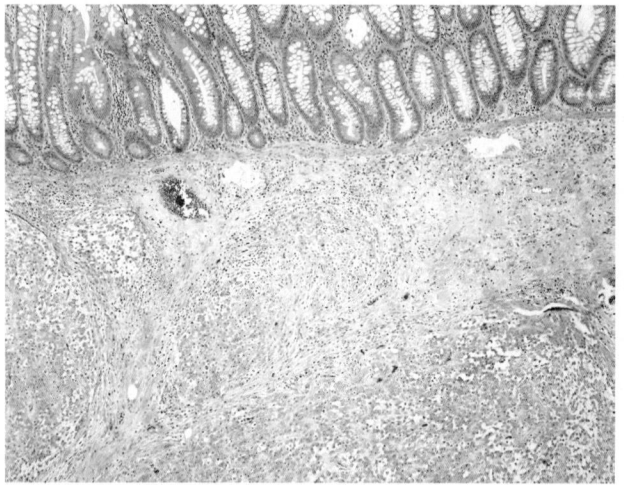

Figure 6-39. Epithelioid inflammatory myofibroblastic sarcoma (high-grade form of inflammatory myofibroblastic tumor). The neoplasm is high grade and has extended from the mesentery into the submucosa.

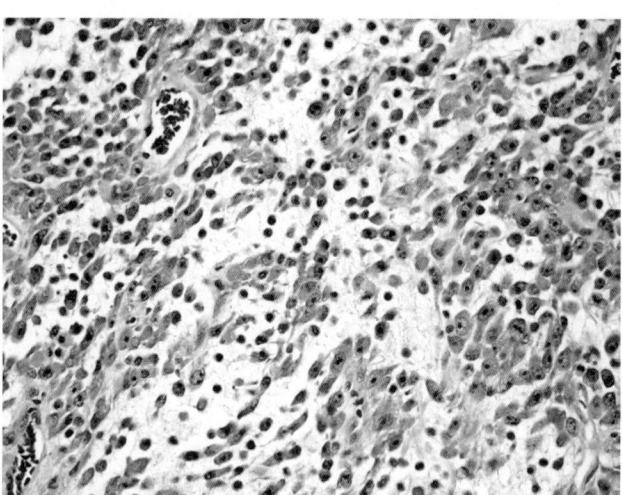

Figure 6-40. Epithelioid inflammatory myofibroblastic sarcoma (high-grade form of inflammatory myofibroblastic tumor). The neoplasm consists of epithelioid malignant cells with macronucleoli. The appearance is similar to that of epithelioid leiomyosarcoma and probably some cases diagnosed as the latter in the past are instead epithelioid inflammatory myofibroblastic sarcoma.

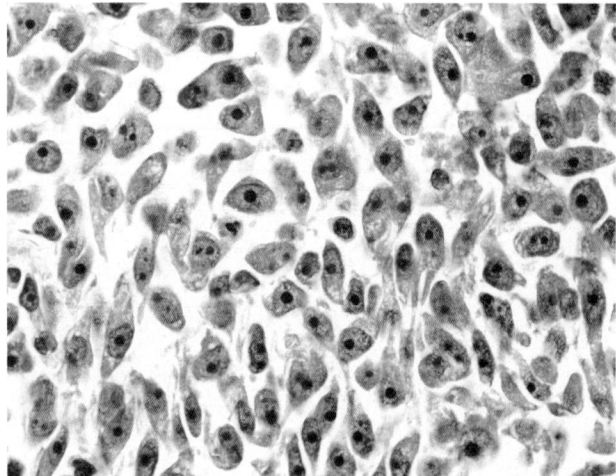

Figure 6-41. Epithelioid inflammatory myofibroblastic sarcoma (high-grade form of inflammatory myofibroblastic tumor). Note the macronucleoli in this mesenteric neoplasm.

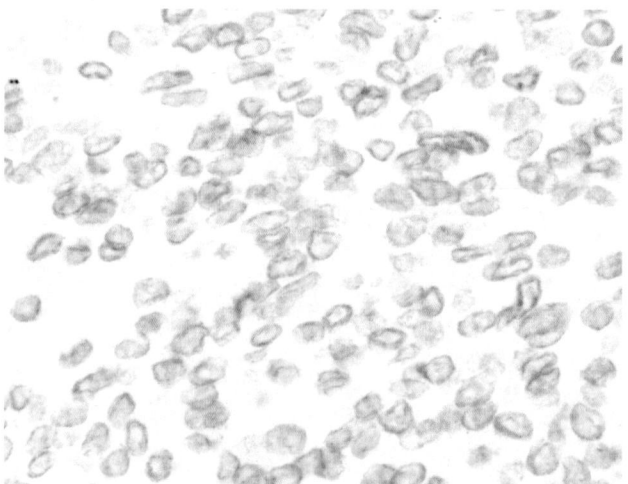

Figure 6-42. Epithelioid inflammatory myofibroblastic sarcoma (high-grade form of inflammatory myofibroblastic tumor). This example shows a peculiar distribution of ALK immunolabeling in a rim around the nuclear membranes.

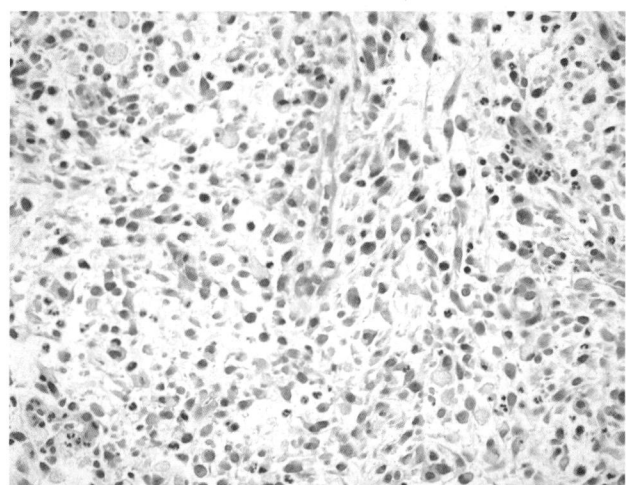

Figure 6-43. Epithelioid inflammatory myofibroblastic sarcoma (high-grade form of inflammatory myofibroblastic tumor). This example shows less distinctive macronucleoli than the example seen in Figs. 6.40–6.42.

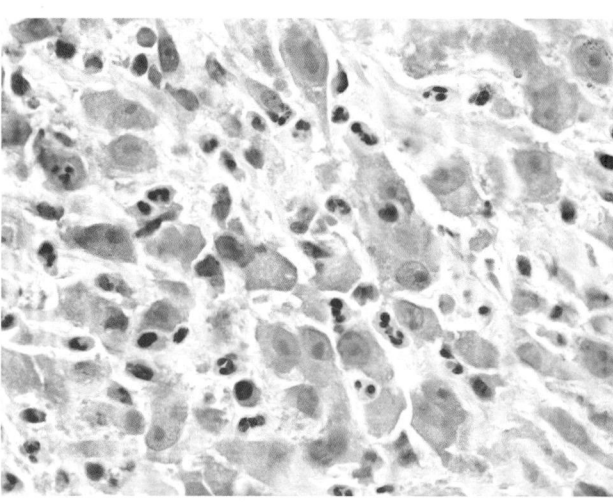

Figure 6-44. Epithelioid inflammatory myofibroblastic sarcoma (high-grade form of inflammatory myofibroblastic tumor). A backdrop that is rich in neutrophils is characteristic of this type of neoplasm.

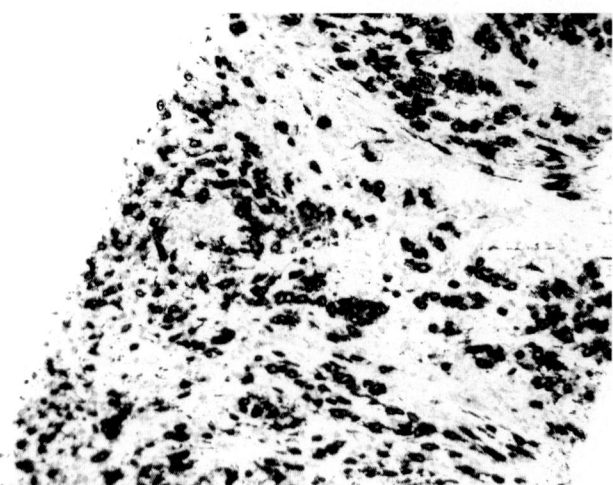

Figure 6-45. Epithelioid inflammatory myofibroblastic sarcoma (high-grade form of inflammatory myofibroblastic tumor). This is an ALK stain from the neoplasm shown in Figs. 6.43 and 6.44. The stain is heavy but note the perinuclear band.

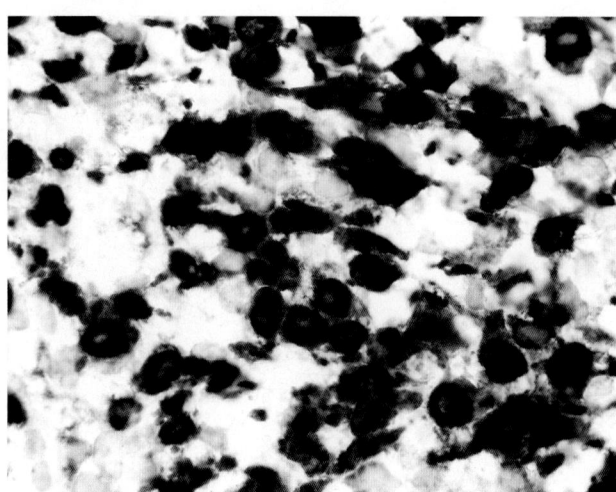

Figure 6-46. Epithelioid inflammatory myofibroblastic sarcoma (high-grade form of inflammatory myofibroblastic tumor). The ALK stain in this case (same as Figs. 6.43–6.45) shows perinuclear labeling forming a dense ring in each malignant cell.

FAQ: Targeted therapy for inflammatory myofibroblastic tumor is great but what if the tumor is ALK-negative?

Answer: Many ALK-negative tumors using immunolabeling are also *FISH* negative and about 60% of inflammatory myofibroblastic tumors harbor *ALK*. As such, 40% are negative, which can be disappointing. However, a sizable percentage of these ALK-negative tumors (on the order of 25%) can be shown to harbor *ROS1* rearrangements, particularly in children. Tumors with this rearrangement also respond to the same targeted therapy as that for *ALK*-rearranged tumors. There is even an immunohistochemical test that has been developed for ROS1.[9,15] Even though it is not practical to offer this testing in small centers, it is good to know about it in the event that a pediatric tumor is encountered.

IgG4-RELATED FIBROSCLEROSING DISEASE

This is a family of disorders unified by the presence of storiform fibrosis, obliterative phlebitis, and the admixture of many IgG4-expressing plasma cells. Years ago, these disorders were believed to reflect a host of separate lesions in various parts of the body until several colleagues studied their unifying association with IgG4-expressing plasma cells and elevated serum IgG4[16] (Fig. 6.47). The remaining mystery is learning the antigen or antigens that trigger the IgG4 response in these people and make them develop tumefactive lesions or retroperitoneal fibrosis.[17] The key findings are the presence of storiform fibrosis and obliterative phlebitis and too many IgG4-labeled cells (Figs. 6.48–6.50).

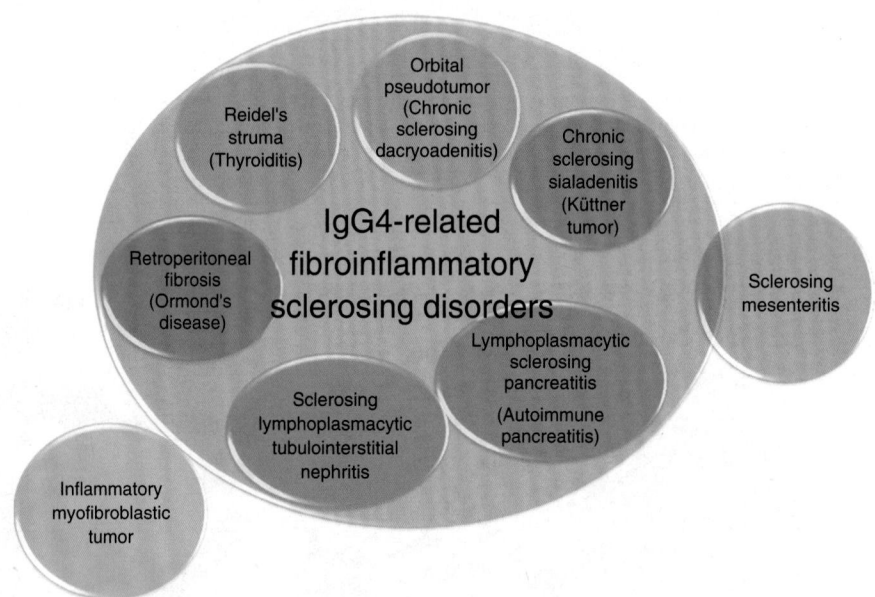

Figure 6-47. Venn diagram showing IgG4-related fibrosclerosing disorders in various organs. Note that inflammatory myofibroblastic tumor is not really a family member!

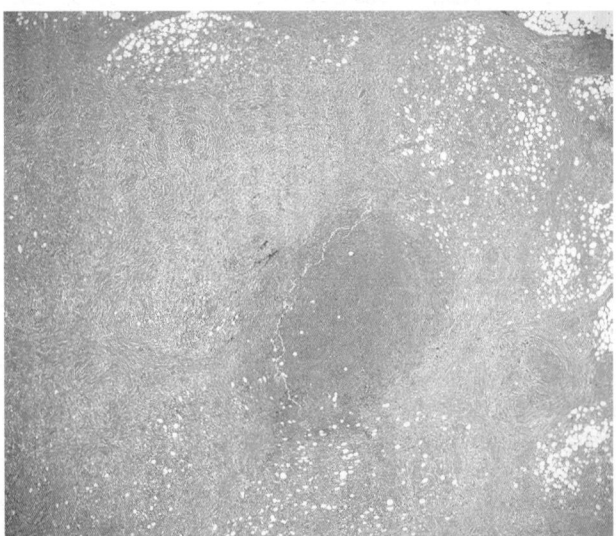

Figure 6-48. IgG4-related fibrosclerosing disease. There is a sclerotic lesion with storiform fibrosis that lacks prominent fat necrosis. A zone in the center shows ischemic injury secondary to vasculitis.

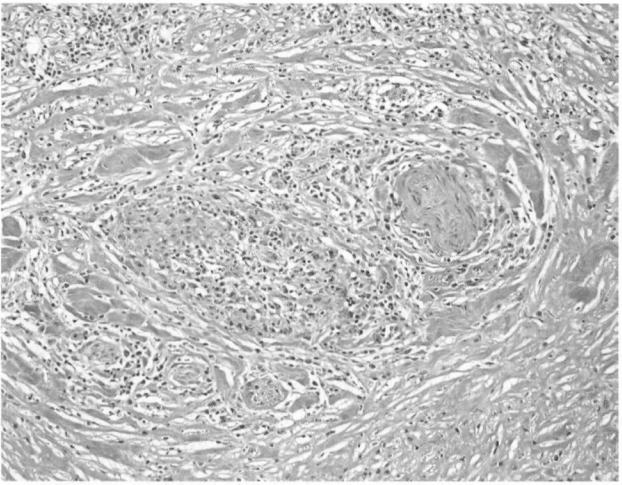

Figure 6-49. IgG4-related fibrosclerosing disease. There is a background of storiform fibrosis in the center of which there is a badly damaged vein with phlebitis and sclerosis. To the right of the destroyed vein is a healthy pink artery!

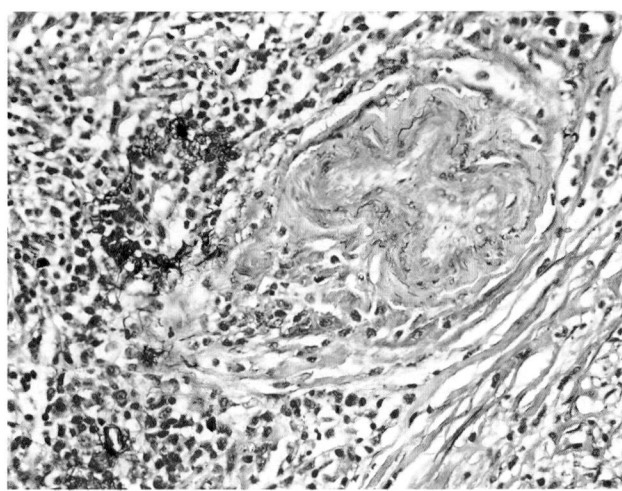

Figure 6-50. IgG4-related fibrosclerosing disease. This is a Movat stain. The remnants of the damaged vein (left) show residual frayed elastic fibrils but the elastic artery is in good shape!

FAQ: How many IgG4-labeled cells are needed for a diagnosis of IgG4-related fibrosclerosing disease?

Answer: There are tables with suggested cutoffs,[16] but using these tables has to be in the context of other features that should be seen and in practice a clinico-pathologic correlation is the order of the day. We do not focus too much on the IgG4 counts in the setting of the appropriate morphology; before the stain was widely available, we diagnosed the condition regularly based on *morphology*! Having the test is simply to *confirm* what we already know based on the H&E morphology. However, generally it should be easy to find fields with >10 labeled cells to confirm an interpretation of IgG4-related fibrosclerosing disease in the correct context. Some authors suggest looking for the ratio of IgG4-labeled cells to total IgG-labeled cells. This sounds great, but in practice, when an IgG stain is performed, the entire slide is dark brown, and counting is therefore impossible to do in an accurate fashion. Additionally, there is nothing specific about these ratios, which can, for example, but identical in inflammatory myo-fibroblastic tumor, as discussed earlier.[10,11] Serum IgG4 can always be checked. The main thing is that it is important to consider whether one is dealing instead with an infection, a lymphoma, or an area that is responding to another type of neoplasm (sampling error; see the following FAQ). In our practices, IgG4/IgG ratios are not reported.

A summary of the similarities and differences between IgG4-related fibrosclerosing disease, sclerosing mesenteritis, and inflammatory myofibroblastic tumor appears in Table 6.2.

TABLE 6.2: Principle Inflammatory Mesenteric Lesions

Condition	IgG4-Related Fibrosclerosing Disease	Sclerosing Mesenteritis	Inflammatory Myofibroblastic Tumor
Usual location	Mesentery, retroperitoneum	Mesentery	Mesentery, retroperitoneum
Mass?	Sometimes	Yes	Yes
Key features	• Cellular lesion • Storiform fibrosis • Minimal fat necrosis • Obliterative phlebitis	• Hypocellular lesion • Prominent fat necrosis	• Cellular lesion • Minimal fat necrosis • Plump myofibroblastic cells with macronucleoli • *ALK* or *ROS1* rearrangements
IgG4 present?	Yes	Often	Often
Steroid responsive?	Yes	No	No

FAQ: What issues can be encountered in needle biopsies of mesenteric fibroinflammatory lesions?

Answer: Sampling error always needs to be considered. An especially important pitfall is the proclivity of ileal neuroendocrine tumors to spread to the mesentery and invoke a brisk fibroinflammatory response that is stuffed with IgG4-reactive plasma cells (Figs. 6.51–6.53). Furthermore, some well-differentiated liposarcomas (atypical lipomatous tumors) and dedifferentiated liposarcomas can have an inflammatory backdrop (Figs. 6.54–6.56). These latter tumors feature scattered large hyperchromatic nuclei that differ from the fibroblastic and myofibroblastic nuclei in inflammatory myofibroblastic tumor, sclerosing mesenteritis, and IgG4-associated fibrosclerosing conditions. In doubtful cases, MDM2 immunolabeling or FISH testing can be added to confirm an interpretation of well-differentiated (atypical lipomatous tumor) or dedifferentiated liposarcoma with prominent inflammation. In fact, some observers have used the term "inflammatory myofibroblastic tumor–like" dedifferentiated liposarcoma to describe this pattern.[18] Because of all these types of sampling issues, we have become total wimps in reporting fibroinflammatory lesions on small needle biopsies and write our reports carefully.

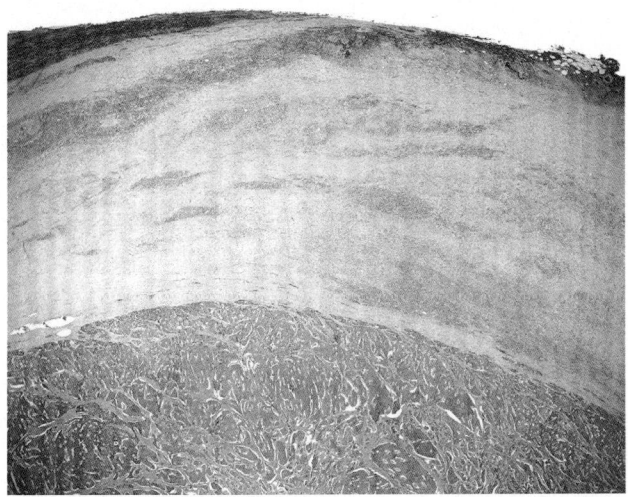

Figure 6-51. Mesenteric well-differentiated neuroendocrine (carcinoid) tumor producing dramatic fibroinflammatory response. There is an obvious neoplasm at the bottom of the image, but it has resulted in a striking fibroinflammatory response. This is a situation that can result in a false negative needle biopsy! This type of response can be rich in IgG4-labeled plasma cells. The vascular changes are absent.

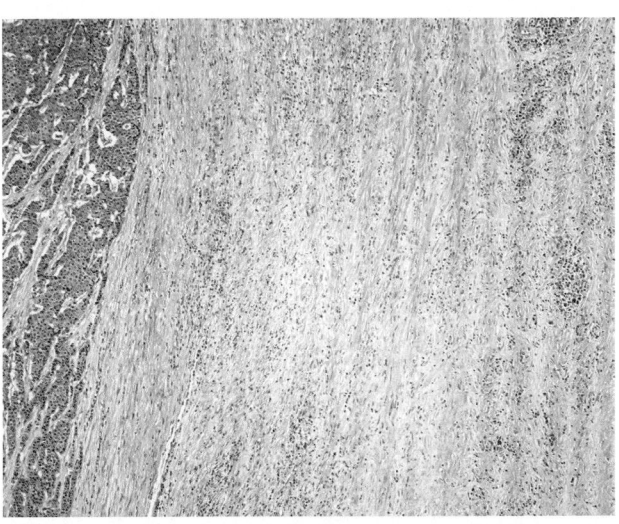

Figure 6-52. Mesenteric well-differentiated neuroendocrine (carcinoid) tumor producing dramatic fibroinflammatory response. This area even features storiform fibrosis!

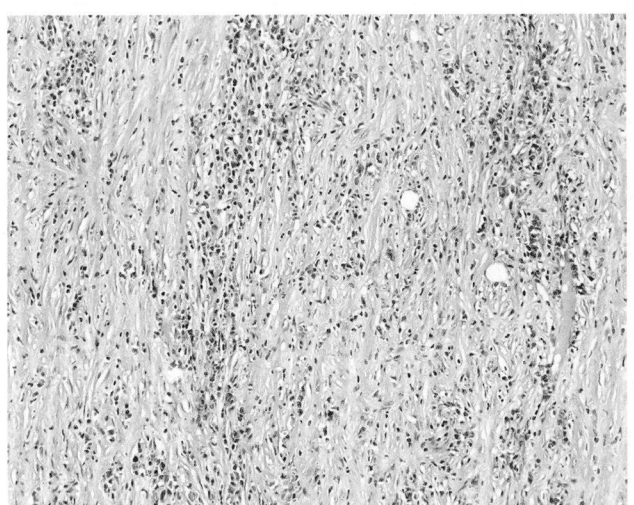

Figure 6-53. Mesenteric well-differentiated neuroendocrine (carcinoid) tumor producing dramatic fibroinflammatory response. Note the storiform fibrosis. The well differentiated neuroendocrine (carcinoid) tumor is not present in this field.

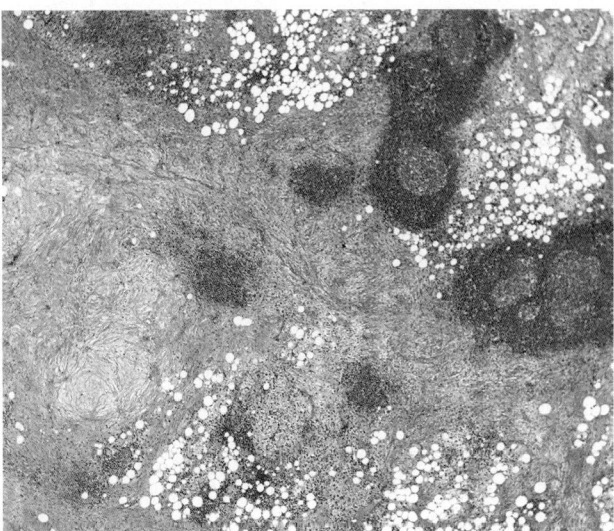

Figure 6-54. Retroperitoneal well-differentiated liposarcoma (atypical lipomatous tumor) with prominent inflammation. The key to diagnosis is noting individual atypical nuclei. Sometimes a lipomalike component is present.

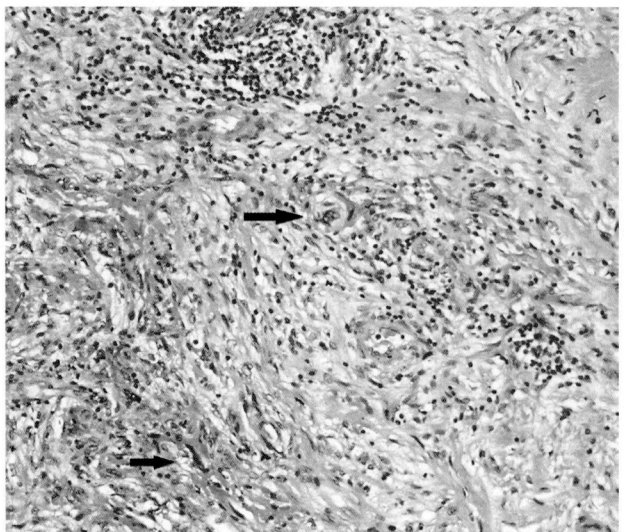

Figure 6-55. Retroperitoneal well-differentiated liposarcoma (atypical lipomatous tumor) with prominent inflammation. Scattered atypical hyperchromatic nuclei (*arrows*) are a diagnostic clue.

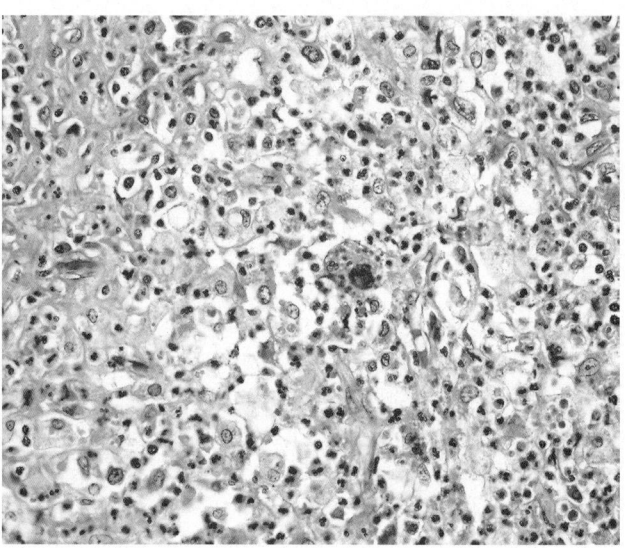

Figure 6-56. Retroperitoneal dedifferentiated liposarcoma with prominent inflammation. These tumors were referred to as "inflammatory malignant fibrous histiocytoma" in the past, but they are dedifferentiated liposarcomas. Note the hyperchromatic nucleus in the center.

SAMPLE REPORTS: Needle Biopsy of Retroperitoneal and Mesenteric Fibroinflammatory Lesions

Small Bowel Mesenteric Mass (Needle Biopsy): Fibroinflammatory Process. See Note

Note: This lesion shows adipose tissue with fat necrosis in an inflammatory backdrop in keeping with sclerosing mesenteritis. Our reservation in the aforementioned interpretation reflects the possibility of sampling error. For example, well-differentiated neuroendocrine tumors that have spread to the mesentery can invoke a prominent fibroinflammatory response.

Small Bowel Mesenteric Mass (Needle Biopsy): Fibroinflammatory Process. See Note

Note: This lesion shows storiform fibrosis in an inflammatory backdrop with prominent plasma cells and areas with up to 15 IgG4-labeled plasma cells per high power field. There are no vessels in the sample to assess for obliterative phlebitis. The findings suggest the possibility of IgG4-related fibrosclerosing disease and it would be worthwhile to consider correlation with IgG4 serology. Our reservation in the aforementioned interpretation reflects the possibility of sampling error. For example, well-differentiated neuroendocrine tumors that have spread to the mesentery can invoke a prominent fibroinflammatory response.

TRANSLOCATION SARCOMAS ASSOCIATED WITH THE GASTROINTESTINAL TRACT

GENERAL COMMENTS

Translocation sarcomas of the gastrointestinal tract are really rare, but they are predictably rare and tend to be found in certain sites. All but the last (low-grade fibromyxoid sarcoma) tend to arise in young adults:

Ewing sarcoma—duodenum; mucosa and submucosa
Synovial sarcoma—stomach; mucosa and submucosa
Clear cell sarcoma–like tumor—ileum; muscularis propria
Low-grade fibromyxoid sarcoma—small bowel and colon; mesentery

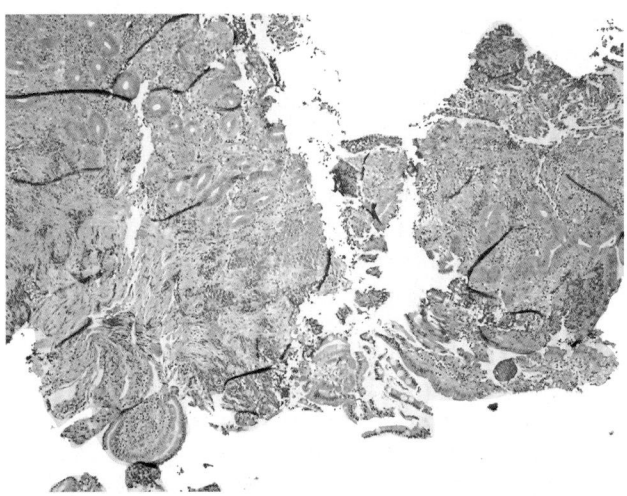

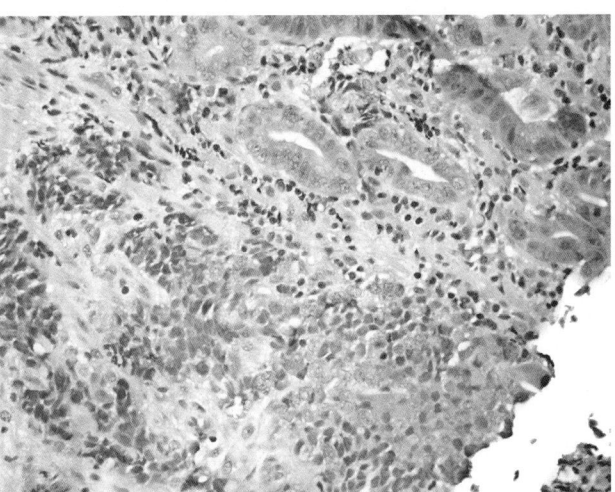

Figure 6-57. Ewing sarcoma involving the duodenum. Such cases are rare and should be considered in young adults. Remember also to consider a germ cell tumor. This neoplasm required molecular techniques to diagnose but note the uniformity of the malignant cells, a feature of translocation-associated sarcomas.

Figure 6-58. Ewing sarcoma involving the duodenum. This tumor features small primitive cells.

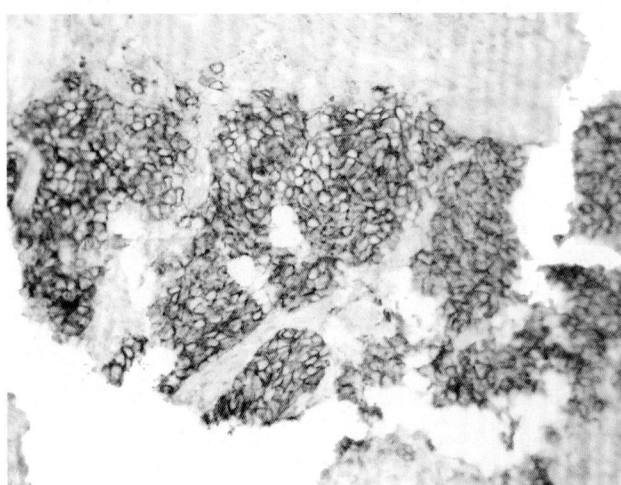

Figure 6-59. Ewing sarcoma involving the duodenum. This is a CD99 immunostain.

An important concept is that sarcomas with characteristic translocations have uniform nuclei rather than lots of nuclear pleomorphism,[19] a characteristic that they share with GISTs. Translocation sarcomas also lack atypical mitoses (another feature shared with GISTs).

EWING SARCOMA

Primary Ewing sarcoma involving the gastrointestinal tract is vanishingly rare such that it is the grist for case reports, and most such reports are of tumors of the small intestine in children and young adults. Rare gastric tumors have also been reported. Ewing sarcoma in the gastrointestinal tract looks like Ewing sarcoma in the bones and soft tissues, but you have to think of it. In the gastrointestinal tract, the first consideration will generally be lymphoma/leukemia and then neuroendocrine tumors and then germ cell tumors based on the youthful age of the patient. The tumor cells are uniform and fairly small and hyperchromatic (Figs. 6-57–6-59). They express CD99 and sometimes can display unexpected expression of S100 protein or even keratins such that molecular techniques may be needed to confirm the interpretation. This is one time when it is worthwhile to arrange molecular testing—Ewing sarcoma responds to treatment protocols!

CLEAR CELL SARCOMA–LIKE TUMOR OF THE GASTROINTESTINAL TRACT

Gastrointestinal type clear cell sarcoma is fairly well delineated as an entity, and it differs a bit from classic clear sarcoma of soft tissues. The typical location is the ileum and the patients tend to be young adults. Tumors consist of sheets of rounded to slightly spindled cells that are uniform (Figs. 6.60–6.67). Some examples have a nodular appearance and some cases show cells with prominent uniform nucleoli. The malignant cells express S100 protein but not typically HMB45 or other melanoma markers. This is different from the staining pattern for clear cell sarcoma of the soft tissues, which usually expresses melanoma markers in addition to S100 protein. Most soft tissue clear cell sarcomas have *EWSR1-ATF1* gene rearrangements, but those in the GI tract tend to have *EWSR1-CREB1* rearrangements.[20] These tumors can have overlapping features with neuroendocrine tumors, a problem that can be compounded by their synaptophysin labeling. Fortunately, they lack keratins and chromogranin expression and show strong S100 protein expression. They also overlap with metastatic melanoma such that some cases require molecular confirmation. They usually lack CD117 expression. The term "malignant gastrointestinal neuroectodermal tumor" has also been suggested for these neoplasms. They have a dismal prognosis.[21]

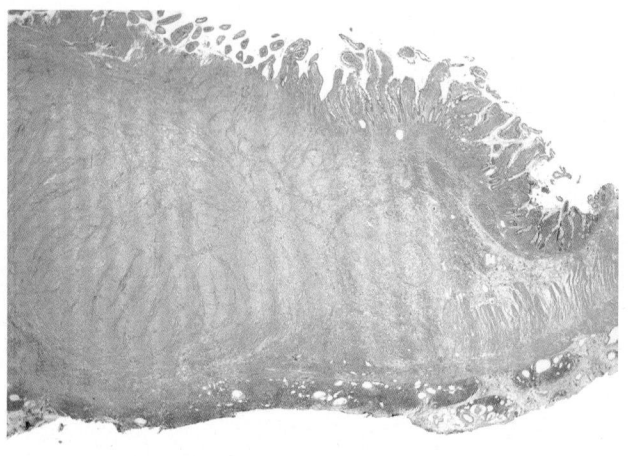

Figure 6-60. Clear cell sarcoma–like tumor of the ileum. At low magnification, the tumor is composed of cells arranged in nests.

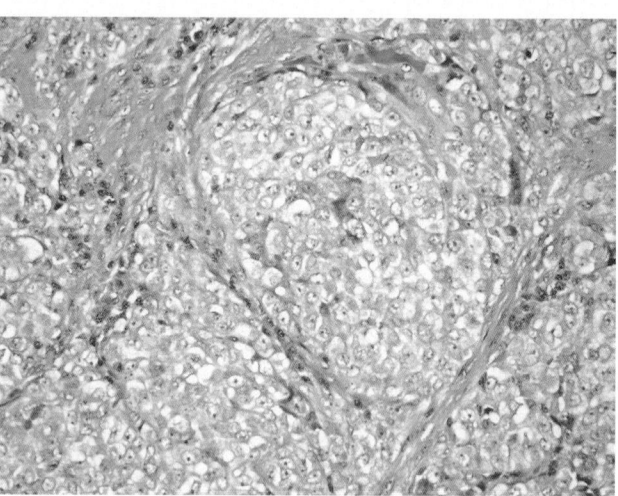

Figure 6-61. Clear cell sarcoma–like tumor of the ileum. Note the prominent nucleoli in each cell. The malignant cells are uniform. Atypical mitoses are not found in translocation-associated sarcomas.

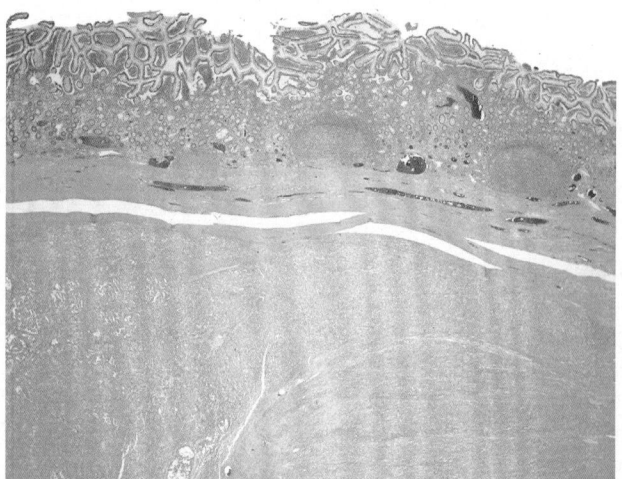

Figure 6-62. Clear cell sarcoma–like tumor of the ileum. This example shows a solid growth pattern with pseudopapillary areas, but this is not a solid pseudopapillary neoplasm of the type found in the pancreas. This is a very aggressive neoplasm.

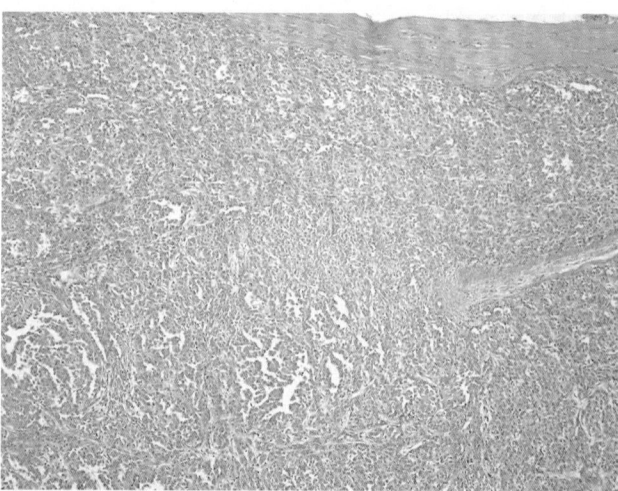

Figure 6-63. Clear cell sarcoma–like tumor of the ileum. This is a higher magnification of the neoplasm seen in Fig. 6.62.

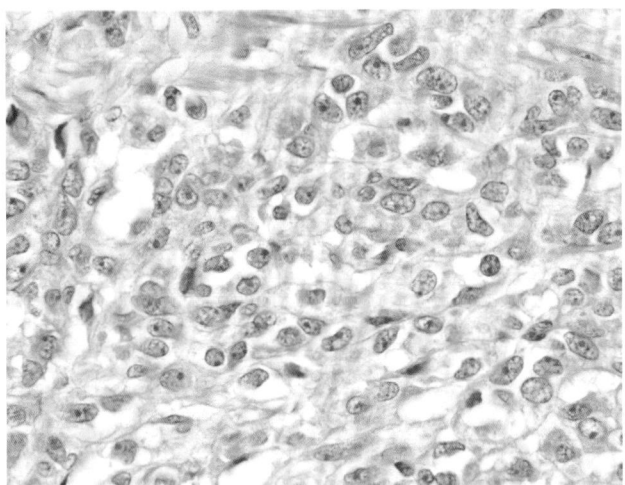

Figure 6-64. Clear cell sarcoma–like tumor of the ileum. High magnification of the tumor seen in Figs. 6.62 and 6.63 shows an area with prominent nucleoli.

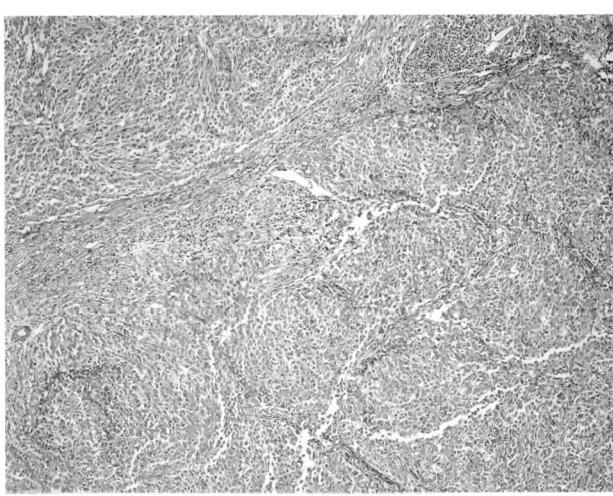

Figure 6-65. Clear cell sarcoma–like tumor of the ileum. This example shows the malignant cells arranged in an overall solid pattern with vague nests.

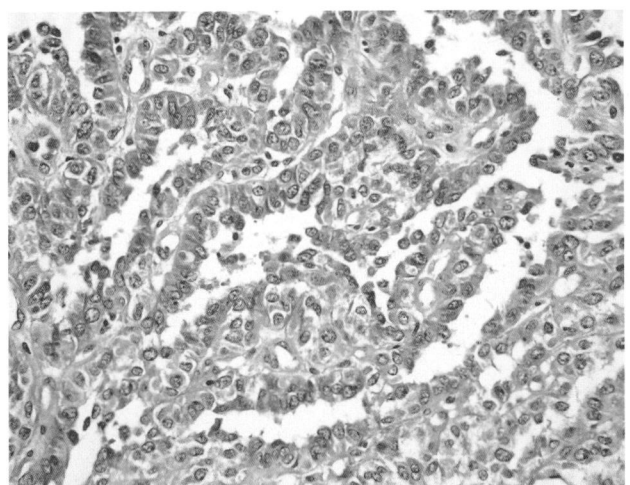

Figure 6-66. Clear cell sarcoma–like tumor of the ileum. This example has a pseudopapillary arrangement. The appearance is reminiscent of that of a well-differentiated neuroendocrine (carcinoid) tumor, and the expression of synaptophysin can lead to an incorrect diagnosis for such tumors, but keratin is nonreactive. Note that the nuclei are uniform.

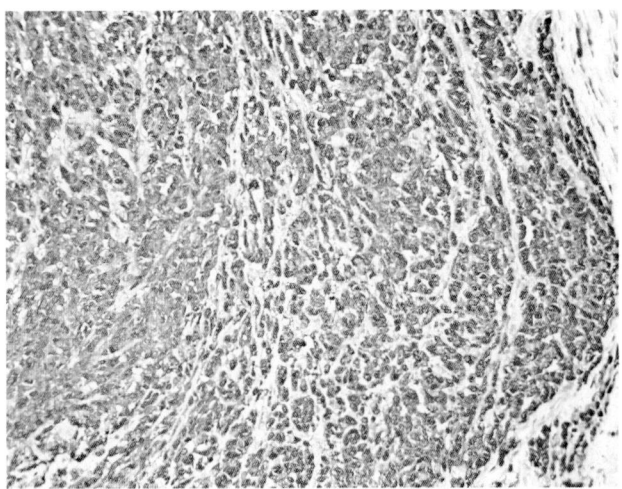

Figure 6-67. Clear cell sarcoma–like tumor of the ileum. There is strong S100 protein expression.

PEARLS & PITFALLS

Clear cell sarcoma–like tumor of the GI tract can have strong synaptophysin expression and mimic a neuroendocrine tumor. Because the mitotic activity is not invariably high, this could result in an interpretation of a well-differentiated neuroendocrine tumor even though these are very aggressive sarcomas. Before diagnosing an ileal well-differentiated neuroendocrine (carcinoid) tumor in a young adult, consider this sarcoma type. Fortunately these sarcomas lack keratin expression.

LOW-GRADE FIBROMYXOID SARCOMA

Low-grade fibromyxoid sarcoma (which has a t(7,16) (q32-34;p11) or t(11,16) (p11;p11) translocation, resulting in *FUS-CREB3L2* or *FUS-CREB3L1*) has been reported in the small bowel[22] and can also be seen associated with the colon. Tumors are centered in the mesentery and unlikely to be encountered in mucosal biopsies (Figs. 6.68–6.71). They appear similar to fibromatoses but differ by featuring more hyperchromatic nuclei and varying cellularity throughout the neoplasm, whereas the cellularity of fibromatoses is uniform throughout the lesion. They can occasionally have areas with the type of vascular changes seen in fibromatosis. These tumors lack nuclear β-catenin immunostaining. The high-grade counterpart, sclerosing epithelioid fibrosarcoma, can also be found in the mesentery (Figs. 6.72–6.74). These sarcomas are tricky to diagnose but, fortunately, there is a confirmatory immunostain—MUC4, which was discovered by using gene profiling studies.[23,24] MUC4 indicates "mucin core protein," so this protein can be found in some carcinomas (for example, prostate carcinoma), but generally even the most sleep-deprived among us can distinguish a sarcoma from a gland forming prostate carcinoma.

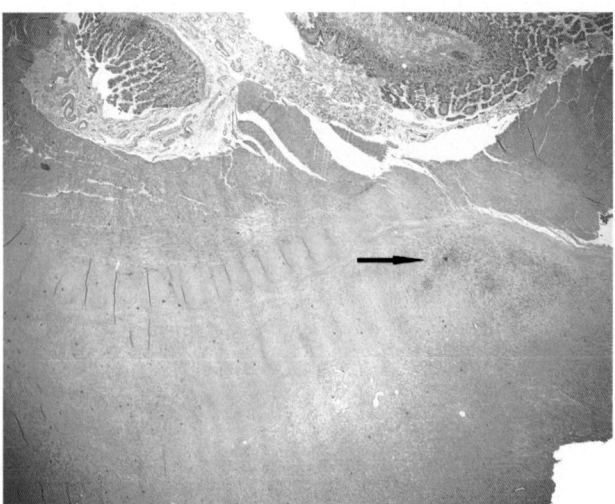

Figure 6-68. Low-grade fibromyxoid sarcoma involving the gastrointestinal tract. The lesion is reminiscent of a fibromatosis but differs from having variable cellularity with a hypocellular area with myxoid features in the center and a hypercellular area indicated by an *arrow*.

Figure 6-69. Low-grade fibromyxoid sarcoma involving the gastrointestinal tract. This area has uniform cellularity but the cells are more hyperchromatic than those in fibromatoses. As such, the vessels do not appear as prominent as they do in fibromatoses.

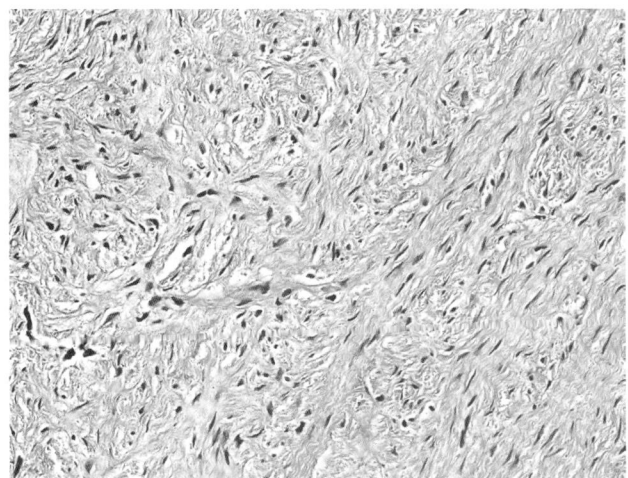

Figure 6-70. Low-grade fibromyxoid sarcoma involving the gastrointestinal tract. This is a high magnification image of the neoplasm seen in Fig. 6.69.

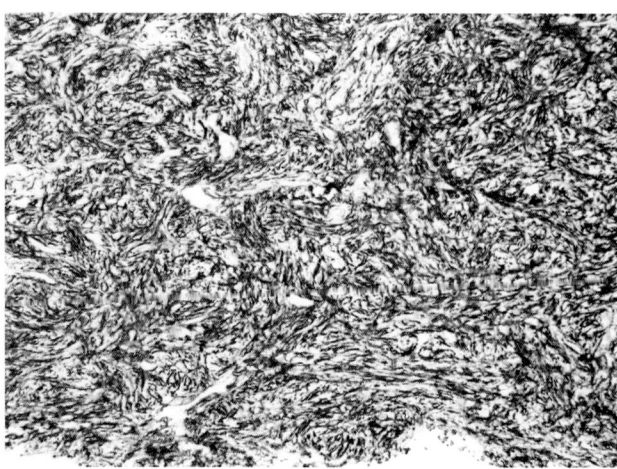

Figure 6-71. Low-grade fibromyxoid sarcoma involving the gastrointestinal tract. This is a MUC4 stain, a useful adjunct for diagnosis of low-grade fibromyxoid sarcoma.

Figure 6-72. Low-grade fibromyxoid sarcoma involving the gastrointestinal tract transforming to a high-grade form (sclerosing epithelioid fibrosarcoma). The low-grade component is at the lower right and the cellular high-grade component is at the upper left.

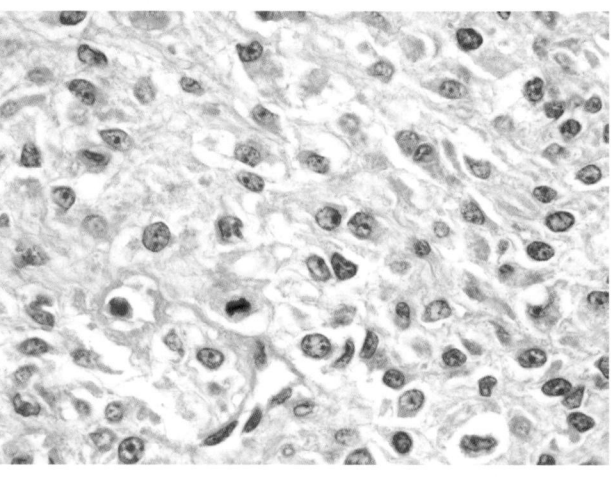

Figure 6-73. Low-grade fibromyxoid sarcoma involving the gastrointestinal tract transforming to a high-grade form (sclerosing epithelioid fibrosarcoma). This is a high magnification image of the lesion seen at the upper left of Fig. 6.72. The cells are uniform and embedded in sclerotic stroma.

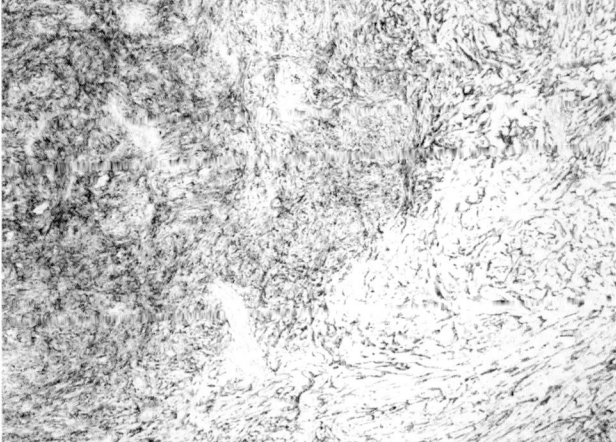

Figure 6-74. Low-grade fibromyxoid sarcoma involving the gastrointestinal tract transforming to a high-grade form (sclerosing epithelioid fibrosarcoma). MUC4 immunostaining labels both the low- and high-grade components.

SYNOVIAL SARCOMA

Gastrointestinal synovial sarcomas are rare. The stomach is the most common site, where these tumors present as polyps or submucosal plaques in young adults, but some examples manifest large transmural masses.[25] Like synovial sarcomas elsewhere, they consist of monotonous spindle cells with minimal cytoplasm, and no abnormal mitoses (Figs. 6.75 and 6.76). They can have expression of various keratins (focally) and epithelial membrane antigen, BCL2, and sometimes CD99 but not CD45or KIT and DOG1. Gastrointestinal tract synovial sarcomas show the characteristic *SS18-SSX1/2* gene fusions.

OTHER SPINDLE CELL LESIONS

GASTROINTESTINAL STROMAL TUMOR

Most GISTs arise in the stomach and they are occasionally diagnosed on mucosal biopsies. Often those that are diagnosed on biopsies are aggressive lesions because GISTs that invade the mucosa are the aggressive ones. GISTs show differentiation toward (and supposedly arise from a precursor of) the interstitial cells of Cajal, which normally govern motility of the gut.[26,27] This discovery, of course, has led to our need to be correct when we diagnose GISTs because the molecular alterations are targetable.

Overall, GISTs are the most common mesenchymal lesions throughout the entire GI tract. There are, however, two exceptions: leiomyomas outnumber GISTs in both the esophagus and the distal colon.[28] Most GISTs have either a *KIT* (CD117, a receptor tyrosine kinase) or a *PDGFRA* (platelet-derived growth factor alpha) mutation. A few points about the mutations in GISTs:

1. *PDGFRA*-mutated GISTs almost always arise in the stomach.[28]
2. Some GISTs lack both *KIT* and *PDGFRA* mutations, especially those found in children and associated with various genetic syndromes.
3. With the exception of those found in patients with neurofibromatosis type 1 (NF1), GISTs that **lack** *KIT* and *PDGFRA* mutations nearly always affect the stomach. The GISTs associated with NF1 classically involve the small intestine.
4. Finding multiple GISTs, especially in the small bowel (including the duodenum), should raise the possibility of neurofibromatosis 1 (NF1).[29-31] NF1-associated GISTs are immunoreactive with CD117 and DOG1, but they lack *KIT* or *PDGFRA* mutations as above.[29] GISTs in NF1 patients tend to be small, without mitotic activity, and they are associated with benign behavior.

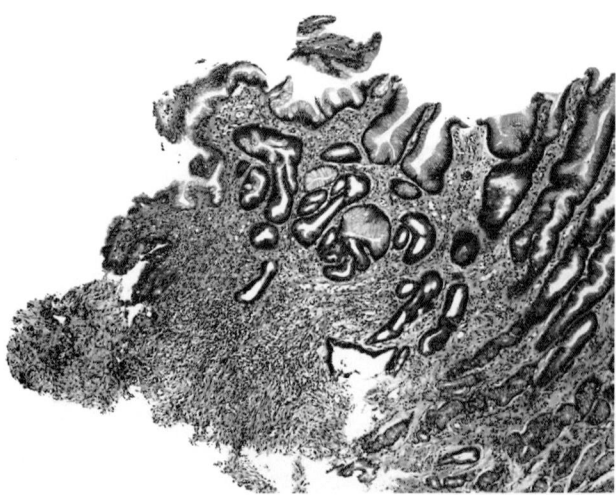

Figure 6-75. Gastric synovial sarcoma. The tumor is at the lower left of the tissue fragment.

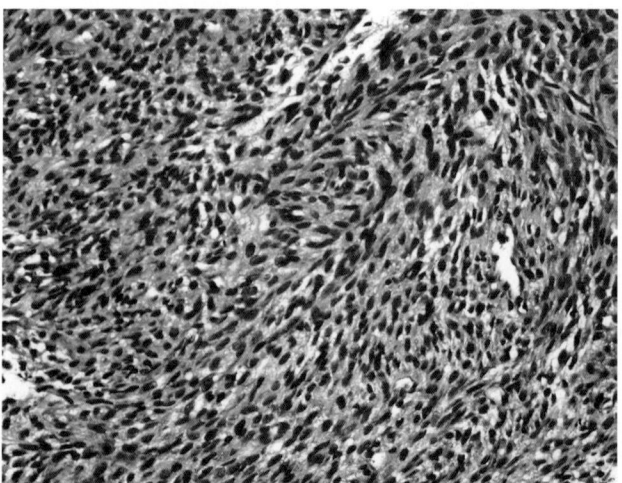

Figure 6-76. Gastric synovial sarcoma. Molecular methods were required to confirm the diagnosis, but note that the cells are highly uniform.

Taking all sites into account, GISTs mostly arise in adults older than 50 years (median age 55-60 years) and are rare in children (<1%).[31,32] There is no gender predilection overall, but there is a male predominance for malignant GISTs. The classic presentation is GI (gastrointestinal) hemorrhage: it can be either acute (melena or hematemesis) or occult (anemia).[31] Symptoms of obstruction may be the presenting issue.

FAQ: What is the distribution of GISTs?

Answer:

Stomach: 60%

Small intestine: 35%

Rectum, esophagus, omentum, and mesentery combined: 5%

Most GISTs found in the mesentery are metastatic rather than primary. About 5% of GISTs are found in patients with neurofibromatosis type 1 (multiple small intestinal tumors[29]) and Carney triad (paraganglioma, GIST, and pulmonary chondroma, usually in young females[33]). Familial GISTs arise in patients with inherited germline *KIT* or *PDGFRA* mutations.

FAQ: What are the sexy "new" types of GISTs?

Most recently, succinate dehydrogenase (SDH)-deficient GISTs have been discussed.[34-48] These GISTs are reactive with KIT and DOG1 immunostains, but they are wild type on mutational analysis for *KIT* and *PDGFRA* mutations. These tumors are only detected in the stomach (including those described in Carney triad as well as in the Carney-Stratakis syndrome [paraganglioma and gastric stromal tumors]).

The types of GISTs that usually arise in the small bowel include those associated with NF1 and those that have *BRAF* mutations.[37]

Rare families with germline mutations in *KIT* or *PDGFRA* are reported in the literature. Patients with germline *KIT* mutations present at an age about 10 years younger than those with sporadic lesions.[49] There is no gender predilection for this autosomal dominant condition. GISTs in these patients arise throughout the gastrointestinal tract (mostly in the stomach and small intestine). The patients also have diffuse hyperplasia of interstitial cells of Cajal, skin pigmentation, and sometimes mast cell disorders. Patients with germline mutations of *PDGFRA* develop both GISTs and inflammatory fibroid polyps; virtually all their GISTs arise in the stomach.

Diagnosing Gastrointestinal Stromal Tumors

Overall, GISTs are either spindle cells lesions or epithelioid lesions. Epithelioid GISTs are the old leiomyoblastomas. Epithelioid GISTs comprise about 10% of gastric GISTs, and overall about 75% to 80% of gastric GISTs behave in a benign fashion. Large tumors in the fundus, cardiac area, or posterior wall are more likely to be malignant. In contrast, about half of small bowel GISTs behave in a malignant fashion.

GISTs can be either spindled or epithelioid (Figs. 6.77–6.94). Most GISTs are spindle cell tumors with variable palisading, peculiar paranuclear vacuoles, and collagen fibrils. They can often be more palisaded than nerve sheath tumors! Epithelioid GISTs (Figs. 6.90–6.92) are most likely to cause diagnostic problems on mucosal biopsies because they are easy to mistake for carcinomas and melanoma. A very important point concerning GISTs is that the vast majority have very little nuclear pleomorphism and atypical mitoses are unusual. This point generally makes them easy to separate from leiomyosarcomas and other pleomorphic sarcomas. However, there are exceptions. Sometimes, after treatment and development of

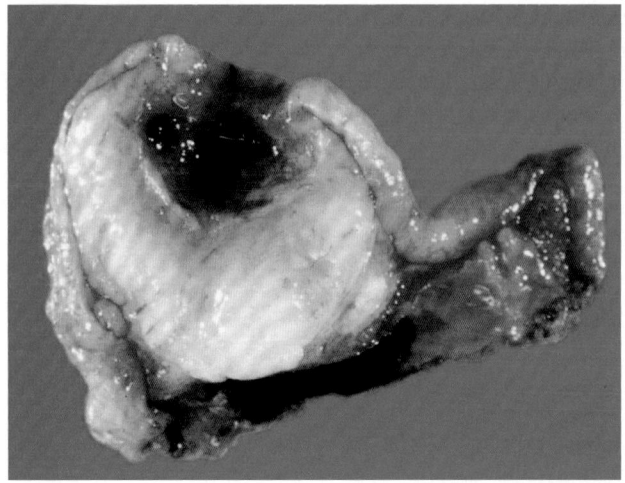

Figure 6-77. Gastrointestinal stromal tumor. This gastric example is centered in the muscularis propria, but the overlying mucosa has become ulcerated.

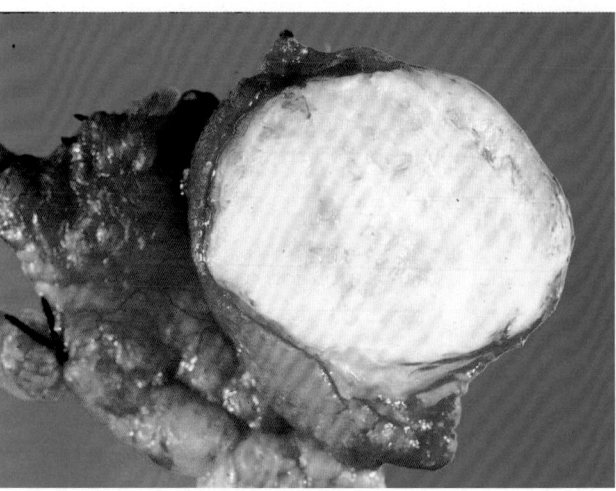

Figure 6-78. Gastrointestinal stromal tumor. This example has not resulted in ulceration. The gross appearance is nonspecific with a fish flesh–type appearance.

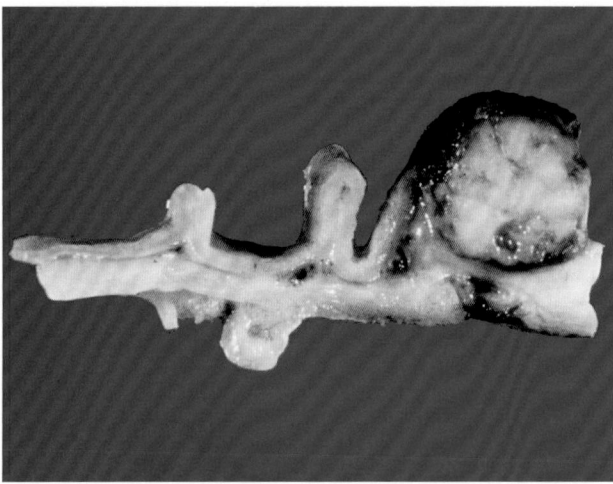

Figure 6-79. Gastrointestinal stromal tumor. Most gastrointestinal stromal tumors are centered in the muscularis propria, but this one involves the gastric submucosa.

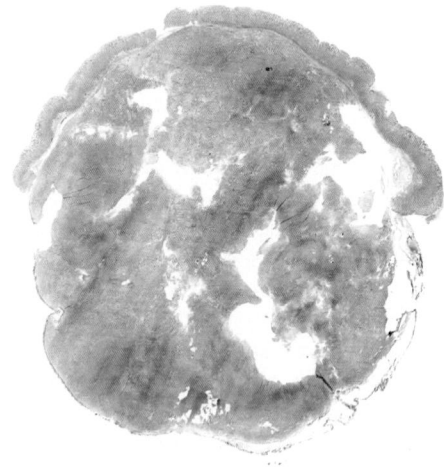

Figure 6-80. Gastrointestinal stromal tumor. This low magnification image of a gastric submucosal example shows the high cellularity of these tumors.

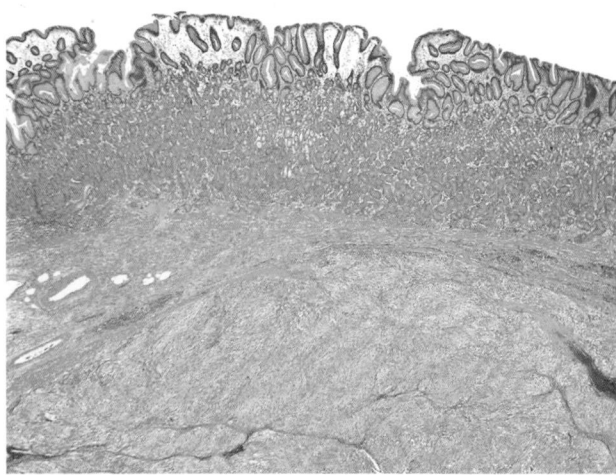

Figure 6-81. Gastrointestinal stromal tumor. This gastric lesion is cellular, but the nuclei have uniform feature.

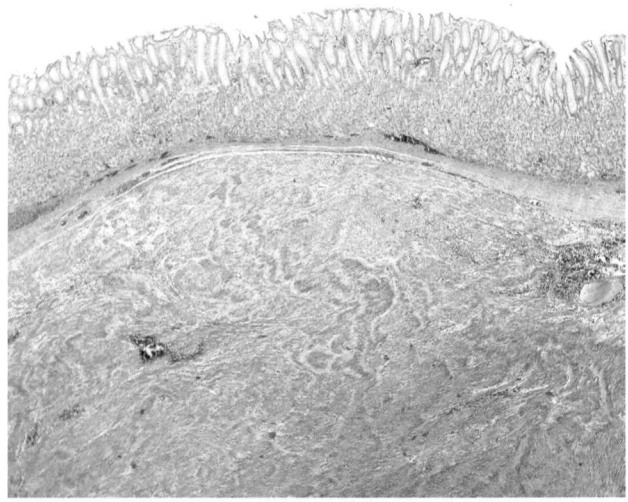

Figure 6-82. Gastrointestinal stromal tumor. Nuclear palisading is often dramatic in gastrointestinal stromal tumors—far more than in most nerve sheath tumors.

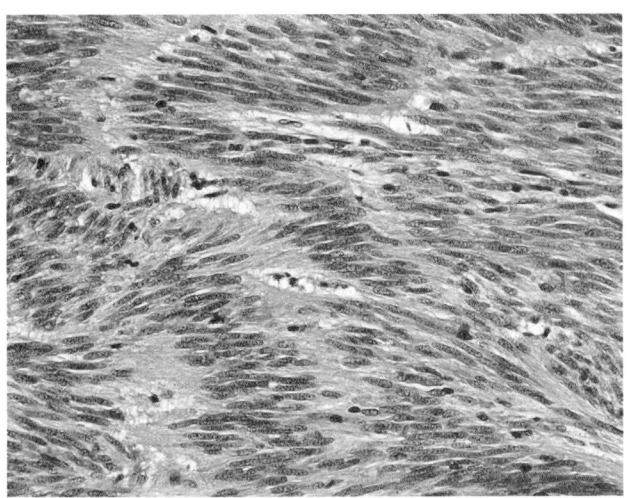

Figure 6-83. Gastrointestinal stromal tumor. This is a high magnification of the neoplasm seen in Fig. 6.82. The nuclear palisading is impressive and the nuclei are highly uniform.

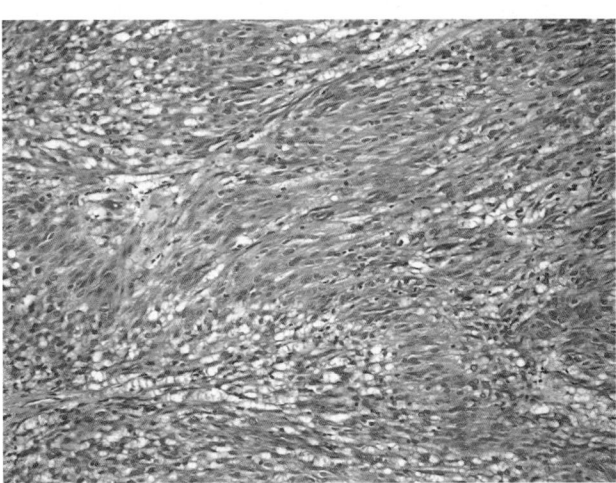

Figure 6-84. Gastrointestinal stromal tumor. This lesion is cellular and mitotic activity was easy to spot. This would be expected to have an aggressive course without treatment. Note that the cells are quite uniform regardless of the cellularity.

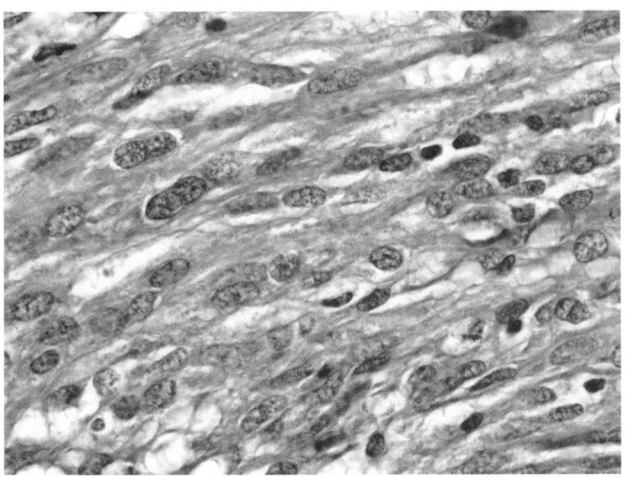

Figure 6-85. Gastrointestinal stromal tumor. The nuclei are uniform and the cytoplasm lacks well-developed longitudinal striations.

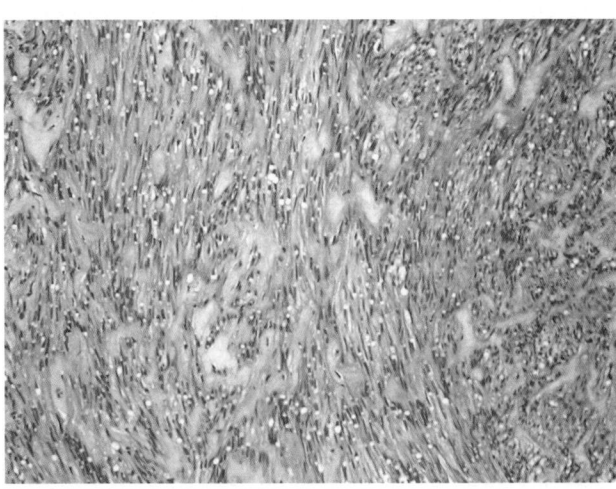

Figure 6-86. Gastrointestinal stromal tumor. Many of the cells have paranuclear vacuoles. Although paranuclear vacuoles are a feature of smooth muscle tumors, finding this many nearly always indicates that the lesion is a gastrointestinal stromal tumor.

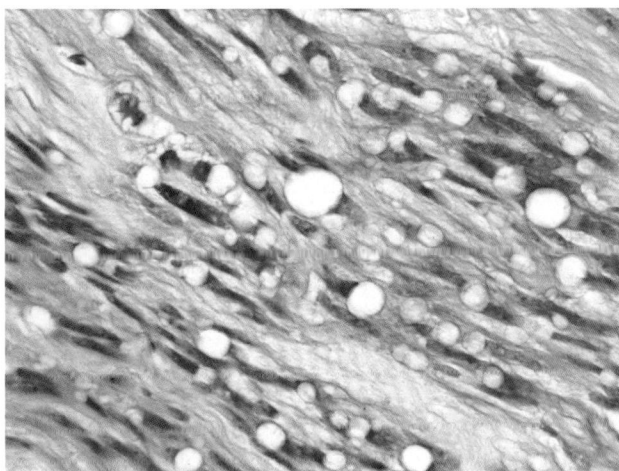

Figure 6-87. Gastrointestinal stromal tumor. This is a high magnification image of the tumor seen in Fig. 6.86.

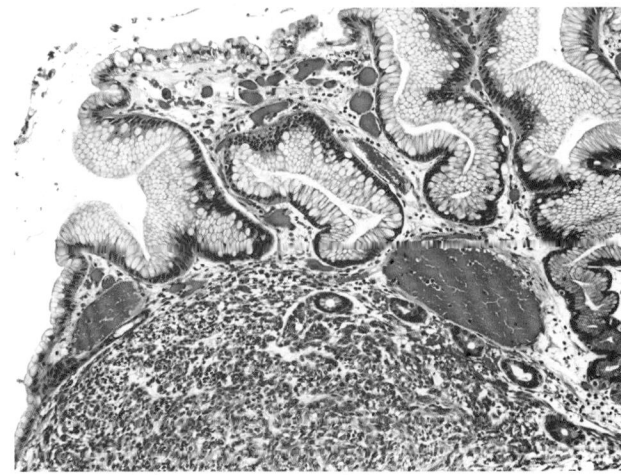

Figure 6-88. Gastrointestinal stromal tumor. This lesion has extended into the gastric mucosa, often an indication of aggressive behavior.

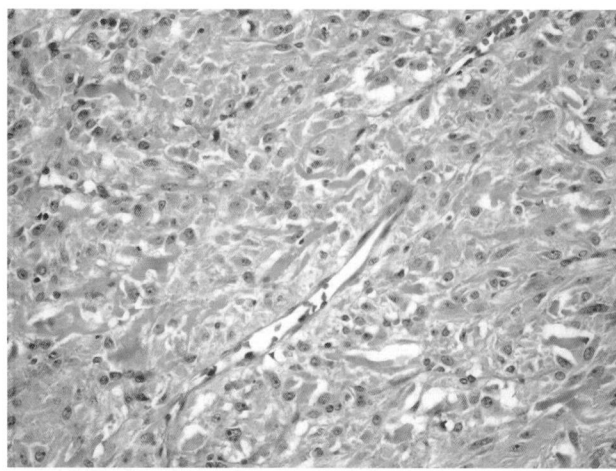

Figure 6-89. Gastrointestinal stromal tumor. The wiry eosinophilic collagen fibrils have been termed skenoid fibrils because their ultra-structural features reminded our forefathers of the appearance of skeins of yarn. They are characteristic of small intestinal gastrointestinal stromal tumors and their presence has correlated with favorable outcome.

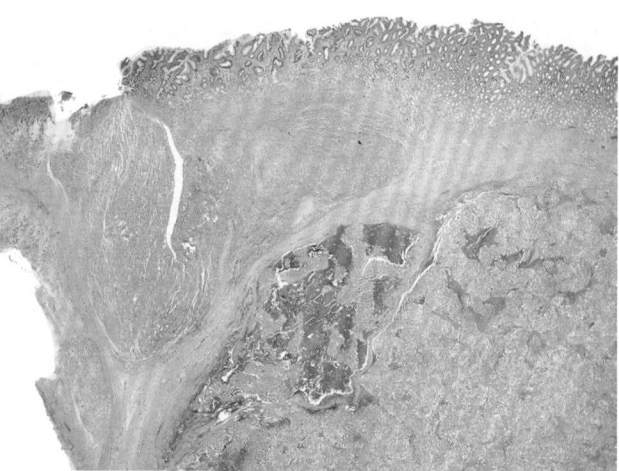

Figure 6-90. Gastrointestinal stromal tumor. This is an epithelioid gastric lesion.

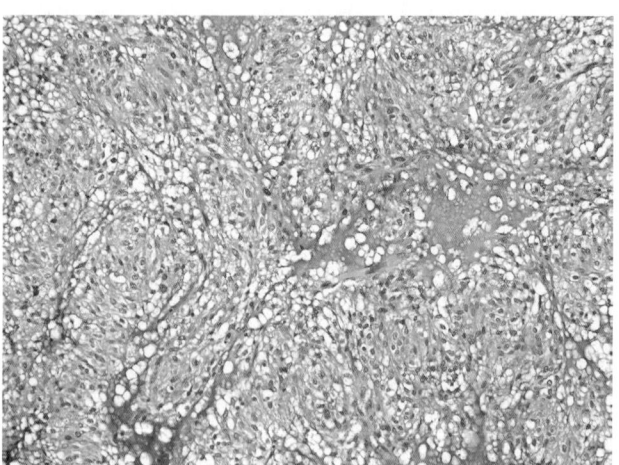

Figure 6-91. Gastrointestinal stromal tumor. Like spindle cell gastrointestinal stromal tumors, epithelioid ones can have many paranuclear vacuoles.

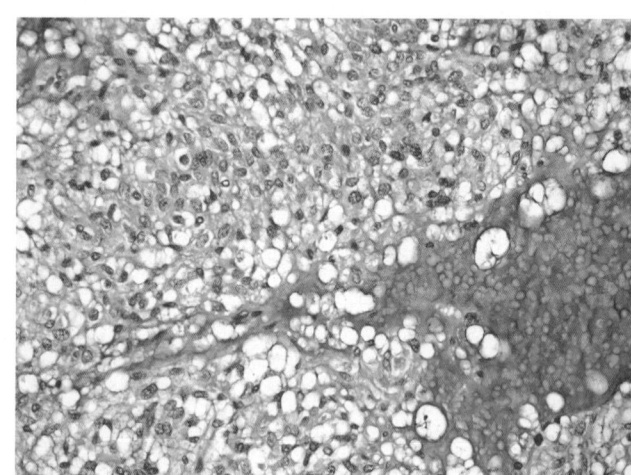

Figure 6-92. Gastrointestinal stromal tumor. The nuclei are uniform in this epithelioid gastrointestinal stromal tumor.

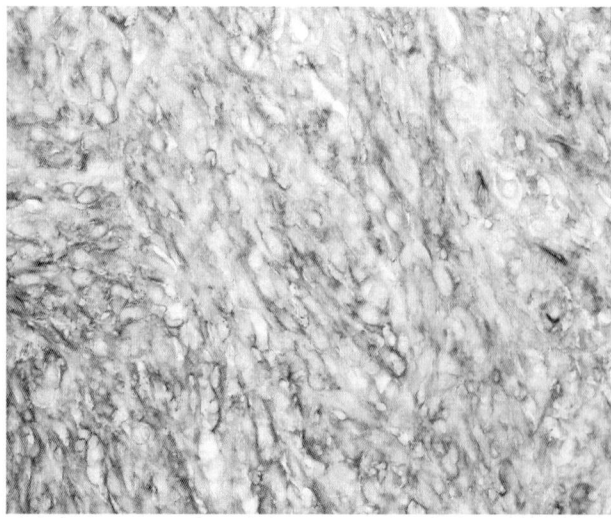

Figure 6-93. Gastrointestinal stromal tumor. This is a CD34 stain.

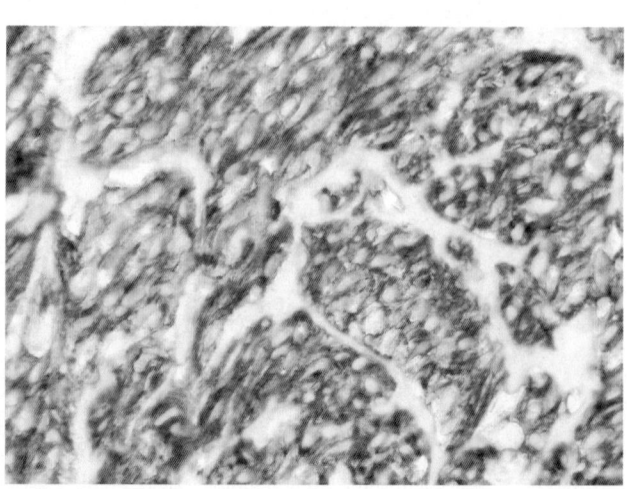

Figure 6-94. Gastrointestinal stromal tumor. This is a CD117/KIT stain.

additional mutations, GISTs can dedifferentiate into pleomorphic sarcomas that lose their characteristic immunolabeling pattern. Additionally, sometimes SDH-deficient GISTs have pleomorphic nuclei. The message is that if a diagnosis of GIST is being entertained for a pleomorphic sarcoma in the GI tract, it is important to consider alternative interpretations such as leiomyosarcoma, sarcomatoid carcinoma, melanoma, and dedifferentiated liposarcoma.

An immunohistochemical panel that can be performed in assessing GISTs might include CD117/KIT, S100 protein (to address melanoma), and a cytokeratin stain to address signet cell carcinoma if the lesion is epithelioid, but the morphology is often so characteristic that such testing is not needed. Of course, in cytologic preparations, KIT testing on cell blocks can be reassuring.

The vast majority of GISTs have *KIT* mutations and are CD117/KIT positive, but about 5% (from all sites) lack *KIT* mutations and many in the CD117 negative subset have alternate mutations of platelet-derived growth factor-α instead.[50-52] Because about 70% of gastric GISTs express CD34, this can also be included in a diagnostic panel. The addition of DOG1 (discovered on GISTs1, also known as anoctin 1 or ANO1 and ORAOV2 or—overexpressed in oral carcinoma) to the diagnostic armamentarium for GISTs has been useful but more so for gastric GISTs than intestinal ones.[37] DOG1 is a chloride channel protein that was found to be overexpressed in GISTs by gene profiling studies.[53-55] It is expressed by about 95% of GISTs. Overall DOG1 is expressed in 36% to 92% of KIT-negative GISTs.[37] This stain has been illustrated in "Esophagus" chapter (Fig. 1.15), and it has a labeling pattern similar to that of CD117/KIT. KIT is more sensitive for intestinal GISTs than DOG1. However, the two markers together[28] capture nearly all GISTs.

PEARLS & PITFALLS: Evaluating Gastrointestinal Stromal Tumors

Be sure to use S100 protein or SOX10 as the immunostain to address spindle cell melanoma rather than one of the so-called melanoma markers. The reasoning is that many spindle cell melanomas do not label with HMB45 or MELAN-A, and, at least in one of our labs, MELAN-A tends to be found in epithelioid GISTs (Fig. 6.95).[56] Another important pitfall is the proclivity of gastric and esophageal adenocarcinomas to express DOG1[57] (Figs. 6.96–6.98).

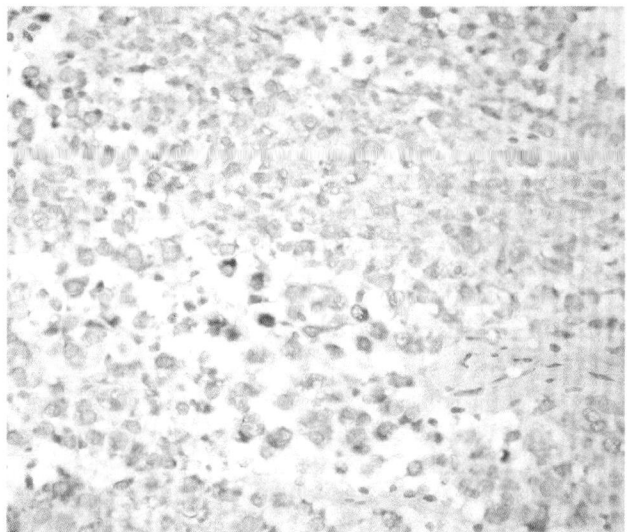

Figure 6-95. Gastrointestinal stromal tumor. This epithelioid gastrointestinal stromal tumor of the stomach shows nonspecific labeling with MELAN-A.

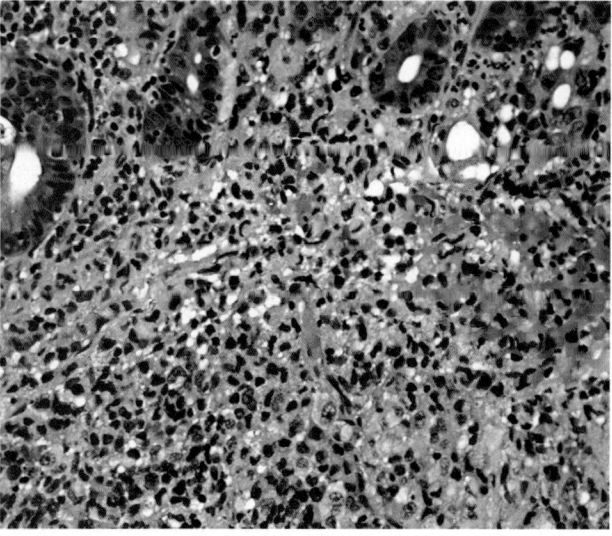

Figure 6-96. Gastric adenocarcinoma. The tumor is poorly differentiated such that an immunolabeling panel was done to address several types of neoplasms.

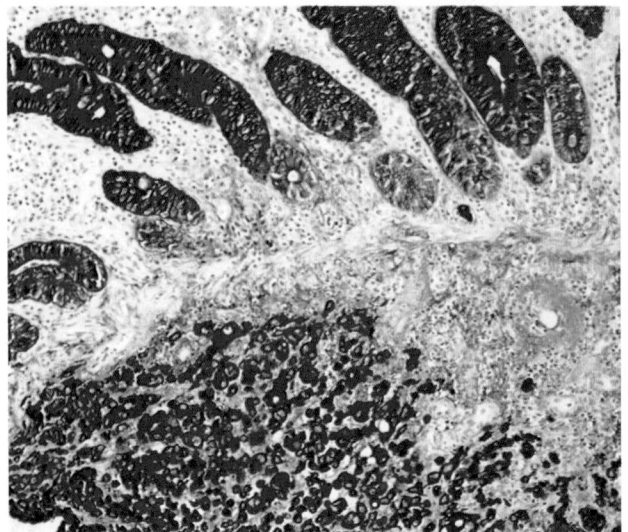

Figure 6-97. Gastric adenocarcinoma. This is a pankeratin stain, which labels the tumor and the overlying gastric mucosa.

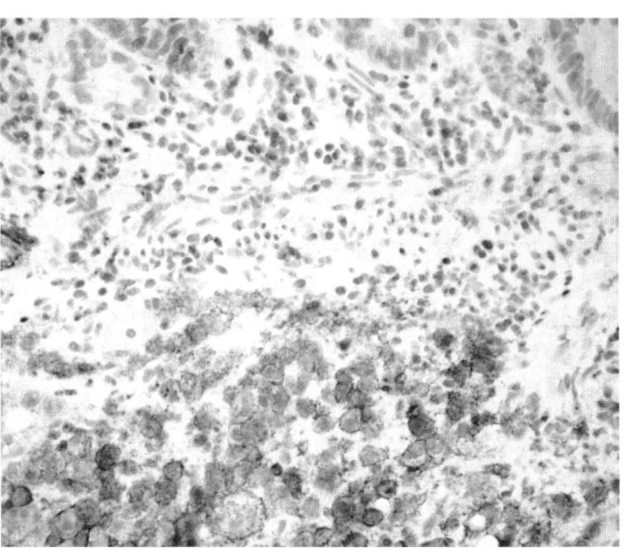

Figure 6-98. Gastric adenocarcinoma. This DOG1 stain is reactive. The gastric epithelium is weakly reactive. DOG1 labeling has been reported in about a third of gastroesophageal adenocarcinomas.

Mutational Analysis in Gastrointestinal Stromal Tumors

The most common mutations in GISTs are those of exon 11 of the *KIT* gene. These mutations are found in GISTs from all sites of the GI tract and their presence correlates with excellent responses to imatinib treatment. About 20% of GISTs have mutations in exon 9 instead, and these usually arise in the intestines (small and large). These are less sensitive to imatinib. Tumors with mutations in exons 13, 17, and 8 also tend to affect the small bowel although there are few data on the latter because they are rare.[28,37] Occasional small intestinal GISTs have *BRAF* V600E mutations. So-called dedifferentiated GISTs have various *KIT* mutations in both the low- and high-grade components.[58]

FAQ: Is it necessary to order mutational analysis on all GISTs?

Answer: Although some have advocated for universal mutational analysis of GISTs, there are situations for which molecular analysis of GISTs is silly, such as in the case of tiny "seedling" GISTs as discussed later. It is probably best to discuss the issue with treating colleagues. Some observers, however, advocate for universal testing so that mutational status is already known should a tumor recur. Testing for large mitotically active lesions is never unreasonable.

Prognostication in Gastrointestinal Stromal Tumors

Essentially it is our job to assess mitotic counts and tumor size to prognosticate. On mucosal biopsies, it is often impossible to assess tumor size and mitotic counts, but it is possible to make a diagnosis in many cases and schedule the patient for an operation to remove the tumor. It is worth looking back on the raw data that are the foundations of the AJCC staging scheme.[59] The former AFIP group had the best studies of gastric stromal tumors and reported 1,765 GISTs confined to the stomach, with follow-up information[60] in the preimatinib era. The group had slight male predominance (55%) and a median age of 63 years. Only 2.7% of the tumors arose in patients before age 21 years, and 9.1% before age 40 years. Outcome was strongly dependent on tumor size and mitotic activity. Only 2% to 3% of tumors <10 cm and <5 mitoses per 50 HPF metastasized, whereas 86% of tumors >10 cm and >5 mitoses per 50 HPF metastasized. However, tumors >10 cm with mitotic activity <5 per 50 HPF and those <5 cm with mitoses >5 per 50 HPF had relatively low metastatic rates (11% and 15%, respectively). A small number of patients survived intra-abdominal metastasis to >20 years. Tumor location in the fundus or the gastroesophageal junction, coagulative necrosis, ulceration, and mucosal invasion were all unfavorable factors ($P < .001$), whereas tumor location in the antrum was favorable ($P < .001$). Probably the key feature of this very large series is that it allowed the separating out of a "benign" category of gastric GISTs, based on large numbers of cases.[60]

After they published their data on gastric GISTs, Miettinen et al. then reported a large series of jejunal and ileal GISTs with long-term follow-up from the preimatinib era. For this cohort, there were 906 patients.[61] Overall tumor-specific mortality was 39%, twice that for gastric GISTs. In general, mortality increased with tumor size and mitotic rate.

The Miettinen data have thus informed the current staging system such that different schemes are used for stomach and omentum versus small bowel and other sites. Furthermore, nomograms and other clinical tools developed for prognostication in GISTs are all based on the Miettinen data.[62,63]

Table 6.3 shows the reporting scheme that can be used based on mitotic activity and tumor size. We would note that the 2018 AJCC has a comment on mitotic counts that is very important:

> The mitotic rate is best expressed as the number of mitoses per 5 mm^2 (using 400x magnification). This value corresponds to 50 HPF in large prognostic studies obtained with older-model microscopes using "conventional" optics (i.e., not using a wide field size). The number of fields required for 5 mm^2 should be determined for individual microscopes. ***Practically, this means counting mitoses in 20-25 HPF with modern microscopes…***[59]

Using the correct counting will not usually matter because GISTs tend to have either almost no mitoses or lots of them!

FAQ: How well do the new targeted treatments work?

Answer: With modern therapy using imatinib (Gleevec) as a first-line drug and sunitinib or regorafenib as second- and third-line drugs, the outcome has improved[64] (Figs. 6.99 and 6.100). Whereas the 5-year survival for malignant GISTs was on the order of 50% before there were targeted treatments, now it is closer to 75%. Unfortunately most (about 80%) of these tumors develop resistance to the available drugs over time.

FAQ: What is the difference in reporting mitotic counts and size versus mutational analysis?

Answer: It is important to remember that the size and mitotic index measurements are used to prognosticate, whereas mutational analysis is best for predicting response to targeted therapy.

TABLE 6.3: Risk Assessment in Gastrointestinal Stromal Tumors

Tumor Size (cm)	T Stage, AJCC	Mitotic Rate[a] <5—Low >5—High	Risk of Progression for Gastric Lesions (With Anticipated Similar Outcome for Omental Lesions)/AJCC Stage Group[b]	Risk of Progression for Small Bowel Lesions (With Anticipated Similar Outcome for Esophagus, Colon, Mesentery, Peritoneum/AJCC Stage Group[b]
<2	T1	Low	0%/IA	0%/IA
<2	T1	High	No data	50%/IIIA
>2–5	T2	Low	0%/IA	0%/I
>2–5	T2	High	16%/II	73%/IIIB
>5–10	T3	Low	3%–4%/IB	24%/II
>5–10	T3	High	55%/IIIA	85%/IIIB
>10	T4	Low	12%/II	52%/IIIB
>10	T4	High	86%/IIIB	90%/IIIB

[a]The mitotic rate is best expressed as the number of mitoses per 5 mm² (using 400× magnification). This value corresponds to 50 HPF in large prognostic studies obtained with older-model microscopes using conventional optics (i.e., not using a wide field size). The number of fields required for 5 mm² should be determined for individual microscopes. ***Practically, this means counting mitoses in 20–25 HPF with modern microscopes....***"[59]

[b]If there are nodes or distant metastases, the lesion is designated as Stage group IV regardless of any other parameter.[59]

Modified from Amin M, Edge S, Greene F, et al. *AJCC Cancer Staging Manual*. 8th ed. Springer International Publishing AG Switzerland; 2017; Miettinen M, Sobin LH, Lasota J. Gastrointestinal stromal tumors of the stomach: a clinicopathologic, immunohistochemical, and molecular genetic study of 1765 cases with long-term follow-up. *Am J Surg Pathol*. 2005;29(1):52-68; Miettinen M, Makhlouf H, Sobin LH, Lasota J. Gastrointestinal stromal tumors of the jejunum and ileum: a clinicopathologic, immunohistochemical, and molecular genetic study of 906 cases before imatinib with long-term follow-up. *Am J Surg Pathol*. 2006;30(4):477-489.

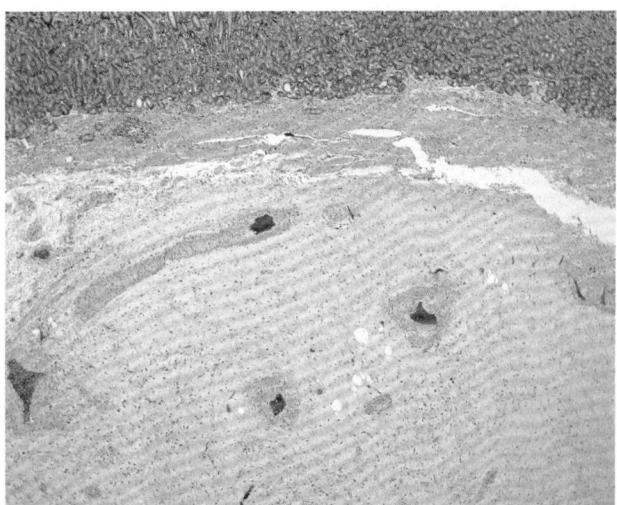

Figure 6-99. Treated gastrointestinal stromal tumor. The lesion has undergone extensive sclerosis.

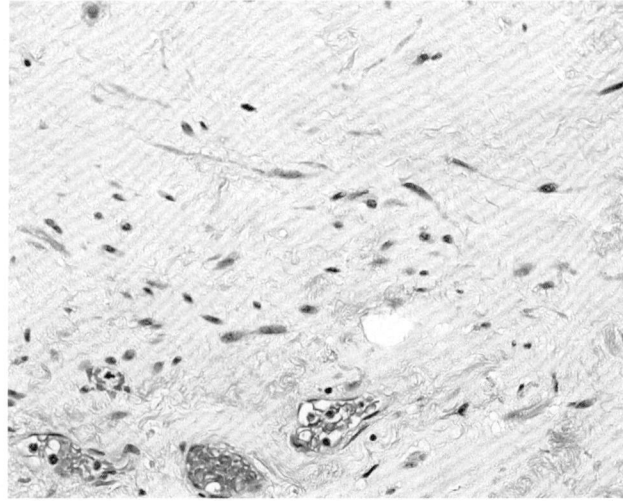

Figure 6-100. Treated gastrointestinal stromal tumor. A few viable nuclei remain.

Succinate Dehydrogenase–Deficient Gastrointestinal Stromal Tumors

SDH-deficient GISTs are fascinating and have wonderfully interesting morphology. There is a female predominance and these special GISTs arise only in the stomach.[38,39,41,44,48,65-69] They are characterized by a plexiform growth pattern and epithelioid morphology, with prominent vascularity (Figs. 6.101–6.109). They express CD117 and DOG1, but they lack *KIT* or *PDGRFA* mutations. They often spread to lymph nodes but yet do not behave aggressively. The usual risk assessments do not predict outcome in these tumors.[70] These tumors have been reviewed in detail by Leona Doyle and Jason Hornick.[37]

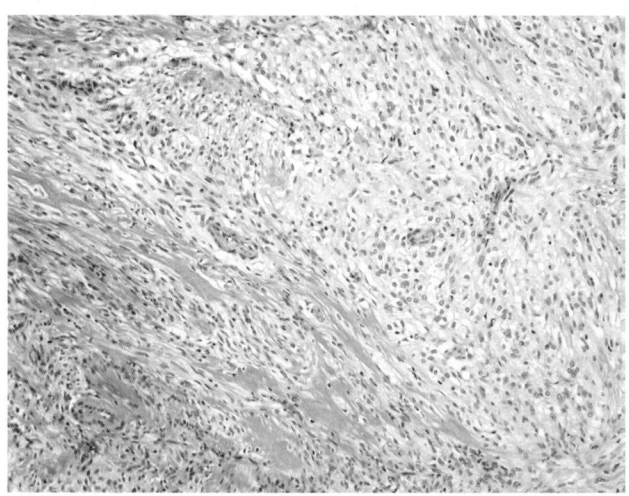

Figure 6-101. Gastrointestinal stromal tumor. This example is epithelioid and had a plexiform pattern such that the possibility of a succinate dehydrogenase–deficient gastrointestinal stromal tumor was considered but this tumor proved proficient.

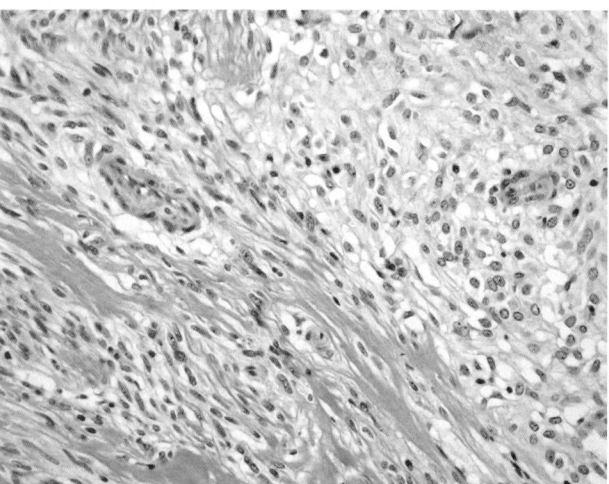

Figure 6-102. Gastrointestinal stromal tumor. This is a high magnification image of the neoplasm seen in Fig. 6.101.

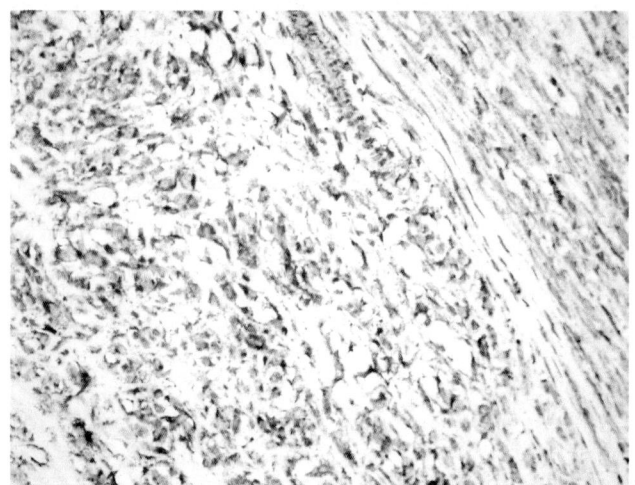

Figure 6-103. Gastrointestinal stromal tumor. This is a succinate dehydrogenase B (SDHB) stain of the lesion seen in Figs. 6.101 and 6.102. The tumor cells and all other cells in the image stain. SDH is a component of the Krebs metabolic cycle such that all cells in the body should contain it. It is thus always easy to find internal positive controls in stained sections.

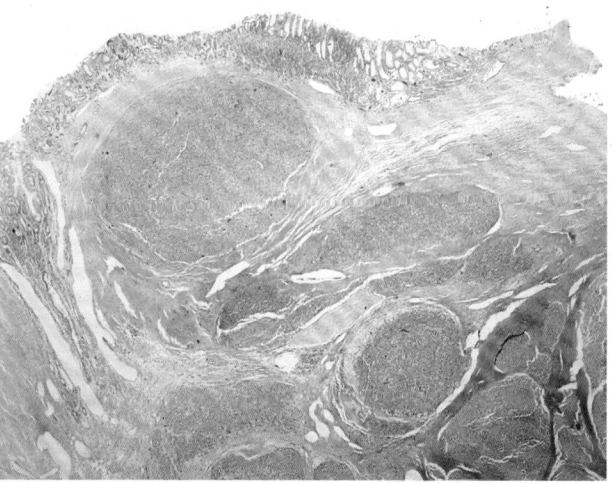

Figure 6-104. Succinate dehydrogenase–deficient gastrointestinal stromal tumor. This tumor arose in the stomach—such tumors reported to date have all been gastric. Note the plexiform architecture with nodules separated by normal muscularis propria. Imagine a worm balled up in the tissue in three dimensions but cut in two dimensions to consider the meaning of plexiform.

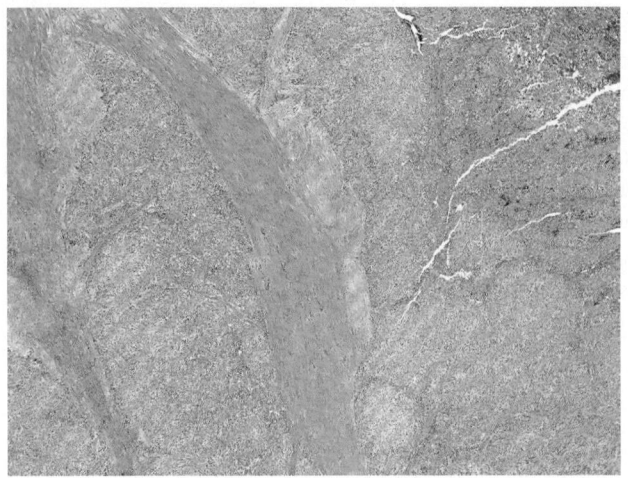

Figure 6-105. Succinate dehydrogenase–deficient gastrointestinal stromal tumor. This example is slightly less plexiform.

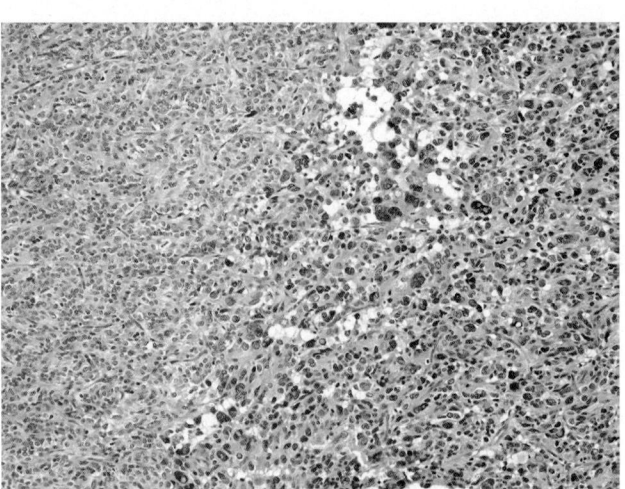

Figure 6-106. Succinate dehydrogenase–deficient gastrointestinal stromal tumor. This type is an exception to the rule of monotonous cytologic features in gastrointestinal stromal tumors. In this example, there are uniform epithelioid cells on the left but larger pleomorphic ones on the right. However, mitoses are sparse.

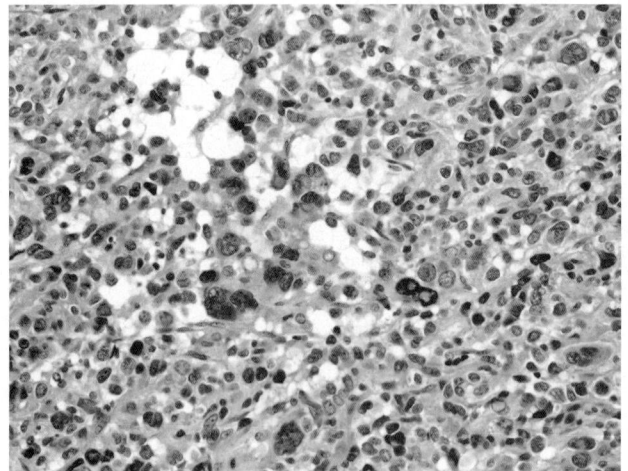

Figure 6-107. Succinate dehydrogenase–deficient gastrointestinal stromal tumor. This field shows dramatic cytologic alterations, but the tumor lacks mitoses.

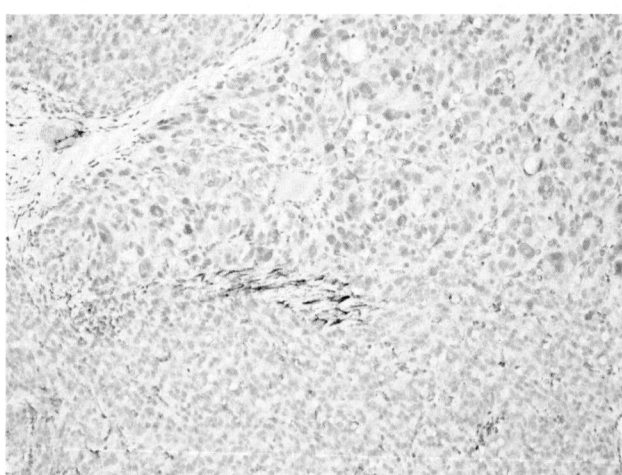

Figure 6-108. Succinate dehydrogenase–deficient gastrointestinal stromal tumor. This is an SDHB stain. Smooth muscle and endothelial cells serve as internal positive controls, but there is loss in the neoplasm.

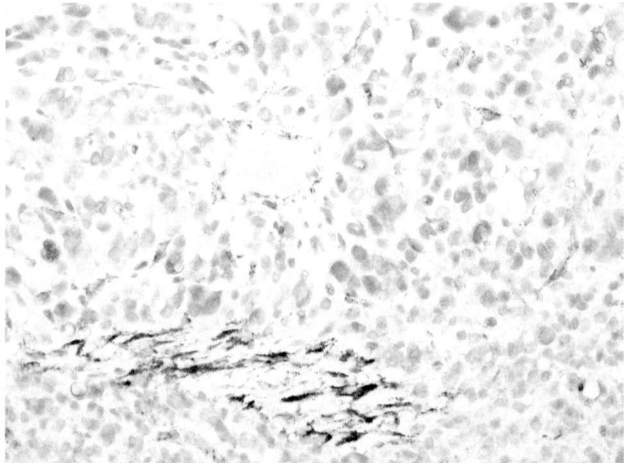

Figure 6-109. Succinate dehydrogenase–deficient gastrointestinal stromal tumor. This is a high magnification image of the SDHB preparation seen in Fig. 6.108.

SDH is an enzyme in the Krebs cycle, which we all forgot about years ago right after learning it. The SDH enzyme complex has four components: SDHA, SDHB, SDHC, and SDHD. The key molecule for diagnostic purposes is SDHB. The SDH complex is found in every cell in the body, but if any component is lost, SDHB will be lost on immunolabeling. On the other hand, loss of SDHA immunolabeling indicates loss of SDHA only. About a third of SDH-deficient GISTs are associated with *SDHA* mutations; these are usually found in adult females and are not usually familial.

Abnormalities of the SDH complex were initially identified in familial paraganglioma syndrome. Affected patients have germline alterations in the genes encoding for SDHB, SDHC, or SDHD. GISTs from patients with Carney-Stratakis syndrome were then found to have similar alterations. Carney-Stratakis syndrome is a variant of familial paraganglioma syndrome in which patients also develop GISTs. It is an autosomal dominant condition with incomplete penetrance that has the same genetic alterations as the familial paraganglioma syndrome. A syndrome with a similar name, Carney triad, consists gastric GIST, paraganglioma, and pulmonary chondroma. Affected patients can also have esophageal leiomyomas and adrenal adenomas. These patients have SDH-deficient GISTs but no germline mutations.

GISTs arising in children are also likely to be SDH deficient and display the plexiform growth pattern and spread to lymph nodes noted earlier.

Microscopic Incidental Gastric Gastrointestinal Stromal Tumors

Tiny (microscopic) GISTs can be found in gastrectomies performed for other indications (for example, in bariatric surgery samples) and in about 3% of stomachs at autopsy[71] and in about 10% of esophagogastric resections performed for carcinomas in which the entirely embedded esophagogastric junction is studied.[72] They can be regarded as incidental benign lesions that do not merit follow-up (Figs. 6.110–6.112). Because clinically detected GISTs are rare, such incidental (seedling[72]) GISTs presumably are highly unlikely to progress to clinically important lesions. The studied seedling tumors have harbored activating *KIT* and *PDGFRA* mutations such that they are neoplasms rather than hyperplasias.

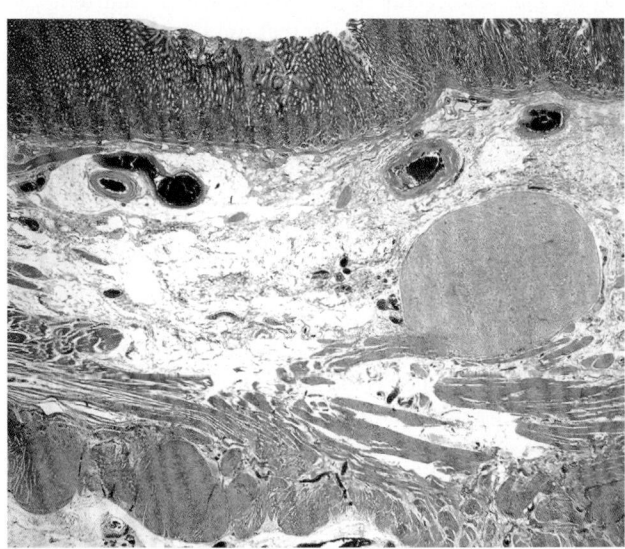

Figure 6-110. Incidental "seedling" gastrointestinal stromal tumors at the gastroesophageal junction. These tiny tumors are probably not destined to progress as they are common in autopsy series.

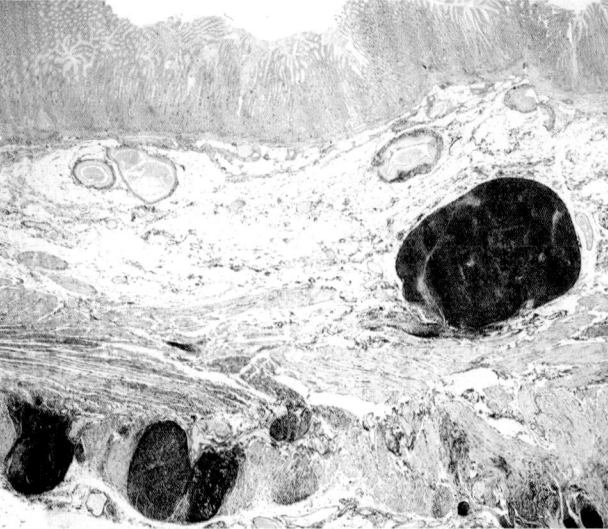

Figure 6-111. Incidental "seedling" gastrointestinal stromal tumors at the gastroesophageal junction. This is a CD34 stain.

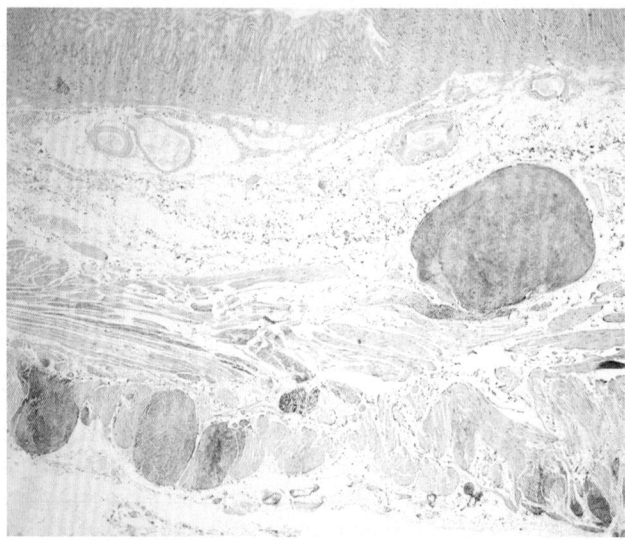

Figure 6-112. Incidental "seedling" gastrointestinal stromal tumors at the gastroesophageal junction. This is a CD117/KIT stain.

INFLAMMATORY FIBROID POLYP

The first description of these tumors was by J. Vaněk and appeared in the *American Journal of Pathology* in 1949,[73] although there were prior case reports. Professor Vaněk was from Pilsen in the Czech Republic, so presumably these tumors were discussed over mugs of Pilsen beer. The present term "inflammatory fibroid polyp" was coined later[74] and has remained despite the fact that we now know that these lesions are benign neoplasms. The vast majority of inflammatory fibroid polyps arise in the stomach, where they account for about 3% to 4% of all gastric polyps after excluding fundic gland polyps,[75,76] but they can be found throughout the gastrointestinal tract. Patients with gastric examples are typically 60 to 80 years old.[75] These polyps are quite rare in children.[77] Most arise in the antrum. The endoscopic appearance is that of a smooth submucosal lesion that can be pedunculated or sessile with surface ulceration/erosion. Small intestinal examples lead to intussusception about half the time[78] or obstruction, and gastric examples are found in patients with pain, nausea, and vomiting. They were believed to be reactive in the past, but they are now known to harbor mutations in the *platelet-derived growth factor receptor alpha (PDGFRA)* gene,[79] akin to a subset of GISTs. However, inflammatory fibroid polyps are always benign, whereas *PDGFRA*-mutated GISTs are not. Presumably, the inflammatory polyps reported in an English family in which three generations of women had Devon polyposis lesions[80,81] arose in the setting of some sort of familial alteration in *PDGFRA*.

Microscopically, inflammatory fibroid polyps are well-marginated, but nonencapsulated, and centered in the submucosa, but they sometimes extend up into the mucosa (Figs. 6.113–6.122). They are formed by uniform spindled cells, mixed inflammatory cells typically with numerous eosinophils, and they have prominent vasculature. The spindle cells have amphophilic elongated cytoplasm and pale nuclei, ranging from ovoid to spindle shaped. Often there is a whorled, "onion skin" proliferation around vessels. Mitoses are infrequent.

On immunolabeling, there is variable actin but no S100 protein or epithelial marker expression, but the key feature is consistent CD34 reactivity in small tumors (Fig. 6.122), which sometimes is diminished as lesions attain larger sizes.[82] The CD34 expression raises the differential diagnostic consideration of GIST, but the morphology is different and inflammatory fibroid polyps lack CD117 and DOG1 expression. In large examples, sarcomas are often considered, especially myxoid liposarcoma, but the bland appearance of the proliferating cells and the inflammatory background argue against this interpretation.

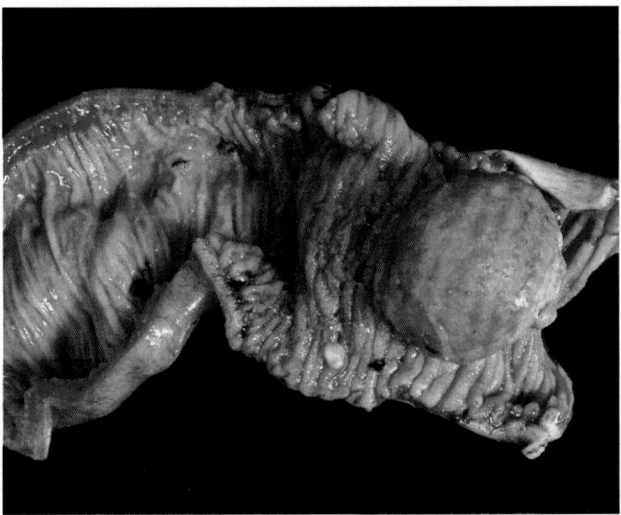

Figure 6-113. Inflammatory fibroid polyp. This small intestinal submucosal tumor resulted in intussusception.

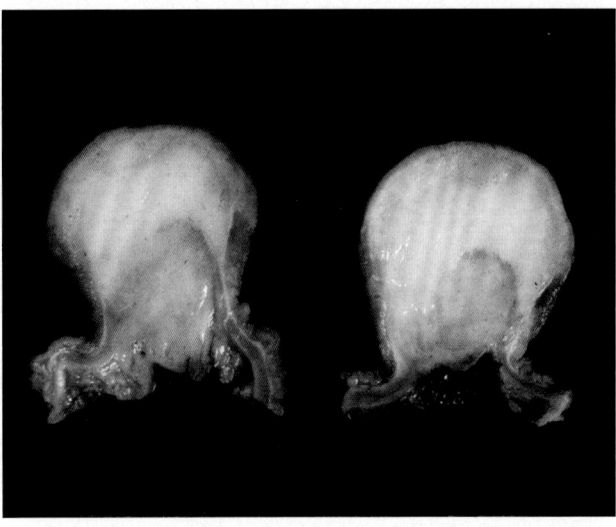

Figure 6-114. Inflammatory fibroid polyp. This is a cross section of the neoplasm seen in Fig. 6.114. The submucosal location of the tumor is apparent.

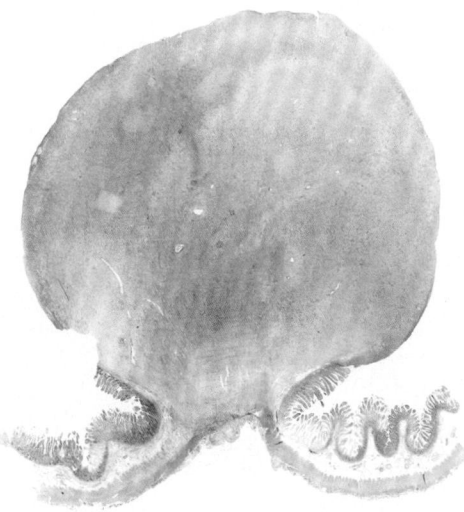

Figure 6-115. Inflammatory fibroid polyp. The neoplasm is centered in the submucosa. Intussusception resulted in surface ulceration.

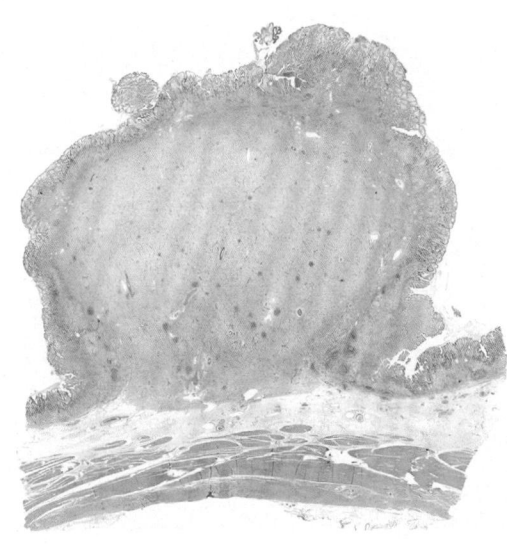

Figure 6-116. Inflammatory fibroid polyp. This gastric example resulted in gastric outlet obstruction. Note that the tumor is centered in the submucosa and contains lymphoid aggregates.

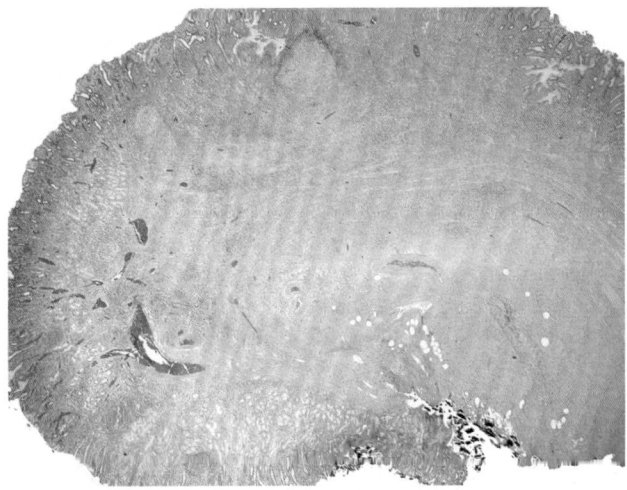

Figure 6-117. Inflammatory fibroid polyp. This is a gastric antral polypectomy. The tumor is centered in the submucosa.

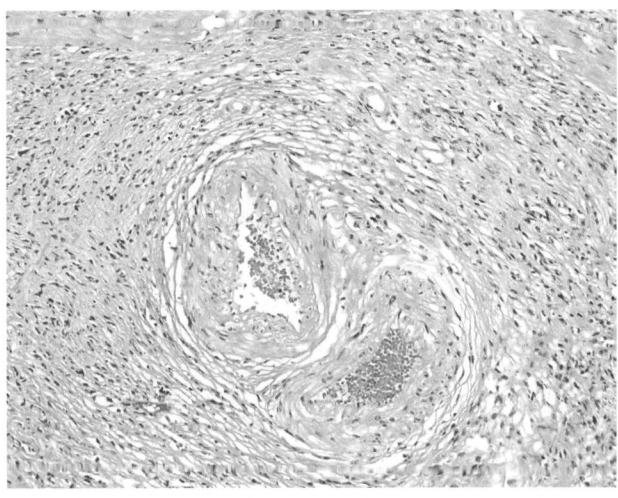

Figure 6-118. Inflammatory fibroid polyp. The tumor cells whorl around submucosal vessels.

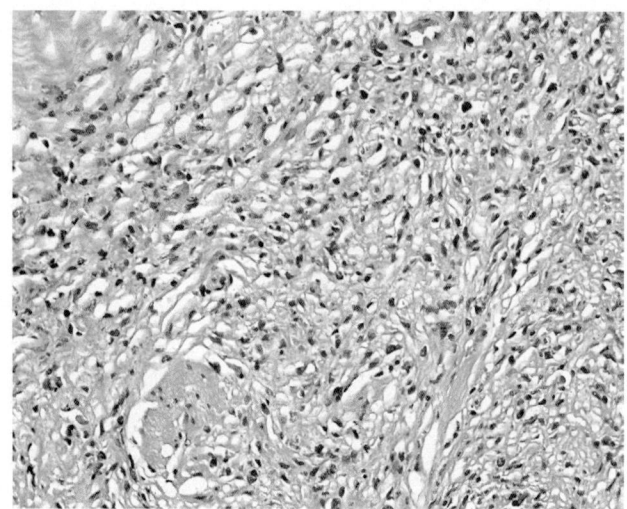

Figure 6-119. Inflammatory fibroid polyp. Note the backdrop of eosinophils and the uniform nuclei of the tumor cells.

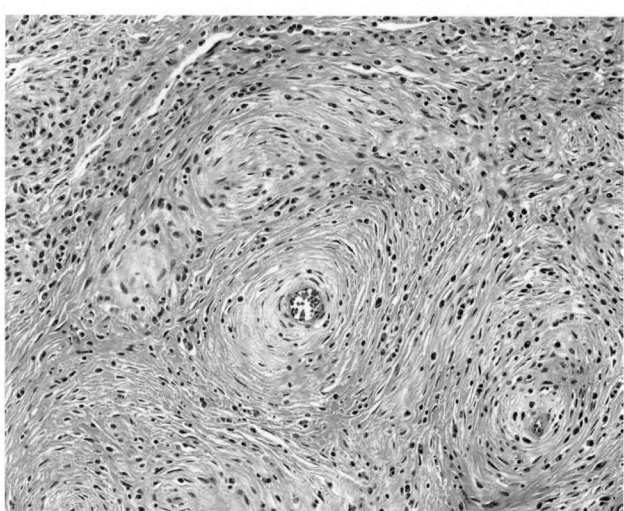

Figure 6-120. Inflammatory fibroid polyp. This example shows a striking "onion skin" appearance, as cells whorl around the submucosal vessels. Many eosinophils are present.

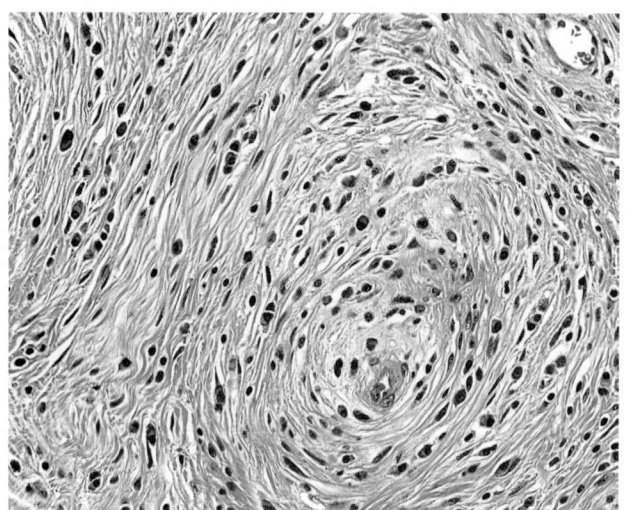

Figure 6-121. Inflammatory fibroid polyp. This is a high magnification image of the lesion shown in Fig. 6.120.

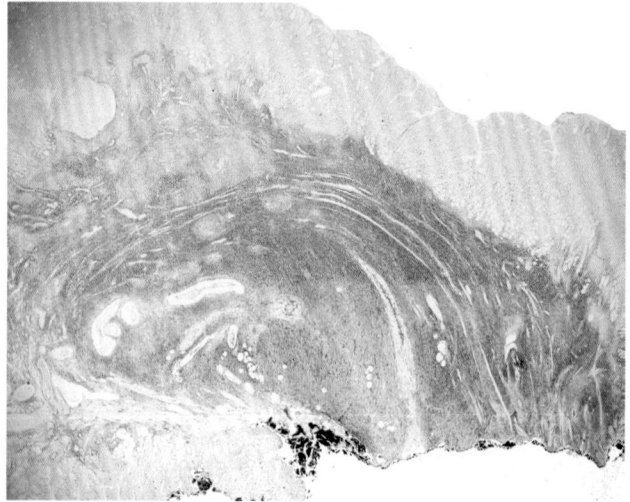

Figure 6-122. Inflammatory fibroid polyp. This is a CD34 stain from the inflammatory fibroid polyp shown in Fig. 6.117.

SMOOTH MUSCLE NEOPLASMS

There is generally no reason to worry about a brightly eosinophilic colorectal spindle cell lesion with bland cytologic features arising in association with the muscularis mucosae because it is an incidental leiomyoma, managed by polypectomy[83] (Figs. 6.123–6.132). However, most spindle cell tumors of the GI tract are GISTs except in the esophagus and superficial distal colon where leiomyomas predominate. Most muscularis mucosae–associated tumors of the colorectum are leiomyomas. Leiomyomas of the colon have a male predominance (overall 2.4:1) and are found in adults. They are typically small (1 to 2 cm) and located predominantly in the rectum and sigmoid colon. If immunolabeling is done, leiomyomas express desmin, but not CD34, CD117, and S100 protein. In daily practice, we do not perform immunohistochemical stains on these lesions, but in any doubtful case, a negative CD117 is reassuring.

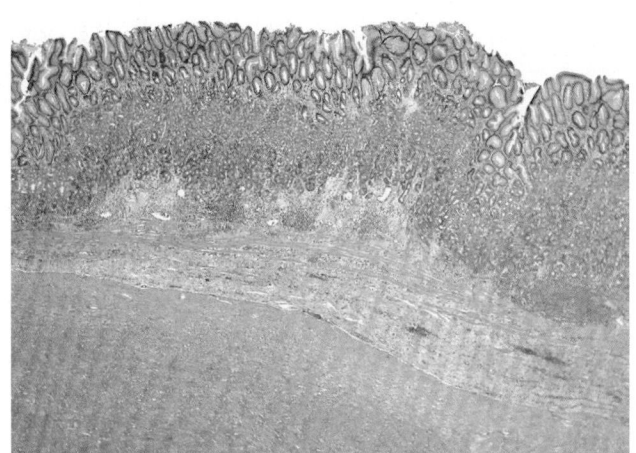

Figure 6-123. Leiomyoma. This is a gastric leiomyoma. It is seen in the muscularis propria and is of the same color as the muscularis mucosae. It is brightly eosinophilic and paucicellular.

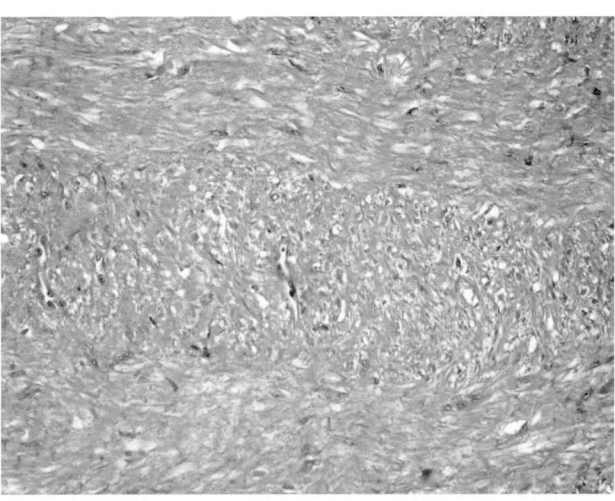

Figure 6-124. Leiomyoma. The cytoplasm is *bright pink* and the nuclei are bland with pale chromatin. The fascicles are perpendicular to one another. The ones at the bottom and top course across the image, whereas the one in the center is seen cut en face with the fibers diving into the image and cut across their bellies. This perpendicular orientation is characteristic of smooth muscle tumor fascicles, whether benign or malignant.

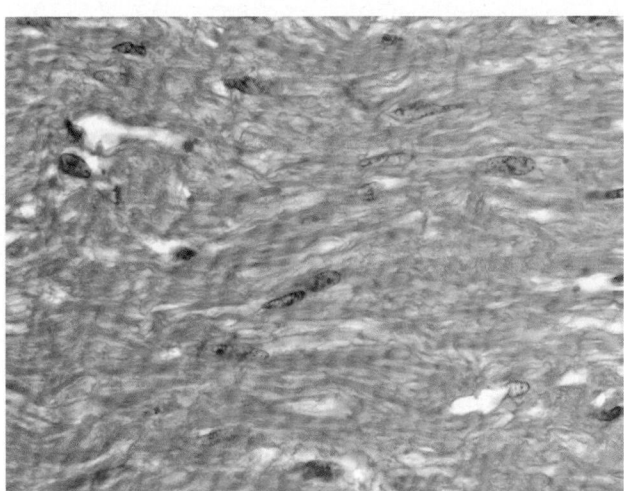

Figure 6-125. Leiomyoma. Note the delicate longitudinal striations and blunted ended nuclei.

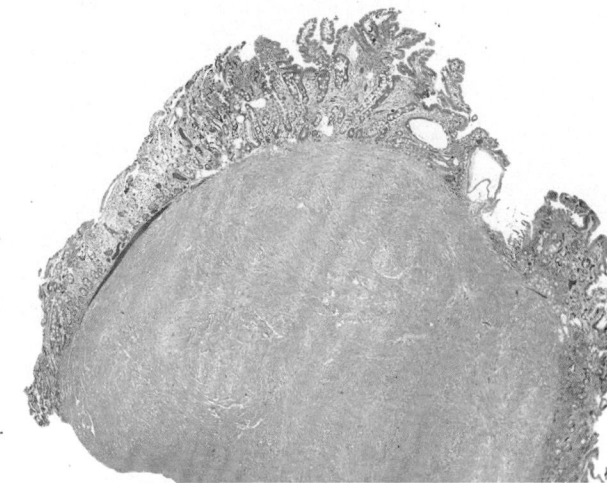

Figure 6-126. Leiomyoma. This lesion has arisen in association with the muscularis mucosae of the small bowel. It has the same appearance as that of the gastric one seen in Figs. 6.123–6.125.

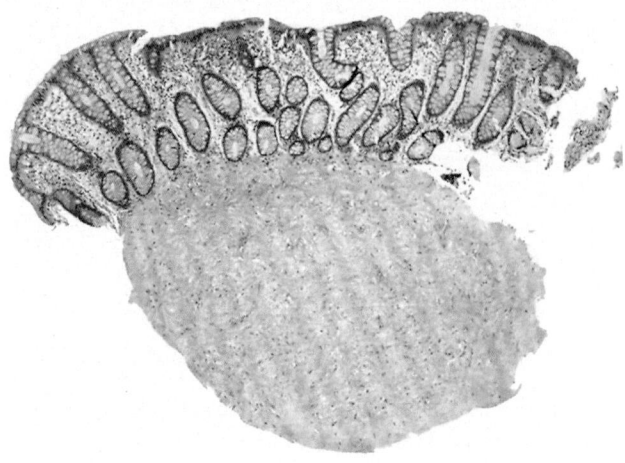

Figure 6-127. Leiomyoma. Colorectal leiomyomas typically are detected on colonoscopy because they arise in association with the muscularis mucosae and present as distal colorectal polyps.

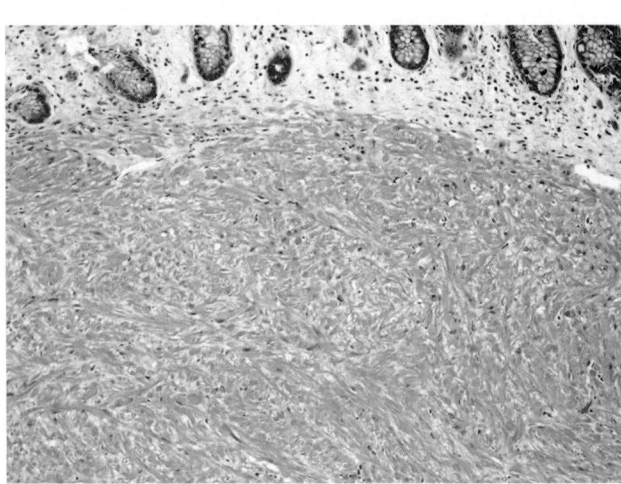

Figure 6-128. Leiomyoma. The lesion drips off the muscularis mucosae of the colon.

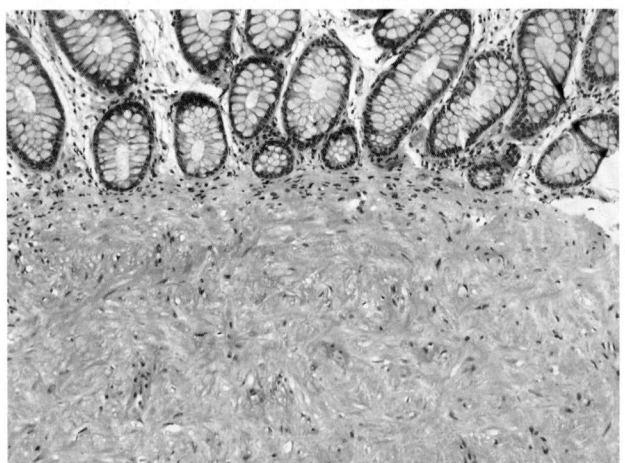

Figure 6-129. Leiomyoma. There is a sliver of residual nonneoplastic muscularis mucosae at the top of the lesion.

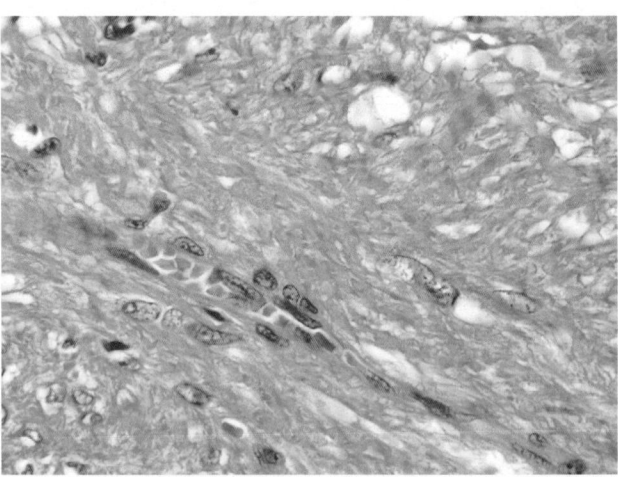

Figure 6-130. Leiomyoma. There is a cell with a paranuclear vacuole at the right. The tumor cell nuclei are paler than those of the endothelial cells in the capillary that tracks through the center of the image.

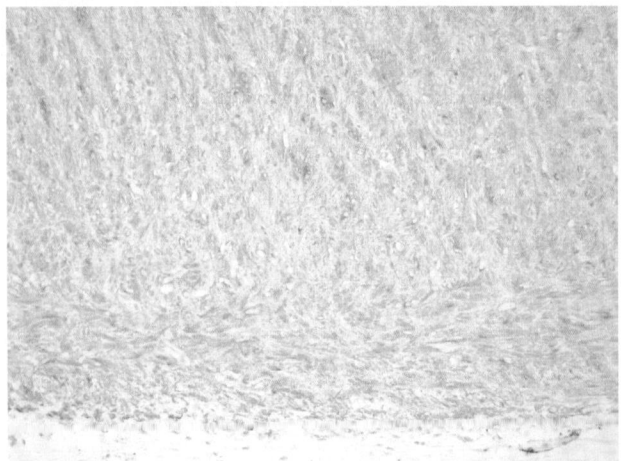

Figure 6-131. Leiomyoma. This is an actin stain. There is really no reason to stain such tumors because they are diagnostic on hematoxylin and eosin.

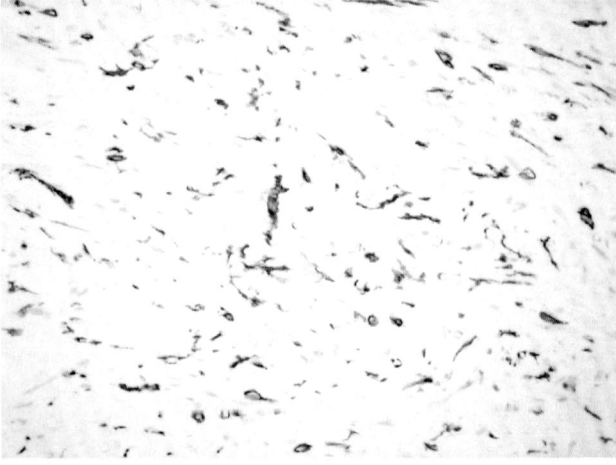

Figure 6-132. Leiomyoma. This CD117 stain highlights Cajal cells that are either entrapped in or proliferate as a subcomponent of these benign lesions. If this staining is performed, it is important to be aware of the possibility of observing this staining pattern in leiomyomas.

Leiomyosarcomas of the gastrointestinal tract display the same features as leiomyosarcomas elsewhere in the body. They have perfectly perpendicular fascicles of spindle cells with brightly pink cytoplasm, pleomorphic blunt-ended nuclei, and paranuclear vacuoles just like leiomyosarcomas elsewhere in the body (Figs. 6.133–6.140). The issue is typically in separating them from GISTs, which is unusually easy because they are usually desmin+, CD117−. They are also more pleomorphic than GISTs.

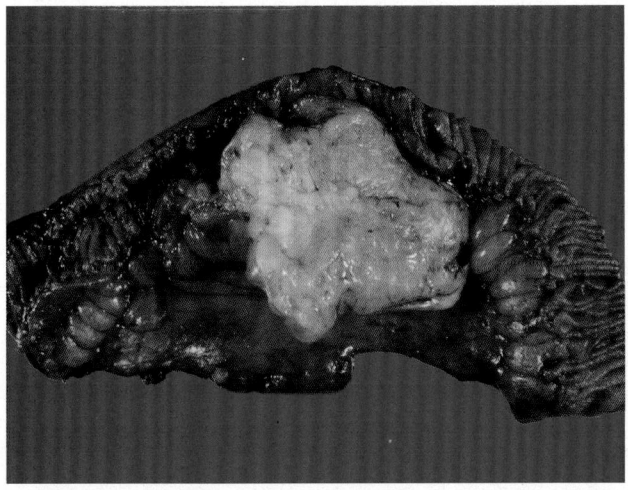

Figure 6-133. Leiomyosarcoma. There is nothing specific about the appearance of this ileal leiomyosarcoma.

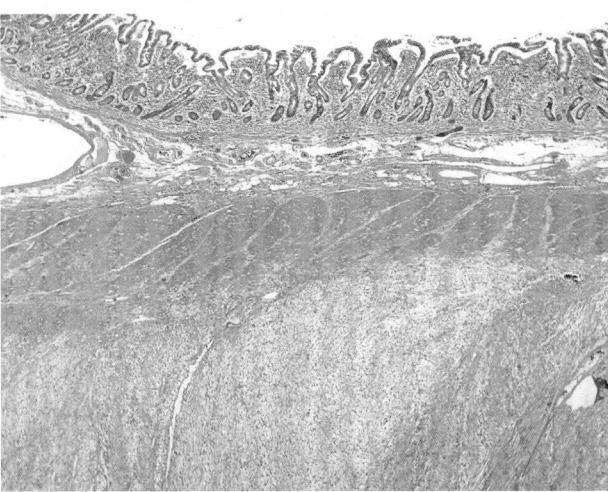

Figure 6-134. Leiomyosarcoma. The cytoplasm of the cells is brightly eosinophilic in keeping with smooth muscle differentiation, but there are plenty of dark enlarged nuclei, so the tumor is clearly not a leiomyoma even at scanning magnification.

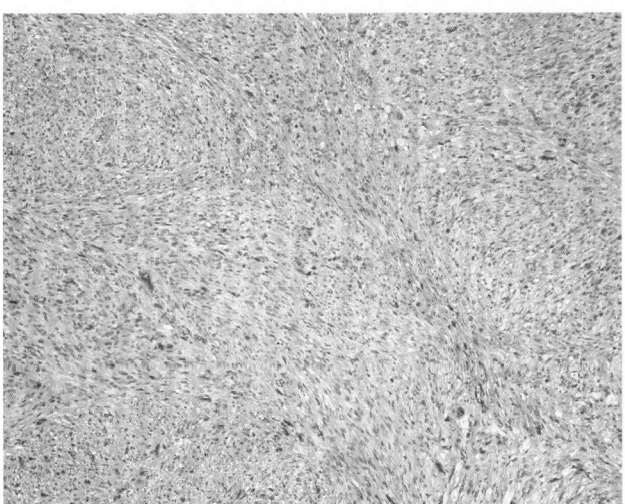

Figure 6-135. Leiomyosarcoma. The fascicles of malignant cells have a perfectly perpendicular arrangement just like those in leiomyomas, but the cellularity argues against a benign interpretation.

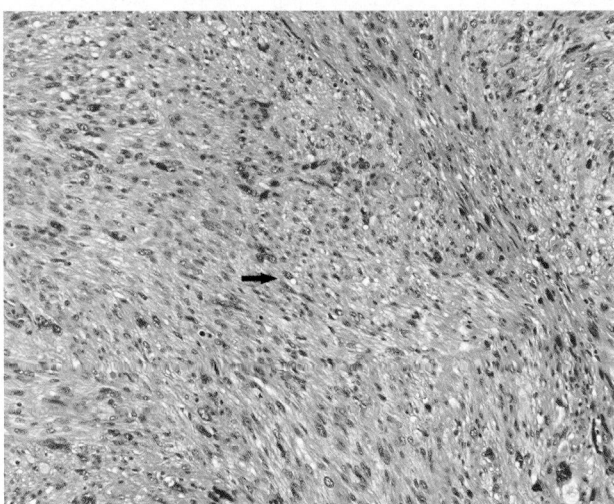

Figure 6-136. Leiomyosarcoma. The cytoplasm is brightly eosinophilic and the fascicles are perpendicularly oriented. There are hyperchromatic nuclei, many with blunt-ended contours. A paranuclear vacuole is indicated by an *arrow*.

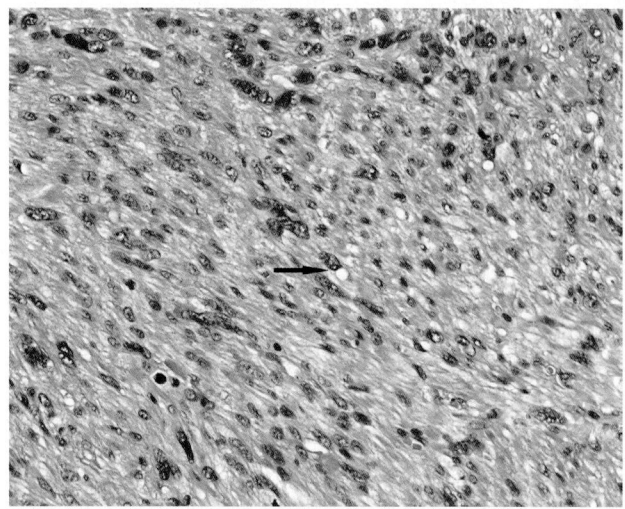

Figure 6-137. Leiomyosarcoma. Note the delicate longitudinal cytoplasmic striations. A paranuclear vacuole is indicated (*arrow*), but there is another to the upper right of the indicated one.

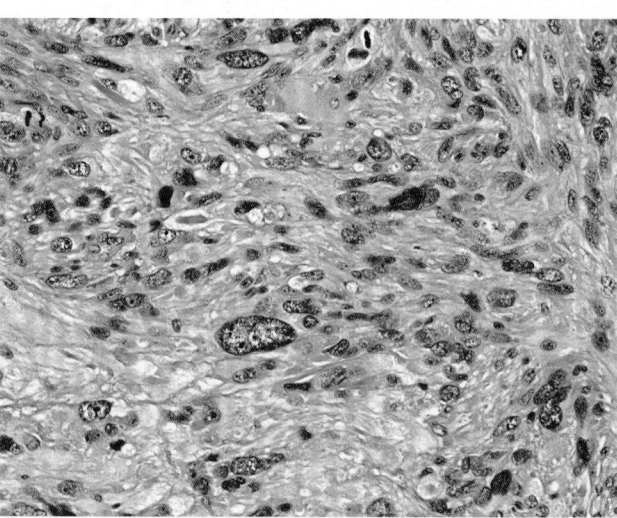

Figure 6-138. Leiomyosarcoma. A blunt-ended hyperchromatic nucleus dominates the image, but a few cells with paranuclear vacuoles and brightly eosinophilic cytoplasm with delicate longitudinal striations can also be appreciated.

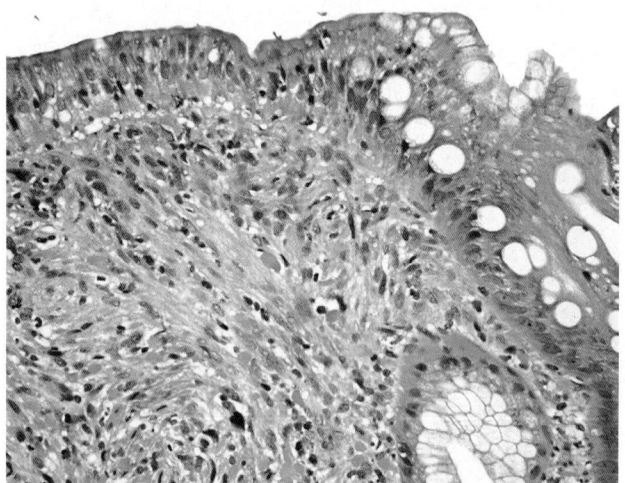

Figure 6-139. Leiomyosarcoma. This tumor has extended into small intestinal mucosa. There is gastric mucin cell metaplasia at the surface as well.

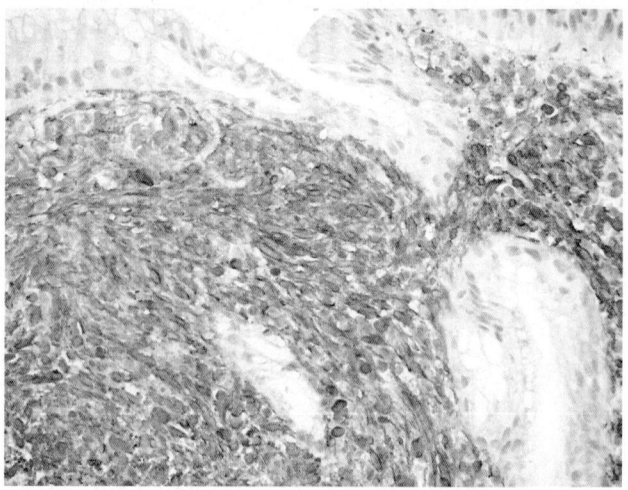

Figure 6-140. Leiomyosarcoma. This is a smooth muscle actin stain from the lesion seen in Fig. 6.139.

PEARLS & PITFALLS: Diagnosing Leiomyomas

Remember that there can be a few delicate labeled Cajal cells in these lesions (Fig. 6.132), as discussed in "Esophagus" chapter in more detail.

FAQ: What are the differences in appearance between GISTs and leiomyosarcomas?

In general, GISTs have monomorphic nuclei, whereas leiomyosarcomas have pleomorphic nuclei. The cytoplasm of leiomyosarcomas is pinker with delicate longitudinal striations. GISTs also can have ropy collagen fibrils ("skeinoid fibers"). Their nuclei are less blunt-ended than those of leiomyosarcomas and there are generally fewer mitoses, all of which are typical rather than atypical. Of course immunolabeling can also be helpful but, for example, believe the morphology if desmin is nonreactive and smooth muscle actin is positive if the lesion has the appearances of a leiomyosarcoma.

PLEXIFORM FIBROMYXOMA

This rare tumor usually arises in the stomach, but examples are found elsewhere (small bowel). In the stomach, most arise in the antrum, sometimes with duodenal extension. There is no reported gender or age predominance, but the number of reported cases is small.[84] Because plexiform fibromyxoma usually involves the muscularis propria, it is unlikely to be encountered on mucosal biopsies. It consists of a plexiform growth of richly vascularized paucicellular nodules of spindle cells with minimal mitotic activity (Figs. 6.141–6.143). The tumor cells express SMA and CD10 but not KIT or DOG1. Some cases have a translocation, t(11;12)(q11;q13), involving the long noncoding gene metastasis-associated lung adenocarcinoma transcript 1 (*MALAT1*) and the gene glioma-associated oncogene homologue 1 (*GLI1*).[85] These tumors have had benign follow-up in reports to date.

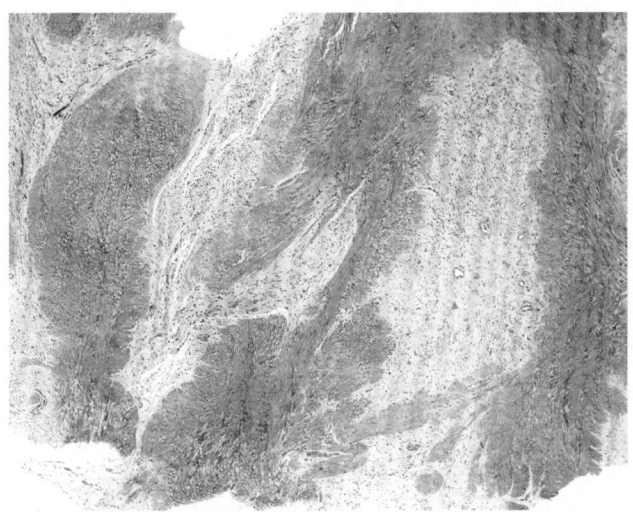

Figure 6-141. Plexiform fibromyxoma. These are rare tumors that primarily arise in the gastric muscularis propria. They express smooth muscle actin but not desmin.

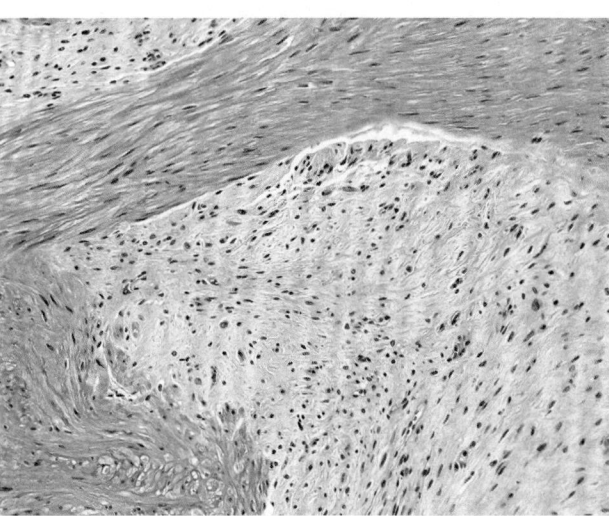

Figure 6-142. Plexiform fibromyxoma. Note the bland cytologic features.

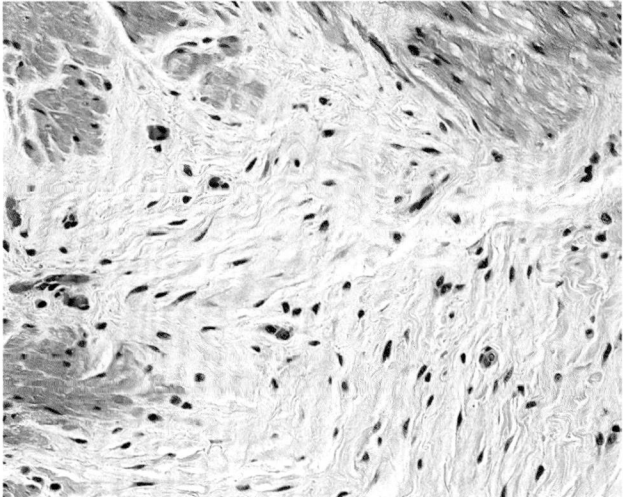

Figure 6-143. Plexiform fibromyxoma. Scant fibrillary collagen is present.

SCHWANNOMA

The gastric muscularis propria is the preferred site for gastrointestinal schwannomas, but sometimes they extend into the submucosa. They sometimes arise in the esophagus or colon and rarely in the small bowel. There is a female predominance; the largest series documents nearly a 4:1 female-to-male ratio.[86] Grossly, schwannomas are similar to GISTs, with a fibrotic, rubbery, white-yellow cut surface and well-circumscribed outline without a capsule. The tumor is surrounded by a lymphoid cuff nearly all the time (>90%), even featuring germinal centers (Figs. 6.144–6.147).

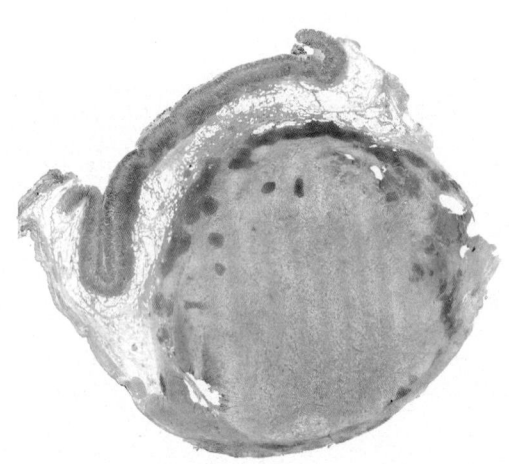

Figure 6-144. Gastric schwannoma. There is an invariable lymphoid cuff encircling these tumors, which arise in the muscularis propria.

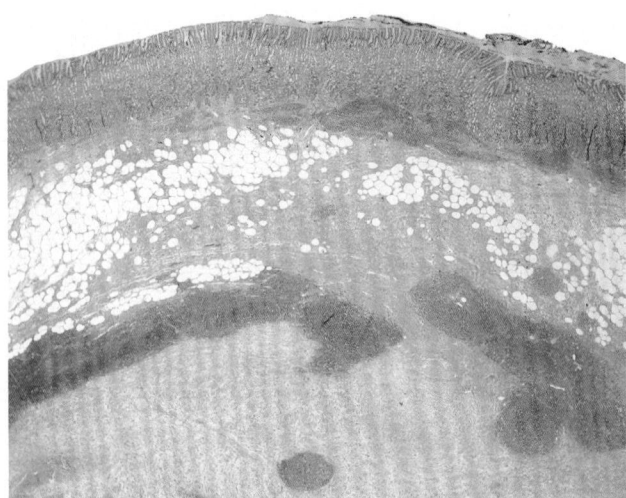

Figure 6-145. Gastric schwannoma. There are lymphoid aggregates cuffing the lesion and also within it.

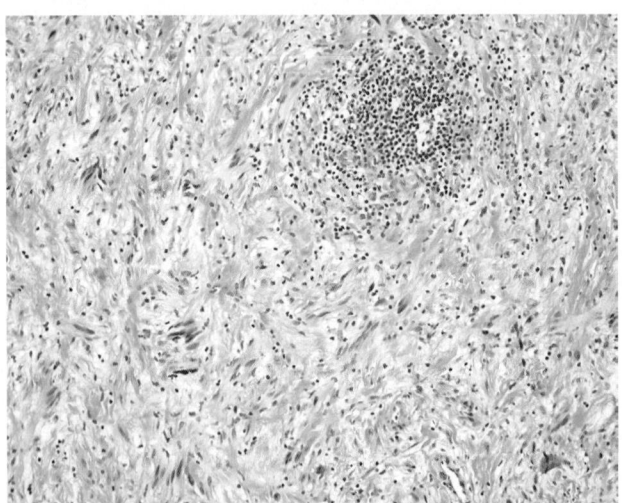

Figure 6-146. Gastric schwannoma. The tumor itself contains plenty of lymphoplasmacytic cells and nuclei that show zones of vague palisading. Note the strands of coarse collagen.

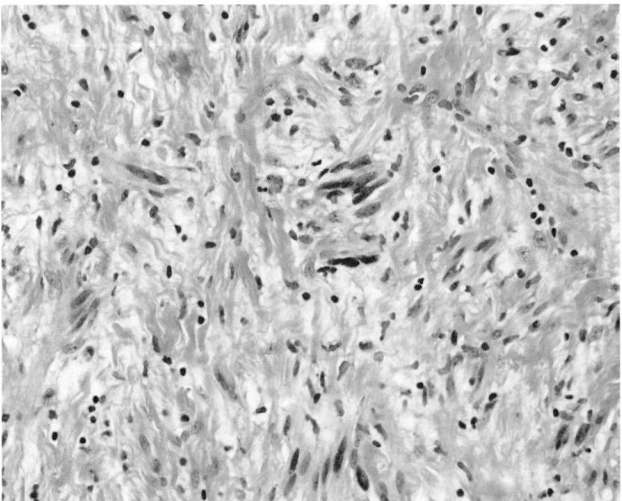

Figure 6-147. Gastric schwannoma. Lymphocytes are easy to find within the lesion. This is not the case with gastrointestinal stromal tumors. Gastric schwannomas are easy to recognize on hematoxylin and eosin, but they are consistently strongly S100 protein reactive if a bit of reassurance is needed.

GI tract schwannomas are typically not encapsulated, distinct from schwannomas in the peripheral nervous system. They can also be plexiform. Intralesional lymphocytes are seen in all cases. The schwannian cells appear as interlacing bundles of spindle cells that are only weakly palisaded (in contrast to GISTs which, ironically, often display striking nuclear palisading). Well-formed Verocay bodies are seldom seen. Occasional cases show epithelioid morphology. Most cases have a few cells with nuclear atypia, but mitotic activity is low. Areas of myxoid change, xanthoma cells, and vascular hyalinization can be encountered. Although schwannomas appear quite similar to GISTs at low magnification, the lymphoid cuff is a tip-off that they are different. Remember that GISTSs usually have scarcely any intralesional inflammatory cells. Schwannomas are all strongly S100 protein-positive and lack muscle markers and CD117. Variable immunoreactivity for GFAP is a common finding. Most examples are negative for CD34. The differential diagnosis is with GIST. The inflammatory background is the main morphologic feature that should prompt diagnostic consideration of a nerve sheath tumor. Schwannomas lack *KIT* and *PDGFRA* mutations. *NF2* mutations, common is soft tissue schwannomas, are rare in gastrointestinal tract examples. Gastrointestinal tract schwannomas are benign.

GLOMUS TUMOR

Glomus tumors are nearly always found in the muscularis propria. They are rare in the GI tract. There is a female predominance and a median age at presentation of 55 years. [87] The vast majority are gastric, but they can arise in the small bowel and colon as well. Gastric lesions often present with severe bleeding producing melena. Ulcerlike pain can also be a feature. Most are circumscribed masses of the muscularis propria with a median diameter of 2.5 cm (Figs. 6.148–6.150).

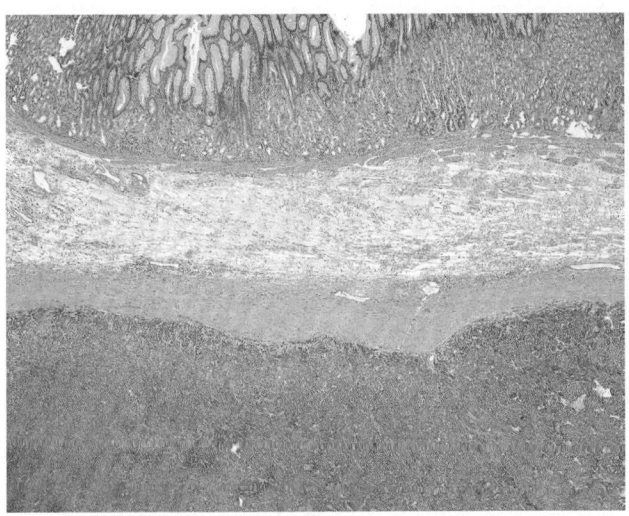

Figure 6-148. Gastric glomus tumor. The neoplasm is in the muscularis propria and very cellular.

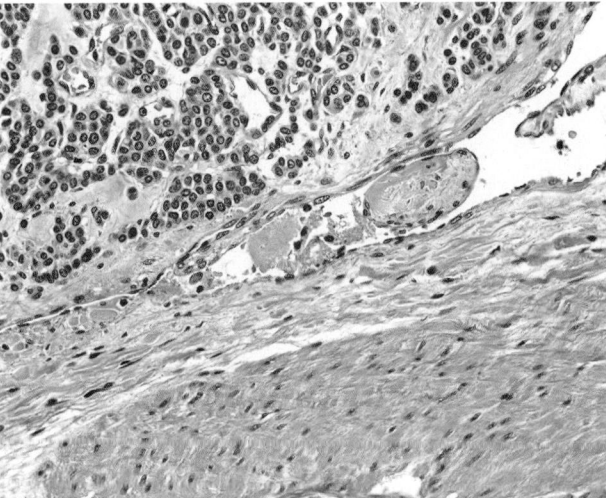

Figure 6-149. Gastric glomus tumor. The tumor cells tend to be found near blood vessels and are evenly spaced with basement membrane between them. Their nuclei are perfectly round such that glomus tumors can be mistaken for well-differentiated neuroendocrine (carcinoid) tumors.

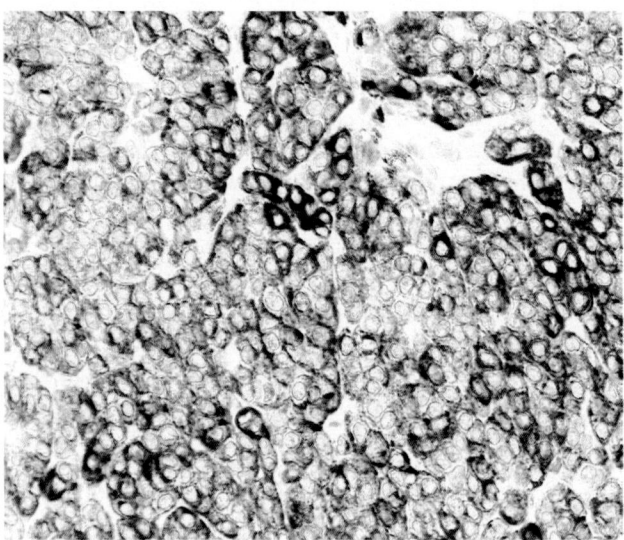

Figure 6-150. Gastric glomus tumor. This is a smooth muscle actin stain. Glomus cells are modified smooth muscle cells and express actin but not desmin.

Glomus tumors have a multinodular appearance at scanning magnification. The nodules are separated by strands of residual muscularis propria. Glomus tumors are composed of solid sheets of cells that surround gaping capillary vessels that have a hemangiopericytoma-like pattern. Tumor cells are also in the muscular walls of larger vessels. Individual tumor cells are very round with sharply defined cell membranes, perfectly rounded nuclei, and delicate chromatin. Some tumors have densely eosinophilic cytoplasm.

Glomus tumors are composed of modified smooth muscle cells. Because of this, on immunolabeling, these tumors express SMA, calponin, and h-caldesmon, but lack desmin. Pericellular net–like arrangements of basement membrane proteins can be highlighted with laminin and collagen type I. Some cases have focal CD34. Glomus tumors are negative for CD117.

Glomus tumors lack *KIT* mutations, but they have been shown to have *MIR143-NOTCH* gene fusions.[88] There is a case report of a lesion with loss of INI1/SMARCB1 alterations.[89]

PEARLS & PITFALLS: Glomus Tumors of the GI Tract

Occasional glomus tumors express synaptophysin (Fig. 6.151). Glomus tumors have very round nuclei: this adds to their mimicry of well-differentiated neuroendocrine tumors. The latter lack the prominent cell borders (basement membrane). In addition, keratin and chromogranin are negative in glomus tumors.

On frozen sections, glomus tumors again mimic well-differentiated neuroendocrine (carcinoid) tumors, but the trick is the rule of the layers—glomus tumors are centered in the muscularis propria rather than the deep mucosa (where the neuroendocrine cells are found). They are also fed by large vessels and the cells cling to them. Fig. 6.152 shows a gastric type 3 well-differentiated neuroendocrine (carcinoid) tumor. Note that it is centered straddling the deep mucosa and the superficial submucosa.

The differential diagnosis of gastric glomus tumors includes endocrine tumors (carcinoids) and GISTs. Their occasional synaptophysin expression may lead to confusion, but a panel approach should exclude this possibility because these tumors lack keratin and express smooth muscle markers (other than desmin).

The vast majority of glomus tumors behave in a benign fashion. However, rare examples are lethal with metastases. It is difficult to predict which will have an unfavorable outcome.

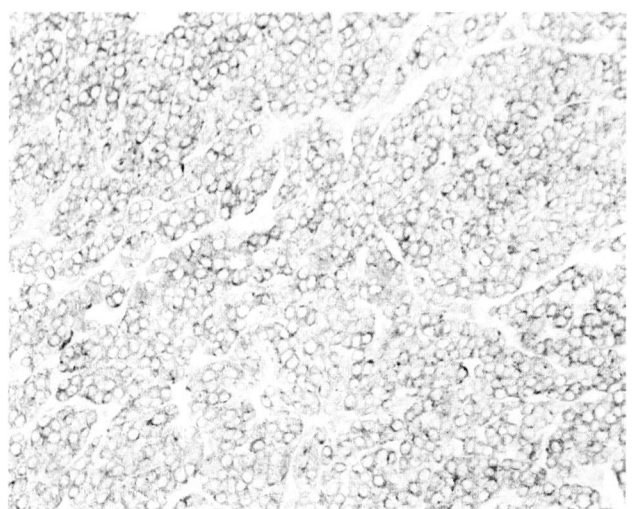

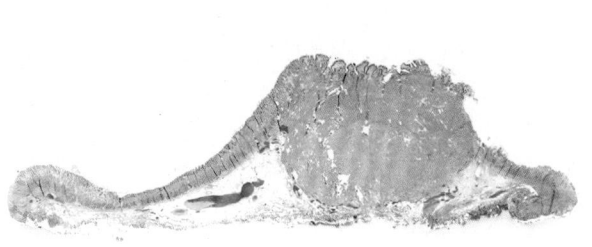

Figure 6-151. Gastric glomus tumor. This is a synaptophysin stain. Glomus tumors sometimes display synaptophysin labeling but are not reactive with keratins or chromogranin. Because they are formed by cells with round nuclei, it is already easy to mistake them for well-differentiated neuroendocrine (carcinoid) tumors.

Figure 6-152. Well-differentiated neuroendocrine (carcinoid) tumor of the stomach arising in normal oxyntic mucosa (type 3 carcinoid tumor). Note that this tumor is centered in the base of the mucosa and submucosa, which contrasts to the mural location of glomus tumor. Just knowing this topography can help with interpretation of frozen sections!

CALCIFYING FIBROUS TUMOR

Calcifying fibrous tumor was initially recognized as a soft tissue tumor of children, termed "Childhood fibrous tumor with psammoma bodies." Calcifying fibrous tumor/pseudotumor is a benign fibrous lesion. Whereas soft tissue examples affect children and young adults without gender predilection, visceral cases usually occur in adults. Notable sites are the mesentery, peritoneum, and pleura (sometimes multiple). Visceral examples may produce site-specific symptoms. Calcifications are seen on CT and may be thick and bandlike or punctate. On MRI, these tumors appear similar to fibromatoses, with a mottled appearance and a signal closer to that of muscle than fat. Although examples have followed trauma and occurred in association with Castleman disease and inflammatory myofibroblastic tumors, the pathogenesis remains unknown. The notion of burned-out inflammatory myofibroblastic tumor as a unifying explanation for them has gained no traction because these tumors are essentially always negative for ALK.

Grossly calcifying fibrous tumors are well marginated but unencapsulated, ranging in size from <1 to >10 cm. Some show indistinct boundaries with infiltration into surrounding tissues. Sometimes a gritty texture is noted on sectioning. Calcifying fibrous tumor consists of well-circumscribed, unencapsulated, paucicellular, hyalinized fibrosclerotic tissue with an inflammatory infiltrate consisting of lymphocytes and plasma cells (Figs. 6.153–6.156). Lymphoid aggregates are often present. Calcifications, both psammomatous and dystrophic, are scattered throughout. The lesional cells express FXIIIa, but usually not actins, desmin, FVIII, S100 protein, neurofilament protein, cytokeratins, CD34, and CD31. As discussed earlier, the immunophenotype differs from that of inflammatory myofibroblastic tumors because most calcifying fibrous pseudotumors lack actin and anaplastic lymphoma kinase (ALK). These tumors are benign, but occasional recurrences are known.

FOLLICULAR DENDRITIC CELL SARCOMA

Follicular dendritic cell sarcoma is the preferred terminology in the latest WHO classification.[90] Wait, this is not a hematopathology book, darn it! Except that this type of tumor is more likely to be extranodal (over half of cases) than to involve lymph nodes (about a third of cases). This is a tumor of adults. For our purposes, it tends to involve the muscularis propria of the small bowel, where it mimics GIST but, like schwannoma, differs by having a lot of lymphocytes in the lesion.

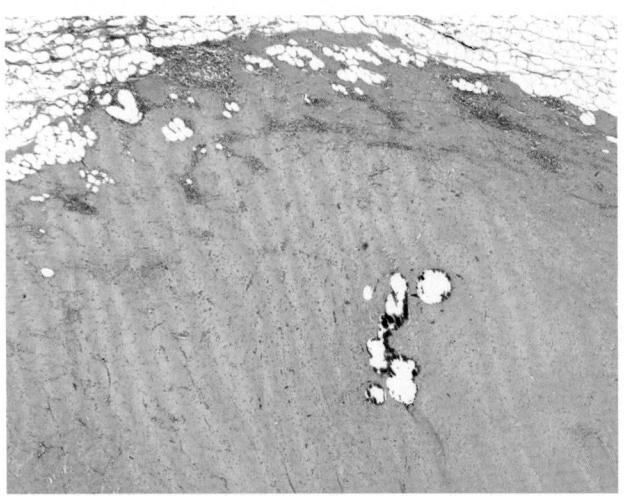

Figure 6-153. Calcifying fibrous tumor. This lesion is hypocellular and contains plasma cells, lymphocytes, and lymphoid aggregates, and calcifications.

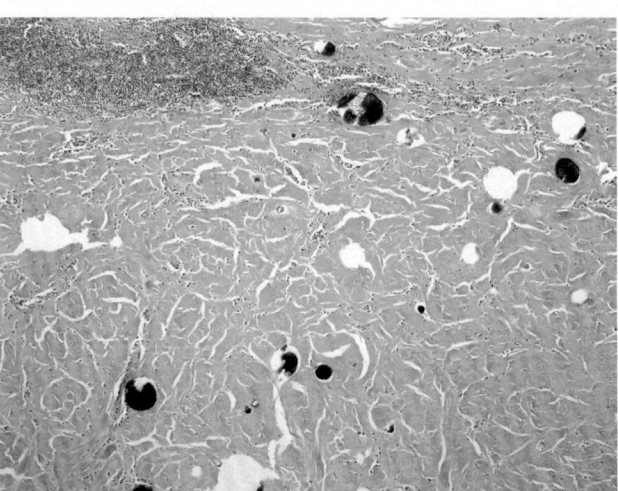

Figure 6-154. Calcifying fibrous tumor. Note the calcifications.

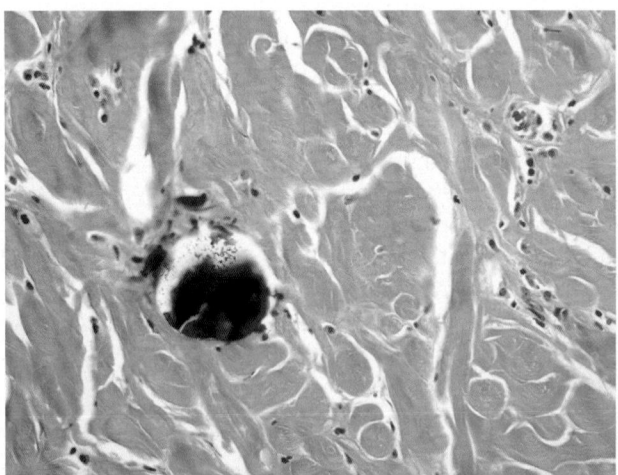

Figure 6-155. Calcifying fibrous tumor. There are a few fibroblastic nuclei and scattered plasma cells and lymphocytes.

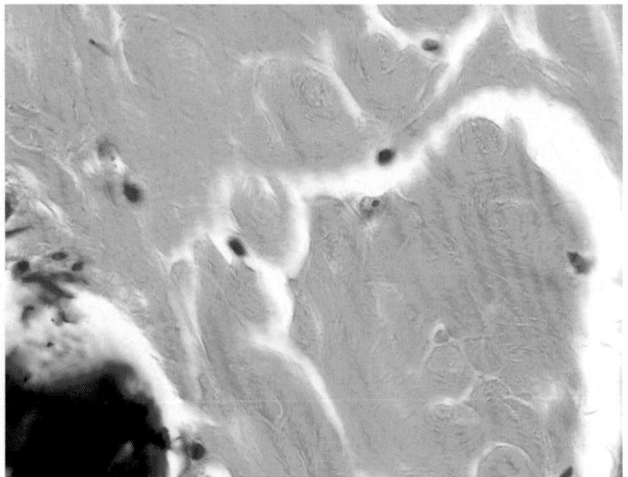

Figure 6-156. Calcifying fibrous tumor. A tumor nucleus at high magnification. Note the delicate nucleolus. The appearance is similar to that of the nuclei in fibromatoses, but the lesion is very calcified, hypocellular, and punctated with inflammatory cells.

The tumors consist of syncytial spindle cells that form bulky masses and have an epithelioid appearance (Figs. 6.157–6.159). There are usually a lot of tumor-infiltrating lymphocytes. When immunolabeling is done, there can be some S100 protein labeling, but you have to consider this diagnosis. This is the desperation diagnosis! Strange tumor and you are clueless—what to do? Try CD21 or CD23 and hope for some relief.

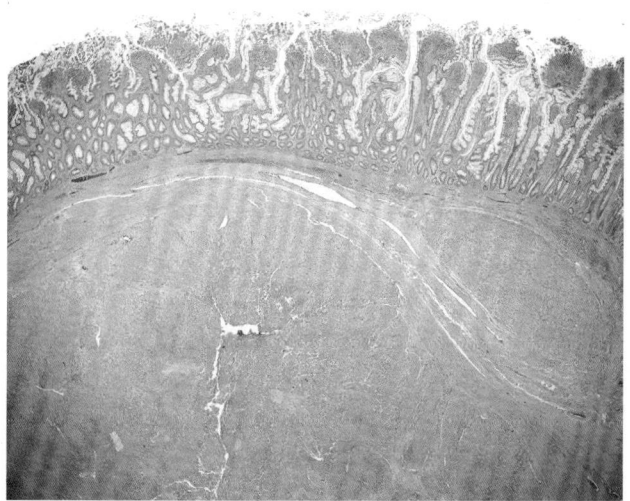

Figure 6-157. Follicular dendritic cell sarcoma. This tumor is cellular and fills the muscularis propria. These can be mistaken for gastrointestinal stromal tumors, but they differ by having intralesional lymphoplasmacytic cells, among other features.

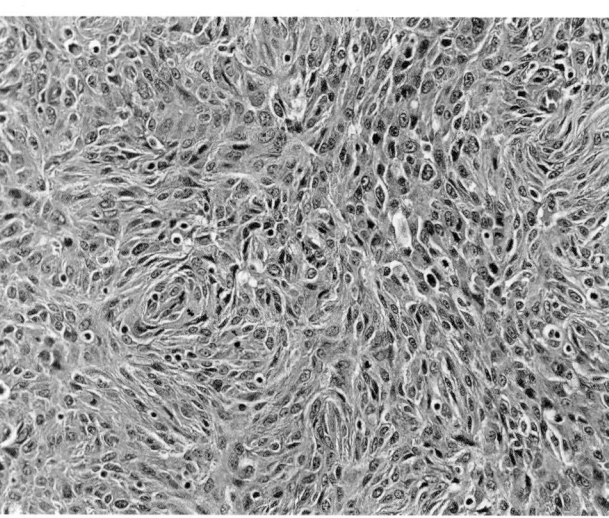

Figure 6-158. Follicular dendritic cell sarcoma. Note the population of inflammatory cells and epithelioid appearance of the tumor cells.

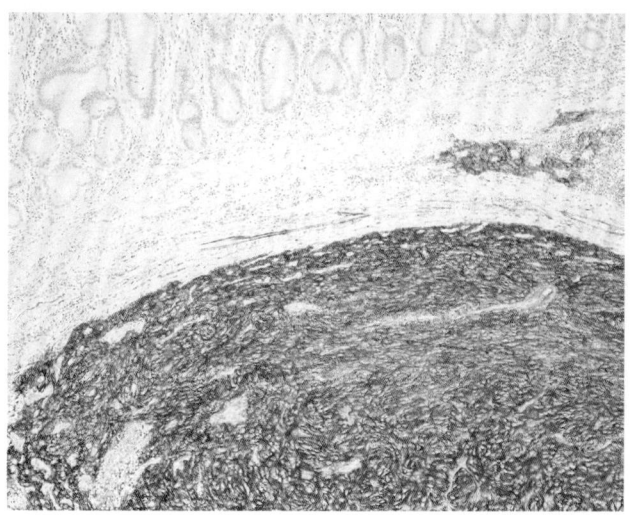

Figure 6-159. Follicular dendritic cell sarcoma. This is a CD21 stain.

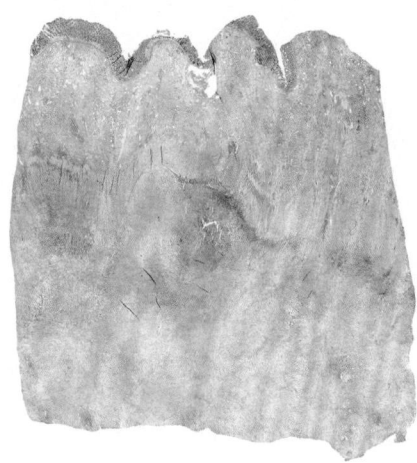

Figure 6-160. Rosai-Dorfman disease. There are dark and light zones in this process that involves the mesentery of the colon with extension into the muscularis propria. The dark areas are lymphoid aggregates and the pale areas are where the abnormal histiocytes are found. This pattern is reminiscent of the pattern of a checkerboard.

ROSAI-DORFMAN DISEASE

This contrasts with Langerhans cell histiocytosis, a histiocytosis with *BRAF* mutations. Rosai-Dorfman disease is a histiocytosis that can be encountered throughout the gastrointestinal tract. It is rare and lacks *BRAF* mutations. The characteristic finding in Rosai-Dorfman disease is the presence of emperipolesis (Figs. 6.160–6.172) in which the abnormal histiocytes ingest other cells but do not destroy them.[91] The disease was initially noted in lymph nodes, where it is called "sinus histiocytosis with massive adenopathy" as described by Drs. Rosai and Dorfman[92,93] but later it was described all over the body, to include the soft tissues[94] and GI tract.[95] The trouble is that it sounds kind of silly to diagnose "sinus histiocytosis with massive adenopathy" in a body part that is not a lymph node, so the term Rosai-Dorfman disease is perfect for the GI tract and other extranodal sites.

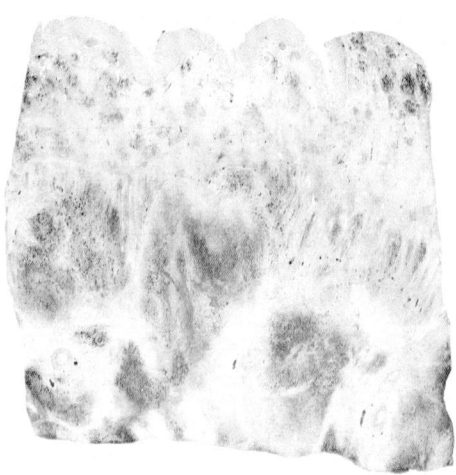

Figure 6-161. Rosai-Dorfman disease. An S100 protein stain labels the light areas seen in Fig. 6.160. Rosai-Dorfman disease is a non-Langerhans cell histiocytosis in which the abnormal histiocytes express S100 protein but lack *BRAF* mutations.

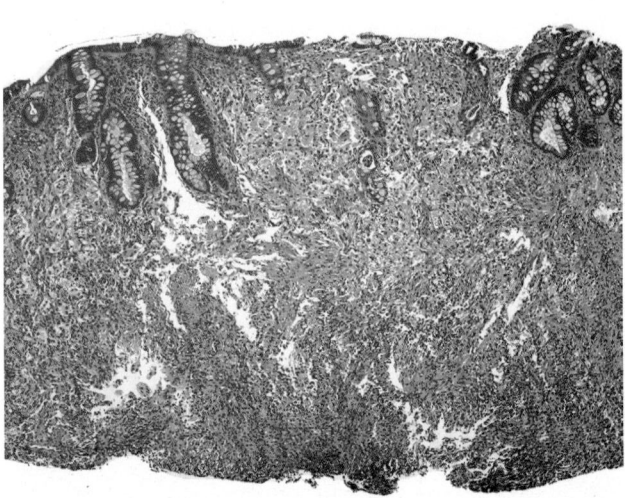

Figure 6-162. Rosai-Dorfman disease. This is a mucosal biopsy that shows a population of pale histiocytes.

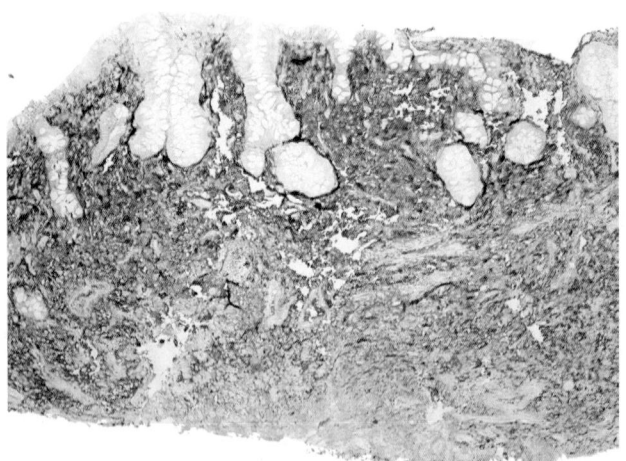

Figure 6-163. Rosai-Dorfman disease. This is an S100 protein stain from the lesion depicted in Fig. 6.162.

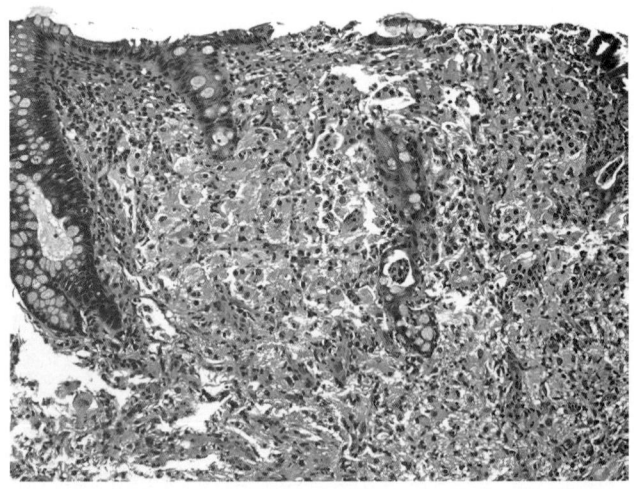

Figure 6-164. Rosai-Dorfman disease. At high magnification, emperipolesis is seen in this example of Rosai-Dorfman disease.

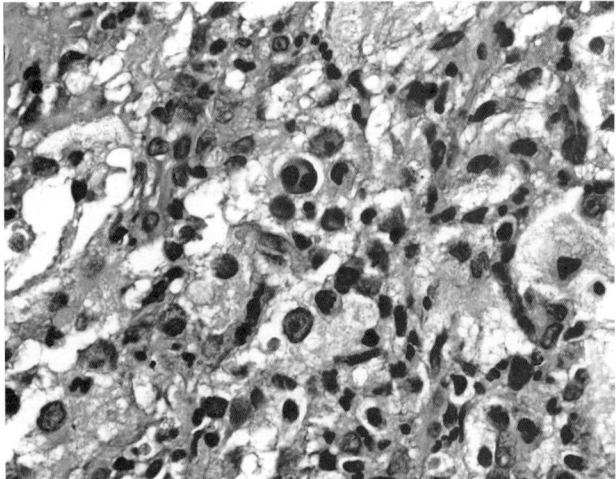

Figure 6-165. Rosai-Dorfman disease. This is a very high magnification showing engulfed lymphocytes and plasma cells within the cytoplasm of the abnormal histiocytes (emperipolesis). The engulfed cells are not destroyed.

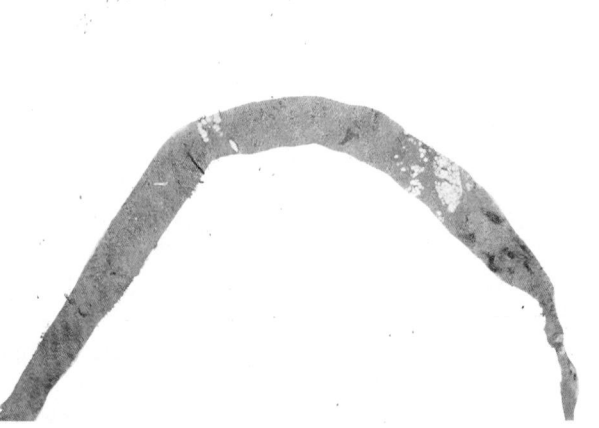

Figure 6-166. Rosai-Dorfman disease. This is a needle biopsy from a mass that involved the colon and pericolic soft tissue. It was interpreted as "malignant fibrous histiocytoma."

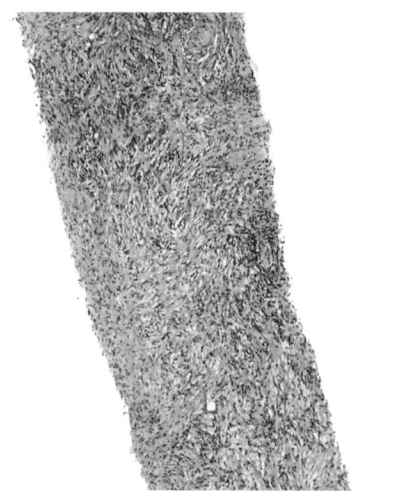

Figure 6-167. Rosai-Dorfman disease. This area shows storiform fibrosis such that the findings overlap with those of IgG4 related fibrosclerosing disease. Rosai-Dorfman disease often contains IgG4-labeled plasma cells. This image is from the same case as that shown in Fig. 6.166.

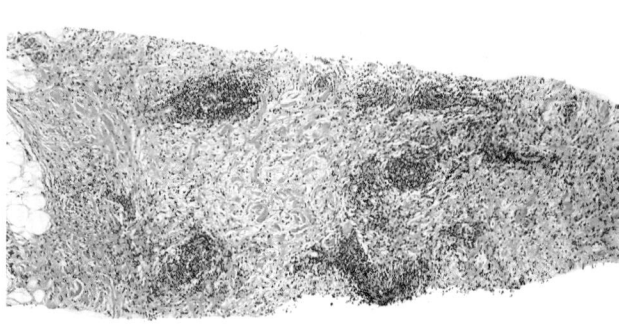

Figure 6-168. Rosai-Dorfman disease. This area, from the case shown in Figs. 6.166 and 6.167, shows nonspecific fibroinflammatory features but the pale color was the clue to search for emperipolesis and add S100 protein staining.

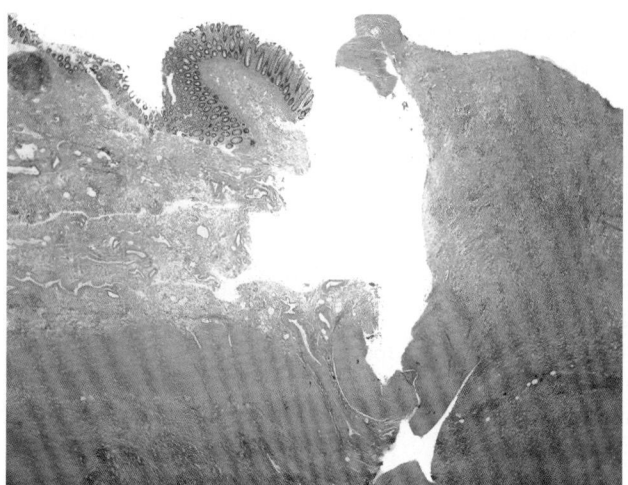

Figure 6-169. Rosai-Dorfman disease. This is a resection specimen from the lesion seen in Figs. 6.166–6.168.

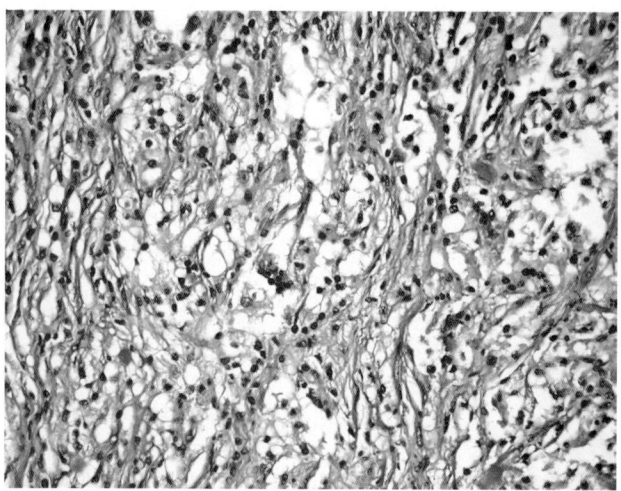

Figure 6-170. Rosai-Dorfman disease. There is a suggestion of emperipolesis in this area (same case as shown in Figs. 6.166–6.169).

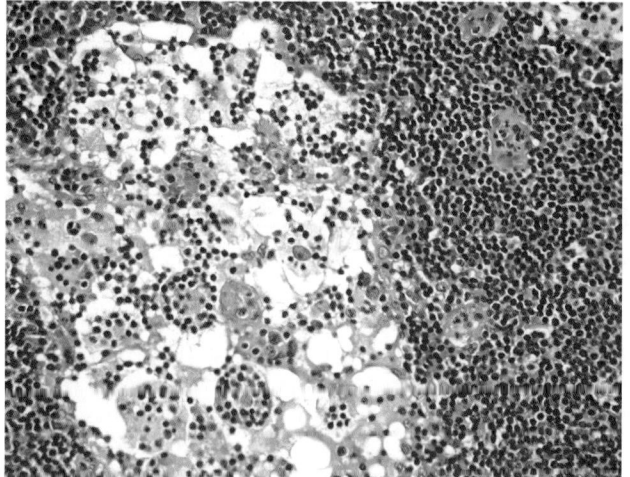

Figure 6-171. Rosai-Dorfman disease. Stunning emperipolesis is present (same case as shown in Figs. 6.166–6.170).

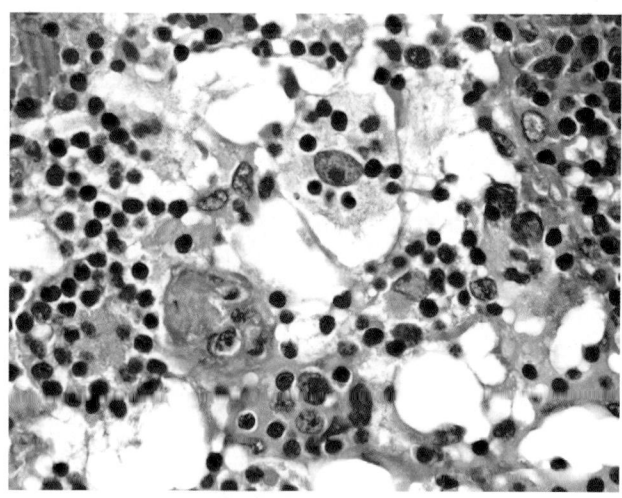

Figure 6-172. Rosai-Dorfman disease. This is a high magnification of the area seen in Fig. 6.171.

Additionally, Rosai-Dorfman disease is easy to diagnose in enlarged lymph nodes because the emperipolesis is easy to spot in the dilated sinuses, but it is trickier in extranodal sites because it has to be considered to be diagnosed and the appearance is simply that of a fibroinflammatory process. An important issue in diagnosing Rosai-Dorfman disease is that it can have areas with an appearance virtually identical to that of IgG4-associated fibrosclerosing disease, namely featuring zones of storiform fibrosis. Rosai-Dorfman disease can also contain many IgG4-labeled plasma cells. If the diagnosis is considered, the abnormal histiocytes express S100 protein, but *considering* extranodal Rosai-Dorfman remains mostly an H&E diagnosis. Look for a checkerboard pattern of light (the histiocytes) and dark (lymphoid aggregates) areas at low magnification and then begin the hunt for emperipolesis. Look for the emperipolesis in the loosest least sclerotic zones. Hunt also in any dilated lymphatic spaces.

Rosai-Dorfman disease is usually treated with surgery, but some patients require immunomodulatory treatment.

SUMMARY OF GASTROINTESTINAL TRACT LESIONS CONTAINING MANY INFLAMMATORY CELLS

Fig. 6.173 highlights the GI tract lesions that tend to have a lot of inflammatory cells:

1. Inflammatory fibroid polyp—submucosal based, uniform cells, many eosinophils, whorled cells around vessels (onion skin pattern), benign.
2. GI tract schwannoma—based in muscularis propria, lymphoid cuff, some enlarged nuclei, slight palisading, plasma cells, and lymphocytes (not very dense) in the lesion, benign.
3. Sclerosing mesenteritis—in the mesentery with plenty of fat necrosis, sometimes calcifications, a bit of lymphohistiocytic inflammation, benign.
4. IgG4-associated fibroinflammatory disease—often in mesentery but in many organs as well, storiform fibrosis, the fibroblasts are very bland appearing, lymphocytes, plasma cells, eosinophils, obliterative phlebitis, prominent IgG4-labeled plasma cells, benign but can be associated with morbidity.
5. Calcifying fibrous tumor—often in mesentery but location quite variable, very hypocellular, plasma cells and lymphocytes, calcifications, may be multifocal, benign.
6. Rosai-Dorfman disease—can arise wherever it likes, extranodal lesions can have a storiform pattern, benign but can be extensive.
7. Inflammatory myofibroblastic tumor—may arise anywhere, but often in retroperitoneum and mesentery, myofibroblastic cells in a prominent inflammatory background with plasma cells and lymphocytes. May harbor *ALK* or *ROS1* rearrangements. Usually low-grade sarcoma type behavior but an aggressive subset termed epithelioid inflammatory myofibroblastic sarcoma.
8. Follicular dendritic cell sarcoma—may arise anywhere but in small bowel is not uncommon. Sheets of spindle cells sprinkled with lymphocytes. Differentiation along the lines of follicular dendritic cells can be confirmed with CD21 or CD23 immunolabeling. Usually low-grade behavior but a subset is aggressive.

SELECT COLORECTAL LESIONS LIKELY TO BE ENCOUNTERED ON BIOPSIES

This section begins with a host of nerve-related lesions that tend to be detected on mucosal biopsies, with a focus on the colon. In the United States, as of 1998,[96] average-risk patients could have screening colonoscopy to detect adenomas and remove them to prevent cancer, all using Medicare funding, which has resulted in the removal of many adenomas as well as many other lesions that have been characterized based on the increase in the number of colonoscopies. Some of these have been neural tumors, which have become better characterized and better recognized. In this section, we discuss nerve-related tumors as well some other lesions with spindle cells that can be encountered.

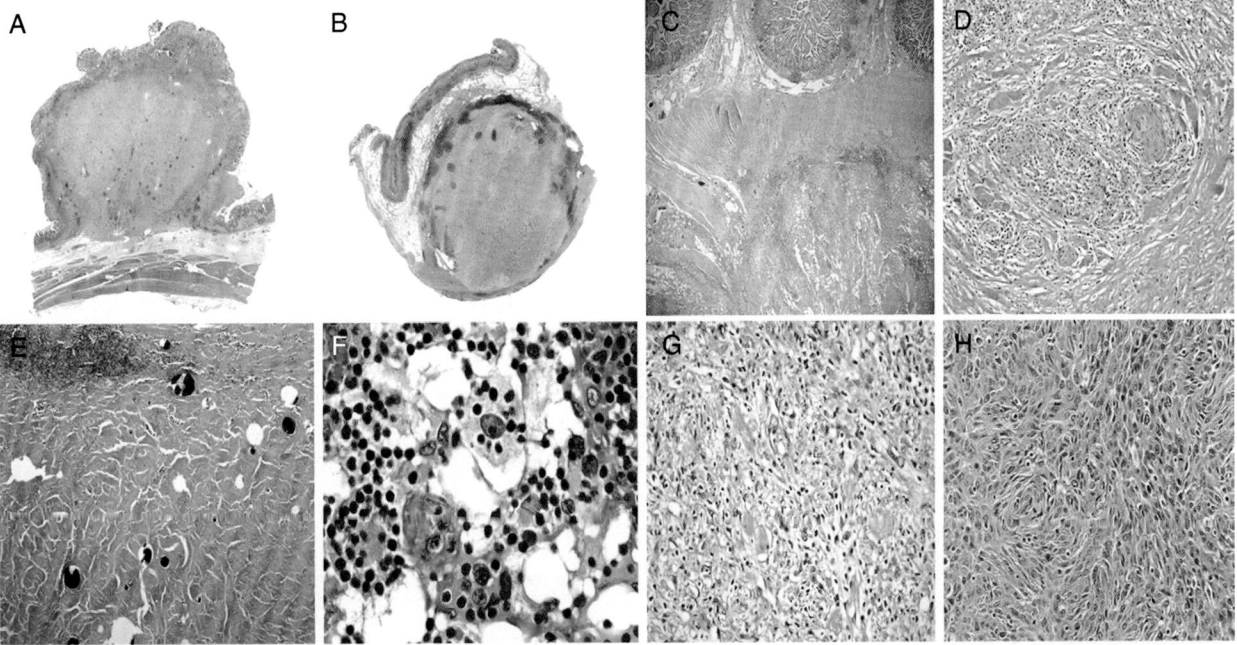

Figure 6-173. Inflammatory cell–rich lesions that can be separated. A: Inflammatory fibroid polyp. The tumor is submucosal based with uniform cells, many eosinophils, whorled cells around vessels (onion skin pattern), and benign. B: GI tract schwannoma. The tumor is centered in muscularis propria, with a lymphoid cuff, some enlarged nuclei, slight palisading, plasma cells, and lymphocytes (not very dense) in the lesion, and is benign. C: Sclerosing mesenteritis. The tumor is in the mesentery with plenty of fat necrosis, sometimes calcifications, a bit of lymphohistiocytic inflammation, and benign. D: IgG4-associated fibroinflammatory disease is often in the mesentery but in many organs as well, with storiform fibrosis. The fibroblasts are very bland appearing, and there are lymphocytes, plasma cells, eosinophils, obliterative phlebitis, and prominent IgG4-labeled plasma cells. This disease is benign but can be associated with morbidity. E: Calcifying fibrous tumor. This lesion is often in the mesentery, but its location is quite variable. The tumor is very hypocellular, with plasma cells and lymphocytes, and calcifications. It may be may be multifocal but is benign. F: Rosai-Dorfman disease can arise wherever it likes; extranodal lesions can have a storiform pattern. The tumor is benign but can be extensive. There is expression of S100 protein. G: Inflammatory myofibroblastic tumor may arise anywhere but is often in the retroperitoneum and mesentery, with myofibroblastic cells in a prominent inflammatory background with plasma cells and lymphocytes. The tumor may harbor ALK or ROS1 rearrangements. There is usually low-grade sarcoma–type, behavior but there is an aggressive subset termed epithelioid inflammatory myofibroblastic sarcoma. H: Follicular dendritic cell sarcoma may arise anywhere, but the small bowel is not uncommon. The tumor consists of sheets of spindle cells sprinkled with lymphocytes. Differentiation along the lines of follicular dendritic cells can be confirmed with CD21 or CD23 immunolabeling. This sarcoma is usually of low-grade behavior, but a subset is aggressive.

GANGLIONEUROMA

Ganglioneuromas occur in two general settings: (1) the more common isolated solitary lesions and (2) syndromic multiple lesions that either produce multiple exophytic polyps ("ganglioneuromatous polyposis") or poorly demarcated transmural proliferations ("ganglioneuromatosis").[97] For solitary examples, there is no gender predominance and lesions have been detected in adults from ages 20 to 90 years, with a peak incidence between the ages of 40 and 60 years (those special colonoscopy years; mean age of 48 years). Most arise in the colon, usually on the left side. Patients are asymptomatic; the lesions are detected during colonoscopy. Solitary lesions are not associated with genetic syndromes. On the other hand, ganglioneuromatous polyposis and diffuse ganglioneuromatosis are associated with multiple endocrine neoplasia (MEN) type IIB and with NF1. Diffuse ganglioneuromatosis is present in virtually all patients with MEN IIB and can antedate the endocrine neoplasms. Patients with MEN IIB and ganglioneuromatosis present with many varying GI symptoms, which may include constipation, diarrhea, difficulty in feeding, projectile vomiting, and crampy abdominal pain. Syndromic GI tract ganglioneuromas arise in the colorectum in patients younger (mean age of about 35 years) than those with sporadic isolated ganglioneuromas.

Isolated ganglioneuromas form small sessile or pedunculated polyps, whereas the polyps in ganglioneuromatous polyposis are multiple (20 to 40). Some are filiform. Rare pediatric examples of ganglioneuromatous polyposis have been reported in association with production of vasoactive intestinal polypeptide producing the watery diarrhea, hypokalemia, and achlorhydria syndrome. Diffuse ganglioneuromatosis forms a poorly demarcated, whitish thickening that may be transmural.

Polypoid sporadic ganglioneuromas resemble juvenile or inflammatory polyps because they have disturbed crypt architecture and expanded lamina propria. The lamina propria is expanded by collections of spindle cells within a fibrillary matrix, and irregular nests and groups of ganglion cells (Figs. 6.174–6.176). Sporadic examples sometimes extend into the submucosa. The ganglioneuromas in ganglioneuromatous polyposis show overlapping features with sporadic ganglioneuromas, but have more numerous ganglion cells and more impressive filiform architecture. In diffuse ganglioneuromatosis, the process is centered in the area of the myenteric plexus, is either diffusely intramural or transmural, and consists of fusiform expansions or confluent transmural ganglioneuromatous proliferations.

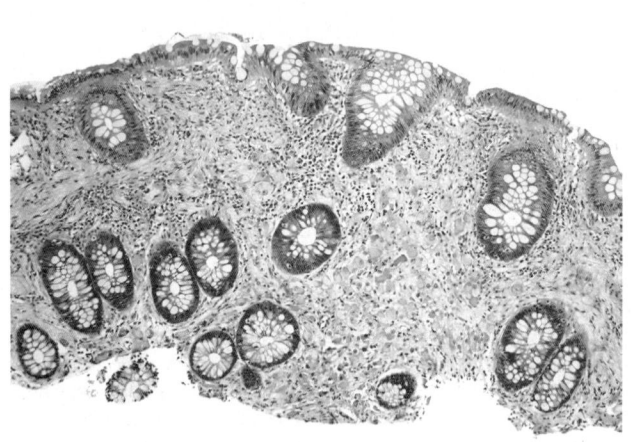

Figure 6-174. Ganglioneuroma. This tumor is expanding the lamina propria of the colon. Schwann cells are seen in the upper left and there are quite a few ganglion cells in the lower right.

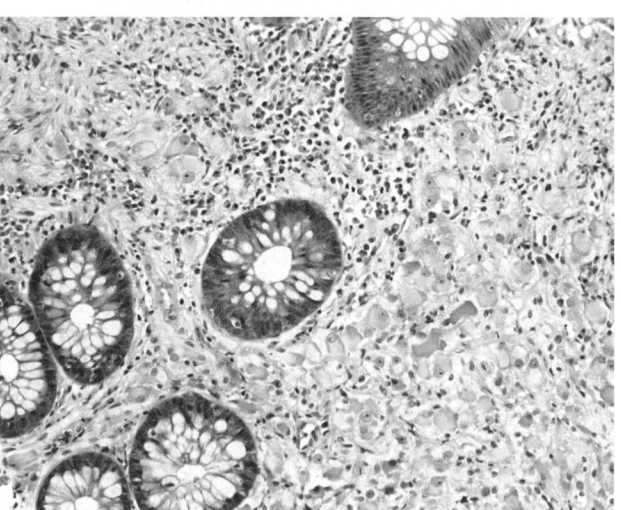

Figure 6-175. Ganglioneuroma. This image shows congeries of lesional ganglion cells.

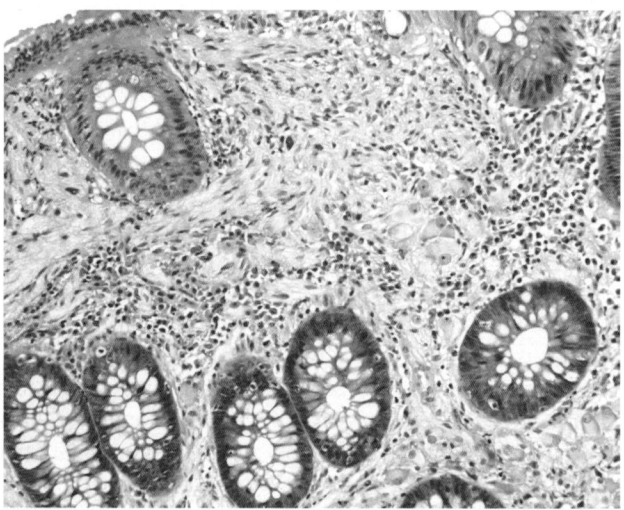

Figure 6-176. Ganglioneuroma. This image shows both Schwann cells and ganglion cells.

Ganglioneuromas are easy to diagnose without immunohistochemistry, but if it is done, the spindle cells react with S100 protein and the ganglion cells with neuron specific enolase (NSE), synaptophysin, and neurofilament protein (NFP).

Of course, in contrast to neurofibromas, ganglioneuromas contain ganglion cells. When ganglion cells are infrequent, NSE or synaptophysin staining may help detect them.

Sporadic ganglioneuromas are treated by polypectomy and seldom recur. Patients with syndromic ganglioneuromas require careful follow-up. Those with NF1 are prone to develop other lesions, including malignant peripheral sheath tumors, GISTs, and somatostatinomas; those with MEN IIB may develop endocrine neoplasms. Polypoid ganglioneuromas may also herald Cowden disease (PTEN hamartoma syndrome), tuberous sclerosis, FAP, and juvenile polyposis, whereas the diffuse type is most likely associated with NF1 and MEN IIB. The ganglioneuromas, themselves, however, are all benign.

Although gangliocytic paraganglioma is discussed in "Small Bowel" chapter, it is worthwhile to review a case that has overlapping features with ganglioneuroma. Figs. 6.177–6.180 show a gangliocytic paraganglioma detected on mucosal biopsy from the duodenum (where nearly all such tumors arise—ganglioneuromas are usually in the colon). The epithelioid nests are the clue, although some zones of the tumor are impossible to separate from ganglioneuroma.

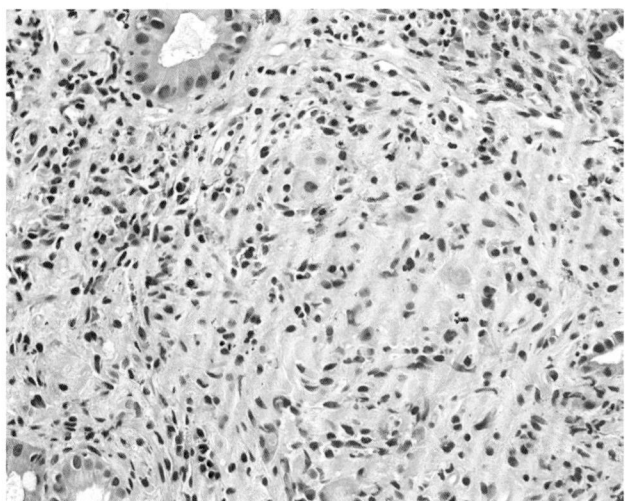

Figure 6-177. Gangliocytic paraganglioma. This field shows findings that are indistinguishable from those in ganglioneuroma. There are spindled schwannian cells and ganglionic cells. The clue to search more was that the tumor was found in the duodenum.

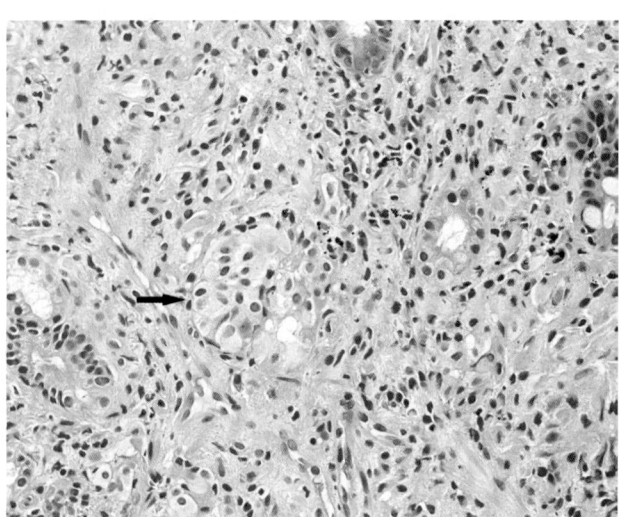

Figure 6-178. Gangliocytic paraganglioma. This is another field from the same tumor as that depicted in Fig. 6.177. Note the nest of epithelioid cells indicated by the *arrow*.

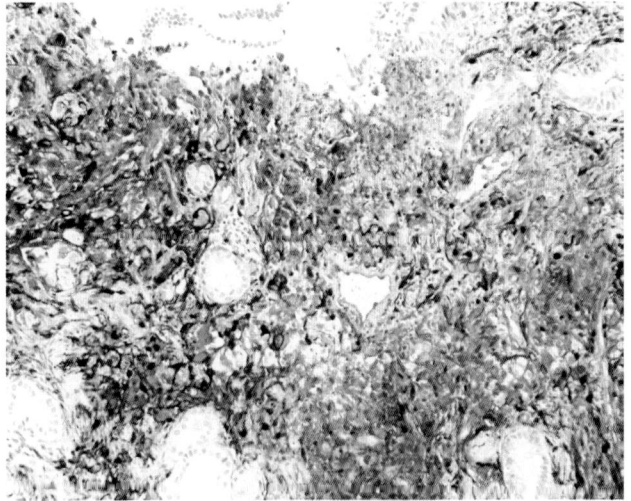

Figure 6-179. Gangliocytic paraganglioma. This is an S100 protein stain, which labels the entire process.

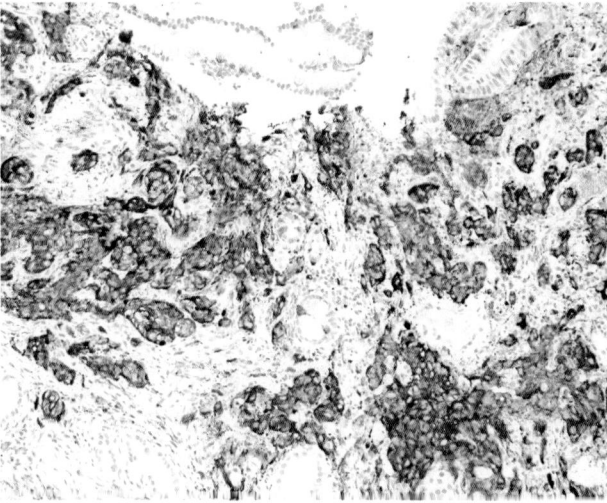

Figure 6-180. Gangliocytic paraganglioma. This is a synaptophysin stain, which labels epithelioid nests and ganglion cells.

MUCOSAL NEUROMAS ASSOCIATED WITH MEN IIB

Anytime other types of benign nerve sheath tumors are encountered, the concern is that the lesion could be a syndromic mucosal neuroma. Such tumors are different from ganglioneuromas. Both ganglioneuromas and mucosal mucosal neuromas are components of MEN IIB/Sipple syndrome, consisting of mucosal neuromas, pheochromocytoma, mesodermal dysplasia, and medullary thyroid carcinoma. Some of the patients with MEN IIB present with disfigured lips/mouths as a hint that there could be neural tumors throughout their gastrointestinal tracts, whereas others present with intestinal obstruction. Neuromas found in patients with MEN IIB are true neuromas; they are composed of coiled and tortuous enlarged nerves in which individual fibers are enrobed by coats of perineurium in a fashion similar to the appearance of a traumatic neuroma (Fig. 6.181). Because of the surrounding perineurium associated with such neuromas, they are easy to distinguish from various nerve sheath tumors in the differential diagnosis that are pointed out later.

NEUROFIBROMAS

Lesions that can be classified as sporadic neurofibromas are difficult to identify because most of the time, careful search demonstrates a few lesional ganglion cells such that a ganglioneuroma is diagnosed. In contrast, the neurofibromas in patients with NF1 are not very cellular and can course through all layers of the bowel or other viscera (Figs. 6.182 and 6.183). They show S100 protein labeling in some but not all of the cells and demonstrate expression of neurofilament protein.[98] Sometimes GI tract neurofibromas contain tactoid bodies (Wagner-Meissner bodies), a feature of so-called diffuse neurofibromas. However, rarely, tactoid bodies can be seen as incidental lesions without an associated neurofibroma (usually at the gastroesophageal junction) and they are unassociated with NF1 (Figs. 6.184 and 6.185).[99]

SCHWANN CELL HAMARTOMA

These tumors are also mentioned in "Colon" chapter, but it is nice to have some compare and contrast images for this section. Mucosal Schwann cell hamartoma consists of an unencapsulated proliferation of spindle cells within the lamina propria that courses between colonic crypts to form a dainty polyp detected at colonoscopy.[98] They are predominantly encountered in the rectosigmoid, but these polyps can arise anywhere in the colon. They are small (1 to 6 mm) and incidental at colonoscopy. The spindle cells show indistinct cell borders and are bland appearing with elongated or wavy nuclei arranged in a vaguely palisading configuration with ample eosinophilic fibrillary cytoplasm. There is no mucosal ulceration, nuclear atypia, or mitotic activity (Figs. 6.186–6.188).

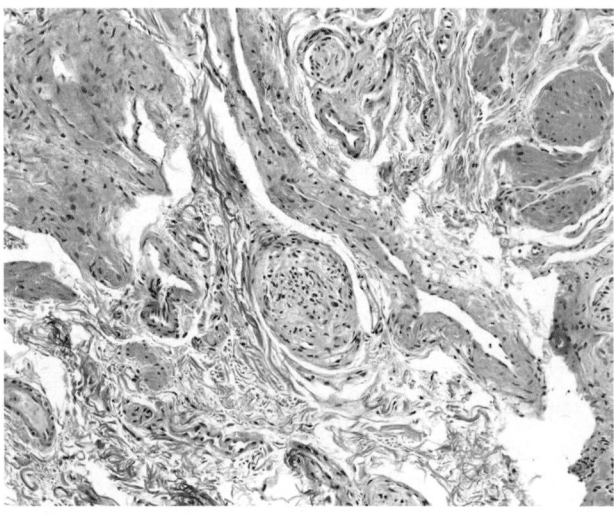

Figure 6-181. Neuroma in a patient with MEN IIB. The lesion is encircled by a ring of perineurium.

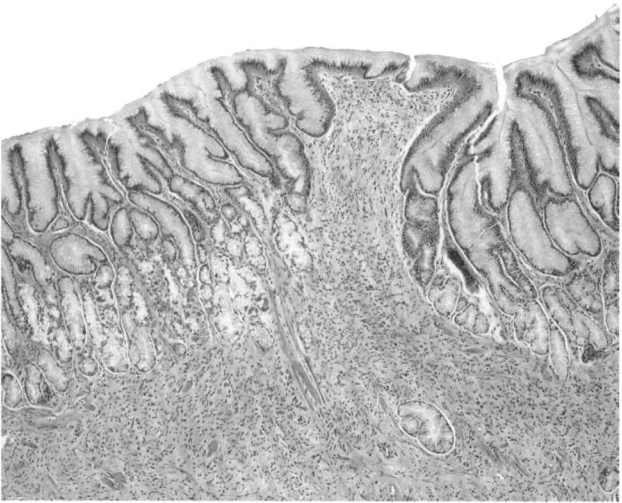

Figure 6-182. Diffuse neurofibroma in a patient with NF1. The tumor replaces the gastric lamina propria.

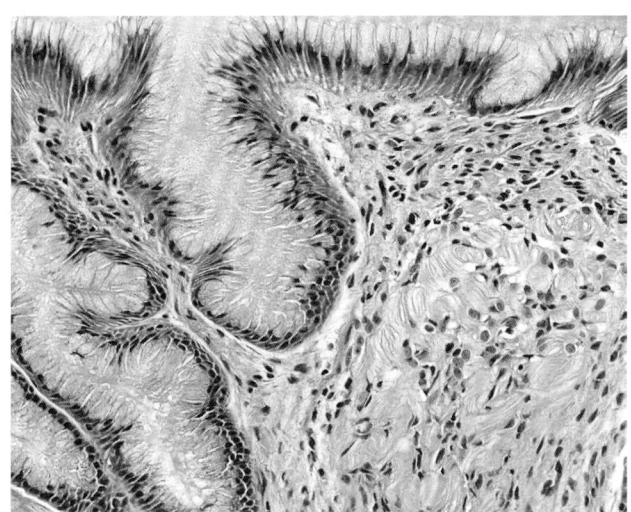

Figure 6-183. Diffuse neurofibroma in a patient with NF1. Note the Wagner-Meissner (tactoid) body.

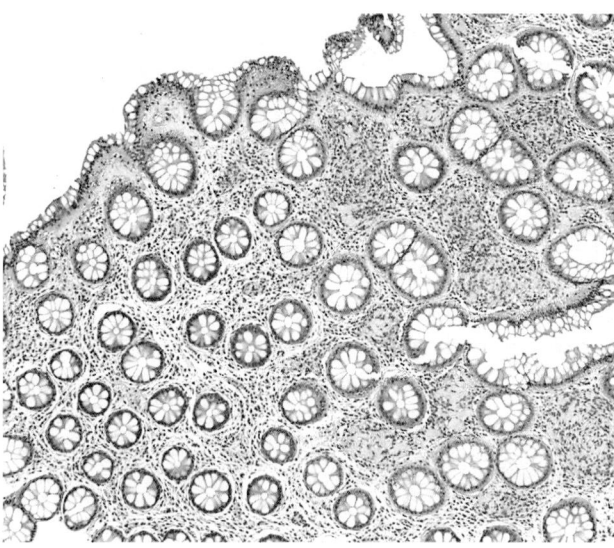

Figure 6-184. Sporadic tactoid bodies unassociated with neurofibroma.

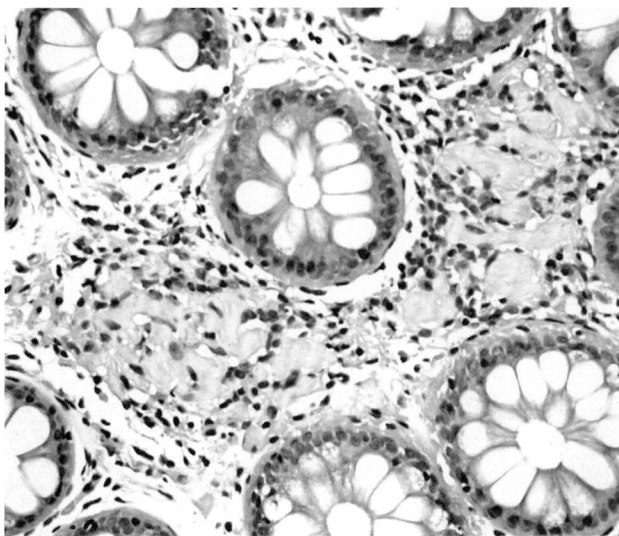

Figure 6-185. Sporadic tactoid bodies unassociated with neurofibroma. These are an incidental findings—the tactoid bodies are naked in the lamina propria with no Schwann cell population to hide them!

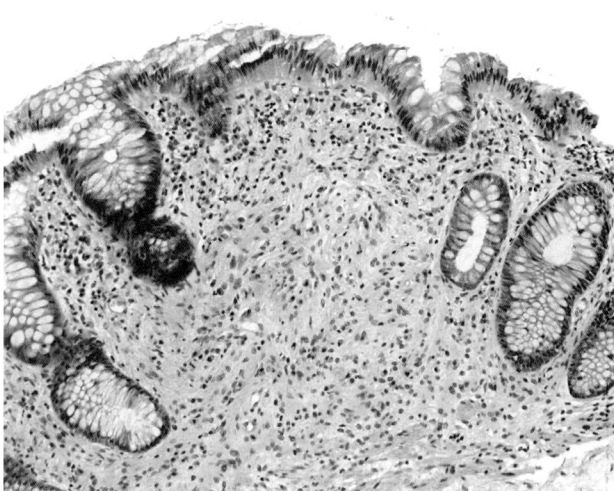

Figure 6-186. Schwann cell hamartoma. This benign sporadic neural proliferation is found in the lamina propria of the colon. There is a suggesting of nuclear palisading.

Schwann cell hamartomas are diffusely immunoreactive for S100 protein. They are negative for CD34, GFAP, EMA, SMA, and CD117. The main differential diagnosis is with colonic neurofibroma, an important distinction given an association between neurofibromas and NF1. Colonic neurofibromas display more cellular heterogeneity with more nuclear variability and varying amounts of cytoplasm; by immunohistochemistry the spindle cells in neurofibromas are only focally immunoreactive with S100 and all contain associated axons, which are highlighted with a neurofilament protein immunostain. Schwann cell hamartomas are unassociated with syndromes. Follow-up is not necessary after diagnosis.

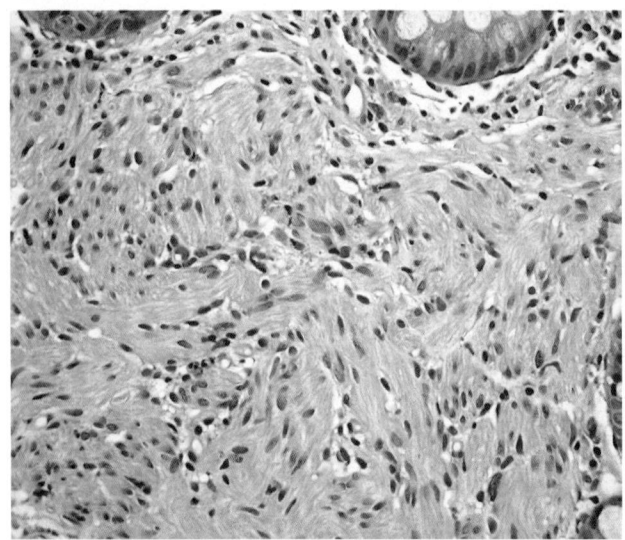

Figure 6-187. Schwann cell hamartoma. Note the fibrillary pink cytoplasm, which is reminiscent of smooth muscle cytoplasm, but the nuclei have more pointy ends than those of smooth muscle lesions.

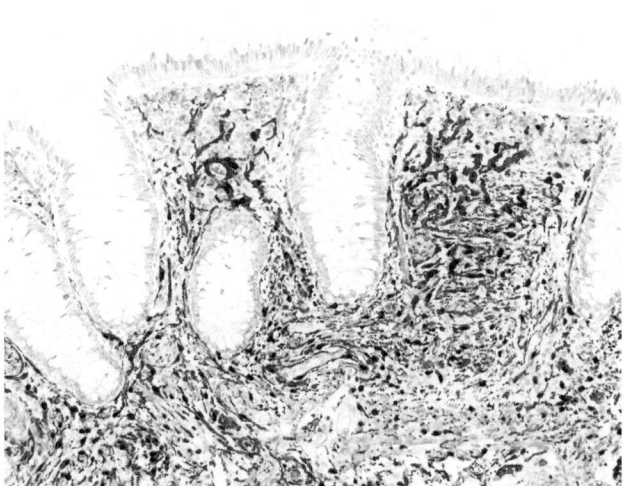

Figure 6-188. Schwann cell hamartoma. There is strong labeling with S100 protein.

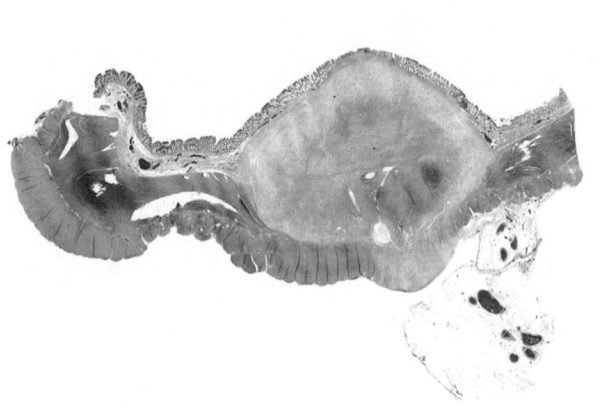

Figure 6-189. Benign epithelioid nerve sheath tumor (epithelioid schwannoma). This lesion has filled the submucosa and is also present in the mucosa and muscularis propria. However, this type of tumor is often restricted to the mucosa and submucosa.

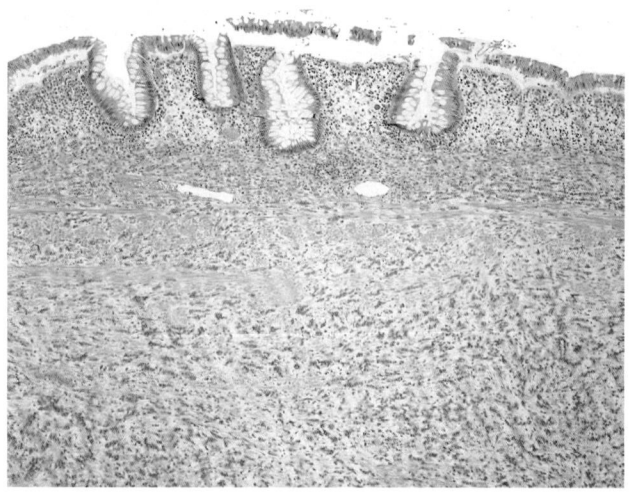

Figure 6-190. Benign epithelioid nerve sheath tumor (epithelioid schwannoma). The tumor consists of plump eosinophilic cells.

EPITHELIOID NERVE SHEATH TUMOR (EPITHELIOID SCHWANNOMA)

Colonic epithelioid nerve sheath tumors (epithelioid schwannomas) are detected at screening colonoscopy as incidental polyps[100] and usually arise in the left colon, attaining a size of up to 1 cm. Most are restricted to the mucosa and submucosa, although we have occasionally encountered transmural large examples. None of the patients that we have studied with these tumors has had a known history of neurofibromatosis or MEN IIB.

These lesions have an infiltrative growth pattern, consisting of spindled to predominantly epithelioid cells arranged in nests and whorls (Figs. 6.188–6.196). They are centered in the lamina propria with extension to the superficial submucosa although, as discussed earlier, we have also reviewed cases that extend into the muscularis propria. The tumor cells have uniform round to oval nuclei with frequent intranuclear pseudoinclusions and eosinophilic fibrillary cytoplasm. Some cases contain cystic spaces and

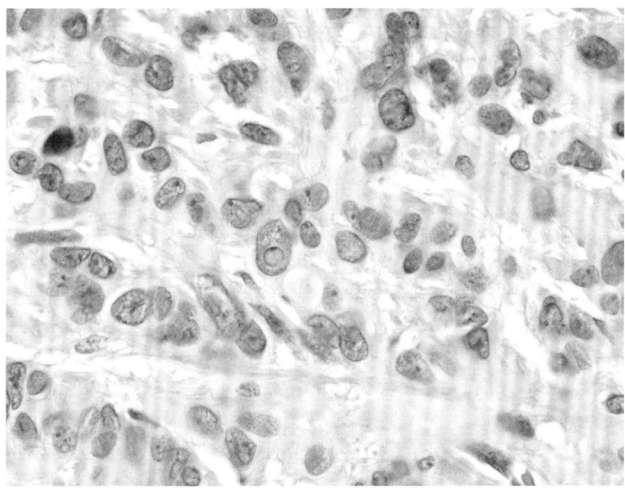

Figure 6-191. Benign epithelioid nerve sheath tumor (epithelioid schwannoma). Note the intranuclear cytoplasmic invagination (inclusion) in the center of the field.

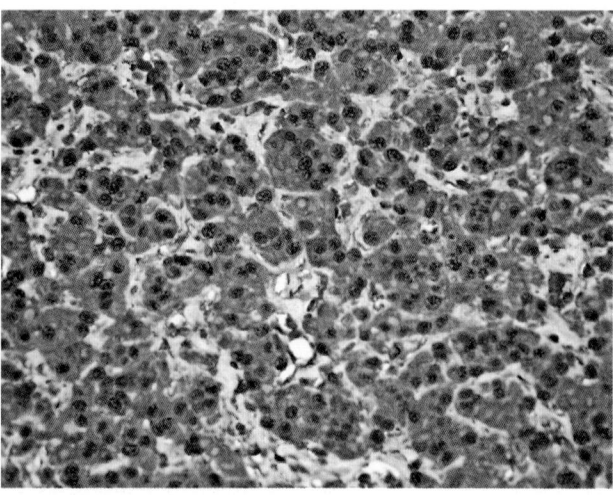

Figure 6-192. Benign epithelioid nerve sheath tumor (epithelioid schwannoma). These tumors have strong diffuse S100 protein expression.

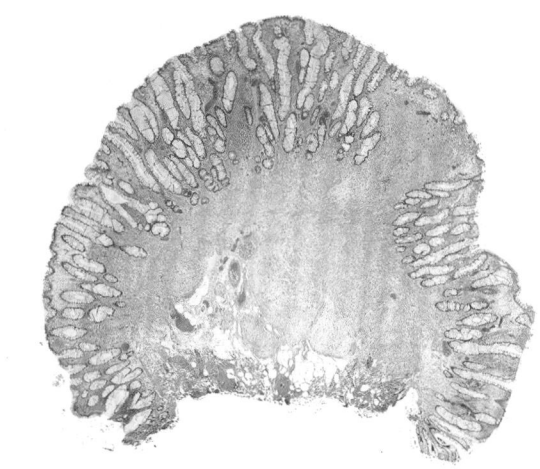

Figure 6-193. Benign epithelioid nerve sheath tumor (epithelioid schwannoma). This example is present in the mucosa and submucosa.

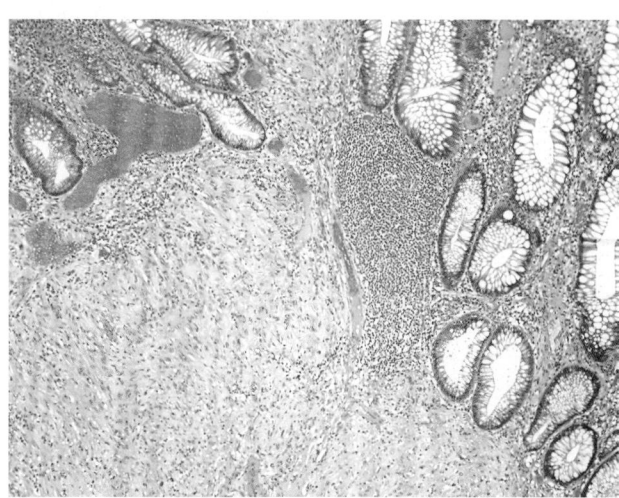

Figure 6-194. Benign epithelioid nerve sheath tumor (epithelioid schwannoma). Note the plump epithelioid cells.

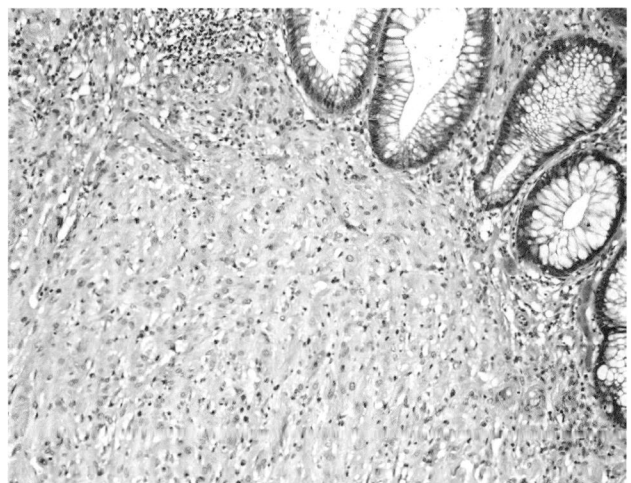

Figure 6-195. Benign epithelioid nerve sheath tumor (epithelioid schwannoma). Many cells have intranuclear pseudoinclusions.

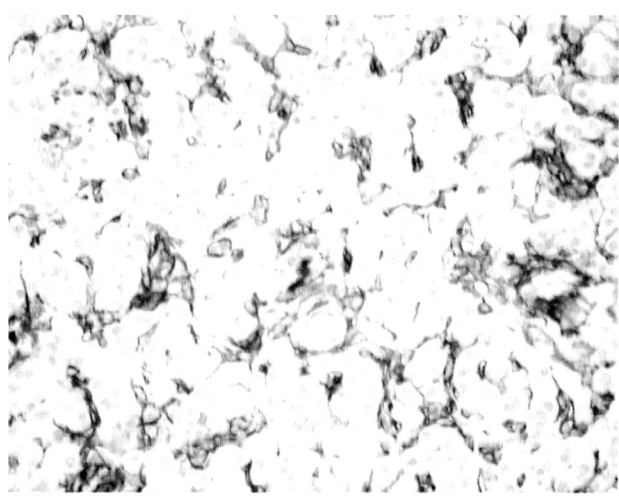

Figure 6-196. Benign epithelioid nerve sheath tumor (epithelioid schwannoma). A CD34 stain highlights supporting cells and blood vessels.

a pseudoglandular pattern. No mitoses are seen. If Ki-67 is performed, there is a low proliferative index. This is sometimes done based on the concern that the patient harbors a melanoma and can be reassuring. These tumors express diffuse S-100 protein but lack other than the faintest blush of melanoma marker expression. They often show focal CD34 labeling in supporting cells. Mercifully, CD117 is negative. Calretinin and SM31 shows no intralesional neuraxons.

GRANULAR CELL TUMOR

Most gastrointestinal granular cell tumors are found in the esophagus, but the colon is the second most common site.[101] Gastrointestinal tract granular cell tumors display the features of granular cell tumors elsewhere (including S100 protein expression) and they are also discussed in "Esophagus" chapter, but they can be sneaky when they are present in the colonic lamina propria, where they can have an appearance similar to that of muciphages (Figs. 6.197 and 6.198). There is an equal gender distribution and a mean age of about 50 years, so these tumors are found in members of the elite screening colonoscopy club.[102] In contrast to granular cell tumors of the esophagus, colorectal granular cell tumors are slightly more common in whites than in African Americans. They are usually incidentally discovered at colonoscopy and most often arise in the right colon. They range in size from less than 1 cm to about 2 cm. Colorectal granular cell tumors can be infiltrative or well-marginated, involving the mucosa, submucosa, or both. Sometimes they are associated with a lymphoid cuff just like schwannomas. An important pitfall is that they can display cytologic atypia and areas of calcification. Some cases underlie reactive surface epithelial changes, which can lead to misdiagnosis as adenoma. Mitoses and areas of necrosis are typically absent. We are aware of rare reports of multicentric granular cell tumors of the colon[103] but found only a single malignant example with histologic documentation arising in the colorectum.[104] Please forgive us if we missed your case report of another one! Benign colorectal granular cell tumors can recur following incomplete excision.

PERINEURIOMA

These tumors were initially described using the term "benign fibroblastic polyp of the colon."[105] These are—like many other entities reported since colonoscopy was endorsed for average-risk patients—incidental lesions detected in adult patients during screening colonoscopy. The mean age in reported series ranges from 56 to 64 years. These tumors present as small, solitary, asymptomatic polyps (size range, 0.2 to 1.5 cm) usually encountered in the rectosigmoid colon.

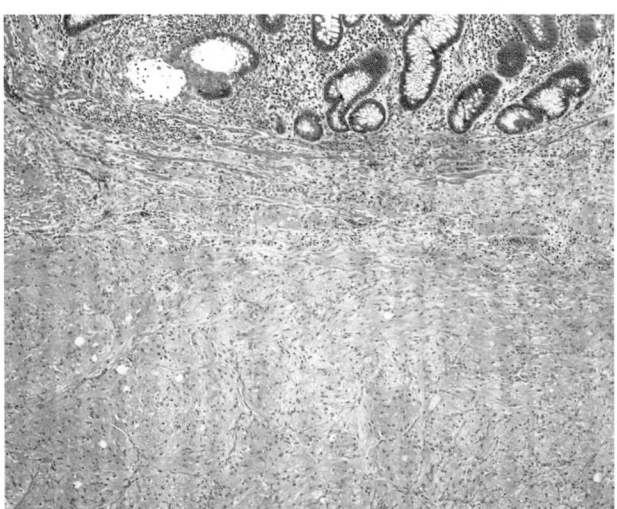

Figure 6-197. Colonic granular cell tumor. The cells are plump and eosinophilic and centered in the superficial submucosa.

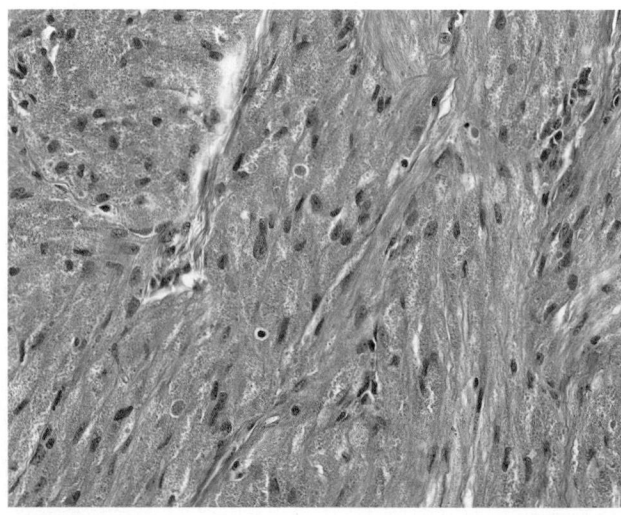

Figure 6-198. Colonic granular cell tumor. Note the granular cytoplasm and mild nuclear atypia, a feature that is common in lesions of the right colon.

Perineuriomas consist of an expansion of the lamina propria by a bland, monomorphic spindle cell population with pale eosinophilic cytoplasm focally arranged in a concentric fashion around vessels and crypts with very delicate fibrillary cytoplasm and no areas of palisading (Figs. 6.199–6.208). There is no mitotic activity or necrosis. Some are found in the lamina propria of serrated polyps (Figs. 6.206–6.208) (either sessile serrated adenomas or hyperplastic polyps), which allows authors to discuss "epithelial stromal interactions," but the whole shootin' match is incidental and benign.[106]

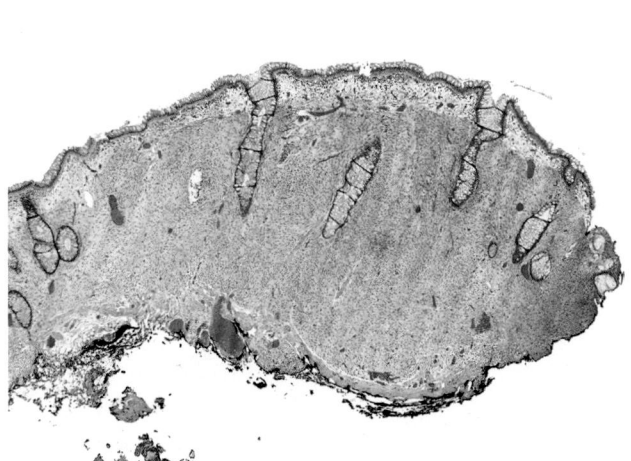

Figure 6-199. Perineurioma. The tumor proliferates between the colonic crypts.

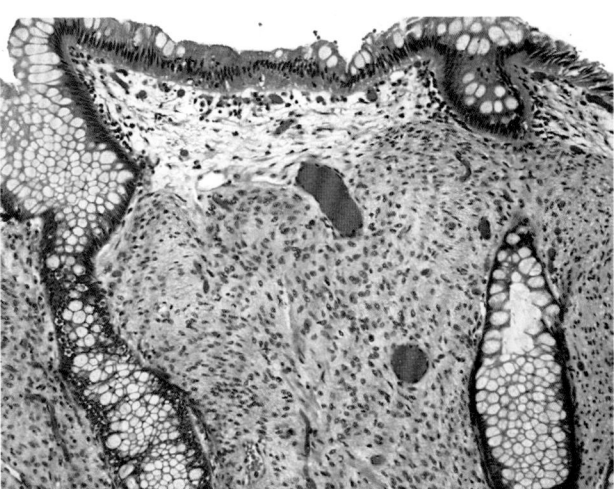

Figure 6-200. Perineurioma. The cytoplasm is paler than that of epithelioid schwannomas and more scant than that of granular cell tumors.

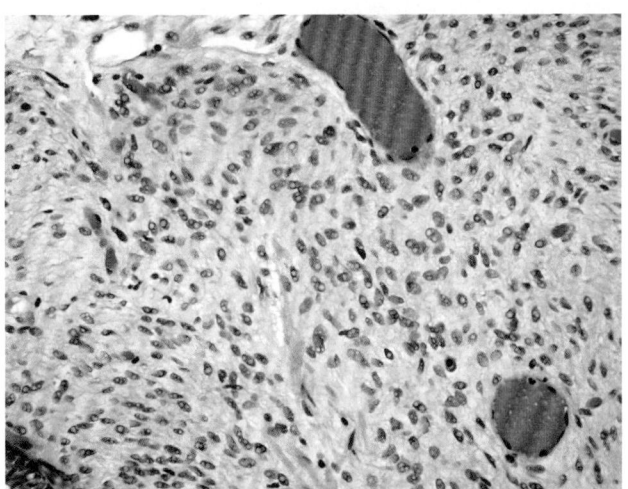

Figure 6-201. Perineurioma. This example has intranuclear pseudoinclusions akin to those in meningiomas. There are cells with long cytoplasmic processes at the left part of the image.

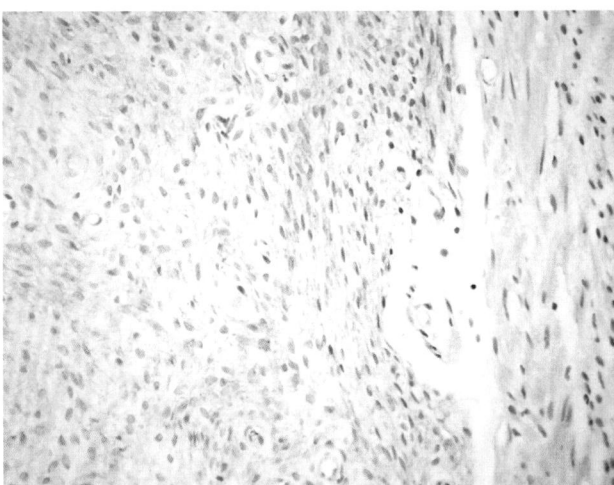

Figure 6-202. Perineurioma. This is an epithelial membrane antigen (EMA) stain. Do not expect intense labeling. EMA highlights the cytoplasmic processes, which are quite slim and dainty.

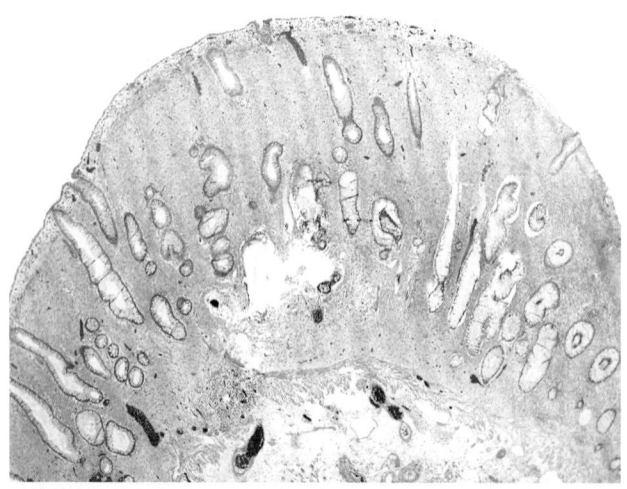

Figure 6-203. Perineurioma. This lesion has filled much of the lamina propria without disturbing too many of the crypts.

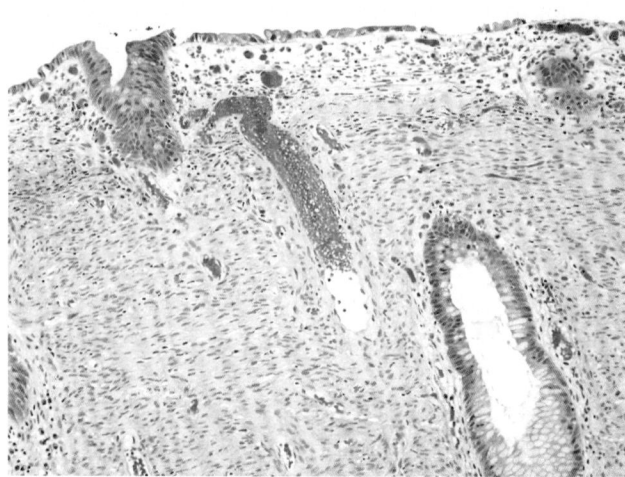

Figure 6-204. Perineurioma. High magnification shows bland cytologic features of the lesion.

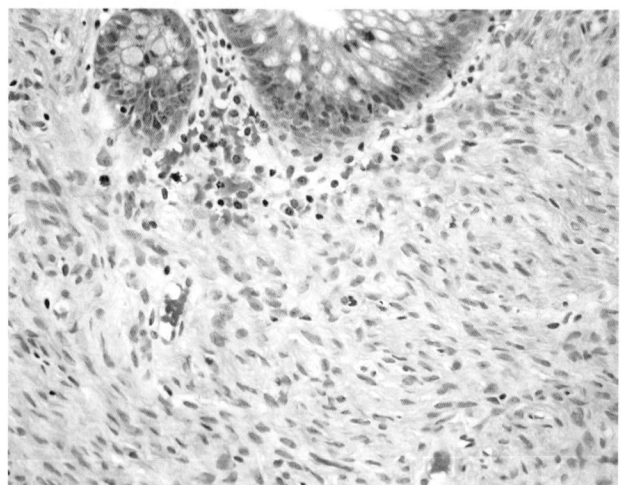

Figure 6-205. Perineurioma. Many of the nuclei have pointy ends.

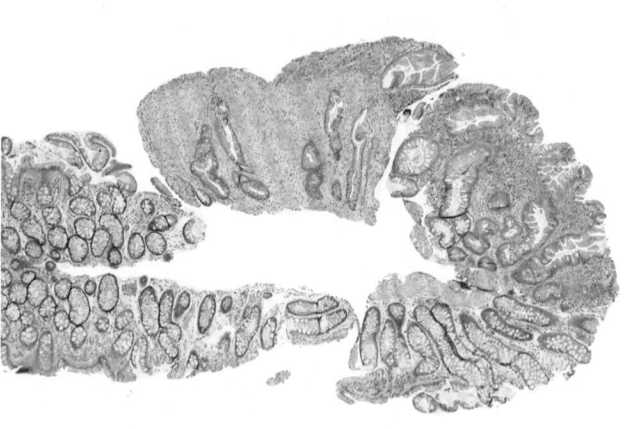

Figure 6-206. Perineurioma. Many are associated with serrated polyps (either hyperplastic polyps or sessile serrated adenomas). This one is associated with a hyperplastic polyp.

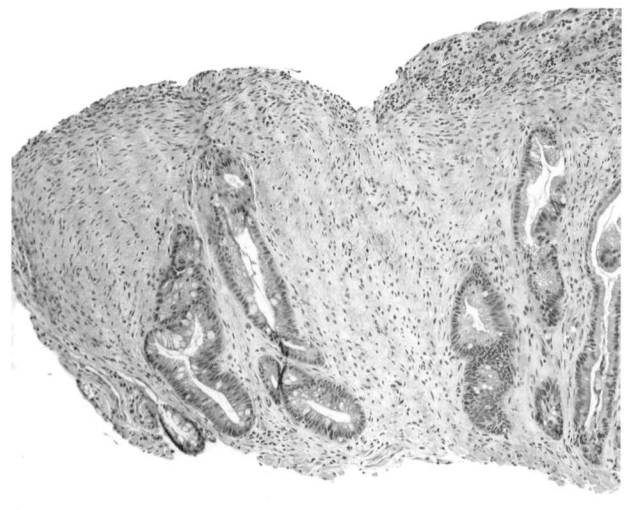

Figure 6-207. Perineurioma. This is a high magnification image of the lesion seen in Fig. 6.206.

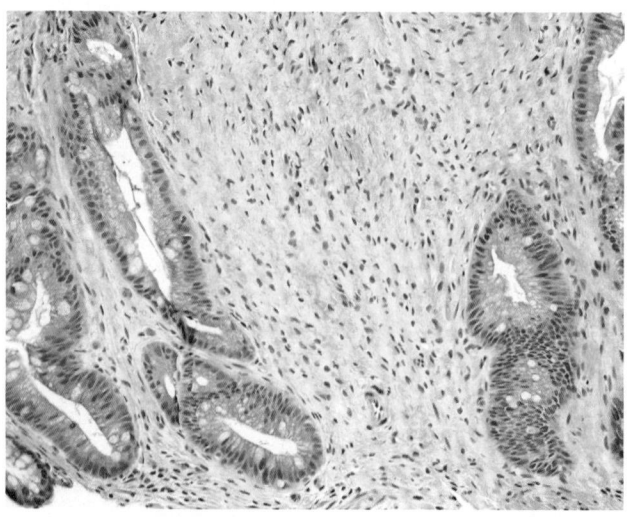

Figure 6-208. Perineurioma. This is a very high magnification image of the lesion seen in Figs. 6.206 and 6.207.

If immunolabeling is performed, there is no CD31, S100, CD117/KIT, Bcl-2, and desmin expression. Most of these polyps express at least one perineurial marker (EMA, claudin 1, and glucose transporter-1/GLUT1).[107-109] There can be focal CD34 or actin labeling, as is the case with most benign neural related lesions. The Ki67 labeling index is consistently low (about 1%). In one study of 22 cases associated with serrated polyps, the authors detected *BRAF* and *KRAS* mutations in 63% and 4% of cases, respectively, in the serrated polyp but not in the perineurioma.[106]

Perineuriomas are benign and managed by polypectomy and require no endoscopic follow-up. Of course if there is an associated sessile serrated polyp/adenoma, it drives the follow-up, as discussed in "Colon" chapter.

SUMMARY OF NEURAL POLYPS

See Fig. 6.209.

1. *Ganglioneuroma*
   Can be syndromic (MEN IIB, NF1, Cowden syndrome/PTEN hamartoma syndrome) but usually sporadic. Schwann cells and scattered ganglion cells. Syndromic lesions are large or multifocal.
2. *Mucosal neuroma*
   Syndromic—characteristic of MEN IIB. Schwann cell proliferation coated by perineurium. Can traverse the layers of the bowel or present as "mucosal neuromas."

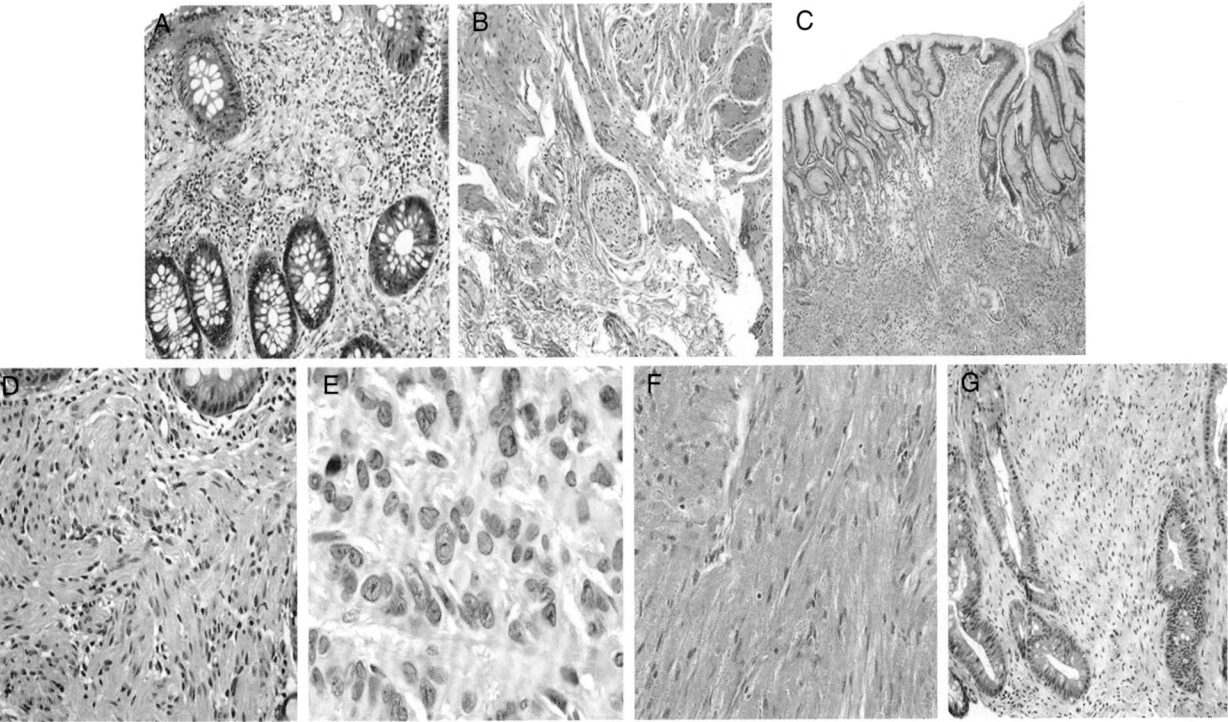

Figure 6-209. Summary of neural polyps. **A:** Ganglioneuroma can be syndromic (MEN IIB, NF1, Cowden syndrome/PTEN hamartoma syndrome) but is usually sporadic. It consists of Schwann cells and scattered ganglion cells. **B:** Mucosal neuroma is syndromic and characteristic of MEN IIB. Lesions consist of a Schwann and axonal cell proliferation coated by perineurium. **C:** Neurofibroma of the mucosa is rare as a sporadic lesion and associated with NF1. It consists of a Schwann cell proliferation with lesional axons. **D:** Schwann cell hamartoma is sporadic and consists of a Schwann cell proliferation in the mucosa with fibrillary pink cytoplasm. Every cell labels with S100 protein. **E:** Epithelioid nerve sheath tumor (epithelioid schwannoma) is sporadic and formed by epithelioid cells with prominent intranuclear pseudoinclusions. There is strong diffuse S100 protein expression. **F:** Granular cell tumor is sporadic and composed of granular cells usually seen in the lamina propria and submucosa of esophagus and colon. Mild nuclear atypia is acceptable. **G:** Perineurioma (benign fibroblastic polyp of the colon) is sporadic. It is sometimes associated with serrated polyps. It is centered in lamina propria, proliferating between glands. The cells have long cytoplasmic processes. On immunolabeling it is characterized by negative S100 protein and expression of perineurial markers (EMA, claudin 1, GLUT1).

3. *Neurofibroma*

Rare as a sporadic lesion—If encountered, consider NF1. Schwann cell proliferation with lesional axons. Can be found in any layer. Not all lesional cells express S100 protein.

4. *Schwann cell hamartoma*

Sporadic—Schwann cell proliferation in mucosa with fibrillary pink cytoplasm. Every cell labels with S100 protein.

5. *Epithelioid nerve sheath tumor (epithelioid schwannoma)*

Sporadic—Epithelioid cells with prominent intranuclear pseudoinclusions in lamina propria and submucosa. Strong diffuse S100 protein expression.

6. *Granular cell tumor*

Sporadic—Granular cells usually seen in lamina propria and submucosa of esophagus and colon. Mild nuclear atypia is acceptable.

7. *Perineurioma (benign fibroblastic polyp of the colon)*

Sporadic—Sometimes associated with serrated polyps. Centered in lamina propria, proliferating between glands. Long cytoplasmic processes. Negative S100 protein, expression of perineurial markers (EMA, claudin 1, GLUT1).

NEAR MISS

CASE

The biopsies shown in Figs. 6.210–6.214 were taken from a colorectal polyp from a 40-year-old woman. A diagnosis of adenocarcinoma invading the submucosa was made, and the patient was scheduled for a limited resection and asked for a second opinion on her slides. Fortunately the pathologist who re-reviewed the case spotted an issue.

What Went Wrong?

There is no adenocarcinoma, just endometriosis! Endometriosis is tough to recognize outside its usual locations.

Endometrial Lesions (Endometriosis and Endometrial Stromal Sarcoma)

Endometriosis can be a real pitfall—it is known to present in a variety of sites. It involves the GI tract in up to 40% of patients with pelvic endometriosis; about a third of these patients have mucosal lesions that can be encountered on biopsies.[110] The secret weapon for diagnosing endometriosis is to think of it! Ouch. The sigmoid colon is the most likely site.

Most of the time, endometriosis affects the serosa or muscularis propria and is accompanied by abundant fibrosis and adhesions, although submucosal examples are also reported.

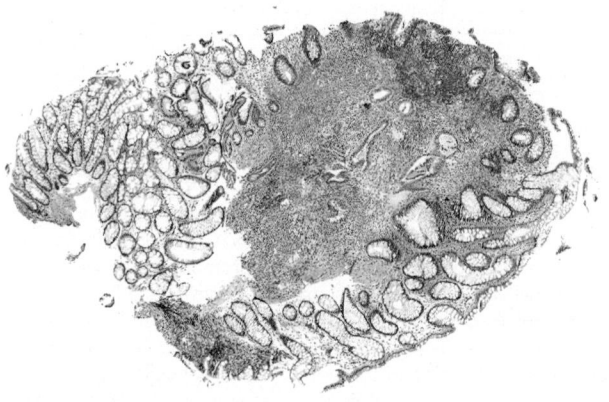

Figure 6-210. Endometriosis. The lesion consists of endometrial-type glands and stroma. The key to diagnosis is to consider it.

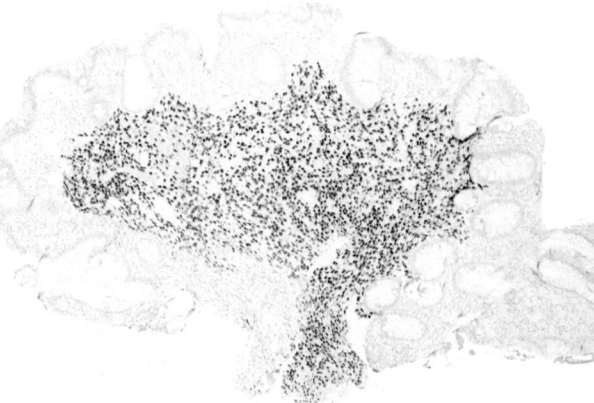

Figure 6-211. Endometriosis. This is an estrogen receptor stain.

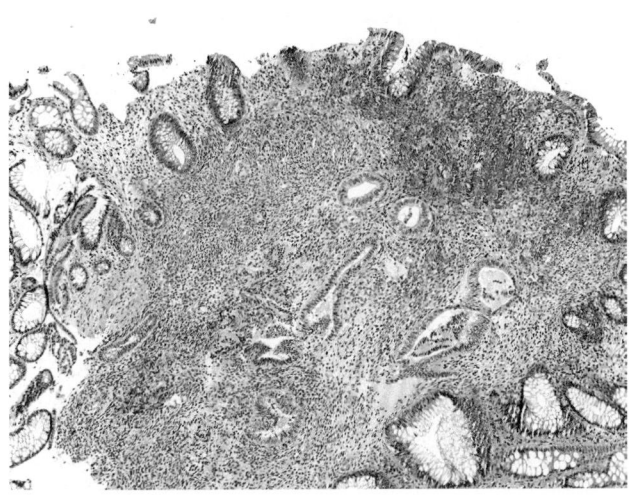

Figure 6-212. Endometriosis. In this example, both endometrial glands and stroma are present. Cases lacking the glands can be difficult and a sarcoma can be considered.

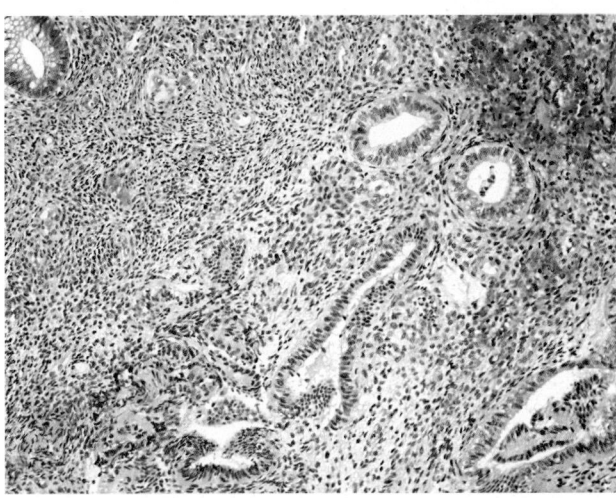

Figure 6-213. Endometriosis. The glands lack goblet cells.

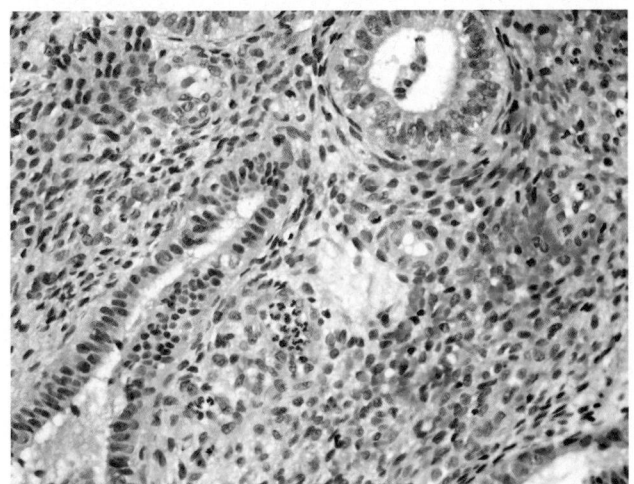

Figure 6-214. Endometriosis. High magnification highlights the stromal cells.

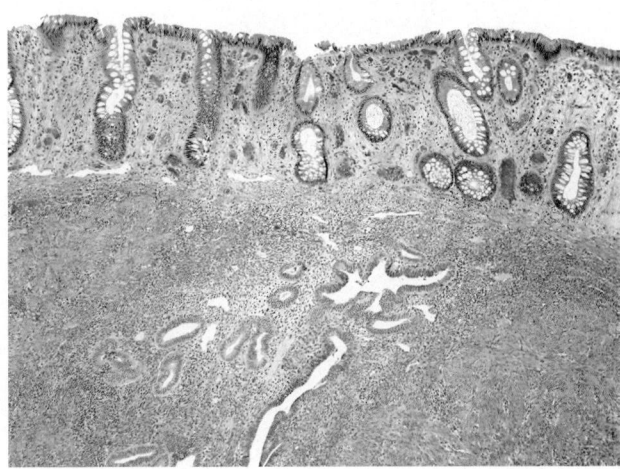

Figure 6-215. Endometriosis. In this example, there is brightly eosinophilic smooth muscle metaplasia in the stroma in the areas at the upper left and lower right.

Of course once you think of it, the diagnosis is easy—colonic endometriosis has the same appearance as found elsewhere, consisting of endometrial-type glands, stroma associated with some hemosiderin deposition, and a fibroblastic response (Figs. 6.210–6.214). Some examples develop smooth muscle metaplasia in the stromal component (Figs. 6.215 and 6.216)! A stromal decidual reaction can be found in endometriotic foci in pregnant patients.

Endometriosis can mimic Kaposi sarcoma, and if only the stromal component is present, this can raise the possibility of a sarcoma. Additionally, reactive epithelial changes in endometriosis can simulate colonic neoplasms. Rarely, endometrial stromal sarcomas can spread to the colon or even arise in association with colorectal endometriosis—because these are translocation sarcomas, they have monotonous nuclei such that synovial sarcoma (see earlier discussion) can be considered. A special clue: look for the starburst pattern of collagen deposition (Figs. 6.217–6.220).[111] Adding CD10 and hormone receptor protein immunolabeling seals the diagnosis. Fortunately, KIT labeling is unlikely in low-grade endometrial stromal sarcomas, but PDGFRA immunolabeling is often reactive.[112] Unfortunately, KIT immunolabeling is likely in high-grade endometrial stromal sarcomas with *YWHAE* gene rearrangements, and it is the high-grade ones that lose their hormone receptors.[113] However, these appear far more malignant (small round blue cell tumors) than GISTs or the usual endometrial stromal sarcoma and can require molecular testing to diagnose.

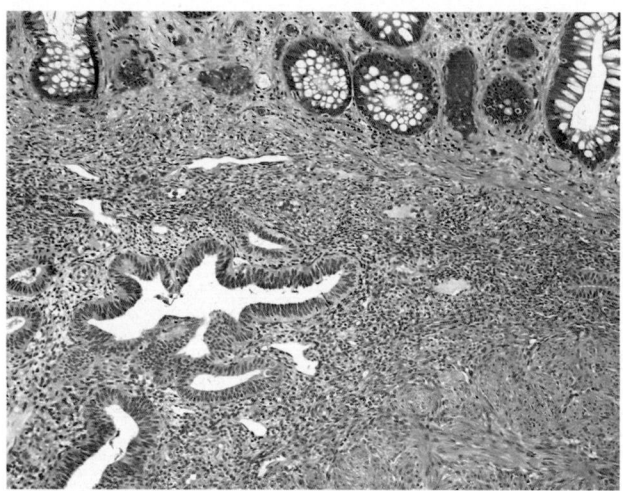

Figure 6-216. Endometriosis. This high magnification image of the lesion seen in Fig. 6.215 shows smooth muscle metaplasia in the stroma at the lower right.

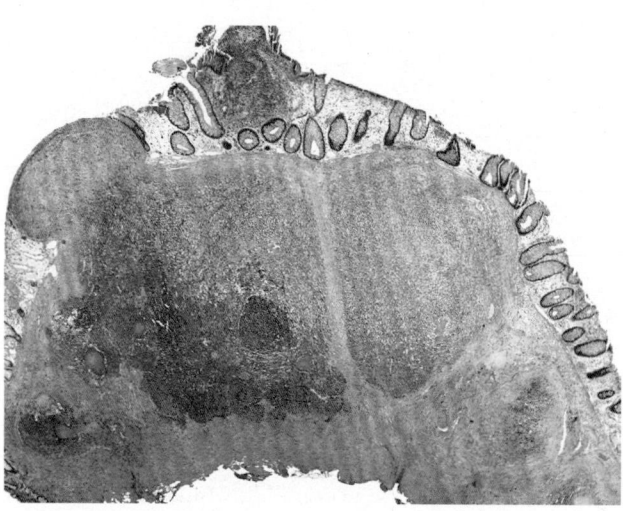

Figure 6-217. Endometrial stromal sarcoma presenting as a colorectal polyp. Note the peculiar pattern of collagen deposition at the lower left of the image.

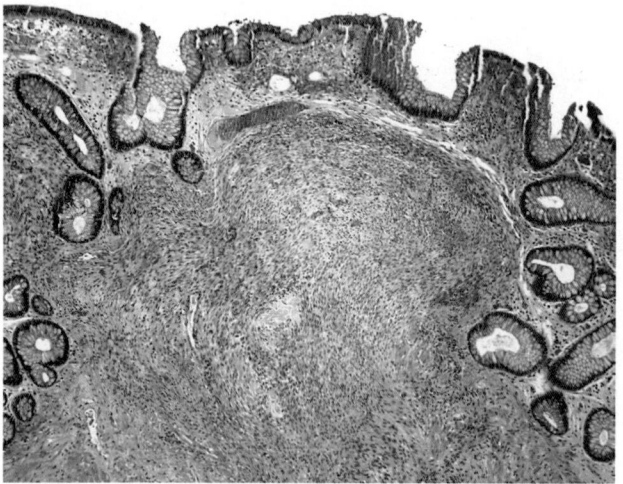

Figure 6-218. Endometrial stromal sarcoma presenting as a colorectal polyp. These are translocation-associated sarcomas, so they are appearing monotonous.

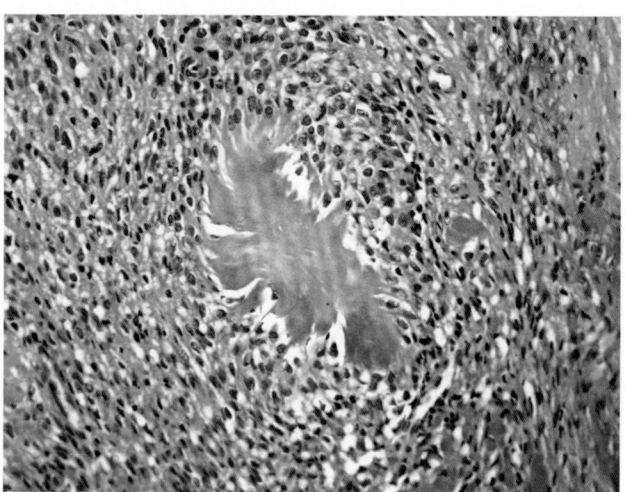

Figure 6-219. Endometrial stromal sarcoma presenting as a colorectal polyp. This image shows the "starburst collagen" pattern that characterizes low-grade endometrial stromal sarcoma.

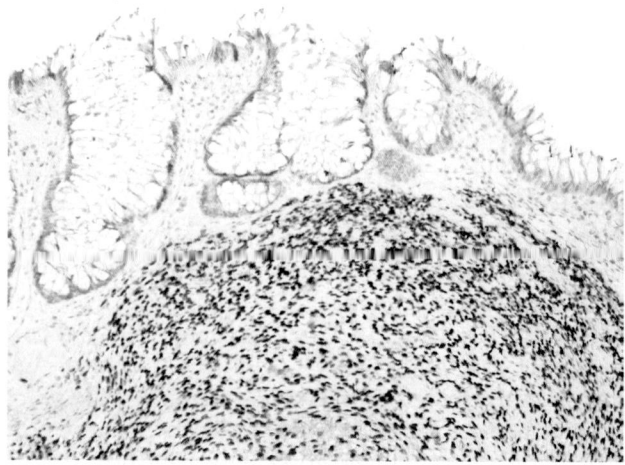

Figure 6-220. Endometrial stromal sarcoma presenting as a colorectal polyp. This is an estrogen receptor stain.

A FEW VASCULAR TUMORS

ANASTOMOSING HEMANGIOMA

These are rare lesions and mainly of importance because they can be mistaken for angiosarcoma.[114,115] They were initially reported in the male genital tract and kidney but can be found anywhere in the body, so far reported in adults. They occasionally arise in the colon, mesentery, and liver!

Overall, anastomosing hemangiomas are well marginated even though this can be tough to discern on a needle biopsy (Figs. 6.221–6.223). Like angiosarcomas, they have an anastomosing pattern (vessels that are not round tubes through which blood passes but vessels with irregular outlines that snake into the tissue). However, unlike in angiosarcomas, the endothelial cells in anastomosing hemangiomas line spaces, but there is a rim of cells that are not endothelial cells that support the vessels such that the spaces are basically forming in the way that normal vessels form. So, not only are the vessels held up with their own special supporting tissues, but also the endothelial cells that line them are not particularly large and mitoses are not there. There can be some mitoses in the supporting cells around the lumina and this is acceptable. The endothelial cells in anastomosing hemangiomas have a hobnail appearance (they pooch out into the lumina) but they are small. Many examples contain hyaline globules and extramedullary hematopoiesis.

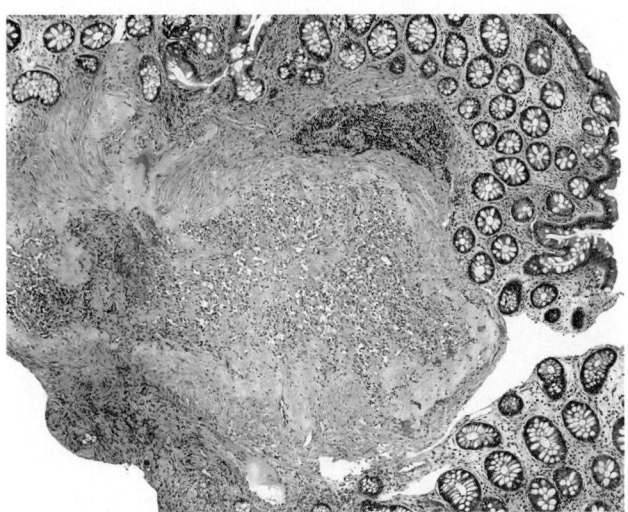

Figure 6-221. Anastomosing hemangioma. This lesion presented as a colorectal polyp. It is small and relatively well marginated.

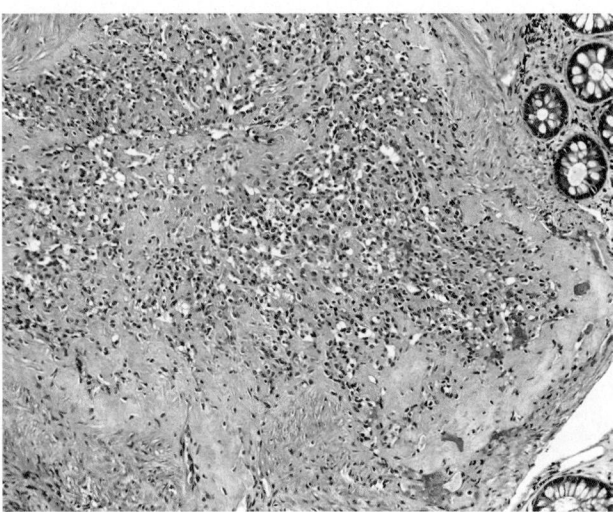

Figure 6-222. Anastomosing hemangioma. The vessels have an anastomosing pattern, but they are cuffed by supporting cells.

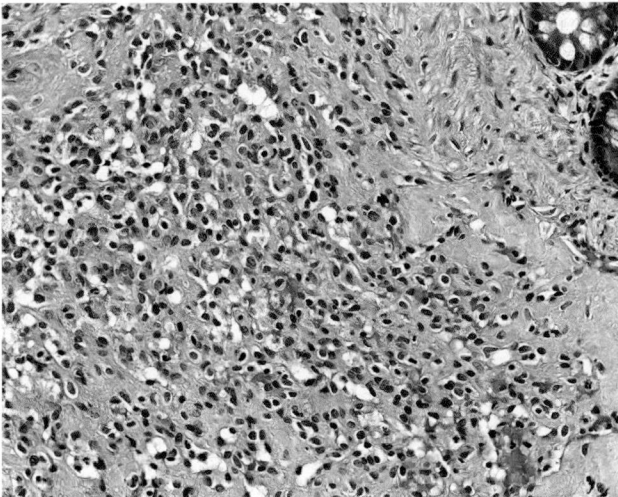

Figure 6-223. Anastomosing hemangioma. The nuclei of the lesional cells are small and not particularly atypical.

MALIGNANT VASCULAR LESIONS

GI tract angiosarcomas are rare and tend to be epithelioid. They can involve the GI tract as a primary or metastatic sarcoma. The tendency to epithelioid morphology in GI tract angiosarcomas means that they are easily confused with carcinoma. They usually are found in the small bowel or mesentery thereof. Grossly they are often red, polypoid mucosal- or serosal-based hemorrhagic, friable lesions. They are infiltrative, growing in diffuse sheets of epithelioid cells with areas of clefting. They typically consist of uniform, epithelioid cells with eosinophilic cytoplasm and hyperchromatic nuclei with very prominent nucleoli (Figs. 6.224 and 6.225). Some cells have intracytoplasmic lumina that hold red blood cells. Immunohistochemical staining can lead to trouble, as the epithelioid variant of angiosarcoma is immunoreactive to AE1/AE3 and may also show immunoreactivity using other keratins such as Cam5.2, CK19, and CK7 and using EMA. These tumors, for whatever reason, lack CK20 expression and are immunoreactive with vascular markers (ERG, CD31, CD34, or Factor VIII). This tumor has aggressive behavior and recognizing it is important, sadly mostly to prognosticate.[116]

Kaposi's sarcoma can be found anywhere in the GI tract, usually in the setting of severe immunosuppression as a result of HIV infection. Histologic exam shows a proliferation of HHV8/LAN1+, CD34+, CD31+ spindle cells usually associated with extravasated erythrocytes (Figs. 6.226–6.231).

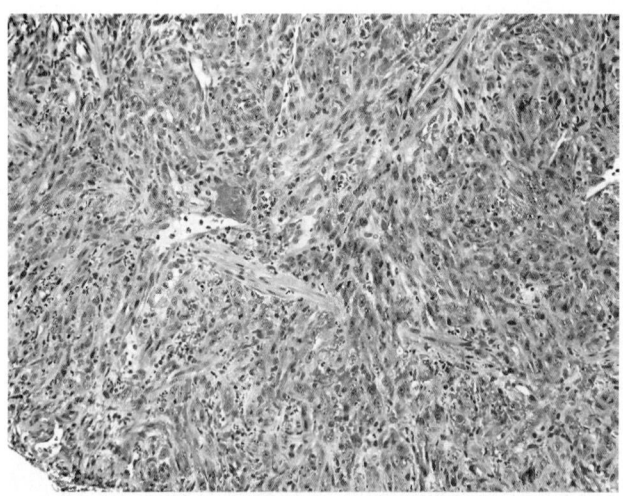

Figure 6-224. Angiosarcoma. There are sheets of endothelial cells that are scarcely vasoformative.

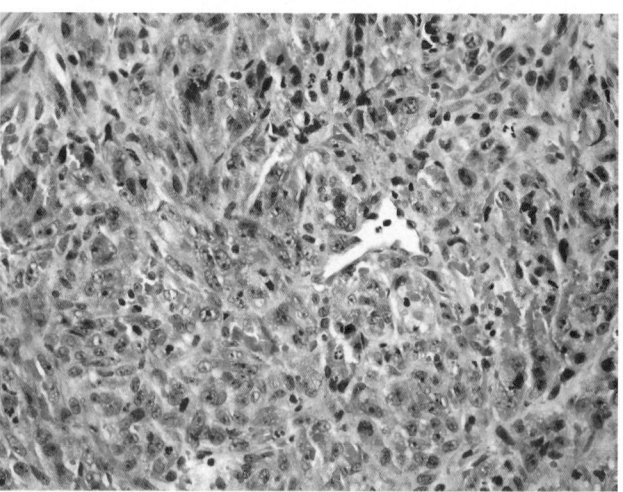

Figure 6-225. Angiosarcoma. There are enlarged atypical cells with macronucleoli.

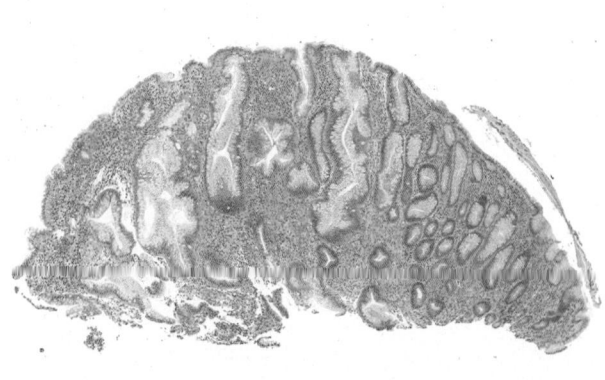

Figure 6-226. Kaposi sarcoma. The tumor has replaced the gastric lamina propria.

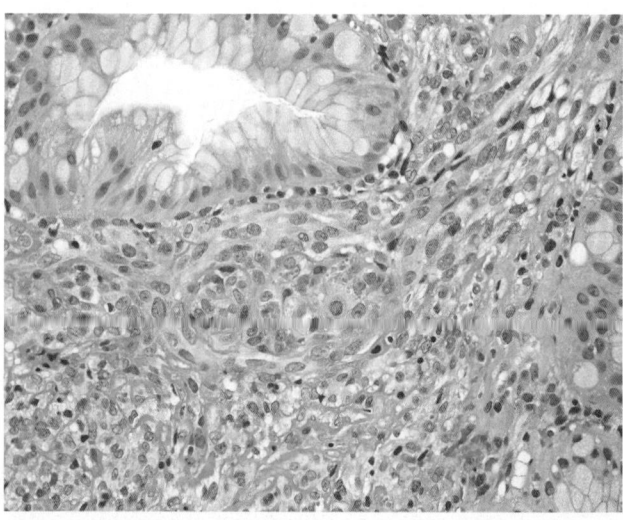

Figure 6-227. Kaposi sarcoma. There is a spindle cell population replacing the lamina propria. Note the hyaline globules (erythrophagolysosomes) in the center of the image.

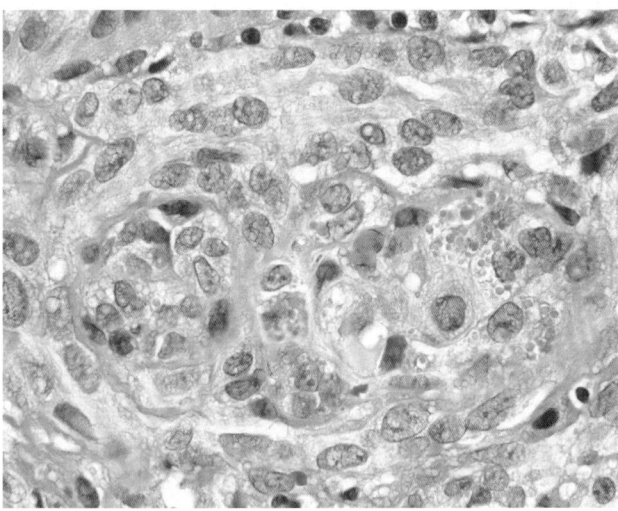

Figure 6-228. Kaposi sarcoma. This high magnification image highlights the hyaline globules.

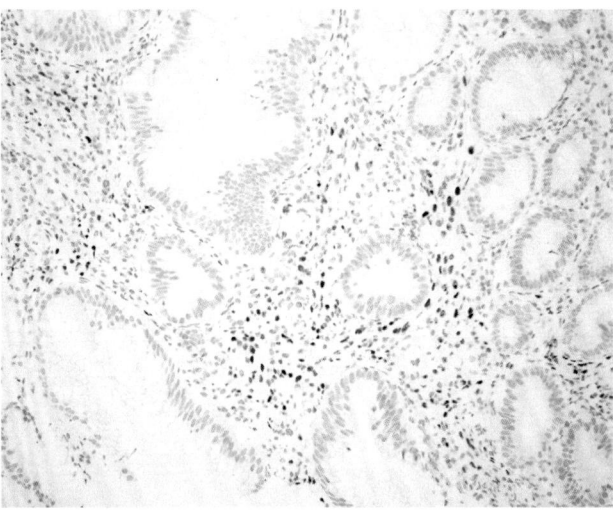

Figure 6-229. Kaposi sarcoma. The nuclei are highlighted by immunolabeling for LANA (human herpes virus 8/HHV8).

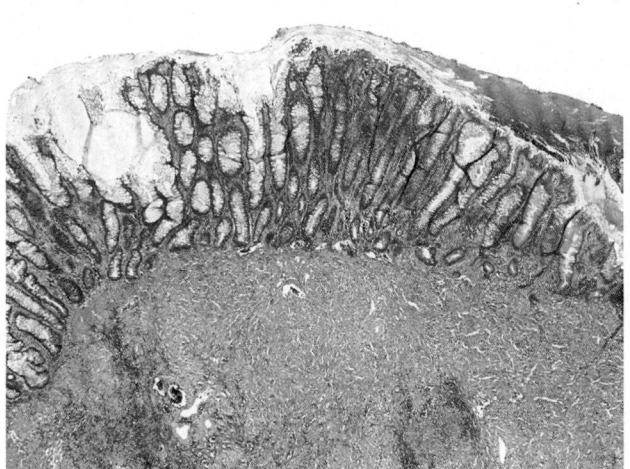

Figure 6-230. Kaposi sarcoma. This lesion has a more vasoformative appearance than many examples.

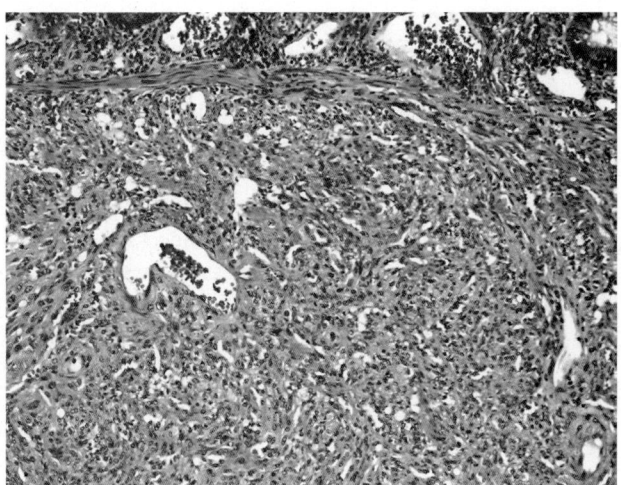

Figure 6-231. Kaposi sarcoma. On high magnification of the lesion seen in Fig. 6.230, extravasated erythrocytes are a prominent feature.

PEARLS & PITFALLS: Kaposi Sarcoma

An important pitfall is that Kaposi sarcoma is often KIT reactive but, mercifully, not DOG1 reactive.[117]

NEAR MISS

CASE

The lesion shown in Figs. 6.232 and 6.233 was resected from a 76-year-old man's colon and retroperitoneum and diagnosed as a GIST based on CD117 immunolabeling. The patient sought an oncology opinion, and the oncologist requested *KIT* and *PDGFRA* mutational analysis, which prompted review of the slides to choose a block for testing. The diagnosis was revised.

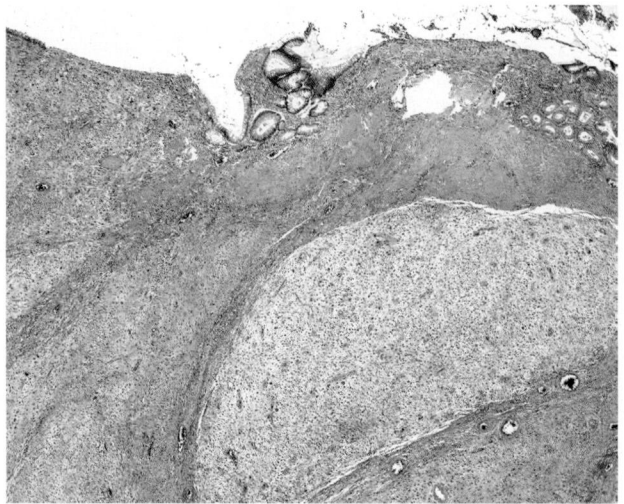

Figure 6-232. Dedifferentiated liposarcoma extending into the gastrointestinal tract. Note the nuclear pleomorphism, which is evident even at low magnification.

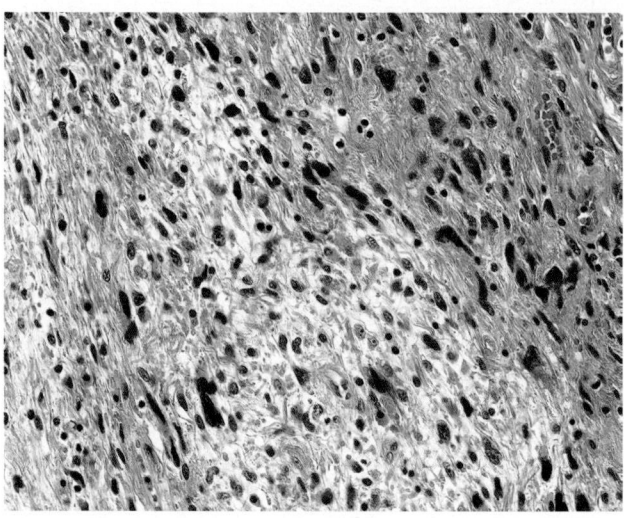

Figure 6-233. Dedifferentiated liposarcoma extending into the gastrointestinal tract. High magnification shows striking nuclear alterations.

What Went Wrong?

This is not a GIST. The clue is the degree of nuclear atypia. Of course, the oncologist was a bit naïve as well as the pathologist because GISTs outside the stomach seldom harbor *PDGFRA* mutations. Just when we thought it was safe to come out of the water after going through this book, look what crawled into the GI tract. Figs. 6.232 and 6.233 show a dedifferentiated liposarcoma that has extended from the retroperitoneum all the way to the colonic mucosa. It is impossible to diagnose the lesion as dedifferentiated liposarcoma on the basis of these images alone, and the case is exceptional in that most extracolonic sarcomas do not extend onto the mucosa. However, the important pitfall is that many lesions can display KIT/CD117 immunolabeling, and we must always ask ourselves if the KIT confirms the morphology. In this case the pleomorphic morphology and involvement of both the GI tract and retroperitoneum should result in consideration of a retroperitoneal sarcoma, and the most common pleomorphic one is dedifferentiated liposarcoma, so this tumor was tested for *MDM2* amplification and had it, supporting the diagnosis.

Regardless of exceptional cases such as this, we hope that we have offered some helpful information for approaching GI tract neoplasms in daily practice.

References

1. Reitamo JJ, Hayry P, Nykyri E, Saxen E. The desmoid tumor. I. Incidence, sex-, age- and anatomical distribution in the Finnish population. *Am J Clin Pathol.* 1982;77(6):665-673.

2. Gurbuz AK, Giardiello FM, Petersen GM, et al. Desmoid tumours in familial adenomatous polyposis. *Gut.* 1994;35(3):377-381.

3. Yantiss RK, Spiro IJ, Compton CC, Rosenberg AE. Gastrointestinal stromal tumor versus intra-abdominal fibromatosis of the bowel wall: a clinically important differential diagnosis. *Am J Surg Pathol.* 2000;24(7):947-957.

4. Bhattacharya B, Dilworth HP, Iacobuzio-Donahue C, et al. Nuclear beta-catenin expression distinguishes deep fibromatosis from other benign and malignant fibroblastic and myofibroblastic lesions. *Am J Surg Pathol.* 2005;29(5):653-659.

5. Montgomery E, Folpe AL. The diagnostic value of beta-catenin immunohistochemistry. *Adv Anat Pathol.* 2005;12(6):350-356.

6. Chen TS, Montgomery EA. Are tumefactive lesions classified as sclerosing mesenteritis a subset of IgG4-related sclerosing disorders? *J Clin Pathol.* 2008;61(10):1093-1097.

7. Yantiss RK, Nielsen GP, Lauwers GY, Rosenberg AE. Reactive nodular fibrous pseudotumor of the gastrointestinal tract and mesentery: a clinicopathologic study of five cases. *Am J Surg Pathol.* 2003;27(4):532-540.

8. Wilson JD, Montague CJ, Salcuni P, Bordi C, Rosai J. Heterotopic mesenteric ossification ('intraabdominal myositis ossificans'): report of five cases. *Am J Surg Pathol.* 1999;23(12):1464-1470.

9. Hornick JL, Sholl LM, Dal Cin P, Childress MA, Lovly CM. Expression of ROS1 predicts ROS1 gene rearrangement in inflammatory myofibroblastic tumors. *Mod Pathol.* 2015;28(5):732-739.

10. Chougule A, Bal A, Das A, Agarwal R, Singh N, Rao KL. A comparative study of inflammatory myofibroblastic tumors and tumefactive IgG4-related inflammatory lesions: the relevance of IgG4 plasma cells. *Appl Immunohistochem Mol Morphol.* 2016;24(10):721-728.

11. Saab ST, Hornick JL, Fletcher CD, Olson SJ, Coffin CM. IgG4 plasma cells in inflammatory myofibroblastic tumor: inflammatory marker or pathogenic link? *Mod Pathol.* 2011;24(4):606-612.

12. Marino-Enriquez A, Wang WL, Roy A, et al. Epithelioid inflammatory myofibroblastic sarcoma: an aggressive intra-abdominal variant of inflammatory myofibroblastic tumor with nuclear membrane or perinuclear ALK. *Am J Surg Pathol.* 2011;35(1):135-144.

13. Butrynski JE, D'Adamo DR, Hornick JL, et al. Crizotinib in ALK-rearranged inflammatory myofibroblastic tumor. *N Engl J Med.* 2010;363(18):1727-1733.

14. Mansfield AS, Murphy SJ, Harris FR, et al. Chromoplectic TPM3-ALK rearrangement in a patient with inflammatory myofibroblastic tumor who responded to ceritinib after progression on crizotinib. *Ann Oncol : Official Journal of the European Society for Medical Oncology.* 2016;27(11):2111-2117.

15. Antonescu CR, Suurmeijer AJ, Zhang L, et al. Molecular characterization of inflammatory myofibroblastic tumors with frequent ALK and ROS1 gene fusions and rare novel RET rearrangement. *Am J Surg Pathol.* 2015;39(7):957-967.

16. Deshpande V, Zen Y, Chan JK, et al. Consensus statement on the pathology of IgG4-related disease. *Mod Pathol.* 2012;25(9):1181-1192.

17. Stone JH, Zen Y, Deshpande V. IgG4-related disease. *N Engl J Med.* 2012;366(6):539-551.

18. Lucas DR, Shukla A, Thomas DG, Patel RM, Kubat AJ, McHugh JB. Dedifferentiated liposarcoma with inflammatory myofibroblastic tumor-like features. *Am J Surg Pathol.* 2010;34(6):844-851.

19. Montgomery E, Argani P, Hicks JL, DeMarzo AM, Meeker AK. Telomere lengths of translocation-associated and nontranslocation-associated sarcomas differ dramatically. *Am J Pathol.* 2004;164(5):1523-1529.

20. Antonescu CR, Nafa K, Segal NH, Dal Cin P, Ladanyi M. EWS-CREB1: a recurrent variant fusion in clear cell sarcoma–association with gastrointestinal location and absence of melanocytic differentiation. *Clin Canc Res.* 2006;12(18):5356-5362.

21. Stockman DL, Miettinen M, Suster S, et al. Malignant gastrointestinal neuroectodermal tumor: clinicopathologic, immunohistochemical, ultrastructural, and molecular analysis of 16 cases with a reappraisal of clear cell sarcoma-like tumors of the gastrointestinal tract. *Am J Surg Pathol.* 2012;36(6):857-868.

22. Laurini JA, Zhang L, Goldblum JR, Montgomery E, Folpe AL. Low-grade fibromyxoid sarcoma of the small intestine: report of 4 cases with molecular cytogenetic confirmation. *Am J Surg Pathol.* 2011;35(7):1069-1073.

23. Doyle LA, Moller E, Dal Cin P, Fletcher CD, Mertens F, Hornick JL. MUC4 is a highly sensitive and specific marker for low-grade fibromyxoid sarcoma. *Am J Surg Pathol.* 2011;35(5):733-741.

24. Doyle LA, Wang WL, Dal Cin P, et al. MUC4 is a sensitive and extremely useful marker for sclerosing epithelioid fibrosarcoma: association with FUS gene rearrangement. *Am J Surg Pathol.* 2012;36(10):1444-1451.

25. Bosman F, Carneiro F, Hruban R, Theise N, eds. *WHO Classification of Tumours of the Digestive System.* Lyon: IARC; 2010. Bosman F, Jaffee E, Lakhani S, Ohgaki H, eds. *World Health Organization Classification of Tumours.*

26. Kindblom LG, Remotti HE, Aldenborg F, Meis-Kindblom JM. Gastrointestinal pacemaker cell tumor (GIPACT): gastrointestinal stromal tumors show phenotypic characteristics of the interstitial cells of Cajal [see comments]. *Am J Pathol.* 1998;152(5):1259-1269.

27. Sircar K, Hewlett BR, Huizinga JD, Chorneyko K, Berezin I, Riddell RH. Interstitial cells of Cajal as precursors of gastrointestinal stromal tumors. *Am J Surg Pathol.* 1999;23(4):377-389.

28. Miettinen M, Lasota J. Gastrointestinal stromal tumors. *Gastroenterol Clin North Am.* 2013;42(2):399-415.

29. Miettinen M, Fetsch JF, Sobin LH, Lasota J. Gastrointestinal stromal tumors in patients with neurofibromatosis 1: a clinicopathologic and molecular genetic study of 45 cases. *Am J Surg Pathol.* 2006;30(1):90-96.

30. Hirashima K, Takamori H, Hirota M, et al. Multiple gastrointestinal stromal tumors in neurofibromatosis type 1: report of a case. *Surg Today*. 2009;39(11):979-983.

31. Miettinen M, Lasota J. Gastrointestinal stromal tumors: review on morphology, molecular pathology, prognosis, and differential diagnosis. *Arch Pathol Lab Med*. 2006;130(10):1466-1478.

32. Miettinen M, Lasota J. Gastrointestinal stromal tumors: pathology and prognosis at different sites. *Semin Diagn Pathol*. 2006;23(2):70-83.

33. Carney JA, Sheps SG, Go VL, Gordon H. The triad of gastric leiomyosarcoma, functioning extra-adrenal paraganglioma and pulmonary chondroma. *N Engl J Med*. 1977;296(26):1517-1518.

34. Belinsky MG, Rink L, von Mehren M. Succinate dehydrogenase deficiency in pediatric and adult gastrointestinal stromal tumors. *Front Oncol*. 2013;3:117.

35. Bolland M, Benn D, Croxson M, et al. Gastrointestinal stromal tumour in succinate dehydrogenase subunit B mutation-associated familial phaeochromocytoma/paraganglioma. *ANZ J Surg*. 2006;76(8):763-764.

36. Celestino R, Lima J, Faustino A, et al. Molecular alterations and expression of succinate dehydrogenase complex in wild-type KIT/PDGFRA/BRAF gastrointestinal stromal tumors. *Eur J Hum Genet*. 2013;21(5):503-510.

37. Doyle LA, Hornick JL. Gastrointestinal stromal tumours: from KIT to succinate dehydrogenase. *Histopathology*. 2014;64(1):53-67.

38. Doyle LA, Nelson D, Heinrich MC, Corless CL, Hornick JL. Loss of succinate dehydrogenase subunit B (SDHB) expression is limited to a distinctive subset of gastric wild-type gastrointestinal stromal tumours: a comprehensive genotype-phenotype correlation study. *Histopathology*. 2012;61(5):801-809.

39. Dwight T, Benn DE, Clarkson A, et al. Loss of SDHA expression identifies SDHA mutations in succinate dehydrogenase-deficient gastrointestinal stromal tumors. *Am J Surg Pathol*. 2013;37(2):226-233.

40. Janeway KA, Kim SY, Lodish M, et al. Defects in succinate dehydrogenase in gastrointestinal stromal tumors lacking KIT and PDGFRA mutations. *Proc Natl Acad Sci U S A*. 2011;108(1):314-318.

41. Jove M, Mora J, Sanjuan X, et al. Simultaneous KIT mutation and succinate dehydrogenase (SDH) deficiency in a patient with a gastrointestinal stromal tumour and Carney-Stratakis syndrome: a case report. *Histopathology*. 2014;65(5):712-717.

42. Killian JK, Kim SY, Miettinen M, et al. Succinate dehydrogenase mutation underlies global epigenomic divergence in gastrointestinal stromal tumor. *Canc Discov*. 2013;3(6):648-657.

43. Mason EF, Hornick JL. Succinate dehydrogenase deficiency is associated with decreased 5-hydroxymethylcytosine production in gastrointestinal stromal tumors: implications for mechanisms of tumorigenesis. *Mod Pathol*. 2013;26(11):1492-1497.

44. Miettinen M, Killian JK, Wang ZF, et al. Immunohistochemical loss of succinate dehydrogenase subunit A (SDHA) in gastrointestinal stromal tumors (GISTs) signals SDHA germline mutation. *Am J Surg Pathol*. 2013;37(2):234-240.

45. Miettinen M, Lasota J. Succinate dehydrogenase deficient gastrointestinal stromal tumors (GISTs) - a review. *Int J Biochem Cell Biol*. 2014;53:514-519.

46. Nannini M, Astolfi A, Paterini P, et al. Expression of IGF-1 receptor in KIT/PDGF receptor-alpha wild-type gastrointestinal stromal tumors with succinate dehydrogenase complex dysfunction. *Future Oncol*. 2013;9(1):121-126.

47. Pantaleo MA, Nannini M, Astolfi A, Biasco G, Bologna GSG. A distinct pediatric-type gastrointestinal stromal tumor in adults: potential role of succinate dehydrogenase subunit A mutations. *Am J Surg Pathol*. 2011;35(11):1750-1752.

48. Wang JH, Lasota J, Miettinen M. Succinate dehydrogenase subunit B (SDHB) is expressed in neurofibromatosis 1-associated gastrointestinal stromal tumors (Gists): implications for the SDHB expression based classification of Gists. *J Canc*. 2011;2:90-93.

49. Ricci R. Syndromic gastrointestinal stromal tumors. *Hered Cancer Clin Pract*. 2016;14:15.

50. Heinrich MC, Corless CL, Demetri GD, et al. Kinase mutations and imatinib response in patients with metastatic gastrointestinal stromal tumor. *J Clin Oncol*. 2003;21(23):4342-4349.

51. Heinrich MC, Corless CL, Duensing A, et al. PDGFRA activating mutations in gastrointestinal stromal tumors. *Science*. 2003;299(5607):708-710.

52. Yamamoto H, Oda Y, Kawaguchi K, et al. c-kit and PDGFRA mutations in extragastrointestinal stromal tumor (gastrointestinal stromal tumor of the soft tissue). *Am J Surg Pathol*. 2004;28(4):479-488.

53. Espinosa I, Lee CH, Kim MK, et al. A novel monoclonal antibody against DOG1 is a sensitive and specific marker for gastrointestinal stromal tumors. *Am J Surg Pathol.* 2008;32(2):210-218.

54. Gomez-Pinilla PJ, Gibbons SJ, Bardsley MR, et al. Ano1 is a selective marker of interstitial cells of Cajal in the human and mouse gastrointestinal tract. *Am J Physiol Gastrointest Liver Physiol.* 2009;296(6):G1370-G1381.

55. West RB, Corless CL, Chen X, et al. The novel marker, DOG1, is expressed ubiquitously in gastrointestinal stromal tumors irrespective of KIT or PDGFRA mutation status. *Am J Pathol.* 2004;165(1):107-113.

56. Guler ML, Daniels JA, Abraham SC, Montgomery EA. Expression of melanoma antigens in epithelioid gastrointestinal stromal tumors: a potential diagnostic pitfall. *Arch Pathol Lab Med.* 2008;132(8):1302-1306.

57. Miettinen M, Wang ZF, Lasota J. DOG1 antibody in the differential diagnosis of gastrointestinal stromal tumors: a study of 1840 cases. *Am J Surg Pathol.* 2009;33(9):1401-1408.

58. Antonescu CR, Romeo S, Zhang L, et al. Dedifferentiation in gastrointestinal stromal tumor to an anaplastic KIT-negative phenotype: a diagnostic pitfall: morphologic and molecular characterization of 8 cases occurring either de novo or after imatinib therapy. *Am J Surg Pathol.* 2013;37(3):385-392.

59. Amin M, Edge S, Greene F, et al. *AJCC Cancer Staging Manual.* 8th ed. Springer International Publishing AG Switzerland; 2017.

60. Miettinen M, Sobin LH, Lasota J. Gastrointestinal stromal tumors of the stomach: a clinicopathologic, immunohistochemical, and molecular genetic study of 1765 cases with long-term follow-up. *Am J Surg Pathol.* 2005;29(1):52-68.

61. Miettinen M, Makhlouf H, Sobin LH, Lasota J. Gastrointestinal stromal tumors of the jejunum and ileum: a clinicopathologic, immunohistochemical, and molecular genetic study of 906 cases before imatinib with long-term follow-up. *Am J Surg Pathol.* 2006;30(4):477-489.

62. Bischof DA, Kim Y, Behman R, et al. A nomogram to predict disease-free survival after surgical resection of GIST. *J Gastrointest Surg.* 2014;18(12):2123-2129.

63. Gold JS, Gonen M, Gutierrez A, et al. Development and validation of a prognostic nomogram for recurrence-free survival after complete surgical resection of localised primary gastrointestinal stromal tumour: a retrospective analysis. *Lancet Oncol.* 2009;10(11):1045-1052.

64. Jakhetiya A, Garg PK, Prakash G, Sharma J, Pandey R, Pandey D. Targeted therapy of gastrointestinal stromal tumours. *World J Gastrointest Surg.* 2016;8(5):345-352.

65. Celestino R, Lima J, Faustino A, et al. A novel germline SDHB mutation in a gastrointestinal stromal tumor patient without bona fide features of the Carney-Stratakis dyad. *Fam Cancer.* 2012;11(2):189-194.

66. Gaal J, Stratakis CA, Carney JA, et al. SDHB immunohistochemistry: a useful tool in the diagnosis of Carney-Stratakis and Carney triad gastrointestinal stromal tumors. *Mod Pathol.* 2011;24(1):147-151.

67. Gill AJ, Chou A, Vilain R, et al. Immunohistochemistry for SDHB divides gastrointestinal stromal tumors (GISTs) into 2 distinct types. *Am J Surg Pathol.* 2010;34(5):636-644.

68. Killian JK, Miettinen M, Walker RL, et al. Recurrent epimutation of SDHC in gastrointestinal stromal tumors. *Sci Transl Med.* 2014;6(268):268ra177.

69. Urbini M, Astolfi A, Indio V, et al. SDHC methylation in gastrointestinal stromal tumors (GIST): a case report. *BMC Med Genet.* 2015;16:87.

70. Mason EF, Hornick JL. Conventional risk stratification fails to predict progression of succinate dehydrogenase-deficient gastrointestinal stromal tumors: a clinicopathologic study of 76 cases. *Am J Surg Pathol.* 2016;40(12):1616-1621.

71. Muenst S, Thies S, Went P, Tornillo L, Bihl MP, Dirnhofer S. Frequency, phenotype, and genotype of minute gastrointestinal stromal tumors in the stomach: an autopsy study. *Hum Pathol.* 2011;42(12):1849-1854.

72. Abraham SC, Krasinskas AM, Hofstetter WL, Swisher SG, Wu TT. "Seedling" mesenchymal tumors (gastrointestinal stromal tumors and leiomyomas) are common incidental tumors of the esophagogastric junction. *Am J Surg Pathol.* 2007;31(11):1629-1635.

73. Vanek J. Gastric submucosal granuloma with eosinophilic infiltration. *Am J Pathol.* 1949;25:397-411.

74. Helwig E, Ranier A. Inflammatory fibroid polyps of the stomach. *Surg Gynecol Obstets.* 1953;96:355-367.

75. Stolte M, Finkenzeller G. Inflammatory fibroid polyp of the stomach. *Endoscopy*. 1990;22(5):203-207.

76. Stolte M, Sticht T, Eidt S, Ebert D, Finkenzeller G. Frequency, location, and age and sex distribution of various types of gastric polyp. *Endoscopy*. 1994;26(8):659-665.

77. Righetti L, Parolini F, Cengia P, et al. Inflammatory fibroid polyps in children: a new case report and a systematic review of the pediatric literature. *World J Clin Pediatr*. 2015;4(4):160-166.

78. Liu TC, Lin MT, Montgomery EA, Singhi AD. Inflammatory fibroid polyps of the gastrointestinal tract: spectrum of clinical, morphologic, and immunohistochemistry features. *Am J Surg Pathol*. 2013;37(4):586-592.

79. Schildhaus HU, Cavlar T, Binot E, Buttner R, Wardelmann E, Merkelbach-Bruse S. Inflammatory fibroid polyps harbour mutations in the platelet-derived growth factor receptor alpha (PDGFRA) gene. *J Pathol*. 2008;216(2):176-182.

80. Allibone RO, Nanson JK, Anthony PP. Multiple and recurrent inflammatory fibroid polyps in a Devon family ('Devon polyposis syndrome'): an update. *Gut*. 1992;33(7):1004-1005.

81. Anthony PP, Morris DS, Vowles KD. Multiple and recurrent inflammatory fibroid polyps in three generations of a Devon family: a new syndrome. *Gut*. 1984;25(8):854-862.

82. Hasegawa T, Yang P, Kagawa N, Hirose T, Sano T. CD34 expression by inflammatory fibroid polyps of the stomach. *Mod Pathol*. 1997;10(5):451-456.

83. Miettinen M, Sarlomo-Rikala M, Sobin LH. Mesenchymal tumors of muscularis mucosae of colon and rectum are benign leiomyomas that should be separated from gastrointestinal stromal tumors–a clinicopathologic and immunohistochemical study of eighty-eight cases. *Mod Pathol*. 2001;14(10):950-956.

84. Miettinen M, Makhlouf HR, Sobin LH, Lasota J. Plexiform fibromyxoma: a distinctive benign gastric antral neoplasm not to be confused with a myxoid GIST. *Am J Surg Pathol*. 2009;33(11):1624-1632.

85. Spans L, Fletcher CD, Antonescu CR, et al. Recurrent MALAT1-GLI1 oncogenic fusion and GLI1 up-regulation define a subset of plexiform fibromyxoma. *J Pathol*. 2016;239(3):335-343.

86. Voltaggio L. Gastric schwannomas. 2011.

87. Miettinen M, Paal E, Lasota J, Sobin LH. Gastrointestinal glomus tumors: a clinicopathologic, immunohistochemical, and molecular genetic study of 32 cases. *Am J Surg Pathol*. 2002;26(3):301-311.

88. Mosquera JM, Sboner A, Zhang L, et al. Novel MIR143-NOTCH fusions in benign and malignant glomus tumors. *Genes Chromosomes Cancer*. 2013;52(11):1075-1087.

89. Dabek B, Kram A, Kubrak J, et al. A rare mutation in a rare tumor–SMARCB1-deficient malignant glomus tumor. *Genes Chromosomes Cancer*. 2016;55(1):107-109.

90. Swerdlow SH, Campo E, Pileri SA, et al. The 2016 revision of the World Health Organization classification of lymphoid neoplasms. *Blood*. 2016;127(20):2375-2390.

91. Detlefsen S, Fagerberg CR, Ousager LB, et al. Histiocytic disorders of the gastrointestinal tract. *Hum Pathol*. 2013;44(5):683-696.

92. Rosai J, Dorfman RF. Sinus histiocytosis with massive lymphadenopathy. A newly recognized benign clinicopathological entity. *Arch Pathol*. 1969;87(1):63-70.

93. Rosai J, Dorfman RF. Sinus histiocytosis with massive lymphadenopathy: a pseudolymphomatous benign disorder. Analysis of 34 cases. *Cancer*. 1972;30(5):1174-1188.

94. Montgomery EA, Meis JM, Frizzera G. Rosai-Dorfman disease of soft tissue. *Am J Surg Pathol*. 1992;16(2):122-129.

95. Lauwers GY, Perez-Atayde A, Dorfman RF, Rosai J. The digestive system manifestations of Rosai-Dorfman disease (sinus histiocytosis with massive lymphadenopathy): review of 11 cases. *Hum Pathol*. 2000;31(3):380-385.

96. Mobley LR, Subramanian S, Koschinsky J, Frech HE, Trantham LC, Anselin L. Managed care and the diffusion of endoscopy in fee-for-service Medicare. *Health Services Research*. 2011;46(6 Pt 1):1905-1927.

97. Shekitka KM, Sobin LH. Ganglioneuromas of the gastrointestinal-tract - relation to Von-Recklinghausen-disease and other multiple tumor syndromes. *Am J Surg Pathol*. 1994;18(3):250-257.

98. Gibson JA, Hornick JL. Mucosal Schwann cell "hamartoma": clinicopathologic study of 26 neural colorectal polyps distinct from neurofibromas and mucosal neuromas. *Am J Surg Pathol*. 2009;33(5):781-787.

99. Celeiro-Munoz C, Huebner TA, Robertson SA, et al. Tactile corpuscle-like bodies in gastrointestinal-type mucosa: a case series. *Am J Surg Pathol*. 2015;39(12):1668-1672.

100. Lewin MR, Dilworth HP, Abu Alfa AK, Epstein JI, Montgomery E. Mucosal benign epithelioid nerve sheath tumors. *Am J Surg Pathol*. 2005;29(10):1310-1315.

101. Johnston J, Helwig EB. Granular cell tumors of the gastrointestinal tract and perianal region: a study of 74 cases. *Dig Dis Sci*. 1981;26(9):807-816.

102. Singhi AD, Montgomery EA. Colorectal granular cell tumor: a clinicopathologic study of 26 cases. *Am J Surg Pathol*. 2010;34(8):1186-1192.

103. Saleh H, El-Fakharany M, Frankle M. Multiple synchronous granular cell tumors involving the colon, appendix and mesentery: a case report and review of the literature. *J Gastrointestin Liver Dis*. 2009;18(4):475-478.

104. Choi SM, Hong SG, Kang SM, et al. A case of malignant granular cell tumor in the sigmoid colon. *Clin Endosc*. 2014;47(2):197-200.

105. Eslami-Varzaneh F, Washington K, Robert ME, Kashgarian M, Goldblum JR, Jain D. Benign fibroblastic polyps of the colon: a histologic, immunohistochemical, and ultrastructural study. *Am J Surg Pathol*. 2004;28(3):374-378.

106. Agaimy A, Stoehr R, Vieth M, Hartmann A. Benign serrated colorectal fibroblastic polyps/intramucosal perineuriomas are true mixed epithelial-stromal polyps with frequent BRAF mutations. *Am J Surg Pathol*. 2010;34(11):1663-1671.

107. Groisman G, Amar M, Alona M. Early colonic perineurioma: a report of 11 cases. *Int J Surg Pathol*. 2010;18(4):292-297.

108. Groisman GM, Polak-Charcon S. Fibroblastic polyp of the colon and colonic perineurioma: 2 names for a single entity? *Am J Surg Pathol*. 2008;32(7):1088-1094.

109. Groisman GM, Polak-Charcon S, Appelman HD. Fibroblastic polyp of the colon: clinicopathological analysis of 10 cases with emphasis on its common association with serrated crypts. *Histopathology*. 2006;48(4):431-437.

110. Yantiss RK, Clement PB, Young RH. Endometriosis of the intestinal tract: a study of 44 cases of a disease that may cause diverse challenges in clinical and pathologic evaluation. *Am J Surg Pathol*. 2001;25(4):445-454.

111. Oliva E, Clement PB, Young RH. Endometrial stromal tumors: an update a protean phenotype. *Adv Anat Pathol*. 2000;7(5):257-281.

112. Abeler VM, Nenodovic M. Diagnostic immunohistochemistry in uterine sarcomas: a study of 397 cases. *Int J Gynecol Pathol*. 2011;30(3):236-243.

113. Lee CH, Hoang LN, Yip S, et al. Frequent expression of KIT in endometrial stromal sarcoma with YWHAE genetic rearrangement. *Mod Pathol*. 2014;27(5):751-757.

114. Lin J, Bigge J, Ulbright TM, Montgomery E. Anastomosing hemangioma of the liver and gastrointestinal tract: an unusual variant histologically mimicking angiosarcoma. *Am J Surg Pathol*. 2013;37(11):1761-1765.

115. Montgomery E, Epstein JI. Anastomosing hemangioma of the genitourinary tract: a lesion mimicking angiosarcoma. *Am J Surg Pathol*. 2009;33(9):1364-1369.

116. Allison KH, Yoder BJ, Bronner MP, Goldblum JR, Rubin BP. Angiosarcoma involving the gastrointestinal tract: a series of primary and metastatic cases. *Am J Surg Pathol*. 2004;28(3):298-307.

117. Parfitt JR, Rodriguez-Justo M, Feakins R, Novelli MR. Gastrointestinal Kaposi's sarcoma: CD117 expression and the potential for misdiagnosis as gastrointestinal stromal tumour. *Histopathology*. 2008;52(7):816-823.

CHAPTER 1 ESOPHAGUS—QUIZ QUESTIONS

1-1. **Which statement is true concerning the lesion seen in Fig. 1.1?**

A. This squamous cell carcinoma would be staged as T1a.

B. This esophageal gastrointestinal stromal tumor would be expected to behave in an indolent fashion.

C. This granular cell tumor has elicited pseudoepitheliomatous hyperplasia.

D. This esophageal rhabdomyoma would be expected to express keratin.

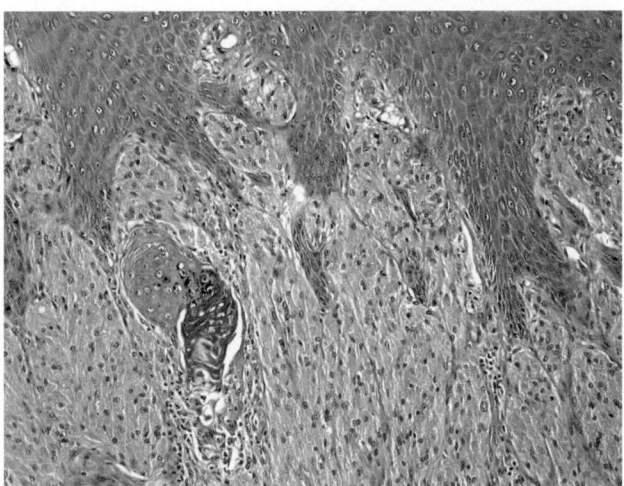

Figure 1-1.

1-2. **Fig. 1.2A is from a hematoxylin and eosin–stained section of a 2 cm mass that was found in the esophagus, and Fig. 1.2B is a CD117/KIT stain from the same lesion. Which statement is true?**

A. This esophageal gastrointestinal stromal tumor would be expected to behave in an aggressive fashion.

B. This granular cell tumor would be expected to express S100 protein.

C. This esophageal leiomyoma shows scattered Cajal cells, a common finding.

D. This leiomyosarcoma is likely to spread to the lungs.

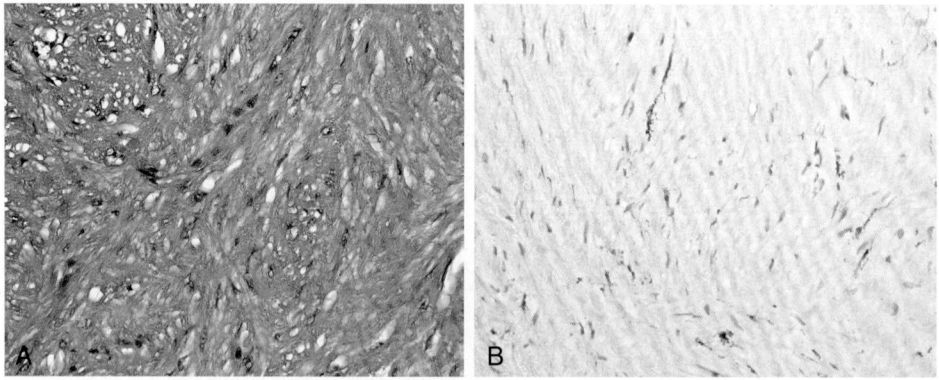

Figure 1-2.

1-3. **There is a nodular lesion in Fig. 1.3A and B. Which statement is true?**

A. This well-differentiated neuroendocrine (carcinoid) tumor has invaded the lamina propria.

B. Pancreatic acinar cell heterotopia is not infrequently encountered in esophageal samples.

C. This well-differentiated neuroendocrine (carcinoid) tumor has invaded the submucosa.

D. This is a pancreatic carcinoma that has spread to the esophagus.

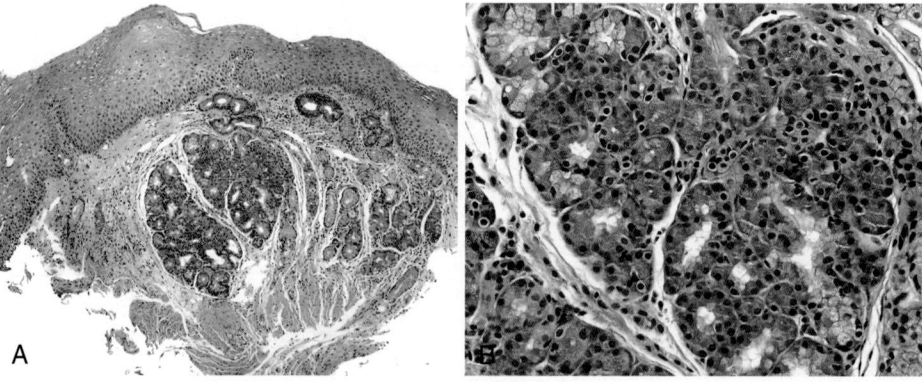

Figure 1-3.

1-4. Which statement applies to the findings in the biopsy seen in Fig. 1.4?

A. High-grade dysplasia is managed by esophagectomy.

B. Early adenocarcinoma (T1a) is managed by esophagectomy.

C. Nondysplastic Barrett esophagus is managed with mucosal ablation, usually radiofrequency ablation.

D. Low-grade dysplasia is managed with endoscopic ablation procedures (endoscopic resection for visible lesions and radiofrequency ablation for others).

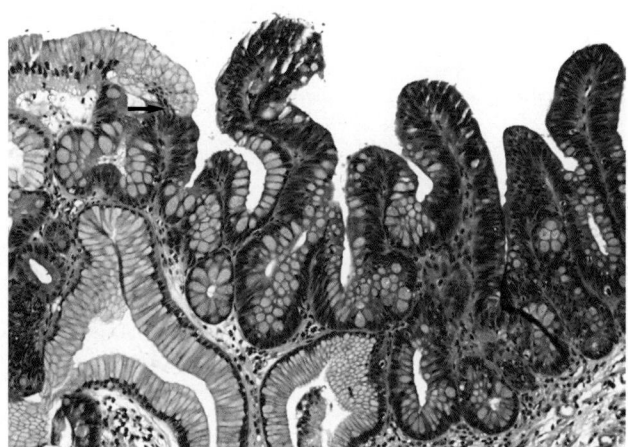

Figure 1-4.

1-5. Fig. 1.5A and B is from an esophageal biopsy. The immunostain (5B) is a P53 stain. Which statement is correct?

A. The P53 labeling in the glands in the center is abnormal and confirms an interpretation of basal pattern dysplasia.

B. The negative P53 in the cells at the surface confirms that the findings are reactive.

C. The P53 labeling pattern is noncontributory.

D. The P53 shows a null pattern of labeling and is an abnormal finding that can confirm an interpretation of dysplasia/early carcinoma.

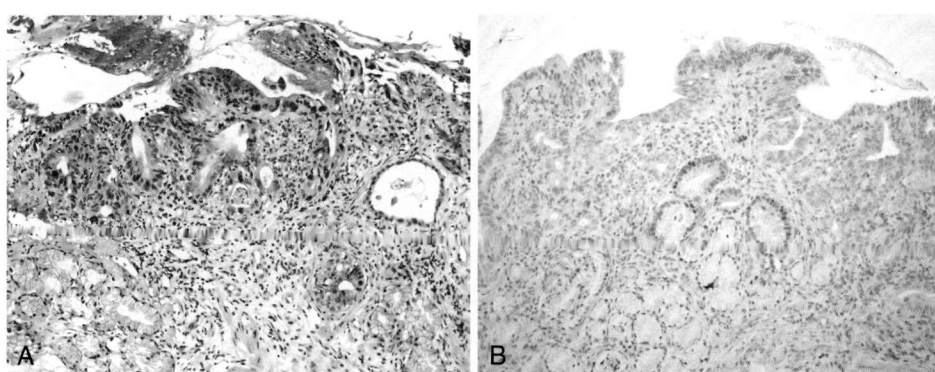

Figure 1-5.

1-6. Fig. 1.6 shows a biopsy of an esophageal mass. Which statement is true?

A. Finding pagetoid invasion of single cells into squamous epithelium is an indication of an associated deeply invasive adenocarcinoma.

B. The atypical cells are reactive and can be ignored.

C. Because there is no associated Barrett mucosa in the sample, this cannot be an adenocarcinoma.

D. The atypical cells most likely reflect a metastasis from another site.

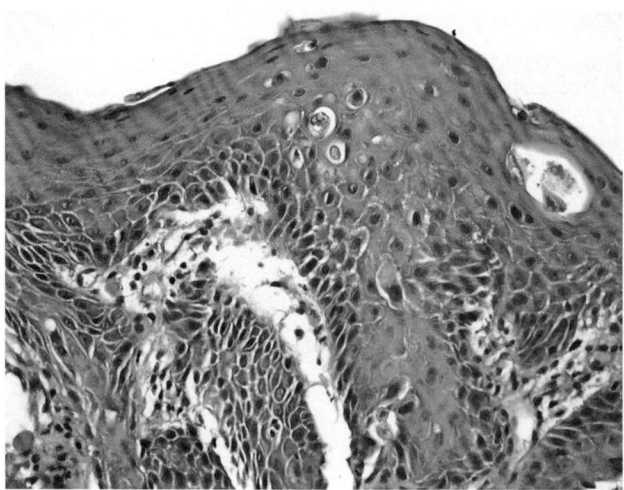

Figure 1-6.

1-7. Fig. 1.7 shows the base of an endoscopic mucosal resection (EMR) performed to excise a lesion associated with Barrett esophagus. Which statement is true?

A. This early carcinoma has invaded the submucosa and is present at the submucosal margin indicated by the blue line.

B. This early carcinoma has invaded the lamina propria and is present at the lateral mucosal margin indicated by the blue line.

C. This deeply invasive carcinoma will require follow-up esophagectomy.

D. Low-grade dysplasia is present.

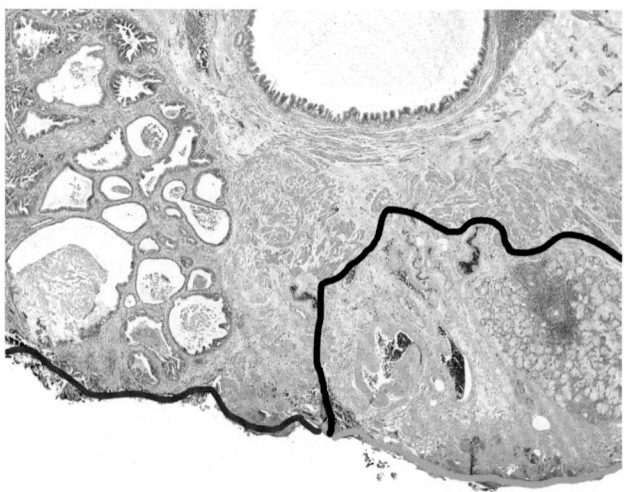

Figure 1-7.

1-8. **Which statement is true about the process seen in an esophageal biopsy and depicted in Fig. 1.8?**

A. This is normal squamous epithelium.

B. This is epidermoid metaplasia.

C. This finding suggests that the patient has *Candida* infection.

D. This finding suggests that the patient has herpes esophagitis.

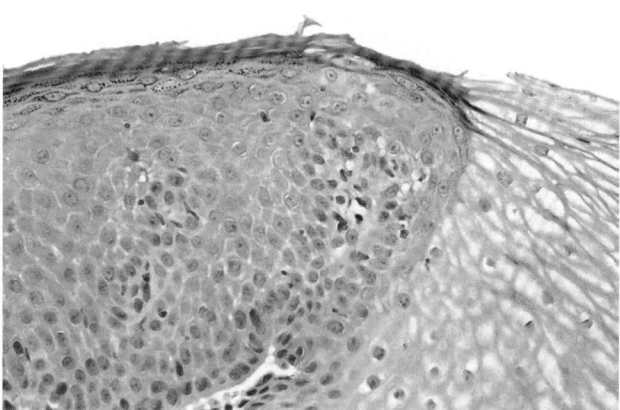

Figure 1-8.

1-9. **Fig. 1.9 shows a malignant-appearing spindle cell neoplasm that was bi-opsied in the distal esophagus. A CD117/KIT stain (not shown) was strongly reactive. Which statement is true?**

A. This is a gastrointestinal stromal tumor.

B. This is probably a sarcomatoid carcinoma.

C. This is most likely a spindle cell lymphoma.

D. Additional immunolabeling may better characterize this neoplasm.

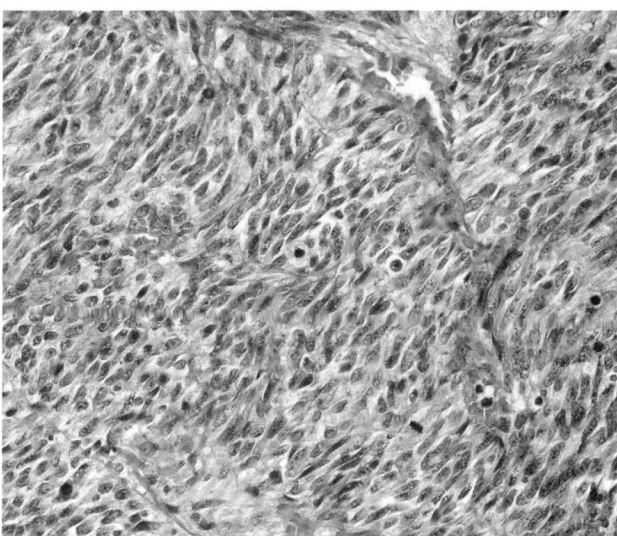

Figure 1-9.

1-10. Fig. 1.10 depicts a field from the superficial eroded area overlying an intramucosal adenocarcinoma of the esophagus. Which of the following best describe the findings?

A. Cytomegalovirus esophagitis

B. Nonsteroidal anti-inflammatory drug (NSAID)– associated injury

C. Taxane-associated changes

D. Herpes simplex virus cytopathic effect

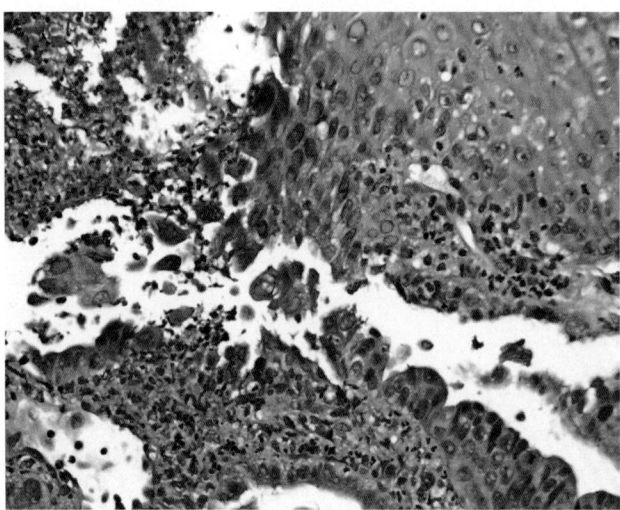

Figure 1-10.

CHAPTER 2 STOMACH—QUIZ QUESTIONS

2-1. This patient presents with severe diarrhea, and the endoscopist describes the stomach, small bowel, and colon as diffusely polypoid. Biopsies from both polypoid and nonpolypoid areas show similar changes, pictured. What is the most likely diagnosis?

A. Cowden syndrome

B. Cronkhite-Canada syndrome

C. Juvenile polyposis syndrome

D. Peutz-Jeghers syndrome

E. Familial adenomatous polyposis syndrome

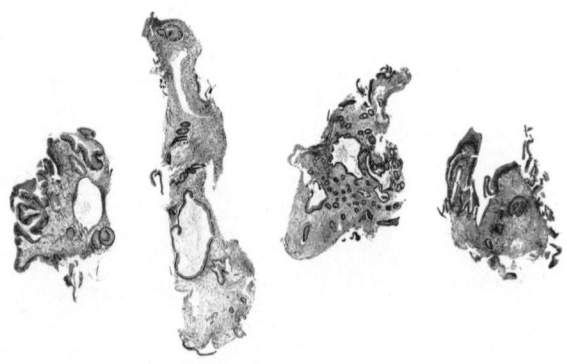

2-2. A gastric polyp with back-to-back glands of the type seen in the photo is best classified as:

    A. Gastric adenoma, intestinal type

    B. Gastric adenoma, foveolar type

    C. Gastric adenoma, pyloric gland type

    D. Gastric adenoma, oxyntic gland type

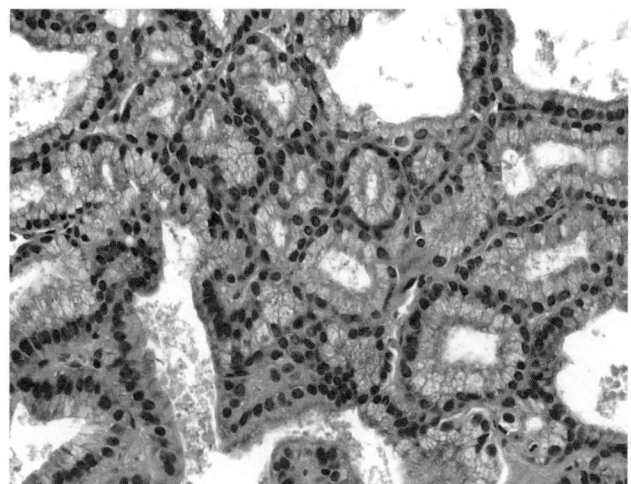

2-3. Which of the tumors pictured should be staged as an esophageal tumor?

    A.

    B.

    C.

    D.

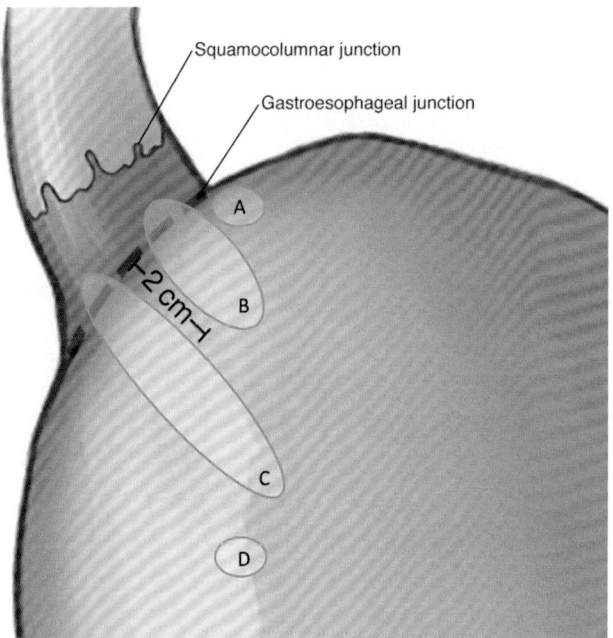

2-4. The pictured tumor is identified in a 35-y/o patient. What genetic or environmental risk factors should be discussed?

A. Familial adenomatous polyposis syndrome (FAP)

B. CDH-1 gene mutation

C. Vinyl chloride exposure

D. Gastric adenocarcinoma and proximal polyposis syndrome (GAPPS)

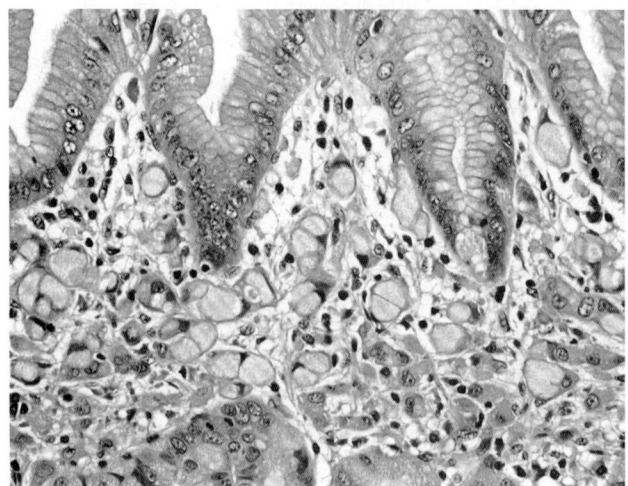

2-5. A gastric well-differentiated neuroendocrine tumor is found in the body/fundus with the pictured backdrop. Given the associated background mucosal changes, which of the following gastric neuroendocrine tumors is most likely?

A. Type 1, arising in autoimmune metaplastic atrophic gastritis

B. Type 2, associated with a gastrinoma

C. Type 3, sporadic

D. Type 4, neuroendocrine carcinoma

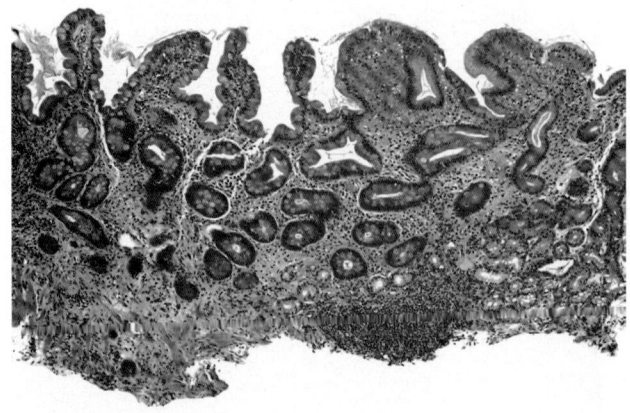

2-6. A gastric well-differentiated neuroendocrine tumor is found in the body/ fundus with the pictured backdrop, and the patient has a history of recurrent ulcers. This patient most likely has which of the following syndromes:

    A. Zollinger-Ellison syndrome and MEN type I

    B. Zollinger-Ellison syndrome and neurofibromatosis type I

    C. Cronkhite-Canada syndrome and neurofibromatosis type I

    D. Neurofibromatosis type I and MEN type I

    E. Neurofibromatosis type II and MEN type II

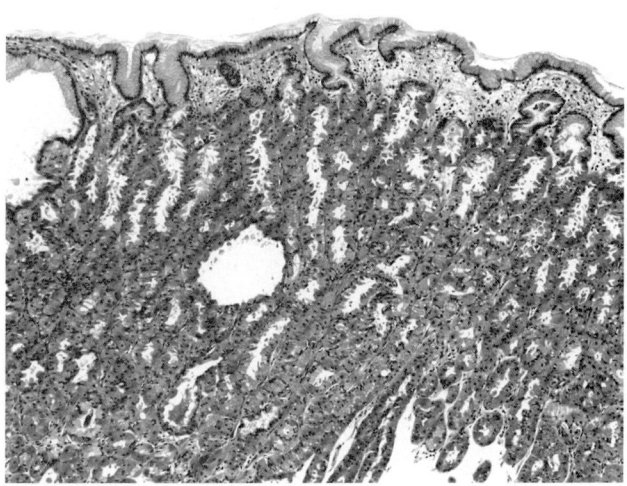

2-7. The most effective way to type the pictured tumor is to assess which of the following:

    A. Mitotic activity

    B. KI-67 proliferation index

    C. Background mucosa

    D. Chromogranin reactivity

    E. Synaptophysin reactivity

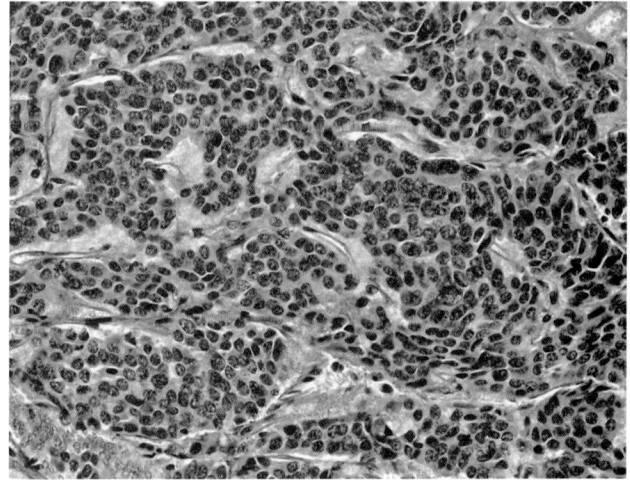

2-8. **Type 1 and Type 2 gastric neuroendocrine tumors arise from the cells pictured in this chromogranin stain. These tumors can only arise in the gastric:**

    A. Pylorus
    B. Antrum
    C. Incisura
    D. Body/fundus
    E. Cardia

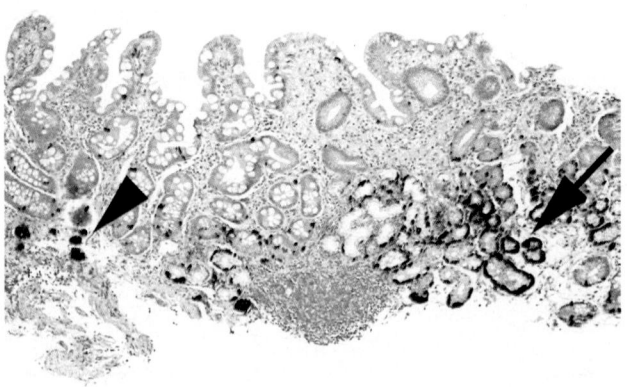

2-9. **Staging of the pictured gastric tumor (synaptophysin stain) is dependent on:**

    A. Tumor type (1, 2, 3, or 4)
    B. Location (antrum vs. body/fundus)
    C. Size—greatest dimension
    D. Depth of invasion
    E. Both size and depth

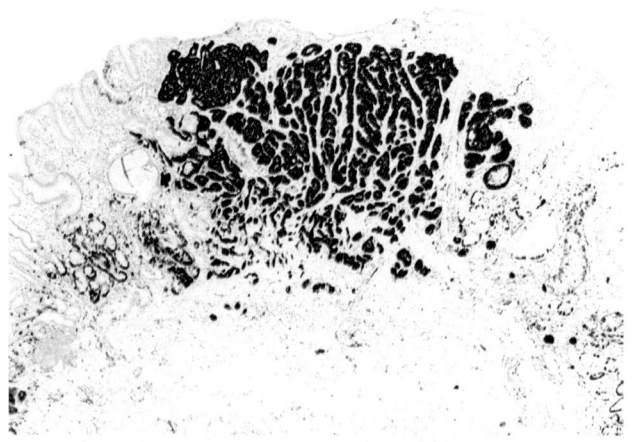

**2-10. The pictured gastric neuroendocrine tumor has 15 mitoses per 2 mm²
and Ki-67 index of 35%. It is best reported as:**

    A. Well-differentiated neuroendocrine tumor, G1
    B. Well-differentiated neuroendocrine tumor, G2
    C. Well-differentiated neuroendocrine tumor, G3
    D. Poorly differentiated neuroendocrine carcinoma

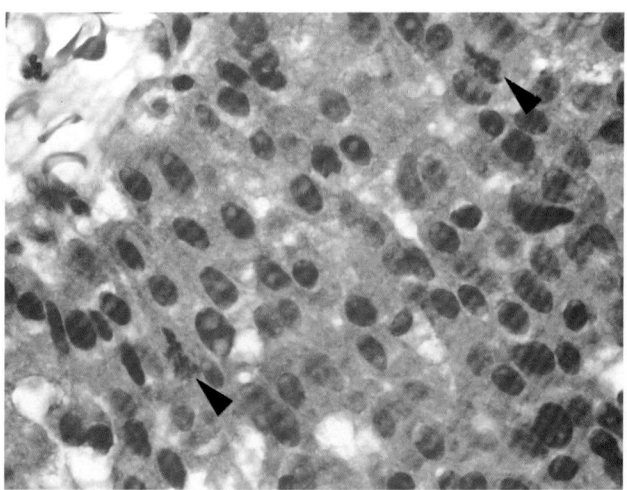

**2-11. The lesion pictured is found in a backdrop of gastric MALT lymphoma.
Which statement is true?**

    A. The intraepithelial cells are benign T-cells.
    B. The intraepithelial cells are benign B-cells.
    C. The intraepithelial cells are malignant T-cells.
    D. The intraepithelial cells are malignant B-cells.
    E. The intraepithelial cells must show co-expression of CD20 and CD43.

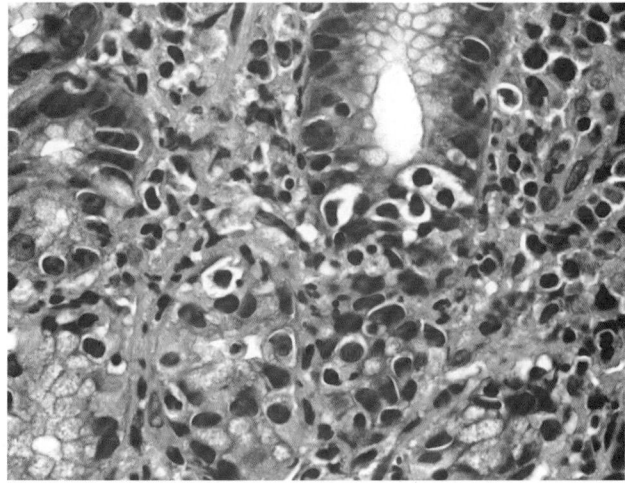

CHAPTER 3 SMALL BOWEL—QUIZ QUESTIONS

3-1. **The small bowel polyp pictured is resected from a patient with which syndrome?**

    A. Cowden syndrome

    B. Cronkhite-Canada syndrome

    C. Juvenile polyposis syndrome

    D. Peutz-Jeghers syndrome

    E. Familial adenomatous polyposis syndrome

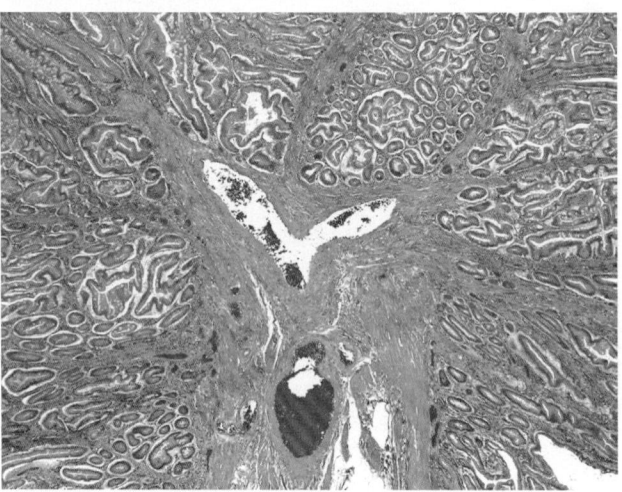

3-2. **A duodenal polyp with back-to-back glands of the type seen in the photo is best classified as:**

    A. Brunner gland hyperplasia

    B. Brunner gland hamartoma

    C. Brunner gland adenoma

    D. Brunner gland proliferative lesion

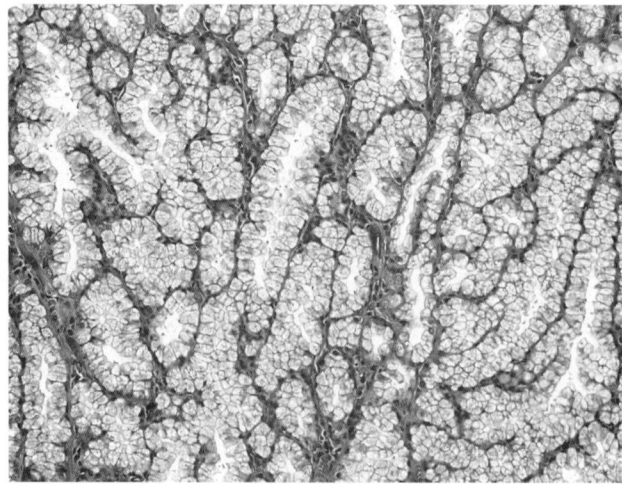

3-3. Which of the tumors pictured should be staged as a small bowel tumor?

   A.

   B.

   C.

   D.

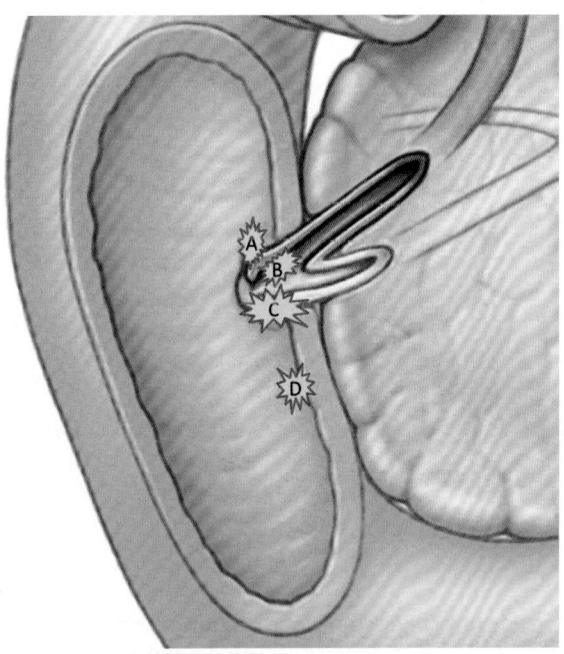

3-4. Multiple polyps of the type pictured are identified in a 35-y/o patient. What genetic or environmental risk factors should be discussed?

   A. Familial adenomatous polyposis syndrome (FAP)

   B. Juvenile polyposis syndrome

   C. PTEN hamartoma tumor syndrome

   D. Exposure to benzene

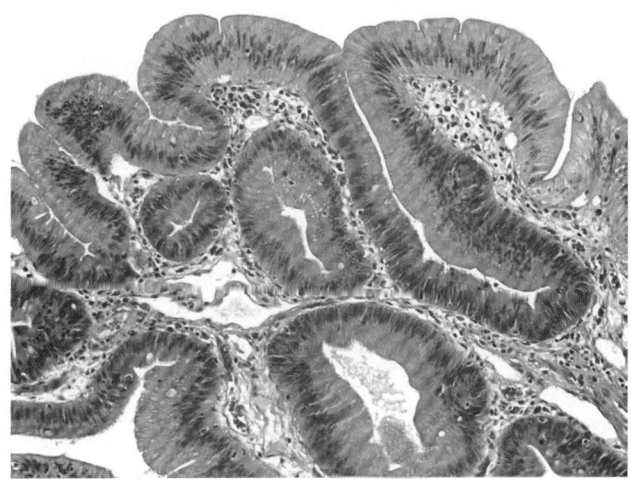

3-5. The lesion pictured is from the proximal duodenum, in the periampullary area. It is strongly and diffusedly reactive for synaptophysin. Among the following neuroendocrine tumors, which is most likely?

    A. Gastrinoma

    B. Somatostatinoma

    C. Insulinoma

    D. Serotonin-secreting tumor

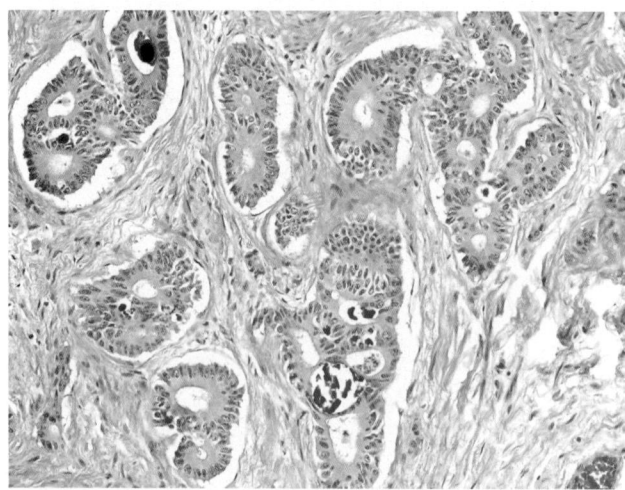

3-6. A well-differentiated neuroendocrine tumor is found in the small bowel in a patient with a history of Zollinger-Ellison syndrome and multiple endocrine neoplasia (MEN) type I. This small bowel tumor most likely secretes which of the following hormones:

    A. Gastrin

    B. Somatostatin

    C. Insulin

    D. Serotonin

    E. Peptide-YY

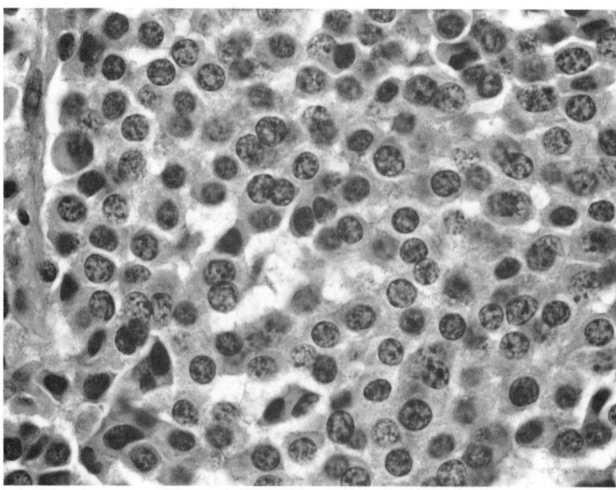

3-7. This lesion is strongly and diffusely reactive for synaptophysin. Its histologic grading relies upon which of the following:

A. Mitotic activity

B. Ki-67 proliferation index

C. Both mitotic activity and Ki-67 proliferation index

D. Cytologic atypia

E. Depth of invasion

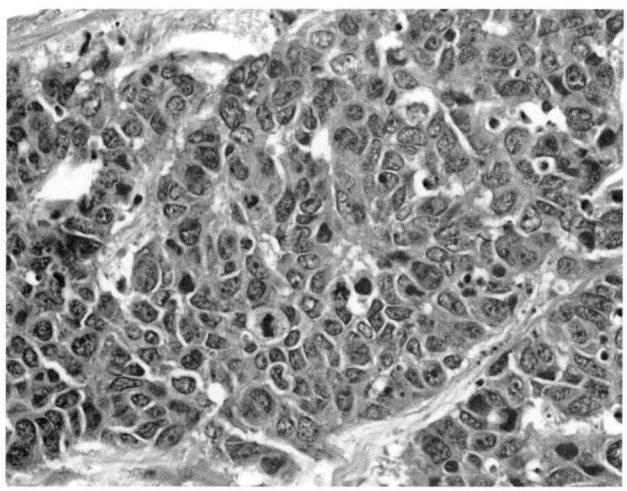

3-8. The arrow in this photo is pointing to which of the following?

A. Capillary vessel

B. Lymphatic channel

C. Calcium deposits

D. Injected saline

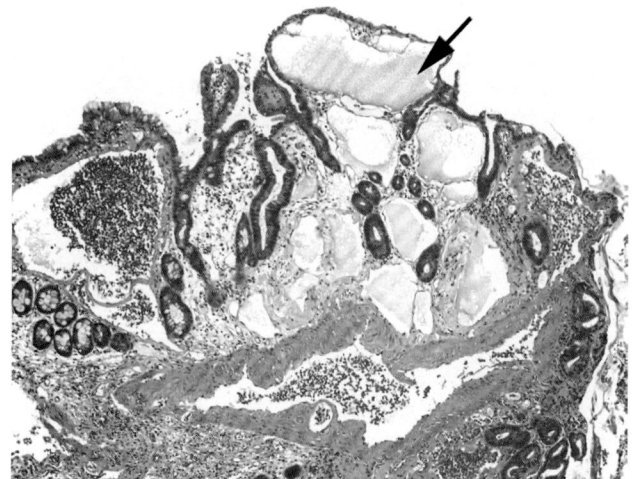

3-9. **At low magnification, what is the most reassuring feature that these lymphoid aggregates are benign?**

A. The villi are expanded.

B. The aggregates are top-heavy and hang into the lumen.

C. The germinal centers have polarized mantle zones.

D. The muscularis mucosae is splayed apart.

E. Tingible body macrophages are not identifiable.

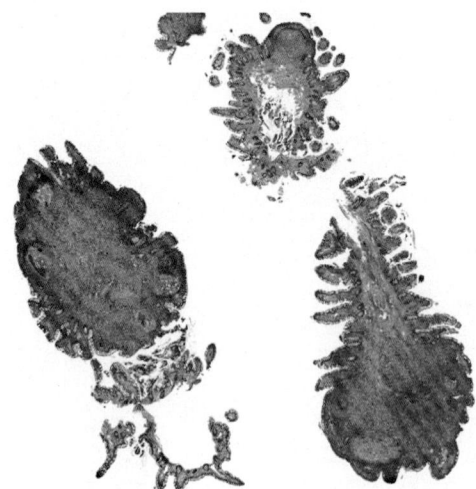

3-10. **The cells filling this lamina propria show immunoreactivity for CD117 and CD25. What is the diagnosis?**

A. Poorly differentiated carcinoma with signet ring cell features

B. Metastatic squamous cell carcinoma

C. Metastatic clear cell renal cell carcinoma

D. Systemic mastocytosis.

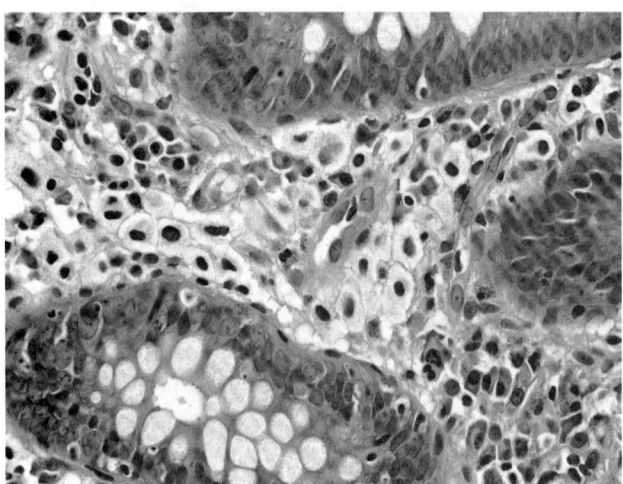

CHAPTER 4 COLON—QUIZ QUESTIONS

4-1. **A colonic biopsy of a mass shows individual cells infiltrating through the basement membrane into the lamina propria. There is no desmoplasia or submucosal invasion seen. Select the correct stage.**

A. Intramucosal carcinoma, pTis
B. Intramucosal carcinoma, pT1
C. Invasive adenocarcinoma, pTis
D. Invasive adenocarcinoma, pT1

4-2. **Select the best classification of a conventional adenoma with 5% villous component:**

A. Tubular adenoma
B. Tubulovillous adenoma
C. Villous adenoma
D. Sessile serrated adenoma with cytologic low-grade dysplasia

4-3. **Which of the following favors a diagnosis of epithelial misplacement over true invasion?**

A. Angulated glands
B. Single cell infiltration
C. Presence of lamina propria
D. Desmoplasia

4-4. **Select the correct feature of squamous morules:**

A. Also known as carcinoid
B. Display strong cytoplasmic β-catenin
C. The grade is determined by Ki67 and mitotic counts
D. Variably stain for neuroendocrine markers

4-5. **What is the minimum diagnostic criterion for an SSA/P?**

A. There are no firm criteria
B. 1 unequivocal dilated crypt
C. 2 to 3 consecutive unequivocal dilated crypts
D. 2 to 3 consecutive equivocal dilated crypts

4-6. **A spindly S100–, EMA+ lesion is seen admixed with an SSA/P. Identify the most likely diagnosis:**

A. SSA/P with perineuriomalike stromal proliferation
B. SSA/P and Schwann cell hamartoma
C. SSA/P and leiomyoma
D. SSA/P and prolapse

4-7. **A proximal hyperplastic polyp of which minimum size will trigger SSA/P clinical management?**

A. There is no size criteria
B. >0.5 cm
C. >1.0 cm
D. >2.0 cm

4-8. A 0.1 cm rectal ugly cauterized polyp (UCP) shows a thickened subepithelial collagen table. This feature alone favors which of the following diagnosis?

A. SSA/P

B. Hyperplastic polyp

C. TA

D. Normal colon

4-9. Identify the correct pairing of syndrome and underlying defect:

A. Lynch syndrome: mutations of mismatch repair genes

B. Familial adenomatous polyposis (FAP): MSI-high

C. MUTYH-associated polyposis: APC

D. Serrated polyposis syndrome: PTEN

4-10. Identify the correct description of the typical findings in patients with Cronkhite-Canada syndrome:

A. Mucosal freckling

B. Small bowel and colorectal carcinomas

C. The intervening nonpolypoid mucosa showing identical findings as the polyps

D. PTEN genetic defects

4-11. Which of the following is true regarding IBD?

A. Serrated epithelial change is synonymous with low-grade dysplasia in some centers.

B. It is critical for management to distinguish colitis-associated dysplasia from sporadic tubular adenomas.

C. "Flat dysplasia" is a term that should be abandoned because such lesions are unassociated with the development of carcinoma.

D. "DALM" is a term that should be abandoned by pathologists and clinicians

4-12. Identify the correct statement:

A. The precursor polyp in Lynch syndrome is the SSA/P

B. The precursor polyp in FAP is the SSA/P

C. Universal screening for Lynch syndrome is recommended for all CRC

D. A cutoff of 50% is suggested for MMR IHC interpretation

CHAPTER 5 ANUS—QUIZ QUESTIONS

5-1. Select the correct statement:

A. Staging of anal cancers is based on the depth of invasion.

B. Staging of anal cancers is based on size.

C. The landmarks of the anus are determined histologically.

D. The landmarks of the anus are determined by the grosser in the pathology laboratory.

5-2. Select the correct statement:

A. Staging of anal cancers and perianal skin cancers is different.

B. Treatment of anal cancers and perianal skin cancers is similar.

C. Treatment of perianal skin and skin cancers is similar.

D. Staging of anal cancers and skin cancers is the same.

5-3. **Select the appropriate context for ordering p16:**

A. Differential diagnosis is LSIL versus HSIL.

B. Differential diagnosis is reactive versus LSIL.

C. Differential diagnosis is -IN2 versus -IN3.

D. When the H&E morphology shows unequivocal HSIL.

5-4. **What is the correct interpretation of a positive p16 immunolabeling in an anal biopsy with LSIL H&E morphology and a tandem LSIL cytology specimen.**

A. HSIL

B. Indefinite for dysplasia

C. Condyloma acuminatum

D. LSIL

5.5. **What is the correct next step in a case with a cytology diagnosis of HSIL and a surgical pathology diagnosis of LSIL?**

A. Review the cytology specimen.

B. Order p16 on the cytology specimen.

C. Order p16 on the surgical specimen.

D. Disregard the cytology specimen because surgical pathology specimens are prioritized over cytology.

5-6. **Identify the correct statement about the 2012 LAST consensus recommendations.**

A. It allows for harmonization of cytology and surgical grading systems of HPV-associated squamous proliferations of the anogenital tract.

B. It allows for a site-specific grading scheme whereby the anus, vulva, and penis are separately graded according to the available site-specific literature.

C. It is a three-tiered system: low-grade squamous intraepithelial lesion, intermediate-grade squamous intraepithelial lesion, and high-grade squamous intraepithelial lesion.

D. Condyloma acuminatum remains an acceptable top-line diagnosis.

5-7. **Identify the correct statement about superficially invasive squamous cell carcinoma (SISCCA):**

A. SISCCA of the anus and perianus are defined by the same criteria.

B. Definitions of SISCCA of the anus were defined after extensive literature review of the anus.

C. The depth of invasion is measured from the most superficial aspect of the normal mucosa to the deepest point of invasion.

D. SISCAA of the anus requires a depth ≤3 mm, a horizontal spread ≤7 mm in maximal extent, absence of lymphovascular invasion, and complete excision.

5-8. **An anal biopsy shows H&E morphologic features concerning for HSIL and a p16 is ordered. The p16 shows diffuse cytoplasmic reactivity in the full-thickness area of atypia. What is the correct interpretation?**

A. P16 reactive, LSIL

B. P16 reactive, HSIL

C. P16 nonreactive, LSIL

D. P16 nonreactive, HSIL

5-9. **How often is anal Paget disease associated with an internal malignancy?**

A. Almost 100%

B. 75%

C. 50%

D. Almost 0%

5-10. Which is the expected immunoprofile of anal Paget disease that represents extension from an adjacent colorectal adenocarcinoma?

    A. CK7–, CK20+, CDX2+, GCDFP–

    B. CK7–, CK20+, CDX2+, GCDFP+

    C. CK7+, CK20–, CDX2–, GCDFP+

    D. CK7+, CK20–, CDX2–, GCDFP–

5-11. Identify the correct statement about malignant melanoma:

    A. Anal melanomas commonly have *BRAF* mutations.

    B. Cutaneous melanomas commonly have *KIT* mutations.

    C. Strong CD117 excludes a diagnosis of melanoma.

    D. Anal melanomas are not staged in the AJCC, 8th edition.

5.12. Identify the correct statement about EBV mucocutaneous ulcer:

    A. It is a self-limited lesion with an indolent course.

    B. It is an aggressive form of PTLD that requires chemotherapy.

    C. Clonal immunoglobulin studies exclude the diagnosis.

    D. Patients are typically immunocompetent.

CHAPTER 6 MESENCHYMAL LESIONS—QUIZ QUESTIONS

6-1. Fig. 6.1A is from a mesenteric mass. Fig. 6.1B is a β-catenin stain. Which statement is true concerning the lesion seen in Fig. 6.1?

    A. This is a melanoma.

    B. This esophageal gastrointestinal stromal tumor would be expected to behave in an indolent fashion.

    C. This granular cell tumor is unusual in involving the mesentery.

    D. This is a mesenteric fibromatosis.

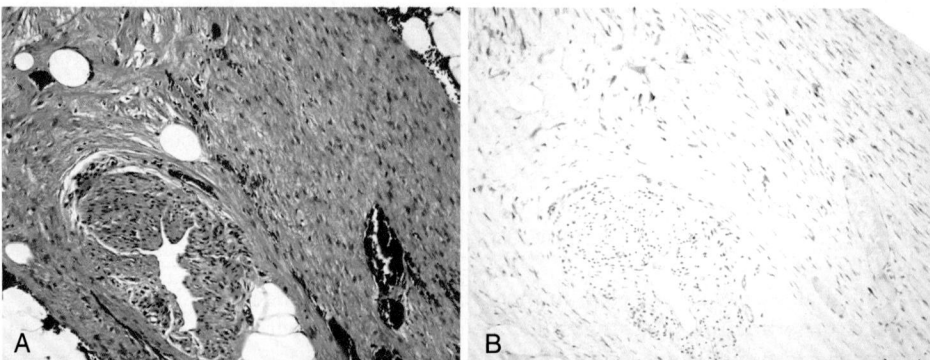

Figure 6-1.

6-2. **Fig. 6.2A is from a hematoxylin and eosin stained section of a large mesenteric mass, and Fig. 6.2B is an ALK stain from the same lesion. Which statement is true?**

    A. This epithelioid inflammatory myofibroblastic sarcoma can be considered a high-grade form of inflammatory myofibroblastic tumor.

    B. This gastrointestinal stromal tumor contains many neutrophils.

    C. Melanomas often express ALK protein.

    D. This leiomyosarcoma is likely to spread to the lungs.

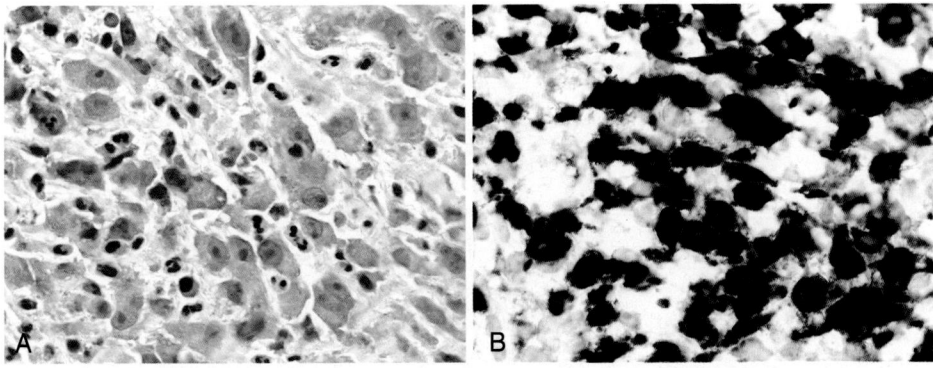

Figure 6-2.

6-3. **Fig. 6.3A and B is from an ileal lesion that arose in a 22-year-old patient. Fig. 6.3B shows an S100 protein stain. Which is the best diagnosis?**

    A. Synovial sarcoma

    B. Low-grade fibromyxoid sarcoma

    C. Clear cell sarcoma–like tumor of the gastrointestinal tract (malignant gastrointestinal neuroectodermal tumor)

    D. Ewing sarcoma

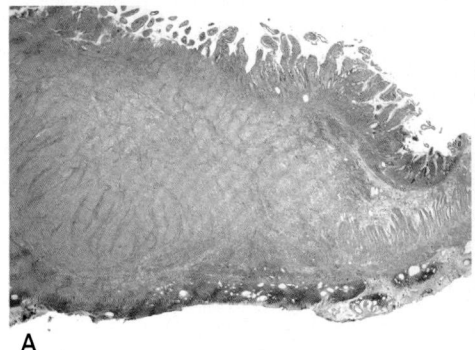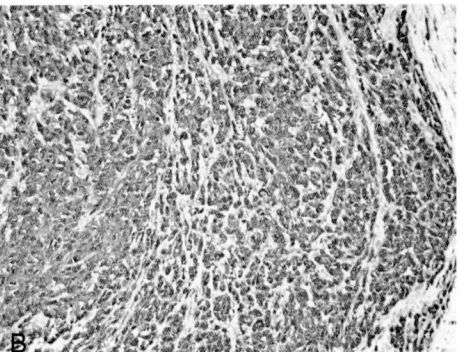

Figure 6-3.

6-4. Which statement applies to the findings in the biopsy seen in Fig. 6.4?

A. Gastrointestinal stromal tumors often have many paranuclear vacuoles.

B. The uniform nuclei make this a fibromatosis.

C. This is a spindle cell melanoma based on the presence of paranuclear vacuoles.

D. This is a leiomyoma because of the paranuclear vacuoles.

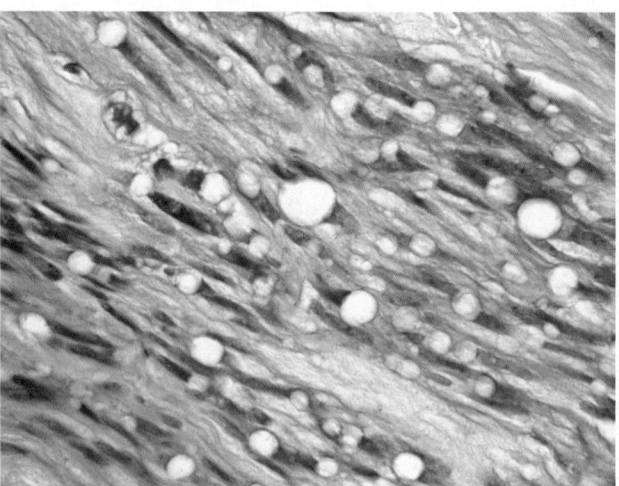

Figure 6-4.

6-5. This is a gastrointestinal stromal tumor that arose in the stomach of a 10-year-old girl. Which statement applies? (Fig. 6.5)

A. The plexiform pattern raises the possibility of a succinate dehydrogenase deficient tumor.

B. The patient probably has neurofibromatosis.

C. The patient probably has MEN IIB.

D. The patient probably has familial adenomatous polyposis.

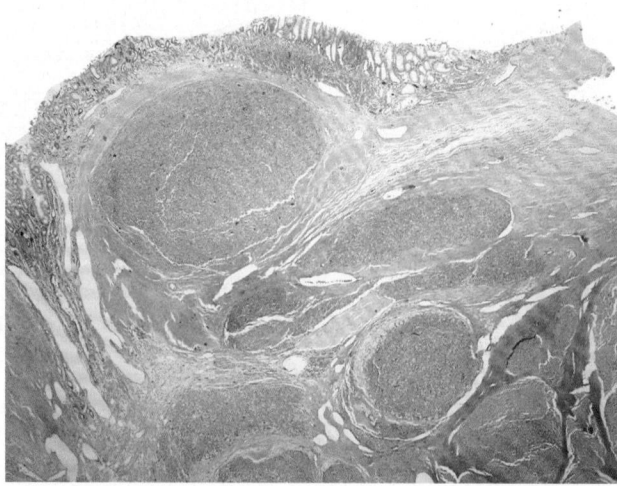

Figure 6-5.

6-6. Fig. 6.6 shows a resection of a stomach mass. Which is the best diagnosis?

A. Gastrointestinal stromal tumor

B. Fibromatosis

C. Schwannoma

D. Gangliocytic paraganglioma

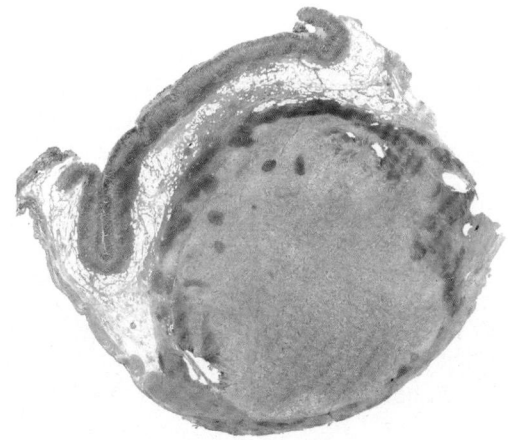

Figure 6-6.

6-7. What is the best diagnosis for the colon polyp shown in Fig. 6.7?

A. Gastrointestinal stromal tumor

B. Mucosal neuroma of the type found in MEN IIB

C. Perineurioma associated with serrated polyp

D. Schwann cell hamartoma

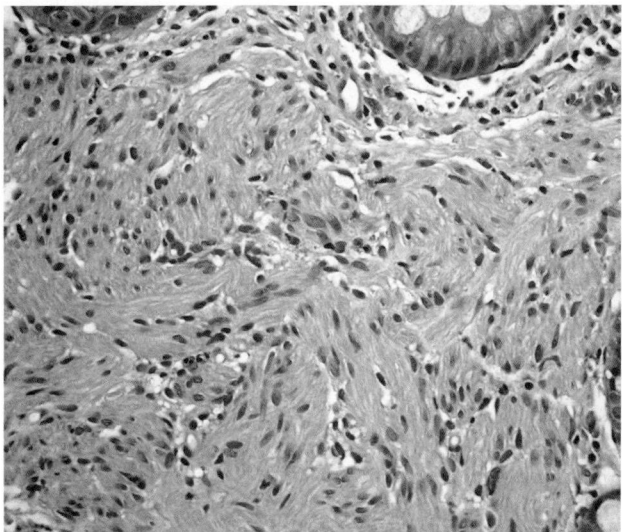

Figure 6-7.

6-8. **Which diagnosis is best for the colon polyp depicted in Fig. 6.8?**

   A. Gastrointestinal stromal tumor
   B. Mucosal neuroma of the type found in MEN IIB
   C. Perineurioma
   D. Schwann cell hamartoma

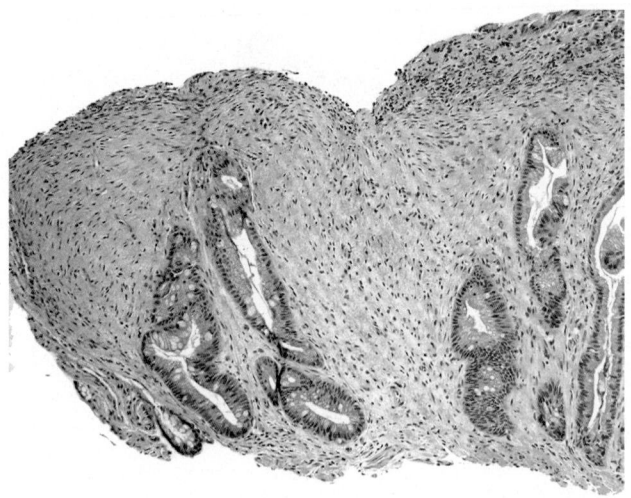

Figure 6-8.

6-9. **Fig. 6.9 shows a colon polyp. Which diagnosis is best?**

   A. Biphasic synovial sarcoma
   B. Carcinosarcoma
   C. Sarcomatoid carcinoma
   D. Endometriosis

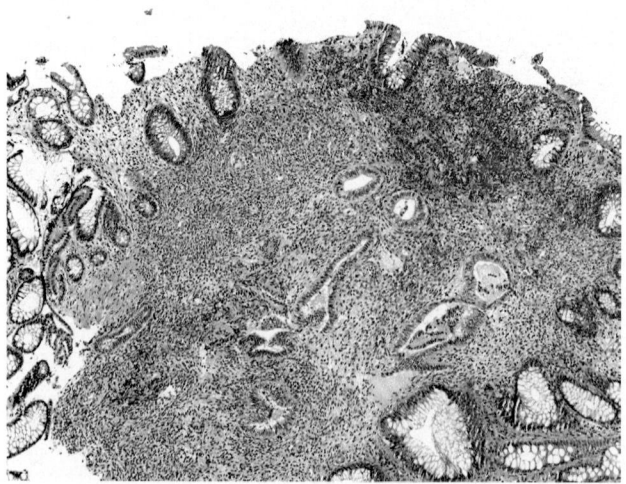

Figure 6-9.

6-10. **Fig. 6.10 depicts a field from a stomach biopsy in an immunosuppressed person. What is the diagnosis?**

A. Cytomegalovirus gastritis

B. Nonsteroidal anti-inflammatory drug (NSAID)–associated injury

C. Kaposi sarcoma

D. Herpes simplex virus cytopathic effect

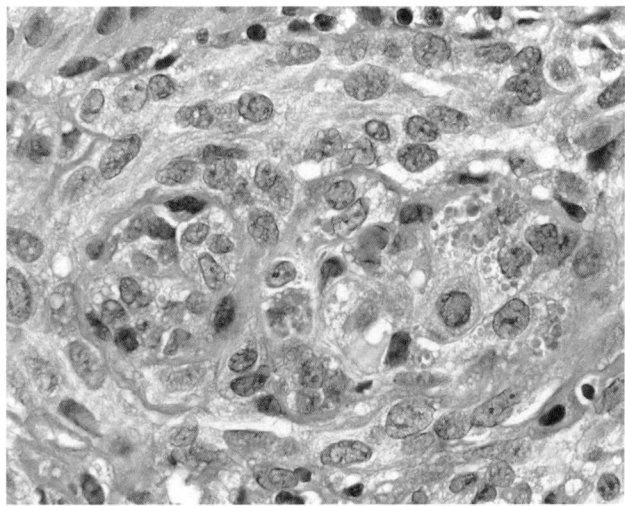

Figure 6-10.

CHAPTER 1 ESOPHAGUS—QUIZ ANSWERS

1-1. Answer: C. This granular cell tumor has elicited pseudoepitheliomatous hyperplasia.

This is not a squamous cell carcinoma (A) and the squamous epithelium is not particularly atypical, but granular cell tumors are known to produce pseudo-epitheliomatous hyperplasia.[1] Most are benign, but rare malignant behavior is known.[2] Gastrointestinal stromal tumors (B) that arise in the esophagus tend to be aggressive (in contrast to gastrointestinal stromal tumors of the stomach).[3] Rhabdomyomas (D) appear similar to granular cell tumors, but their cytoplasm has striations rather than a granular appearance as in this case.[4,5]

1-2. Answer: C.

This is an esophageal leiomyoma based on the morphology. The immunolabeling for KIT can be ignored (or not added in the first place). The presence of pre-sumed Cajal cells in leiomyomas in the GI tract has been interpreted as coloniza-tion and hyperplasia by nonneoplastic interstitial cells of Cajal[6] and is a common finding. The lesion shown is far too hypocellular to be either a gastrointestinal stromal tumor or a leiomyosarcoma (A and D). Of course, granular cell tumors express S100 protein, but the lack of granular cytoplasm in the tumor cells argues against this interpretation (B).

1-3. Answer: B. Pancreatic acinar cell heterotopia is not infrequently encountered in esophageal samples.

This is not a carcinoid tumor (A and C). The granules in the lesional cells are plump and red. If granules are encountered in well-differentiated neuroendocrine (carcinoid) tumors, they are tiny and darker red and essentially never seen in esophageal examples but rather in ileal lesions. The layer in which the process is seen is the lamina propria rather than the submucosa. The cytologic alterations are minimal and the cells appear benign. Pancreatic carcinoma that has spread to distant sites usually shows overtly malignant features or mucinous ones (D).

1-4. Answer: D. Low-grade dysplasia is managed with endoscopic ablation proce-dures (endoscopic resection for visible lesions and radiofrequency ablation for others). This image shows low-grade dysplasia. Current management strategy includes review by an expert pathology consultant followed by endoscopic treat-ment.[7,8] The depicted lesion is low-grade dysplasia because it is adenomalike but has not lost nuclear polarity. Neither high-grade dysplasia nor early carcinoma is managed by esophagectomy (A and B), and ablation of nondysplastic is generally discouraged because the likelihood of complications (strictures) is higher than the likelihood of progression to carcinoma (C).

1-5. Answer: D. The P53 shows a null pattern of labeling and is an abnormal finding that can confirm an interpretation of dysplasia/early carcinoma.

The H&E shows hyperchromatic nuclei at the surface and atypical glands in the lamina propria, some of which have luminal necrosis and have begun to efface the lamina propria. These are the features of the earliest invasion (intramucosal carcinoma, T1a).[9] The glands in the center that show light labeling show a wild-type pattern (A). The completely negative cells in fact have lost their ability to make any P53 at all, and this finding is abnormal (B and C). The total absence of P53 is distinctly abnormal, and this finding confirms an interpretation of dyspla-sia/early carcinoma if reactive areas show light staining (internal control).[10]

1-6. Answer: A. Finding pagetoid invasion of single cells into squamous epithelium is an indication of an associated deeply invasive adenocarcinoma.

Finding pagetoid extension of adenocarcinoma is indeed an indication that the patient has a deeply invasive esophageal adenocarcinoma.[11,12] Of course, in theory, a metastasis could produce this pattern, but that is simply not usually the case (D). Of course any given sample might lack a precursor lesion (C). There is no reason to encounter atypical glandular cells in esophageal squamous epithelium other than neoplasia (B)!

1-7. Answer: B. This early carcinoma has invaded the lamina propria and is present at the lateral mucosal margin indicated by the blue line.

When EMR samples are plunked into formalin, they curl such that the muscularis mucosae forms a convex shape and the mucosa (with any lesion) ends up at the same level as the deep (submucosal margin). In this image, a black line is seen between the muscularis mucosae and submucosa. To the left of it, the muscularis mucosa curls around and ends up continuous with the deep mucosal margin indicated by the green line. The carcinoma itself, characterized by glands with prominent luminal necrosis (and thus not low-grade dysplasia, D), have only invaded the lamina propria, not the submucosa or any deeper structures (A and C).

1-8. Answer: B. This is epidermoid metaplasia.

This finding is poorly understood in terms of its biologic potential, but it is associated with squamous dysplasia and neoplasia.[13,14] Essentially, it simply means that there is a granular layer in the esophagus. It does not seem to be associated with infections (C and D).

1-9. Answer: D. Additional immunolabeling may better characterize this neoplasm.

This is a spindle cell melanoma. Such tumors are sometimes KIT reactive and they may even harbor *KIT* mutations[15,16] but the distinction is important. This is not a gastrointestinal stromal tumor (A). Adding an S100 protein or SOX10 immunostain can confirm the diagnosis of melanoma. Do recall that often spindle cell melanomas lack labeling with so-called melanoma markers (HMB45, MART1). Lymphomas are quite rare in the esophagus and sarcomatoid carcinomas typically lack KIT expression (B and C).

1-10. Answer: D. Herpes simplex virus cytopathic effect.

This one is fun! It reminds us to be on guard for additional findings once we establish a key diagnosis. Of course NSAIDs can be associated with ulcers and erosions, but there are no intranuclear inclusions (B). Cytomegalovirus cytopathic effect is essentially never encountered in squamous epithelial cells but instead in endothelial cells and sometimes columnar cells (A). Taxanes are associated with apoptosis and ring mitoses (C).[17]

References:

1. Johnston J, Helwig EB. Granular cell tumors of the gastrointestinal tract and perianal region: a study of 74 cases. *Dig Dis Sci.* 1981;26(9):807-816.

2. Christopher PR, Kingsley PA, Singh BH, Singh KK, Rathore S, Das KC. Large mid-esophageal granular cell tumor: benign versus malignant. *Rare Tumors.* 2015;7(2):5772.

3. Miettinen M, Sarlomo-Rikala M, Sobin LH, Lasota J. Esophageal stromal tumors: a clinicopathologic, immunohistochemical, and molecular genetic study of 17 cases and comparison with esophageal leiomyomas and leiomyosarcomas. *Am J Surg Pathol.* 2000;24(2):211-222.

4. Pai GK, Pai PK, Kamath SM. Adult rhabdomyoma of the esophagus. *J Pediatr Surg.* 1987;22(11):991-992.

5. Roberts F, Kirk AJ, More IA, Butler J, Reid RP. Oesophageal rhabdomyoma. *J Clin Pathol.* 2000;53(7):554-557.

6. Deshpande A, Nelson D, Corless CL, Deshpande V, O'Brien MJ. Leiomyoma of the gastrointestinal tract with interstitial cells of Cajal: a mimic of gastrointestinal stromal tumor. *Am J Surg Pathol.* 2014;38(1):72-77.

7. Greene CL, Worrell SG, Attwood SE, et al. Emerging concepts for the endoscopic management of superficial esophageal adenocarcinoma. *J Gastrointest Surg.* 2016;20(4):851-860.

8. Shaheen NJ, Falk GW, Iyer PG, Gerson LB, American College of Gastroenterology. ACG clinical guideline: diagnosis and management of Barrett's esophagus. *Am J Gastroenterol.* 2016;111(1):30-50; quiz 51.

9. Amin M, Edge S, Greene F, et al. *AJCC Cancer Staging Manual.* 8th ed. Springer International Publishing AG Switzerland; 2017.

10. Voltaggio L, Montgomery EA. Diagnosis and management of Barrett-related neoplasia in the modern era. *Surg Pathol Clin.* 2017;10(4):781-800.

11. Abraham SC, Wang H, Wang KK, Wu TT. Paget cells in the esophagus: assessment of their histopathologic features and near-universal association with underlying esophageal adenocarcinoma. *Am J Surg Pathol.* 2008;32(7):1068-1074.

12. Zhu W, Appelman HD, Greenson JK, et al. A histologically defined subset of high-grade dysplasia in Barrett mucosa is predictive of associated carcinoma. *Am J Clin Pathol.* 2009;132(1):94-100.

13. Singhi AD, Arnold CA, Crowder CD, Lam-Himlin DM, Voltaggio L, Montgomery EA. Esophageal leukoplakia or epidermoid metaplasia: a clinicopathological study of 18 patients. *Mod Pathol.* 2014;27(1):38-43.

14. Singhi AD, Arnold CA, Lam-Himlin DM, et al. Targeted next-generation sequencing supports epidermoid metaplasia of the esophagus as a precursor to esophageal squamous neoplasia. *Mod Pathol.* 2017;30(11):1613-1621.

15. Carvajal RD, Hamid O, Antonescu CR. Selecting patients for KIT inhibition in melanoma. *Meth Mol Biol.* 2014;1102:137-162.

16. Carvajal RD, Lawrence DP, Weber JS, et al. Phase II study of nilotinib in melanoma harboring KIT alterations following progression to prior KIT inhibition. *Clin Cancer Res.* 2015;21(10):2289-2296.

17. Daniels JA, Gibson MK, Xu L, et al. Gastrointestinal tract epithelial changes associated with taxanes: marker of drug toxicity versus effect. *Am J Surg Pathol.* 2008;32(3):473-477.

CHAPTER 2 STOMACH—QUIZ ANSWERS

2-1. Answer: B. Cronkhite-Canada syndrome.

Cronkhite-Canada syndrome is a rare, noninherited clinical condition characterized by gastrointestinal hamartomatous polyposis and the dermatologic triad of alopecia, onychodystrophy, and hyperpigmentation. Consider this syndrome when numerous biopsies show juvenile-polyp-like features: cystically dilated and tortuous glands containing proteinaceous fluid or inspissated mucus with a background lamina propria showing marked edema and chronic inflammation. At first glance, the changes resemble inflammatory-type polyps and are nonspecific in the absence of clinical information, but the tip-off will be the diffuse nature of the changes and the lack of intervening normal mucosa.

2-2. Answer: C. Gastric adenoma, pyloric gland type.

The cells of the pyloric gland adenoma are deceptively bland and resemble normal pyloric glands. The small back-to-back glands are composed of uniform cuboidal or low columnar cells arranged in a monolayer. The cells have abundant clear cytoplasm and uniform nuclei evenly distributed along the basement membrane. These lesions, despite their bland morphology and absence of conventional dysplasia (like that seen in tubular adenomas), are regarded as low-grade dysplastic.

2-3. Answer: B.

Tumors entirely proximal or entirely distal to the GEJ are simply classified as esophageal or gastric, respectively. For tumors that involve the GEJ, the distance of the tumor's midpoint is taken into account. A somewhat arbitrary distance of 2 cm is the cutoff: the tumor is considered esophageal if its *midpoint* is ≤2 cm into the stomach, and gastric if >2 cm.

2-4. Answer: B. **CDH-1 gene mutation.**

Pictured is a signet ring cell carcinoma. The young age of this patient requires screening for hereditary diffuse gastric cancer (HDGC). HDGC is inherited in an autosomal dominant pattern with high penetrance. Nearly 50% of HDGC is associated with germline truncating mutations of the CDH1 gene. The lifetime risk of gastric cancer in individuals from these families is 70% for men and 56% for women, and the average age of onset is 38 years (range 14 to 82). Asymptomatic carriers of the mutation are recommended prophylactic total gastrectomy generally between ages 20 and 30 years.

2-5. Answer: A. **Type 1.**

Type 1 gastric neuroendocrine tumors arise in a background of autoimmune metaplastic atrophic gastritis, characterized by body-predominant changes of oxyntic gland atrophy, intestinal metaplasia, pyloric metaplasia, and inactive chronic gastritis. These tumors arise biologically as endocrine cell *hyperplasia*, which is reversible. They rarely metastasize to lymph nodes and have an excellent prognosis.

2-6. Answer: A. **Zollinger-Ellison syndrome and MEN type I.**

Type 2 gastric neuroendocrine tumors arise in the setting of unopposed gastrin secretion from a gastrinoma, typically found in the small bowel or pancreas. These gastrin-secreting tumors are associated with multiple endocrine neoplasia (MEN) type I with Zollinger-Ellison syndrome. Patients suffer from increased acid secretion and resulting gastric ulcers. Histologically, there is marked oxyntic gland hyperplasia and usually PPI effect.

2-7. Answer: C. **Background mucosa.**

The pictured tumor is a well-differentiated neuroendocrine tumor. Of the answer choices, the background mucosa will provide the most information about the gastric NET type. For example, type I tumors arise in a backdrop of autoimmune metaplastic atrophic gastritis. Type 2 tumors arise in a backdrop of oxyntic gland hyperplasia owing to Zollinger-Ellison syndrome. Type 3 tumors may arise in an otherwise unremarkable gastric environment. Mitotic activity and Ki-67 may provide histologic grading, prognostic information, but not typing. Chromogranin and synaptophysin may be reactive in any of the gastric NET types.

2-8. Answer: D. **Body/fundus.**

Type 1 and Type 2 tumors arise from endocrine cell hyperplasia as a result of hypergastrinemia. More specifically, the cells affected are enterochromaffinlike cells that are found only in the gastric body/fundus. As a result, type 1 and type 2 gastric NETs only arise in the gastric body or fundus.

2-9. Answer: E. **Both size and depth.**

Staging of gastrin neuroendocrine tumors (AJCC 8th edition) is independent of tumor type or location but does take into account both the size and depth of tumor, as follows:

pTX: Primary tumor cannot be assessed

pT0: No evidence of primary tumor

pT1: Invades the lamina propria or submucosa and less than or equal to 1 cm in size

pT2: Invades the muscularis propria or greater than 1 cm in size

pT3: Invades through the muscularis propria into subserosal tissue without penetration of overlying serosa

pT4: Invades visceral peritoneum (serosa) or other organs or adjacent structures

2-10. Answer: C. **Well-differentiated neuroendocrine tumor, G3.**

It is important to note that there are a small group of well-differentiated neuroendocrine tumors with a Ki-67 index >20% and a mitotic rates usually <20 per 10HPF. In the WHO 2010, these tumors were considered as "G3 poorly differentiated neuroendocrine carcinomas (NECs)" despite their typical well-differentiated morphology. However, these well-differentiated tumors with high mitotic rate are unlike G3 NECs because they are less responsive to platinum-based chemotherapy and they lack genetic abnormalities seen in poorly differentiated NECs. Studies done on this subset of tumors in the pancreas show these tumors have a worse prognosis than grade 2 (Ki-67 3% to 20% and mitosis <20/10HPF) neuroendocrine tumors, but they are not as aggressive as poorly differentiated NECs. For these reasons, the WHO-2017 blue book of endocrine tumors and the AJCC 8th edition classify these tumors as "well-differentiated neuroendocrine tumor" based on their morphology and are grade 3 based on mitotic count and Ki-67 proliferation index.

2-11. Answer: D. The cells are intraepithelial malignant B-cells.

The lesion pictured is a lymphoepithelial lesion typical of gastric MALT lymphoma. These are malignant B-cells with a highly characteristic halo surrounding each cell. Although MALT lymphoma cells often co-express CD20 and CD43, up to half are negative for CD43 and a minority of MALT lymphomas may be CD20 negative.

CHAPTER 3 SMALL BOWEL—QUIZ ANSWERS

3-1. Answer: D. Peutz-Jeghers syndrome.

Polyps from patients with Peutz-Jeghers syndrome show highly characteristic morphology in the small bowel. These polyps have an intact lamina propria with a core of arborizing smooth muscle bundles extending from the muscularis mucosae. In some cases, this smooth muscle framework may result in a characteristic lobulated appearance of the otherwise normal appearing background mucosa. Characteristic histology is less frequently seen in small (<1 cm) polyps, and these lesions can be indistinguishable from other hamartomatous lesions such as juvenile polyps or inflammatory/retention polyps. Dysplasia is rarely found in these polyps, but patients with the syndrome have significant risk for malignancy elsewhere, including gastric adenocarcinoma outside of the polyp. These patients are important to recognize because of their high life-time risk of malignancy, including tubular gastrointestinal carcinomas, pancreatic carcinoma, Sertoli cell tumors of the testes, minimal deviation adenocarcinoma (adenoma malignum) of the uterine cervix, sex cord tumor with annular tubules (SCTATs) of the ovaries, and breast carcinomas.

3-2. Answer: D. Brunner gland proliferative lesion.

Under normal conditions, Brunner glands are found in the submucosa of the duodenum and are composed of cuboidal cells with abundant foamy clear cytoplasm and contain basally located nuclei, which may be round or slightly flattened; the appearance is similar to pyloric glands. Polyps or nodules composed predominantly of Brunner glands fall into several categories that are frequently indistinguishable histologically. The literature on this subject has divided Brunner gland proliferations into hyperplasia, hamartoma, and adenoma groupings, but there is considerable histologic overlap resulting in difficulty at the scope. To address this problem, it is best to use an encompassing term like "Brunner gland proliferating lesion" or "Brunner gland polyp." This sensible approach eases sign-out aggravation and is supported by follow-up studies showing no recurrence after local excision among lesions without overt high-grade dysplasia or malignancy.

3-3. Answer: D.

Tumors with epicenters in the duodenum are staged as duodenal tumors (D). Ampullary carcinomas are defined as those that arise within the ampullary complex, distal to the confluence of the distal common bile duct and the pancreatic duct. They may arise on the duodenal surface of the papilla (periampullary type) (A), within the ampulla (intra-ampullary type) (B), or may involve both the intra-ampullary and periampullary regions (mixed type) (C).

3-4. Answer: A. Familial adenomatous polyposis syndrome (FAP).

Pictured is a small bowel adenoma. Small bowel adenomas are rare, and when encountering multiple, always consider the familial syndrome FAP. This autosomal dominantly inherited defect in the *APC* gene imparts a 100% risk of CRC if prophylactic colectomy is not performed. Most of the colon and small intestine polyps are conventional tubular adenomas, and gastric polyps include fundic gland polyps with or without dysplasia, gastric foveolar adenomas, and pyloric gland adenomas. Patients are also at risk for small bowel and thyroid malignancies. Diagnostic criteria for FAP include (1) at least 100 or more colorectal adenomas, *or* (2) a germline pathogenic-causing mutation of the *APC* gene, *or* (3) a family history of FAP and any number of adenomas at a young age. FAP screening involves genetic testing with a definitive FAP diagnosis requiring confirmation of a germline *APC* gene mutation, and the absence of the mutation excludes the diagnosis of FAP.

3-5. Answer: B. Somatostatinoma.

Clues to the answer are the psammomatous calcifications, which are frequently seen in somatostatinomas, and the proximal location. NETs of the small bowel exhibit site-related differences (proximal vs. distal). In the foregut, NETs mainly produce somatostatin and gastrin, similar to ampullary and pancreatic neoplasms. In this location, NETs producing serotonin are rare. These tumors may be functional or nonfunctional. The somatostatinoma syndrome is found almost exclusively in pancreatic somatostatinomas and includes diabetes mellitus, diarrhea, steatorrhea, hypo- or achlorhydria, anemia, and gallstones.

3-6. Answer: A. Gastrin.

Patients with MEN1 have an autosomal dominant syndrome best known for the predisposition to the tumors of the "3Ps": parathyroid glands, pituitary gland, and pancreas. This mnemonic is catchy, but the clinical spectrum of this disorder is broad and includes duodenal gastrinomas, adrenal adenomas, and lipomas. Up to 30% of gastrinomas are found in association with MEN1. These gastrin-secreting tumors cause increased acid secretion and subsequent gastric ulcers, known as Zollinger-Ellison syndrome. Consider MEN1 in the setting of any duodenal gastrinoma.

3-7. Answer: C. Both mitotic activity and Ki-67 proliferation index.

The pictured tumor is a poorly differentiated neuroendocrine carcinoma (PD-NEC). WD-NETs and PD-NECs are distinguished by their morphology; cytologic atypia of this degree combined with the synaptophysin reactivity classifies the tumor as a PD-NEC. Grading requires both mitotic count (50 HPFs) and Ki-67 index (500 to 2000 cells), with final grade being the higher of the two. Depth of invasion is a criterion of staging.

3-8. Answer: B. Lymphatic channel.

The pictured lesion is a lymphangioma, which shows anastomosing "empty" lymphatic channels juxtaposed with blood vessels filled with red blood cells. Lacteals are blind-ended lymphatic channels and normal constituents of the small bowel lamina propria. Normally these delicate structures are difficult to discern at low power; on high power they appear as slightly expanded "slits" containing pale eosinophilic serum. When dilated, the engorged structures are more readily apparent and are a clue to underlying pathology such as lymphangioma, as seen in this case. Lymphangiomas are rare benign congenital malformations causing mass lesions in which the lymphatic channels fail to drain properly into the venous system. The pink acellular material within this lymphatic space is proteinaceous lymphatic fluid.

3-9. Answer: C. The germinal centers have polarized mantle zones.

Reactive lymphoid follicles can impart a nodular endoscopic appearance and raise concern for a hematolymphoid malignancy, especially for those us lacking in hematopathology experience. When encountering lymphoid nodules, look for reassuring features of benign reactive follicles, including germinal centers with variation in size and shape, with a polarized mantle zone. The presence of tingible body macrophages at higher magnification is also reassuring. The other answer choices listed are features concerning for malignancy and warrant further workup.

3-10. Answer: D. Systemic mastocytosis.

Patients with infiltration of the GI tract mucosa by mastocytosis fulfill the WHO criteria for the diagnosis of systemic mastocytosis, which requires the presence of either 1 major and 1 minor criterion, or ≥3 minor criteria:

- Major criterion: Multifocal dense aggregates of mast cells (≥15) detected in bone marrow or other extracutaneous organs (e.g., the gastrointestinal tract, lymph nodes, liver, or spleen) and confirmed by special stains.

- Minor criteria: ≥25% of mast cells have atypical morphology or spindle shapes
  - Mast cells co-express CD117 with CD2 and/or CD25
  - Detection of KIT point mutation at codon 816 in bone marrow, blood, or other extracutaneous organs
  - Serum total tryptase persistently >20 ng/mL

In this case, the biopsy shows a mast cell aggregate of ≥15 mast cells confirmed by CD117 and with aberrant expression of CD25. Mucosal involvement can be remarkably subtle and easily overlooked, and the first clue to a neoplastic process may be a prominent eosinophilic infiltrate, found in nearly half of all cases. These nonneoplastic bystanders are drawn in by chemokines released from the neoplastic cells and warn pathologists to stay attentive. Histologically, look for ovoid to spindled cells with abundant pale granular cytoplasm aggregated in the lamina propria or forming a confluent band beneath the surface epithelium.

CHAPTER 4 COLON—QUIZ ANSWERS

4-1. Answer: A. Intramucosal carcinoma, pTis.

In the colon, intramucosal carcinoma is staged as pTis because of a lack of sufficiently large lymphovascular spaces to support metastasis.[1-3] The term "invasive adenocarcinoma" is reserved for colorectal carcinoma cases with invasion beyond the muscularis mucosae into at least the submucosa and is staged as at least pT1. This staging approach differs from that used for the rest of the tubular GI tract for which a diagnosis of intramucosal carcinoma is associated with metastatic potential and is, accordingly, staged as pT1.[4]

4-2. Answer: A. Tubular adenoma.

The subjective amount of villous component determines the subclassification of the conventional adenoma as tubular adenoma (less than 25% villous, A), tubulovillous adenoma (between 25% to 75% villous, B), or villous adenoma (greater than 75% villous, C).[5] Answer choice D is a distractor.

4-3. Answer: C. Presence of lamina propria.

Epithelial misplacement occurs as a polyp enlarges and bits of its associated smooth muscle and submucosa are dragged into the floppier aspects of the polyp. Epithelial misplacement can mimic invasive adenocarcinoma when the adenomatous glands are displaced into the submucosa or between prolapsed smooth muscle bundles. Typical histologic features of epithelial misplacement include a lobular glandular architecture surrounded by lamina propria, hemosiderin-laden macrophages, a lack of desmoplasia, and cytologic atypia similar to that of the overlying (nonmisplaced) adenomatous epithelium.[6-8] Although we do not routinely use adjunct stains, cutting deeper sections and sharing with a colleague resolves most diagnostic dilemmas.

4-4. Answer: D. Variably stain for neuroendocrine markers.

Squamous morules (also known as squamous metaplasia or microcarcinoids) are one of several mimics of invasive adenocarcinoma. They are not synonymous with "carcinoids" (A) because they are only microscopic collections of cells with neuroendocrine and squamous differentiation (D). Hence, they are not graded (C), although their mitotic count and Ki67 index are invariably negligible. They are most commonly encountered intermingled within large, colonic tubulovillous adenomas with high-grade dysplasia, epithelial misplacement, and serrated features,[9] and they can be a mimic of invasive adenocarcinoma. Typical features of squamous morules include their distinctly bland morphology compared with that of the associated adenoma. They consistently immunolabel with **nuclear** β-catenin (B) and have variable staining for neuroendocrine (synaptophysin and chromogranin) and squamous markers (p63 and CK 5/6) with negligible p53 and Ki67 immunolabeling (D).[9]

4-5. Answer: B. According to the discussed 2012 expert recommendations, the minimum diagnostic criterion for an SSA/P is 1 unequivocal dilated crypt.[10]

4-6. Answer: A. Perineuriomalike stromal proliferations are associated with serrated lesions.

Perineuriomas are S100−/EMA+. Schwann cell hamartomas are *not* associated with serrated lesions; they are S100+/EMA−. Leiomyomas and mucosa prolapse-associated smooth muscle proliferation would be EMA−.

4-7. Answer: C. > 1.0 cm.

According to the discussed 2012 expert recommendations, a proximal HP at least 1.0 cm in greatest dimension will result in SSA/P clinical management.[10]

4-8. Answer: B. A thickened subepithelial collagen table is a clue to a hyperplastic polyp.

4-9. Answer: A. **Lynch syndrome:** mutations of mismatch repair genes.

Lynch syndrome is an autosomal dominantly inherited defect in the genes encoding for mismatch repair proteins, namely: *MLH1, PMS2, MSH2, MSH6,* and *EpCAM* (A). As a result, the colorectal carcinomas are microsatellite unstable/microsatellite instability-high (MSI-high) (B). FAP is an autosomal dominantly inherited defect in the *APC* gene and the colorectal carcinomas are microsatellite stable (MSS) (B). *MUTYH*-associated polyposis is an autosomal recessively inherited defect in the *MUTYH* gene. Patients must lack *APC* gene germline mutations (C). The underlying genetic defect and the mode of inheritance of serrated polyposis syndrome remain unknown. The *PTEN* hamartoma tumor syndrome refers to a group of syndromes molecularly defined by an autosomal dominantly inherited defect in *PTEN*: Cowden, Bannayan-Riley-Ruvalcaba (BRRS), and Lhermitte-Duclos (LDS) syndromes (D).

4-10. Answer: C. The intervening nonpolypoid mucosa shows identical findings as the polyps.

Patients with Cronkhite-Canada syndrome present with malabsorption, protein-losing gastroenterocolopathy, diarrhea, and ectodermal changes such as alopecia, onychodystrophy, and hyperpigmentation. This syndrome is generally unassociated with neoplasia, but it is important to recognize because of a potentially high mortality of up to 50%[11] (B). GI polyps can be seen throughout the GI tract, sparing only the esophagus, and consist of hamartomatous/inflammatory-type polyps. The intervening nonpolypoid mucosa shows identical findings to the polyps (C). Mucosal freckling is a typical clinical feature of Peutz-Jeghers syndrome (A), and *PTEN* genetic defects are the defining feature of the *PTEN* hamartoma tumor syndrome, which refers to a group of syndromes molecularly defined by an autosomal dominantly inherited defect in *PTEN*: Cowden, Bannayan-Riley-Ruvalcaba (BRRS) and Lhermitte-Duclos syndromes (LDS) (D).

4-11. Answer: D. "DALM" is a term that should be abandoned by pathologists and clinicians.

Serrated epithelial change is a controversial, emerging concept in IBD synonymous with *indefinite for dysplasia* in some centers (A). According to the 2015 SCENIC guidelines,[12] the issue today should be if the lesion is endoscopically visible (resectable) or invisible (nonresectable). If the dysplasia has distinct margins, it has endoscopic and histologic confirmation that it was completely removed, and biopsies immediately adjacent to the resection site are free of dysplasia histologically, then the lesion should be fully resected regardless if it was colitis-associated or sporadic (B). According to the 2015 SCENIC guidelines, the terms "dysplasia-associated lesion or mass" (DALM) should be abandoned by pathologists and clinicians (D), and the term "flat dysplasia" should be abandoned by pathologists (C). "DALM" and "flat dysplasia" were terms historically considered an indication for resection. However, today's improved endoscopic techniques allow for some flat dysplasia to be endoscopically visible and, therefore, amenable to endoscopic surveillance or even endoscopic removal. Hence, the critical issue today is to determine if the lesion is endoscopically visible, regardless if the architecture of the lesion is polypoid, ulcerated, sessile, pedunculated, superficially elevated, flat, depressed, or ulcerated.

4-12. Answer: C. Universal screening for Lynch syndrome is recommended for all CRC.

The precursor polyp in Lynch syndrome and FAP is the conventional adenoma (A and B). A cutoff of 5% is suggested for MMR IHC interpretation (D).

References:

1. Fenoglio CM, Kaye GI, Lane N. Distribution of human colonic lymphatics in normal, hyperplastic, and adenomatous tissue. Its relationship to metastasis from small carcinomas in pedunculated adenomas, with two case reports. *Gastroenterology*. 1973;64(1):51-66.

2. Fogt F, Zimmerman RL, Ross HM, Daly T, Gausas RE. Identification of lymphatic vessels in malignant, adenomatous and normal colonic mucosa using the novel immunostain D2-40. *Oncol Rep*. 2004;11(1):47-50.

3. Robert ME. The malignant colon polyp: diagnosis and therapeutic recommendations. *Clin Gastroenterol Hepatol*. 2007;5(6):662-667.

4. *American Joint Committee on Cancer Staging Manual*. 8th ed. Switzerland: Springer International Publishing; 2017.

5. Hamilton SR, Bosman F, Boffetta P, et al. Carcinoma of the colon and rectum. In: Bosman FT, Carneiro F, Hruban RH, Theise ND, eds. *WHO Classification of Tumours of the Digestive System*. Switzerland: Stylus Publishing; 2010:134-146.

6. Muto T, Bussey HJ, Morson BC. Pseudo-carcinomatous invasion in adenomatous polyps of the colon and rectum. *J Clin Pathol*. 1973;26(1):25-31.

7. Muto T, Bussey HJ, Morson BC. The evolution of cancer of the colon and rectum. *Cancer*. 1975;36(6):2251-2270.

8. Panarelli NC, Somarathna T, Samowitz WS, et al. Diagnostic challenges caused by endoscopic biopsy of colonic polyps: a systematic evaluation of epithelial misplacement with review of problematic polyps from the bowel cancer screening program, United Kingdom. *Am J Surg Pathol*. 2016;40(8):1075-1083

9. Salaria SN, Abu Alfa AK, Alsaigh NY, Montgomery E, Arnold CA. Composite intestinal adenoma-microcarcinoid clues to diagnosing an under-recognised mimic of invasive adenocarcinoma. *J Clin Pathol*. 2013;66(4):302-306.

10. Rex DK, Ahnen DJ, Baron JA, et al. Serrated lesions of the colorectum: review and recommendations from an expert panel. *Am J Gastroenterol*. 2012;107(9):1315-1329.

11. Daniel ES, Ludwig SL, Lewin KJ, Ruprecht RM, Rajacich GM, Schwabe AD. The Cronkhite-Canada Syndrome. An analysis of clinical and pathologic features and therapy in 55 patients. *Medicine (Baltimore)*. 1982;61(5):293-309.

12. Laine L, Kaltenbach T, Barkun A, et al. SCENIC international consensus statement on surveillance and management of dysplasia in inflammatory bowel disease. *Gastroenterology*. 2015;148(3):639-651.e628.

CHAPTER 5 ANUS—QUIZ ANSWERS

5-1. Answer: B. Staging is based on size.

The anal canal begins at the point where the rectum enters the puborectalis sling at the apex of the anal sphincter complex, and it terminates at the squamous mucocutaneous junction. Tumors that originate in the anal canal that cannot be completely visualized with gentle retraction of the buttocks are classified as "anal cancers."[1] Tumors that arise at or distal to the squamous mucocutaneous junction within 5.0 cm of the anus and that can be entirely visualized with gentle retraction of the buttocks are classified as "perianal cancers." "Skin cancers" refer to tumors that are more than 5.0 cm distal to the anus. Although correct classification is important for staging and therapy, these exact landmarks are impossible to discern by the pathologist (C and D). As such, relying on the surgeon's in vivo impressions provides the most help in distinguishing anal, perianal, and skin cancers. The 2017 American Joint Committee on Cancer (AJCC) staging is based on size: pT1 = tumor ≤2 cm; pT2 = tumor >2 cm but ≤5 cm; pT3 = >5 cm; pT4 = tumor of any size invading adjacent organ(s) (B).[1]

5-2. Answer: C. Treatment of perianal skin and skin cancers is similar.

Anal cancers are rarely resected because they are usually successfully treated with a combination of chemoradiation therapy. Irradiation of anal cancers targets the primary tumor and reginal node groups. In contrast, tumors designated perianal and skin cancers are treated similarly (B and C) with focused irradiation without inclusion of regional lymph node groups, assuming there is no deep invasion. Stage criteria for anal and perianal cancers are lumped together in the 2017 American Joint Committee on Cancer (AJCC) and CAP based on size (A): pT1 = tumor ≤2 cm; pT2 = tumor >2 cm but ≤5 cm; pT3 = >5 cm; pT4 = tumor of any size invading adjacent organ(s).[1] Direct invasion of perianal skin, subcutaneous tissue, sphincter muscle, or rectal wall is not classified as pT4. Tumors involving the skin more than 5.0 cm distal to the anus are staged as skin cancers (D).

5-3. Answer: A. Differential diagnosis is LSIL versus HSIL.

LAST includes recommendations for the use of biomarkers as diagnostic aides. After identifying almost 2,300 relevant articles, p16 was named the only recommended biomarker based on its ability to act as a surrogate marker for HPV-16, predict which patients are at higher risk for malignant transformation, and reduce interobserver variability in assessment of the -IN2 category. According to the LAST recommendations, p16 should only be ordered in two narrowly defined contexts: (1) when the diagnostic issue is HSIL versus an HSIL mimic, *or* (2) when there is a discrepancy between the cytology and surgical biopsy (A).[2] Because p16 can be a tricky stain to interpret, avoid ordering p16 up front on all cases, when the differential diagnosis is non-HSIL lesions (B), and for unequivocal HSIL on H&E (C and D). For unclear reasons, a small subset of HSIL is p16 nonreactive. Avoid ordering p16 on unequivocal HSIL on H&E to avoid incorrectly down-grading an HSIL lesion, resulting in clinical undertreatment.

5-4. Answer: D. LSIL.

According to the 2012 LAST Consensus Recommendations, p16 should *not* be ordered when the H&E shows unequivocal LSIL and there is LSIL tandem cytology, as in this case. This is because p16 is unreliable outside of the HSIL setting. A diagnosis of HSIL is only appropriate when the case satisfies the morphologic criteria for HSIL on the H&E (A). Indefinite for dysplasia is generally not used in the anus (B). Condyloma acuminatum (C) is a distractor. It is by definition a papillary proliferation with low-grade dysplasia and should be reported as LSIL, formerly "condyloma acuminatum."

5-5. Answer: C. Order p16 on the surgical specimen.

According to the 2012 LAST Consensus Recommendations, p16 should be ordered on the biopsy when there is a discrepancy between the cytology and surgical biopsy to ensure that a small focus of HSIL was not overlooked (C).[2] The other answers are distractors and are not appropriate next steps (A, B, and D).

5-6. Answer: A. It allows for harmonization of cytology and surgical grading systems of HPV-associated squamous proliferations of the anogenital tract.

LAST introduces a single grading system that is applicable to all anogenital sites, including the anus, perianus, penis, cervix, vulva, and vagina (A and B). This provides for uniform reporting while simplifying the diagnostic process in anatomic sites difficult to discern, i.e., it can be difficult for clinicians (and almost impossible for pathologists) to accurately distinguish the vulva, perianus, and anus. It is a *two*-tiered system: LSIL (formerly "-IN 1") or HSIL (formerly "-IN 2" and "-IN 3") (C). Condyloma acuminatum is by definition a papillary proliferation with low-grade dysplasia and should be reported as LSIL, formerly "condyloma acuminatum" (D).

5-7. Answer: A. SISCCA of the anus and perianus are defined by the same criteria.

According to the 2012 LAST Consensus Recommendations, SISCCAs of the anus and perianus are defined by the same criteria (A).[2] Definitions of SISCCA of the anus were *not* defined after extensive literature review; they were defined to parallel the criteria for the cervix to allow for uniform reporting (B). The depth of invasion is a measurement from the nearest discernable nonneoplastic epidermal-dermal junction to the deepest point of invasion (C). SISCCA defines a subset of patients eligible for conservative, local excision. Criteria include all of the following: invasion with a depth ≤3 mm from the basement membrane of the point of origin, invasion with a horizontal spread ≤7 mm in maximal extent, and completely excised (D). At this time, the presence or absence of lymphovascular invasion does *not* affect the classification of SISCCA in the anus and perianus.[2] In contrast, SISCCA in the penis requires the absence of lymphovascular space invasion.

5-8. Answer: C. P16 nonreactive, LSIL.

A positive p16 supports a diagnosis of HSIL only if the case satisfies the morphologic criteria for HSIL on the H&E (B and D). Positive p16 requires diffuse, block immunolabeling that highlights the *nucleus and cytoplasm* of the basal layer and at least the continuous one-third of the epithelial thickness in the atypical foci seen on H&E (A and B). Full-thickness reactivity is not required for positive p16 immunolabeling. Negative p16 can be entirely negative, focal, patchy, or *only cytoplasmic* (C and D).

5-9. Answer: C. 50%.

Although Paget disease of the breast is almost always associated with an underlying breast malignancy, only 50% of patients with extramammary Paget disease of the anus have an associated underlying malignancy.[3]

5-10. Answer: A. CK7−, CK20+, CDX2+, GCDFP−.

Anal Paget disease is divided equally into two groups:

1. Anal Paget disease associated with synchronous or metachronous malignancies, usually colorectal primary adenocarcinoma. The immunoprofile of this type reflects the typical immunoprofile of the underlying colorectal adenocarcinoma (CK7−, CK20+, and nonreactive for the apocrine marker GCDFP).[4-6]
2. The other half of patients with anal Paget disease has no underlying malignancy. This type has a higher rate of local recurrence and progression to invasive adenocarcinoma.[3] The immunoprofile of this type reflects its derivation from the apocrine glands (CK7+, CK20−, and reactive for the apocrine marker GCDFP).[3,4,6] The cytoplasmic mucin can be highlighted with a mucicarmine or PAS special stain.

5-11. Answer: D. Anal melanomas are not staged in the AJCC, 8th edition.

Anal melanoma is an aggressive neoplasm with a 5-year survival of 19.8%.[7] In contrast to cutaneous melanoma, which is caused by UV light exposure and associated with *BRAF* mutations, anal melanoma is not linked to UV light exposure and more often has c-*kit* mutations (A and B). KIT is a transmembrane tyrosine kinase receptor that promotes growth-activating pathways when bound to its ligand or mutated. As a result, KIT inhibitory therapies can be beneficial for a subset of patients with metastatic melanoma and *KIT* mutations.[8,9] Melanotic pigment is a clue when present, but up to 30% are amelanotic. A primary diagnosis of malignant melanoma is only rarely an H&E diagnosis owing to the morphologic overlap with a wide variety of lesions. Following is a suggested immunohistochemical panel approach for such cases. Beware that up to 75% of anal melanoma display CD117 reactivity and these cases should not be confused for GIST (C).[10,11] In these cases the panel approach is reassuring with anal melanomas displaying strong reactivity for multiple melanoma markers, and reactivity with only one of the GIST makers (CD117). Similarly, beware that focal cytokeratin expression can be seen in up to 10% of anal melanoma, which should not be confused for a carcinoma (D).[10] Again the panel approach is helpful with anal melanomas displaying strong reactivity for multiple melanoma markers and only focal cytokeratin expression.

CHECKLIST: Anal Melanoma Immunohistochemical Panel Approach

☐ Three melanoma markers: S100 protein, SOX10, and MITF

☐ S100 protein also evaluates for neural processes, such as a schwannoma

☐ AE1/3 to evaluate for a sarcomatoid carcinoma (focal reactivity can be seen in melanoma)

☐ CD117 and DOG1 to evaluate for a GIST (strong CD117 is common in anal melanoma)

☐ SMA and desmin to evaluate for a smooth muscle tumor

5-12. Answer: A. It is a self-limited lesion with an indolent course.

EBV MCU is an isolated lesion seen in the skin, oral cavity, or GI tract in patients with a history of iatrogenic or age-related immunosuppression (D). It is a self-limited lesion with an indolent course that responds well to conservative management, such as decreased immunosuppression (A and B). Its etiology is presumed transient immunosuppression that facilitates the EBV-induced mucocutaneous ulcer. Histologically, a heavy polymorphous infiltrate is seen admixed with large B-cell blasts with Reed-Sternberg-like appearance, necrosis, and ulceration.[12,13] The B-cells label with CD30 and EBER and appear in a background of prominent, small T-cells. Clonal immunoglobulin heavy chain gene rearrangements are seen in up to 39%, and clonal T-cell patterns are seen in up to 31% (C).[13] As a result, an evaluation from a pathologist with hematopathology expertise is worthwhile in these wildly atypical morphologic cases in precarious patients. The differential diagnosis is the more clinically aggressive posttransplant lymphoproliferative disease (PTLD). Distinguishing features of EBV MCU include its presentation as an isolated ulcer (not a mass) and the absence of circulating EBV DNA in the peripheral blood. Correct classification is important because EBV MCU responds to conservative therapy, whereas PTLD often requires chemotherapy. In the small series available, the ulcers resolved over a period of weeks with no EBV MCU-related fatalities.[12,13] A CMV immunohistochemical stain is suggested in all cases based on the intense lymphoid infiltrate.

References:

1. Welton ML, Steele S, Goodman K, et al. *American Joint Committee on Cancer*. 8th ed. Chicago, Illinois: Springer Nature; 2017:275-284.

2. Darragh TM, Colgan TJ, Cox JT, et al. The lower anogenital squamous terminology standardization project for HPV-associated lesions: background and consensus recommendations from the College of American Pathologists and the American Society for Colposcopy and Cervical Pathology. *Arch Pathol Lab Med*. 2012;136(10):1266-1297.

3. Welton M, Lambert R, Bosman F. Tumours of the anal canal. In: Bosman F, Carneiro F, Hruban R, Theise N, eds. *WHO Classification of Tumours of the Digestive Tract*. 4th ed. Lyon, France: International Agency for Research on Cancer; 2010:185-193.

4. Goldblum JR, Hart WR. Perianal Paget's disease: a histologic and immunohistochemical study of 11 cases with and without associated rectal adenocarcinoma. *Am J Surg Pathol*. 1998;22(2):170-179.

5. Goldblum JR, Hart WR. Vulvar Paget's disease: a clinicopathologic and immunohistochemical study of 19 cases. *Am J Surg Pathol*. 1997;21(10):1178-1187.

6. Yang EJ, Kong CS, Longacre TA. Vulvar and anal intraepithelial neoplasia: terminology, diagnosis, and ancillary studies. *Adv Anat Pathol*. 2017;24(3):136-150.

7. Chang AE, Karnell LH, Menck HR. The National Cancer Data Base report on cutaneous and noncutaneous melanoma: a summary of 84,836 cases from the past decade. The American College of Surgeons Commission on Cancer and the American Cancer Society. *Cancer*. 1998;83(8):1664-1678.

8. Guo J, Si L, Kong Y, et al. Phase II, open-label, single-arm trial of imatinib mesylate in patients with metastatic melanoma harboring c-Kit mutation or amplification. *J Clin Oncol*. 2011;29(21):2904-2909.

9. Carvajal RD, Antonescu CR, Wolchok JD, et al. KIT as a therapeutic target in metastatic melanoma. *J Am Med Assoc*. 2011;305(22):2327-2334.

10. Tariq MU, Ud Din N, Ud Din NF, Fatima S, Ahmad Z. Malignant melanoma of anorectal region: a clinicopathologic study of 61 cases. *Ann Diagn Pathol*. 2014;18(5):275-281.

11. Chute DJ, Cousar JB, Mills SE. Anorectal malignant melanoma: morphologic and immunohistochemical features. *Am J Clin Pathol*. 2006;126(1):93-100.

12. Hart M, Thakral B, Yohe S, et al. EBV-positive mucocutaneous ulcer in organ transplant recipients: a localized indolent posttransplant lymphoproliferative disorder. *Am J Surg Pathol*. 2014;38(11):1522-1529.

13. Dojcinov SD, Venkataraman G, Raffeld M, Pittaluga S, Jaffe ES. EBV positive mucocutaneous ulcer—a study of 26 cases associated with various sources of immunosuppression. *Am J Surg Pathol*. 2010;34(3):405-417.

CHAPTER 6 MESENCHYMAL LESIONS—QUIZ ANSWERS

6-1. Answer: D. **This is a mesenteric fibromatosis.**

This is not a melanoma (A) and the lesional cells are not as atypical as those in melanomas. Gastrointestinal stromal tumors lack β-catenin nuclear immunolabeling (B).[1,2] Granular cell tumors have plump granular cytoplasm (C).

6-2. Answer: A. **This epithelioid inflammatory myofibroblastic sarcoma can be considered a high-grade form of inflammatory myofibroblastic tumor.**

The peculiar pattern of ALK labeling is typical of these lesions.[3] The lesion shown is far too atypical for most gastrointestinal stromal tumor (B). Melanoma might be considered, but they lack ALK expression (C). With the off ALK labeling, epithelioid leiomyosarcoma is unlikely but some such tumors were probably misinterpreted in the past as epithelioid leiomyosarcoma.

6-3. Answer: C. **Clear cell sarcoma–like tumor of the gastrointestinal tract (malignant gastrointestinal neuroectodermal tumor).**

This is not a synovial sarcoma, which can have focal but not diffuse S100 protein expression (A). It is too cellular to be a low-grade fibromyxoid sarcoma and the S100 protein expression would be again that interpretation.[4] It is not Ewing sarcoma (D) based on the growth pattern in nests and strong S100 protein expression, which leaves clear cell sarcoma–like tumor.[5]

6-4. Answer: A. **Gastrointestinal stromal tumors often have many paranuclear vacuoles.**

Gastrointestinal stromal tumors of the stomach often have large numbers of paranuclear vacuoles. Together with the appearance of the nuclei (uniform) and cytoplasm, this is the best diagnosis in this case. Indeed fibromatoses (B) have uniform nuclei but not paranuclear vacuoles. Paranuclear vacuoles are not a feature of spindle cell melanomas (C). Leiomyomas (D) have paranuclear vacuoles but never in so many of the cells.

6-5. Answer: A. The plexiform pattern raises the possibility of a succinate dehydrogenase–deficient tumor.

Succinate dehydrogenase–deficient gastrointestinal stromal tumors arise in the stomach and often affect young persons.[6-10] Those that arise in neurofibromatosis tend to affect the small bowel and are not plexiform (B).[10-12] Gastrointestinal stromal tumors are not a major component of MEN IIB and familial adenomatous polyposis (C and D).

6-6. Answer: C. Schwannoma.

The lymphoid cuff is the 1× giveaway to the diagnosis of the gastric neoplasm.[13] Gastrointestinal stromal tumors tend to arise in the muscularis propria but contain little inflammation (A). Fibromatoses (B) arise in the mesentery and usually have little inflammation, and gangliocytic paragangliomas (D) are found in the duodenum and are generally uninflamed.

6-7. Answer: D. Schwann cell hamartoma.

This lesion shows fibrillary cytoplasm and is seen in the lamina propria and the cells lack much atypia. These are features of Schwann cell hamartoma.[14] Gastrointestinal stromal cell tumor (A) is unlikely because these typically invade the mucosa when they are malignant. Mucosal neuromas in MEN IIB have cuffs of perineurium (B), and perineuriomas have less eosinophilic cytoplasm (C).

6-8. Answer: C. Perineurioma.

Gastrointestinal stromal cell tumor (A) is unlikely because these typically invade the mucosa when they are malignant. Mucosal neuromas in MEN IIB have cuffs of perineurium (B). The cytoplasm is less eosinophilic than that seen in Schwann cell hamartomas (D). The associated serrated polyp is a clue to the diagnosis of perineurioma, which has also been called benign fibroblastic polyp of the colon.[15,16]

6-9. Answer: D. Endometriosis.

The diagnosis of endometriosis is easy as long as it is considered.[17] Biphasic synovial sarcoma is highly unlikely to present in this fashion (A) and the lesion is not atypical enough for sarcomatoid carcinoma (C), which is the same thing as carcinosarcoma (B); the latter term is out of favor.

6-10. Answer: C. Kaposi sarcoma.

These are hyaline globules of Kaposi sarcoma, which are erythrophagolysosomes. They are less eosinophilic than the inclusions of cytomegalovirus (A) and they are in the cytoplasm, which is against herpes simplex virus (D). NSAIDs result in erosions and scarring rather than inclusions!

References:

1. Bhattacharya B, Dilworth HP, Iacobuzio-Donahue C, et al. Nuclear beta-catenin expression distinguishes deep fibromatosis from other benign and malignant fibroblastic and myofibroblastic lesions. *Am J Surg Pathol.* 2005;29(5):653-659.

2. Montgomery E, Torbenson MS, Kaushal M, Fisher C, Abraham SC. Beta-catenin immunohistochemistry separates mesenteric fibromatosis from gastrointestinal stromal tumor and sclerosing mesenteritis. *Am J Surg Pathol.* 2002;26(10):1296-1301.

3. Marino-Enriquez A, Wang WL, Roy A, et al. Epithelioid inflammatory myofibroblastic sarcoma: an aggressive intra-abdominal variant of inflammatory myofibroblastic tumor with nuclear membrane or perinuclear ALK. *Am J Surg Pathol.* 2011;35(1):135-144.

4. Laurini JA, Zhang L, Goldblum JR, Montgomery E, Folpe AL. Low-grade fibromyxoid sarcoma of the small intestine: report of 4 cases with molecular cytogenetic confirmation. *Am J Surg Pathol.* 2011;35(7):1069-1073.

5. Stockman DL, Miettinen M, Suster S, et al. Malignant gastrointestinal neuroectodermal tumor: clinicopathologic, immunohistochemical, ultrastructural, and molecular analysis of 16 cases with a reappraisal of clear cell sarcoma-like tumors of the gastrointestinal tract. *Am J Surg Pathol.* 2012;36(6):857-868.

6. Celestino R, Lima J, Faustino A, et al. Molecular alterations and expression of succinate dehydrogenase complex in wild-type KIT/PDGFRA/BRAF gastrointestinal stromal tumors. *Eur J Hum Genet.* 2013;21(5):503-510.

7. Doyle LA, Hornick JL. Gastrointestinal stromal tumours: from KIT to succinate dehydrogenase. *Histopathology.* 2014;64(1):53-67.

8. Miettinen M, Killian JK, Wang ZF, et al. Immunohistochemical loss of succinate dehydrogenase subunit A (SDHA) in gastrointestinal stromal tumors (GISTs) signals SDHA germline mutation. *Am J Surg Pathol.* 2013;37(2):234-240.

9. Miettinen M, Lasota J. Succinate dehydrogenase deficient gastrointestinal stromal tumors (GISTs) - a review. *Int J Biochem Cell Biol.* 2014;53:514-519.

10. Wang JH, Lasota J, Miettinen M. Succinate dehydrogenase subunit B (SDHB) is expressed in neurofibromatosis 1-associated gastrointestinal stromal tumors (Gists): implications for the SDHB expression based classification of Gists. *J Cancer.* 2011;2:90-93.

11. Agaimy A, Vassos N, Croner RS. Gastrointestinal manifestations of neurofibromatosis type 1 (Recklinghausen's disease): clinicopathological spectrum with pathogenetic considerations. *Int J Clin Exp Pathol.* 2012;5(9):852-862.

12. Miettinen M, Fetsch JF, Sobin LH, Lasota J. Gastrointestinal stromal tumors in patients with neurofibromatosis 1: a clinicopathologic and molecular genetic study of 45 cases. *Am J Surg Pathol.* 2006;30(1):90-96.

13. Voltaggio L, Murray R, Lasota J, Miettinen M. Gastric schwannoma: a clinicopathologic study of 51 cases and critical review of the literature. *Hum Pathol.* 2012;43(5):650-659.

14. Gibson JA, Hornick JL. Mucosal Schwann cell "hamartoma": clinicopathologic study of 26 neural colorectal polyps distinct from neurofibromas and mucosal neuromas. *Am J Surg Pathol.* 2009;33(5):781-787.

15. Groisman G, Amar M, Alona M. Early colonic perineurioma: a report of 11 cases. *Int J Surg Pathol.* 2010;18(4):292-297.

16. Groisman GM, Polak-Charcon S. Fibroblastic polyp of the colon and colonic perineurioma: 2 names for a single entity? *Am J Surg Pathol.* 2008;32(7):1088-1094.

17. Yantiss RK, Clement PB, Young RH. Endometriosis of the intestinal tract: a study of 44 cases of a disease that may cause diverse challenges in clinical and pathologic evaluation. *Am J Surg Pathol.* 2001;25(4):445-454.

CCS0120